MUIR'S
TEXTBOOK OF PATHOLOGY

NINTH EDITION

Revised by

D. F. CAPPELL, C.B.E.

M.D., LL.D., F.R.C.P.(Glas.Edin.Lond.)
F.R.C.Path., F.R.S. Edin.

Emeritus Professor of Pathology, University of Glasgow

and

J. R. ANDERSON

B.Sc., M.D., F.R.C.P.(Glas.), M.R.C.P.(Lond.), F.R.C.Path.,
F.R.S. Edin.

Professor of Pathology, University of Glasgow
Pathologist to the Western Hospitals Group, Glasgow
Consultant Pathologist to the Western Regional Board

EDWARD ARNOLD

© D. F. CAPPELL and J. R. ANDERSON, 1971

First published 1924
by Edward Arnold (Publishers) Ltd.
25 Hill Street,
London, W1X 8LL

Reprinted	1924, 1926, 1927
Second edition	1929
Reprinted	1930, 1932
Third edition	1933
Fourth edition	1936
Fifth edition	1941
Reprinted	1944, 1946
Sixth edition	1951
Reprinted	1956
Seventh edition	1958
Eighth edition	1964
Reprinted	1968
Ninth edition	1971
Reprinted	1972

ISBN: 0 7131 4179 4

Printed in Great Britain by Richard Clay (The Chaucer Press), Ltd., Bungay, Suffolk

PREFACE TO THE NINTH EDITION

In preparing this book we have retained the objective of previous editions, namely, to meet primarily the needs of medical students but also to provide an account which we hope will be useful to graduates training in various branches of medicine. The ever increasing expansion of knowledge has made necessary extensive revision of the text and careful selection from the wealth of information that has become available in the last few years. It has not been our intention to provide the bare minimum, and the text contains considerably more than will be assimilated by most medical students during their formal course in pathology. We believe that certain new and exciting developments should be presented in some detail, and that this is likely to catch the interest of the student. Methods in teaching are becoming less rigid, and the student reading this book should receive guidance from his teachers in deciding which aspects of the subject deserve most attention.

We have followed the general pattern established by Sir Robert Muir of arranging the text into two sections, the first a general section which presents the major types of disease process—inflammation, hypersensitivity, neoplasia, etc., and the second a systematic account of the more important disease processes as they affect the various tissues and systems of the body. This division into general and systematic pathology accords with the curricula of most medical schools and we believe that it remains the best method of presentation.

The section on general pathology has been very largely re-written and has been arranged in twelve chapters in place of the previous seven. The first chapter, on mechanisms and features of cell injury, has been compiled very largely by Professor R. B. Goudie who has also contributed the first half of Chapter 4 on the immune response. A whole chapter has been devoted to the inflammatory reaction and two chapters have been provided on infection, one dealing with host-parasite relationships and the other with the features of various types of infection. The chapter on healing, repair and hypertrophy has been re-written mainly by Dr. Mary E. Catto. Because of the advances in immunology and the increasing realisation of the importance of immune reactions in disease processes, a new chapter is devoted to the features of normal specific immune responses and another to hypersensitivity reactions and immunological deficiencies. The chapters on disturbances of the circulation and on various degenerations and pigmentations have been very extensively revised and re-arranged. The general account of tumours now comprises three chapters, the first on the nature, origin and causation of tumours, the second and third on the general features of epithelial and other types of tumours respectively: they have been revised mainly by Professor Bernard Lennox who has also contributed to the sections on lymphoid and skin tumours. These considerable changes, and the addition of approximately 120 illustrations, are largely responsible for an increase in the length of the book of approximately 100 pages.

In revising the systematic chapters, we have been careful not to lose sight of the fact that the descriptions of structural changes of diseases in the previous editions were based to a large extent on cumulative personal experience and observation. In general, we have retained these accounts. We have, however, introduced or enlarged on topics which have gained in importance, have reduced or eliminated others which are now of less consequence, and have expanded many of the accounts of clinical features and their correlation with pathological changes. We have also sought to maintain Sir Robert Muir's policy of avoiding dogma on controversial subjects. Recent advances in our understanding and classification of renal diseases has necessitated almost complete re-writing of the chapter on the urinary system, and much of the chapters on the alimentary tract and liver are also new. Various sections of the other systematic chapters have been replaced, and the inclusion of all this new material has prompted us to scrutinise the whole text and to introduce a uniformity of style which differs somewhat from that of previous editions. We have not dwelt at length on diseases which occur mainly in tropical countries. Authoritative books on the pathology of diseases of the tropics, complementary to general pathology texts, are now available and should be used where appropriate.

At the end of the text there is a brief bibliography which is not intended to be exhaustive but to introduce to the student a selection of literature which may be read with interest and profit. Some of the works cited are of great historical interest and are included in order to give the actual words of those who made the original discoveries; others provide further details of the present state of knowledge on particular subjects. In the latter category we have thought it more helpful to quote mainly authoritative reviews, from which the references to original articles may be obtained.

The following colleagues have been very largely responsible for revision of the chapters indicated. Drs. H. E. Hutchison and F. D. Lee (haematological chapters), F. D. Lee (gastro-intestinal tract), M. E. Catto (orthopaedic pathology), J. Hume Adams (neuropathology), and Professor J. A. Milne (diseases of the skin and various illustrations in other chapters). Much valued help and advice has also been provided by Drs. A. J. Cochran (male reproductive system and pancreas), A. A. M. Gibson (respiratory system), W. A. Harland (atheroma, ischaemic heart disease and thrombosis), C. H. W. Horne (chronic infections), W. R. Lee (emphysema), R. F. Macadam (pyelonephritis and also various photomicrographs and electron micrographs), R. N. M. MacSween (liver diseases), Professor D. K. Mason (oral pathology), Drs. A. T. Sandison (female reproductive system and endocrines), Morag C. Timbury (virus infections), J. M. Vetters (amyloid disease, pigmentations, myasthenia gravis and also numerous photomicrographs) and R. B. Goudie (thyroid gland).

Valuable contributions have also been made by the following clinical colleagues: Messrs. A. Litton, F.R.C.S. and M. A. Turner, F.R.C.S., who have helped with the section on shock, Dr. G. P. McNicol, who is largely responsible for the account of haemostatic and clotting mechanisms, Drs. J. J. Brown, A. F. Lever and J. I. S. Robertson (M.R.C. Hypertension Research Unit), who have helped in the revision of the section on hypertension and have provided accounts of the renin-angiotensin system and of Conn's syndrome, and Mr. J. Stewart Orr (Principal Physicist, Regional Department of Clinical Physics and Bio-engineering) who has provided most of the section on cellular injury by radiation. The account of fluid and electrolyte balance was re-written for the eighth edition with the help of Professor D. A. K. Black and has required little change. It is a pleasure to acknowledge our indebtedness and gratitude to all these colleagues for their help and also to members of the Department and particularly Drs. A. B. Busuttil, W. G. S. Spilg and P. G. Toner for their painstaking help with proof reading.

A number of diagrams have been introduced to illustrate the text and for these we are indebted to Mr. R. Callander, F.F.PH., M.M.A.A. We are greatly indebted also to the various colleagues who have provided photographs and histological sections: those supplied from outwith this Department are acknowledged in the text. To Mr. William Carson, F.I.M.L.T. and Mr. Norman Russell, F.I.M.L.T., sincere thanks are due for a very large amount of fine technical work, also to Mr. David McSeveney, F.I.M.L.T. for his outstanding preparations for electron microscopy, and to Mr. Peter Kerrigan and Mr. Robin Ewart for the large amount of painstaking work involved in the preparation of the many new photographs.

We are grateful to Mrs. Margaret Morton, M.A.M.S. and Mrs. Norma McCulloch for efficient typing of many untidy and often barely legible manuscripts. To Mrs. Margaret Morton we are also deeply grateful for her untiring aid in many ways, but above all for her help with proof reading, for her efficiency in co-ordinating our efforts with those who have helped us and with the publishers, and for her assistance in the preparation of the index.

We are glad to take this opportunity of expressing our thanks to Messrs. Edward Arnold and particularly to Miss Barbara Koster for their helpful co-operation and for making every effort to overcome delays in the production of this edition.

Finally, we offer our grateful thanks to our respective wives, who have borne with understanding, if not in silence, our pre-occupation and irritability over the past three years.

D. F. CAPPELL
J. R. ANDERSON

CONTENTS

INTRODUCTION

What is Pathology?

Pathology is the study of disease by scientific methods. Disease may be defined as any abnormal variation in structure or function of any part of the body. It is an acceptable principle that disease does not occur spontaneously but only as the consequence of some abnormality induced in cells of the body by specific causal factors, and in studying a particular disease we have not only to discover and define the abnormalities—structural or functional or both—and observe how these change throughout the course of the disease, but also we have to discover what factors have caused the disease to develop. Although some diseases can be treated successfully on an empirical basis, logical methods of prevention can be applied only when the cause is known, and rational treatment is possible only when the nature of the changes in structure and function is understood.

The methods used to study the changes of a disease include observation of both the gross and microscopic structural abnormalities (*morbid anatomy* and *histopathology* respectively) and the *physiological* and *biochemical* disturbances. Special methods are applied to the investigation of *genetic factors* in disease and the importance of *immunological disturbances* in many diseases is becoming increasingly apparent. Parasitic organisms are an important cause of disease—in this country, mainly micro-organisms (bacteria, viruses, fungi, etc.)—and accordingly *microbiology* is an important aspect of pathology. The wide range of methods applicable to the study of disease has inevitably led to the division of the science of pathology into an ever-increasing number of specialties, and pathology laboratories of human and veterinary hospitals include departments of biochemistry, microbiology, and morbid anatomy and histopathology. The study of diseases of the blood and haemopoietic tissues has also developed into the specialty of *haematology*. The relative importance of the various branches of pathology varies for different types of disease. In some instances, for example in diabetes mellitus, biochemical investigations provide the best means of diagnosis and are of the greatest value in the control of therapy. By contrast, recognition of the nature of many diseases, for example tumours, and the choice of the most appropriate therapy, depend very largely on examination of the gross and histological features. For most diseases, diagnosis is based on a combination of pathological investigations. To give an example, biochemical tests may indicate that a patient is suffering from impairment of renal function, but the nature of the renal disease responsible for this commonly requires histological examination of renal tissue (*renal biopsy*). Another example is provided by the condition of anaemia, which may have many causes. The changes in the cells of the blood and the bone marrow may suggest deficiency of a factor essential for erythropoiesis, and biochemical and physiological tests are then indicated to confirm the deficiency, e.g. of vitamin B_{12} or folic acid. Alternatively, anaemia may result from blood loss and this may be due to a structural lesion of the gastro-intestinal tract or of the endometrium, diagnosis of which may require histological examination. Examination of body fluids, faeces, or excised pathological tissue by microbiological techniques, or examination of the serum for the presence of antibodies to particular micro-organisms, are essential to the accurate diagnosis of many types of infection.

Why learn Pathology?

Most medical students are not going to become pathologists. It is nevertheless essential that the medical school curriculum should include a course of pathology which provides a clear account of the causes, where these are known, and of the pathological changes, of the more important diseases. Most disease processes bring about structural changes and these usually provide a logical explanation for the symptoms and signs and commonly also for the biochemical changes. An appreciation of the pathological processes of disease thus aids the doctor in the correct interpretation of the clinical features of the patient's illness. This applies not only to the clinical diagnostician but also to the surgeon who must recognise the nature of the structural changes exposed at operation and act accordingly, and to the radiologist who can only interpret the significance of shadows on an x-ray film on the basis of the structural changes of disease. To the research worker, histopathology and electron microscopy are superb techniques; both can be adapted to enzymic and other chemical investigations (*histochemistry*), and such methods continue to rank high in the solution of many problems in medical research.

From what has been said above, pathology is important to the medical student, regardless of the branch of medicine he intends to pursue. It is apparent also that the pathologist is not a "dead meat merchant". His most important duties are in diagnosis and in elucidating the nature and causes of disease. He must co-operate fully with his clinical colleagues, both in the diagnosis of individual patients, and in the conduct of clinicopathological meetings for teaching purposes. One of the best places to learn pathology and to correlate the patient's illness with the structural changes of his disease is the post-mortem room, and a well-conducted necropsy, attended by the clinicians who looked after the patient during life, is unsurpassed as a teaching method.

Pathological processes

It was first pointed out by Virchow that all disturbances of function and structure in disease are due to cellular abnormalities and that the phenomena of a particular disease are brought about by a series of cellular changes. Pathological processes are of a dual nature, consisting firstly of the changes of the injury induced by the causal agent, and secondly of reactive changes which are often closely similar to physiological processes. If death is rapid, as for example in cyanide poisoning, there may be little or no structural changes of either type. Cyanide inhibits the cytochrome-oxidase systems of the cells and thus halts cellular respiration before histological changes can become apparent. Similarly, blockage of a coronary artery cuts off the blood supply to part of the myocardium and death may be immediate, when no structural changes will be found: if, however, the patient survives for some hours or more, the affected myocardium shows the structural changes which occur subsequent to cell death and the lesion becomes readily visible. Reactive changes may be exemplified by enlargement of the myocardium in the patient with high blood pressure. In this condition, there is an increase in the resistance to blood flow through the arterioles and consequently the normal rate of circulation can be maintained only by a rise in blood pressure. Reflex stimulation of the heart results in more forcible contractions of the left ventricle, and in accordance with the general principle that increased functional demand stimulates enlargement (hypertrophy) and/or proliferation (hyperplasia) of the cells concerned, the myocardial cells of the left ventricle increase in size. Although part of a disease state, the reactive hypertrophy of the myocardium in hypertension is closely similar to the physiological hypertrophy of the skeletal muscles in the trained athlete. To give another example, the invasion of the body by micro-organisms, in addition to causing injury, stimulates reactive changes in the lymphoid tissues, with the development of immunity. The distinction between the changes due to injury and those due to reaction are not usually so well defined as in the above examples. In many instances where cell injury persists without killing the cells, the cytological changes are complex and those due to injury often cannot be distinguished from those due to reaction. Some examples of the various types of cell injury and reaction are provided in Chapter 1.

In order to facilitate the understanding of pathological processes, it is helpful to group together those which have common causal factors and as a consequence exhibit similarities in their structural changes. For example, bacterial infections have certain features in common, and may with advantage be further sub-divided into *acute* and *chronic* infections. The features and behaviour of neoplasms or tumours are sufficiently similar to classify most tumours into two categories, benign and malignant, and to provide a general account of each group. The changes resulting from a deficient blood supply are similar for all tissues. Accordingly, the first twelve chapters of this book are of a general nature and deal with the commoner pathological processes. The remaining chapters are systematic and go on to describe the special features of disease processes as they affect the various organs and systems.

The causes of disease

Causal factors in disease may be of a genetic nature or acquired. *Genetically-determined disease* is due to some abnormality of base sequence in the DNA of the fertilised ovum or the cells derived from it, or to reduplication or loss of a whole or part of a chromosome. Such abnormalities are often inherited from one or both parents. *Acquired disease* is due to effects of some environmental factor, e.g. malnutrition or micro-organisms. Most diseases are acquired, but very often there is more than one causal factor and there may in fact be many. Genetic variations may, for example, influence the susceptibility of an individual to environmental factors. Even in the case of infections, where the cause is clearly a micro-organism, there is considerable individual variation in the severity of the disease. Of the many individuals who become infected with poliovirus, most develop immunity without becoming ill; some have a mild illness and a few become paralysed from involvement of the central nervous system. This is a good example of variation in susceptibility to disease and illustrates also the importance of *host factors* as well as causal agents. Spread of tuberculosis is favoured by poor personal and domestic hygiene, by overcrowding, malnutrition and by various other diseases. Accordingly, disease results not only from exposure to the major causal agent but also from the existence of *predisposing* or *contributory factors*.

Congenital disease. Diseases may also be classified into those which develop during fetal life (congenital) and those which arise at any time thereafter during post-natal life. Genetically-determined diseases are commonly congenital, although some develop many years after birth, a good example being polyposis coli, which is transmitted by a dominant abnormal gene (see below) and is characterised by multiple tumours of the colonic mucosa, appearing in adolescence or adult life. Congenital diseases may also be acquired, an important example being provided by transmission of the virus of rubella (german measles) from mother to fetus during the first trimester of pregnancy. The early fetus lacks specific immunological responsiveness to this and other pathogens and, depending on the stage of fetal development at which infection occurs, it may result in fetal death, or involvement of various tissues leading to mental deficiency, blindness, deafness, or structural abnormalities of the heart. The mother may also transmit to the fetus various other infections, including syphilis and toxoplasmosis, with consequent congenital disease. Ingestion of various chemicals by the mother, as in the thalidomide disaster, may induce severe disorders of fetal development and growth. Another cause of acquired congenital disease is maternal–fetal incompatibility. Fetal red cells, containing antigens inherited from the father, may enter the maternal circulation and stimulate antibody production: the maternal antibody may pass through the placenta and react with the fetal red cells, causing a haemolytic anaemia.

Genetically-determined disease

As already mentioned, this results from abnormalities, inherited from one or both parents, in the DNA which forms the genome. In some instances the alteration consists of gain or loss of a whole chromosome or of part of a chromosome. Such gross abnormalities can now be detected by cell culture techniques: most of them probably arise by non-disjunction of chromosomes in the meiosis which precedes germ-cell formation, and only a few appear to be compatible with life, e.g. an additional chromosome 21, which is the usual cause of Down's syndrome (mongolism).

A very large number of diseases result from abnormal genes, commonly termed *mutations*. These may be provoked by irradiation, mutagenic chemicals and probably by viruses, but in most instances the cause of mutations in man remains unknown. Examples of the many conditions resulting from abnormal genes are colour blindness, albinism, haemophilia, sickle-cell anaemia, dystrophia myotonica and polyposis coli. The abnormal gene may be dominant, i.e. may induce an abnormality in spite of the presence of a normal corresponding gene from the other parent, or it may be recessive, i.e. causing disease only in the absence of a corresponding normal gene. The latter circumstance arises most usually in abnormalities of genes on the X chromosome, males being thus affected, or from the presence of two abnormal corresponding genes, the likelihood of which is enhanced by inbreeding.

In addition to those diseases due to mutations or recognisable chromosomal anomalies, there are many which show a familial tendency, but in which the mode of inheritance has not been elucidated. Examples include diabetes mellitus, chronic thyroiditis (see (6) below), and some of the commoner cancers, e.g. of the breast and of the bronchus. It is likely that both genetic and environmental factors are of causal importance in these conditions.

Acquired disease

The major causal factors may be classified as follows:

(1) *Deficiency diseases*. Inadequate diet still accounts for poor health in many parts of the world. It may take the form of deficiency either of major classes of food, usually high-grade protein, or of vitamins or elements essential for specific metabolic processes, e.g. iron for haemoglobin production. Often the deficiencies are multiple and complex. In acute states of privation arising from earthquakes, famine or drought, and from warfare, fluid and electrolytes are of particular importance. Disturbances of nutrition are by no means restricted to deficiencies, for in the more affluent countries obesity, due to over-eating, has become increasingly common, with its attendant dangers of arterial hypertension and heart disease.

(2) *Physical agents*. These include mechanical injury, heat, cold, electricity, irradiation, and rapid changes in environmental pressure. In all instances, injury is caused by a high rate of transmission of particular forms of energy (kinetic, radiant, etc.) to or from the body. Important examples in this country are mechanical injury, particularly in road accidents, and burns. Exposure to ionising radiations cannot be regarded as entirely safe in any dosage. While radiation is used with benefit in various diagnostic and therapeutic procedures, any pollution of the environment with radio-active material is potentially harmful to those exposed to it and probably to subsequent generations.

(3) *Chemicals*. All chemical substances are harmful if administered in sufficient amount, and with the use of an ever-increasing number of chemical agents as drugs, in industrial processes, and in the home, chemically-induced injury has become very common. The effects vary. At one extreme are those substances which have a general effect on cells, such as cyanide (see above) which causes death almost instantaneously, with little or no structural changes. Many other chemicals, such as strong acids and alkalis, cause local injury accompanied by an inflammatory reaction in the tissues exposed to them. A third large group of substances produces a more or less selective injury to a particular organ or cell type, for example the barbiturate drugs affect especially the neurones, paraquat causes severe injury to the lungs, while many substances cause death of the cells of the liver and of the renal tubules.

(4) *Parasitic micro-organisms*. These include bacteria, protozoa, lower fungi and viruses. In spite of the advances in immunisation procedures and the extensive use now made of antibiotics, many important diseases still result from infection by micro-organisms, and the danger of widespread epidemics, e.g. of influenza, cholera and smallpox, has been enhanced by air travel. The disease-producing capacity of micro-organisms depends on their ability to invade and multiply within the host, and on the possibility of their transmission to other hosts. The features of the disease produced by infection depend on the specific properties of the causal organism. Bacteria bring about harmful effects mainly by the production of chemical compounds termed *toxins*, and the biological effects of these, together with the response of the host, determine the features of the disease. Viruses colonise host cells, and have a direct cytopathic effect: features of virus diseases depend largely on which cells are colonised, the rate of viral replication, the nature of the cytopathic effect, and the response of the host. Of the protozoa, the malaria parasite is of enormous importance as a cause of chronic ill health in whole populations.

(5) *Metazoan parasites* are also an important cause of disease in many parts of the world. Hookworm infestation of the intestine and schistosomiasis are causes of ill health prevalent in many tropical countries.

(6) *Immunological factors.* Harmful effects, both local and general, can result from the reaction of antibody or sensitised cells with foreign antigenic material. Asthma, hay fever, and skin rashes following contact with various chemicals, are examples of such hypersensitivity reactions, but they are many and complex, and hypersensitivity to penicillin and other drugs sometimes causes a fatal reaction. Disease may result also from the development of *auto-immunity:* the immunity system develops antibodies and sensitised cells which react specifically with constituents of normal cells or tissues, and injury results from such reactions. Examples are chronic thyroiditis, commonly progressing to myxoedema, and the excessive destruction of red cells in auto-immune haemolytic anaemia.

In another group of disorders, the immunity system is deficient, and the patient lacks defence against micro-organisms: this may result from abnormalities of fetal development or may be induced by immuno-suppressive therapy.

(7) *Psychogenic factors.* The mental stresses imposed by conditions of life, particularly in technologically advanced communities, are probably largely responsible for three important and overlapping groups of diseases. First, acquired mental diseases such as schizophrenia and depression, for which no specific structural or biochemical basis has yet been found. Second, diseases of addiction, particularly to alcohol, various drugs and tobacco: these result in their own complications, for example alcohol predisposes to cirrhosis of the liver and causes various neurological and mental disturbances, while cigarette smoking is the major cause of lung cancer and chronic bronchitis, and is concerned also in peptic ulceration and coronary artery disease. The third group of diseases is heterogeneous, and includes peptic ulcer, high blood pressure and coronary artery disease. In these three important conditions, anxiety, overwork and frustration appear to be causal factors, although their modes of action are obscure.

CHAPTER 1

CELL DAMAGE

The metabolic activities of the body are carried out and regulated by the cells of the tissues, and since the time of Virchow cell injury has been recognised as a central problem in pathology. It is clearly important to know what factors cause cell damage and how these lead to the cellular disorders which result in the states we recognise as diseases. Unfortunately our knowledge of this large and important subject is still in its infancy because of the slow development of methods for investigating it, and the extremely complex interrelationship of biological activities within the cell. Nevertheless progress in biochemistry and molecular biology is now bringing the pathology of cell damage within our grasp.

In at least one disease, sickle-cell anaemia, we probably know the entire sequence of events leading to cellular destruction and this can be taken as an illustration of the kind of understanding which is our object for the future in other forms of cellular injury. The sickle-cell abnormality is an inherited defect characterised clinically by rapid destruction of red blood cells. Apparently an error has occurred in copying one base in the sequence of 146 base triplets in the DNA constituting the gene for the beta polypeptide chain of the protein moiety of haemoglobin. This error, transcribed through messenger RNA, results in the insertion of the amino-acid valine instead of glutamic acid in position 6 from the N terminal end of the beta polypeptide chain and the shape of that end of the chain is altered. The change in structure is of no account when haemoglobin is oxygenated, but as the haemoglobin molecule gives up oxygen it expands and the abnormal parts of the two beta chains come to project from the surface of the molecule. Accordingly the beta chains of deoxygenated sickle haemoglobin can unite with alpha chains of adjacent molecules. Masses of long helical fibres of polymerised deoxygenated

haemoglobin form and these impart to the red cells abnormal rigidity and a characteristic sickle shape which make them unduly prone to mechanical injury and subsequent phagocytosis within the spleen. It should be noted that, compared with most cells, red cells have a very simple structure and are easily obtained for study; furthermore, haemoglobin is one of the few proteins whose molecular structure is known in detail.

The mechanism of most other forms of cell damage is much less clear. For example, the mode of action of carbon tetrachloride on liver cells has been the subject of much study. In liver cells of rats poisoned with this substance there are abnormalities of protein, fat and carbohydrate metabolism, and electron microscopy shows damage first to the granular endoplasmic reticulum and later to other cellular organelles. Attempts to establish the primary site of action of carbon tetrachloride by study of liver cell homogenates have not been successful. Several other poisons, e.g. thioacetamide, cause similar effects on liver cells and it is evident that various different injuries lead to a train or trains of common secondary effects preceding cell death. McLean *et al.* (1965) compare the structure and chemistry of a cell to a net. When a net is pulled, all the links are disturbed, and the weaker links will tend to break no matter where the stress is applied. A distorted area of the cell, detected by methods currently available, may likewise be only indirectly related to the cause of the injury.

In the following account only a few of the many possible examples of cellular damage have been selected. The topic is frequently mentioned in later chapters and our superficial treatment of this important subject is merely a reflection of our present basic ignorance.

It is convenient to consider the effects of cellular injury under two main headings: (1) *cell death* or *necrosis*, in which irreversible changes take place in the cell so that no further integrated function such as respiration or maintenance of selective membrane permeability is possible; (2) *lesser forms of damage* (sometimes described as degenerations) in which functions important for the economy of the cell or body are diminished or lost but in which integrated vital functions such as respiration and selective membrane permeability remain possible. Many lesser forms of cellular damage are reversible when the cause is withdrawn, for example the injury to neurones by anaesthetic drugs given in therapeutic doses. Others, not resulting in cell death, are irreversible, e.g. radiation damage to chromosomes resulting in non-lethal genetic mutation.

NECROSIS

Necrosis means the death of cells or groups of cells while they still form part of the living body, and implies permanent cessation of their integrated function. Necrosis may occur suddenly, for example when cells are exposed to heat or toxic chemicals, or cell death may be preceded by gradual and potentially reversible damage in which case the term *necrobiosis* is occasionally used.

Causes of necrosis

(a) **Marked impairment of blood supply,** usually the result of obstruction of an end-artery (that is, one without adequate collaterals) is a common and important cause of necrosis, the necrotic area being known as an *infarct* (p. 173). Different cells can withstand anoxia resulting from impaired blood flow for different periods, nerve cells, for example, dying after only a few minutes, while fibrocytes survive much longer periods of anoxia.

(b) **Toxins.** Certain bacteria, plants, and animals such as snakes and scorpions, produce toxic organic compounds which even in very small quantities can cause cell damage amounting to necrosis. Some toxins have identifiable enzyme activity; for example, the causal organism of gas gangrene, *Clostridium welchii*, forms a lecithinase which acts directly on the lipoprotein of cell membranes. Diphtheria toxin appears to inhibit cellular protein synthesis by indirect interference with the transfer of aminoacyl–tRNA to ribosomes. Certain bacterial toxins, including those mentioned above, exert their effects not only in the proximity of the bacteria but also in organs remote from the infection due to dissemination of toxins by the blood stream and other routes. The necrosis accompanying bacterial infection may be partly due to interference with the circulation brought about by severe inflammation in addition to the effect of toxins.

(c) **Immunological injury.** As will be described in Chapter 5, cell injury results in various ways from immune reactions. This is a feature of many infections, including tuberculosis in which tuberculoprotein, a nontoxic derivative of the tubercle bacillus, evokes an immune reaction which, though possibly protective in function, paradoxically leads to necrosis of cells in the neighbourhood of the organism.

(d) **Infection of cells.** In certain infections, notably by viruses, the infecting agent proliferates within cells. Most viruses kill infected cells in tissue culture (cytopathic effect) and an analogous destructive effect *in vivo* is probably the cause of necrosis of the anterior horn cells of the spinal cord in poliomyelitis.

(e) **Chemical poisons.** Many chemicals in high concentration cause necrosis by non-selective denaturation of the cellular proteins (e.g. strong acids, strong alkalis, carbolic acid, mercuric chloride). Cyanide and fluoroacetate are much more selective poisons and in low concentrations quickly cause cell death by interfering with oxidative production of energy from glucose, fatty acids and amino-acids. As shown in Fig. 1.1 cyanide inhibits the enzyme cytochrome oxidase, thereby preventing the use of oxygen, while fluoroacetate forms a powerful competitive inhibitor of the enzyme aconitase which normally converts citrate to isocitrate in the Krebs citric acid cycle. Necrosis of liver or other specialised cells results from poisoning with such substances as carbon tetrachloride but detail of the mode of interaction between poison and cell is usually obscure.

(f) **Physical agents.** Cells are very sensitive to the action of heat and, depending on the origin of the cells, they die after variable periods of exposure to a temperature of 45°C. Low temperatures are much less injurious and, provided certain precautions are taken, cell suspensions and even whole animals can be frozen without being killed. Necrosis after frostbite is due to

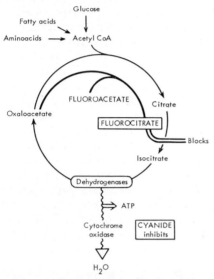

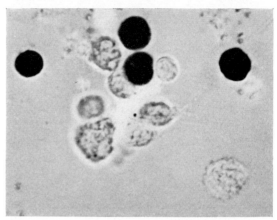

FIG. 1.1.—The effects of fluoroacetate and of cyanide on cellular metabolism. Note that fluoroacetate is converted to fluorocitrate which inhibits aconitase.

FIG. 1.2.—A suspension of lymphocytes treated with cytotoxic iso-antibody and complement. Some of the cells have been killed, and have become stained by trypan blue dye present in the suspending fluid: other cells have survived and are unstained. (Phase microscopy.) (Miss Patricia Bacon.)

of permeability of cell membranes to dyes such as neutral red or trypan blue. These dyes are normally excluded from the nucleus but when cells die, the nuclei become stained due to increased permeability of the membranes of the cell (Fig. 1.2). Alternatively, membranous components of the living cells may be labelled with radioisotopes such as Cr^{51} or P^{32}; subsequent

damage to capillaries which results in thrombosis that may even extend to the arteries. Radiation damage, also a cause of necrosis, is considered on p. 22. Mechanical trauma such as crushing may cause direct disruption of cells. Certain disorders of the nervous system are sometimes accompanied by necrotic lesions in the limbs; these "trophic" lesions were previously attributed to an ill-defined effect of denervation on tissue nutrition but are now thought to result from unnoticed mechanical trauma consequent upon sensory loss.

The recognition of necrosis

As a rule it is not possible to determine exactly when a particular cell becomes necrotic— i.e. when the disintegration of its vital functions has reached an irreversible stage. Many of the changes by which necrosis is recognised occur *after* cell death and are due to the secondary release of lytic enzymes normally sequestrated within the cell, e.g. in the lysosomes; this process of *autolysis* is described below.

Necrosis of cell suspensions in tissue culture can be studied conveniently by observing changes

severe injury to the cell, probably lethal, is recognised by release of the radioactive label from the cells into the culture medium.

In organised tissues such as liver or kidney, necrosis is usually recognised by secondary changes seen on histological examination. In preparations stained with haematoxylin and eosin, the nuclei may gradually lose their characteristic staining with haematoxylin so that the whole cell stains uniformly with eosin (Fig. 1.3), although the nuclear outline may persist; this change, the result of hydrolysis of chromatin within the cell after its death, is called *karyolysis*. Sometimes the chromatin of necrotic cells, especially those with already dense chromatin such as polymorphonuclear leukocytes, forms dense haematoxyphilic masses (*pyknosis*) and these may break up (*karyorrhexis*) to form granules inside the nuclear membrane or throughout the cytoplasm (Fig. 1.5). In many necrotic lesions the outlines of swollen necrotic cells can be recognised but the cytoplasm is abnormally homogeneous or granular and frequently takes up more eosin than normal. In other tissues, e.g. the central nervous system,

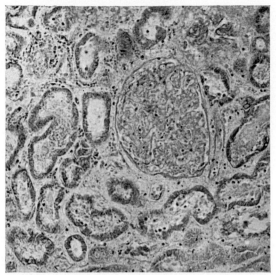

FIG. 1.3.—Portion of infarct of kidney, showing coagulative necrosis.

A glomerulus and tubules are seen, but the nuclei have disappeared and the structural details are lost. × 200.

necrotic cells absorb water and then disintegrate, leaving no indication of the architecture of the original tissue; the lipids derived from myelin etc. persist in the debris of the necrotic tissue. The activities of certain enzymes, e.g. succinic acid dehydrogenase, diminish rapidly after cell death and appropriate tests provide useful indicators of recent tissue necrosis.

Electron microscopy of cells which have undergone necrosis shows severe disorganisation of

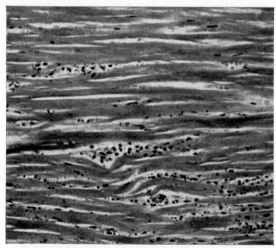

FIG. 1.4—Coagulative necrosis in infarction of heart muscle.

The dead fibres are hyaline and structureless; remains of leukocytes are present between them. × 125.

structure. Gaps are seen in the various membranes and abnormal polymorphic inclusions presumably derived from membranes, lie in the ground substance. Fragmentation and vacuolation of endoplasmic reticulum and mitochondrial membranes precedes the disappearance of these structures. Curious lamellar structures with concentric whorling form from the cell membrane especially where there have been microvilli. Ribosomes and Golgi apparatus are unrecognisable from an early stage. There is loss of density of the nucleoplasm and large chromatin granules accumulate just inside the nuclear membrane before it disappears.

Necrosis can often be recognised macroscopically when large groups of cells die. The necrotic area may become swollen, firm, dull and lustreless, and is yellowish unless it contains much blood. This appearance is often found in kidney, spleen and myocardium. Histologically the outlines of the dead cells are usually visible (Figs. 1.3 and 1.4) and the firmness of the tissue

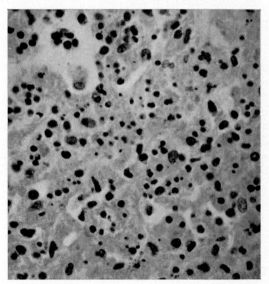

FIG. 1.5—Spreading necrosis with karyorrhexis in lymph node in typhoid fever. × 400.

Note destruction of nuclei and numerous deeply-stained granules of chromatin.

may be due to the action of tissue thromboplastins on fibrinogen which together with other plasma proteins has been shown to diffuse through the damaged membranes of necrotic cells. This type of necrosis is appropriately described as *coagulative necrosis*. By contrast, necrotic brain tissue, which has a large fluid component, becomes "softened" and ultimately turns into a turbid liquid (*colliquative necrosis*) with profound loss of the previous histological architecture.

Certain necrotic lesions develop a firm cheese-like appearance to the naked eye and microscopy shows amorphous granular eosinophilic material lacking in cell outlines; a varying amount of finely divided fat is present and there may be minute granules of chromatin. Because of its appearance this lesion is described as "*caseation*". It is very common in tuberculosis but essentially similar changes are occasionally seen zymes is largely responsible for the softening of necrotic tissues and the associated loss of histological structure. In the intact cell, the enzymes concerned do not have general access to the protoplasm. For example, various hydrolytic enzymes are associated with microsomes, mitochondria and lysosomes. The hydrolases confined within the lysosomal membranes include proteases which are most effective at low pH, a state which prevails in necrotic cells due to acid production from anaerobic glycolysis and the action of phosphatases and proteolytic enzymes.

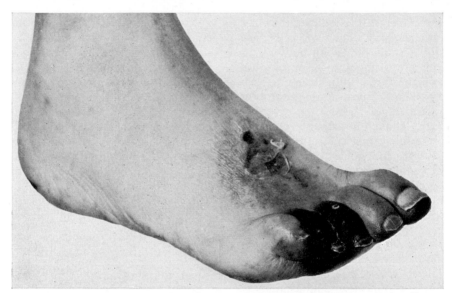

FIG. 1.6.—Gangrene of the third and fourth toes, with more recent changes in the adjacent part of the foot and fifth toe (Mr. Gabriel Donald).

in infarcts, necrotic tumours and in inspissated collections of pus.

Necrotic lesions affecting skin or mucosal surfaces are frequently infected by organisms which cause putrefaction, i.e. the production of foul-smelling gas and brown, green or black discoloration of the tissue due to alteration of haemoglobin. Necrosis with putrefaction is called *gangrene* (Fig. 1.6). It may be primarily due to vascular occlusion, e.g. in the limbs or bowel where the necrotic tissue is exposed to putrefactive bacteria, but it may also result from infection with certain bacteria, namely the clostridia which cause gas gangrene (p. 139) or fusiform bacilli which result in *noma* (p. 140).

The special features of *fat necrosis* are described on pages 595 and 859.

Autolysis. The structural disintegration of cells as a result of digestion by their own en-

The small molecules produced by hydrolysis of macromolecules lead to osmotic swelling of the necrotic cells and their organelles provided that the membranes are sufficiently intact.

It should be noted that when many polymorphonuclear leukocytes are present in necrotic tissue the enzymes from their abundant lysosomes may contribute to the hydrolysis of other cells. This is an important factor in the liquefaction of pus and in the softening seen in infected organs at necropsy.

If tissue is killed by heating, e.g. to 55°C, or by immersion in fixative such as formalin, the enzymes and other proteins are denatured and the histological features of necrosis attributable to autolysis do not develop. On the other hand if a piece of tissue is deprived of its blood supply by removal from the living body and kept at 37°C the development of autolysis can be observed, with marked osmotic swelling of membrane-bounded structures.

With the above points in mind consideration must now be given to two practical aspects in the recognition of necrosis. First, signs of necrosis will not be apparent until enough time has elapsed (12–24 hours) for autolysis to develop in the necrotic tissue. Second, following death of the individual (somatic death), all cells of the body will in time die due to lack of blood supply and post-mortem autolysis will gradually take place. This is particularly marked in the epithelium of the liver and kidney and when seen at necropsy does not necessarily indicate that true necrosis has occurred, i.e. that these cells have died while still part of the living body. This problem is of great importance in electron microscopy which shows ultra-structural evidence of necrosis and of post-mortem autolysis within a very short time.

Somatic death. Though not strictly related to cell necrosis, the interesting subject of somatic death (death of the individual) deserves some consideration. Until recently, somatic death has been defined as complete and persistent cessation of respiration and circulation. For legal purposes the persistence of the state is arbitrarily taken as five or more minutes, by which time irreversible anoxic damage will have developed in the neurones of the vital centres. However, it is now possible to restore the circulatory and respiratory functions of heart and lungs in many cases of somatic death as defined above, and integrated function both of cells and of organs (excluding those of the central nervous system) can then continue for prolonged periods with the aid of special equipment. This fact is of great importance in obtaining organs for transplantation from cadaveric donors and a legal redefinition of somatic death in terms of extensive and irreversible brain damage is now necessary.

Effects of necrosis

By definition, necrotic cells are functionless. The effect of cell necrosis on the general well-being of the body accordingly depends on the functional importance of the tissue involved, the extent of the necrosis, the functional reserve of the tissue, and on the capacity of surviving cells to proliferate and replace those which have become necrotic. For example, the spleen is not an essential organ for health in man and extensive splenic necrosis is apparently of little importance. On the other hand extensive necrosis of renal tubular epithelium results in the serious clinical condition of renal failure which is likely to be fatal unless the patient is kept alive (e.g. by haemodialysis) until there is regeneration of tubules by proliferation of surviving cells. Necrosis of a relatively small number of motor nerve cells may produce severe paralysis which persists because nerve cells cannot proliferate to replace others which are necrotic. Since myocardial cells have not only a contractile but also a conducting function quite small necrotic lesions may result in striking alterations in the electrical activity of the heart.

The breakdown of necrotic cells results in escape of their contents. Enzymes such as transaminases released into the plasma from necrotic liver or myocardial cells form the basis of clinical tests for necrosis in these tissues though it should be emphasised that abnormal enzyme release occurs from cells with damage short of necrosis (e.g. in muscular dystrophy). In poisoning by alloxan, which affects the β cells of the pancreatic islets, discharge of stored insulin from the necrotic cells results in hypoglycaemia which may be fatal (Dunn).

Sequels to necrosis

Neutrophil polymorphs frequently accumulate in small numbers around necrotic cells (Fig. 1.4). Occasionally infarcts and caseous lesions are invaded by large numbers of these cells and this leads to softening as already described. Such softening is a notable feature in a small proportion of myocardial infarcts (which usually show coagulative necrosis) and may lead to rupture of the heart; it is also common in tuberculosis of the lumbar vertebrae where the caseous material liquefies and tracks down beneath the psoas fascia to form a "cold abscess" in the groin.

Individual cells killed by toxins rapidly undergo autolysis and are absorbed, especially when the circulation is maintained. They may be quickly replaced by proliferation of adjacent surviving cells. When a large mass of tissue undergoes necrosis, e.g. in an infarct, the necrotic material may be gradually replaced by ingrowth of capillaries and fibroblasts from the surrounding viable tissue so that a fibrous scar results. If this process is incomplete the necrotic mass becomes enclosed in a fibrous capsule, may persist for a long time, and may become calcified. Areas of necrotic softening in the brain are usually invaded by microglial phagocytes and eventually become cyst-like spaces containing clear liquid and surrounded by proliferated astroglia.

Old caseous lesions and necrotic fat have a marked affinity for calcium and frequently become heavily calcified.

CELL DAMAGE SHORT OF NECROSIS

Many forms of injury may cause cellular abnormalities short of necrosis, which may have profound and serious effects on the welfare of the body. Such cellular abnormalities may be detected as disorders of function, i.e. the impairment of a physiological activity such as conduction of a nerve impulse; by chemical or histochemical means (diminished or excessive enzyme activity or storage or depletion of a chemical substance); by structural abnormality revealed by microscopy of one kind or another, or by a combination of these methods. Some of these forms of cellular damage lend themselves to scientific study because they can be accurately, if arbitrarily, defined in contrast to necrosis, the time of onset of which cannot be precisely established.

The following discussion deals with very heterogeneous topics. First we consider damage to the membranes and organelles of the cell, then give examples of damage resulting in abnormal storage of metabolites. Next, the important problem of irradiation damage, both to single cells and cell populations, is discussed and finally, shrinkage of cells (*atrophy*) and alteration of cell structure to a form more resistant to injury (*metaplasia*).

Damage to Membranes and Organelles

Electron microscopy reveals membranous structures which form the boundary wall around the cell and various compartments (organelles) within. The membranes are composed of lipoprotein (protein combined with phospholipid, predominantly lecithin) and have the general properties of semipermeable membranes. The important definition of cellular compartments depends to a large extent on this property since soluble proteins of different types can thereby be sequestered within the cell; for example, hydrolases, potentially harmful to the cell, are confined within the lysosomes. As a result of the semipermeability of the membrane, the cell and its organelles tend to be subject to swelling and shrinkage depending on the relative osmotic pressures of the solutions in their various compartments and in the extracellular fluid. The membranes are not, however, inert but actively regulate the transport of crystalloids, including electrolytes, by enzymatic action which constantly modifies the chemical structure of the membrane and requires the provision of energy from ATP. Thus although K^+ and to a smaller extent Na^+ can passively diffuse through cell membranes, the intracellular concentration of K^+ is much higher and of Na^+ lower than that of the extracellular fluid; these differences are due to the outward "pumping" of sodium by the cell membrane.

An additional important function of the membranes of the cell is that they form a cytoskeleton. This to some extent determines the shape of the cell and provides supporting structures for arrays of enzymes which form sequential functional units, such as those involved in the citric acid cycle and the flavoprotein and cytochrome systems of the cristae of the mitochondria.

Cell membranes. It has been shown by microsurgery that cells can survive incision of the surface membrane, and presumably self-sealing gaps develop in membranes when particulate material (e.g. nuclear fragments from normoblasts) is extruded from cells. However, most forms of reversible injury to surface membranes are not associated with demonstrable structural lesions. Blebs and holes in the membranes (Fig. 1.7) due to activation of the esterases of complement by interaction of antibody with antigen associated with cell membrane (p. 81) are followed by lethal osmotic injury to the affected cells.

An indication of surface membrane dysfunction frequently encountered following anoxia and certain poisons is osmotic swelling of the

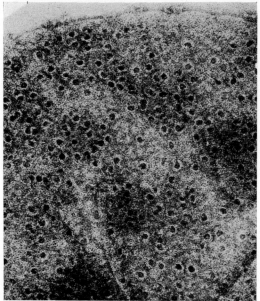

FIG. 1.7.—Electron micrograph of part of the cell membrane of *Esch. coli* treated with antibody and complement, followed by treatment with trypsin. Activation of complement at the sites of antigen–antibody reaction has resulted in lesions—apparently holes—in the cell membrane, and these are accentuated by trypsin. × 140,000. (Dr. R. Dourmashkin.)

cell with accumulation of water in the cytoplasm and resulting separation of organelles (Fig. 1.8 and 1.9). Such intracellular oedema when reversible is probably in most cases due to increased permeability of the surface membrane to sodium, to failure to remove sodium from the cell consequent upon diminished supply of ATP or to poisoning of the enzymes involved in the sodium pump.

Hereditary spherocytosis, an anaemia in which the erythrocytes become smaller and more spherical and are unduly prone to destruction in the spleen, illustrates some of the consequences of a lesion of the cell membrane. According to Jacob (1966) the basic defect is an abnormal permeability of the red cell membrane to sodium which tends to accumulate within the cell and stimulates the activity of the sodium pump, the energy being provided by increased glycolysis. The accelerated sodium transport is effected by cell membrane phospholipid whose metabolism is increased, and this in turn leads to loss of lipid from the cell with diminution of its surface area. Accordingly the volume of the cell is reduced and the cell becomes spherical (giving maximum volume for available surface area). The abnormal permeability of the membrane

to sodium and the spherical shape of the red cells both contribute to their excessive osmotic fragility in saline *in vitro*, a property long known to be characteristic of hereditary spherocytosis.

Damage to *desmosomes*, the adhesion points of cell membranes which bind epithelial cells together, apparently caused by antibody and complement, is seen in the skin disease pemphigus. The desmosomes of the stratified squamous epithelium of the skin and mucous membranes (the "prickles" of the prickle cell layer) disappear and the resulting loss of cellular adhesion (acantholysis) is expressed in the formation of large intraepidermal blisters (bullae) containing viable disaggregated prickle cells.

Endoplasmic reticulum. Loss of parallel arrays of endoplasmic reticulum and vacuolation due to accumulation of water within the membrane-lined spaces are frequently encountered as reversible lesions in anoxia and various poisonings, again presumably due to alterations in membrane permeability (Fig. 1.10). The swelling may be so severe in carbon tetrachloride poisoning as to give the cells a ballooned appearance. A marked proliferation of smooth endoplasmic reticulum in liver cells, seen following administration of phenobarbitone for a few days, is interesting in view of the fact that these organelles contain the enzymes responsible for metabolising this drug.

Disaggregation of polyribosomes, presumably associated with decreased production of mRNA, has been noted in ischaemic cell damage and with certain poisons, some of which also cause loss of ribosomal particles from the rough endoplasmic reticulum. The resulting failure of protein synthesis has been corrected in experimental situations by the provision of a synthetic mRNA, but when the outlines of the ribosomal particles, as seen by electron microscopy, become indistinct there is irreversible failure of protein synthesis.

Mitochondria. Diminished oxygen supply quickly interferes with the important mitochondrial function of oxidative phosphorylation—the production of high energy phosphate bonds in ATP by combination of oxygen with hydrogen through the flavoprotein—cytochrome enzyme systems. One minute of ischaemia causes a tenfold decrease in the ATP : ADP ratio. Mitochondrial function can be restored by a return of adequate oxygenation even after lethal changes have occurred elsewhere in the cell.

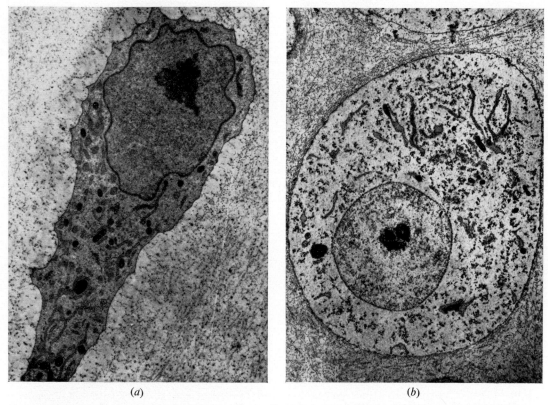

(a)   (b)

FIG. 1.8.—Electron micrographs of chicken cartilage cells (a) before and (b) after injury by glutamyl-aminoaceto-
nitrile. The damaged cell is swollen due to accumulation of water. × 2500. (Dr. Morag McCallum.)

Anoxia and many poisons cause reversible
osmotic swelling of mitochondria which gives
the cell cytoplasm a swollen, cloudy and granular
appearance in light microscopy (Fig. 1.11). This
change, long known as "cloudy swelling", is seen
especially in metabolically active tissues such as
liver, kidney and myocardium, and is exactly the
same as that which develops within a few minutes
of cessation of the circulation after death of the
body or excision of the tissue. For this reason,
pathological significance can be attached to its
finding only if pieces of tissue small enough to be
permeated rapidly are promptly placed in
fixative. Isolated mitochondria can be made to
swell and contract *in vitro* by adding calcium ions
and ATP respectively to the medium in which
the mitochondria are suspended.

Electron microscopy of injured mitochondria,
in addition to showing in detail the site of swelling, reveals other abnormalities. A very early
indication of anoxic damage is the disappearance
of the dense granules occasionally seen in the
matrix of normal mitochondria. These bodies

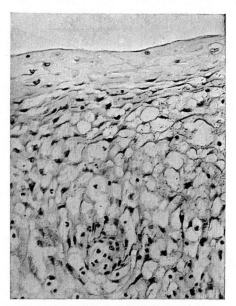

FIG. 1.9.—Ballooning of epithelial cells in acute
laryngitis. × 250.

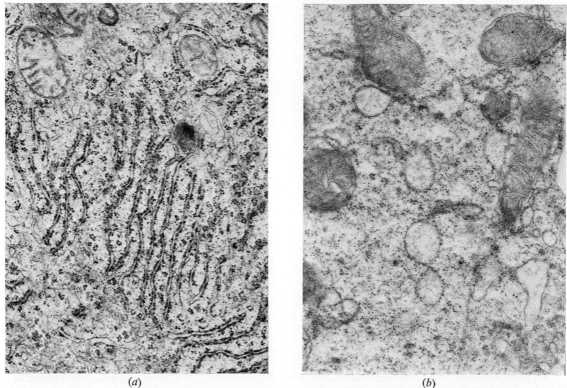

(a)   (b)

FIG. 1.10.—Effect of carbon tetrachloride on the liver cells. (*a*) Part of normal centrilobular cell of mouse liver: note the regular parallel plates of granular endoplasmic reticulum and discrete clusters of ribosomes. (*b*) Part of centrilobular mouse liver cell 4 hours after oral administration of carbon tetrachloride. The plates of granular endoplasmic reticulum appear to have segregated into smaller oval vesicles from which many of the ribosomes have become detached and are dispersed singly in the cytoplasmic matrix. Mitochondria show no abnormality. × 21,700. (Dr. Alasdair M. Mackay.)

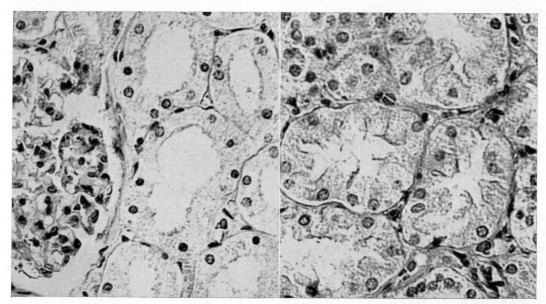

FIG. 1.11.—Left, normal kidney. Right, cloudy swelling of renal tubular epithelium, showing cytoplasmic granularity. × 500.

are thought to represent lipid-bound calcium which accumulates under the influence of respiration and ATP. A later structural change, characteristic of mitochondrial damage following various types of cell injury, is development in the matrix of dense poorly defined aggregations of unknown composition. A second type of abnormal mitochondrial inclusion apparently composed of calcium (sometimes as hydroxyapatite) is found in very varied circumstances, e.g. in renal tubular epithelium in nephrocalcinosis due to vitamin D poisoning or to hyperparathyroidism, and in cardiac mitochondria in magnesium deficiency. Dense

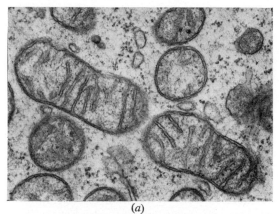

(a)

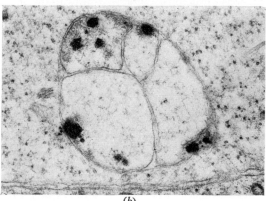

(b)

FIG. 1.12.—Electron micrographs of human erythroblasts. Above, mitochondria of normal erythroblast. Below, mitochondrion of erythroblast from a patient with sideroblastic anaemia. The mitochondrion is swollen and has an electron-lucent matrix in which lie electron-dense masses of iron-containing material. × 37,400. (Dr. A. M. Mackay.)

mitochondrial inclusions (Fig. 1.12) containing iron are found in the red cell precursors in sideroblastic anaemia (p. 428).

Lysosomes. These are cytoplasmic organelles limited by a single membrane. They contain various hydrolase enzymes which act on proteins, fats, carbohydrates, etc. Under the electron microscope they present very varied appearances and can be recognised with certainty only when there is histochemical evidence of acid hydrolase activity. The enzymes have a low pH optimum and become active when the membrane of the *primary lysosome* is altered, e.g. by fusion with a phagocytic vacuole to form a *secondary lysosome*, *phagosome*, or *phagolysosome*.

Lysosomal hydrolases seriously impair the biochemical function and structure of subcellular particles *in vitro* and there has been much speculation on the importance of lysosomal damage in cell injury *in vivo* (see Dingle and Fell, 1969). Damage to the lysosomal membrane leading to release of lysosomal enzymes into the cytoplasm of living cells results in various degrees of cell damage up to necrosis. This happens in certain bacterial infections, e.g. by streptococci, and appears to result from the action of bacterial toxins. It is also encountered in hypervitaminosis A where it is attributed to the surfactant effect of the vitamin on the lysosomal membranes. Another example is the necrosis of macrophages which have ingested silica particles; some of the silica of the particles within phagolysosomes is converted to silicic acid and this forms hydrogen bonds with the phospholipids of the lysosomal membrane which then ruptures and releases the enzymes into the cytoplasm. Some photosensitivity reactions are due to lysosomal membrane damage when certain pigments, e.g. porphyrin, taken up by lysosomes, release energy on exposure to light of appropriate wavelength. Cortisol and chloroquine, drugs known to stabilise lysosomal membranes, diminish cell damage in vitamin A poisoning and some photosensitivity reactions. In many forms of cellular injury, however, the "suicidal" release of lysosomal enzymes into the cytoplasm does not seem to be an important factor. For example, autolysis by lysosomal enzymes in cells injured by hypoxia, carbon tetrachloride and many other poisons occurs only after the cells have become necrotic.

Lysosomes containing membranous structures (e.g. damaged mitochondria) are commonly encountered in cells with focal cytoplasmic damage such as follows irradiation (Fig. 1.13). The damaged parts of the cell are taken into an autophagic vacuole which coalesces with a primary lysosome to form a phagosome, and the activated hydrolases digest the contents of the vacuole. Material resistant to digestion sometimes remains within a lysosome and forms one variety of *residual body* seen on electron microscopy. Lipofuscin pigment (p. 205) seems to originate from undigested lipid-rich material in this way. The hydrolysis of effete membranous structures and the re-utilisation of the

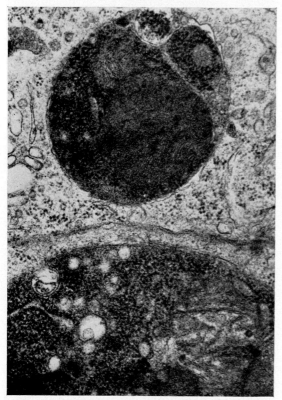

Fig. 1.13.—Electron micrograph showing two autophagic vacuoles in adjacent cells of intestinal mucosa of mouse following radiation injury. Mitochondria and glycogen granules can be identified in the large, electron-dense vacuoles. × 57,000.

products of digestion are probably of considerable importance in cellular economy.

Several inborn errors of lysosomal function have been described. Most of these involve deficiency of an enzyme and are characterised by progressive accumulation of the appropriate substrate within greatly swollen lysosomes. Some examples of the resulting "storage diseases" are given on p. 19 and p. 21.

Nuclear damage

The importance of nuclear damage depends on the fact that the cell nucleus contains the genetic information upon which all the vital activities of the cell ultimately depend. Indeed, as already explained, severe nuclear damage indicated by pyknosis and karyolysis are customarily taken as evidence of cell necrosis. It should be remembered, however, that red blood cells, although devoid of a nucleus, maintain selective membrane permeability, produce energy by anaerobic respiration and perform their vital specialised function of oxygen transport in the blood for over 100 days in man. Protozoa such as *Amoeba proteus* survive at least for several days following microsurgical removal of their nucleus. Motility and phagocytic activity are arrested but these return together with the ability to reproduce when the nucleus from another amoeba is introduced. It is therefore clear that cells can survive despite total cessation of nuclear function; their metabolic versatility will, however, be greatly reduced and their ability to multiply lost.

Gene mutation. Perhaps the best understood form of nuclear damage is that due to irradiation or to mutagenic chemicals such as nitrogen mustards. These and other unidentified factors may result in errors in the sequence of purine and pyrimidine bases on DNA molecules. If the damage is sufficiently localised, e.g. affecting only one base, it is most unlikely to lead to an alteration in the nucleus demonstrable by available chemical or morphological techniques. Its presence may be inferred if there is an inherited abnormality, e.g. an enzyme deficiency due to incorporation of a "wrong" amino-acid at a functionally important part of the enzyme molecule. For example in phenylketonuric oligophrenia, a form of mental deficiency affecting 1 in 20,000 of the population and inherited as a Mendelian recessive, there is deficiency of an enzyme which converts phenylalanine to tyrosine in the liver; in consequence there is a raised concentration of phenylalanine in the blood and cerebrospinal fluid and this results in brain damage. Sickle-cell disease, as already described, is another example of inherited disease due to a single mutation.

In the above examples the mutation has occurred in a germ cell and the resulting abnormality becomes apparent in the descendants of the individual in whom the mutation took place. It is believed that mutation also occurs in cells other than germ cells—*somatic mutation*—but this is likely to be apparent only when the geneti-

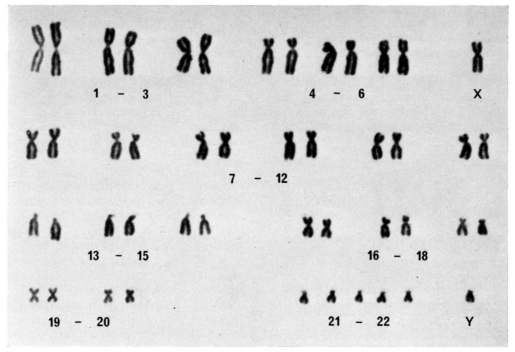

FIG. 1.14.—Karyotype in Down's syndrome, showing three No. 21 chromosomes instead of the normal two. (Dr. M. A. Ferguson Smith.)

cally altered cell proliferates to form a large family or clone of similar cells, e.g. when a tumour forms (p. 224) or, in the lymphoid tissues, during stimulation by antigens (p. 82).

Chromosomal abnormalities. Damage to the genetic apparatus more gross than that described above can sometimes be seen when the chromosomes of dividing cells are examined microscopically. An extra chromosome may be found, e.g. three instead of the normal pair of No. 21 chromosomes are commonly present in mongolism (Down's syndrome), (Fig. 1.14), but it is not understood how the chromosome abnormality leads to the physical and mental defects found in this condition. Total absence of one chromosome from all body cells is almost invariably incompatible with survival, with the notable exception of the Y sex chromosome, present in males (XY) but not in normal females (XX). Individuals with one X and no Y chromosome are phenotypically female but have a group of physical abnormalities including dwarfism and failure of ovarian development known as Turner's syndrome. Structural abnormality of chromosomes in the form of deleted portions or added pieces derived from other chromosomes, or unusual shapes such as rings are sometimes

found and may be associated with characteristic clinical syndromes (Fig. 1.15). In a familial variety of Down's syndrome the two No. 21 chromosomes are normal but there is an abnormal No. 13 chromosome with an attached extra piece derived from a No. 21. This arises from a reciprocal exchange of fragments between two chromosomes during meiosis.

As would be expected, the above chromosomal abnormalities affecting all the cells of the body lead to complex abnormalities since many genes must be involved. They arise during meiotic division of germ cells, the presence of an extra chromosome or absence of a chromosome being due to failure of separation of a pair of homologous chromosomes (*non-disjunction*); one of the resulting gametes will have an extra chromosome and the other will be correspondingly defective. Structural chromosomal abnormality is due to chromosome breakage with re-arrangement of fragments during repair. The reciprocal exchange of unequal fragments between non-homologous chromosomes (*translocation*) accounts for the occurrence of abnormally large or small chromosomes.

Abnormal chromosome numbers (*aneuploidy*) and structural chromosomal aberrations are invariably found in the cells of malignant tumours. The best known example of a consistent structural chromosomal aberration in neoplasia (the occurrence of tumours) is the small G chromosomal deletion, the "Philadelphia" chromosome, present in the granulocytes in chronic myeloid leukaemia (a neoplastic proliferation of leukocytes). Radiation damage is known to cause chromosomal abnormalities in

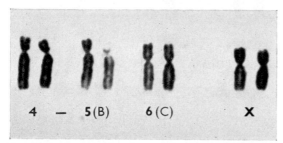

Fig. 1.15.—Structural chromosome abnormality: deletion of the short arms of one chromosome 5. (Dr. M. A. Ferguson Smith.)

somatic cells and the frequency of chromosomal breakage has been used to assess exposure to radiation. Aneuploidy and structural abnormalities in individual chromosomes are also found in other circumstances e.g. in thyroid epithelial cells which have proliferated following stimulation by pituitary thyrotrophic hormone, and in cells damaged by viruses.

Nutritional nuclear damage. An interesting and clinically important form of nuclear damage is encountered in patients deficient in vitamin B_{12} or folic acid. The nuclei are larger than normal but contain less than optimal amounts of DNA for cell division. The chromatin of the

large nuclei is arranged in a fine threadlike fashion (Fig. 16.2, p. 388) compared with the condensed masses seen normally (Fig. 16.1, p. 388), and when mitosis occurs the chromosomes in affected individuals are longer and less tightly coiled than normal. These changes occur in many tissues but are best known in the precursors of red cells in the bone marrow which is said to exhibit *megaloblastic erythropoiesis*. In addition to nuclear enlargement in megaloblasts there is increased amount of cytoplasm, cytoplasmic basophilia due to excessive RNA and apparently premature haemoglobinisation as judged by the immature state of the nucleus.

The mechanism of these changes is incompletely understood. Folate plays an essential role in the synthesis of purine bases and of thymine and deficiency of these substances presumably impairs nucleic acid synthesis, especially DNA which, unlike RNA, contains thymine. This could explain the delay of nuclear growth prior to cell division together with prolonged cytoplasmic growth and apparently premature haemoglobinisation. Vitamin B_{12} is thought to influence nuclear structure by affecting folate metabolism (see Chanarin, 1969). Methyl folate is inactive in purine and thymine biosynthesis and one of the main functions of vitamin B_{12} is the transfer of methyl groups from methyl folate for the synthesis of choline. Accordingly, when there is severe vitamin B_{12} deficiency megaloblastic change occurs due to accumulation of methyl folate, and is reversed temporarily by the administration of folic acid, and permanently by life-long administration of vitamin B_{12}.

Abnormal Storage of Triglyceride Fat

Triglycerides (or neutral fats) are glycerol esters of long-chain fatty acids and their storage in excess is a common and conspicuous feature of cell damage. One of the first manifestations of sublethal cellular injury to be recognised, its mode of development has been a centre of interest for many years. Perhaps of chief importance now is its relationship to dietary excess and to nutritional deficiency. It is important to distinguish between an abnormal increase in the cells of adipose tissue (*pathological obesity*—or, when the condition is localised, *pathological adiposity*) and the accumulation of fat in other

types of cell (*fatty change*). The two processes are quite distinct although in pathological obesity fat also commonly accumulates in the liver cells.

Over 95 per cent of the triglyceride in the diet is normally absorbed in the small intestine: much of it is hydrolysed in the gut into free fatty acids and monoglycerides, but these are re-esterified in the jejunal mucosal cells and passed into the lymphatics and thence to the plasma as microscopically visible particles of complex composition termed *chylomicrons*. Reduction in size of the particles, and some hydrolysis, is effected by lipoprotein lipase; the resulting glycerol and fatty acids are removed from the plasma by the cells of various tissues, including the liver. Some of the fatty acid is oxidised to provide energy, but much of it is re-esterified to triglyceride which is combined with protein, phospholipids, cholesterol and cholesterol esters to form the pre-beta lipoproteins which are then secreted into the plasma, and provide the means of transporting triglyceride in water-soluble form. These pre-beta plasma lipoproteins rich in triglyceride are of very low density (0·95–1·006): they recycle through the liver, but are also taken up by the cells of the fat depots and of other tissues, where the triglyceride is either used for energy or stored. Triglyceride stored in adipose tissue is continuously being hydrolysed, and the fatty acids secreted into the plasma where they are carried in combination with albumin. These so-called free fatty acids are taken up by muscle for the production of energy and by the cells of the liver, where they are either oxidised or re-esterified with glycerol to form triglyceride.

The control of these major metabolic processes is influenced by food intake and also by various hormonal and emotional factors: insulin stimulates the deposition of triglyceride in the adipose tissue depots; adrenal hormones (probably catecholamines and corticosteroids acting together) stimulate hydrolysis in the depots and release of fatty acids into the plasma, as does growth hormone and also thyroxine. The rate of uptake of triglyceride and fatty acids by various other tissues, particularly the liver, is dependent on their concentrations in the plasma. Starvation results in release of fatty acids from the depots, and this is suppressed after a fatty meal. In addition to that provided by the diet, triglyceride is synthesised within the body, particularly in the liver and adipose tissues, from glucose, amino-acids and fatty acids, and enters the metabolic pathways outlined above.

Fatty change

This is the accumulation of fat in cells other than adipose tissue cells, and was previously subdivided into fatty infiltration and fatty degeneration. It is due to imbalance between fat and fatty acids entering the cell and the rate of utilisation or release of fat by the cell. Probably all parenchymal cells which accumulate an abnormal amount of fat are injured. Even the gross fatty change seen in the liver in obesity (p. 548) can be regarded as a form of injury to the liver cells due to the disturbed fat metabolism resulting from overeating.

Because of its major role in fat metabolism, the liver requires special consideration in fatty change. However, fatty change is seen not only in the liver cells, which are usually most seriously affected, but also in various other organs and tissues. The cells most prone to undergo fatty change are the parenchymal cells of the various organs, and skeletal and heart muscle cells, i.e. the cells which because of their specialised functions have a high metabolic activity. Part of their energy is normally supplied by the oxidation of fatty acids, provided largely by uptake from the plasma of free fatty acids released from the fat depots, and lipoproteins secreted mainly by the liver.

Microscopic appearances. In fatty change of most organs, small droplets, consisting mainly of triglyceride, appear in the cytoplasm of the affected cells. Even in an advanced stage the droplets remain small and discrete, and do not greatly enlarge the cell (Fig. 1.16). In the liver, however, they may fuse to form much larger droplets (Fig. 1.17) and the liver cells may be greatly distended.

Electron microscopy shows the fat globules to lie free in the cytoplasmic matrix, without a limiting membrane. The distribution of fatty change induced in the liver has not been fully explained. In most instances, the centrilobular cells are affected first and most severely, but in phosphorus poisoning the change may be very severe and yet confined to the cells in the outer part of the lobules.

Causes of fatty change. The three major causes of fatty change are (*a*) hypoxia, (*b*) starvation and wasting diseases, and (*c*) numerous chemicals and bacterial toxins.

(*a*) *Hypoxia.* The hypoxia resulting from chronic anaemia is a common cause of fatty change in the various organs and tissues. In the liver it occurs especially in the central zone of the lobules, which receives the poorest supply of oxygenated blood, while in the heart it is more marked in parts farthest from the arterioles, that is, it is pararterial in distribution. The change may be seen through the endocardium as a fine mottled pallor ("thrush breast") of the myocardium of the left ventricle and papillary muscles.

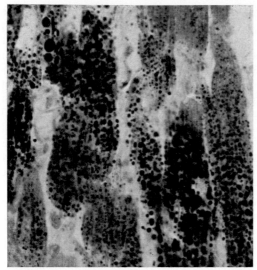

FIG. 1.16a.—Fatty change of heart muscle,
stained with osmic acid.

Note the very numerous minute intracellular droplets
arranged in rows.   × 500

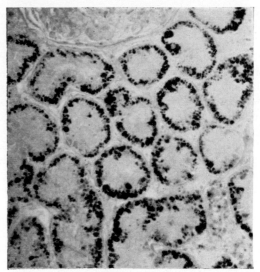

FIG. 1.16b.—Fatty change of tubules of kidney,
stained with osmic acid.   × 500.

Another example of fatty change in hypoxia is in the centrilobular liver cells in chronic venous congestion (p. 158). The fatty change commonly present in the cells of rapidly growing tumours is probably of the same nature, although in both these instances there is inadequate blood supply or flow, and not just hypoxia.

(b) *Starvation and wasting diseases.* Fatty change is observed in the liver and to a smaller extent in the myocardium and elsewhere in some patients who, previously well nourished, have died of a wasting disease such as gastric carcinoma or pulmonary tuberculosis. In other instances of equally or even more severe wasting, fatty change is not found. This has been explained by Dible and his co-workers (1941) who demonstrated experimentally that fat accumulates in the cells of the liver and other tissues under conditions of near-starvation so long as some adipose tissue remains. Once the fat depots are depleted, the fatty change disappears. The low food intake in wasting diseases leads to excessive lipolysis in the depots and release of fatty acids into the blood: these are taken up in increased amounts by the cells of various tissues and converted to triglyceride. Failure of carbohydrate metabolism resulting from the low caloric intake may also be of importance by interfering with intracellular oxidative breakdown of fatty acids, particularly in the liver.

The fatty change in uncontrolled *diabetes mellitus* is attributable mainly to excessive release of fatty acids from the fat depots and impaired carbohydrate metabolism, both of which are a consequence of deficiency of insulin. The situation is thus similar to that in starvation, and in both conditions oxidation of fatty acids in the liver is incomplete and partial breakdown products, aceto-acetic and hydroxybutyric acids, escape into the blood, resulting in ketosis. The subject is discussed more fully on p. 897.

Where a wasting disease is attributable to a toxic condition or complicated by severe infection, this may further impair hepatic fat metabolism, as explained below: a good example is provided by infantile gastro-enteritis due to certain strains of *Esch. coli*, in which dietary intake is severely impaired by anorexia, vomiting and diarrhoea, and the liver is subjected to toxins absorbed from the infected gut. The liver usually shows gross fatty change in fatal cases.

(c) *Chemical and bacterial toxins.* Of the many simple chemicals which can cause fatty change, phosphorus, carbon tetrachloride and puromycin are well-known examples. As in fatty change from other causes, the liver is usually most severely affected, but the changes are widespread, and may involve not only parenchymal cells, but also vascular endothelium and connective tissue cells. Fatty change is also a feature of severe infections, e.g. typhoid, smallpox and septicaemias.

Two factors are involved in the production of fatty change by chemicals and toxins. Firstly, they directly injure the cells; secondly they produce anorexia and often vomiting, and the low calorie intake results, as described above, in increased mobilisation of fatty acids from the depots. The nature of the cell injuries by many chemicals and toxins and the way these cause fatty change is by no means fully understood.

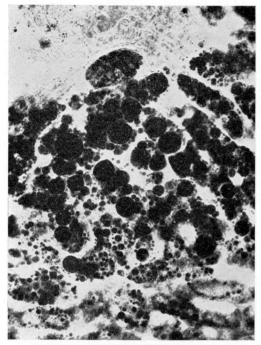

FIG. 1.17.—Fatty change of liver.
The cells are filled with large globules of fat. (Stained with Sudan IV.) × 190.

As a result of recent experimental investigations, it has been established that fatty change in the liver is attributable largely to reduced production of lipoprotein. The triglyceride which would normally have been released as lipoprotein thus accumulates in the liver cells. This applies to fatty change induced in rats by administration of chlorinated hydrocarbons, ethionine, phosphorus, puromycin, orotic acid, or a diet deficient in choline. The fatty change induced by these agents is preceded by a fall in the low-density lipoproteins which carry triglyceride and the reduced amount of lipoprotein present in the plasma shows a diminution of protein:fat

ratio. The nature of the impaired lipoprotein production has not been established with certainty, but the present evidence suggests that some of the agents responsible, e.g. carbon tetrachloride, phosphorus, puromycin and ethionine, impair the hepatic production of proteins. This has not, however, been demonstrated following administration of orotic acid or a diet deficient in choline, and the mechanisms of fatty change induced by these agents are unknown. There is some evidence that choline deficiency impairs the production of phospholipids, which are an essential constituent of lipoproteins.

It still remains to explain how the various chemicals and toxins which cause fatty change in the liver affect also the cells of various other tissues. With the exception of the intestinal mucosa, which shares with the liver the property of converting fat to lipoprotein, tissue cells in general expend fat mainly by oxidative breakdown. It therefore seems likely that the various chemicals and toxins which produce widespread fatty change interfere in some way with this latter process.

Effects. Fatty change results from cell injury, but the degree of fatty change does not necessarily parallel the severity of the injury. For example, liver cell necrosis in virus hepatitis is not accompanied by any significant degree of fatty change, but there is severe fatty change associated with liver cell necrosis in phosphorus poisoning. Also the gross fatty change in the liver which may accompany obesity or alcoholism is not itself associated with severely impaired hepatic function.

Fat accumulates less rapidly in the other organs than in the liver, but as in the liver, the important factor is the severity of the cell injury which has caused the fatty change.

Fatty change in the heart may indicate severe myocardial injury, and heart failure may result from any undue strain. For example, in severe anaemia attributable to a lesion requiring surgical intervention, such as recurrent haemorrhage from a peptic ulcer, it is important that, when practicable, the anaemia should be treated and time allowed for the myocardium to return to normal before any major operation is undertaken. The administration of a large volume of blood or packed red cells over a short period carries a risk of overloading the impaired myocardium, especially if followed immediately by major surgery.

Pathological obesity

Obesity, the accumulation of excessive amounts of adipose tissue, is a subject in which it is difficult, if not impossible, to draw a sharp dividing line between the physiological and pathological states. However, there is no doubt that gross obesity is harmful, and must be regarded as pathological.

Basically, obesity is very simply explained, being due to a dietary intake of calories beyond those expended to provide energy for the body's metabolism. It is thus attributable to overeating, particularly of carbohydrates and fats, often combined with lack of exercise. Attempts to demonstrate metabolic differences between fat and thin people, e.g. in efficiency in intestinal absorption or basal metabolic rate have, in general, been unsuccessful and the problem of obesity appears to reside mainly in the elucidation of the factors which result in overeating, a subject involving psychological factors which will not be discussed here. Despite lack of scientific evidence, however, some individuals seem to be predisposed to obesity more than others, and genetic factors may be involved. It has been observed that when healthy young adults are given a high calorie diet and kept at rest in bed, those who are overweight gain more weight than the thinner subjects. The activity of the thyroid gland, by influencing the rate of general metabolism, has an important influence on energy expenditure, and the pituitary, adrenals and gonads all influence the amount of fat deposited. Damage to the hypothalamus with deficiency of pituitary secretion in early life leads to adiposity along with failure of sexual development, and there is evidence that some forms of obesity in the adult are of similar causation. Extreme degrees of adiposity can be induced in rats by small precisely placed experimental lesions in the tuber cinereum, the mode of action of which appears to be the development of a voracious appetite.

Gross abnormalities of the hypothalamus or of endocrine function have not been demonstrated in the great majority of obese subjects investigated, but it may be that more subtle variations in the functioning of these organs are of importance.

Structural changes. Apart from the increase in size of the normal depots, e.g. the subcutaneous tissue, the omentum, retroperitoneal tissues and epicardium, adipose tissue in obesity may extend to tissue where it is normally absent. For example, in pathological adiposity of the heart, fat extends along the lines of connective tissue through the heart wall (Fig. 1.18), and leads to atrophy of the muscle fibres and consequent weakening

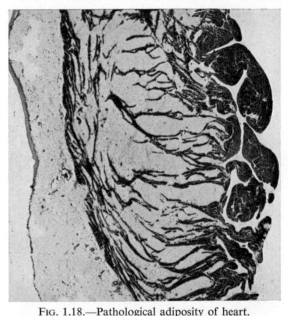

FIG. 1.18.—Pathological adiposity of heart.
The whole thickness of the wall of the right ventricle is infiltrated with adipose tissue extending from the epicardial layer between the muscle fibres which are consequently atrophied. Even the columnae carneae are involved. × 6.

of the wall to such an extent that the right ventricle may rupture. A similar accumulation of stromal fat occurs in the pancreas.

In obese individuals, the liver may be grossly enlarged by accumulation of large droplets of fat in the liver cells. This is discussed on p. 548.

Effects. Apart from the limitations imposed on physical activity by obesity, it has long been recognised, and notably by life insurance companies, that obesity is associated with a reduced expectation of life attributable to an increased incidence of high blood pressure, coronary artery disease, heart failure, chronic bronchitis and respiratory infections, and late-onset diabetes mellitus. The high and increasing incidence of obesity in affluent societies poses a major health problem.

Abnormal Storage of Other Lipids

The lipids of the body other than triglyceride are chemically very heterogeneous and include sterols (cholesterol and its esters), phospholipids and complex lipids (e.g. glycolipids). These substances are frequently united with proteins to form lipoproteins some of which constitute the insoluble membranes of cells while others are soluble and play an important part in the transport of triglyceride in suspension in the plasma. Many diseases are known in which one or some of these substances accumulate in cells in abnormal amounts. By far the most important is *atheroma*, a poorly understood disorder in which various lipids including sterols, phospholipids and triglyceride accumulate in the intima of arteries and cause narrowing or occlusion of the lumen with consequent impairment of blood flow.

Most of the other disorders are much less common but illustrate interesting principles. Pathological accumulation of lipids other than triglycerides within cells may develop in the following ways.

Inherited deficiency of lysosomal enzymes

Cells may be overloaded following autophagy of their structural lipids or lipids derived from their neighbours. A good example is the rare disease due to inherited deficiency of the lysosomal sulphatase enzyme responsible for the hydrolysis of cerebroside sulphate. As might be expected, the predominant lesions are found in the nervous system where the substrate is particularly abundant. The acid cerebroside sulphate gives a metachromatic reaction with such stains as acidified cresyl violet, and since the lesion is most obvious in the white matter of the brain the disease is known as "metachromatic leukodystrophy". Electron microscopy shows lamellated inclusion bodies within lysosomes of affected nerve and glial cells, and similar material lying in extracellular spaces. Other comparable cerebral lipidoses are described on p. 651.

In Gaucher's disease, an inherited deficiency of a lysosomal β-glucosidase leads to intracellular accumulation of glucocerebroside. Neurones and reticulo-endothelial cells of liver and bone marrow are frequently affected but the most striking changes are found in the spleen which may be enormously enlarged probably due to storage of lipid from effete erythrocytes which are removed from the circulation by the spleen as part of its normal function. Gaucher cells present a typical histological appearance (p. 455) and electron microscopy shows large vacuoles containing tubular material. Probably as a result of the lysosomal enlargement, there is a marked increase in acid phosphatase in the spleen and in the serum in this disease.

Metachromatic leucodystrophy and Gaucher's disease illustrate the great differences between lesions due to inherited deficiency of enzymes responsible for intracellular breakdown of lipids and demonstrate some of the reasons for these differences.

Disordered plasma lipid transport

Several inherited abnormalities of plasma lipoproteins are known which lead to massive accumulation of lipid in histiocytes. These cells become spherical and enlarged due to the presence of numerous lipid vacuoles which give the cytoplasm a foamy appearance (Fig. 1.19). The

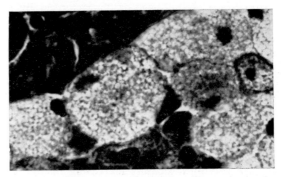

FIG. 1.19.—Histiocytes distended with multiple fine droplets of doubly-refractile lipid. Photographed through crossed polarising films. × 500.

predominant lipids stored are cholesterol esters which are seen to be doubly refractile when viewed under the microscope with polarised light (Fig. 1.20). Large accumulations of these cells (often accompanied by extracellular lipid deposits) may form nodules called *xanthomas* because of their yellow and tumour-like appearance.

In the rare **familial α-lipoprotein deficiency**

there is a moderate increase in the plasma level of triglyceride which is associated with β-lipoproteins as unstable complexes. These are phagocytosed by reticulo-endothelial cells in spleen, liver and lymph nodes, all of which become enlarged due to accumulation of cholesterol esters which are presumably derived from the β-lipoprotein. Great enlargement of the tonsils, orange in colour due to the stored lipid, is a unique finding in this disease.

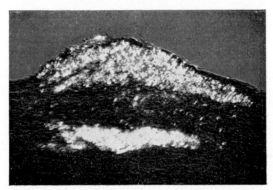

F𝗂𝗀. 1.20.—Deposition of doubly-refractile lipid in early atheroma of aorta, photographed by polarised light.

Familial hyperchylomicronaemia (Type 1 hyperlipoproteinaemia of Frederickson *et al.* (1967)), apparently due to inherited deficiency of serum lipoprotein lipase, is characterised by a milky appearance of the serum due to chylomicrons which are not cleared from the plasma at the normal rate. There is lipid storage in the enlarged liver and spleen and xanthomas may be found in the dermis. It is of interest that in both of the above diseases the stored lipid is predominantly cholesterol ester although the main elevation in serum lipid affects the triglycerides. Presumably the latter are broken down following phagocytosis by the macrophages, leaving a steadily increasing residue of less digestible esters of cholesterol. The steroid nucleus cannot readily be broken down and is mainly disposed of by excretion.

Familial hyperbetalipoproteinaemia (Type II familial hyperlipoproteinaemia) is a relatively common disorder, inherited as a Mendelian dominant, in which the plasma β-lipoprotein is greatly increased. Cholesterol, an important integral part of the lipoprotein molecule, is correspondingly raised, hence the old name "familial hypercholesterolaemia". There is little elevation in triglycerides and the plasma is not milky. Atheroma, fatal even in childhood in rare homozygous individuals, and in many cases xanthomas affecting skin and tendon sheaths, increase with time and parallel in severity the plasma lipoprotein abnormality.

These, and several other inherited lipoprotein disorders, illustrate the varied metabolic abnormalities underlying excessive storage of cholesterol esters in foam cells in different parts of the body. Hyperlipoproteinaemia also develops secondary to other diseases; for example, transitory hyperchylomicronaemia is encountered sometimes when severe diabetes mellitus is inadequately controlled and secondary hyperbetalipoproteinaemia, reversible by thyroxine therapy, is seen in hypothyroidism. These and other disorders (e.g. obstructive jaundice, pancreatitis, alcoholism and nephrotic syndrome) may be associated with various forms of hyperlipoproteinaemia.

Accumulation of lipids in absence of clearly defined metabolic abnormality

Submucosal aggregates of foam cells are often found in the gallbladder giving it a "strawberry" appearance (Figs. 19.47, 19.48, p. 585); presumably this results from intracellular storage of part of the cholesterol that is normally reabsorbed from the bile.

The important subject of atheroma will be considered later (p. 264). Suffice it to say here that pressure filtration of lipoprotein from the plasma into the intimal layer of the arteries leads to a difficult problem in disposing of the associated cholesterol by the local population of modified smooth muscle cells. At first the filtered lipid is found within these cells but these are quickly overwhelmed and most of the accumulated lipid eventually lies in an extracellular position. As already indicated atheroma is particularly prone to develop in individuals with certain of the inherited lipoprotein abnormalities; it seems to result also from modern western dietary habits which lead to alterations in serum lipoproteins and lipids.

Abnormal Glycogen Storage

The normal human body contains approximately 500 grams of glycogen, present mainly in muscle and liver cells, but also found in small amounts in the other tissues. Glycogen is a water-soluble branched polymer, composed exclusively of glucose units, and is broken down by enzymes (glycogenolysis) when reserves of glucose are needed to meet the body's energy requirements, e.g. during muscular exercise. The depolymerisation is effected mainly by phosphorylase enzymes which liberate glucose 1-phosphate, and this in turn is converted into glucose 6-phosphate which can be used for the intrinsic metabolic needs of the cell. For the maintenance of blood glucose levels during fasting and exercise, glucose 6-phosphate must be converted to glucose before release from the cell, and this happens almost exclusively in the liver, but also in the kidney, both of which contain the necessary enzyme, glucose 6-phosphatase.

Largely as a result of the brilliant biochemical studies of G. E. Cori, at least six distinct inherited *glycogen storage diseases* have been recognised, each associated with a different single enzyme deficiency. In several forms of the disease, the affected organs are enlarged due to an increased content of glycogen. Histological examination of sections stained by haematoxylin and eosin reveals clear unstained material distending the affected cells (Fig. 1.21); histochemical confirmation of the nature of the material is given by Best's carmine, or the periodic acid Schiff (PAS) stain (with and without prior hydrolysis of the section with diastase), and this is most satisfactorily obtained with tissue fixed promptly in alcohol in which glycogen is insoluble. Glycogen also has a characteristic appearance on electron microscopy, occurring as dense particles larger than ribosomes; these sometimes form rosette-like clusters (Fig. 1.22).

In *von Gierke's disease* (Cori Type 1) there is deficiency of glucose 6-phosphatase, an enzyme which is associated with the endoplasmic reticulum. The resulting failure to convert glucose 6-phosphate to glucose for release into the circulation leads to hypoglycaemia and a tendency to increased glycogen storage in liver and kidney, the organs which normally contain glucose 6-phosphatase. As a consequence of the excessive glycogen storage, these organs become enormously enlarged. The disordered

carbohydrate metabolism leads to increased lipogenesis and raised serum levels of triglyceride (in the form of low density pre β-lipoprotein), xanthomatosis, obesity, fatty change in the liver

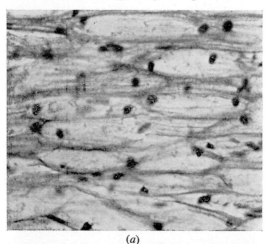

(a)

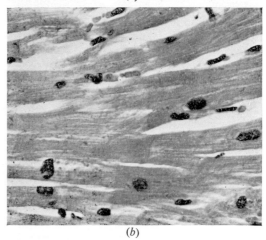

(b)

FIG. 1.21.—Myocardium in Pompe's disease (*a*), compared with normal myocardium (*b*). The affected muscle fibres are distended with glycogen and appear vacuolated. × 460.

and ketoacidosis. The affected children also show retarded growth.

Pompe's disease (Cori Type 2) has recently been shown to result from an inherited deficiency of the lysosomal enzyme acid α-glucosidase which is normally present in all tissues and presumably hydrolyses the small amount of glycogen which enters lysosomes during autophagy. In Pompe's disease, the glycogen taken into α-glucosidase-deficient lysosomes persists and accumulates, being inaccessible to the general cytoplasm with its normal complement of phosphorylase and other enzymes in the major glycogenolytic pathway. Accordingly much of the stored glycogen is seen by electron microscopy to be within greatly enlarged lysosomes, and it seems likely that the serious cellular dysfunction encountered in Pompe's disease is the result of lysosomal rupture and spilling of harmful hydrolases into the general cytoplasm of the cell. This explains most of the features of Pompe's disease, namely generalised glycogen storage—e.g. in myocardium, skeletal muscle, nervous and lymphoid tissue, and peripheral blood leukocytes—enlargement of organs, cardiac failure, mental deficiency, severe muscle weakness and absence of hypoglycaemia.

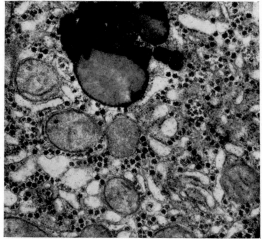

FIG. 1.22.—Electron micrograph of normal liver showing the characteristic small, dense, round particles of glycogen. The large dense organelle at the top of the field is a residual body. × 16,000.

Other extremely rare forms of glycogen storage disease include deficiency of muscle phosphorylase (*McArdle's syndrome*) which results in rapid muscle fatigue without hypoglycaemia, and deficiency of liver phosphorylase which causes hepatomegaly and hypoglycaemia.

Of great interest is the deficiency of the enzyme responsible for the branching of the tree-like glycogen molecule during its synthesis: in this condition the stored glycogen has an abnormal structure which impairs the effectiveness of phosphorylase by steric hindrance.

In contrast to the rare disorders described above in which deficiency of a particular enzyme satisfactorily explains most of the observed pathological findings, increased glycogen storage is found in many other disorders but the mechanisms involved are usually obscure. In diabetes mellitus, a serious disorder of carbohydrate metabolism characterised by diminished ability to utilise glucose, there is increased glycogen deposition in cardiac muscle, in Henle's tubules in the kidney, in liver cell nuclei, in polymorphonuclear leukocytes and in the hydropic β-cells seen in acute cases in young subjects in the pancreatic islets; the glycogen content of skeletal muscle is, however, reduced. More glycogen than normal is found in polymorphs in acute inflammation, in recently formed pus and in the peripheral blood when there is a leukocytosis. Glycogen is abundant in embryonic tissues and in some malignant tumours but in these its occurrence is more closely related to the tissue of origin than to the growth activity. It is particularly constant in clear cell carcinoma of kidney.

Cell Damage Due to Ionising Radiation

Because of the widespread use of radiation and radioactive materials in industry and medicine the study of their effects on living matter is now of great importance. Of all the branches of radiation biology—molecular, sub-cellular, cellular, organ and whole animal—cellular radiation biology is the most instructive in the present state of knowledge. This is firstly because the measurement of effects in terms of cellular units makes quantitation fairly easy. Secondly, it is mainly by the study and analysis of cellular effects that information can be obtained on molecular and sub-cellular processes in the

development and repair of radiation damage. Thirdly, it appears that effects at the level of whole organs or whole animals can often, to a first approximation at least, be described or explained on the basis of cellular injury. This third principle will be illustrated below in terms of the impaired ability of sub-lethally irradiated cells to divide, although the properties which actually characterise a multicellular organism will result in effects which cannot be explained purely by the known properties of individual cells.

Radiation causes its effects by transferring

energy to the substance through which it passes. This energy can produce two changes, excitation or ionisation. Excitation is a change in the energy state of some electrons or charged parts of molecules. Radiations which, like ultra-violet light, produce excitations only, are of very low penetrating power and are not discussed in this section. Other radiations produce mixtures of ionisations and excitations.

No widely useful and accurate biological method of measuring radiation dose has so far been developed. This is because the ultimate biological effects produced are very complex. The standard methods of measuring radiation dose are purely physical. The first is based on the application of a voltage to an air-filled chamber through which the ionising radiation passes. This voltage has the effect of separating the positive and negative electric charges produced by the ionisations. The flow of these charges under the influence of the applied voltage constitutes a small electric current which can be measured with great sensitivity and accuracy. The unit of dose measured by ionisation in air is the *roentgen*. This method neglects the excitations produced by the radiation.

The second method of measuring radiation dose is based on the measurement of the total energy absorbed from a beam of radiation by a solid material. The material must be one in which no radiation-produced chemical energy can be stored, all of it being transformed into heat which can be measured by sensitive calorimetry. The unit of absorbed dose is the *rad*.

Much research has been done on the effects of radiation on aqueous solutions; these are mediated primarily through the decomposition products of the water, and probably reflect the initial damage produced in living biological material. However, this initial damage has never been directly observed. The effects which are observed are the result of an interaction, one side of which is the disruption of the complex of normal biochemical processes arising from the initial molecular damage; the other is the response of the cell or organism in trying to overcome the disruption. From an analysis of these effects much has been learned about the nature of the disruption and repair, but very much more still remains unknown.

Ionising radiations fall into three categories; electromagnetic radiation, charged particles and uncharged particles. The ionisation is caused by the charged particles—electrons, protons or heavy nuclei—which are produced by the electromagnetic radiation and uncharged particles.

All of these radiations can be administered to animals and human beings externally or internally. External sources include X-ray machines, electron or other charged particle accelerators, high activity γ-ray sources, neutron generators, nuclear reactors and atomic bombs. Internal irradiation arises from the ingestion of any of the hundreds of known radionuclides (radioactive isotopes) many of which are used for medical diagnostic or therapeutic purposes, for commercial non-destructive testing and for irradiating materials for industrial purposes; they are produced in nuclear reactions. The best known severe radiation damage produced by accidental ingestion of radioactive material is the damage produced by radium which was once used extensively in luminising paints. Some sufferers from radium poisoning have been under medical supervision for up to fifty years and the effects are well documented. Today, in spite of strict regulations and control, occasional accidents occur in nuclear reactors, industry and hospitals, which result in significant radiation of personnel. Ionising radiation for diagnosis and therapy, however, has a secure and important place in modern medicine and has been essential for many research purposes.

Cellular radiation effects

The foundation of the quantitative study of cellular radiation effects is the survival curve, based on the ability of cells to produce clones of daughter cells in appropriate environmental conditions. One of the most marked effects of radiation is the destruction of this ability. The number of cells in which the ability survives can be readily measured by counting the number of clones in cultures of the irradiated cells.

The percentage "survival", that is, the percentage of cells which still retain the ability to produce clones after irradiation, is plotted on a logarithmic scale and the radiation dose is plotted on a linear scale (Fig. 1.23). Since log percentage survival decreases continuously with increasing dosage, the origin is placed in the top left corner of the figure. The resultant curve usually approximates to a straight line after an initial shoulder. This shoulder shows that an accumulation of sub-lethal damage is necessary before an observable effect is produced. After sufficient dose has been given to reach the straight portion of the survival curve, no further accumulation of sub-lethal damage occurs. If, however, the cells are allowed to recover for some hours, it is found that once again a considerable accu-

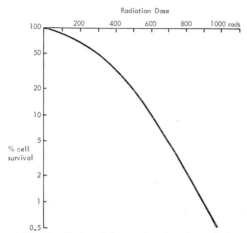

Fig. 1.23.—Radiation injury, showing the relationship between percentage cell survival and dose of ionising radiation.

mulation of sub-lethal damage is necessary before the radiation effects are produced with maximum efficiency. It appears that the shoulder therefore represents the repair process by which the cells can overcome some of the damage.

The slope of the portion of the survival curve which is almost straight on the log-linear plot of Fig. 1.23—the exponential part—represents the rate at which additional lethal damage is produced as additional dose is administered. The fact that this portion of the curve is almost straight means that, irrespective of the damage already created, a given amount of irradiation always reduces the survival by the same fraction. This kind of relationship is indicative of an effect controlled by probability. In this case it is usually regarded as the probability of the track of ionisations, produced by charged particles, causing damage to small discrete targets in the cells.

In the light of existing evidence it is reasonable to accept that, for each type of radiation, no great differences exist in the slopes of survival curves for various types of mammalian cells. The magnitude of the shoulder, however, is dependent on the history, the environment, and the biochemical condition of the cells.

Survival curves referring to different types of radiation have different shapes. The reason for this is that although the total number of ionisations, or the total energy deposited by equal doses of different radiations, are equal, the geometrical distribution of these ionisations in the cell can vary greatly. These large variations in distribution have a considerable effect on the mean number of ionisations necessary to produce the kind of biological damage which, after complex development, results in a cell losing its ability to continue to divide.

Heavy charged particles moving relatively slowly produce dense columns of ionisations, while electrons produce sparse lines of ionisations with occasional small clumps (Fig. 1.24).

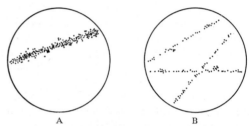

FIG. 1.24.—The distribution of ionisations for high LET radiation (A) and low LET radiation (B).

The average amount of energy deposited per micron of track of a particle or photon is called the linear energy transfer (LET) and can be used to characterise the quality of the radiation. A number of ionisations grouped closely together are more likely to initiate a lethal chain of biological events than the same number of ionisations widely separated. The dense group of ionisations also prevents the cellular repair mechanisms from acting effectively. Thus the survival curves for high LET radiation such as α-particles show no shoulder, and have a steeper slope than those for low LET radiation such as X-rays or electrons (Fig. 1.25). For both these reasons a dose of high LET radiation produces far more biological damage than an equal dose of low LET radiation.

Another factor which has a striking effect on survival curves is the presence or absence of oxygen. Oxygen has the ability to combine with freshly severed ends of molecular structures thus preventing them from rejoining, which they commonly do if the opportunity presents itself. Oxygen thus interferes with a natural recovery process—a different one from that which produces the shoulder—and causes a given dose of radiation to be much more damaging than it would be in hypoxic or anoxic conditions. The ratio of the doses required to reduce the survival

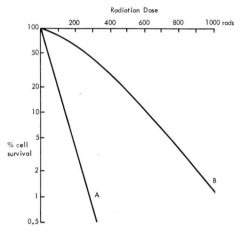

FIG. 1.25.—The comparative cytotoxic effects of α particles (A) and electrons (B).

to the same level in anoxic and normal conditions is called the oxygen enhancement ratio (OER) (Fig. 1.26).

There are many other radio-sensitisers and radio-protectors which affect different levels of recovery and repair processes. Estimation of the biological damage produced by a given dose of radiation must therefore take into account both the type of radiation, the environment in which it is administered and the time allowed for repair and recovery.

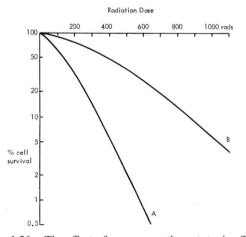

FIG. 1.26.—The effect of oxygen on the cytotoxic effect of X-irradiation. A, high oxygen tension; B, low oxygen tension.

Tissue radiation effects

The effect of radiation in destroying the ability of cells to continue dividing has been discussed above in relation to individual cells. It is important because it plays a major part in causing tissue effects. Cell function which is not related to mitosis and division is relatively insensitive to radiation. Much higher doses of radiation are required to produce gross changes in such function than are required to inhibit cell division. Hence the typical radiation effect on tissues arises from an inhibition of division.

Tissues whose cells are undergoing continuous controlled division, and whose integrity requires a continual flow of new cells are therefore the first tissues to show the effects of radiation. The most obvious are the skin, the intestinal tract, the bone marrow and the immunity system. Similar considerations apply to the therapeutic use of radiation for malignant tumours, in which there is excessive division of cells. The initial effect upon a tissue is a reduction in cell numbers as the supply of new cells falls below the normal rate. The drop in cell numbers leads via homoeostatic feedback mechanisms to a build up of the population of viable stem-cells from which new cells are produced, and to an increase in the rate of cell division. If this compensation is successful, then in due course enhanced production of cells not only restores the depleted population but commonly results in a temporary hyperplasia or overshoot before the cell numbers return to normal (Fig. 1.27).

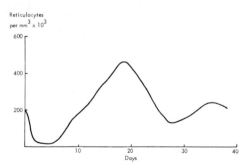

FIG. 1.27.—Changes in the numbers of reticulocytes in the blood following 200 rads whole-body irradiation.

The fall, rise, overshoot and return to normal of the cell populations exhibiting such behaviour after irradiation can be understood and explained in cellular terms if the appropriate homoeostatic feedback mechanisms are known. The normal cell turnover controls the rate at which the cell population falls following irradiation. The extent of the fall depends on the percentage of surviving cells and the rate at which they can divide.

If the cell population of a tissue falls below a critical value the tissue can lose its functional effectiveness. In the cases of the intestinal tract and the bone marrow the result is death of the individual. A rapidly administered X-ray dose of about 800 rads to the bone marrow and 1200 rads to the intestinal tract reduces the number of surviving cells to such low levels that the delay before an adequate production of cells can be re-established is long enough to allow the cell population to fall below the critical value.

The cells whose reproductive ability has been destroyed by the irradiation often remain in the tissue for some time. Their abortive attempts to divide or prepare to divide can produce gross abnormalities in cytological appearance (Fig. 1.28). Toxic products of cell disintegration can increase the damage. However, the damaged cells are no longer directly relevant to the course of events leading to permanent damage or repair. This course is determined by the number of

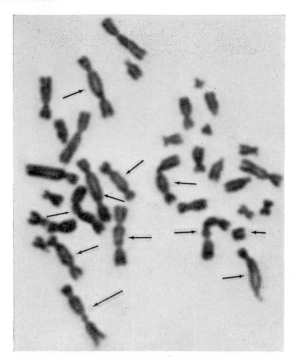

FIG. 1.29.—Dividing lymphocyte in peripheral blood culture from a patient with bronchial carcinoma and spinal metastases, treated by five 500 r doses of Co^{60} radiation to the lumbar spine. This cell shows the result of extensive chromosome breakage followed by random fusion of broken ends due to radiation. There are nine dicentric chromosomes, one possible tricentric, one acentric fragment and at least three other abnormal chromosomes. 44 centromeres can be counted, indicating elimination of two chromosomes. Aceto-orcein × 2,000. (Dr. M. A. Ferguson Smith.)

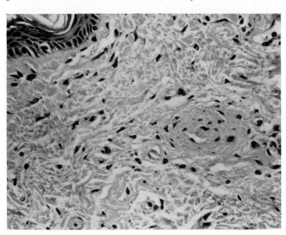

FIG. 1.28.—Variations in the size and shape of cell nuclei following radiation, seen in the cells of the dermis 5 years after destruction of an epithelial tumour by radiation. × 160.

surviving cells still capable of division and by the kinetics of proliferation in the tissue.

Tissues whose cells are long-lived and therefore are not normally dividing show very little effect after doses of several hundred rads. Damage has been done, however, and becomes apparent if the cells are stimulated to divide, even after long intervals of time. Examples of such tissue are the adult liver, adult thyroid, and long-lived lymphocytes. Again the major effect is that many of the cells are unable to divide when called upon to do so, and in the course of their abortive attempts they show highly abnormal appearances (Fig. 1.29).

Radiation damage to the gonads may lead to infertility due to impairment of germ cell division. Errors also occur in copying the base sequence of DNA in the germ cells, the number of errors—mutations—being related to the radiation dosage as shown in Fig. 1.30. A given dose of radiation insufficient to cause infertility gives rise to the same total number of mutations irrespective of the number of individuals among whom it is distributed. As a corollary there is no "safe" level of background radiation. It is known that radiation induces the development of malignant tumours, possibly by causing mutations in somatic cells (p. 217).

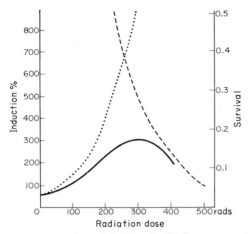

FIG. 1.30.—The effect of dosage of radiation on mutation rate in mice. As the dose is increased, the mutation rate rises (dotted line), but the survival rate diminishes (interrupted line). The incidence of mutation-dependent abnormality, in this case leukaemia, is dependent on mutation and survival rates, and is shown by the continuous line.

Microscopic appearances. Following a substantial dose of radiation there is a latent interval of hours or days before histological evidence of tissue injury is seen. As already explained, the damage depends on the dose and type of radiation, on the interval following exposure and on the tissue exposed. Early changes in the skin include dilatation of blood vessels and other signs of acute inflammation and these reflect acute tissue injury. With a single dose of 1500 rads mitotic activity of the basal cells is arrested, with subsequent loss of the epidermis and epilation. The walls of the dermal vessels are infiltrated with fibrin; later a characteristic concentric proliferation of intimal fibrous tissue is seen (endarteritis obliterans) and large bizarre fibrocytic nuclei are present in the dermal connective tissue (Fig. 1.28). With repeated exposure to radiation the dermal collagen becomes very dense and there is a tendency for the dermal connective tissue to become necrotic even years after the exposure; persistent melanin pigmentation and vascular dilatation are also noted. Comparable changes found in other tissues following irradiation are described later in the appropriate chapters; the detailed findings depend, of course, upon the radio-sensitivity of the various types of cells present and the architectural features of the tissue.

ATROPHY

By atrophy is meant diminution in size of a cell or reduction in the essential tissue of an organ due to decrease in the size or numbers of its specialised cells. Pathological atrophy has its prototype in the physiological atrophy of old age, which affects all the tissues, and notably the bones, lymphoid tissue, and the sexual glands; and although some of the changes occurring in old age are the result of atrophy of the gonads, this atrophy in its turn cannot be explained. The cause of *senile atrophy* is of course merely part of the larger question of what limits the duration of life. Atrophic specialised epithelial cells tend to lose their special features and to become dedifferentiated, as may be seen in local atrophic changes in the liver and kidneys. Senile atrophy is not infrequently accompanied by accumulation of the yellowish-brown pigment lipofuscin and the term *brown atrophy* is then applied. As already indicated (p. 12) lipofuscin represents indigestible lipid which forms residual bodies and is often the product of cellular autophagia.

An organ may be undersized as the result of imperfect development; the term *hypoplasia* is then applied. For example, the hypoplasia of the genital glands which results from deficiency of the pituitary secretion at an early period of life.

Causes of atrophy

1. Defective nutrition. This may be produced locally by arterial disease interfering with the blood supply to a part, when the reduction is not so severe as to cause necrosis. The functioning parenchymatous elements of the tissue then undergo atrophy, and sometimes there is also a concomitant overgrowth of connective tissue. This is often seen in the myocardium and in the kidneys, in which small atrophic depressions result from narrowing of the lumina of the small arteries. When there is atrophy of the muscle cells of the walls of arteries, the overgrowth of connective tissue becomes very marked, and this is possibly of compensatory nature since it gives support and minimises dilatation. *General atrophy* is seen in cases of *starvation*; emaciation depends chiefly upon utilisation of the fat of the adipose tissue but there is also a general wasting of the tissues. The various organs may thus diminish in weight, the liver and spleen are markedly affected, the kidneys and heart to a less though distinct degree, whilst the central nervous system is only slightly affected. In most cases of wasting disease, however, such as malignant tumours of the alimentary tract, chronic tuberculosis or suppuration, a toxic element is concerned in the production of the wasting. Various other forms of cellular damage and diminished cell production may thus come

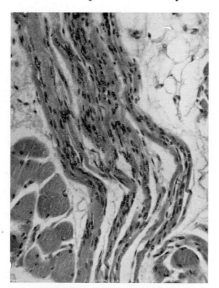

FIG. 1.31.—Neuropathic atrophy of muscle fibres of tongue.

A group of unaffected fibres on the left, contrasts with the atrophied fibres crossing the field. × 154.

to be associated with atrophy; secondary anaemia, for example, is present, although slight or absent in wasting due to starvation alone. The term *cachexia* is often applied to a combination of wasting, anaemia and weakness.

2. Diminished functional activity. It is a general law that diminution in the catabolic processes leads to reduced anabolism and thus to diminution in the size of cells. When the function of a part is in abeyance the blood supply also diminishes. *Disuse atrophy*, as it is sometimes called, is seen when a gland, for example, the pancreas, has its duct obstructed; its functional activity is thus stopped and the exocrine glandular tissue undergoes atrophy. The muscles around a joint which has been immobile for some time undergo marked atrophy and the bones also are affected. Unless such atrophy has become extreme it is

reversible and full functional activity may be restored.

3. Interference with the nerve supply. This form of atrophy is seen where there is any destructive lesion of the lower motor neurons or their axons. In this type, *neuropathic atrophy*, there is not only a simple wasting, but also more active degenerative changes in the muscles (Fig. 1.31). For at least a few weeks after nerve section, during which the muscle fibre mass may be reduced by half, anabolic processes take place at a normal rate: catabolism due to increased lyso-

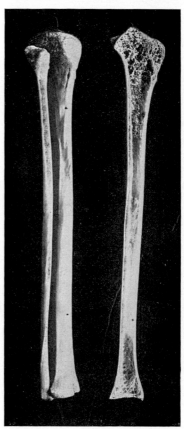

FIG. 1.32.—Tibia and fibula from a longstanding case of poliomyelitis, showing marked atrophy. × ⅓.

some numbers and activity is greatly accelerated. That this form is different in nature from disuse atrophy is shown by the electrical "reactions of degeneration" which are given by the muscles and indicate that a complete return to normal is no longer possible. Sometimes marked atrophy occurs also in the bones from the same cause; for example, in cases of poliomyelitis the bones of the limb may become thin and light and this appears to be due simply to inactivity (Fig. 1.32). In some forms of inherited muscular atrophy, however, no nerve lesion is present and the terms *primary myopathy* or *muscular dystrophy* are often applied (p. 809).

4. Deficiency of the endocrine glands. Atrophy of thyroid, gonads and adrenal cortex are seen when destruction of the pituitary results in diminished secretion of trophic hormones. In thyroid deficiency (myxoedema) there occurs marked atrophy of the structures of the skin, hair follicles, sweat glands and sebaceous glands, but structure and function may be restored by oral administration of thyroid hormone.

5. Toxic action. The best example of this is probably the wasting of the muscles in fevers. No doubt inactivity and interference with nutrition also play a part, but the wasting is probably due mainly to utilisation of proteins, as is indicated by the increased excretion of nitrogen. This increased protein catabolism is one of the characteristic features of fever and is generally attributed to toxic action. Other tissues may suffer atrophy in a corresponding way, but in the parenchymatous organs other expressions of cellular injury are more common.

6. Pressure atrophy is also described. The pressure must be continuous, and it acts mainly by interfering with the blood supply and also the functions of a tissue. Thus atrophy of the organs may be brought about by the pressure of simple tumours and cysts. When bone is subjected to pressure there is active absorption by osteoclasts.

Examples of atrophy are provided in the later chapters on diseases of the different systems.

METAPLASIA

An interesting cellular response to injury is the phenomenon of metaplasia—the transformation of one type of differentiated tissue into another. An example is provided by the surface epithelium of the bronchi which commonly changes from the normal ciliated pseudostratified columnar type to squamous (Fig. 1.33). In this example it appears that chronic injury or irritation, often due to cigarette smoke, results in adaptive changes in the surface epithelium to a type likely to be more resistant to the cause of the irritation. Similarly stratified squamous epithelium may form as a result of chronic irritation in the mucous membrane of the nose, salivary ducts, gallbladder, renal pelvis and urinary bladder. In some cases the injurious stimulus is apparent, e.g. when there is a stone in the renal pelvis or in cases of extroversion of the urinary bladder, while in others the cause is obscure. In vitamin A deficiency, in addition to xerophthalmia, stratified squamous epithelium may replace the transitional and columnar epithelia of nose, bronchi, urinary tract, and the specialised secretory epithelia of the lacrimal and salivary glands. In auto-immune chronic gastritis, a condition in which the lymphoid cells attack the mucosa of the fundus of the patient's own stomach, the specialised surface-lining cells and chief and parietal cells of the gastric glands are often replaced by tall columnar cells with striated

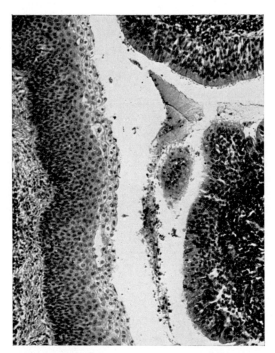

Fig. 1.33.—Metaplasia of bronchial epithelium to stratified squamous type is seen on the left side, persistence of columnar ciliated epithelium on the right. × 200.

borders, goblet cells and Paneth cells—*intestinal metaplasia*.

In the connective tissues, metaplasia occurs between fibrous tissue, myxoid tissue, bone and cartilage. Bone formation occasionally follows the deposition of calcium salts in such tissues as arterial walls (Fig. 1.34), bronchial cartilage and the uveal tract of the eye. In healing fractures cartilaginous metaplasia may occur especially when there is undue mobility. The flattened serosal endothelium of the rabbit pleural cavity becomes cubical, columnar, transitional or even squamous following injection of the dye Sudan III with sodium cholate in olive oil and the lining of adjacent alveoli also becomes cubical or columnar. Similar changes, which are rapidly reversible, follow the injection of strontium chloride.

Metaplasia is to be distinguished from a mere loss of the special characters of cells, for example the dedifferentiation which is encountered when there is interference with the function of glands. Developmental epithelial abnormalities e.g. squamous epithelium within the thyroid, arising from the thyroglossal duct, do not constitute metaplasia nor does encroachment of one tissue upon another. Thus the fatty marrow of the long bones is replaced in certain types of anaemia by red haemopoietic marrow: in this case the haemopoietic tissue has spread by proliferation of haemopoietic stem cells and not by metaplasia of the adipose tissue cells originally present.

It is believed that all nucleated cells carry a complete list of the genetic information required for bodily development, including all types of cellular differentiation and function, but little is yet known about the factors which determine the differentiation of cells in an orderly manner to form the various tissues. The way in which the many different stimuli producing metaplasia act within the cell is correspondingly obscure. It seems likely that a change in gene repression and activation takes place in serosal endothelium when it undergoes metaplasia to squamous epithelium. On the other hand in surfaces lined by columnar epithelium, metaplasia may result from gradual atrophy of the columnar cells and proliferation and maturation of the less well differentiated basal or reserve cells to form squamous epithelium. It is noteworthy that many stimuli which bring about metaplasia are also capable of inducing neoplasia, and indeed tumour formation is relatively common in some metaplastic epithelia; conversely metaplasia is frequently encountered in malignant tumours. Indeed metaplasia may represent a cellular change in response to injury intermediate between the kind we have been considering earlier in this chapter and that which underlies the development of tumours.

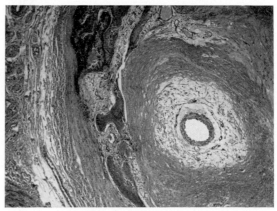

FIG. 1.34.—Metaplastic bone formation in the wall of a partially obliterated artery. × 50.

CHAPTER 2

INFLAMMATION

Introduction

The term inflammation has been used since the earliest days of medicine. Celsus (30 B.C. to A.D. 38) gave as its cardinal signs; heat, redness, swelling and pain, and to these Galen (A.D. 130–200) added impairment of function, such as limitation of movement of an inflamed limb. These changes are most commonly the result of infection with micro-organisms, but even before the discovery of bacteria inflammation had been produced experimentally, e.g. by Lister, by the application of irritating chemicals to the tissues, and the underlying processes had been studied in detail. Cohnheim (1882) first emphasised the important part played by damage to the small blood vessels in producing the changes of inflammation, and it has become increasingly apparent that vascular changes dominate the picture of inflammation, and that they are induced by tissue injury which may be brought about in many different ways. Physical agents such as heat, mechanical trauma, ultraviolet and X-irradiation, and a very wide range of chemicals, both organic and inorganic, and including the metabolic products (toxins) of many bacteria, are all capable of causing inflammation in the tissues to which they are applied. We may define inflammation as the series of changes which takes place following injury to a living tissue provided that the injury is not of such a nature as at once to destroy its structure and vitality. Depending on the degree and duration of tissue injury, all grades of inflammatory changes are observed, and they may subside within a few hours or may persist, even for months or years. There is, of course, a limit to the severity of injury to which the tissues can be subjected without producing cessation of blood flow and necrosis, but even in such serious injuries, the adjacent tissues will be less severely damaged,

and inflammatory change commonly surrounds the area of central necrosis.

As it results from tissue injury, inflammation cannot be regarded as a physiological change. Nevertheless, it has, in general, beneficial effects in combating infection and in limiting the extent of injury caused by toxic compounds, and it is appropriate to refer to inflammation as being a *response* or *reaction* to tissue injury. Like other beneficial processes, it is not without disadvantages and, as explained later, it may lead to the production of scar tissue. Moreover, the changes of inflammation can occur as a result of hypersensitivity reactions, i.e. immunological reactions occurring within the tissues, and in these circumstances the entry of normally harmless substances into the body can induce inflammatory changes which appear to serve no useful function.

The changes of inflammation are conveniently grouped into two major classes which may be termed *exudative* and *formative* respectively. Exudative changes result from acute tissue injury, are mainly vascular, and are responsible for the cardinal signs of heat, redness, swelling and pain, described by Celsus. The major processes involved include (1) dilatation of blood vessels in the affected tissues; (2) increase in the permeability of the walls of capillaries and venules; (3) escape of protein-rich fluid from the blood plasma, and (4) migration of phagocytic leukocytes from the blood vessels into the interstitium of the tissues. While this group of changes, which provide the main topic of this chapter, may suitably be termed the *acute inflammatory reaction*, they may continue for long periods and are observed throughout chronic infections with various types of bacteria. Formative changes in inflammation consist mainly in the production of young connective (*granulation*) tissue which matures into collagenous or scar tissue: the processes involved are closely similar to those of healing and repair which are discussed in the next chapter. Although formative changes may occur without much exudation, both processes are often pre-sent in marked degree, particularly in prolonged infections with certain bacteria. It is therefore incorrect to regard chronic inflammation as *solely* formative, as is sometimes done.

THE ACUTE INFLAMMATORY REACTION

The gross and microscopic appearances of inflamed tissues vary greatly depending on the structure of the tissues affected, the nature of the injurious agent, and the dose and duration of its application. Nevertheless, the under-lying processes are the same in all instances, and may be grouped together as the acute inflammatory reaction. For various reasons, these processes are studied most readily in inflammation produced experimentally by thermal or chemical injury, and much of our knowledge stems from observing the changes occurring in tissues during the few hours follow-ing such injuries. The available evidence suggests that the findings obtained from this work are applicable also to the inflammatory changes produced by infections.

The mild inflammatory changes which result from firm stroking of the skin were described in 1927 by Sir Thomas Lewis. After transient initial pallor a line of dull redness (the flush) appeared along the stroke. This was followed by reddening of the surrounding skin (the flare) and if the stroke was sufficiently firm by swelling of the skin (the weal). Lewis recognised these three components of this mild inflammatory reaction, which he termed the *triple response*. The changes illustrate two of the cardinal signs of inflammation, namely redness and swelling, and even in such mild transient in-flammation careful measurement will show a rise in the temperature of the reddened skin, a feature which is more readily detected by simply palpating more severely inflamed skin, as in acute bacterial infections. The triple response can be elicited also by mild injury induced by application of certain chemicals to the skin or other tissues. In such mild inflammations, the tissues return to normal by a process termed *resolution*. In more severe inflammation caused by thermal injury, various severely toxic chemicals and many bacterial infections, the changes are more widespread and persistent, and pain and partial immobilisation of the affected tissues are experienced. The most severely injured tissues may also be destroyed and the dead tissue is either separated and dis-charged if superficial (as in the common boil) or if deeper is gradually digested and replaced by young connective (granulation) tissue, scar tissue being the end result. Another regular feature of acute inflammation, migration of phagocytic cells of the blood into the interstitial spaces of the affected tissues, is particularly marked in infections with certain bacteria. When accompanied by death of tissue, the phagocytes, and particularly neutrophil poly-morphs, migrate into and digest the dead tissue, leaving a space filled with fluid exudate rich in polymorphs (*pus*). Such a space is termed an *abscess cavity* and by formation of new con-nective tissue comes to be enclosed in a capsule or *pyogenic membrane*; scarring results and may be extensive. The production of granulation tissue eventually maturing into scar tissue, i.e. formative changes, occurs also when the inflam-matory exudate is rich in fibrinogen which, on leaving the blood vessels, coagulates to form insoluble fibrin. In inflammation of serous membranes a thick layer of fibrin is commonly deposited on the surface, e.g. of the pleura or pia-arachnoid, and is eventually replaced by fibrous tissue. Both the fibrin and the sub-sequently formed fibrous tissue may give rise to adhesions and may have deleterious mechanical effects.

The changes of the acute inflammatory reaction together with mediating factors and effects must now be considered in more detail. The processes involved have been elucidated mainly in tissues which are suitable for micro-scopic examination in the living state, for example in the web of the frog's foot, the frog's tongue, the mammalian mesentery, and by means of a transparent chamber implanted in the rabbit's ear.

Vascular hyperaemia

Dilatation of the arterioles, capillaries and venules is an essential and early feature of acute inflammation (Figs. 2.1, 2.2). Before considering the mechanisms involved, it is appropriate to describe some of the features of the normal microcirculation.

Normal microcirculatory control. The smallest arterioles are connected to the smallest venules by thoroughfare channels containing muscle cells at their arterial end. Off these the true capillaries open, usually with a backward loop, their mouths being guarded by muscular sphincters; after a short course, in which they anastomose freely, they rejoin the thoroughfare channel towards the venous end at an acute angle. The capillary walls consist of a single layer of endothelial cells, the overlapping edges of which, as revealed by electron microscopy, appear to correspond to the so-called cement lines. These cells are surrounded externally by a basement membrane which splits to enclose here and there smaller peri-endothelial cells, the function of which is unknown.

Under normal resting conditions, at any one time only some of the true capillaries contain red cells, the entry of which is controlled by the precapillary sphincters. In the functional sense, capillaries have independent powers of contraction and relaxation, but the capacity for rapid contractility appears to be restricted anatomically to the precapillary sphincters, and, during periods when entry of red cells is restricted, the capillaries may retain their usual diameter although filled only with plasma. The rapid flow of blood across their venous junctions exercises a certain suction effect and drains their plasma back into the general circulation. During this phase the true capillaries take up fluid from the tissue spaces whereas during their active perfusion with red cells fluid is given out. No doubt this alternation of activities plays an important part in fluid exchange. When the precapillary sphincters are closed and the return of plasma to the venules is greater than the uptake of fluid from the tissues, the true capillaries may be collapsed. When, therefore, we speak of *dilatation* of the capillaries we really refer to the filling of these channels with red cells. When we speak of *contraction* we refer to their emptying owing to the action of precapillary sphincters restricting the entry of red cells, without implying that the capillary wall as a whole undergoes contraction throughout its length. Capillary endothelial cells in general are able to contract only feebly and slowly, and this property is not apparently concerned in

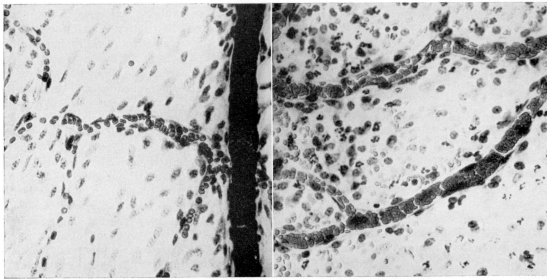

FIG. 2.1.—Surface view of normal omentum of guinea-pig. × 300.

FIG. 2.2.—Inflamed omentum of guinea-pig, showing emigration of leukocytes, increased cellularity, and engorgement of small vessels. × 300.

the normal control of the circulation through the tissues.

Microcirculatory changes in inflammation. As illustrated in Lewis's triple response there are two phases of tissue reddening in early inflammation. Firstly the flush, which is dull red and confined to the area of tissue directly injured. Secondly the flare, which is bright red and extends into the surrounding tissue. Microscopically the flush is seen to be due to dilatation of venules and capillaries. This is independent of local nerves and still occurs following section and degeneration of these. It is seen also in tissues in which the arterial flow has been temporarily arrested by means of a tourniquet, and indeed persists during the period of arrest of blood flow. The flush is therefore not dependent on raised intravascular pressure. Lewis showed that these features were mimicked by an intradermal injection of histamine and considered that the flush was due to a chemical mediator, which he termed "H" or histamine-like substance, produced by tissue injury. The role of histamine in inflammation will be considered later (p. 37). The flare is attributable to dilatation of arterioles outwith the area of tissue injury. This results in increased hydrostatic intravascular pressure

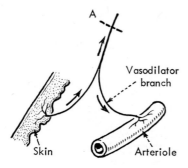

FIG. 2.3.—Diagram of peripheral end of sensory nerve fibre with vasodilator axon branch. Stimulation of sensory nerve ending in the skin results in an antidromic reflex along vasodilator branch, with resulting arteriolar dilatation. Section of the nerve fibre at A does not abolish this reflex until the fibre distal to A has degenerated.

which extends to the capillaries and even venules, resulting in their mechanical dilatation and a great increase in blood flow. There is evidence that this arteriolar dilatation is mediated by an axon reflex, stimulation of the sensory nerve endings, probably by histamine, providing impulses which pass up the axon and then along its vasodilator branch (see Fig. 2.3) to an

adjacent arteriole. This explanation is supported by experiments in which it has been shown that section of the nerve (at point A) does not prevent production of the flare unless time has been allowed for degeneration of the axon to occur. Stimulation of the peripheral end of the recently cut nerve or of the sensory ending both cause a flare, but this is also inhibited by first allowing time for degeneration of the nerve to take place.

The autonomic nerve supply to arterioles can influence the degree of their dilatation in the inflammatory reaction but does not appear to play a basic role in the process.

The effects of the vascular dilatation in acute inflammation are considered on p. 35 in relation to exudation: briefly, the consequent rise in intravascular pressure increases the amount of fluid and electrolytes which pass from the blood to the interstitium of the surrounding tissues but has little effect on the escape of macromolecules, such as plasma proteins.

Changes in blood flow

During the early stages of acute inflammation, microscopic examination shows a great increase in rapidity of blood flow through the dilated arterioles, capillaries and venules. This may persist for some hours and is followed by a gradual slowing of blood flow although the vessels remain dilated: complete stasis of flow may ensue, and in intense inflammation there may even be coagulation of the stagnant blood. As explained below, there is escape of a considerable portion of the plasma fluid from the dilated capillaries and venules and this results in haemoconcentration of the red cells, which become aggregated into rouleaux. These changes increase the viscosity of the blood and result in slowing of the blood stream. The effect of haemoconcentration on blood flow can be demonstrated by an application of hypertonic solution to living tissue: this withdraws fluid from the small vessels and blood flow slows dramatically. It may be that changes in the capillary and venular endothelium also impede blood flow by increasing frictional resistance, but although the endothelial cells may enlarge, specific changes in their luminal surface have not been observed by light or electron microscopy.

Slowing of the blood flow will tend to impair

the supply of oxygen, glucose, etc., to the tissues, and also the removal of metabolites, but these effects are likely to be counteracted by the increased flow of fluid from the plasma into the tissues and increased lymphatic drainage (see below). In fact, it is only when the vascular stagnation is extreme that it appears to impair tissue nutrition seriously and in this circumstance it may contribute to the necrosis which is commonly observed in severe inflammatory reactions.

Exudation of fluid

Microscopic examination of inflamed tissues reveals an accumulation of extracellular fluid, i.e. interstitial oedema (Fig. 2.4). This can only

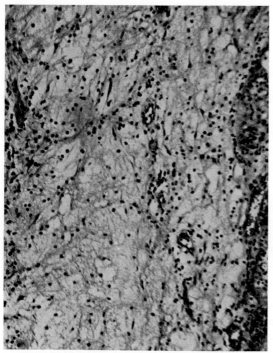

FIG. 2.4.—Meso-appendix in acute appendicitis, showing inflammatory oedema with early leukocytic emigration. × 100.

the walls of the small vessels were elucidated largely by Starling, who pointed out that the main force driving fluid out of vessels is the difference between the hydrostatic pressure within the vessels and that in the extravascular space, and that this was opposed by the difference between the osmotic pressure of the plasma and that of the interstitial fluid. He envisaged the vascular endothelium as behaving like a semipermeable membrane across which fluid and electrolytes moved according to the relative effects of these two forces. This hypothesis is supported by the demonstration that there is a rise in the hydrostatic pressure within the capillaries and a rise in the osmotic pressure of the interstitial fluid in inflamed tissues: both these changes will tend to increase the amount of fluid leaving the vessels and reduce the amount returning to them (Fig. 2.5). The hydrostatic pressure in the small vessels in normal and inflamed tissues was investigated by Landis

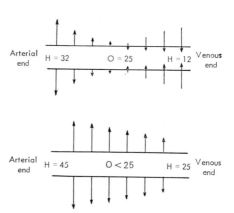

FIG. 2.5.—Exchange of fluid across the walls of capillaries and venules. H and O represent the heights of the hydrostatic and osmotic pressures respectively (mm. Hg.) of the plasma above the corresponding pressures of the extravascular space. The arrows indicate the net movement of fluid into and out of the vessels along their length. Upper figure, normal tissue: fluid movement across vessel walls approximates to equilibrium. Lower figure, acute inflammation: much more fluid leaves the vessels than returns to them.

The values of H and O are approximations. In inflammation, H may be less than indicated by rise of pressure in the extravascular space, and O will be reduced by escape of plasma proteins into the inflammatory exudate.

have come from the plasma of the blood and since it has been shown that the amount of fluid draining away from inflamed tissues by the lymphatics is also greatly increased, it is apparent that there is a considerable rise in the amount of fluid leaving the blood vessels. The factors involved in the passage of fluid through

(while he was a medical student). The pressure in the arteriolar and venular ends of the capillaries of small mammals is normally 32 and 12 mm. Hg. respectively above that of the extravascular fluid, which approximates to atmospheric pressure. The osmotic pressure of the plasma is normally about 25 mm. Hg., and is exerted mainly by the plasma proteins, while the extravascular fluid, being poor in proteins, exerts a very low osmotic pressure. Consequently, there will be loss of fluid from the arteriolar end of capillaries and re-absorption into the venular end and into venules. The result is an equilibrium in which most of the fluid leaving the blood is normally re-absorbed: the remainder, as measured by regional lymph flow, varies in amount for different tissues. In the limbs it is very small but is increased by movement, whereas much larger amounts of lymph drain from some of the internal organs and particularly from the liver. In inflammation induced by chemicals and also by injection of histamine, Landis demonstrated by means of fine cannulae attached to manometers that the hydrostatic pressure of the blood in the capillaries rose to over 40 and over 20 mm. Hg. at the arteriolar and venular ends respectively.

The second major factor in the production of inflammatory oedema is a rise in osmotic pressure of the extravascular fluid. This is due mainly to an increase in the permeability of the walls of the capillaries and venules, resulting in escape of increased amounts of plasma proteins into the extravascular fluid. Accordingly the lymph draining from inflamed tissues increases greatly, not only in volume, but also in its protein concentration. Drinker showed, for example, that the protein concentration of lymph flowing from the leg of a dog was increased from approximately 2% to over 4% when sterile inflammation was induced in the tissues of the leg. Similar observations have been made by many workers using various experimental models. The same principles apply to fluid loss from the small vessels in man: both the overall capillary pressure and the osmotic pressure of the plasma are normally greater than in small mammals, but a similar balance is maintained with normally only a small net loss of plasma fluid, and the changes leading to exudation in inflamed tissues are the same.

The proportions of the various proteins in the inflammatory exudate differ from those in the plasma; the amount of each escaping does not depend solely on its concentration in the plasma but is related inversely to its molecular size.

There is thus a disproportionately high concentration of albumin in the exudate, as compared with the relatively larger molecules of globulins and fibrinogen. Nevertheless, all the plasma proteins are present in the exudate, and where the increase in vascular permeability is considerable, there may be escape of fibrinogen in sufficient amounts for a fibrin coagulum to be produced by the action of tissue thromboplastin (p. 163) (Figs. 2.6, 2.7). It is not known whether this molecular sieving effect is exerted by the vascular endothelial layer, or by the basement membrane.

Two important questions relate to the increased vascular permeability of inflammation. Firstly, what are the mediating agents? Secondly, what is the route of escape of the exudate? Both have long been controversial and are discussed below.

Mediators of increased vascular permeability. It has long been known that the inflammatory

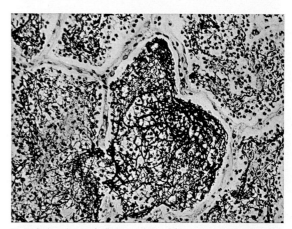

FIG. 2.6.—Acute inflammation of lung, showing network of fibrin and numerous polymorphonuclear leukocytes (Weigert's fibrin stain).   × 150.

exudate contains, in solution, agents which are capable of inducing an inflammatory reaction, including increased vascular permeability, when injected into the tissues of normal animals. This raises the probability that chemical mediators are responsible for the increased vascular permeability, and since heat or mechanical trauma can cause inflammation it appears that endogenous humoral factors resulting from tissue damage are involved. The nature of these factors has been investigated extensively, but progress has been slow. Of many substances, both real and hypothetical, which have been suspected, only histamine has been convincingly implicated, and it is by no means solely responsible for increasing vascular permeability. Most of the suspected substances are highly labile, particularly *in vivo*, and are difficult to investigate.

A useful method of studying increased vascular permeability is to introduce readily visualised macromolecular or particulate material, such as a colloidal suspension of carbon, into the circulation of an animal at intervals after the application of an inflammatory stimulus. The escape of the macromolecules or colloidal particles from individual capillaries and venules can then be observed microscopically, both in the living tissue and in fixed material. By this and similar experimental procedures, it has been shown that during the early stages of the inflammatory reaction, increased vascular permeability occurs mainly in venules; this subsides and is followed by a later phase of increased permeability of both the capillaries and venules. During the early phase, histamine is known to be released in effective amounts; the phase is suppressed by various histamine antagonists in realistically low dosage, or by prior treatment of the animal with histamine-releasing agents which deplete the tissue stores. Moreover, injection of histamine brings about rapid and short-lived increase in the permeability of venules but not of capillaries. There is thus good evidence that histamine is mainly responsible for the early phase of increased vascular permeability of the venules. Histamine is believed to be produced mainly by mast cells, which are widely distributed throughout most tissues, and the available evidence indicates that tissue injury results in release of free (active) histamine by mast cells and that this reacts directly on the walls of venules, increasing their permeability to macromolecules. As mentioned earlier, there is evidence also that histamine is responsible for capillary dilatation, as in the flush of Lewis's triple response (p. 34), and that it probably also stimulates sensory nerve endings and thus triggers off the axon reflex responsible for arteriolar dilatation. Little is known of the mechanism of histamine release or of the nature of its direct action on small blood vessels.

Other suspected endogenous mediators of the inflammatory reaction include 5-hydroxytryptamine, various polypeptides including kinins, a globulin permeability factor, ribonucleic acid, nucleosides, prostaglandins and mono-amine oxidases. The role of these agents in the inflammatory reaction is inconclusive, and it is unnecessary to discuss them in detail. It is

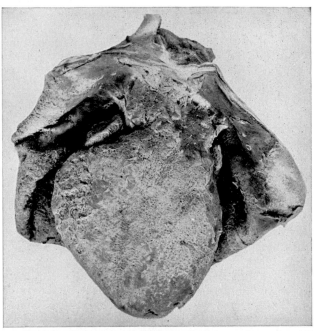

FIG. 2.7.—Acute pericarditis, showing irregular layer of fibrin on the surface of the heart. × $\frac{2}{3}$.

unlikely that 5-hydroxytryptamine is of importance in inflammation in man, but in rats it causes increased vascular permeability in remarkably low concentrations and may play a role in inflammation. *Kinins* are produced by the action of proteolytic enzymes (e.g. kallikrein) upon certain plasma globulins: the enzymes are normally present in the plasma in inactive form but may become activated by tissue injury. Kinins are capable of inducing increased vascular permeability in the small vessels in various species, including man, and also cause local pain: they are inactivated rapidly by normal plasma. The *globulin permeability factor* is present in plasma in an inactive form: it also is activated during inflammation and appears to be distinct from the kinin mechanism. Both the kinin and globulin permeability factor systems are activated by simple dilution of plasma or by its contact with glass, and they are thus very difficult to investigate. Their action appears to be mainly on venules rather than capillaries.

In 1940 Menkin described a series of experiments in which he induced acute inflammation by injection of turpentine, and investigated the chemical and biological properties of the inflammatory exudate. He claimed to have isolated polypeptides with specific biological activity. One polypeptide, *leukotaxin*, was claimed to be responsible for increased vascular permeability and also for leukocyte emigration, while a second, termed *leukocytosis promoting factor*, was regarded as responsible for increasing the production of neutrophil leukocytes by the bone marrow (p. 124). Tissue injury was regarded as being brought about by a third polypeptide, termed *necrosin*. While of considerable importance in emphasising the role of endogenous substances in the inflammatory reaction, Menkin's views went too far in denying the role of histamine, and also of bacterial products, in influencing the inflammatory reaction. Moreover, the isolation of polypeptides with the above-mentioned specific activities has not been confirmed, and it is a criticism of his work that he obtained tissue extracts for analysis usually 24 hours or more after the induction of inflammation.

The role of complement (p. 81) in mediating histamine release and leukocyte emigration in antigen-antibody reactions is considered on pp. 103, 104: it may have a wider significance in acute inflammation in general.

Lymph-node permeability factor. Lymphocytes which accumulate at the site of a delayed hypersensitivity reaction release a factor, known as lymph-node permeability factor, which increases the permeability of the small blood vessels and thus promotes exudation. This is considered in more detail in Chapter 5.

Route of exudation from small vessels. It has long been considered likely that macromolecules escape from the blood vessels of inflamed tissues by passing between adjacent vascular endothelial cells. Electron-microscopic studies have provided support for this view by demonstrating that intercellular spaces appear, and when particles of colloidal carbon or macromolecules such as ferritin, which are recognisable in electron micrographs, are injected

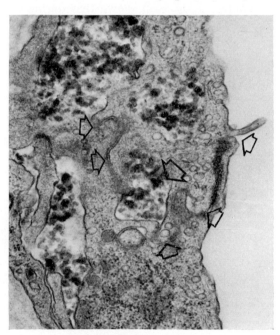

Fig. 2.8.—Electron micrograph of a venule in rat skin, showing escape of carbon particles between endothelial cells. Carbon suspension was injected intravenously, followed by histamine intradermally (to increase vascular permeability). The lumen is at the right, and the endothelial cell junction (small arrows) has separated to form a space (large arrow) containing carbon particles. Carbon is also seen lying in a subendothelial space, limited by basement membrane and pericytes. × 30,000. (Lady Florey.)

intravascularly, they can be observed to leave the venules and capillaries by way of the intercellular spaces (Fig. 2.8). There is also some evidence to suggest the passage of macromolecules through the endothelial cell cytoplasm.

A normal feature of these cells is the presence of *caveolae intracellulares* (Fig. 2.9): these are blind-ending channels in the cytoplasm, opening onto the luminal or outer surface of the cell and lined by plasma membrane. Vesicles with a lining membrane of similar appearance, but apparently separate from the cell surface, have also been described. The functions of these structures are unknown, and it has been suggested that they may transmit fluid across the endothelium. In some experiments macromolecules injected into the blood stream have been observed shortly afterwards in the endothelial caveolae, but the findings have been in-

without validity, and that transcytoplasmic flow may be important.

Emigration of leukocytes

The passage of leukocytes, and particularly of neutrophil polymorphs and monocytes, from the blood into the tissue spaces is a most important feature of acute inflammation and of particular significance in the defence against bacteria. The process involves two stages: firstly, the leukocyte must become arrested on the surface of the vascular endothelium, and secondly it must pass through the vessel wall.

In acute inflammatory lesions, neutrophil polymorphs migrate earlier and in much greater numbers than monocytes. This account relates mainly to migration of polymorphs, although much of it applies also to monocytes.

Margination of polymorphs. Arrest of neutrophil polymorphs on the vascular endothelium is often conspicuous in acute inflammation (Fig. 2.10) and is known as *pavementing* or *margination* of leukocytes. It is seen mainly in venules, but also in capillaries, and occurs when the blood flow in the dilated vessels becomes slow. In the

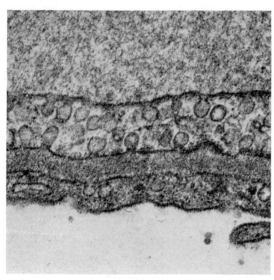

FIG. 2.9.—Electron micrograph of lung, showing part of a pulmonary capillary, the lumen of which occupies the upper part of the field. Note the caveolae intracellulares of the vascular endothelium. × 56,000.

consistent, and there is no evidence of increase in number or size of the caveolae to account for the increased escape of macromolecules in inflammation. It therefore seems more likely that the main loss is by the intercellular spaces.

It is likely that some of the increased loss of water and electrolytes from the small vessels also results from the development of intercellular spaces, but increased flow across the endothelial cell cytoplasm is another possibility. Admittedly, the control of fluid passing into and out of cells is complex, and not strictly comparable to passage across a semipermeable membrane, but the importance of hydrostatic and osmotic pressures suggests that the comparison is not

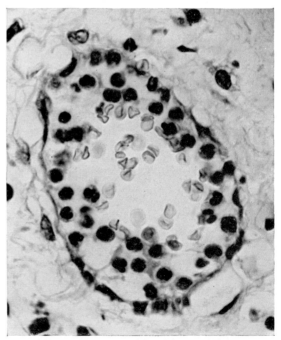

FIG. 2.10.—Section of venule in acute inflammation, showing pavementing of polymorphonuclear leukocytes. × 1000.

earlier stage of rapid flow, blood in the arterioles and venules shows *axial streaming*, the cells being mainly in the central or axial column of blood, separated from the vessel wall by a clear layer of plasma containing only occasional cells. This streaming is dependent on the rapid flow of blood: when the rate of flow decreases in acutely inflamed tissues, loss of axial streaming and aggregation of the red cells into rouleaux favour margination by increasing the chance contacts between leukocytes and endothelium. The nature of the adhesion of neutrophil polymorphs to the endothelium is not understood. *In vivo* observation has shown that, as the blood flow in the dilated venules slows down, polymorphs making contact with the endothelium tend to become arrested momentarily and then become detached and move on, or roll slowly along the endothelial surface. Eventually more and more of them come to rest for longer periods in contact with the endothelium and they may form an almost continuous layer or may even become heaped up on one another (Fig. 2.10). These appearances suggest stickiness between the leukocytic and endothelial cell surfaces. The process of pavementing has been shown to be inhibited by trisodium ethylenediamine tetra-acetic acid (EDTA), a calcium chelating agent, suggesting that calcium ions play a role in the process.

Emigration of polymorphs. Migration of pavemented neutrophil polymorphs through the vessel wall occurs almost exclusively in venules. The stationary leukocyte pushes out pseudopodia of clear cytoplasm, and if one of these encounters the junction between two endothelial cells, it extends between the cells, disrupting the junction by some unknown mechanism, and comes into contact with the basement membrane. The pseudopodium is followed by the remainder of the cell, which may pass directly through the basement membrane and adjacent reticulin fibres to reach the interstitium of the tissue, or may remain for a time between the endothelium and basement membrane. The junction between the endothelial cells re-forms rapidly after passage of a polymorph, although there is a tendency for immediate use of the same gap to be made by other migrating polymorphs. The breach in the vascular basement membrane caused by the emergence of a leukocyte is rapidly sealed off, the membrane regaining its continuity almost immediately: the mechan-

ism of this repair process is not understood. Cells which have emigrated wander through the tissues (Fig. 2.11) and play a role in digestion and phagocytosis of fibrin and degenerate tissue and cell fragments, and, most important in infections, in the destruction and removal of bacteria. The phagocytic function of leukocytes is considered on pp. 43 and 122.

The migration of leukocytes through the walls of venules has been widely assumed to be mediated by *chemotaxis*, a process whereby the movement of the cell is influenced by the concentration gradient of certain substances termed *chemotactic agents*. By observing the movements of leukocytes *in vitro* in fibrin clot, the chemotactic effect of various substances can be detected, and by this means it has been found that many bacteria release substances which attract leukocytes, i.e. positive chemotactic agents. Some substances, including the products of certain bacteria, have been regarded as exerting negative chemotaxis, i.e. of repelling leukocytes, but this may be largely dependent on a high concentration of the substances concerned. Time-lapse cine-photography of inflamed tissues within rabbits' ear chambers

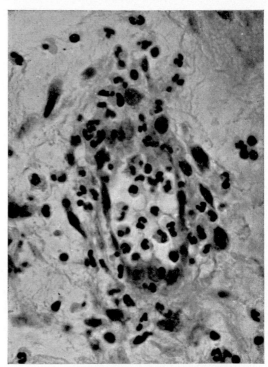

Fig. 2.11.—Inflammatory change. Emigration of neutrophil polymorphs from a venule in the inflamed tissue. × 375.

has revealed that the movements of polymorphs in pursuit of bacteria are as purposeful as a dog following a scent, and there can be no reasonable doubt that bacterial products exert chemotactic effects *in vivo*, as they have been shown to do *in vitro*. Extracts of thermally injured skin, neutrophil polymorphs, or of minced tissue, e.g. liver, have all been observed to induce inflammatory changes, including emigration of leukocytes, when injected into normal tissues, and incubation with serum or plasma has been shown to enhance the capacity of minced tissue to promote emigration of leukocytes. The endogenous agents responsible for these effects have not been isolated and their chemical nature is unknown. Histamine and the other possible mediators of increased vascular permeability (p. 37) do not appear to be strongly chemotactic, although some of them are weakly active.

Intensity of leukocyte emigration in acute inflammation depends both upon the severity of tissue injury and upon the nature of the injurious agent. Insignificant numbers of polymorphs emigrate into the tissues in Lewis's triple response induced by a firm stroke of the skin. In more severe tissue injury, illustrated on a small scale by a scratch, emigration of leukocytes is more conspicuous; if the scratch is covered with a glass coverslip, polymorphs in the exudate adhere to the glass and may be studied supravitally (i.e. in the living state but removed from the body). In general, polymorph emigration is of only moderate intensity in physical injury to the tissues, such as burning or mechanical trauma, unless infection supervenes. Some chemicals, e.g. turpentine, promote intense leukocytic emigration progressing even to pus formation, whereas with other chemicals, fluid exudation is much more prominent than emigration of leukocytes. In the mild inflammatory reaction which occurs around tissue dying from acute ischaemia, i.e. an infarct (p. 173), the degree of polymorph emigration varies with the tissue affected and also in different examples affecting the same tissue. In myocardial infarction, for example, there may be virtually no polymorph infiltration of the dead muscle, or large numbers may be present, particularly near the margin. The outstanding examples of intense emigration of polymorphs are provided by bacterial infections: bacteria which, like *Strep. pyogenes*, *Staph. aureus* and *Strep. pneumoniae* are particularly active in this respect, are accordingly termed *pyogenic* (pus inducing) bacteria. Other bacteria, such as *B. anthracis* responsible for anthrax, bring about an intense inflammatory reaction with escape of large numbers of red cells into the exudate, but much less conspicuous polymorph emigration (p. 138). These special features are considered in more detail below and in Chapter 6, but it is worth noting here that the variations in the composition of the exuded fluid and in leukocyte emigration indicate that agents which cause tissue injury not only induce inflammation, but also determine, to some extent, variations superimposed on the basic processes involved. This suggests that certain chemical agents, including bacterial products, have a direct action on the vascular endothelium and on the behaviour of leukocytes, and that they do not operate wholly by activating or releasing endogenous mediators, as was proposed by Menkin.

Emigration of monocytes. The origins (p. 47) and appearances (Fig. 16.8, p. 399) of monocytes are described elsewhere. Like neutrophil polymorphs, they become arrested on vascular endothelium and migrate into inflamed tissues. Also they show chemotactic responses *in vitro* to the same substances which attract polymorphs. Emigration of monocytes is, however, slower and at first nearly all the cells in the inflamed tissues are polymorphs; after a day or so monocytes appear in small but increasing numbers. The life of a neutrophil polymorph which has left the blood vessels is very short, possibly less than 24 hours, but emigrated monocytes can live for very much longer; accordingly their proportion in the exudate is high in prolonged inflammation and they may even outnumber polymorphs. Following its migration into the tissues, the monocyte enlarges and becomes actively phagocytic. In this enlarged active form monocytes are known as *macrophages* (c.f. polymorphs, termed by Metchnikoff *microphages*). Not all of the macrophages in inflamed tissues are derived from blood monocytes: some arise from reticuloendothelial cells in the tissues (*histiocytes*). In inactive form, the histiocytes are inconspicuous, but they enlarge, develop an increased amount of cytoplasm containing numerous lysosomes, and the nucleus assumes a more open, vesicular structure. The excitation, and conferment upon the macrophage of lethal properties for other cells and bacteria in immunological reactions, is described on p. 106.

Further stages of acute inflammation

The three most important sequelae to acute inflammation are:

(a) Reversal of the inflammatory processes with return of the tissues to normal, i.e. *resolution*. This is considered below.

(b) Progression to *suppuration* (p. 135).

(c) Progression to a *chronic phase* with formative inflammatory processes closely similar to healing and repair (p. 44).

Resolution. In this process the various inflammatory phenomena are reversed and the tissues return to normal. The stagnation gradually passes off and the blood flow is restored, though vascular dilatation often persists for some time, as illustrated by persistent redness following an acute inflammatory lesion of the skin. Fluid exudate is removed chiefly by the lymphatics, and fibrin is digested by leukocytes and absorbed. If, however, the fibrin is abundant or dense, it is replaced by fibrous tissue, i.e. organised (p. 60). Connective tissue cells which have become swollen and separated in an inflamed part diminish in size and become related again to fibres, or form new fibres, and defects in endothelial linings may be completely restored by the surviving cells.

Healthy leukocytes may pass back through the endothelium of the venules to the blood stream, but those that are damaged, and also the extravasated red cells, are taken up by phagocytes, either locally or in the draining lymph nodes. This scavenging process may be studied in rabbits injected intraperitoneally with a suitable suspension of staphylococci. The resulting inflammatory reaction resolves rapidly. Within an hour or two after the injection, polymorphonuclear leukocytes emigrate in large numbers from the vessels and rapidly ingest the cocci. The emigration of these cells continues until the organisms are destroyed. Some non-granular cells also appear early, and at first these can be identified as of two main kinds, viz. monocytes which have emigrated from the blood vessels and cells of local origin, mainly of the histiocyte class (p. 48) which have become enlarged, spherical and motile. Later, the monocytes also enlarge, and the histiocytes and monocytes thus change into macrophages of identical appearance.

During the process of destruction of the cocci,

many of the polymorphonuclear leukocytes undergo degeneration and die: their nuclear lobes first become shrunken and stain densely (pyknosis) and then fragment. Phagocytosis of these damaged polymorphonuclear leukocytes by macrophages then follows (Fig. 2.12) and macrophages are sometimes seen to contain several polymorphs, which are gradually digested and disappear. Extruded red cells are also taken

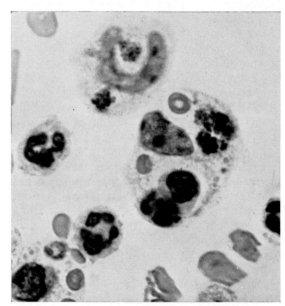

Fig. 2.12.—Exudate from peritoneal cavity of guinea-pig in resolving acute inflammation of three days' duration. Note polymorphonuclear leukocytes, also macrophages which have ingested leukocytes and red cells. × 1000.

up by these phagocytes and destroyed. Phagocytosis is seen also in the sinuses of the draining lymph nodes, the damaged leukocytes and red cells carried to the node by the lymph stream being ingested by the macrophages lining the sinuses. The same process occurs in the splenic pulp when bacteria enter the blood. As a sequel to this process of phagocytosis by macrophages, there is a marked diminution of the cells in the inflammatory lesion, and ultimately those left are almost all macrophages: these then become smaller, lymphocytes appear relatively increased in number, and there is a gradual return to normal. There thus occurs first of all a destruction of the organisms by the polymorphonuclear leukocytes, and these cells are in their turn taken up and digested by macrophages.

The most striking example of resolution on a large scale in man is provided by acute lobar pneumonia, an infection of the lung alveoli in which all the phenomena described above are well seen (Figs. 15.21, 15.22, p. 350). After the destruction of the organisms, usually within several days, there is a gradual softening and digestion of the fibrin in the alveoli, brought about by enzymes released by neutrophil polymorphs. The degenerate leukocytes and escaped red cells are taken up by macrophages locally or in the bronchial lymph nodes, and they undergo intracellular digestion. The lymph tracts and sinuses of these nodes are packed with macrophages containing degenerate polymorphs and cell fragments. With the absorption of the fluid contents of the air vesicles, these once more become air-containing, and the part returns practically to normal. Some of the liquefied exudate is expectorated but the amount may not be large, and in every case a large proportion of the exudate is absorbed.

Effects of acute inflammation

In the acute inflammatory reaction, the environment within the affected tissue is altered (a) by an increased flow of protein-rich extra-vascular fluid—the inflammatory exudate, and (b) by migration of neutrophil polymorphs and monocytes into the extravascular spaces. Controversy over the relative importance of these two major features, the humoral and cellular factors in defence mechanisms, is long past, and it is clear that both factors are important and that they augment one another in eliminating infection and lessening the harmful effects of toxic agents.

The inflammatory exudate

The harmful effects of bacteria are caused by their toxic products which are usually proteins or complex protein-containing compounds. Apart from some highly specialised toxins which affect mainly the nervous system, the effect of toxin is usually most marked in the infected tissue, for it is here that it reaches its highest concentration. By increasing the flow of fluid through the tissue, the process of exudation dilutes the toxin and so prevents or diminishes local tissue injury.

Secondly, the inflammatory exudate brings the various plasma proteins into contact with the invading bacteria. If the patient's plasma contains antibody reactive with the organism, it will promote destruction by the action of complement and by phagocytosis: this is considered further in Chapter 6.

Thirdly, the inflammatory exudate may be rich in fibrinogen which, by clotting to form a network of fibrin in the inflamed tissues, may form a mechanical obstruction to the spread of bacteria through the tissues.

Fourthly, the inflammatory exudate tends to carry bacteria and their toxins, either free or in phagocytes, to the regional lymph nodes where, being antigenic, they promote specific defensive mechanisms in the form of an immune response which will become effective a week or so after development of infection, and may persist for years (see Chapter 4).

Lastly, the inflammatory exudate increases the supply of oxygen, glucose, etc. to the infected tissues and removes the products of metabolism of the greatly increased number of cells in the area of infection.

Phagocytosis

Phagocytosis of bacteria by neutrophil polymorphs and macrophages is a most important factor in the defence against bacteria. This is illustrated by the condition of *agranulocytosis*, in which there is a deficiency of neutrophil polymorphs in the blood. Affected individuals are especially prone to infections, particularly of the pharynx and intestines, and although the invading bacteria are not of unusually high virulence, they tend to cause deep lesions with extensive necrosis, and to spread rapidly both locally and to the regional lymph nodes. Other defects of the neutrophil polymorphs are known and they also increase the susceptibility to infection (p. 396).

The phagocytic activity of leukocytes is almost identical to the engulfing of food particles by amoebae and other protozoa. When the particle to be ingested, e.g. a bacterium, comes into contact with the phagocyte, the plasma membrane of the latter extends over the surface of the particle which comes to lie at first in a depression on the cell surface and then is completely enveloped. Finally, the plasma membrane surrounding the particle breaks away from the surface and the particle is thus included in a vesicle (phagosome) lined by plasma membrane within the cell cytoplasm. Digestion of the engulfed particle is brought about by various enzymes which are normally present in the lysosomes of the phagocyte. These organelles fuse with the plasma membrane lining the phagosome and empty their contents into it, and the ingested particle is thus bathed in fluid rich in active enzymes. As already mentioned, invading bacteria may be destroyed by antibody and complement and then phagocytosed and digested. Both neutrophil polymorphs and macrophages are also capable of phagocytosing live bacteria and, depending on their virulence, these may then be killed and digested. Bacteria of high virulence, however, both resist phagocytosis and, if they are phagocytosed, are relatively resistant to the killing and digestive properties of the phagocyte. They may indeed multiply within the cell and may bring about its destruction. The factors determining the outcome of the struggle between bacteria and phagocytes are numerous and complex and are discussed in Chapter 6.

Polymorphs and macrophages also engulf droplets of the fluid inflammatory exudate. The process is similar to phagocytosis of particles but is sometimes termed *pinocytosis*, and the contained proteins, including bacterial toxins, are similarly exposed to the digestive lysosomal enzymes. As already stated, the neutrophil polymorph has a short extravascular life. Dead polymorphs are present in the inflammatory exudate and are particularly numerous in pus. They may undergo auto-digestion by their own lysosomal enzymes, and these are also released into the exudate where they play an important role in the digestion of damaged tissue, dead bacteria, cell fragments, red cells and fibrin.

The phagocytic and digestive activities of macrophages are closely similar to those of polymorphs, but they are capable of ingesting larger particles, including whole cells, and also they have a much longer extravascular life than the polymorph: indigestible materials such as haemosiderin derived from the breakdown of red cells or inhaled or injected particles of extraneous materials may persist within macrophages for months or even years (Fig. 9.7, p. 201).

CHRONIC INFLAMMATION

The essential feature of chronic inflammation is the proliferation of tissue cells to produce vascular granulation tissue, which matures into fibrous tissue. Such *proliferative* or *formative* changes are in contrast to the exudative changes of the acute inflammatory reaction, but when acute inflammation fails to resolve, chronic inflammation supervenes and the two processes are thus commonly associated.

Even in an early stage of acute inflammation, some proliferation of the connective tissue cells occurs and, in general, the more chronic the inflammatory reaction, the more pronounced are the proliferative changes, and the greater the degree of ultimate fibrous scarring. This is well illustrated in the kidneys, in which an acute bacterial infection produces exudative changes with congestion, inflammatory oedema, and emigration of leukocytes. If the infection is overcome quickly these changes may resolve without residual damage, but if it persists, the exudative changes are accompanied by formation of granulation tissue and the kidneys eventually show fibrous scarring. Similarly, acute bacterial infection of the gallbladder stimulates an acute inflammatory reaction, but persistent infection results in fibrosis of the wall. In these examples, fibrosis is dependent on persistence of the causal agent, but even when this is rapidly removed, fibrosis may follow either by organisation of the inflammatory exudate or by fibrous replacement of destroyed tissue. Thus the fibrinous exudate in pleurisy is organised, i.e. replaced by fibrous tissue, and failure of resolution of the fibrinous exudate in acute pneumonia results in organisation, with fibrous tissue formation in the alveoli (p. 351). Strictly speaking, such changes should be distinguished from chronic inflammation, although both processes result in fibrosis. Loss of tissue is a common feature of intense acute inflammation, and when polymorph emigration is pronounced, the dead tissue may be digested, leaving an abscess cavity (Fig. 2.13): at this stage, resolution is no longer possible, and if the causal agent (usually bacterial) is eliminated, granulation tissue grows from the surrounding tissue and extends into the space, with eventual fibrosis.

In the lesions described above, fibrosis ensues on acute, exudative inflammatory lesions, but chronic inflammation commonly arises without preceding acute inflammation, and is thus a primary change from the outset.

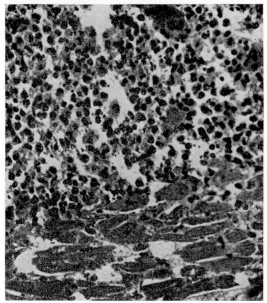

FIG. 2.13.—Margin of an abscess cavity in the myocardium. In the upper part of the field the myocardial cells have been killed and digested, leaving a space filled with purulent exudate. × 250.

Primary chronic inflammation is caused by many types of irritants, and these fall into the following four main classes.

(a) Bacterial and fungal infections. Various types of bacteria and fungi produce infections in which acute inflammation is minimal, and the most prominent change is formation of granulation and fibrous tissue. Such lesions are termed the *infective granulomas*: classical examples are provided by tuberculosis (p. 141) and syphilis (p. 147). The factors which induce the proliferative changes are usually obscure, and while the various micro-organisms concerned may be directly responsible, tissue injury may result also from hypersensitivity reactions to the microbial antigens: this latter mechanism appears to be particularly important in the lesions of tuberculosis (p. 142).

(b) Chemical irritants. Many chemical compounds are mildly irritating, and when they persist within the tissues, chronic inflammatory changes result. Inhalation of certain particulate materials, e.g. silica (quartz), fibrous silicates (asbestos), and dust or fumes of beryllium compounds produces chronic inflammation of the lungs. Similarly, granulomatous lesions may result from these and other particulate irritants gaining entrance to the tissues in dirty wounds; also from suture materials, and from the talc formerly used to lubricate the surgeon's gloves. Chronic inflammation may occur also around organic material, both foreign and endogenous, e.g. cholesterol crystals.

(c) Auto-immune reactions. Chronic inflammation of the thyroid, adrenals, gastric mucosa, and possibly certain other organs results from hypersensitivity reactions due to the development of immune responses against constituents of these organs (pp. 110–112).

(d) Unknown agents. In some granulomatous reactions, the causal agents remain unknown. One of the most important examples is *sarcoidosis* (p. 152), which produces lesions in the lymph nodes and various internal organs, resembling somewhat those of tuberculosis.

Histological features. Chronic inflammation is characterised by formation of new connective tissue: in the early stages this may be highly cellular and vascular, the cells being plump spindle-cells (fibroblasts), and the collagen fibres are delicate and scanty (Fig. 2.14). As it ages, such young connective (granulation) tissue matures into tougher fibrous tissue: the cellularity and vascularity diminish and thickening of the fibres results from further collagen deposition. When the inflammatory process is very low grade throughout, there may be formation of dense collagen without the preliminary stage of granulation tissue. These processes are described in more detail in relation to healing and repair in the next chapter.

In addition to the above changes, the area becomes infiltrated with leukocytes and histiocytes. When the chronic process supervenes on an acute inflammatory lesion, e.g. a persistent pyogenic bacterial infection, polymorphs and monocytes may continue to emigrate from the blood vessels, but plasma cells and lymphocytes also accumulate in the inflammatory focus (Fig. 2.15), their proportions depending on the nature of the causal agent. In other instances of chronic inflammation not associated with a marked exudative reaction, polymorphs may be scanty or absent and lymphocytes or plasma cells usually predominate. In all instances, macrophages, derived from emigrating mono-

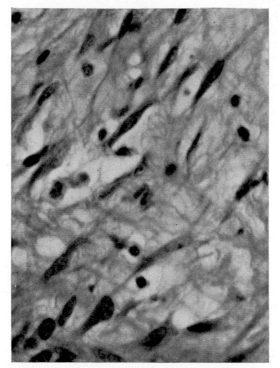

FIG. 2.14.—Fibroblasts in young fibrous tissue.   × 600.

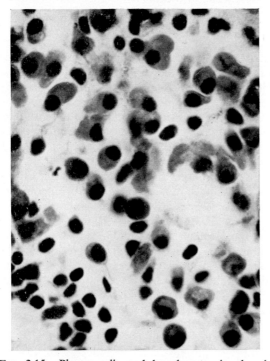

FIG. 2.15.—Plasma cells and lymphocytes in chronic inflammation, from a case of chronic otitis media. × 1000.

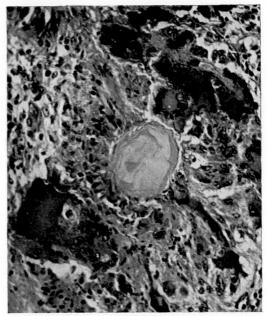

FIG. 2.16.—Section of nodule from peritoneal cavity, showing large foreign-body giant cell and proliferation of macrophages around a lentil starch grain, which is seen in the centre of figure.   × 240.

cytes and tissue histiocytes, are present, and they may be very numerous. In some chronic bacterial infections, e.g. actinomycosis (p. 151), the macrophages may become enlarged, with abundant cytoplasm which appears foamy owing to numerous droplets of lipid. In chronic inflammation due to particulate material of low solubility, multinucleate cells, termed *foreign-body giant cells*, may form by fusion of macrophages, and tend to phagocytose or surround the particles (Fig. 2.16). Giant cells of similar origin, but of somewhat different morphology, may appear in chronic inflammation due to infections, and are particularly prominent in tuberculosis (Fig. 7.11, p. 144).

Variations in the histological features of chronic inflammation are illustrated by the examples of infective granulomas described in Chapter 7. It is often possible to make a provisional diagnosis from the histological features, but there are dangerous pitfalls. For example, several agents can give rise to changes readily mistaken for tuberculosis, and a firm diagnosis is usually dependent on detection and recognition of a specific causal agent, or on other procedures such as serological tests for a particular infection. The morphology and staining reactions are, in some instances, sufficiently characteristic for the identification of the causal bacteria or fungi, while examination in polarised light may afford recognition of anisotropic foreign material, e.g. silica, talc, starch, suture material.

Results. The tendency of the newly formed tissue to contract may induce serious effects by narrowing orifices and tubes—for example, stenosis of the mitral valve in chronic endocarditis, or stenosis of the small intestine in regional ileitis. Chronic inflammation of internal organs is usually accompanied by loss of parenchymal cells, and this, together with irregular fibrosis, results in shrinkage, irregular scarring and distortion. Commonly the surface becomes uneven, with a fine or coarse granularity: this is particularly well seen in cirrhosis of the liver (Fig. 19.18, p. 561), where the irregularity is accentuated by proliferation and enlargement of surviving liver cells.

In some instances, the fibrous tissue produced in chronic inflammation may have a useful function: for example, weakening of the aorta results from destruction of elastic tissue and muscle of the media as a result of syphilitic aortitis, but fibrous tissue is laid down and may delay or prevent abnormal stretching and rupture.

Other causes of fibrosis. While fibrosis is a common feature of chronic inflammation, it may result from other causes. For example, when the blood supply to a part is gradually diminished by arterial disease, atrophy of the specialised cells may be accompanied by overgrowth of the supporting tissue. Similarly, death of tissue resulting from sudden occlusion of an artery, e.g. by thrombosis, is followed by replacement of the dead tissue by supporting tissue. Thus, in the brain, patches of neuroglial overgrowth from which the nervous elements have disappeared are common in chronic arterial disease, and patches of fibrosis are frequently encountered in the myocardium and in the kidneys. Such changes may be termed *replacement fibrosis.* As in chronic inflammation, replacement fibrosis sometimes has a useful supporting function: thus the fibrosis which accompanies loss of a patch of myocardium from arterial insufficiency usually prevents rupture.

TYPES OF CELLS IN INFLAMMATORY LESIONS

Neutrophil polymorphs. The origin and morphology of these cells are described on pp. 125 *et seq*. Their migrating activity has already been discussed, and their roles in the defence against micro-organisms and in Arthus-type hypersensitivity reactions are considered in later chapters.

Macrophages: the reticulo-endothelial system. The term macrophage was applied by Metchnikoff to the large mononuclear phagocytes, to distinguish them from the smaller neutrophil polymorphs, which he termed microphages. The participation of macrophages in inflammation and their immediate origin from blood monocytes has been outlined in the preceding account, and their role in hypersensitivity reactions and infections are discussed in Chapters 5 and 6. Macrophages belong to an ill-defined and widely dispersed system of cells termed the reticulo-endothelial system, and this is described below. Macrophages are not a homogeneous class but include cells of various origins, e.g. blood monocytes, histiocytes, derivatives of the endothelium of lymph channels and certain blood sinusoids, reticulum cells, etc. The source of such cells may sometimes be traced by histological methods, especially under experimental conditions. But after a time they may lose their characteristic features and in many naturally-occurring lesions it is impossible to discriminate different kinds of macrophages and to assign their origin. The use of some general term, such as macrophages or non-granular wandering cells, is thus often convenient in describing them.

The method of vital staining—that is, the staining which results from the injection of certain dyes, e.g. trypan blue, *intra vitam*—has been used extensively to elucidate the origins and behaviour of these cells. When a vital dye is injected intravenously certain cells are coloured deeply, others faintly, others not at all. The cells which stain deeply have therefore the property of taking up the stain in solution without being damaged, and the stain is then deposited in granules in their cytoplasm. Aschoff and Landau observed that the property of deep staining was shown especially by certain endothelial cells and reticulum cells and by some of the macrophages derived from them; they accordingly applied the term *reticulo-endothelial system* to the tissue cells which are vitally stained and also to their derivatives which show the same property. The phagocytic property of reticulo-endothelial cells can also be demonstrated by injecting colloidal particles (Fig. 2.17).

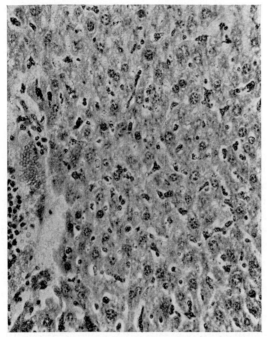

Fig. 2.17.—Mouse liver showing uptake of carbon by Kupffer cells following intravenous injection of colloidal carbon. × 250.

The cells of this system comprise both relatively fixed cells and also wandering cells. The chief examples of the former are (*a*) the reticulum cells of the splenic tissue, of the bone-marrow, and of the nodes and cords of lymphoid tissue, and (*b*) the endothelial cells of the splenic sinuses, lymph channels, and of the sinusoids of the liver (Kupffer cells), bone-marrow, adrenals and hypophysis. The distinction between reticulum cells and endothelial cells is convenient but must not be sharply maintained, for certain endothelial cells, e.g. those of the hepatic sinusoids and splenic venous sinuses, may also be capable of forming reticulin. In addition to the cells mentioned as constituting the reticuloendothelial system, there occur also, widely distributed in the tissues, oval or spindle-shaped cells with branching processes and lumpy cytoplasm which stains more deeply and is more defined than that of the fibrocytes. They have a

wide distribution in the connective tissues, and are generally believed to be migratory cells of mesenchymal origin which in the resting phase are known as *histiocytes*. In inflammatory conditions they rapidly assume the round form of macrophages and become actively phagocytic. They take up vital stains readily and are included in the reticulo-endothelial system. In contrast, fibrocytes stain only faintly by *intra-vitam* methods, and any stained granules in them are small. Inflammatory foci become deeply stained by vital dyes owing to the presence of the large numbers of cells which take up the dye. This fact has been found of service in aiding the recognition of small foci of inflammation in experimental conditions.

The conception of the reticulo-endothelial system has been of great service in bringing into prominence a group of cells with special properties in relation to the storage of chemical substances and to phagocytosis. It is not a sharply defined system either anatomically or physiologically and its cells have great powers of proliferation and regeneration, so that its functions as a whole cannot readily be abrogated by stuffing the cells with inert materials—so-called reticulo-endothelial blockade. While the functions of the system come into prominence chiefly in abnormal states, it is the main site of formation of bile pigment. In various disease states the reticulo-endothelial cells may accumulate large quantities of lipids, iron compounds, pigments, etc.

Plasma cells. The presence of plasma cells in inflamed tissues, as elsewhere, is indicative of antibody production: they usually appear about a week after onset and are present in greatest numbers in persistent lesions caused by bacteria. The origin, function and morphology of the plasma cell is discussed in Chapter 4 (Figs. 4.10, 4.11, p. 82).

Lymphocytes accumulate in chronic inflammatory lesions and their presence in large numbers suggests a delayed hypersensitivity reaction (see Chapters 4, 5). Their presence in acute inflammation is usually obscured by much larger numbers of polymorphs.

Eosinophil polymorphs. The accumulation of these cells in inflammatory lesions is closely associated with hypersensitivity reactions. They are observed particularly in the lesions of bronchial asthma, in the tissues around metazoan parasites, in certain skin diseases, and in

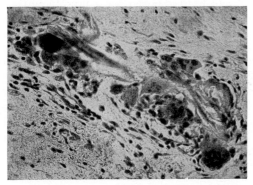
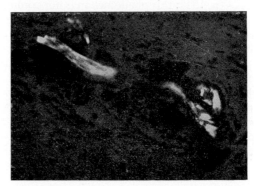

FIG. 2.18.—Foreign-body giant cells around particles of surgical talc accidentally introduced at operation. On the right as seen through crossed polarising screens which render the birefringent particles brilliantly visible. × 200. (Prof. J. B. Gibson.)

various lesions of the gastro-intestinal tract. Intense local accumulation of eosinophils is commonly associated with eosinophil leuko-cytosis in the blood and there is recent evidence to suggest that this is mediated by an immune response. The thymic-derived lymphocytes which respond to antigenic stimulation, e.g. by a parasitic worm, in some way stimulate the proliferation of eosinophil precursors in the bone marrow. The function of eosinophil polymorphs is obscure: it is discussed on p. 397.

Giant cells. The multinucleated or giant cells seen commonly in inflammatory lesions are formed from macrophages, usually by fusion of many cells, less commonly by repeated nuclear division without separation of the cytoplasm. The number of nuclei ranges from a few to over 200 and cell size from around 40μ to 500μ. The individual nuclei and the appearance of the cytoplasm resemble those of macrophages. Giant cells develop particularly in relation to

material which is not readily removed or digested: they are seen around crystals of cholesterol or urates and around the fat released from degenerated adipose tissue as in "fat necrosis" (p. 859). They are common in relation to foreign material, and in old wounds are seen around catgut or silk sutures, and around surgical talc embedded in the tissues (Fig. 2.18). Like the macrophage their function is phago-cytic and, as illustrated, they can ingest and surround much larger particles.

In acute infections giant cells are not usually conspicuous, although small examples with two or more nuclei are often seen in suppurating lesions. They are, however, more numerous and much larger in certain chronic infections and are particularly conspicuous in tuberculous lesions (Fig. 7.12, p. 144). They occur also in syphilitic lesions but are usually smaller and less numerous. Multinucleated giant cells also form by cell fusion brought about by infection with certain

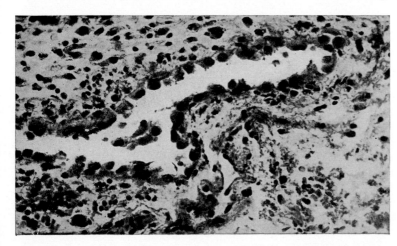

FIG. 2.19.—Omentum in acute in-flammation, showing swelling and desquamation of the serosal cells. × 390.

viruses (p. 131): this phenomenon is not confined to cells of the reticulo-endothelial system, and is observed to occur in epithelial cells. Fusion of cells of different species has been shown to occur in tissue cultures infected with *Sendai* virus, and the behaviour of such hybrid cells, and of hybrid-cell tumours, when implanted into experimental animals is of considerable interest.

Serosal cells. In acute inflammation of a serous surface the serosal lining cells enlarge and usually desquamate at an early stage (Fig. 2.19).

They can be recognised for a time lying free in the exudate, and appear to be non-phagocytic but in more chronic inflammation may form sheets of several cells thickness or small hollow spheres containing mucus. They may also differentiate into fibroblasts.

Fibroblasts. These may be seen in most acute inflammatory lesions but their presence in large numbers is associated with formative inflammatory changes and reparative processes. They are considered in the next chapter.

CHAPTER 3

HEALING, REPAIR AND HYPERTROPHY

HEALING AND REPAIR

Reaction of tissues to injury varies greatly in different species of animals and in different tissues. *Regeneration*, i.e. the replacement of a single type of parenchymatous cell by multiplication from the surviving cells of the same kind may be seen in man but differs greatly from one tissue to another. A helpful guide to the expected reaction to damage of any tissue is given by the division of somatic cells into three types.

(*a*) *Labile cells* are those which under normal conditions continue to multiply throughout life and include epidermis, alimentary, respiratory and urinary mucous membranes, uterine endometrium and the haemopoietic bone marrow and lymphoid cells.

(*b*) *Stable cells* normally cease multiplication when growth ceases but retain mitotic ability during adult life so that some regeneration of damaged tissues may occur. This group includes liver, pancreas, renal tubular epithelium, thyroid and adrenals.

(*c*) *Permanent cells* lose their mitotic ability in infancy and the classic example of this group is the neurone.

In many instances injury to an organ or tissue is followed by complete restoration, the cells lost being replaced by proliferative activity of those remaining. However, when the injury involves a cell type inherently incapable of this or when other factors, e.g. interruption of blood supply, prevents restoration, healing occurs by the formation of a fibrous scar the development of which is best illustrated by the healing of a wound of skin and subcutaneous tissue.

Healing of wounds by first intention (primary union)

Primary union occurs in uninfected surgical incisions and in other clean wounds sutured without undue delay. It is characterised by the formation of only minimal amounts of granulation tissue.

The wound clot and its removal. When an incision is made in the skin and subcutaneous tissue, blood escaping from cut vessels clots on the wound surface and fills the gap between the wound edges which, in sutured wounds, is narrow. The blood clot with its fibrin meshwork was once thought to be vital as a scaffold for connective tissue cells and a support to epithelium migrating into the wound from adjacent tissue, but it is now regarded primarily as a wound adhesive and protective cover. Excessive and deeply situated blood clot (haematoma) delays healing. During the first 24 hours, there is a mild inflammatory reaction at the wound edges with exudation of fluid and migration of polymorphs and later of monocytes and lymphocytes. Blood clot is digested by enzymes from disintegrated polymorphs and this is aided from about the third or fourth day by macrophages, derived from blood monocytes and tissue histiocytes which ingest and digest any remaining fibrin, red cells and cellular debris. Within a few days haemoglobin from the red cells may be converted to haemosiderin and haematoidin (bilirubin). These changes represent the exudative (acute inflammatory) phase of response to injury and are usually mild unless infection supervenes.

Epithelial repair. The first tissue to bridge the incisional gap is the squamous epithelium of the epidermis. Within 24 hours and extending from 3—4 mm. around the wound edge there is enlargement of the cells of all layers of the skin. Two processes then contribute to the closure of the gap. Close to the cut edge, cells from the deeper part of the epithelium begin to slide over each other, *migrate* out over the wound surface and become flattened to form a continuous ad-

C

vancing sheet. *Proliferation* also plays a part:
cells divide at first in a localised zone in the epidermis and pilosebaceous follicles close to the
wound edge and later in the new epithelium but
mitoses are rarely seen in actively migrating cells.
While the advancing edge of the sheet of new
epidermis consists of a single layer of flat cells,
the older part at the periphery of the wound becomes stratified so that there is a gradient of
thickness. The cells grow beneath the surface clot
and sometimes also down the cut edges into the
dermis (Figs. 3.1 and 3.2). The wound may be
bridged by epithelium within the first 2 or 3 days
and this is often followed rapidly by stratification
but usually there is imperfect development of
rete ridges (Fig. 3.3). Any epithelium which has
grown down into the dermis later becomes resorbed (Fig. 3.1).

Suture tracks. Epithelium also tends to grow
down suture tracks, in some instances meeting
epithelium growing down from the opposite end
of the stitch wound. Often much of the epithelium is avulsed when stitches are removed but
some may remain and is later either resorbed
with a mild associated foreign body granulomatous reaction or occasionally gives rise to a
small implantation cyst. Each suture track is
another wound in that there is haemorrhage,
death of cells and injury to skin appendages, and
in consequence there is a slight inflammatory
reaction and fibroblast proliferation (Fig. 3.4).
Because of the continuity with the skin surface
bacterial contamination of suture tracks is
particularly likely and "stitch abscesses" are
commoner than sepsis of the incision.

Vascular proliferation. The productive phase
of the response to injury is represented by the
proliferation of new blood vessels and fibroblasts to form "granulation tissue". From about
the third day, new vascular sprouts grow from

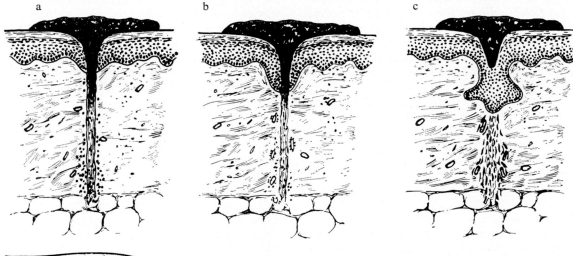

FIG. 3.1.—Primary wound healing. a.—The first day after wounding. Blood clot,
dead tissue and squames have formed the dark scab on the surface and
there are strands of fibrin and polymorphs between the wound margins.
The skin edges are inverted and there is hypertrophy of epithelial cells at the
edge of the wound. There is slight polymorph infiltrate around the wound.

b.—Around day 2–3. Proliferating tongues of epithelium, one cell thick at the
advancing edge, have grown down under the scab and cover part of the dermal
collagen. The wound gap now contains mononuclear leukocytes rather than
polymorphs, mixed with some fibrin strands. There is slight cellular cuffing of
blood vessels in the dermal collagen and subcutaneous fat.

c.—Around day 4 or 5. The incision is bridged by epithelium and the scab
has begun to loosen. Fibroblasts have grown into the wound gap from loose
areolar tissue around blood vessels in the dermis and subcutaneous fat. A
few vertical fibrils of collagen have also formed. There is minimal proliferation
of blood vessels.

d.—About 14 days or later. The healed epithelium may be thinner or thicker
than normal, is lacking in rete ridges and slightly raised above the surface.
Fibroblasts and collagen are now running parallel to the skin surface. Slightly
increased vascularity and cellularity remain to mark the wound site.

blood vessels at the wound margins (Fig. 3.5), and advance up to 2 mm. per day into the wound: the capillary sprouts are produced partly by rearrangement and migration of pre-existing endothelial cells and partly by prolifera-

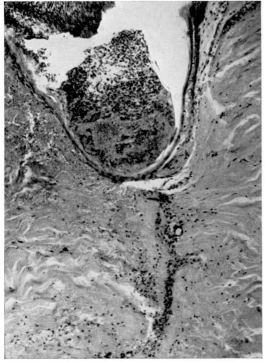

FIG. 3.2.—Aseptic abdominal wound with healing after five days.

The incision is represented merely by a vertical cellular line. The round body on the surface is a small scab. Note that the epithelium has extended down into the dermis. × 105.

tion just behind the advancing tip. The sprouts are at first often solid, but they unite with one another or join a capillary already carrying blood and develop a lumen. These newly formed vessels are more delicate (Fig. 3.12) and more permeable than normal so that they tend both to leak fluid and to allow the escape of leukocytes and red cells. It has been observed in rabbits that if blood flow is not soon established through a new vessel then the lumen disappears, the vessel reverting to a solid cord which then breaks and the ends retract by sliding back of endothelial cells to the nearest vessel carrying blood. Within a few days of the establishment of circulation some of the new vessels differentiate into arterioles and venules by the acquisition of muscle cells either by migration from

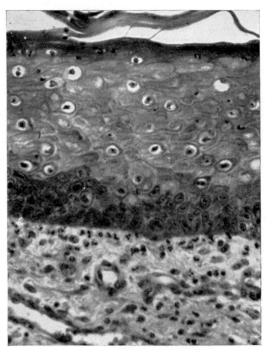

FIG. 3.3.—Newly formed epithelium on healed ulcer.

The cells are in several layers but there is little differentiation, and there is no formation of rete ridges. A similar appearance is seen in a healed surgical incision. × 400.

pre-existing larger blood channels or by differentiation from mesenchymal cells.

Lymphatic channels are re-established in the same manner as blood channels but there is no anastomosis between the two systems.

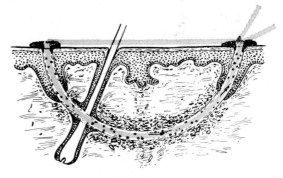

FIG. 3.4.—Diagram of suture track before removal of sutures about 9 days after wounding. In the centre of the picture the healed epithelium still forms a small projection into the dermis and beneath it the more cellular vertical line of the healing wound is seen.

The surface epithelium and that from a damaged hair follicle have grown down and line the suture track which is open to the skin surface and contains fibrin and polymorphs. There is more vascular and fibroblastic proliferation around the suture track than around the original wound.

Fibrous tissue proliferation. After the removal of blood, fibrin and dead cells from the wound and simultaneously with the development of new blood vessels, long, spindle-shaped fibroblasts (Fig. 3.6, a and b) begin to proliferate and to move into the incisional area. These cells appear to derive chiefly from fibrocytes or their precursors in the loose fibrous tissue of the dermal papillary layer, around blood vessels and from deep tissues rather than from the dense dermal collagen. Within 4 or 5 days fibroblasts mingle in the incision and produce randomly arranged reticulin fibres which are soon converted into mature collagen. The fibres come to lie across the incision and probably unite the cut edges from about the end of the first week after injury. During the second week there is a great increase both in reticulin fibres and also in the mature collagen bundles on which the tensile strength of the healing wound depends.

At 14 days the strength is not greatly below that of normal skin but the full strength is more slowly acquired in the ensuing weeks.

It seems likely that fibroblasts are derived chiefly from resting, locally resident fibrocytes or undifferentiated mesenchymal cells around blood vessels. On electron microscopy the fibroblast is seen to contain much endoplasmic reticulum studded with ribosomes and a substantial Golgi apparatus,

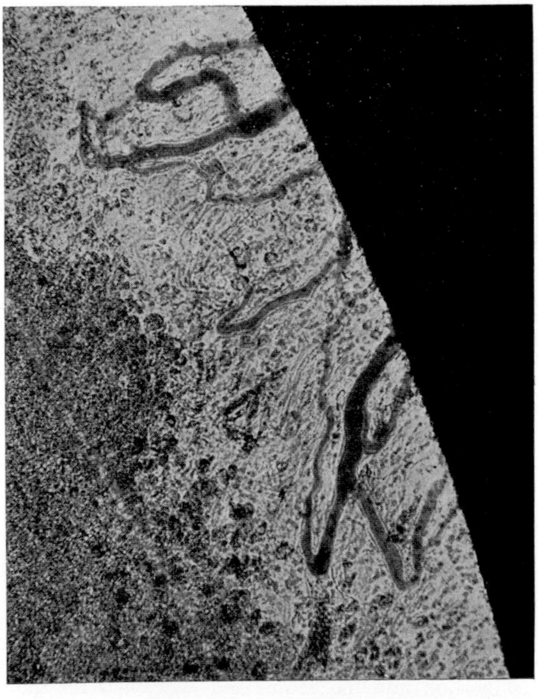

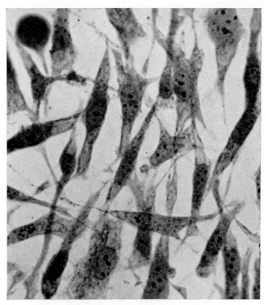

Fig. 3.6a.—Fibroblasts as seen in a culture *in vitro*. (Dr. Janet S. F. Niven.) × 300.

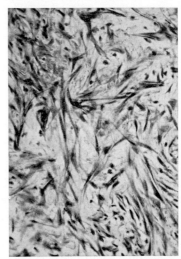

Fig. 3.6b.—Fibroblasts in healing wound, showing the characteristic shape and early formation of collagen fibrils. × 250.

Fig. 3.5.—Capillary loops growing into thin blood clot, as seen in special chamber attached to rabbit's ear. Similar but less marked vascular proliferation is seen in the healing of a simple surgical incision. (Photograph taken during life.) Note large numbers of macrophages in advance of growing vessels. (the late Prof. Lord Florey.)

features characteristic of a secretory cell. The initial steps of collagen synthesis are probably associated with the ribosomes, with later transfer from the endoplasmic reticulum to the Golgi apparatus and a soluble form of collagen is then discharged from the cell surface. Most of this precipitates extracellularly as typical fibres. The tropocollagen molecule, which is the basic building block of collagen, forms a triple helix and these macromolecules become aggregated laterally and longitudinally to form the typical collagen fibre with a regular 64 nm. periodic cross banding (Fig. 3.7). These collagen fibres become

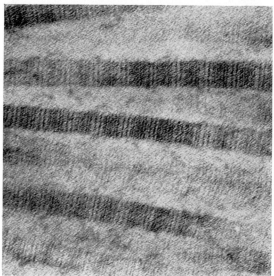

FIG. 3.7.—Collagen fibres are seen here in longitudinal section. The characteristic, regular cross banding is evident. × 100,000 approx.

grouped together extracellularly, producing the argyrophil fibres recognised under the light microscope as one form of reticulin, the other being basement membrane reticulin which is a very stable lipomucoprotein chemically and antigenically distinct from collagen. The argyrophil reticulin fibres become thicker by further accretion of tropocollagen and develop the histological staining reactions of mature collagen. Further thickening may occur later by bonding of fibres, and this, rather than continuing fibroblast proliferation, accounts for the smaller and slower increase in strength of a healing wound after 14 days.

Events following primary wound healing. Once the wound has healed the young scar is raised above the surface due to the underlying proliferative processes and is red as a result of increased vascularity. The blood vessels gradually decrease in number, probably in the manner

already described, and excess fibrous tissue may slowly disappear. Elastic fibres regenerate much later than collagen and their method of formation is not known (Fig. 3.8). Sensory nerves may reach the scar in about three weeks but specialised nerve endings such as Pacinian corpuscles do not reform. The end result of healing by first intention should be a pale, linear scar level with the adjacent skin surface, but sometimes a hypertrophic scar or *keloid* forms (p. 245).

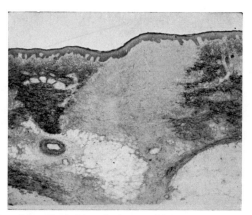

FIG. 3.8.—Healed surgical wound of skin of 14 days' duration. × 4.

Note that the line of incision is soundly healed but that the elastic tissue (stained black) has not regenerated.

Healing by second intention (secondary union)

Healing of an open wound or an infected closed wound occurs by the formation of granulation tissue which grows from the base of the wound to fill the defect. The vascular and fibroblastic proliferation which together make up the granulation tissue are much more abundant than in healing by first intention.

Clean open wounds. As in the closed wound there is haemorrhage and exudation of fibrin from the cut surfaces. This is soon followed by a much greater emigration of polymorphs and by macrophages which together, by enzymic action and phagocytosis, soften and remove the fibrin and other debris. As in the incised wound, epithelial cells at the margins enlarge and from there begin to migrate down the walls of the wound in the first day or two after injury. Migration and proliferation together produce a sheet of cells which advances in a series of tongue like projections beneath any remaining blood clot or exudate on the wound surface. As the single layer of cells moves inwards towards the wound centre there is stratification of the cells near to the wound margin (Fig. 3.9). Since the denuded area is large the advancing epithelial sheet does not completely cover the wound until the granulation tissue from the base (see below) has started to fill the wound space. Care should always be taken, in removing dressings from an open wound, that the delicate epithelium, which at first has a relatively tenuous hold on the underlying tissue, is not ripped off. As soon as the wound surface is covered, epithelial cell migration ceases and stratification and keratinisation are rapidly completed.

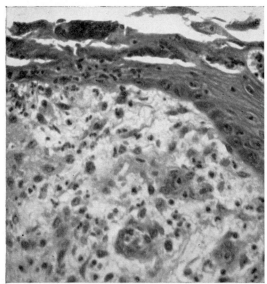

FIG. 3.9.—Granulating wound with early growth of epithelium over the surface.

The epithelium is growing from the right-hand side and tapers off as a thin layer. × 400.

Delay in epithelial spread occurs in a deep burn since the cells must burrow their way, probably helped by the production of collagenases, beneath the thick eschar of dead coagulated dermal collagen. Less delay is occasioned by a thick dry scab of exudate and as this acts as a barrier against infection and possibly also helps, by contracting, to reduce the size of the wound, it is usually best left *in situ*. In a superficial wound, a partial thickness ("second degree") burn and the site of removal of a split thickness skin graft, re-epithelialisation is relatively rapid as proliferation of epithelium occurs not only from the wound edge but also from the cut mouth of each pilosebaceous follicle. In man,

little epithelial regeneration occurs from sweat gland ducts. If skin appendages are destroyed they are not reformed.

Although epithelium shows the first evidence of reparative activity, within a few days the pre-existing vessels in the wound bed produce vascular sprouts which grow upwards forming loops and coils at right angles to the wound surface (Fig. 3.10) and giving it a red, granular

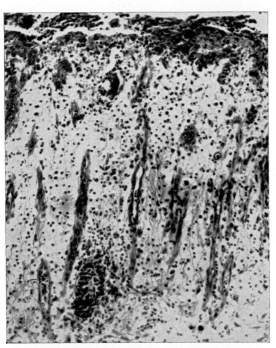

FIG. 3.10.—Granulating wound showing the vertical lines of newly formed blood vessels. × 150.

appearance (Fig. 3.11). From these new, more permeable vessels (Fig. 3.12), small haemorrhages occur and polymorphs migrate, reinforcing those already present in the exudate on the wound surface and helping to keep down bacterial growth. At the same time as the new capillaries form, fibroblasts, some of which are in mitosis, are seen in the base and walls of the wound, often running parallel to the new capillary walls. Later the fibroblasts become orientated parallel to the wound surface (Fig. 3.13) and about the end of the first week collagen is produced and rapidly increases in amount. This fibrovascular granulation tissue continues to proliferate and to fill the wound space only until epithelium grows over its surface when the exudative inflammatory changes and the migration of polymorphs also subside. If epithelialisa-

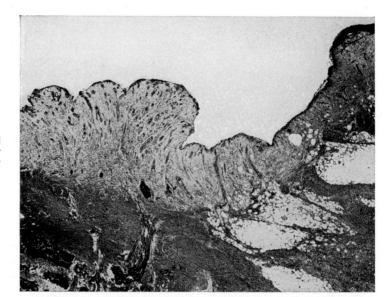

Fig. 3.11.—Granulating wound of 12 days' duration.

On the right, the advancing epithelial margin; in the floor the "granules" composed of new capillary loops and fibroblasts. × 10.

tion is delayed e.g. by further trauma or infection, granulations may pout from the wound surface forming so-called "proud flesh". Following healing, there is gradual resorption and retraction of some of the new vascular channels and further maturation of collagen which, over a period of months, becomes progressively less cellular.

One of the striking features of a healing open wound is the shrinkage of its surface area. This has the immediate advantage of reducing the time required for re-epithelialisation but may later result in unwanted contracture and deformity. While the cause of the shrinkage is not fully understood early skin grafting is found to reduce contracture.

Infected wounds. The repair of infected wounds is accomplished by the same processes already described for clean, open wounds; that is, by the production of granulation tissue. This is accompanied by a more pronounced acute inflammatory reaction, with more exudation of fluid and migration of leukocytes and also by formation of larger and more numerous blood vessels.

Open wounds, apart from those produced under aseptic surgical conditions, are almost always contaminated by bacteria, and for this reason a careful surgical toilet should include removal of devitalised tissue because it promotes bacterial growth; this is an important part of treatment. The granulation tissue itself provides a good defence against excessive bacterial multi-plication because, being rich in small blood vessels, it can mount an effective inflammatory response. These local defensive factors may be aided by systemic or local chemotherapy, which may even permit early suture or skin grafting. If infection continues however, more leukocytes pour into the surface exudate which then becomes purulent. The result of acute infection

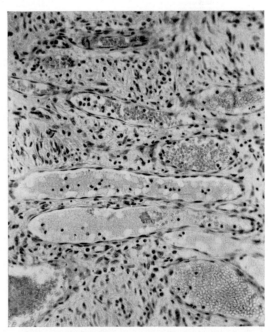

Fig. 3.12.—Newly formed thin-walled blood vessels in granulating wound, the surface of which is to the right. × 150.

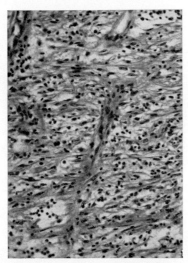

FIG. 3.13.—Deeper part of granulating wound.

Below, the collagen fibrils are being formed parallel to the surface; above, the vessels are seen running in a vertical direction. × 150.

on the healing processes is to inhibit both epithelial growth on the surface and also the production of fibroblasts, so that healing is delayed. This longer period and the greater tissue destruction results eventually in increased fibrous tissue and a more bulky and denser scar (Fig. 3.14).

Factors controlling repair

While the morphological changes of wound healing are well known, the factors controlling the various observed processes are controversial or unknown.

Control of cell movement. The covering of a wound surface by epithelium cannot be explained as due simply to movement by "*growth pressure*". While a burst of mitoses may displace adjacent cells by a concerted nudge, it is known that healing may occur without cell division and, in the skin, epithelial cell migration over the wound surface appears to precede proliferation. There is evidence from tissue culture that virtually all cells have the ability to move along a surface to which they can adhere. If two cultures of fibroblasts are made on a plane surface the cells grow out from each explant until they collide, when movement virtually ceases because the cells will almost never cross over each other, perhaps as a result of adhesion between them. This phenomenon is known as *contact inhibition*. The same phenomenon may govern the covering of the surface of a wound by epithelial cells from around the margin. This "contact inhibition" appears to be tissue specific in some degree, for if skin and oeso-

phageal epithelium meet, although both are squamous, cell movement and proliferation continue and cells heap up at the junction. How a sheet of cells comes to a halt when the site of re-established contact is some distance from the moving cells remains a mystery. The concept of contact inhibition in regard to epidermal cells and fibroblasts is sufficient to explain in part not only initiation of movement but also the direction of cells into the wounded area especially since there is no evidence that chemotaxis applies to any cell other than the leukocytes.

Explantation of a fragment of adult tissue into a culture medium does not result in rapid migration, although the cells at the free edge of the fragment now lack contact with similar cells. If the tissue is first wounded however, migration is greatly increased and it seems that some factor in addition to loss of contact inhibition may be involved. There is some evidence to suggest that there is a change in the cell surface causing a diminution of its adhesive properties and that this permits mobilisation.

The stimulus to migration and proliferation. It has been suggested that the stimulus to wound healing and enhanced mitotic activity is mediated by a growth promoter, "*trephone*" or "wound hormone" liberated by damaged cells. In the 1920s it was observed that chick embryo extracts added to tissue

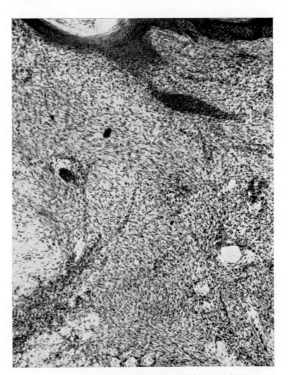

FIG. 3.14.—Healed abdominal wound.

There has been irritation and healing has been protracted. Note that the line of cellular tissue is much broader than in Fig. 3.2. × 75.

culture promoted their growth, but it was later shown that normal adult and embryonic tissue, autolysed and inflamed tissue, and protein degradation products had much the same effect and the action of all may simply have been to increase the nutrition of the culture. More recent tissue culture work still suggests that there may be a stimulating substance but this has never been shown *in vivo* to initiate cell migration or multiplication and at the moment the existence of a wound hormone derived from damaged cells and promoting healing in animals remains no more than a possibility.

It has been postulated that epidermal cells and other tissues normally secrete a diffusible tissue-specific depressor of cell mitosis and that a wound, by removing some of this depressor substance or "*chalone*", allows an increase in mitotic activity. The experimental finding that removal of skin from one side of a mouse's ear provoked a burst of mitotic activity in the intact epidermis of the other side, maximal opposite the middle of the defect rather than opposite the wound edges, supports this possibility. The concept of the "chalone" has interesting implications apart from those related to wound healing. Their inhibitory action on mitoses in skin cultures is apparently potentiated by adrenalin and glucocorticoids and the known cyclical fluctuation in adrenal function may thus account for the diurnal mitotic rhythm seen in many organs. There is some evidence also to suggest that tumours may fail to synthesise or release adequate concentrations of tissue specific "chalones" and so allow uncontrolled mitotic activity.

Factors influencing healing

Healing may be influenced to some extent by local factors. Infection delays healing (p. 57) as does a poor local blood supply; wounds of the relatively avascular shin tend to unite more slowly than those of the highly vascular scalp or face. Recently it has been found that heterologous cartilage fragments particularly from young animals may stimulate the connective tissue elements in wound repair but the mechanism is not known. Defects in collagen formation may result from generalised deficiency in vitamin C or of sulphur-containing amino-acids and also from an excess of cortisone. In severe trauma these metabolic disturbances appear to be inter-related.

Deficiency of vitamin C (ascorbic acid) and sulphur containing amino-acids. Man, monkey and guinea-pig are unable to synthesise vitamin C, and in the guinea-pig deficiency in wound collagen results from a diet lacking in the vitamin even when this is of very short duration. In man, however, a much longer period of dietary deficiency is necessary before collagen formation is affected although this may occur before scurvy is clinically apparent (p. 759). Patients with multiple injuries or extensive burns may have diminished serum and tissue levels and low urinary output of ascorbic acid and this is corrected readily by giving extra vitamin C. Deficiency of the vitamin appears to disturb the synthesis of collagen within the fibroblast and also to arrest the maturation of much of the collagen at the stage of the argyrophil fibre. As a result the tensile strength of the wound is low and there is a tendency, after re-epithelialisation of the wound and apparent healing, for it to break down again, this being a well known complication of naval surgery in the old days. In addition to the reduced amount of collagen formation, capillary endothelial cell proliferation may be diminished so that the blood vessels are fewer and abnormal. Deficient galactosamine may alter the properties of the ground substance. Similar alteration in collagen production with loss of wound strength may be seen in starving animals deficient in the sulphur-containing amino-acids such as methionine, which are essential for collagen synthesis. Even when starvation continues some of the methionine required for wound healing may be obtained from already existing tissue proteins but wound strength is increased by instituting an adequate diet. In well nourished individuals protein and vitamin supplements will not speed healing or improve wound strength.

Excess of adrenal glucocorticoid hormones. A large excess of cortisone given to susceptible experimental animals has much the same effect on wound healing as ascorbic acid deficiency. In addition to diminished blood vessel formation and ground substance abnormalities, fewer fibroblasts appear in the wound and collagen formation is both delayed and deficient. The usual therapeutic doses used in man probably have, however, no appreciable effect on wound healing. The tendency of cortisone to inhibit vascular endothelial proliferation has been useful in the treatment of corneal injuries: topical cortisone will allow healing without the formation of the permanent corneal opacities which result from formation of blood vessels and connective tissues.

Organisation

The processes involved in wound healing are also concerned in the removal, and replacement by fibrous tissue, of inert material such as thrombus, fibrinous exudate, haematoma (Fig. 3.15) or of dead tissue (p. 177). Organisation is illustrated by the two following examples.

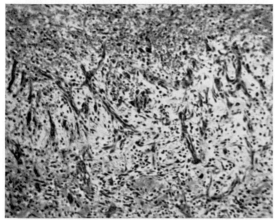

Fig. 3.15.—Organisation of a haematoma after 12 days. Numerous capillary sprouts are growing into the mass of clot, seen above. × 85.

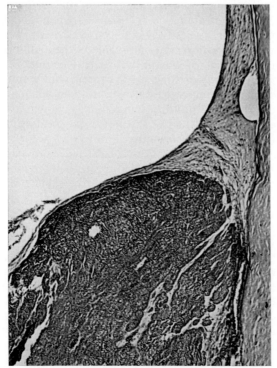

Fig. 3.16.—Section of thrombus in artery, showing growth of endothelium over the surface. × 65.

Organisation of thrombus. Endothelial cells from the lining of the vessel rapidly migrate and proliferate to cover the surface of mural thrombi (Fig. 3.16) and penetrate into any clefts, forming small vascular channels in continuity with the lumen. Similar capillaries, derived in arteries from the vasa vasorum of the deep part of the media and in veins from a vascular plexus just deep to the internal elastic lamina, grow into the thrombus at its site of attachment to the vessel wall. Phagocytes also enter and begin to remove the various constituents of the thrombus (Fig. 3.17). At the same time as the thrombus begins to become vascularised, connective tissue cells penetrate the clot. These

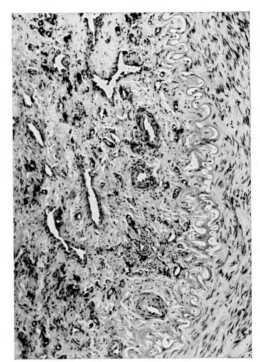

Fig. 3.17.—Advanced organisation of a thrombus in an artery. The thrombus is permeated by new capillaries, some of which have acquired muscular walls and become small arterioles. Many phagocytes with broken-down haemoglobin pigments lie in the young fibrous tissue. × 115.

cells are morphologically similar to the smooth muscle cells of the vessel wall and are said to be capable of producing both collagen and elastica so that the thrombus begins to be converted into connective tissue. Delayed or incomplete organisation is more likely to occur when the thrombus is dense and slowly formed or when arteries are affected. The necessary preliminary vascularisation of the artery wall may be inhibited both by haemodynamic factors and by intimal degeneration due to atheroma (p. 264). An atheromatous vessel may be further narrowed by organisation of mural thrombi.

Restoration of the lumen following occlusion occurs chiefly as a result of shrinkage of the thrombus by fibrinolysis but sometimes partly by recanalisation which, especially if the thrombus is short, links up the endothelial lined clefts and spaces traversing the clot.

Organisation of exudate. Organisation of fibrinous exudate on a serous membrane such as pleura, pericardium or peritoneum follows a similar pattern. If the fibrin is abundant and dense, glueing together the visceral and parietal surfaces, capillaries and fibroblasts grow in from the underlying tissue on each side and finally meet, the fibrin being absorbed or phagocytosed by accompanying macrophages. This mass of granulation tissue which binds the opposing surfaces together then becomes less vascular and forms fibrous adhesions. If the fibrin forms a more open meshwork there may be effective digestion of it by leukocytes with some repair of the mesothelial surface. Fibrous tissue may also replace intra-alveolar fibrin in unresolved pneumonia (Fig. 15.23, p. 351).

Fracture healing

Healing by callus formation

Healing in bones bears many resemblances to healing in soft tissues; there is initial haemorrhage and exudative inflammation, followed by a proliferative or productive stage in which osteogenic cells play a vital part. The first need is to re-establish continuity between the bone fragments and to this end a mass of new bony and sometimes cartilaginous tissue (*provisional callus*) is formed: once continuity is re-established, this undergoes slow remodelling, with resorption and replacement so that under favourable conditions, firm bony union is achieved. Sometimes restoration is so good that the fracture site is later hardly identifiable.

Early stages. A good deal of force is normally required to break a bone, the fragments are usually displaced, and in addition to a relatively small amount of haemorrhage between the bone ends from torn medullary vessels much blood may seep into the soft tissues from ruptured extra-osseous vessels. The fibrin mesh of the blood clot between the bone ends has, as in soft tissue wounds, been claimed to provide an essential scaffolding effect for migrating cells. However, fracture healing is not delayed either in haemophiliacs or in rats given short term courses of heparin which inhibits coagulation. Indeed a large amount of clot and debris between the bone fragments almost certainly delays healing until its removal is complete. In addition to haemorrhage, local exudative inflammatory changes take place with hyperaemia and exudation of protein-rich fluid from which fibrin may be deposited. Polymorphs are scanty unless there is infection and this is common only in compound fractures, i.e. with breach of the overlying skin or mucous membrane. Macrophages also invade and phagocytose clot and tissue debris. Red blood cells often disappear rapidly from the fracture site leaving a homogeneous mass of fibrin.

Bone necrosis occurs partly from direct injury but chiefly as a result of tearing of blood vessels in the medullary cavity, cortex and periosteum: the first recognisable histological evidence is observed within a day or two, the haemopoietic marrow cells showing loss of nuclear staining. Fat released from dead adipose marrow may be taken up by macrophages, and fat "cysts" form surrounded by foreign body giant cells. Damage to the adipose marrow may have serious results when globules enter marrow venules and produce *fat emboli* in the pulmonary bed, brain, heart or kidneys (p. 171). The bone tissue itself also dies and the cortex, because of its more restricted vascularity, tends to be more extensively affected than the spongy medullary bone. The amount of bone death depends especially on the local peculiarities of the blood supply; the talus, carpal scaphoid, and femoral head following subcapital fracture are particularly liable to undergo extensive ischaemic necrosis. When there is splintering of bone (*comminuted fracture*) some of the fragments may lose their blood supply; they become necrotic and are eventually resorbed. Bone death is recognisable histologically by loss of osteocytes from the bone lacunae (Fig. 3.18) but some cells may still remain after many days.

Provisional callus formation. (*a*) *Periosteal reaction.* The cells of the inner or cambium layer of the undamaged periosteum proliferate

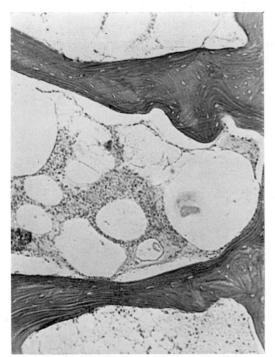

FIG. 3.18.—The bone is necrotic and empty of osteocytes. Cell ghosts can be seen in the necrotic haemopoietic marrow. × 100.

in a fairly wide zone overlying the living cortex of each fractured bone end. A cuff of bone trabeculae is formed at right angles to the cortex and anchored to it (Fig. 3.19). Further woven bone trabeculae (p. 751), less well orientated, form an irregular meshwork whose pattern at this stage is uninfluenced by stress. This is dependent on the blood supply which derives partly from surviving periosteal vessels but largely from muscle and other surrounding soft tissues. Mixed with this cuff of new bone there are often nodules of hyaline cartilage which usually do not appear until bone formation is well under way (Fig. 3.19). The amount of cartilage which is formed in provisional callus varies greatly from one species to another. Small mammals such as mice, rats and rabbits tend to form chiefly cartilaginous callus while in man the amount, though variable, is less. Cartilage formation is thought to be promoted by a poor blood supply and by shearing strains and stresses so that it is particularly abundant in poorly immobilised fractures: bone gradually replaces the cartilage by endochondral ossification. The two enlarging cuffs of bony and cartilaginous callus advance towards each other and finally

unite to bridge the fracture line leaving a gap between the bone ends (Fig. 3.19). This "bandage" of *external callus* helps to immobilise the bone ends in an unstable or poorly fixed fracture. The amount of bridging periosteal callus varies greatly in different sites and under different circumstances. In intracapsular fractures such as subcapital fractures of the femoral neck the periosteum is lacking and union is wholly dependent on *internal callus* formed by osteoblasts lying in the medullary cavity. By contrast, fracture of the diaphysis of large tubular bones such as the femur and humerus tend to form much external callus, internal callus in the relatively small medullary cavity not being striking. The formation of bulky external callus probably depends on plenty of surrounding undamaged muscle as a source of blood supply, for one of the causes of the difficulty in healing of fractures of the tibia is that they are partially covered by relatively avascular subcutaneous tissue and tend to form little callus. Poorly aligned fractures and those with much movement at the fracture site (e.g. the ribs and clavicle) are liable to produce a wealth of external callus, whereas fractures which are well immobilised by external or internal surgical fixation may unite with relatively little callus formation.

(*b*) *Medullary reaction.* The first evidence of healing is the advance of capillaries from the viable into the necrotic marrow closely followed by fibroblasts and macrophages (Fig. 3.20). The latter cells phagocytose and remove dead material. Osteoclasts also develop and proliferate and begin to resorb dead spongy bone and the endosteal surface of the necrotic cortex. The osteogenic cells covering the medullary trabeculae and the endosteal surface of the cortex become plump and new woven bone begins to form in the marrow spaces, partly on the surface of dead trabeculae which, when surrounded by new bone, may remain unresorbed for months or even years (Fig. 3.21). In contrast with external callus, cartilage is rare in the medullary cavity, perhaps because it is a relatively vascular site and is protected from mechanical stress. It may form, however, when the process reaches the fracture gap (see below).

(*c*) *Cortical reaction.* The most striking reaction in the living cortex adjacent to the fracture is an increase in osteoclastic resorption with widening of the canals, presumably partly the result of immobilisation (p. 768). This may

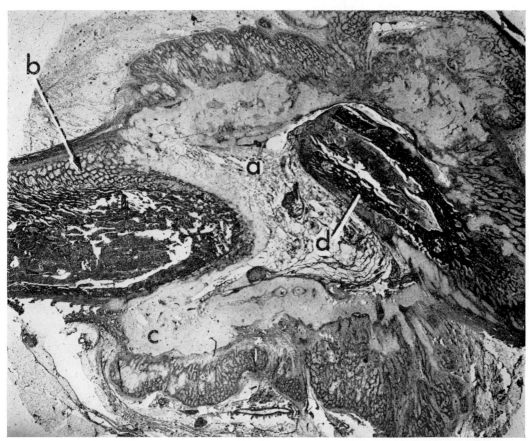

Fig. 3.19.—Healing of displaced birth-fracture in the femur of a premature infant. The bone ends are cut obliquely. Bridging periosteal callus has formed but around the bone ends there is still a gap (a) which contains a meshwork of fibrin. The subperiosteal cuff of new bone is well seen at (b). The bridging callus consists partly of woven bone and partly of pale hyaline cartilage (c). The Haversian canals of the living cortex (d) are slightly enlarged by osteoclasis. × 5.

be followed later by some osteoblastic activity. Similar changes are seen in the dead cortex of the bone ends once there has been revascularisation of the Haversian canals from adjacent vessels in viable bone or from periosteal and medullary vessels. The resorption of necrotic bone may widen the fracture gap.

The fracture gap. The periosteal (external) callus unites the bone ends externally but the aim is for extension of union directly across the bone ends. As already stated, immediately after fracture, blood clot, exuded fibrin and bony debris fill the gap and this is attacked by macrophages and by osteoclasts, polymorphs being scanty. The fibrin clot, which usually persists between the bone ends, is finally invaded by blood vessels and cellular tissue and bony union may occur in either of two ways. Direct ossification is brought about by osteogenic cells spread-

ing from medullary and periosteal callus. Cartilage may also be formed and is converted into bone. This direct process is relatively rapid and effective but sometimes union is brought about first by fibrous tissue which grows in from medulla or periosteum or both, becomes densely collagenised and only then much more slowly becomes ossified. Instability, distraction or marked resorption of the bone ends, massive necrosis, a poor blood supply, comminution and infection all predispose to this slower type of union. Sometimes following fibrous union conversion to bone is very slow (*delayed union*) and occasionally it fails to occur (*non-union*). In non-union the fibrous tissue may become very dense, hyaline, and finally fibrocartilaginous. The appearance of an area of eosinophilic fibrinoid necrosis is followed by a linear split which may enlarge and eventually develop a

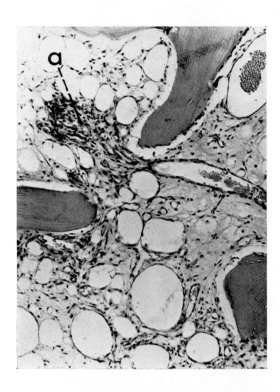

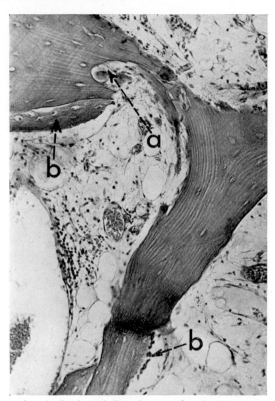

FIG. 3.20a.—Dead fatty marrow in the medullary cavity is being revascularised. A knot of proliferating capillaries is seen at (a). × 100.

b.—A dead medullary bone trabecula is being removed by osteoclasts at (a) and new bone is being laid down on the surface of dead bone at (b). × 120.

lining similar to synovium, thus forming a false joint (*pseudarthrosis*) (Fig. 3.22). The bone ends buried in the dense fibrous tissue tend to become very sclerotic.

Final remodelling. Once bony union has occurred and function has been regained, the bone begins to be remodelled in response to mechanical stresses. Excessive callus is resorbed, slowly formed lamellar bone begins to replace the hastily laid down woven bone, and any remaining necrotic bone is removed and replaced (Fig. 3.23). The cortex is reformed across the fracture gap and gradually medullary callus is removed and retubulation of the bone occurs. The whole process may take about a year.

Primary union

Although primary union of soft tissues is the rule in clean sutured surgical incisions, primary union in fractures is a curiosity and has only fairly recently been described. It entails bony union with the formation of only minimal amounts of callus and was first described in compression arthrodesis (i.e. obliteration of the joint) of the knee, the cancellous surfaces of femur and tibia being held together by compression clamps. Bony union occurs in about 4 weeks and biopsy shows only a thin line of new bone at the contact points of opposing trabeculae. While compression forces probably play some part, a major factor may be the rigid fixation and close apposition of surfaces. Cortical fractures in dogs, produced by a very fine saw with minimal necrosis, and fixed by a compression plate have united without periosteal callus, but although union of similarly treated long bone fractures in man occurs quickly and without radiologically apparent periosteal callus, it seems doubtful, in view of the probable amount of bone necrosis, that they can truly be described as undergoing primary union.

General factors affecting bone healing

Some of the local factors affecting bone healing have already been mentioned but, as in wound healing, general factors are also operative. Lack of vitamin C results in depression of

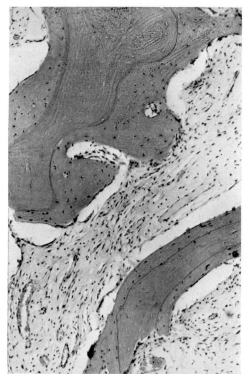

FIG. 3.21.—Months after fracture dead bone trabeculae are still recognisable, covered by new living bone. × 70.

both fibroblastic and osteogenic activity so that collagen and bone production are both deficient. Cortisone administered to animals with fractures also retards healing but it seems that it has little effect when given to patients in the usual therapeutic doses. In vitamin D deficiency (p. 760) abundant callus may form, but it fails to calcify, remaining soft until the deficiency is made good.

Transplantation of bone (bone grafting)

Bone grafting is a relatively common surgical operation. Grafts may be used to bridge a bony gap, e.g. in a fracture with much bone loss such as may occur following a gunshot wound or in reconstructive plastic surgery; to fill a space within a bone, e.g. following curettage of a

benign intraosseous tumour, and to promote bony union whether of an un-united fracture or across a diseased joint (arthrodesis). The bone used may come from the patient himself, an *autograft*; from another human, an *allograft or homograft* or from another animal species, a *xenograft or heterograft* (see p. 77). It may consist of cancellous or cortical bone and may be fresh, or in the case of allografts or xenografts may have been stored under sterile conditions following a variety of treatments.

Autogenous compact bone is used chiefly when strength and rigidity are required. The removal of the graft cuts off its blood supply and due to

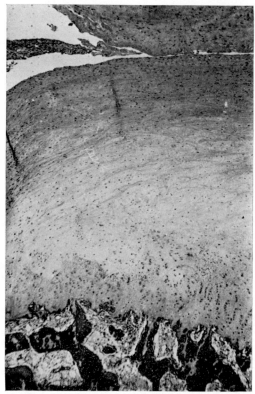

FIG. 3.22.—Pseudarthrosis following fracture of the clavicle. The bone ends have become covered by cartilage. At the top of the picture a split in the cartilage has occurred giving a false joint. There is endochondral ossification of the proliferated cartilage in the lower part of the picture. × 40.

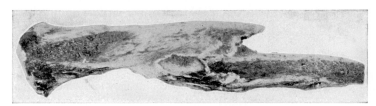

FIG. 3.23.—Malunited fracture of clavicle.

the difficulty of transmission of nutrition from tissue fluid through the canalicular system only a few superficially placed osteocytes survive along with some periosteal and endosteal cells. These surviving cells may proliferate and form some new bone but the major contribution is probably made by invading "host" osteoblasts which accompany blood vessels from the tissue bed in which the graft is implanted. These vessels grow into the marrow spaces, Haversian canals, and along the surfaces of the graft; osteoclasts resorb some of the dead bone and new bone also forms so that the dead graft is first united with the "host" bone and then gradually replaced over a period of months by new living bone (Fig. 3.24). At first the new bone is woven and forms an open meshwork; later it is remodelled to become lamellar and compact. The osteocytes in *autogenous cancellous bone* almost all die following transplantation but there is a much larger surface area of bone so that more endosteal cells are available for proliferation, and more importantly there is a greater stimulation of new bone formation by "host" cells. This type of graft is *par excellence* a stimulator of osteogenesis although the dead graft bone is, as in the compact type, resorbed.

In fresh bone allografts in animals there is, as in the fresh autograft, necrosis of most of the transplant, invasion by host capillaries and some proliferation of surviving graft osteoblasts with new bone formation. About 7 to 10 days after transplantation, however, lymphocytes appear around blood vessels which become obliterated and any surviving transplanted cells and new bone which has proliferated die. The dead graft is then either completely resorbed or acts as a scaffolding for "host" cells and is slowly replaced by living bone. Second grafts from the same donor undergo accelerated rejection. The rejection process is a delayed hypersensitivity reaction (p. 112). The strongest antigen in the foreign bone seems to be the haemopoietic marrow cells. *Allografts used therapeutically in man* are not fresh, they do not contain living cells but have been treated, sterilised and stored. The aim in selecting methods of treatment, sterilisation and storage is to provide a graft which has low antigenicity, high powers of induction of new bone formation by the "host" cells and the ability to be actively remodelled. So far it seems that frozen, freeze dried or decalcified bone both encourages more new bone formation and is less antigenic than boiled,

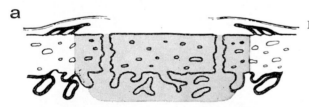

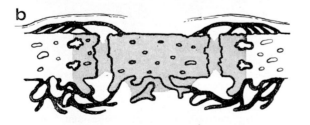

Fig. 3.24.—Incorporation of a bone graft (after Ham). a.—The graft, seen in the centre, consists of cortex with some attached spongy bone trabeculae and marrow. Both the graft and the margins of the bony bed into which it is laid are dead (hatched). New living bone (black) is forming under the "host" periosteum and around living (white) endosteal trabeculae.

b.—The amount of new living bone has increased and the graft bone is now attached to the "host" bone by new trabeculae which have formed partly on the surface of dead bone. Haversian canals in the dead "host" bone have been revascularised and widened by osteoclastic resorption. Some living bone is also proliferating around the margins of the canals. Union has occurred between the "host" bone and the graft.

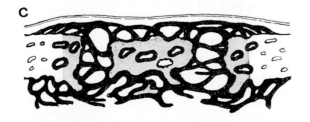

c.—The remaining amount of dead graft bone is much diminished by osteoclastic resorption and there is also some resorption of the remaining dead bone of the "host" bed. The dead graft is being replaced by living new bone.
The type of reaction illustrated occurs no matter what type of graft is used. There tends to be rather more graft osteoblast contribution to the final amount of new bone when fresh autograft bone is used.

autoclaved or deproteinised bone or bone stored in merthiolate. The "host" response to grafting is enhanced by the removal of soft tissue from Haversian systems and intertrabecular spaces leaving an open channel for the ingrowth of vessels and cells and by implantation of the graft at sites of maximum osteogenesis, e.g. in cancellous bone or haemopoietic marrow.

While *xenografts* have seldom been used, some success has been reported using freeze dried, fat-free calf bone. Autografts, especially of cancellous bone, remain the first choice for transplantation.

Aseptic necrosis of bone

The processes of revascularisation, laying down of new bone and gradual resorption of dead bone involved in the replacement of bone grafts also come into play in the replacement of aseptic necrotic bone whether this follows fracture, caisson disease (p. 661), sickle-cell anaemia (p. 408), Gaucher's disease, the long term administration of steroids or is of unknown etiology. The femoral and humeral heads appear particularly susceptible to aseptic necrosis and if revascularisation and reossification is incomplete or fails to occur necrotic trabeculae may eventually collapse with resultant deformity of the joint surface and disabling secondary degenerative changes. Aseptic necrosis is thought to be the cause of a number of eponymous conditions affecting the epiphyses of children (*osteochondritis juvenilis*) e.g., the femoral head (*Perthes' disease*), navicular (*Kohler's disease*), head of second or third metatarsal (*Freiberg's disease*) and the lunate in adults (*Kienbock's disease*).

Repair and regeneration of nervous tissue and nerves

Central nervous tissue. Once mature nerve cells are destroyed, they are not replaced by the proliferation of other nerve cells. There is also no useful regeneration of axons in the central nervous system: indeed when an axon in the central nervous system is severed at any point, the entire axon and the nerve cell body degenerate. In contrast peripheral nerves, because of the presence of Schwann cells, have consider-able regenerative capacity (see below). Of the neuroglial cells, proliferation in response to tissue damage is restricted to astrocytes, this being referred to as gliosis (p. 608).

Regeneration of peripheral nerves. When a nerve is transected the axis cylinders distal to the cut undergo Wallerian degeneration, i.e. the axon and its myelin sheath are broken down and are absorbed by macrophages (p. 47). At the same time the Schwann cells proliferate within the neurilemmal sheath to form pathways along which the axons may regrow. Proximal to the level of transection myelin degeneration extends upwards only to the first or second node of Ranvier and the nerve cell body characteristically shows central chromatolysis (p. 606). Axonal sprouts soon emerge from the proximal ends of the interrupted axis cylinders and, if the cut ends of the nerve are in close apposition, they grow into the distal part of the nerve and along the spaces formerly occupied by axis cylinders and now filled with proliferated Schwann cells. The axons grow at a rate of about 3 mm. per day. These new axons, which at first are very thin, increase in diameter and develop a new myelin sheath. In addition to growth and maturation of the axon, time is also needed for the re-inervation of motor end plates and sensory end organs so that restoration of function is always slow and often imperfect.

When the cut ends of the nerve are not in close apposition there may be intense proliferation of axonal sprouts and Schwann cells from the proximal end of the nerve to form a bulbous swelling—the so-called amputation or traumatic neuroma (Fig. 3.25).

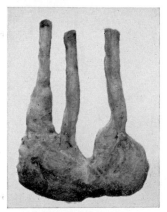

Fig. 3.25.—Amputation neuroma at severed proximal ends of nerves of arm.

If a nerve is crushed so that the axons are severed but the continuity of the endoneurium and perineurium is preserved, the distal portion undergoes Wallerian degeneration as before. Owing to the persistence of continuity of the framework of the nerve the regenerating axons can grow more easily into the distal part of the nerve. Restoration of function also tends to be more satisfactory. Secondary suture of severed nerves up to 6 months after injury is often satisfactory but if it is performed later than this it may give poor results. Attempts at restoration of function by nerve suture should therefore not be postponed too long.

Repair and regeneration of muscle

(a) Skeletal muscle. In man muscle loss in injuries and usually also in surgical wounds is repaired by the ingrowth of fibrovascular tissue which later matures to form a collagenous scar. Regeneration of muscle, however, may occur in two ways. It is generally accepted that once dead muscle is removed by invading macrophages, several or single sarcoplasmal sprouts with multiple nuclei (Fig. 3.26) may form from the viable end of a damaged fibre and advance, especially if an intact sarcolemmal tube or well orientated endomysium remains to act as a guide line. More controversial is the suggestion that new muscle fibres may form by the fusion of mononuclear cells which may have originated

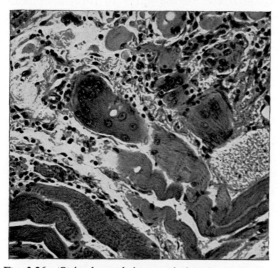

FIG. 3.26.—Striped muscle in granulation tissue, showing sarcoplasmal sprouts with multiple nuclei. × 200.

from the sarcolemma of the original fibre, or possibly from other or additional sources.

Effective muscle regeneration depends greatly on the preservation of the supporting structures but even in the most advantageous circumstances the slow advance of fibres, probably at less than 1 mm./day, may at any time be halted by ingrowing fibrous tissue. The most successful and extensive regeneration in man occurs when individual muscle fibres are damaged, as in Zenker's hyaline degeneration. This condition may accompany severe infections and toxaemias, especially typhoid fever, and tends to involve most severely the muscles of the abdominal wall, diaphragm and intercostals. Regeneration by the two methods already mentioned has been described, and because of the intact sarcolemma is usually complete. Worthwhile functional recovery may also occur by regeneration in polymyositis (p. 810).

Where there is extensive muscle damage in man only abortive attempts at regeneration may be seen. For instance at the margin of a mass of necrotic muscle in Volkmann's ischaemic contracture (p. 805) multinucleate muscle sprouts may be seen but fibrous replacement eventually results, the endomysial framework being colonised by fibroblasts (Fig. 22.66, p. 805).

(b) Visceral muscle (smooth, non-striped muscle). The healing of visceral muscle, e.g. in surgical incisions in the bowel, occurs by fibrous repair and although smooth muscle may be seen in recently differentiated arterioles (p. 53) and in atheromatous plaques (p. 265), its origin is uncertain and it may arise by migration or by differentiation from other mesenchymal cells. Proliferation with mitotic activity is said to occur in the early months of the physiological uterine enlargement of pregnancy.

(c) Cardiac muscle. Destruction of cardiac muscle by infarction is repaired by fibrous tissue (Fig. 14.11, p. 304). Effective regeneration occurs in young patients with Coxsackie virus infections or diphtheria, where there is damage to individual fibres with preservation of the endomysium, a situation similar to that of Zenker's degeneration in skeletal muscle.

Repair of tendon

When a tendon is injured or cut, regardless of whether it has a synovial sheath, fibroblasts and blood vessels migrate from surrounding connective tissue into the fibrin meshwork between the ends. The cells, at first more or less randomly arranged, later become orientated along the line of the tendon and produce reticulin fibres and then more mature collagen. Suitable cell orientation and so healing is promoted by bringing together tendon stumps. As in skin healing (p. 53), the rate of collagen formation increases until the end of the second week after injury and then slows down. The cells of the dense collagen of the tendon, like those of the dense dermal collagen, play little part in the process. The good functional results of tendon healing depend on the resorption of fibrovascular adhesions between the tendon and the surrounding tissues. While these adhesions appear to be increased by clumsy handling at operation little is known of the factors which influence their removal.

Healing of mucosal surfaces

The cells which line mucosal surfaces, like those of the epidermis, are being lost and replaced continuously throughout life and have a good potential for regeneration (Fig. 3.27). In general, the first aim is to cover the raw surface

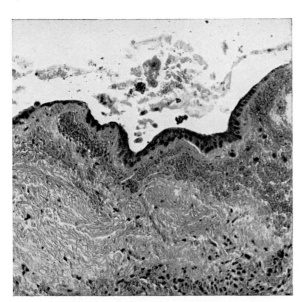

FIG. 3.27.—Repair of lining of gallbladder after acute inflammatory desquamation.

The epithelial cells extend as a thin flattened layer to reline the viscus. × 150.

and only later is there differentiation of more specialised cells.

(a) Gastro-intestinal tract mucosa. Physiological replacement of lost surface cells takes place by proliferation of the more protected cells of the mucosal glandular necks. Experimental excision of an area of mucosa, in the stomach for instance, is rapidly followed by re-epithelialisation: epithelial cells of the mucous neck type migrate over the exposed connective tissue, forming first a layer of thin, flattened epithelium which later becomes cubical or columnar. The epithelium of glands adjacent to the wound undergo mitosis as do surface cells and this proliferation keeps up the supply of migrating cells until the surface is covered. Gland crypts reform by mucous cells growing down into the underlying granulation tissue and some weeks later, specialised cells, e.g. parietal cells, differentiate from the mucous cells in the crypts. While delay in, or complete failure of, re-epithelialisation of chronic peptic ulcers in man has been attributed to the necrotic slough forming the ulcer base and to the narrowing of blood vessels by endarteritis, the cause is not fully understood. Even when the ulcer does heal the mucosa tends to be thin or of intestinal type. Wounds of the mucous membranes following surgical anastomoses heal readily and the line between the two different types of mucosa remains sharp.

The small and large bowel mucosae have a similar capacity for regeneration (Fig. 18.46d, p. 509). Repeated ulceration and repair as, for instance, in ulcerative colitis and bilharzial infestation, may lead to overgrowth of the reparative mucosa, producing polypoid projections (Fig. 18.64, p. 522).

(b) Respiratory tract mucosa. The basal cells of the tracheal and bronchial lining epithelium proliferate throughout life and replace loss of the surface ciliated epithelium. Many bacterial injuries involve the loss of only part of the thickness of the pseudostratified columnar epithelium and this, as in physiological regeneration, is readily replaced by basal cell proliferation. Full thickness destruction of the mucosa is followed by the usual pattern of migration and proliferation from surviving cell islands as is seen in the epidermis. Repeated damage, as for instance in chronic bronchitis, may result in a less physiologically effective regeneration, the ciliated cells being replaced by columnar non-

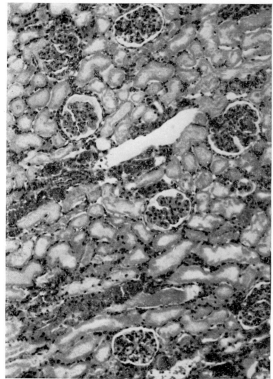

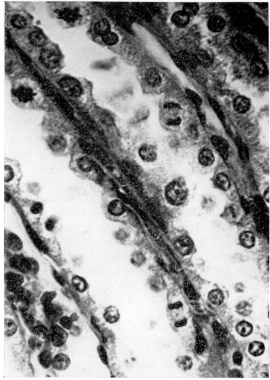

Fig. 3.28a.—Acute tubular necrosis in the rat. Note the anatomical normality of the glomeruli and the absence of nuclei in the dead tubular epithelial cells. × 150.

b.—Regeneration of renal tubular epithelium following acute tubular necrosis in the rat. Four mitotic figures are present. The adjacent regenerated cells are still of subnormal size. × 450.

ciliated cells and under very unfavourable circumstances, metaplastic change of the regenerating epithelium to squamous type may be seen.

(c) Urinary tract mucosa. The urinary tract mucosa like the epidermis responds to injury by movement and proliferation of cells. The transitional cell mucosa of the bladder has particularly good powers of rapid regeneration.

Repair of kidney

The nephron is a highly specialised unit and there is little effective regeneration following damage. Loss of renal substance is repaired by fibrous tissue. If the basement membrane of the tubules remains intact, damage to tubular epithelium may be followed by proliferation (Fig. 3.28) and slow migration of surviving cells to restore continuity. It is doubtful, however, whether, when the damaged cells are highly specialised, as in the proximal convoluted tubule, the regenerated cells have the same degree of functional efficiency.

Repair and regeneration of the liver

The hepatic parenchymal cells form a fairly stable population, and few mitotic figures are seen in the normal liver. Replacement of normal "wear-and-tear" cell loss is by division of neighbouring cells. Some replacement is effected by amitotic division and this probably explains the occurrence of binucleate and multinucleate liver cells, particularly in elderly individuals.

Wounds of the liver are repaired by formation of connective tissue, although there is some replacement of destroyed cells by proliferation of parenchymal cells around the margin of the wound. New liver "lobules" (see p. 546) are never formed.

The outcome of liver cell necrosis depends on the distribution of the cells affected and also upon the presence or absence of an intact vascular system. Occlusion of hepatic arterial branches may be followed by infarction of liver tissue. As in most other tissues the infarct undergoes coagulative necrosis and is repaired by a process of organisation, leaving a fibrous scar. Necrosis of individual liver cells scattered throughout the lobules, as in the typical attack of virus hepatitis, is followed by autolysis of the dead cells, which disappear and are replaced by proliferation of surviving cells (Fig. 19.3, p. 546). The liver may thus be restored to normal. Necrosis of all or most of the liver cells in the centres or mid-zones of the lobules is also followed by autolytic change in the dead cells: cell plates, often more than one cell thick, are formed by proliferation of neighbouring hepatocytes and extend into the surviving vascular framework so that normality is once again achieved. If, however, there is loss of most or all of the hepatocytes in whole or major parts of lobules, and particularly when those cells lying peripherally in the lobules are lost, the vascular framework collapses and while the surviving hepatocytes still proliferate, regeneration is incomplete and irregular. Scarring occurs in the collapsed areas and regeneration produces a nodular pattern (Fig. 19.11, p. 554).

The very high regenerative capacity of liver cells has been demonstrated by subjecting animals to excision of various amounts of liver tissue. After excision of two-thirds of the rat's liver, hypertrophy and hyperplasia in the remaining third result in restoration of a normal liver mass in 15–20 days. The capacity of the liver to regenerate in this way is maintained even when partial hepatectomy is performed monthly for up to one year.

When partial hepatectomy is performed upon one member of a pair of parabiotic rats, hepatocyte proliferation occurs in both animals. This and similar experiments suggest that a chemical mediating factor is responsible for hepatic regeneration, but it is not clear whether proliferation results from release of stimulatory factors or from removal of growth inhibiting factors. The establishment of a porto-caval vascular shunt may impair the rate of regeneration and it thus seems that portal venous flow through the liver is more important than arterial blood flow in determining the degree of restoration. Diet, age, hormones and biliary obstruction may modify, but do not specifically impair the regenerative process.

HYPERTROPHY

This term is used by custom to denote increase in the specialised protoplasm of an organ, e.g. the muscle cells of the heart and the hepatic cells of the liver. The increase may depend on enlargement of individual cells—true or cell *hypertrophy*—or on proliferation of cells—*hyperplasia*. While the two processes may occur together, hypertrophy alone signifies that the cells concerned have lost their capacity for mitosis and while capable of synthesising more protein and RNA are unable to reduplicate DNA. The term hypertrophy is sometimes loosely and wrongly used as synonymous with enlargement. For example retention of secretion in the thyroid gland, amyloid infiltration in the liver or venous engorgement of the spleen may produce an enlargement of the organ but this is not due to hypertrophy. Each organ and tissue seems to have a pattern of response which, although it may alter with age, is largely uninfluenced by the type of stimulus which promotes it. For instance hyperplasia and hypertrophy of the renal tubular epithelial cells, affecting especially the proximal tubule, may be seen in the compensatory hypertrophy of the remaining kidney following unilateral nephrectomy (see below) and also associated with the increased production of growth hormone in the generalised enlargement of organs in acromegaly. Hypertrophy in a tissue is brought about by two main factors, (a) an increase in the amount of work which it is called upon to perform, and (b) an alteration in hormonal balance.

(a) The response to increased functional demand may be clearly seen in *muscular tissues* which usually undergo true hypertrophy without hyperplasia. The physiological hypertrophy of skeletal muscle in manual labourers or athletes is a good example, the individual fibres increasing in thickness and length but not in number. Similarly when extra work is demanded of the heart as a result of valvular disease or high blood pressure (Fig. 3.29) there may be much thickening of the muscular walls, those chambers which bear the brunt of the extra work being most severely affected, e.g. narrowing of the mitral valve produces chiefly left atrial and right ventricular hypertrophy whereas systemic hypertension gives rise predominantly to left ventricular hypertrophy (Fig. 14.2, p. 298). The heart weight may rise to twice the normal or more, the degree of hypertrophy being limited by the

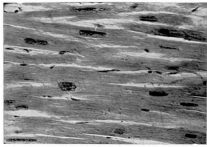

FIG. 3.29a.—Hypertrophied muscle fibres of heart in a case of arteriosclerosis with high blood pressure. × 185.

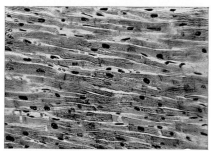

FIG. 3.29b.—Slightly atrophied heart muscle; to compare with Fig. 3.29a. × 185.

waning capacity of oxygen and nutrients to diffuse sufficiently from the capillaries, now widely separated by thick fibres. While an adequate blood supply is required to allow hypertrophy to occur there is no evidence that an increased vascular bed will, of itself and without an increased demand, produce hypertrophy. Smooth muscle may also undergo hypertrophy, as is seen in the muscle of a hollow viscus, for example in the stomach behind a stenosed pylorus, in large bowel proximal to a carcinoma (Fig. 18.75, p. 536), or in the bladder when the outflow is obstructed by an enlarged prostate (Fig. 23.5, p. 821). The muscle in arterial walls also hypertrophies in response to long continued high blood pressure (Fig. 13.13, p. 271). The most striking hypertrophy is seen in the pregnant uterus, where a combination of increased functional demand and hormonal stimuli results in enlargement of fibres to more than a hundred times their original volume. In early pregnancy, in contrast to the other conditions, there may be

some proliferation (hyperplasia) of muscle fibres. After parturition the fibres return to a normal size and this is seen also in hypertrophied heart muscle when the increased work stimulus is removed.

Response to an increased demand may be met sometimes by pure hyperplasia, for instance blood loss is followed by proliferation of the red cell and leukocyte precursors of the haemopoietic marrow and not by their hypertrophy (Fig. 16.10b, p. 402).

Compensatory hypertrophy may occur in the survivor of a pair of organs when one is removed. Following nephrectomy the remaining kidney enlarges and particularly in young patients may double its weight. This is not brought about by the formation of new nephrons, but by an increase in nephron size as a result of both hypertrophy and hyperplasia of the component cells. Both glomeruli and tubules increase in volume. Loss of one testis in childhood probably results in accelerated growth of the remaining one but in adult life there is little evidence to suggest any compensatory enlargement. Functional hyper-

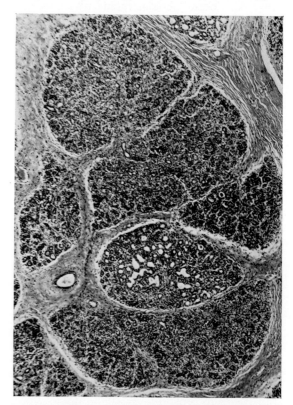

FIG. 3.30.—Breast lobule in pregnancy showing marked hypertrophy and hyperplasia. × 40.

trophy does not occur in the adult rat subjected to unilateral orchidectomy, the number of spermatozoa produced being reduced to half. Removal of one adrenal leads to increase in size of the cells of the opposite cortex, the medulla remaining unchanged. The enlargement of the contralateral lung following pneumonectomy, however, is chiefly caused by over-distension which produces a lasting enlargement of the alveoli; only when it occurs in early life is there any formation of new alveoli. Compensatory hypertrophy may also occur when part of an organ is removed, for instance following partial hepatectomy (p. 71).

(b) Hypertrophy associated with hormonal changes. A balanced activity of certain of the endocrine glands is essential for the normal growth and nourishment of the tissues and many of the examples of hypertrophy and hyperplasia already mentioned require the continued physio-logical action of the growth hormone of the anterior pituitary as well as an adequate blood supply. An increase in the growth hormone produced by the oxyphil cells of the anterior pituitary results in adults in acromegaly (p. 877) with increase in bone mass and generalised organ and tissue hypertrophy. This is even more strikingly seen when the excess of hormone occurs in adolescence, before the skeleton matures; the result is gigantism (p. 878). A physiological example of hormonal hypertrophy is the enlargement of the breasts in pregnancy, when the formation of mammary gland acini is stimulated chiefly by hormones from the corpus luteum or placenta (Fig. 3.30).

It may be that some examples of unexplained pathological hypertrophy such as that occa-sionally seen in the breasts of adolescents and commonly in the prostate gland in the elderly will ultimately prove to be of endocrine origin.

CHAPTER 4

THE IMMUNE RESPONSE

Introduction

The invasion of the body by living organisms, including viruses, bacteria, and protozoan and metazoan parasites, presents a major threat to the stability of the internal milieu upon which Claude Bernard placed such importance. To counter this threat certain general defence mechanisms have evolved—a relatively impermeable epidermis, methods of ridding the body of noxious material, such as vomiting, diarrhoea and coughing, the dilution of irritants by increased flow of interstitial fluid in inflammatory oedema, and the ingestion of particulate matter by phagocytic cells. In addition, there exists in vertebrates a special defence mechanism of immense potentiality which is mobilised when the body is invaded by foreign organisms and which is expressly and specifically adapted to overcome the effects of the particular invader in question. The special mechanism is called *acquired specific immunity* and its study—the science of *immunology*—is of great importance in the understanding and prevention of disease.

The phenomenon of acquired specific immunity has been recognised for centuries in that individuals who had survived an attack of certain clearly recognisable infectious diseases such as smallpox were known to be much less susceptible to the disease during a later epidemic. Such individuals could be said to show *immunity* (i.e. protection) against the disease, *acquired* inasmuch as it did not apparently exist before the first infection, and *specific* inasmuch as an attack of smallpox protected the individual against a further attack of smallpox but had no bearing on his susceptibility to later attacks of measles, diphtheria, etc.

This knowledge has been applied with great success to the prevention of infectious disease by prophylactic immunisation, a procedure in which a relatively harmless variant or metabolic product of a pathogenic organism is purposely introduced into the body, and which results in the development of specific immunity such as would be encountered following recovery from the natural disease. The principle is well illustrated by Edward Jenner's use of fluid from the lesions of cowpox (vaccinia) to vaccinate against smallpox; it was known to Jenner that milkmaids who had had natural cowpox infection had developed not only markedly altered reactivity to reinfection with cowpox but also resistance to a first infection by smallpox, a closely related but much more serious disease. In this case the two viruses are so similar that immunity to one is effective also against the other.

When an individual has become immune following natural infection or prophylactic exposure to a pathogenic organism or its toxin he is said to be *actively immunised* against that organism. Specific resistance to infection can in many instances be conferred upon a non-immune individual by an alternative method, namely the injection of *serum* or *lymphoid cells* from an actively immune individual. The state of *passive immunity* so conferred is not due to transfer of the infecting organism or its toxin but to the transfer of the products of immunisation developed by the actively immunised donor of the serum or lymphoid cells. The *passive transfer* of immunity thus provides a way of analysing the factors which contribute to the immune state, and by transfer experiments it has been shown that in some instances specific immunity results from the presence in the serum of special globulins known as *antibodies*, while in other cases the immune state seems to be mediated directly by *specifically altered (sensitised) lymphocytes* without the participation of serum antibody. Serum containing one or more antibodies produced by active immunisation is termed *antiserum* or *immune serum*.

There is obviously considerable survival

advantage in having the ability to acquire specific immunity to pathogenic organisms or their toxins. Unfortunately the specifically altered reactivity produced by an immune response can lead to reactions which result in tissue injury. This can happen following exposure even to relatively harmless substances, such as grass pollen, which on subsequent contact causes a harmful and seemingly unnecessary inflammatory reaction in certain individuals. Such *acquired specific hypersensitivity* has in many cases been shown to be due to reactions of an immunological nature although with its connotation of protection the word "immune" appears unsuitable. Because of this difficulty and the gradual way in which knowledge of the complex processes involved has unfolded, an elaborate but imprecise jargon relating to immunology has developed and many authors have used the same terms with different meanings. Von Pirquet, for example, coined the word *allergy* as a unifying term to indicate *altered* specific reactivity of all kinds, including both protective immune responses and also hypersensitivity. Despite this the words allergy and hypersensitivity are frequently used interchangeably.

In this book we follow the current common practice of using the words "immune" and "immunity" in two distinct ways: in one they are general terms to embrace all forms of specifically altered reactivity (i.e. allergy in von Pirquet's sense) and in the other they refer to the specific protection against disease; we believe that the meaning implied will be evident from the context.

ANTIGENS

An antigen is a substance capable of evoking an immune response, i.e. the series of changes in an individual leading to specifically altered reactivity to the substance which has been introduced into the body.

The immune response to a given antigen may take three main forms.

(1) Antibody production, i.e. the appearance of globulin molecules which have the property of combining specifically with and remaining attached to antigen of the same kind as that which has led to their formation.

(2) Delayed hypersensitivity, i.e. the production of specifically sensitised lymphocytes whose presence can be demonstrated *in vivo* by the development of a local inflammatory reaction appearing about 24 hours after intradermal injection of the antigen. An antigenic stimulus commonly evokes both delayed hypersensitivity and antibody production. These responses take place in the lymphoid tissues, and their products, specifically sensitised lymphocytes and antibody, both capable of reacting with the antigen, are released into the blood stream.

(3) Specific immunological tolerance, i.e. the production of incapacity to develop antibody or delayed hypersensitivity on subsequent exposure to the specific antigen. Such acquisition of specific non-reactivity has been recognised as a form of immunological response only since 1948.

The term "*immunological reaction*" should not be confused with "*immune response*" as described above. An immunological reaction is the effect observed when the products of the immune response—antibody or sensitised lymphocytes—encounter and combine with the appropriate antigen *in vitro* or *in vivo*.

Factors affecting the immune response

The form taken by the immune response depends upon several factors including the nature of the antigen, the genetic constitution of the individual exposed to the antigen, the route by which the antigen enters the body and the dose administered. These factors are discussed below.

The nature of the antigen. It is difficult to define precisely the properties which make a substance capable of evoking an immune response, but in general terms antigens are large molecules, usually of molecular weight exceeding 3,000, fairly rigid in structure, and either protein or carbohydrate, with or without associated substances such as lipids. Antigen–antibody reactions appear to be the result largely of stereochemical interactions of molecules of complementary configurations, analogous to the interaction of lock and key. For this reason floppy molecules such as gelatin are poor antigens. Presumably molecular size determines the way in which substances are metabolised and only large molecules follow a metabolic pathway which brings them into appropriate contact with the cellular machinery of the immune response.

Although some small molecules, such as para-aminobenzoic acid, are not by themselves antigenic, they may become so if they are attached to larger molecules. Injection of *p*-aminobenzoic acid attached by diazotisation to serum albumin may result in formation of some antibody molecules which combine specifically with the *p*-aminobenzoic acid moiety and not with the albumin carrier protein. In these circumstances, *p*-aminobenzoic acid is said to be a *hapten* i.e. a substance which is antigenic inasmuch as it can take part in an immunological reaction (in this case antigen–antibody combination) but which cannot by itself evoke an immune response (in this example, the formation of specific antibody) unless it is conjugated with macromolecular material. The existence of such simple haptens suggests that the antigenic specificity of large molecules may be determined by the three-dimensional configuration of small parts of these molecules (*antigenic determinant sites* or *groups*). Study of synthetic polypeptide and polysaccharide antigens has confirmed that specific antigenic determinant sites do consist of a few amino-acids or monosaccharides, and it has been shown that macromolecules such as plasma albumin contain several antigenic determinant sites of differing specificity. There is evidence that determinant sites participating in delayed hypersensitivity responses are larger than those concerned in antibody production: thus production of delayed hypersensitivity to a simple chemical depends not solely upon the specific antigenicity of the chemical, but also on that of the adjacent part of the macromolecular protein carrier to which the chemical is bound.

Genetic constitution of the individual. Inheritance of immunological responsiveness to simple synthetic oligopeptide antigenic determinant groups has been demonstrated in mice and other rodents. For example, some inbred strains of guinea-pigs have a genetically determined inability to respond immunologically to certain determinant groups which are immunogenic for other strains. This is presumably true also for natural antigens, though less easily demonstrated because of the multiplicity and variety of determinant sites on natural macromolecules.

Genetic factors also play a large part in determining the antigenicity of tissues, and this field has become particularly important in the practice of blood transfusion and of tissue transplantation. The structure of tissues, including potential antigenic sites, is, of course, genetically determined. In general, when tissues are injected or transplanted from one individual to another, the more genetically dissimilar or foreign the two individuals towards one another, the easier it is to induce antibody formation or delayed hypersensitivity. For example, human red cells injected into rabbits evoke a wide variety of antibodies reacting with a corresponding variety of antigenic determinants on the human red cell; when, as in this case, the antigen is derived from a species other than that of the immunised animal (and this would include bacteria, etc.), it is called a *hetero-antigen* and the antibodies are *hetero-antibodies*. Injection or transplantation of one human with the red cells or tissue cells of another may result in the formation of antibodies to antigenic groups not shared by both individuals; e.g. human red cells containing the Rhesus antigen D (Rhesus positive cells) into a person whose cells do not contain this antigen (Rhesus negative) may result in the development of antibodies specific for D antigen; antigens which differ within a species are called *iso-antigens* and the corresponding antibodies *iso-antibodies*. In general, iso-antigens are much less numerous and less likely to evoke an immune response than hetero-antigens. Finally it should be noted that injection of an individual with his own cells (*auto-antigen*) results in *auto-antibody* formation or delayed hypersensitivity only in exceptional cases; the subject of *auto-immunity* is considered further on p. 110. Unfortunately the prefixes used to indicate the relationship between individuals providing antigen and forming antibody are, by usage, different from those used in the more recent field of tissue transplantation, in which graft rejection is effected mainly by delayed hypersensitivity reactions. Table 4.1 summarises this confusing and irrational situation.

As stated above, the cells and tissues of an individual are antigenic when injected or grafted into an animal of another species or even into a different individual of the same species, yet with certain exceptions the individual does not react to the antigens of his own cells by the development of auto-antibody or delayed auto-hypersensitivity. Non-reactivity to auto-antigen is a general physiological principle described by

Ehrlich as "horror autotoxicus". It may reflect absence of lymphoid cells with the genetic coding necessary for the synthetic processes associated with formation of antibody or delayed hypersensitivity against "self" components, analogous to the inherited non-reactivity of certain strains of animals to synthetic polypeptide antigens. Burnet has, however, suggested an attractive alternative explanation, that the various potential antigens in an individual's tissues do act on the cells responsible for immune reactions but that, instead of causing antibody formation or delayed hypersensitivity, they lead during fetal life to the third form of immune response mentioned above, namely, an acquired state of specific immunological tolerance. Whatever its explanation, "horror autotoxicus" is clearly an important safeguard which prevents immunological destruction of an individual's own tissues.

Route of administration of antigen. In most cases antigens elicit an immunological response only when they are introduced parenterally (i.e. not through the alimentary canal) so that their macromolecular state and the configuration of their antigenic determinants are not destroyed by digestion in the gut. Traces of certain proteins, such as those in heterologous milk, may, however, be absorbed from the gut and bring about specific sensitisation, especially in infants.

Table 4.1. Terminology of antigens, antibodies and tissue grafts

Relationship between donor and recipient	Genetic terminology	Antibody, antigen	Transplantation terminology
Same animal	—	Auto-antibody Auto-antigen	Autograft
Identical twins and inbred strain	Syngeneic (Isogeneic)	—	Isograft
Same outbred species or different inbred strains	Allogeneic	Iso-antibody Iso-antigen	Allograft (Homograft)
Different species	Heterogeneic Xenogeneic	Hetero-antibody Hetero-antigen	Xenograft (Heterograft)

ANTIBODIES

Antibody molecules have the special property of combining specifically with antigen or hapten. In so doing they may cover up harmful areas on molecules of toxin, in which case they are said to be *antitoxins*, or their combination with cells such as bacteria may lead (with the help of complement—p. 81) to their dissolution (*bacteriolytic effect*) or phagocytosis by polymorphonuclear leukocytes (*opsonic effect*). Chemically antibodies belong to the immunoglobulin (Ig) proteins of the plasma (sometimes called γ-globulins because of their electrophoretic mobility); and there are five classes: IgG (γG), IgM (γM), IgA (γA), IgD (γD) and IgE (γE). All immunoglobulins are composed of one or more similar units, each unit consisting of two pairs of identical polypeptide chains (Fig. 4.1); one pair termed the *heavy chains* are about twice the size (molecular weight) of the other pair, which are termed the *light chains*. Digestion of an im-

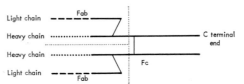

FIG. 4.1.—Structure of monomeric immunoglobulin molecule. In any one molecule the two light chains have an identical amino-acid sequence and so also have the heavy chains. Each immunoglobulin class has a distinctive Fc piece (C terminal end of heavy chains). The amino-acid sequence of the interrupted portions of the light chains and dotted portions of heavy chains (the N-terminal ends) vary greatly among immunoglobulin molecules even of the same class and constitute the specific antigen-binding (Fab) sites, of which there are two on each molecule. (The light lines indicate separation of the molecules into an Fc and two Fab fragments by papain digestion.)

munoglobulin molecule by papain breaks it into three fragments, of which two are identical and are termed Fab (antigen-binding fragments) because each contains a combining site for antigen. The third fragment consists of the C-terminal ends of the heavy chains, and is termed Fc fragment; it is readily obtained in crystalline (hence Fc) form. Heavy chains differ structurally for each class immunoglobulin, and the letters γ, μ, α, δ, ε, are used to indicate the heavy chains of IgG, IgM, IgA, etc. respectively. By contrast, light chains are the same in different classes of immunoglobulins. Differences in the behaviour of antibodies of different immunoglobulin classes are determined by the properties of their heavy chains.

The combination of antibody with antigen is believed to be achieved by van der Waal's forces which are effective over a very short range and hold separate molecules together only when they fit snugly. The specificity of antigen–antibody union therefore depends on the antibody-combining-site having a complementary shape to the antigenic determinant which permits the necessary close fit. The shape of the combining site is determined by the amino-acid sequence of the N-terminal ends of the heavy and, to a lesser extent, of the light chains. In view of what is now known of protein synthesis this is of great interest and of fundamental importance in elucidating how antigenic stimulation gives rise to specific antibody formation. In contrast to most other proteins, each one of which in a given individual is of uniform amino-acid sequence, the immunoglobulins in a serum show marked heterogeneity at the N-terminals, the number of variations amounting to millions. This variety allows for the great range of antigens, natural and synthetic, against which antibody may be formed.

Some idea of the specificity of antibody–antigen union can be gained from study of antibody against chemically defined haptens. Landsteiner, for example, showed that antibody raised against para-aminobenzene sulphonic acid does not combine with the ortho- form but gives a weak reaction with meta-aminobenzene sulphonic acid (Fig. 4.2). The latter is called a cross-reac-

tion and it implies immunological reactivity with an antigen different from that which has led to the production of antibody. It results from the production of some antibody molecules which fit the cross reacting antigen sufficiently well to permit intermolecular attraction by van der Waal's forces.

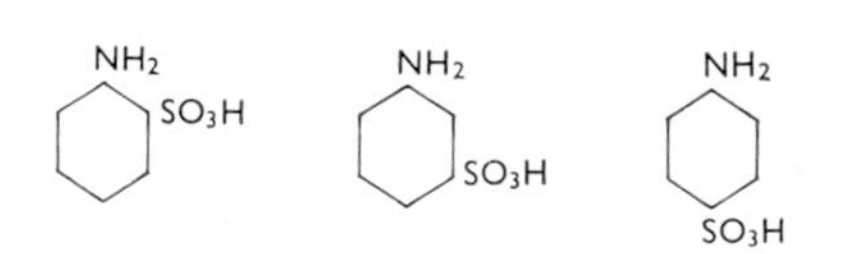

Properties of the immunoglobulin classes

The various immunoglobulin classes have different functions (beyond that of specific combination with antigen, which is common to all) and this is determined by the structure of the part of the heavy chains included in the Fc fragment.

Table 4.2. Size and serum concentrations of immunoglobulins

Class	Molecular weight	Degree of polymerisation	Concentration (normal serum) mg./100 ml.
IgG	150,000	Monomer	900–1500
IgM	1,000,000	Pentamer and hexamer	40–120
IgA	Mainly 150,000	Mono- and polymer	110–180
IgD	150,000	Monomer	0·3–30
IgE	200,000	Monomer	$1–14 \times 10^{-5}$

When immunoglobulin of a particular class is injected into animals of another species it acts as an *antigen*, and antibody specific for the particular immunoglobulin class appears in the serum of the injected animal. Combination of such antibody with immunoglobulin *in vitro* provides a simple method of demonstrating the class to which a particular immunoglobulin belongs, for example by immunoelectrophoresis (p. 79).

Table 4.2 compares some of the features of the five known immunoglobulin classes. **IgG** is present in the serum in the largest amount and is the most widely studied immunoglobin. IgG antibodies to various bacterial toxins (*antitoxins*) are of importance because they combine with and neutralise the toxin, thus protecting the individual from its harmful effects. The reaction of IgG antibody with the corresponding antigen can usually be demonstrated *in vitro* (see below): it can cross the human placenta and in this way passive immunity is transferred from mother to child. **IgM,** a macroglobulin consisting of pentameres and hexameres of the basic four-chain unit (each of which has two antigen-combining sites), is the immunoglobulin class of the first antibody to be produced following the

FIG. 4.2.—Isomeric forms of aminobenzene sulphonic acid.

initial introduction of an antigen. It is especially effective in destroying bacterial cells and its reactions are readily demonstrated *in vitro*. **IgA** is present in the plasma, and the intestinal mucosa is particularly rich in IgA-producing plasma cells. It is secreted into colostrum, saliva, tears, respiratory-tract mucus and especially into intestinal mucus. The glandular cells concerned in these secretions take up IgA from the extracellular fluid and couple it with a carbohydrate "transport piece", which may render it resistant to digestive enzymes. The function of IgA is not known, but it may form a protective coating over mucous membranes, and an analogy to "antiseptic paint" has been made. **IgE** has the special property of attaching to tissue cells (probably to mast cells) by means of its Fc fragment, leaving the specific combining sites (on the Fab fragments) available for union with antigen. If such union takes place, pharmacologically active substances such as histamine are released, with the production of a so-called "immediate hypersensitivity reaction" within a few minutes (p. 99). The biological properties of **IgD** are unknown.

Demonstration of antigen–antibody reactions

In vivo

Antigen–antibody reactions may be demonstrated *in vivo* in two ways.

(1) A potentially harmful antigenic substance may be rendered harmless by union with antibody and not have the expected effect. For example, in the Schick test, intradermal injection of a small amount of diphtheria toxin into the skin of a non-immune individual results in an area of inflammation. The diphtheria antitoxin present in an immunised individual neutralises the toxin and so suppresses the inflammation.

(2) A normally harmless stimulus may result in tissue injury i.e. a hypersensitivity reaction. For example, inhalation of grass pollen may induce an attack of hay fever or asthma, mediated by its reaction with antibody specific for grass pollen. In this instance, the antibody is usually of IgE class, but hypersensitivity reactions may result from the union *in vivo* of other classes of antibody with antigen: they are of considerable importance in disease processes and are described in Chapter 5.

In vitro

Antigen–antibody combination may be demonstrated *in vitro* in various ways, depending on the nature of the antigen and the type and amount of antibody present.

(1) Visible aggregation of antigen. Since each antibody molecule has at least two combining sites it can bind with two or more antigen molecules. If the antigen molecules contain several antigenic determinants, and if they are in solution, antibody can cause the formation of a lattice of antigen and antibody molecules, cross-linked together (Fig. 4.3); if enough molecules

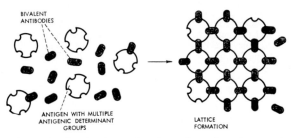

Fig. 4.3.—Lattice formation by union of antigen and antibody. If the antigen is soluble, an insoluble precipitate may form: if it is particulate, e.g. bacteria, the aggregation is termed agglutination.

are aggregated in this way, the aggregates will be visible as an insoluble precipitate (*precipitin reaction*). Lattice formation and therefore precipitation can be inhibited when an excessive amount of antigen saturates the combining sites on all the antibody molecules, and complexes as small as three molecules (Ag-Ab-Ag) may then be formed. When gross excess of antibody is present, each antigen combining site may fix a separate antibody molecule, and, once again, the complexes may be too small to form a visible precipitate (*prozone effect*). Optimum antigen–antibody proportions for lattice formation can readily be achieved by allowing antibody and antigen to diffuse towards each other through agar (Ouchterlony technique, Fig. 4.4). The interpretation of agar diffusion tests involving antiserum raised against a complex mixture of antigens (as when human serum is injected into rabbits) is facilitated by partial separation of the constituent antigens by electrophoresis prior to the precipitin reaction; this method, called immunoelectrophoresis, is illustrated in Fig. 4.5.

When the antigen molecules are associated with a large particle, e.g. the antigenic deter-

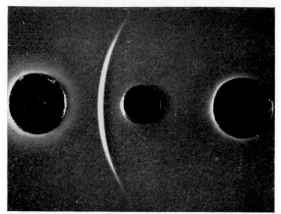

FIG. 4.4.—Ouchterlony technique. The central well contains a solution of antigen. The well on the left contains the corresponding antiserum, and that on the right a negative control serum. A white line of insoluble precipitate, composed of antigen–antibody complex, has formed between the antigen and antibody wells.

minants of the surface of a red cell or bacterium, or are adsorbed artificially on to red cells or latex particles, antibody causes aggregation of the particles (*agglutination reaction*). The visible aggregation of large particles such as bacteria can be effected by minute amounts of antibody.

(2) Demonstration of antibody attached to antigen by anti-immunoglobulin reagent. In certain circumstances antibody combines with antigen without causing aggregation. This may occur if the spatial arrangement of the antigen

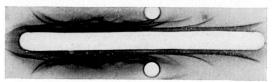

FIG. 4.5.—Immunoelectrophoresis. Complex mixtures of antigens have been placed in the circular well in the slab of agar and subjected to electrophoresis. Subsequently an antiserum containing antibodies to the various antigens is placed in the longitudinal trough and discrete lines of precipitate formed by the various reactions can be identified. In this example, the wells contain specimens of human serum and the trough contains antiserum to human serum prepared in a rabbit.

(e.g. the Rhesus antigen on the surface of red cells) prevents the divalent IgG antibody molecule from combining simultaneously with antigenic determinant groups on two different red cells. In these circumstances, exposure of the Rhesus positive red cells to anti-Rhesus antibody merely results in their being coated with IgG.

However, the coated cells can be agglutinated by antibody against IgG (*antiglobulin* or *Coombs'* *reagent*) (Fig. 4.6).

A similar principle is used in the *indirect immunofluorescence* (*indirect fluorescent antibody*)

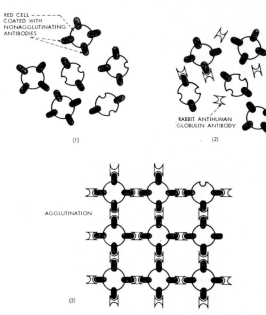

FIG. 4.6.—Agglutination of antibody-coated particles by antibody to immunoglobulin (antiglobulin reagent).

technique. Here the antigen molecules (e.g. bacterial capsular polysaccharide) are present in a histological section or smear. When this is exposed to antiserum the antibody combines with antigen without visible effect. The slide is washed to remove the antiserum, leaving only the specific antibody which is, of course, an immunoglobulin, attached to the antigen present in the section. Antibody to immunoglobulin, conjugated with a fluorescent dye such as fluorescein isothiocyanate, is then applied to the section or smear and the site of antigen-antibody combination is visualised by the presence of the fluorescent antiglobulin when the section is examined microscopically with ultraviolet light (Figs. 4.7, 4.8). (In the *direct immunofluorescence technique* the antibody against the antigen in the histological section or smear is directly conjugated with fluorescent dye and its attachment to the section is demonstrated as above but without the use of an antiglobulin reagent.)

(3) Methods involving damage to cells. Antibody combined with antigen on the surface of intact cells such as bacteria or erythrocytes can

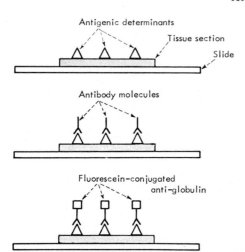

FIG. 4.7.—The indirect immunofluorescence technique performed on a tissue section. *Top*, tissue section on slide. *Middle*, section treated with antibody (人) to a tissue constituent and washed: antibody molecules adhere to the tissue antigen. *Bottom*, section treated with fluorescein-conjugated antibody (☐) to immunoglobulin: sites of antigen–antibody reaction fluoresce in ultra-violet light.

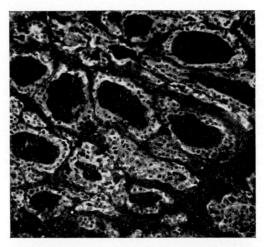

FIG. 4.8.—A positive indirect immunofluorescence test for antibody to thyroid epithelium. A frozen section of thyroid tissue has been treated with the serum undergoing test (from a patient with chronic thyroiditis), followed by treatment with fluorescein-conjugated anti-human-IgG. Note the staining of the thyroid epithelial cytoplasm. (U.V. microscopy.)

damage the cell membrane and cause lysis (partial dissolution) of the cells which is readily demonstrable. The lysis is mediated by a complex group of at least nine factors present in fresh normal serum and known collectively as *complement*. These factors are activated by the Fc portions of antibody molecules which have combined with antigen, and once activated they give rise to a chain of enzyme reactions culminating in digestion of the cell membrane where the antibody is attached. In the course of the reaction complement is used up, or "fixed".

(4) Complement fixation. Complement is fixed in many antigen–antibody reactions in addition to those involving cell-surface antigens. Invisible antigen–antibody reactions can often be demonstrated indirectly by allowing them to occur in

the presence of a measured amount of complement and subsequently adding an indicator system, namely red cells coated with an antibody (haemolysin) which will cause red cell lysis only in the presence of complement. Fixation of complement by the invisible antigen–antibody reaction prevents haemolysis in the indicator system (Fig. 4.9). One of the best known practical applications of the complement fixation reaction is the Wassermann test for syphilis.

The production of antibody

Injection of an antigen to which an individual has not previously been exposed results in a *primary antibody response*, i.e. the transient

	Mix antigen and antibody	Add complement (C)	Add sensitised RBC
Positive test	$Ag^x + Ab^x \longrightarrow Ag^x\!\!-\!\!Ab^x$ (union)	$+ C \longrightarrow Ag^x\!\!-\!\!\underset{C}{\overset{\mid}{}}\!\!Ab^x$ (complement used up)	No lysis
Negative test	$Ag^x + Ab^y \longrightarrow Ag^x + Ab^y$ (no union)	$+ C \longrightarrow Ag^x + Ab^y + C$ (complement not used)	Lysis

FIG. 4.9.—The complement fixation reaction depends on the "fixation" of complement by an antigen–antibody complex (upper line). The fixation of complement is demonstrated by non-lysis of subsequently added red cells coated with a haemolytic antibody. If there is no antigen–antibody reaction (lower line), complement is not used up and lyses the sensitised red cells.

appearance in the blood of a small amount of specific antibody of IgM class, about seven days after the injection. Re-injection of the same antigen at a later date leads to a *secondary* or *anamnestic* (remembering) *response* in which large amounts of specific antibody, usually of IgG class, appear in the blood rapidly (in four days or so) and continue to be produced, although in gradually diminishing amounts, for weeks, months or even years. The greatly enhanced antibody production of the secondary response is the reason for the repeated injections of antigens (vaccines) widely used in prophylactic immunisation.

Most of the antibody found in serum is produced by plasma cells in lymph nodes, spleen and bone marrow but some may also be formed by plasma cells in the lymphoid tissue of the gut and in the inflammatory lesion which forms around injected antigenic material. Plasma cells (Fig. 4.10) are somewhat larger than small lymphocytes, of ovoid shape with a small round nucleus in which granules of chromatin are regularly spaced around the periphery, giving a "cart-wheel" or "clock-face" appearance. Their

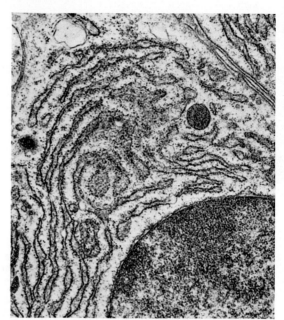

FIG. 4.11.—Electron micrograph showing parts of two adjacent plasma cells. Note the abundant rough endoplasmic reticulum. × 15,750.

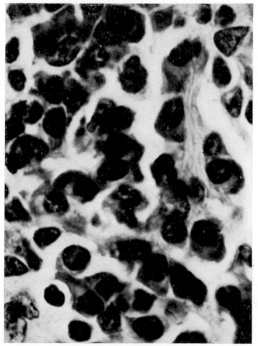

FIG. 4.10.—Plasma cells in the medulla of a lymph node. Note the small round, eccentric nucleus with clumping of chromatin, the basophilic cytoplasm and, in some cells, the perinuclear crescent of paler cytoplasm. × 1000.

cytoplasm is basophilic and also pyroninophilic, indicating a high content of ribonucleic acid, and electron microscopy (Fig. 4.11) reveals a large amount of complex granular endoplasmic reticulum of the type found in cells which produce a protein secretion. It has been shown by immunofluorescence that each plasma cell at any given time produces light chains together with heavy chains of only one immunoglobulin class (e.g. IgG or IgM). Furthermore, following stimulation with two distinct antigens (e.g. diphtheria and tetanus toxins) individual plasma cells will produce antibody to one or the other but not to both of these antigens.

The clonal selection theory of antibody production. It is uncertain how plasma cells are induced to produce antibody molecules whose combining sites appear to be tailor-made to fit the corresponding antigenic determinant groups. The most widely accepted hypothesis is the clonal selection theory proposed by Burnet. He suggests that during the continuous proliferation of lymphoid cells from fetal life onward there occurs a huge number of mutations affecting the parts of the genes which control the structure of antigen-combining sites of the antibody molecule. As a result there develops a large heterogeneous population of plasma cell precursors differing in that part of their DNA which codes for the N-terminal ends of immunoglobulin polypeptide chains. We thus have a heterogeneous assembly of cells, each type containing the DNA code to produce immunoglobulin with a distinctive sequence of amino-acids at the antibody combining site for antigen, i.e. immunoglobulins with distinctive specificity. Such cells are conveniently termed *specifically responsive*. When antigen comes into contact with such a population of cells it combines with cells whose immunoglobulin is of appropriate specificity, and this induces selective proliferation of these cells leading to *clones* (families of identical descendants) which mature to become plasma cells producing the appropriate specific antibody. In the clonal selection theory the secondary antibody response owes its magnitude and rapidity to the presence of appropriate clones which have multiplied during the slowly developing primary response. Strong support for the clonal production of antibody comes from the observation that the immunoglobulin produced by a tumour composed of plasma cells (all of whose cells are presumably descended from a single plasma cell precursor which has undergone malignant proliferation) is completely homogeneous in amino-acid sequence and appears on electrophoresis as a narrow "myeloma" band in contrast to the usual wide electrophoretic band formed by the heterogeneous immunoglobulin molecules found in normal serum (p. 438). Although first applied to the cells concerned in antibody responses, the development of delayed hypersensitivity (see below) is also initiated by specifically-responsive cells (pp. 85 et seq.), and Burnet's hypothesis is equally applicable to this type of immune response.

DELAYED HYPERSENSITIVITY

Many antigenic stimuli lead to the production of lymphocytes which, like antibody, are capable of reacting specifically with the antigen: this is the *delayed hypersensitivity response*, and in spite of its name it is as normal a feature of the immune response as is antibody production. The state of delayed hypersensitivity to an antigen is demonstrated classically by intradermal injection of the antigen, which leads to an indurated erythematous lesion in the dermis maximal 24–72 hours later. During development of the lesion there is early emigration of polymorphonuclear leukocytes but this phase is transient, and the polymorphs soon disappear from the site: there follows an increasing accumulation of mononuclear cells (mainly lymphocytes, but with some macrophages), around small veins, hair follicles and sweat glands and accompanied by inflammatory oedema (Fig. 5.8, p. 108). Delayed hypersensitivity can also be demonstrated in animals by injecting antigen into the cornea, which results in a similar reaction with corneal opacity 24–48 hours later. These sites are convenient for the elicitation of delayed hypersensitivity reactions, but all tissues are reactive, i.e. the state of delayed hypersensitivity is generalised.

Evidence is accumulating that the state of delayed hypersensitivity may be demonstrated *in vitro* by observing the effect of the appropriate antigen on living cells from the sensitised individual. For example, it has been shown that tuberculoprotein inhibits the migration from a capillary tube of macrophages obtained from a sensitised guinea-pig. This type of experiment has also been performed using blood leukocytes, and it has been shown that when circulating small lymphocytes from a sensitised individual are exposed to the antigen in tissue culture, a small proportion of them *transform* into larger cells with basophilic cytoplasm, synthesise DNA and undergo mitosis. Such tests are being used increasingly to demonstrate delayed hypersensitivity to various micro-organisms and other antigens. The mechanism of delayed hypersensitivity reactions is considered in Chapter 5.

A classical example of delayed hypersensitivity is that which develops to tuberculoprotein in most individuals who have been infected by *Mycobacterium tuberculosis* or inoculated with BCG. The Mantoux test, in which more or less purified tuberculoprotein is injected intradermally, is a classical delayed hypersensitivity reaction. It has been found that injection of protein antigens, which in ordinary circumstances merely evoke an antibody response, can also lead to the development of delayed hypersensitivity provided that the antigen is injected emulsified in an oily "adjuvant" containing *M. tuberculosis* (Freund's adjuvant), other myco-

D

bacteria, or a peptidoglycolipid extracted from the cell wall of these organisms. Delayed hypersensitivity is also a prominent feature of the immunological response to living allografts and xenografts. When certain simple chemicals, for example picryl chloride, are applied to the skin, they combine with skin proteins to act as haptens and delayed hypersensitivity results: on subsequent application to the skin these substances give rise to the lesion known as contact dermatitis which is simply a delayed hypersensitivity reaction. It has been suggested by Medawar that delayed hypersensitivity develops when antigen is fixed in the peripheral tissues so that it is encountered mainly by wandering lymphocytes (see p. 87) and is carried only later to the regional lymph nodes in significant amounts. It should be noted that although delayed hypersensitivity is usually demonstrated by tests leading to an apparently exaggerated and harmful reaction, there is strong evidence that it plays an important role in the body's defence against infection. Thus in children with congenital hypogammaglobulinaemia, resistance to most virus infections is diminished only when there is co-existing failure of responsiveness of the delayed hypersensitivity type.

ACQUIRED IMMUNOLOGICAL TOLERANCE

This is the third form of immune response which may result from exposure to a potentially antigenic substance. In this case the individual becomes non-reactive to the antigen, being incapable of developing antibody or delayed hypersensitivity to it. This non-reactivity is specific, i.e. applying only to the antigen to which tolerance has developed and not to other, unrelated antigens. Acquired tolerance can be overcome by injecting the tolerant animal with "immunologically competent" lymphocytes of a normal (non-tolerant) animal of the same strain and this shows that tolerance is due to failure of the central machinery of the immune response i.e. the lymphoid cells, rather than to an alteration in the metabolic processing of antigen before it reaches the lymphoid tissues.

Immunological tolerance is most readily produced in fetal and neonatal animals and lasts only so long as the tolerising antigen persists in the tolerant animal. In adult animals it may be induced by very large doses of soluble antigens, or in certain circumstances by minute doses i.e. either more or less than the dose required to stimulate antibody production and/or delayed hypersensitivity. A state of partial tolerance may occur, characterised by the development of weak delayed hypersensitivity or subnormal amounts of antibody, and a condition of "*split*

tolerance" or "*immune deviation*" is sometimes encountered in which specific non-reactivity of the delayed hypersensitivity response is induced while antibody production to the same antigen is normal. Strongly established acquired immunological tolerance towards a particular antigen can sometimes be broken down by immunisation with a closely related cross-reacting antigen or by incorporation of the antigen in Freund's adjuvant.

According to Burnet's clonal selection theory (p. 82) acquired immunological tolerance is the consequence of inactivation or even destruction by antigen of the cells which can produce the complementary specific receptors, thus preventing the clonal proliferation of the type proposed in antibody formation. Apart from dose effects it is uncertain how antigen sometimes causes elimination of potentially reactive lymphoid cells whereas in other circumstances antigenic stimulation causes antibody production and/or delayed hypersensitivity. As already mentioned on page 77, elimination of potentially auto-reactive clones in fetal life and thereafter, with the acquisition of immunological tolerance to auto-antigens, is now thought to be the explanation of "horror autotoxicus", i.e. the physiological unwillingness to develop auto-immune responses to "self" antigens.

THE CELLULAR BASIS OF IMMUNE RESPONSES

So far, this account has been concerned with defining the different types of immune response to an antigenic stimulus and describing their products—antibodies, specifically sensitised lymphocytes, and a state of non-reactivity (tolerance). We must now consider the mechanisms of immune responses and in particular the parts played by the various types of participating cells.

Specifically responsive cells

As already stated, the specific reactivity of antibodies is determined by the sequence of amino-acids in the N-terminal ends of their heavy and light chains. Assuming that antibody production conforms to the general principles of protein synthesis, then production of a particular antibody requires the participation of cells with the DNA coding sequence for the antigen-combining sites of that antibody. It is apparent that antigenic material must stimulate a genetically appropriate cell to proliferate, to provide cells similarly responsive to the particular antigen. This is really another way of stating Burnet's clonal selection theory (p. 82). It is apparent also that production of specifically sensitised lymphocytes in a delayed hypersensitivity response likewise requires the stimulation, by antigenic material, of a genetically appropriate cell. Thus production of both antibody and specifically sensitised lymphocytes is initiated by *specifically-responsive cells* (sometimes termed *immunologically-competent cells*), capable of recognising a particular antigenic determinant group and responding to it. The nature of these cells—the keystones of the immune response—has long been a subject of controversy, but there is now an impressive weight of evidence implicating **the small lymphocyte**. Recognition of antigenic material by such cells is believed to be mediated by their production of immunoglobulin-like material which has been demonstrated on the cell surface, and union of antigenic material with this fixed "recognition factor" triggers off the cell to initiate the specific immune response.

It has, however, become apparent that there are two types of specifically responsive cell; one of these, the circulating small lymphocyte, is derived from the thymus, while the other is a lymphoid cell of similar morphology, which is independent of the thymus.* We may thus speak of *thymus-dependent* and *thymus-independent immune responses*. These concepts are based on recent developments relating to the origin, life-cycle and properties of populations of lymphoid cells and the changes in the lymphoid tissues which accompany immune responses. The cytology of the immune response is complex, and by no means fully elucidated: the origins, functions and inter-relationships of the various cells which participate in delayed hypersensitivity and antibody responses will be appreciated more readily if the following basic points are kept in mind.

1. The immune response (delayed hypersensitivity response and antibody production) is initiated by lymphoid cells capable of recognising and responding to a particular antigenic stimulus, i.e. by *specifically-responsive cells*.

2. The specifically-responsive cells which mediate delayed hypersensitivity responses are small lymphocytes which are produced in, and released from, the thymus. They are long-lived and circulate continuously between the blood and certain lymphoid tissues (lymph nodes, spleen and lymphoid tissue in the wall of the alimentary canal). These cells constitute the *recirculating pool of small lymphocytes*.

3. On encountering an antigen to which it can respond, the recirculating small lymphocyte enlarges to become an *immunoblast*, which undergoes sequential mitotic divisions to provide a clone of small lymphocytes which are capable of reacting directly with the antigen. It is likely that these cells have three functions: (a) on encountering the antigen they react with it and bring about the changes of the delayed hypersensitivity reaction; (b) some of them persist (without encountering the antigen) for long periods and are responsible for immunological memory; (c) they do not themselves give rise to antibody-producing cells but they co-operate with the precursors of plasma cells (which are of non-thymic origin) in the production of antibodies to some antigens (*thymic-dependent antibody production*).

4. Production of antibody to other antigens is *not dependent on thymus-derived lymphocytes*, but

---

* In current jargon the thymic-derived cells and their descendants are termed **T cells** and the thymic-independent cells **B cells**, the latter because of their origin, in the fowl, from the Bursa of Fabricius, (p. 87).

is mediated by lymphoid cells of unknown morphology which lie in the lymph nodes, spleen and lymphoid tissues in the wall of the alimentary canal; they include specifically responsive cells which, on encountering an antigen to which they can respond, multiply to produce (a) plasma cells which elaborate and secrete the corresponding antibody, and probably (b) memory cells responsible for the anamnestic or secondary response.

5. Thymic small lymphocytes and plasma cell precursors are derived from stem cells produced throughout life in the haemopoietic bone marrow: these stem cells are released into the blood and supply the thymus and other lymphoid tissues.

The thymus-dependent immune response

(a) The recirculating pool of small lymphocytes

Among the many contributions to our understanding of the functions of lymphocytes, the studies of Gowans and his colleagues, working in Oxford, are of particular importance. Gowans used techniques in which rats were subjected to thoracic-duct cannulation, the cells (virtually all lymphocytes) contained in the lymph being removed, the fluid being returned to the animal. By combining this procedure with radio-isotope labelling of thoracic-duct lymphocytes, he showed that most of the small lymphocytes have a life span of many weeks, i.e. they survive *in vivo* for this period without further differentiation or division. Gowans also demonstrated that the long-lived small lymphocytes circulate repeatedly between the blood and most lymphoid tissues, including the lymph nodes, white pulp of the spleen, and lymphoid tissues along the wall of the alimentary tract. In the lymph nodes, these cells leave the blood and enter the deep cortex, sometimes termed paracortex, by migrating through the cytoplasm of the unusually tall endothelial cells which line the venules in this part of the node (Fig. 4.12). The recirculating small lymphocytes then filter into the medulla of the lymph nodes, and enter the lymph sinuses, whence they pass to the efferent lymphatic and eventually back into the blood via the major lymphatics (Fig. 4.13). Migration occurs similarly through the gut-associated lymphoid tissues (Peyer's patches, solitary follicles and tonsils). In the white pulp of the

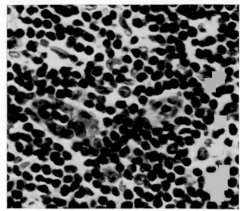

Fig. 4.12.—Two venules in the deep cortex of a human lymph node. Note the prominent endothelium and small lymphocytes in the lumina and walls of the venules. × 400.

spleen, the lymphocytes pass from the blood into the lymphoid sheath around the central arteriole, and from there presumably enter the vascular sinuses of the red pulp. As would be expected, the lymph leaving a lymph node by the efferent lymphatics contains many more small lymphocytes than does the lymph in the afferent lymphatics: nevertheless some are present in the afferent lymph, indicating that lymphocytes leave the blood to filter through the various non-lymphoid tissues and then enter the lymphatic channels, returning to the blood via the lymph nodes. Their number is, however, small compared with those recirculating as described above.

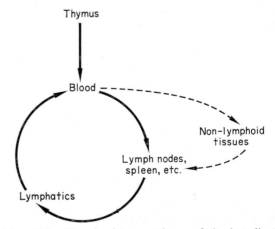

Fig. 4.13.—The circulatory pathway of the long-lived small lymphocytes. Note that although the recirculating small lymphocytes are supplied by the thymus, they do not recirculate through it, but through the lymph nodes, spleen and lymphoid tissues in the wall of the alimentary canal—the secondary lymphoid tissues. Circulation through non-lymphoid tissues involves fewer lymphocytes.

In the rat, the rate of recirculation is such that the time taken for complete replacement of small lymphocytes in the blood is less than one hour. Good opportunity is thus provided for surveillance of antigen, in almost any part of the body, by large numbers of recirculating small lymphocytes.

The lymphoid tissues which are included in the circulating pathway of the long-lived small lymphocytes are also those in which immune responses take place: they are sometimes grouped together as the **secondary lymphoid tissues** to distinguish them from the **primary lymphoid organs** which supply specifically-responsive lymphocytes, but are not sites of immune responses. As explained later, the thymus is the only primary lymphoid organ so far identified in man and other mammals, although in fowls there is another primary organ, the *bursa of Fabricius* in the wall of the cloaca: there is now strong evidence that the thymus supplies most of the recirculating small lymphocytes.

Depletion of the pool of small lymphocytes may be achieved by thoracic-duct drainage for several days, by injections of a heterologous antiserum to lymphocytes, or by neonatal thymectomy (see below). These procedures all result in a profound fall in the number of small lymphocytes in the blood, in the deep cortex of lymph nodes, the equivalent areas of Peyer's patches, etc., and in the peri-arteriolar lymphocytic sheath of the splenic white pulp. The lymphocyte depletion is accompanied by suppression of the capacity of the animal to develop delayed hypersensitivity responses and to produce antibody to some antigens. These deficiencies can be made good by injection of thoracic-duct small lymphocytes from a normal animal of the same inbred strain. Moreover, when the donor animal has been immunised by injection of an antigen or by an incompatible skin graft, primary challenge of the restored animal with the same antigenic material results in a secondary type of immune response (p. 82). By these and other experimental procedures it has been established that small lymphocytes of the recirculating pool include specifically responsive cells. When there has been no previous exposure to a particular antigen, the appropriate specifically-responsive cells are present in small numbers, and are capable of initiating a primary immune response. "Primed" or "memory" cells, derived from a previous immune response, are present in larger numbers and lead, on appropriate antigenic stimulation, to a secondary response.

In man, the evidence for a recirculating lymphocyte pool with these properties is necessarily less complete; it is nevertheless convincing, and study of the persistence of human lymphocytes with chromosomal abnormalities induced by X-irradiation suggests that the human small lymphocyte has a life span of many years.

It has been shown that, when small lymphocytes obtained from human blood are maintained in contact with antigenic material *in vitro*, antigen adheres to some of the cells. This appears to be due to the presence of antibody-like material on the cell surface, for such material has been demonstrated by means of fluorescent anti-IgG, and addition of anti-IgG inhibits their transformation by antigen (see below), presumably by blocking the cell-surface receptors. Addition of antigen to cultures of human or animal small lymphocytes also induces, in a proportion of cells, transformation to a larger type of cell—the *immunoblast*—with an enlarged nucleus and increase in the cytoplasm, which becomes basophilic and pyroninophilic due to production of RNA (Fig. 4.14). These changes are accompanied by synthesis of DNA in the nucleus, and some of the transformed cells divide. The

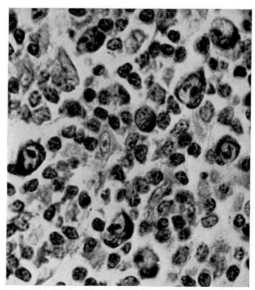

FIG. 4.14.—Large lymphoid cells with enlarged nucleus and pyroninophilic cytoplasm (*immunoblasts*) in a human lymph node removed 6 days after a skin allograft. Methyl green pyronin stain. × 480. (Drs. D. M. V. Parrott and M. A. B. de Sousa.)

immunoblast resembles an immature plasma cell (plasmablast), but differs from it in being poor in endoplasmic reticulum, the cytoplasmic RNA being mainly in the form of free ribosomes. In delayed hypersensitivity responses, the immunoblasts divide successively to produce smaller cells, finally providing clones of small lymphocytes capable of recognising, and reacting with, the particular antigen which has stimulated their proliferation. It is probable that these small lymphocytes are the cells which react with antigen to bring about delayed hypersensitivity *reactions*, and that they release humoral factors which are responsible for the various features of such reactions: this is dealt with more fully on pp. 106–109. Some of the small lymphocytes produced by delayed hypersensitivity *responses* join the recirculating pool of small lymphocytes, while others may possibly remain sessile for long periods in the secondary lymphoid tissues. These "primed" cells form the basis of "immunological memory" whereby a second stimulus by the same antigen is followed by the rapid and powerful secondary type of immune response. The functions of the recirculating small lymphocytes are summarised in Fig. 4.15.

Lymphocytes of the recirculating pool also initiate immune responses leading to the production of antibody to certain antigens. This involves co-operation with B cells in the secondary lymphoid tissues which are not derived from the recirculating long-lived lymphocytes, and which proliferate to provide the antibody-producing plasma cells (p. 92).

(b) The role of the thymus

Development. The thymus develops as a paired organ from epithelial ingrowths, probably of endodermal origin, of the 3rd and 4th branchial arches. During fetal development, the two lobes pass medially and caudally to form a single organ. Although initially composed of epithelium, at an early stage of development the thymus becomes converted to a predominantly lymphoid tissue and differentiates further into a lobulated structure in which each lobule has a central core of medullary tissue with finger-like projections, capped by cortical tissue. Both cortex and medulla consist predominantly of small lymphocytes, but their ratio to other cells is far higher in the cortex, and they are much more closely packed there, than in the medulla (Fig. 4.16). The other cells in the thymus include

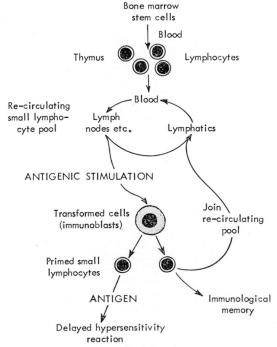

FIG. 4.15.—Functions of the recirculating small lymphocyte.

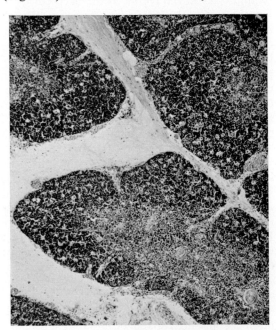

FIG. 4.16.—Thymus of child, showing lobulation and division into cortex (darker areas) and medulla. × 50.

epithelial cells, which are scattered singly as large plump cells in both cortex and medulla, and also reticulo-endothelial cells, distinguishable from the epithelial cells only by electron microscopy. The medulla also contains the collections of squamous epithelial cells known as Hassall's corpuscles, which often show central degeneration and cystic change.

Production of the recirculating lymphocyte pool. Until recently, the function of the thymus has remained a mystery: unlike the lymph nodes and spleen, it does not act as a filter of lymph or blood. Furthermore, it neither enlarges nor shows the morphological changes of an immune response following parenteral antigenic challenge, and unlike other lymphoid tissues it is excluded from the pathway of the recirculating small lymphocytes. It has long been known, however, that the thymic cortex is a very active site of lymphopoiesis. This is especially pronounced from fetal life up to puberty, but continues during the process of thymic involution which follows puberty (p. 469). It is apparent, from more recent morphological and kinetic studies employing radio-isotope cell labelling, that huge numbers of small lymphocytes (some-times termed thymocytes) are produced in the cortex of the thymus of the young animal, and that these pass into the medulla, where most of them die. Some do escape, however, into the blood, and although this is only a small percentage of the total produced, it represents a large contribution in terms of absolute numbers of cells.

Our understanding of the function of the thymus arose largely from the original work of Miller and his colleagues (see Miller and Osoba, 1967) who showed that thymectomy in neonatal mice results in their failure to thrive, and in the development of a wasting disease with a high mortality. Animals surviving thymectomy show severe impairment of their capacity to develop delayed hypersensitivity responses, e.g. to reject incompatible skin allografts, and also impaired production of antibodies to some antigens. Athymic mice also fail to develop the recirculating pool of long-lived small lymphocytes; there is severe lymphopenia and deficiency of lymphocytes in the deep cortex of lymph nodes (Fig. 4.17), Peyer's patches, etc., and in the lymphoid tissue around the central arterioles of the splenic white pulp. These areas of the lymphoid tissues are accordingly sometimes termed

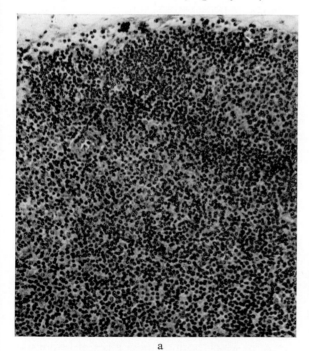 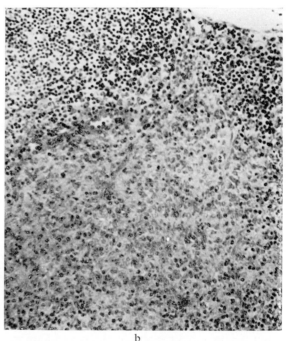

a   b

FIG. 4.17.—Mouse lymph nodes, showing the influence of the thymus on the histological appearances. a, normal lymph node, showing a cortical follicle (top right), and the deep cortex which occupies the lower two thirds of the field. b, lymph node from an athymic mouse: the superficial cortex shows little abnormality, but the deep cortex is almost devoid of lymphoid cells and consists largely of reticulum cells. × 150. (Drs. D. M. V. Parrott and M. A. B. de Sousa.)

the *thymic-dependent areas.* There is thus strong evidence that the thymus supplies the lymphocytes of the recirculating pool, and this has been supported by more direct studies in which isotopically-labelled small lymphocytes leaving the thymus have been demonstrated mainly in the thymic-dependent areas of the lymphoid tissues. The immunological and morphological deficiencies of neonatally-thymectomised mice are corrected by grafts of normal neonatal or fetal mouse thymus.

These findings in mice have been confirmed by other workers, and similar observations have been made in rats, hamsters and in chicks: it thus appears that, in these species, the thymus is essential for the formation of the recirculating lymphocyte pool. Other species of mammal are born in a state of relative immunological maturity, the pool being largely formed before birth. The immunological deficiencies and morphological changes in the secondary lymphoid tissues of young children with defective development of the thymus (p. 114) indicate that, as in various other species, the human thymus has an important role in supplying the specific antigen-responsive small lymphocytes of the recirculating pool.

In adult animals, including man, thymectomy is not followed by obvious impairment of the immune responses, but there is a significant fall in the number of circulating small lymphocytes, and deficiency of delayed hypersensitivity responses has now been shown to develop in mice some months after thymectomy in adult life. The inference is that the supply of thymic cells becomes less important with age because the immunological experience of the individual is stored in the "primed" or "memory" cells of the recirculating pool and in sessile cells in the secondary lymphoid tissues.

Production of a humoral lymphopoietic factor. The immunological role of the thymus is not confined to the production and release of specifically-responsive small lymphocytes, for *partial* restoration of the secondary lymphoid tissues and of immunological responsiveness in the thymectomised animal has been shown to result from implantation of thymic tissue enclosed in a cell-proof millipore membrane. It thus appears that the thymus is capable of secreting a humoral factor which stimulates lymphopoiesis in other lymphoid tissues, and since most of the lymphocytes in such thymic implants die rapidly, the

thymic epithelial cells, some of which normally contain PAS-positive material, are the probable source of the humoral factor, the chemical nature of which is not yet known.

Thymus-independent antibody production

Although the thymus-derived recirculating small lymphocytes are the specific antigen-responsive cells in delayed hypersensitivity responses, and in production of antibodies to some antigens, the antibody response to other antigens is not seriously impaired by neonatal thymectomy, nor by depleting the recirculating pool of small lymphocytes by thoracic duct drainage or heterologous antilymphocyte serum. It is thus apparent that there is a source of specific antigen-responsive cells in addition to the thymus. This second primary lymphoid organ has been shown in fowls to be the bursa of Fabricius, an accumulation of lymphoid tissue within and around a pouch-like outgrowth of the surface epithelium of the cloaca. Removal of the thymus in newly-hatched chicks has the same effect as in mammals, namely depression of delayed hypersensitivity and of some antibody responses: removal of the bursa leads to deficient antibody production and scarcity of plasma cells in the secondary lymphoid tissues, but has little or no effect on delayed hypersensitivity responses.

In mammals, the homologue of the avian bursa has not been identified: the appendix, Peyer's patches and tonsil have all been suggested, but attempts at their removal have not resulted in deficiency of plasma cells or of antibody production comparable with the pronounced effects of bursectomy in chicks. It seems most likely that the function of the avian bursa—the production of thymus-independent specific antigen-responsive cells—is not restricted to a special organ in mammals, but is vested in the various secondary lymphoid tissues, including those in the wall of the alimentary tract. If this is so, these tissues subserve both the primary function of producing specifically-responsive plasma cell precursors, analogous to the production of specifically-responsive small lymphocytes in the thymus, and the secondary function of providing the environment in which both of these types of responsive cell undergo the proliferative and other changes of immune responses.

The thymus-independent specific antigen-responsive (B) cells are small lymphocytes of similar morphology to thymus-derived (T) lymphocytes, but are mainly sessile cells in the secondary lymphoid tissues, lying in the lymphoid follicles of the superficial cortex; stimulation by antigen results in their proliferation, and thus provides the plasma cells which produce the appropriate antibody (Fig. 4.18). Some of the proliferated cells pass via the efferent lymphatic to the blood, and settle in other secondary lymphoid tissues, and especially in the wall of the intestine, where they become antibody-producing plasma cells; they do not, however, join the recirculating small lymphocyte pool. It is uncertain whether any of them become "memory" cells, although it is known that the thymic-independent antibody response does produce memory cells (p. 82) which remain in the lymphoid tissues.

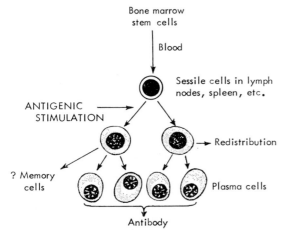

Fig. 4.18.—Thymus-independent antibody production. Stem cells from the bone marrow settle in the lymph nodes, spleen, and lymphoid tissues in the wall of the alimentary canal. These cells, or cells derived from them, are specifically responsive: appropriate antigenic stimulation causes their transformation to large pyroninophilic cells, and these proliferate to provide plasma cells which produce the corresponding antibody. Some of the large pyroninophilic cells pass by the lymphatics and blood to the intestinal mucosa where they lead to production of IgA-class antibody: others settle in the other lymphoid tissues.

The lympho-haemopoietic stem cells

In common with other tissues with a high rate of cell turnover, the lymphoid and haemopoietic tissues require a supply of stem cells, division of which provides the precursors of the specialised differentiated cells. In the embryo,

stem cells for haemopoietic marrow are first detected in the yolk sac and primitive blood; later they appear in the fetal liver, and finally in the haemopoietic marrow, which subsequently maintains its own population of stem cells.

There is evidence that the thymus and secondary lymphoid tissues receive a continuous supply of stem cells from the haemopoietic marrow. Thus in the mouse subjected to a lethal dose of total-body irradiation, and protected by an injection of compatible marrow cells, the donated cells settle not only in the host's marrow, where they provide the progenitors of red cells, granulocytes and megakaryocytes, but they or their descendants also supply, to the thymus, stem cells which multiply and differentiate into small lymphocytes. Donor marrow cells also pass to the secondary lymphoid tissues where they produce the plasma cells responsible for antibody production. The evidence for this is based on experiments in which the donated cells are identified by chromosomal markers, and in similar experiments it has been observed that marrow stem cells with a unique chromosomal abnormality (induced by irradiation) supply both haemopoietic and lymphoid cell progenitors: this suggests that the lympho-haemopoietic stem cells are pluripotent, and that the differentiation of their descendants into the various haemopoietic or lymphoid cells depends on local environmental factors in the marrow and lymphoid tissues respectively (p. 125).

Lymphoid cells from the thymus (the recirculating lymphocyte pool) and from lymph nodes are incapable of replenishing the marrow or the thymus of heavily irradiated animals, and it thus appears that stem cells for these tissues are supplied mainly or wholly by the haemopoietic marrow. It follows also that a supply of stem cells from the marrow is required throughout adult life to sustain lymphopoiesis in the thymus and secondary lymphoid tissues.

Cell co-operation in antibody production

The previous sections have been concerned largely with the origin and behaviour of specific antigen-responsive cells—the so-called immunologically-competent cells which are capable of recognising a particular antigen and initiate the immune *response* to that antigen. We must consider also the nature of the *effector* cells produced by the immune response, namely, the "primed" small lymphocytes which react directly with the antigen in delayed hypersensitivity *reactions*, and the plasma cells which are the main producers of antibody.

As already stated, delayed hypersensitivity responses are mediated by the thymus-derived recirculating small lymphocytes which, on appropriate antigenic stimulation, enlarge into immunoblasts: from these, small lymphocytes are provided by further divisions. It is likely that these last cells are the effector cells of delayed hypersensitivity reactions and that some of them persist in the recirculating lymphocyte pool, and possibly as sessile cells in the secondary lymphoid tissues, and form the basis of immunological memory. Similarly, in antibody responses which are not thymus-dependent, sessile cells of the secondary lymphoid tissues, derived from stem cells provided by the marrow, respond specifically to antigenic stimulation and initiate the events leading to the development of plasma cells which produce and secrete antibody, and possibly also to the development of sessile "memory" cells. There is reason to believe that all plasma cells result from proliferation of marrow-derived stem cells, and not from thymus-derived lymphocytes, and thus it appears that the thymus-dependent and thymus-independent systems can operate separately to provide delayed hypersensitivity and antibodies respectively.

The thymus-dependence of some antibody responses is indicated by the depression of production of antibodies to some antigens following neonatal thymectomy, and also by experiments which indicate the occurrence of synergism between thymus-derived lymphocytes and marrow-derived plasma-cell precursors. For example, when mice which have received a heavy dose of irradiation to the whole body are injected with either thymus cells *or* marrow cells, together with antigen, e.g. sheep red cells, the number of antibody-producing plasma cells which develop is much less than when smaller numbers of thymus *and* marrow cells are administered, together with sheep red cells. In such experiments, it has been shown, by use of thymus and marrow cells from different strains, that all the antibody-producing cells are derived from the donated marrow cells, and not from the thymus cells. The most likely interpretation of these findings is that thymus-dependent antibody responses (in

this case to sheep red cells) involves the co-operation of specifically reactive thymus-derived lymphocytes (probably the immunoblasts or the smaller lymphocytes derived from their division) with marrow-derived plasma-cell precursors (Fig. 4.19).

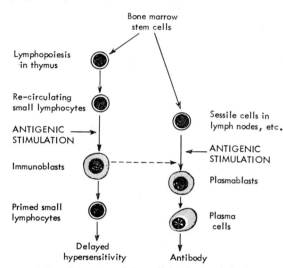

Fig. 4.19.—Summary of the cellular basis of the immune response. Delayed hypersensitivity responses (left) are mediated by antigenic stimulation (? by antigen processed by macrophages) of recirculating lymphocytes of thymic origin. Thymic-independent antibody production (right) is mediated by antigenic stimulation of sessile plasma-cell precursors. Production of antibody to some antigens involves co-operation between the thymic-dependent and thymic-independent systems (interrupted line).

Role of the macrophage in immune responses

Although macrophages are not inherently capable of specific antigen responsiveness, it is possible that they take up and modify antigen in such a way that it is more strongly immunogenic to specifically-responsive lymphoid cells. Undoubtedly, the bulk of an injected antigen is taken up by macrophages. However, this occurs not only in the secondary lymphoid tissues, which are the site of immune responses, but also in the Kupffer cells of the liver, and macrophages of the bone marrow and red pulp of the spleen, tissues which are not important sites of the initiation of immune responses.

The role of the macrophage in immune responses is a complex subject, particularly as it has been shown that macrophages from different tissues behave differently in their treatment of antigen. Experiments in which lymphoid cells are exposed to antigens *in vitro* have yielded conflicting results. Strong antigens, and particularly those which are very large molecules or particulate, appear capable of stimulating immune responses in lymphoid cells in culture without the participation of macrophages, and indeed prior uptake of antigen by macrophages may render it less immunogenic. By contrast, the immunogenicity of weaker antigens may be enhanced by its uptake by macrophages.

There is some evidence, at present inconclusive, that it may be particularly those immune responses initiated by the recirculating small lymphocytes (i.e. thymic-dependent responses) which require modification of the antigen by macrophages.

The possible immunological role of the dendritic cells of lymphoid germinal centres, which may be specialised macrophages, is discussed in the following section.

The Morphological Features of Immune Responses

Immune responses, whether leading to the development of delayed hypersensitivity or production of antibody, take place mainly in the secondary lymphoid organs, i.e. the lymph nodes, white pulp of the spleen and gut-associated lymphoid tissues. In both man and experimental animals, study of the morphological changes of immune responses is not easy, for the large number of micro-organisms in the alimentary and upper respiratory tracts, and in the exposed mucous membranes, provide continual antigenic stimuli which ensure that the immunity system is never completely at rest. The maintenance of animals in a germ-free environment from birth onwards is helpful, but technically exacting, and does not ensure freedom from antigenic stimulation: thus "germ-free" mice are likely to be infected with mouse leukaemia virus, and do, in fact, show evidence of immune responses in their lymphoid tissues. Another variable which must be taken into account is the differences in lymph nodes from various parts of the body, and even between lymph nodes which are anatomically adjacent to one another. The situation is complicated further by the development of both delayed hypersensitivity and antibody in thymus-dependent immune responses, together with thymus-independent antibody production: all three types of response may occur together in the same lymph node, and the precise identification of the morphological change attributable to each one is far from complete. Some progress has been made by studying responses in animals in which the thymic-dependent system has been abolished or suppressed by neonatal thymectomy, anti-lymphocyte serum or thoracic-duct drainage, while in man the morphological features associated with the various immunological deficiency states (p. 114) has helped to clarify the situation.

Lymph nodes

Normal structure (Fig. 4.20). The lymph node consists of cortex, medulla and lymph sinuses. The cortex occupies the superficial part of the node except at the hilar region: the medulla lies centrally, but extends to the hilum. The framework of the node consists of a network of fine reticulin fibrils which are covered by the cytoplasm of elongated, flat reticulum cells with branching cytoplasmic processes. The mesh of the reticular spaces is 15–30μ in diam. in the cortex and 5–10μ in the medulla. The sinuses are simply channels in the reticular framework, and they also are lined and traversed by reticulum cells. Most of the free cells in the node are lymphocytes, and small lymphocytes usually predominate. In the cortex, the lymphocytes are closely arranged, and in *the superficial part of the*

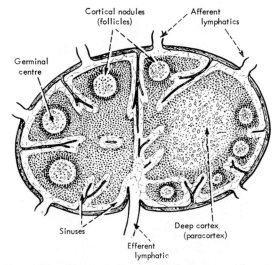

FIG. 4.20.—Diagram of a lymph node, portraying the superficial cortex with nodules and germinal centres, and on the right an ill-defined area of deep cortex.

cortex there are foci, termed *primary nodules*, in which lymphocytes are more closely packed. In a stimulated node, as described below, a focus of lymphopoiesis, termed a *germinal centre*, may develop within the primary nodules: nodules in this state are sometimes referred to as secondary, but it now seems inappropriate to use the terms primary and secondary in this context. The *deeper cortex*, sometimes termed the *paracortex*, consists of ill-defined uniform areas of cortical tissue lying between the superficial cortex and medulla (Fig. 4.21): in the stimulated node, there may be intense proliferation of lymphoid cells here, and this may result in one or more large nodules of tissue which compress the medulla of the node.

Lymph arriving at the node by the afferent lymphatics enters the peripheral sinus which surrounds the lymphoid tissue of the node and communicates at the hilum with the efferent lymphatic. From the peripheral sinus, cortical sinuses pass radially inwards to the medulla, running between the superficial cortical nodules and penetrating the deep cortex. In the medulla, the lymph sinuses are numerous, and the lymphoid tissue lies between them as the *medullary cords*: the medullary sinuses unite to form the efferent lymphatic.

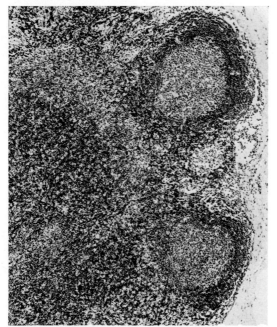

FIG. 4.21.—Part of the cortex of a lymph node, showing two large cortical nodules (follicles) with germinal centres. The ill-defined area to the left of these consists of deep cortex. × 40.

The lymph nodes have two major functions. One of these is the interception and removal of abnormal or foreign material in the lymph stream passing to them, and is described on pp. 457, 459: the other is the production of immune responses, the histological features of which are described below.

Immune responses in lymph nodes

(a) **Delayed hypersensitivity responses.** In lymph nodes draining the site of an antigenic stimulus of a kind which induces a *delayed hypersensitivity response*, e.g. an allogeneic skin graft or application to the skin of the hapten dinitrochlorobenzene, the most conspicuous early change is the appearance of large basophilic (and pyroninophilic) lymphoid cells (immunoblasts) in the deep cortex of the node. These cells appear two days or so after antigenic stimulation; they multiply rapidly and are maximal at about 5 days. Small lymphocytes also increase in number in the deep cortex, which becomes enlarged and conspicuous, causing appreciable increase in size of the node. If the antigenic stimulation is not prolonged, the immunoblasts disappear after a further few days, the main feature then being an increased number of small lymphocytes in the deep cortex.

It will be recalled that delayed hypersensitivity responses are initiated by thymus-derived small lymphocytes of the recirculating pool, and that the deep cortex of the lymph node lies in their pathway (p. 86). It is very likely that the large pyroninophilic cells appearing in the deep cortex are derived by antigen-induced transformation (p. 87) and multiplication of these cells. This implies that recirculating small lymphocytes must have encountered the antigenic stimulus and that they include cells capable of specific response to it. Encounter with the antigen may possibly take place in the antigen-containing tissue, those small lymphocytes capable of specific response to the antigenic material leaving the blood vessels and passing to the draining nodes to settle in the deep cortex and initiate the delayed hypersensitivity response. As an alternative possibility, antigenic material, either free or carried by macrophages, might pass to the draining nodes and there stimulate appropriately responsive cells among the recirculating lymphocytes passing through the deep cortex. If we accept the clonal selection theory of immune responses (p. 82), then only a very small proportion of cells in the recirculating lymphocyte pool could be specifically responsive to an antigen not encountered previously, and recirculation of small lymphocytes can be seen as a phenomenon providing opportunity for very large numbers of specifically responsive cells to "inspect" an antigen. The use of tritiated-thymidine labelling has shown that the immunoblasts in the deep cortex proliferate to produce small lymphocytes, and that these appear in the recirculating lymphocyte pool at about the time of development of delayed hypersensitivity: a second advantage of the recirculation is to allow such "primed" cells to encounter, and react with, the corresponding antigen almost anywhere in the body, a factor of obvious importance in combating infections.

It is not established that *all* the large pyroninophilic lymphocytes which appear in the deep cortex of a node during a delayed hypersensitivity response are cells which are specifically responsive to the particular antigens. There is evidence that the specific reaction between antigen and responsive lymphocytes releases a factor which stimulates transformation and mitosis in other lymphocytes which are not specifically responsive to that antigen. Similarly in delayed hypersensitivity *reactions* (p. 106) only a small percentage of the lymphocytes participating are specifically responsive, although it is possible that the others may have become "passively" sensitised by a transfer factor (p. 107).

(b) Thymus-dependent antibody production. It is unusual for delayed hypersensitivity responses to be unaccompanied by production of some antibody, and this latter response is associated with the additional appearance of plasma cells in the medulla of the draining lymph nodes: these cells have been shown to be the source of the antibody and, as already explained (p. 92), they originate from stem cells provided by the marrow, and they co-operate with thymus-derived, specifically-responsive lymphocytes in thymus-dependent antibody production.

(c) Thymus-independent antibody production. The capacity to develop antibodies to certain antigens has been shown to be independent of the thymus by observations on neonatally-thymectomised animals, and by observations on infants with thymic aplasia. In these circum-

stances, and also in normal animals and man, this type of immune response in the lymph nodes is characterised by the appearance of large numbers of plasma cells in the medullary cords, and the development of prominent germinal centres in the superficial cortex. Both these changes are most prominent in the lymph nodes draining the site of locally-injected antigen; they may persist for weeks after a single injection, and are more pronounced in a secondary than in a primary antibody response.

The plasma cells in the medulla are the main antibody-producing cells, but the morphology and location of the cells from which they originate are not known.

The *germinal centres* (Fig. 4.22) contain

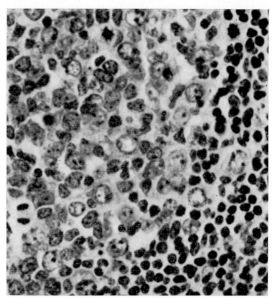

Fig. 4.22.—Segment of a germinal centre, showing the appearances of the cells, some of which are dividing. Note the surrounding tightly-packed small lymphocytes. × 850.

cells of several morphological types, but of uncertain nature. Medium-sized lymphocytes, and larger cells with more basophilic cytoplasm, resembling immunoblasts (p. 87) are numerous, and show intense mitotic activity. Large rounded macrophages containing in their cytoplasm fragments of ingested nuclear material are present in small numbers, and special staining techniques have revealed the presence of dendritic cells with branching cytoplasmic processes. Apart from its association with thymus-independent antibody production, the function of the germinal centre and of its individual cells are not understood. In a primary response, antibody is first detectable, by immunofluorescent techniques, in the medullary plasma cells: it is apparently present in few or none of the germinal-centre lymphoid cells. In secondary responses, medullary plasma cells containing antibody are very numerous, and in some germinal centres antibody may be demonstrable in most of the lymphoid cells. The dendritic cells of the germinal centres may be specialised macrophages: in the germinal centres of antigenically-stimulated rats and chickens, there is evidence that the antigen persists for several weeks on the surface of these cells. This follows the appearance of antigen-containing medullary plasma cells, and as immunoglobulin is also demonstrable on the surface of the dendritic cells, it is probable that these cells are coated with antigen complexed with antibody. The long persistence of antigen in this site may provide a prolonged stimulus, and the proliferating lymphoid cells in the germinal centre may be specifically-responsive cells stimulated by the appropriate antigen. These cells could conceivably differentiate into the antibody-producing plasma cells or into "memory" cells.

Many of the large plasma-cell precursors developing by proliferation of specifically-responsive cells during antibody responses leave their lymph node of origin. They pass by the efferent lymphatic to the blood and settle in other lymph nodes and also in non-lymphoid tissues, such as the marrow, liver, skin, the intestinal mucosa, and particularly in tissues containing the antigen which has stimulated the response. In long-continued antibody responses, plasma cells are commonly present in these non-lymphoid sites, and at least some of them produce antibody.

Immune responses in other lymphoid tissues

Spleen. The structure of the spleen is described briefly on p. 449. Immune responses take place in the white pulp (Malpighian bodies) of the organ, and have been studied in chickens which have the advantage of two well defined lymphoid organs—the thymus and bursa of Fabricius—respective removal of which provides opportunity to study thymus-independent and thymus-dependent immune responses. It appears from such investigations, and also from observations

in rodents, that the area immediately adjacent to the central arteriole is occupied by small lymphocytes of the recirculating pool, and corresponds to the deep cortex of lymph nodes, while the surrounding lymphoid tissue corresponds to the superficial cortex of lymph nodes and is the site of formation of germinal centres during thymus-independent antibody production. Antibody-producing plasma cells appear at the periphery of the Malpighian bodies and pass into the adjacent red pulp.

Immune responses in the spleen occur particularly when antigenic material gains entrance to the blood stream, and present morphological appearances similar to those which have been described for the lymph nodes.

Gut-associated lymphoid tissues. As mentioned previously, it has been suggested, but not established, that the gut-associated lymphoid tissues might subserve the function of a primary lymphoid organ analogous to the bursa of Fabricius of the fowl, producing specifically-responsive precursors of plasma cells. Whether or not this is the case, these tissues resemble the lymph nodes and spleen in being sites of delayed hypersensitivity and antibody responses, and they contain areas corresponding to the superficial and deep cortex of lymph nodes, and also lymph sinuses.

Immune responses in non-lymphoid tissues

When antigenic material persists in the body, e.g. in chronic infections, tissue allografts, and antigen injected in relatively insoluble form, immune responses may occur in the granulation tissue which develops around the antigen. Immunoblasts resembling those developing in the deep cortex of the lymph nodes may be observed, and may participate in both the immune response and in a delayed hypersensitivity *reaction* with the antigenic material. Plasma cells are also commonly present after some days and are derived from precursors produced in the lymphoid tissues and released into the lymphatics from where they reach the blood and settle in the antigen-containing tissues: they are responsible for local antibody production. More concrete evidence of the occurrence of all stages of the immune response in the tissues containing the antigen is provided by the development of lymphoid tissue with germinal centres, and the demonstration of antibody in extracts of the tissue.

In intensive and prolonged antibody responses, plasma cells may be widespread in various tissues, including the haemopoietic marrow, which can be an important site of antibody production. Unless the appearance of plasma cells in the marrow is accompanied by the development of lymphoid tissue, it must be assumed that they originate from plasma cell precursors produced in, and released from, the lymphoid tissues.

The lamina propria of the gut mucosa, and particularly of the intestinal villi, normally contains plasma cells. There is evidence that many of these produce IgA antibody, and that they are derived from the *large* lymphoid cells in efferent lymphatic and thoracic duct lymph, and thus originate in the lymphoid tissues.

CHAPTER 5

IMMUNOPATHOLOGY

This chapter is devoted entirely to disease processes which have an immunological basis. It falls naturally into two parts. First, the *hypersensitivity diseases* due to reactions of an immunological nature. It should be noted that this use of the term hypersensitivity is somewhat restricted. It does not include those conditions in which the subject is abnormally sensitive to a drug as a result of genetically determined deficiency of a catabolic enzyme system or because of disease of the liver or kidneys: this type of undue responsiveness is termed *idiosyncrasy* and is not dealt with here.

The second main section of the chapter describes the *immunological deficiencies*, i.e congenital or acquired conditions in which the subject is incapable of the normal range of immunological responses and as a result is unduly susceptible to infection.

HYPERSENSITIVITY REACTIONS

In most instances, hypersensitivity may be defined as a state in which the introduction of an antigen into the body elicits an unduly severe immunological reaction. It follows previous exposure to the antigen and is a consequence of the development of an immune response, i.e. production of antibodies or sensitised lymphocytes reactive with the antigen. It is this reaction between the antigen and products of the immune response which produces the lesions of the hypersensitivity disease processes.

Hypersensitivity reactions may be localised to the site of entry of the antigen, or generalised: the local reactions are mainly of an inflammatory nature, but may also include spasm of smooth muscle. The generalised effects include fever, shock, gastrointestinal and pulmonary disturbances, and sometimes fatal circulatory collapse. One of the earliest examples of hypersensitivity was provided by Richet and Partier (1902) who observed that intravenous injection of small amounts of extracts of sea anemone into dogs was harmless, but a second injection some weeks later was quickly followed by a violent and sometimes fatal reaction with dyspnoea, vomiting, defaecation, micturition and collapse. Since this early report, which illustrates the acute and severe nature of some hypersensitivity reactions, a great deal has been learned, and hypersensitivity reactions may now be classified into four major types (see below).

The definition of hypersensitivity given above refers solely to foreign antigens entering the body from outside. However, the term includes also the conditions commonly known as the *autoimmune diseases*, in which antibodies or sensitised lymphocytes appear which are capable of reacting with a normal cell or tissue constituent *in vivo*, with consequent pathological changes. Hypersensitivity reactions may result also from passive immunisation, for example when antibody is produced in the mother by active immunisation by fetal red cells, and crosses the placenta in a subsequent pregnancy to gain entrance to the fetal circulation. Another special example of hypersensitivity of increasing importance is *the rejection process in heterogeneic or allogeneic tissue transplants*. The increasing diversity and use of drugs has also provided an important group of "*drug hypersensitivities*" and the same applies to the expanding number of chemicals used domestically and in industry.

The four major types of hypersensitivity reactions are described briefly below and then each is dealt with in more detail. They have been elucidated very largely by animal experiments. Hypersensitivity reactions in man, whether they occur naturally, as a result of transplantation, or from administration of a drug, tend to be complex and often involve more than one of the four types.

Anaphylaxis (atopic or type I hypersensitivity). This occurs in certain individuals who are genetically predisposed to respond to various antigens by the production of unusually large amounts of antibody of the IgE class (p. 79): such antibodies are developed, for example, in response to inhalation of normally harmless substances, such as grass pollens, and they render the individual liable to attacks of hay fever, asthma, or more severe generalised reactions, on further encounters with the antigen. Clearly, the major factor in individuals who exhibit anaphylaxis is an abnormal type of responsiveness to antigenic stimuli.

Cytotoxic antibody (type II) reactions. This results from the development of antibody capable of causing tissue injury by reacting with the surface membrane of the individual's own cells, or with an extracellular tissue constituent. It may occur as an auto-immune reaction, of which a good example is the destruction of circulating red cells by auto-antibody in the auto-immune haemolytic anaemias: also it may result from modification of the antigenicity of cells by an extrinsic agent, e.g. various drugs. In some reactions of this type, complement is fixed by the affected cells or tissue constituents, and may participate in the resulting destructive process; in others, antigen–antibody reactions are non-complement-fixing, and the effects are then mediated solely by the reaction of the antibody.

Immune-complex or Arthus-type (type III) reactions. This type of reaction is brought about by the specific union, within the body, of antigen with the corresponding soluble antibody. The antigen–antibody complexes so formed produce harmful effects, particularly when they are formed in the presence of a relative excess of antigen over antibody. Such complexes are deposited in the walls of small blood vessels, where subsequent fixation of complement leads to inflammatory oedema, neutrophil polymorph infiltration, haemorrhage and necrosis. While Arthus-type reactions result from union of antibody with *soluble* antigen, it is important to appreciate that a similar type of reaction can result from the union of antibody with *particulate* antigens, for example, bacteria; the union of antibody with the bacteria is commonly followed by fixation of complement and this, in turn, provides one of the mechanisms whereby polymorphonuclear leukocytes are attracted to the site. In other words, hypersensitivity comparable to the Arthus reaction can contribute to the inflammatory pyogenic reaction to bacterial infection.

Delayed hypersensitivity (type IV) reactions. As already explained, the development of sensitised lymphocytes, capable of reacting with the antigen, is a normal feature of the immune response to many antigens, and once it has occurred, introduction of the antigen results in an inflammatory reaction which appears after 12 hours or so (hence the term *delayed* hypersensitivity) and increases for 24–48 hours. An excellent example is the tuberculin reaction in which application or injection of tuberculoprotein into the skin is without effect in animals or individuals who have not previously encountered *M. tuberculosis*, whereas infection or immunisation leads to a state of delayed hypersensitivity in which the skin test is positive. Delayed hypersensitivity reactions are mediated by specifically reactive lymphocytes and not by humoral antibodies (p. 83).

Anaphylaxis (atopy; atopic; immediate, or type I hypersensitivity)

This is the type of hypersensitivity which is mainly responsible for hay fever, asthma and infantile eczema: it is also responsible for some cases of hypersensitivity reactions to foods and drugs and for the immediate type of generalised hypersensitivity reactions characterised by dyspnoea, prostration and urticaria, etc., which are sometimes rapidly fatal.

Skin testing. It has long been suspected that anaphylaxis is mediated by antibody (termed *reagin* or *reaginic antibody*) which, in addition to circulating in the plasma, is peculiar in its capacity to become firmly attached to cells and tissues. Moreover, the reaction of such fixed antibody with the corresponding antigen (sometimes termed *allergen*) results in rapid release of histamine and other vasoactive substances which are the effectors of the anaphylactic reaction.

Intradermal injection of a solution of the antigen to which the atopic patient is hypersensitive has long been known to produce, within a few minutes, an acute inflammatory response at the injection site, and this procedure is still widely used clinically to establish the existence of such hypersensitivity (Fig. 5.1). Not only does the

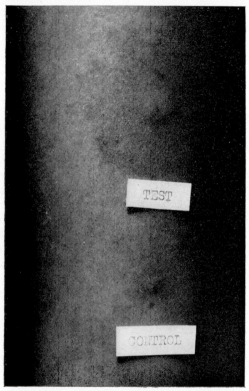

FIG. 5.1.—Skin test showing immediate (type I) hypersensitivity reaction. The patient was an asthmatic and the test was performed by intradermal injection of an extract of house dust. Note the oedema and wide zone of reddening. Photograph taken 10 minutes after injection. (Dr. J. W. Kerr.)

reaction to skin testing develop rapidly, but the sufferer from hay fever or asthma experiences an attack within a few minutes of encounter with the appropriate antigen; for this reason atopic hypersensitivity is sometimes called *immediate type hypersensitivity.*

Passive transfer: the Prausnitz–Küstner reaction. The humoral nature of reagin, the factor responsible for this type of hypersensitivity, and its capacity to become fixed in tissues, was demonstrated beautifully in the classical investigation of Prausnitz and Küstner (1921). Küstner himself regularly experienced a generalised hypersensitivity reaction after eating fish.

Intradermal injection of an extract of fish muscle produced the typical acute inflammatory reaction of atopic hypersensitivity. In attempting passive transfer of the hypersensitivity state, small amounts of Küstner's serum were injected intradermally into Prausnitz, followed 24 hours later by injection of fish muscle extract: the typical acute inflammatory reaction ensued, and was shown to depend on the injection of serum, followed after an interval by fish extract. The experiment was complicated by the fact that Prausnitz had atopic hypersensitivity to pollens, but passive transfer of fish hypersensitivity was achieved also in normal, non-atopic individuals. These findings have since been confirmed repeatedly with serum from subjects with atopic hypersensitivity to various antigens, and it has been shown that the interval between injecting the serum and antigen in the Prausnitz–Küstner reaction may be increased up to 3–4 weeks. Transient atopic hypersensitivity has also been observed to occur in the recipients of blood from atopic donors. Evidence that tissue sensitisation in atopic subjects is generalised, and not restricted to the skin and mucous membranes, has been provided by the demonstration that fresh bronchial tissue removed from an atopic subject undergoes contraction of the smooth muscle when exposed to the appropriate antigen, and it has been shown that normal tissues of various types can be sensitised *in vitro* by the serum of atopic individuals.

Reaginic antibody: IgE. Elucidation of the physico-chemical nature of reagin, and the observation that it is essentially a type of antibody, have been slow, partly because it is present only in trace amounts in the serum, and is less stable than other classes of immunoglobulin, but also because it does not confer atopic hypersensitivity to laboratory animals, and has been demonstrable only by its biological effect in man. Recently, however, investigations have been rendered much easier by the discovery of a patient with a plasma cell myeloma whose myeloma protein was shown to be the same class of immunoglobulin as reagins. The serum of this patient has provided a rich source of reaginic class immunoglobulin, now termed IgE. It has been shown that its propensity to attach to tissues is a property of the Fc part of the IgE molecule (see p. 78), and that injection of relatively large amounts of the Fc fragment into the skin can apparently block the tissue sites of attachment of reaginic antibody, for it inhibits the elicitation of the Prausnitz–Küstner reaction at the same site. The myeloma IgE has been the means of the preparation of antibody to IgE, and use has been made of this to assay *in vitro* the serum levels of IgE in atopic and normal individuals and to assay reaginic antibody *in vitro*.

Chemical mediators: possible role of the mast cell. It is not known which types of cell become coated with human reagin: much of the evidence on this aspect of atopy is derived from studies on guinea-pigs and other animals which can produce antibodies resembling human reagins in binding to tissues and conferring immediate type hypersensitivity. It is known that the reagin-like antibodies of animals can bind onto mast cells in the tissues, and that subsequent exposure to the appropriate antigen results in disruption of the sensitised mast cells, and of their granules. Mast cell granules are rich in histamine, and this is released in active form when the granules are disrupted by the mechanism described above (Fig. 5.2). The major effects of histamine include increase in vascular permeability, and excessive secretion by the nasal, lacrimal, and probably also the bronchial glands. These effects could well account for the features of anaphylaxis in animals and man, and the importance of histamine is also suggested by the suppressive effects of histamine antagonists in human and experi-

mental atopy. However, these agents are only partially effective, and there is evidence that histamine is only one of the effectors of atopy. For example, it has been shown that human lung tissue, removed surgically from an atopic subject who developed a bronchial carcinoma, yielded not only histamine but also SRS-A (the *slow reacting substance* of anaphylaxis) on perfusion with a solution of the antigen to which the individual was hypersensitive. During the first few minutes of perfusion, histamine release predominated, but subsequently SRS-A was released in larger amounts (in terms of pharmacological activity) than histamine. SRS-A is formed by many tissues, and produces increase in vascular permeability and more prolonged spasm of the bronchiolar smooth muscle than does histamine: it could well participate in the bronchospasm of asthma and spasm of the gut in food allergies. It is possible that bradykinin and permeability factors derived from plasma components, which may participate in acute inflammation in general, may also act as mediators in anaphylaxis.

In summary, atopic hypersensitivity occurs in individuals who have developed unusually large amounts of IgE class antibody to a foreign antigen, such as those present in grass pollens, house dust and animal dander. The antibody is present in the circulation, but is also cell-bound —most probably to mast cells and possibly also other types of cell—in various tissues including the conjunctiva, nasopharynx and walls of the bronchi. When the antigen to which hypersensitivity has developed is present in the air, sufficient may be dissolved and absorbed by the mucous membranes to react with the fixed antibody. This releases histamine and other pharmacologically active compounds which bring about the acute inflammatory exudation and glandular secretion characteristic of hay fever and in addition the bronchial muscle spasm of asthma. Some atopic individuals, and particularly children, experience similar reactions in the gastro-intestinal tract on ingestion of antigens in foodstuffs to which they have become hypersensitive. Subjects who have developed a high degree of atopic hypersensitivity may, if they absorb sufficient of the offending antigen by any route, develop generalised anaphylaxis characterised by the features of asthma, hay fever, gastro-intestinal reactions, urticaria and circulatory collapse.

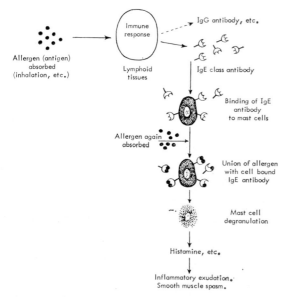

Fig. 5.2.—The probable mechanism of the anaphylactic (type I) hypersensitivity reaction.

This is an over-simplified summary of the subject, and many problems remain to be solved. For example, it is not known why some atopic individuals develop hay fever and others asthma, nor why atopy tends to run in families, although a genetic predisposition to develop IgE class antibodies is the most likely explanation. One method of treatment widely practised is the administration of immunising injections of very small amounts of the antigen to which hypersensitivity has developed ("desensitisation"). This is of value in some patients, and it is likely that its beneficial effect depends upon the production of IgG antibody ("blocking antibody") which reacts with the antigen and thus limits the amount available to react with fixed IgE antibody. An interesting development is the demonstration that the major antigen concerned in atopic hypersensitivity to house dust is a product of the mite *Dermatophagoides pteronyssinus* (Fig. 15.9, p. 335) which lives upon human squames in mattresses. This is extremely common in the home, but is not found in hospitals where the patients' mattresses are sterilised at frequent intervals or enveloped in polythene, and this may explain why children with asthma frequently improve dramatically on admission to hospital. Without doubt, however, psychogenic factors are of importance in some cases of asthma, and it may be that undue responsiveness to histamine and other mediators also plays a role.

The role of blood eosinophilia, and the infiltration of eosinophil polymorphs in hay fever and asthma (p. 335) and other atopic reactions, are unexplained.

Cytotoxic antibody (type II) reactions

Injury of cells by antibody can arise in three ways (Fig. 5.3). Firstly, there may be a breakdown of normal immunological tolerance with the production of auto-antibody capable of reacting with normal constituents of the cell mem-brane and bringing about its destruction. The classical example of this is auto-immune haemolytic anaemia in which red cell injury is brought about by auto-antibody reactive with various antigenic determinants inherent in the surface membrane of red cells. Secondly, the surface membrane of cells may become antigenic as a result of attachment of foreign antigenic or haptenic substances, and when this occurs antibody may develop which is capable of reacting with the modified cell membranes, resulting in cellular injury. An example is provided by the sedative, Sedormid (allyl isopropylacetylurea) which can bind onto platelets: production of antibody to the modified platelets then leads to thrombocytopenia. Thirdly, cell destruction may be brought about by iso-antibodies: this arises in transfusion of incompatible blood, when iso-antibodies in the recipient's plasma may destroy the transfused incompatible cells, or the transfused blood may contain antibodies which react with and destroy the red cells, leukocytes or platelets of the recipient. This third type of reaction, due to iso-antibodies, occurs also in haemolytic disease of the newborn (p. 412), which is due to rhesus or other blood-group incompatibility between mother and fetus: fetal red cells escape into the mother's circulation, usually during labour, and the mother develops antibodies to Rhesus antigens, inherited from the father, and present on the fetal red cells, but absent from her own. During a subsequent pregnancy, the maternal anti-Rhesus antibody passes through the placenta into the fetal circulation, and if the cells of this fetus also contain the corresponding Rhesus antigen, they are destroyed by the maternal iso-antibody (Fig. 5.4). Similarly, the mother can develop iso-antibodies to antigens on the fetal platelets, and thrombocytopenia in the fetus can result. Since the only class of antibody which can cross the placenta is IgG, these examples of cell injury in the fetus are mediated only by IgG iso-antibodies. The iso-antibodies anti-A and anti-

(1) Failure of tolerance to normal cell or $\longrightarrow$ auto-antibodies to normal cells or tissue constituents cells or tissues

(2) Normal cell or tissue constituents rendered $\longrightarrow$ antibody to the altered cell antigenic by union of a foreign hapten or tissue

(3) Iso-antibody (natural, or induced by trans- $\longrightarrow$ reaction with transfused fusion, etc.) (or fetal) cells

Union of antibody results in cell or tissue injury, sometimes with the participation of complement.

G. 5.3.—The ways in which antibody is produced which is capable of reacting directly with cell or tissue constituents, causing a type II hypersensitivity reaction.

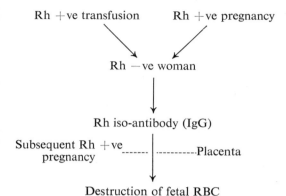

Rh +ve transfusion   Rh +ve pregnancy

Rh —ve woman

Rh iso-antibody (IgG)

Subsequent Rh +ve ------- |----------Placenta
    pregnancy

Destruction of fetal RBC

FIG. 5.4.—Haemolytic disease of the newborn. Fetal red cell destruction is brought about by maternal iso-antibody which has developed as a result of previous Rh +ve pregnancy or transfusion of Rh +ve blood.

B, normally present in the blood of individuals lacking B and A red cell antigens respectively, belong to the IgM class of immunoglobulins and the failure of these to cross the placenta normally protects the fetus from the effects of ABO incompatibility between mother and child.

It will be apparent that the examples given above of cell injury resulting from cytotoxic antibody are all related to cells of the blood. The cytotoxic antibodies are of IgG or IgM classes, and with certain exceptions (e.g. nephro-toxic-antibody nephritis and thyrotoxicosis—see p. 110) these antibodies do not appear capable of injuring the cells or formed elements of organised normal tissues: this is possibly because they do not under normal circumstances gain entrance to the extravascular tissue space in sufficient concentrations to injure target cells, or it may be that some of the antibodies to the cells of organised tissues are reactive with internal cellular constituents and not with the surface membrane. Whatever the explanation, antibodies to cytoplasmic constituents of thyroid and gastric parietal cells are commonly present in the plasma of individuals with chronic thyroiditis and chronic gastritis respectively, but there is evidence that the antibodies do not initiate the destructive changes in these tissues.

Mechanisms of cell injury. Cells of the blood may be injured by the attachment of antibody alone, or by the subsequent fixation of complement. In some instances of auto-immune haemolytic anaemia, for example, the red cells may become coated with antibody of IgG class, and yet there is little or no fixation of complement: in such cases, the union of antibody brings about abnormalities in the metabolism of the red cells, and as a result they age more rapidly than normal cells and become prematurely susceptible to the normal phagocytic process responsible for red cell destruction. Red cells coated with IgG or IgM antibodies also tend to agglutinate, particularly where the circulation is sluggish, as in the sinuses of the spleen, and this probably increases their susceptibility to phagocytosis by splenic macrophages.

Red cells which have become coated with antibody may also be injured by subsequent fixation of complement: this is the rule with antibodies of IgM class, and occurs in some instances with IgG antibodies. It is not fully understood why this latter type of antibody mediates complement fixation in some instances and not in others, but it probably depends, at least in part, on the spacing of the particular antigenic determinant sites on the surface of the cell, for it is known that IgG antibody will not fix complement unless two or more antibody molecules react with closely adjacent sites on the cell surface.

Fixation of complement is an elaborate process involving the sequential activation and reaction of a number of complement factors (at present termed C1–C9). Completion of these reactions is accompanied by a disruptive effect upon the cell surfaces, seen by electron microscopy as holes of approx. 10mμ in the cell membrane (Fig. 1.7, p. 8); in consequence, the cell membrane becomes abnormally permeable and so loses its selective role in the maintenance of the normal environment within the cell. The damaged red cells become spherocytic and haemoglobin leaks out into the plasma (*intravascular haemolysis*): the "ghosts" of the lysed red cells are presumably phagocytosed by cells of the reticulo-endothelial system. A second possible effect of complement fixation, quite apart from cell lysis, is the enhancement of phagocytosis, although, as already stated, the attachment of antibody can promote phagocytosis without the participation of complement. The principles underlying the effect of antibody on living nucleated cells (and on bacteria), and the action of fixed complement, appear to be similar to those outlined above for red cells: antibody alone may interfere with cell metabolism and enhances phagocytosis, while complement fixation kills the cell directly and may also further enhance phagocytosis.

Immune-complex, Arthus-type (type III) reactions

These result from the union of antigen and antibody *in vivo*, to form complexes which are deposited within the walls and lumina of blood vessels. Their occurrence is therefore dependent on the simultaneous presence within the body of antigen and the corresponding antibody. The ensuing tissue injury is an acute inflammation with massive infiltration of neutrophil polymorphonuclear leukocytes, and it may progress to thrombosis, haemorrhage and necrosis; much of the reaction is mediated by the enzymes of complement which are activated and released during the process of fixation of complement to antigen–antibody complexes.

The Arthus reaction is observed when an animal already immunised by injection of foreign protein, e.g. heterologous plasma albumin, and which has developed a high level of circulating antibody, is injected locally, e.g. into the skin, with a small amount of the same foreign protein. Within an hour or so, the injection site becomes red and swollen and this increases for 12 hours or so, after which it subsides slowly. If there is a very high level of circulating antibody, the reaction may be more severe, with haemorrhages and necrosis. Microscopy shows hyperaemia of the small vessels, inflammatory oedema, haemorrhages, and migration of very large numbers of neutrophil polymorphs into the walls of venules and the surrounding tissues. The development and progress of the reaction in the rabbit and other animals have been studied microscopically in the living tissues. The sequence of events is closely similar to that of acute inflammation, but with particularly marked aggregation of neutrophil polymorphs which not only adhere to the endothelium and migrate through the walls of the venules in large numbers, but also, together with platelets, form aggregates which obstruct the flow in some of the venules. When necrosis occurs, it is also seen first, and is most marked, in the walls of venules. Many of the polymorphs which migrate into the affected tissues degenerate rapidly, and their cytoplasmic granules are disrupted.

The mechanism of the Arthus reaction has been elucidated by several techniques. Firstly, the presence of antigen–antibody complexes in the walls of venules, deep to the endothelium, has been demonstrated by immunofluorescence techniques (see p. 80), and phagocytosis of these by neutrophil polymorphs has been observed. Secondly, it has been shown that temporary depletion of neutrophil polymorphs, brought about, for example, by administration of nitrogen mustard, very greatly diminishes or delays the severity of the inflammatory reaction. Thirdly, it has been shown that complement is fixed by the antigen-antibody complexes, and that the reaction may be greatly diminished by various procedures which reduce considerably the level of complement in the plasma. As complement fixation proceeds (p. 103), certain products of the reaction of its components are generated which are of importance in inducing the inflammatory reaction characteristic of the Arthus phenomenon. For example, substances known as *anaphylatoxins* are produced, probably derived from C3 and C5, which increase vascular permeability by effecting the release of histamine from mast cells. (The term anaphylatoxin is unfortunate as it suggests, quite wrongly, a relationship with anaphylaxis.) The products of complement fixation also include factors which are chemotactic for neutrophil polymorphs. From these observations, it appears that the Arthus reaction is triggered off by the formation of antigen–antibody complexes in the walls of venules; complement reacts with the complexes, and this releases pharmacologically active substances which bring about the features of acute inflammation (Fig. 5.5). Many of the neutrophil polymorphs which take part in the reaction are killed and their granules are disrupted, thus releasing lysosomal enzymes which presumably add to the tissue injury.

Serum sickness. This is a condition which results from injection of foreign protein, and was commonly observed in the days when heterologous (usually horse) antitoxic whole serum, or crude preparations of serum globulins, were administered to confer passive immunity to diphtheria, tetanus, etc. Provided the subject has not previously received an injection of serum from a donor of the same or a closely related species, the injection is without immediate harmful effect, but after 7–10 days antibody to the foreign protein appears in the plasma, and if sufficient antigen (foreign serum protein) has been injected for it to be still present in the plasma, then antigen–antibody complexes will be formed in the circulation (Fig. 5.6). At first antigen will be present in relative excess, and in these circumstances the complexes are usually small, i.e. composed of only a few antibody and antigen molecules: within a few days, however, antibody will have increased and will soon be present in relative excess, and the complexes will then usually form large aggregates (Fig. 5.7). The lesions of serum sickness result from the subendothelial deposition of circulating antigen–antibody complexes in the walls of blood vessels, and experimental animal studies have shown that it is the relatively small complexes, forming in antigen excess, which are deposited. The lesions therefore develop during the second week after the initial injection and thereafter subside.

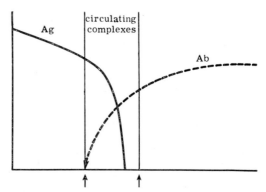

FIG. 5.6.—The formation of antigen–antibody complexes in the circulation. Injection of antigen is followed after some days by the appearance of antibody in the plasma: during the next few days, the concentration of antigen falls sharply and antigen–antibody complexes are present in the serum.

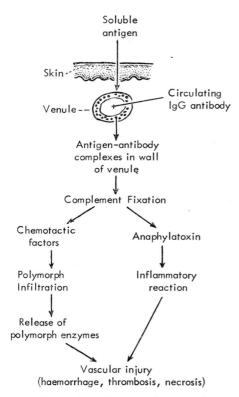

FIG. 5.5.—Mechanism of the Arthus reaction. Local injection of soluble antigen into an animal with a high plasma level of the corresponding antibody of IgG class results in union of antigen and antibody in the walls of venules. Complement reacts with the antigen–antibody complexes, and reaction products of complement induce inflammation and polymorph infiltration. The release of polymorph enzymes brings about vascular and tissue injury.

Deposition of complexes can occur not only in arteries, veins and capillaries in serum sickness, but also in the endocardium, and is accompanied by acute inflammatory change with swelling of the endothelium, inflammatory oedema, neutro-

phil leukocytic infiltration, and sometimes haemorrhage and necrosis. These changes are brought about in a way closely similar to the inflammatory changes of the Arthus reaction (p. 104), mainly by fixation of complement onto the deposited complexes and production of anaphylatoxins and chemotactic factors during the activation of complement.

The factors determining whether or not circulating complexes are deposited in vessel walls, and the sites of their deposition, are not fully understood. In rabbits, complexes formed *in vitro* and injected intravascularly are not deposited to anything like the same extent as complexes formed *in vivo*. However, complex deposition and the production of vascular lesions in serum sickness can be largely prevented by administering antagonists to histamine and to 5-hydroxytryptamine, and it appears that when antigen–antibody complexes are formed in the blood stream (as in serum sickness) they fix

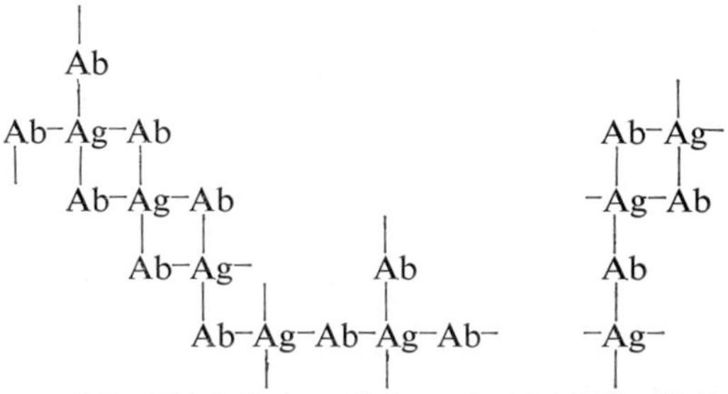

FIG. 5.7.—The influence of the ratio of antigen (Ag) and bivalent (IgG) antibody (Ab) concentrations on the size of the antigen–antibody complexes. Left, part of a large complex found when Ag and Ab are present in equivalent proportions, or when antibody is in excess. In antigen excess (right) small complexes are formed.

larger amounts of complement than do complexes formed *in vitro* and subsequently injected. It is probable that the anaphylatoxins formed during complement fixation play a major role in increasing vascular permeability by releasing histamine and other agents from mast cells or platelets (p. 104) and that the increased permeability allows deposition of the complexes in vessel walls. There is evidence that complexes may fix complement more actively when deposited in vessel walls than when in the circulation; presumably fixation of complement continues at the site of such deposits and thus contributes to the focal inflammatory reactions of serum sickness. Another possible factor in the deposition of circulating complexes is the development of reagin-type antibody capable of attaching to mast cells and of causing them to release histamine, on reacting with the corresponding antigen. Antibody of this type is produced by various species of animals, including man, and it has been noted that serum sickness tends to occur particularly in individuals who, because of a special predisposition to reagin production, suffer from atopy (p. 99), and that it is often accompanied by features of atopy, e.g. bronchospasm, urticarial rash.

So far, this account of Arthus-type reactions has been confined to lesions resulting from the administration of foreign antigens, but the refinement of antitoxins, etc., has greatly diminished the danger of Arthus reactions and of serum sickness, and the importance of this type of hypersensitivity now lies largely in the increasing evidence that, in both animals and man, immune complexes may form in the circulation under natural conditions and from administration of certain drugs, and may be responsible for the lesions of certain diseases. Most of the lesions regarded as being of this nature are in the glomeruli, and are discussed in Chapter 21; another condition which may be attributable to immune complexes is polyarteritis nodosa in which there is very recent evidence suggesting that in some cases the antigen is the SH-antigen of serum hepatitis (p. 558).

Delayed hypersensitivity (type IV) reactions

The *development* of delayed hypersensitivity is a part of the normal immune response to stimulation with various antigens, and as such is described in Chapter 4. The *outcome* of this type of response is the production of small lymphocytes which bear, on their surface, molecules resembling IgG and which, like antibodies, are capable of reacting specifically with the corresponding antigen.

Role of lymphocytes. In a delayed hypersensitivity *reaction*, the lymphocytes release soluble factors which have various effects, including (a) lymph-node permeability factor,* which causes an increase in vascular permeability, resulting in inflammatory oedema; (b) a factor which is chemotactic for other (non-sensitised) lymphocytes; (c) a factor which stimulates proliferation of non-sensitised lymphocytes; (d) a factor which activates macrophages in such a way that, on encountering the antigen, they adhere to one another as though "sticky", and become lethal to bacteria and possibly viruses, which they have engulfed. The nature of these soluble factors released by lymphocytes is still largely unknown; nor is it known whether there are several distinct factors. Activation of macrophages is not solely a specific reaction, for delayed hypersensitivity to the tubercle bacillus can render macrophages lethal not only to tubercle bacilli but also to unrelated microorganisms. In addition to these effects, the sensitised lymphocytes can also react directly with and destroy target cells without the mediation of macrophages: for example in delayed hypersensitivity to transplanted foreign tissue, cells of the transplant may be destroyed by macrophages or lymphocytes. This lethal activity requires close contact between the lymphocyte or macrophage and target cell: its mechanism is not known.

Morphological changes. Delayed hypersensitivity reactions can occur in any part of the body where sensitised lymphocytes encounter the corresponding antigen. In eliciting such reactions, it is convenient to apply the antigen to the skin or, in experimental animals, to the skin or cornea, or to administer it by intradermal injections. The classical example of delayed hypersensitivity is the reaction to intradermal injection of tuberculoprotein (*Mantoux test*). In a non-sensitised individual this produces no local reaction, but in subjects who have been sensitised by a tuberculous infection or by BCG immunisation, the typical "delayed" inflam-

---

* So-called because it was first extracted from lymph nodes.

matory reaction appears within 12–24 hours and persists for 48 hours or more. The skin becomes reddened, and an indurated nodule develops: in a highly sensitised individual, the reaction may progress to necrosis and ulceration, but failing this it subsides within a few days. Microscopically, neutrophil polymorphs migrate into the tissues at the injection site within 2 hours or so, with some accompanying inflammatory oedema, but these changes are mild and the polymorphs disappear within 24 hours. After 6 hours, lymphocytes begin to accumulate in the capillaries and venules, and migrate into the surrounding tissues: this is accompanied by an increase in inflammatory oedema, probably attributable to release of lymph-node permeability factor (see above). At the height of the reaction there is intense accumulation of lymphocytes, together with some macrophages, both in and around the venules and capillaries, and particularly around the sweat glands and hair follicles of the dermis (Fig. 5.8): vascular dilatation, oedema and cellular infiltration account for the macroscopic appearance of the reaction. In experimental studies, in which delayed hypersensitivity to tuberculoprotein has been transferred by injecting lymphocytes from a sensitised to a non-sensitised animal, it has been shown that most of the lymphocytes aggregating at the site of injection of tuberculoprotein are of host origin, and only a small percentage are from the sensitised donor. It is thus apparent that most of the lymphocytes seen in the reaction cannot have become sensitised as a result of the original antigenic stimulus to the donor animal. It is possible that these cells have been attracted by a factor released by the sensitised donor cells on encounter with the antigen, but another possible explanation is suggested by the work of Lawrence et al. (1963) who provided evidence that delayed hypersensitivity can be transferred in man by a cell-free extract of lymphocytes from a sensitised individual. This *transfer factor* might conceivably attach to non-reactive lymphocytes and render them passively sensitised. It is also not known whether these host lymphocytes are "innocent bystanders" or whether they participate in the reaction. There is, however, some evidence that they may activate one of the later components of complement, C8, and that they release this in active form at the site of the reaction with the result that the cytotoxic effects of activated

complement are produced without the earlier steps of complement fixation having occurred.

Delayed hypersensitivity in infections. The effect of delayed hypersensitivity on bacterial and virus infections has not been fully evaluated. In the case of tuberculosis, there is no doubt that partial protection is afforded by a previous infection which has been overcome, or by immunisation with living attenuated *M. tuberculosis* (BCG), and that such protection is accompanied by a state of delayed hypersensitivity demonstrable by the Mantoux test. There is general agreement that antibody has little or no protective role in tuberculosis, and it is therefore likely that the protection is afforded by delayed hypersensitivity. However, there is evidence that guinea-pigs immunised by BCG may be at least partly desensitised by injections of tuberculoprotein without losing their protection: these studies are, however, neither quantitative nor conclusive, and in any case it is difficult to relate them to the human disease, for man has a much greater capacity for developing delayed hypersensitivity to tuberculoprotein than have experimental animals, including the guinea-pig.

While it seems likely that delayed hypersensitivity has a protective effect in tuberculous infection, there is no doubt that it is responsible also for tissue injury. The tubercle bacillus and its products have little or no direct toxic effect on cells, and macrophages in tissue culture may harbour them with little ill-effect unless sensitisation has occurred. Injection of relatively large amounts of tuberculoprotein into an individual already infected with (and sensitised to) tuberculosis brings about a local reaction at the injection site, a systemic reaction with fever, vomiting, malaise, dyspnoea and lymphopenia, and an acute inflammatory reaction at the site of pre-existing tuberculous lesions. These local, systemic and focal reactions are all attributable to delayed hypersensitivity. They are known collectively as the *Koch phenomenon* after Robert Koch, the German bacteriologist who discovered the tubercle bacillus in 1882, and who appreciated the importance of hypersensitivity in tuberculosis. Injection of similar amounts of tuberculoprotein into non-sensitised individuals produces no reaction. In the infected individual, it is likely that most if not all of the features of tuberculosis are attributable to delayed hypersensitivity: fever, malaise and weight loss are

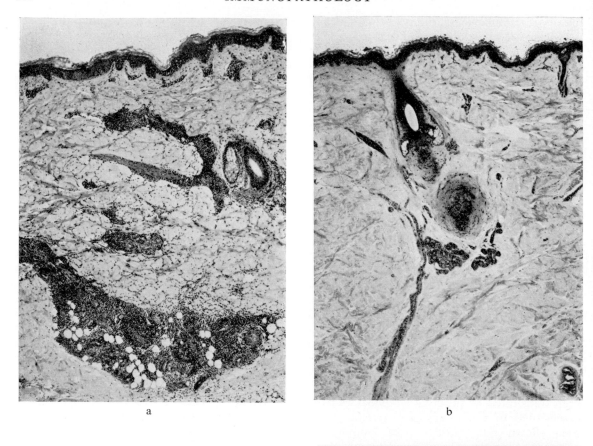

a   b

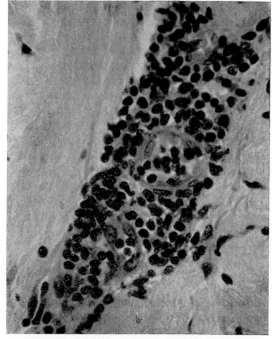

FIG. 5.8.—Positive (a) and negative (b) Mantoux tests. Note the heavy cellular infiltrate around the sweat glands and pilo-sebaceous units in a. This distribution is determined by the vascularity of the skin appendages. × 43. At higher magnification (c), the infiltrating cells are seen to be lymphocytes which are aggregated in and around the capillaries and venules. × 540. (Dr. Janet Niven.)

c

explicable as the systemic reaction, while the features of the lesions—aggregation of macrophages and lymphocytes and necrosis (p. 107)—are all explicable in terms of a localised delayed hypersensitivity reaction. Nevertheless, the delayed hypersensitivity reaction also destroys the bacteria and tends to limit their spread.

Delayed hypersensitivity develops in most bacterial, viral and fungal infections, but in many instances it is accompanied by antibody production, and this often dominates the immunological reaction, particularly in the acute infections. However, delayed hypersensitivity is of particular importance in fungal and chronic bacterial infections: it is well-developed in syphilis and tuberculoid leprosy. Children with congenital agammaglobulinaemia (p. 114), who are incapable of significant antibody responses, are adequately protected by delayed hypersensitivity against the common virus diseases, tuberculosis and fungal infections, etc., but suffer from repeated acute infections, particularly those caused by pyogenic bacteria. The fact that such children recover normally from virus infections, and develop resistance to reinfection, strongly supports the view that delayed hypersensitivity is an important mechanism of eliminating virus infections.

Other examples of hypersensitivity reactions in which delayed hypersensitivity is believed to play a major role are certain of the so-called auto-immune diseases, and the reaction which results in the rejection or destruction of allogeneic or heterogeneic tissue transplants: these are discussed on pp. 110–113.

It is possible also that delayed hypersensitivity reactions are concerned in the lesions of sarcoidosis (p. 152) and for the florid granulomatous reaction sometimes observed around particles of talc embedded in the tissues (p. 45).

Hypersensitivity to drugs and chemicals

Insofar as hypersensitivity of all types develops as a result of antigenic stimulation, antigenic compounds must be involved in all instances. However, hypersensitivity may develop to any of a large number of chemical compounds which are of small molecular size and therefore would not be expected to induce an immune response. There is little doubt that agents of this sort stimulate hypersensitivity by acting as haptens (p. 76) which combine chemically with normal proteins within the body; such complexes are then capable of stimulating an immune response, resulting in production of antibodies or sensitised lymphocytes specifically reactive with the hapten. The type of hypersensitivity reaction which results will then depend on the nature of the immune response, the particular cell or tissue constituent with which the hapten has complexed, the route of administration and dose, etc. In individuals with a tendency to anaphylaxis, reaginic antibodies may develop, and further administration of the hapten can then induce an anaphylactic (type I) reaction, e.g. asthma or hay fever if the hapten is in the form of a gas, vapour, or airborne suspension, an immediate inflammatory reaction if it is applied locally, or a generalised reaction if a large amount of hapten is absorbed by any route. Anaphylactic reactions to penicillin and related compounds are not uncommon, and have resulted in a number of deaths: in most instances the hypersensitivity is directed towards the penicilloyl degradation product of penicillin. The development of IgG class antibody to a haptenic drug or chemical can give rise to local reactions of Arthus type (type III) when the hapten is localised to one particular area within the tissues, or can lead to formation of complexes of hapten and antibody within the plasma, which is liable to produce features closely resembling those of serum sickness. Thirdly, a hapten may complex with a particular type of cell, e.g. red cells or platelets (p. 102), when antibody may develop which has a cytotoxic effect on the cells concerned. An example of a type II reaction of this sort is provided by "Sedormid purpura" (p. 102).

Lastly, a delayed hypersensitivity response may develop towards the hapten–protein complex, and, as described above, subsequent absorption of the haptenic compound gives rise to a delayed hypersensitivity (type IV) reaction. This occurs, for instance, in *contact dermatitis* in which relatively simple chemicals behave as haptens: they are absorbed into the body, often through the skin, and combine with tissue proteins. Delayed hypersensitivity develops against the modified proteins, and subsequent skin contact with the same chemical induces a delayed hypersensitivity reaction (Fig. 5.9), causing inflammatory lesions with cellular infiltration, predominantly lymphocytic, and

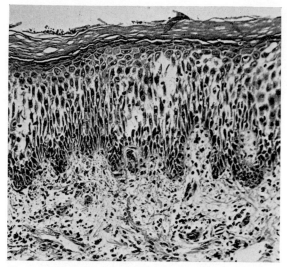

FIG. 5.9.—Contact dermatitis. Note oedema of epidermis and perivascular infiltration of lymphocytes in the dermis. The patient had developed hypersensitivity to chromium salts used as a hardener in cement. × 110.

oedema which affects both the dermis and epidermis and progresses to formation of vesicles. The substances capable to inducing this condition are very numerous, and include particularly chemicals which combine firmly with proteins, e.g. dyes, chrome salts, formalin and various derivatives of benzene. Reactions which appear to be of this type occur commonly in women in relation to nickel fasteners on underclothes, some of the nickel being dissolved by acid sweat and absorbed presumably as nickel salts which can combine with skin proteins. Contact with poison ivy is another common cause in North America, and cases also occur from the use of hair dyes, such as paraphenylene diamine, which, of course, bind firmly to keratin. Contact dermatitis results also from application of various medicaments to the skin. It is noteworthy that any individual can be sensitised to various chemicals, and contact dermatitis can thus be induced, but nevertheless some people appear to develop it more readily than others. This is seen in the use of various adhesive dressings which usually produce no reaction but in some instances lead to contact dermatitis, and a similar effect may result from wearing rubber face masks.

It is important to appreciate that the above account is an oversimplification. In many instances, hypersensitivity to drugs or chemicals is extremely complex and the clinical features often conflict with the results of the various available tests for hypersensitivity. With the ever-increasing number of chemicals used therapeutically and in industry, it is not surprising that hypersensitivity reactions, particularly those manifested in the skin and mucous membranes, are becoming increasingly common. It is not yet possible to state what properties of a substance are related to the likelihood of its stimulating the development of hypersensitivity, nor to predict which individuals are likely to develop it.

Auto-immune hypersensitivity reactions

There are now a number of diseases in which the development of auto-immunity, i.e. of an immune response against normal body constituents, is known to play a part. In some instances, the pathogenic role is attributable to auto-antibodies, while in others, it is suspected that the lesions represent delayed (auto-) hypersensitivity.

The role of cytotoxic auto-antibodies in bringing about injury of cells of the blood and platelets by type II reactions has already been discussed (p. 102). A further example of a type II auto-immune disease is provided by the experimentally-produced *nephrotoxic auto-antibody nephritis*, which is induced by immunising injections of basement membrane material: the resulting antibody reacts with the animal's own glomerular capillary basement membrane, producing a form of glomerulonephritis. This condition, and similar lesions in man, are considered further in Chapter 21. Recent advances in the understanding of the etiology of *thyrotoxicosis* (Graves' disease) are of considerable interest, for they suggest that this condition is caused by a type II hypersensitivity reaction in which auto-antibody of IgG class reacts specifically with elements of thyroid epithelial cells. It has an effect similar to that of thyroid-stimulating hormone, inducing hyperplasia and increased secretory activity: it is doubtful whether an antibody with these effects can justifiably be termed cytotoxic, although there is no doubt as to the harmful effect produced on the individual by this disease (p. 886).

A good example of an immune-complex (type III) reaction resulting from auto-antibody is provided by *systemic lupus erythematosus* (SLE), in which antibodies develop which react with normal cellular constituents. In patients with this disease, and in hybrid (NZB × NZW) mice, which develop a similar disease, it has been demonstrated that antibody to DNA is sometimes detectable in the plasma, while at other times the detection of free DNA has been reported. Immunofluorescence studies on the diseased glomeruli in affected mice and men have shown the presence of deposits of IgG, and it is likely that these represent antigen–antibody complexes, for DNA, anti-DNA and fixed complement have similarly been demonstrated in the deposits. These lesions, and other examples of glomerular injury which may result from antigen–antibody complexes, are also described in Chapter 21.

Systemic lupus erythematosus is one of an ill-defined group of conditions, termed the **connective tissue diseases,** in which auto-antibodies to various cellular constituents occur in the serum. In addition to anti-DNA, auto-antibodies to other nuclear constituents (Fig. 5.10), and to various cytoplasmic constituents of most or all types of cells, may be found. The antibodies are most commonly present, and most numerous, in SLE itself, but not one of them is invariably present in all cases. In rheumatoid arthritis, the commonest member of the group, the so-called rheumatoid factor

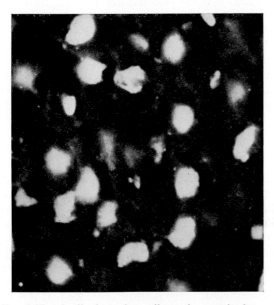

Fig. 5.10.—Antibody to deoxyribonucleoprotein demonstrated by the immunofluorescence technique. Note the diffuse nuclear fluorescence. × 775. (Professor J. Swanson Beck.)

(p. 795) is often demonstrable. It is an IgM antibody which reacts weakly with native IgG, including the patient's own, and more strongly with IgG which has been modified by heat or by attachment to particulate material: it reacts strongly also with IgG antibody complexed with the corresponding antigen (e.g. red cells). There is considerable overlap in both the immunological and the pathological features of the connective tissue diseases; the significance of the various auto-antibodies, and also the etiology of these conditions, are obscure.

Finally, there is the group of **organ-specific auto-immune diseases** in which chronic inflammatory destructive changes in a particular organ are accompanied by the development of auto-immunity to constituents of that organ. The group is exemplified by *chronic thyroiditis*, in which the thyroid gland becomes infiltrated with lymphocytes, plasma cells and macrophages, and there is destruction and fibrosis of the thyroid tissue. Auto-antibodies reacting with various components of thyroid tissue are commonly demonstrable in the serum, but their titres do not correlate closely with the severity and extent of the disease process. As already mentioned, it is probable that thyrotoxicosis is an organ-specific auto-immune disease, mediated by a thyroid-stimulating antibody. Chronic thyroiditis may be induced in animals by administering immunising injections of thyroid tissue preparations incorporated in Freund's adjuvant (p. 83), and from observations made on such animals it appears likely that the thyroid lesion in man is attributable to either delayed hypersensitivity alone, or the combined effects of delayed hypersensitivity and auto-antibody. Similar conditions, accompanied in some cases by organ-specific auto-antibodies, may affect the acid-secreting area of the gastric mucosa, producing *atrophic gastritis* and in some cases *pernicious anaemia*; the cortex of the adrenal glands, causing adrenocortical insufficiency (*Addison's disease*); and the parathyroid glands, leading to "*idiopathic*" *hypoparathyroidism*. In all these diseases, and possibly in certain others, the injury appears likely to be brought about mainly by delayed hypersensitivity. The nature of the defect which leads to auto-immunisation in these conditions is not understood. Clearly there is a breakdown of immunological tolerance to normal body constituents, and the fact that the diseases in this group tend to accompany one another, and to occur in related individuals, suggests that genetic factors are concerned which predispose to abnormal reactivity on the part of the recirculating lymphocytes (p. 86) responsible for delayed hypersensitivity reactions and production of certain antibodies.

The features of the various auto-immune diseases are considered in more detail in the later, systematic chapters.

Rejection of transplanted (grafted) tissues

The treatment of burns by skin grafting is a well-established procedure. The epidermis of autologous grafts extends to cover the denuded area and survives indefinitely, while a graft from another individual becomes established, but invariably undergoes necrosis within two or three weeks. Evidence that this rejection process is mediated by an immunological reaction on the part of the host was first provided by Gibson and Medawar (1943) working in Glasgow. This has since been amply confirmed and the basis of the immunology of transplantation has been established in a beautiful series of experimental studies by Medawar and his colleagues. It is now known that tissue antigens, termed *transplant antigens*, are present on the surface membrane of most, if not all types of nucleated cells, and that these are determined genetically. In man and randomly bred animals, genetic heterogeneity is such that the tissues of one individual are extremely unlikely to be completely compatible with a second individual and accordingly allografts are invariably rejected unless the immunological responsiveness of the host can be suppressed. Grafts between monozygotic twins provide an exception to this rule: being genetically identical, both twins have the same transplant antigens, and grafts between them survive indefinitely. Other exceptions relating to certain tissues and certain transplantation sites are mentioned below.

It is apparent from the investigations of Medawar and others that the rejection of grafts is brought about in most instances by a delayed hypersensitivity reaction. The transplant antigens of the graft cells stimulate the development of a delayed hypersensitivity response in the host, and specifically reactive lymphocytes appear in the blood and migrate into the grafted tissue where they set up a delayed hypersensitivity reaction which destroys the graft (p. 106). If, however, the host has already developed antibodies to transplant antigens of the graft at the time of grafting, as may result from a previous graft, from blood transfusion or from immunisation to fetal transplant antigens during pregnancy, then the antibodies may react with the graft and bring about vascular lesions which result in immediate ischaemia and necrosis of the graft. The mechanism of this effect is not understood, and recent reports indicate that, under certain experimental conditions, antibody to the graft may actually delay or prevent its rejection by the host, a phenomenon which is termed *enhancement*.

Renal transplantation. The success of renal transplantation depends very largely upon immunosuppression of the host by glucocorticoids, azathioprine, etc. These agents are cytotoxic, and suppress the host's capacity to develop delayed hypersensitivity responses. Accordingly, he is unduly susceptible to infections, both by common pathogens and by "opportunistic" micro-organisms (p. 154). Immediately following transplantation, large doses of immunosuppressants are necessary to prevent graft rejection, but the dose can be reduced gradually, in some instances to very low levels, and this suggests that the host has developed a degree of immunological tolerance to the transplant antigens of the graft.

Another approach to the avoidance of graft rejection is to select a kidney donor with relatively few transplant antigens incompatible to the host. This involves tissue typing the recipient and potential donors, i.e. determining which transplant antigens are present in their respective cells, and selecting the least incompatible donor. Since human red cells do not have demonstrable transplant antigens on their surface, leukocytes are usually used for typing, and antisera are obtained from individuals who have developed antibodies from previous grafting, pregnancy or blood transfusion. The transplant antigens are numerous and complex, and specific antisera are in short supply; accordingly, tissue typing is still a somewhat crude method of matching recipient and donor. Nevertheless, there is some evidence that it is of value, and that a well matched graft is less liable to induce severe rejection reactions than a poorly matched one.

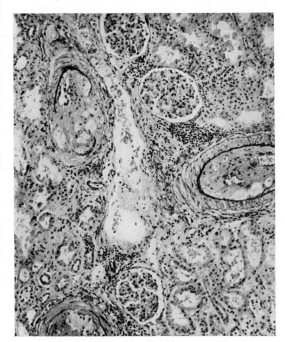

Fig. 5.11.—Chronic rejection of a human renal allotransplant. Note the obliterative arterial changes and disruption of the arterial walls. (Professor K. A. Porter.)

The pathological changes of rejection of a grafted kidney are complex, and not fully understood. In acute rejection, immunoblasts (p. 87) accumulate in and around the peritubular capillaries, accompanied by haemorrhage and tubular necrosis. In human allotransplants this is unusual owing to immunosuppression, and necrosis and thrombosis of arterioles is more common. In chronic rejection, vascular obliteration (Fig. 5.11) is often prominent, and after some years, thickening of the glomerular capillary basement membrane may develop (Porter, 1966).

Immunological rejection of the transplant is not, of course, the only problem in renal transplantation. Liability of the immunosuppressed host to infections has already been mentioned. Another difficulty, which complicates the use of cadaver kidneys, is the rate at which degenerative changes take place in the kidney following death of the donor. In spite of these and other problems, the results of renal transplantation are most encouraging, although the procedure has not been widely used for long enough to assess the long-term results.

Transplantation of other tissues. Successful *corneal allografting* has long been practised without immunosuppression of the recipient. This is because the cornea is avascular and therefore a "protected site" in which the graft does not induce an immune response in the recipient. If, as sometimes happens, blood vessels extend into the grafted cornea, then rejection occurs.

In allografts of *blood vessels* and *tendon*, the cells either die from ischaemia or are destroyed by a rejection reaction, but the collagen and elastic fibres persist, and are repopulated with host cells and vessels: thus the use of stored vessel or tendon is equally, if not more effective. Similarly, the cells of *bone grafts* die, but the matrix may provide the desired mechanical effect (p. 65). The use of *cartilage grafts* in plastic surgery is of considerable interest: both the cells and the matrix of allografts may survive for long periods without inducing a rejection reaction. This is due to the avascular nature of cartilage, and to the matrix which allows diffusion of nutrients and metabolites between graft chondrocytes and host, but acts as an "immunological barrier" between them.

The transplant antigens are not demonstrable on the surface of human red cells, and are distinct from the ABO, Rh, etc. iso-antigens. Blood transfusion may, however, result in the development of antibodies to transplant antigens derived from leukocytes and platelets in the transfused blood.

Another exception to the general phenomenon of allograft rejection is provided by nature's allograft, pregnancy. The trophoblast, of fetal origin, is bathed in maternal blood, and yet it is tolerated for nine months, in spite of the presence of incompatible (paternal) transplant antigens in the fetal cells. There is no significant depression of maternal immune responsiveness during pregnancy, nor does the mother develop specific immunological tolerance to the fetus. The most likely explanation of failure to reject the fetus appears to be that the cells of the syncytiotrophoblast are coated with a layer of mucopolysaccharide, which provides an "immunological barrier". As already mentioned, pregnancy commonly results in the development of maternal antibodies to the transplant antigens of the fetus, but this is without apparent effect.

IMMUNOLOGICAL DEFICIENCY STATES

There are a large number of conditions in which the normal defence mechanisms against invasive micro-organisms are impaired. For most purposes it is useful to classify such deficiencies into two major groups. Firstly, deficiencies of non-specific resistance, as in diabetes, malnutrition, impaired function of neutrophil polymorphs (p. 396), etc. This miscellaneous group is dealt with under the appropriate diseases: it includes also lesions which impair resistance locally, for example obstruction of hollow viscera, as in the urinary tract or air passages, and ischaemia of the lower limb leading to gangrene.

In the second major group, which is discussed below, impaired resistance is due to defects in specific immunological responsiveness. These are best classified into primary and secondary types, and also in relation to the type of immunological defect present.

In the group of *primary conditions*, the immunological deficiency becomes manifest usually, but not always, in early childhood, and in most of the conditions there is good evidence that the defect is genetically determined. Other abnormalities, e.g. thrombocytopenia in the Wiskott–Aldrich syndrome, or hypoparathyroidism in the Di George syndrome, may accompany the immunological defect, giving rise to characteristic disease complexes, but the immunological deficiency is not secondary to the other parts of the syndrome. By contrast, the *secondary immunological deficiencies* occur at any age, are not genetically-determined, and the immunological defects are the result of injury to the lymphoid tissues, either by various disease processes, particularly lymphoid neoplasia, or by immunosuppressive agents.

The type of immunological defect present is of major importance, for it determines the clinical picture and the effectiveness of therapeutic administration of immunoglobulins. The division of the lymphoid tissues and cells, and of immune responses, into two major classes, namely those which are dependent on the presence of a normal thymus, and those which are independent of the thymus, has been dealt with in Chapter 4. Such a division is based largely on experimental studies in animals, and in man its validity is demonstrated mainly by the features of the different immunological deficiencies, particularly those of the primary type. There is thus a group of conditions in which thymic function is not seriously suppressed, and in which the defect appears to reside mainly in the thymic-independent system; consequently there is deficient production of antibodies in response to most or all antigenic stimuli, while delayed hypersensitivity responses are relatively normal. In a second group of conditions, the thymic-dependent system is mainly at fault, and delayed hypersensitivity responses are severely impaired or absent, while antibody responses to some antigenic stimuli are normal, and others (the thymic-dependent antibody responses) are deficient. In a third group of conditions, there is deficiency of both the thymic-dependent and the thymic-independent systems, and failure of both delayed hypersensitivity and antibody production.

Examples of immunological deficiency which support the above scheme are given below, but it must be emphasised that there are other, less well-defined syndromes, in which the nature of the deficiency is not yet understood.

Primary immunological deficiencies

(1) Deficient antibody production. This group is exemplified by *infantile sex-linked agammaglobulinaemia*, which was the first to be described and is sometimes known as the *Bruton type of agammaglobulinaemia* after its discoverer. The major abnormality is a virtually complete inability to produce the three major classes of immunoglobulins—IgG, IgM and IgA. In consequence, there is little or no antibody production in response to infections or immunisation procedures, and the normal blood group iso-antibodies are usually not detectable. The condition is observed nearly always in boys, being transmitted by a gene defect in the X chromosome (sex-linked recessive). Symptoms usually arise in the second year of life, protection before that being provided by maternal antibodies of IgG class transmitted to the fetus. The defect results in unusually frequent and serious bacterial infections, particularly those due to the pyogenic bacteria, and including respiratory and pulmonary infections, meningitis and septicaemia. The infections respond to antibiotics, and diagnosis depends upon the demonstration of the near-absence of serum IgG (below 100 mg. per 100 ml.), IgM and IgA (below 3 mg. per 100 ml.). Deficiency of IgG cannot be demonstrated until the maternal IgG has fallen to a low level—usually about 8 months old, although very low levels of the other two immunoglobulins are observed before this time, since they do not cross the placenta.

The lymph nodes and tonsils are small, and biopsy reveals an absence of germinal centres and plasma cells, while plasma cells are also absent from the rectal mucosa. The thymus is normal, the blood lymphocytes are not reduced in number, and delayed hypersensitivity reactions are not impaired. Accordingly, the responses to BCG and vaccinial immunisation are normal and afford protection, and virus infections in general occur with the same frequency and clinical features as in normal children. However, boys with this condition are said to be particularly likely, as they grow older, to suffer from anaphylactic hypersensitivity, including infantile eczema, hay fever, asthma, and reactions to penicillin and other drugs; chronic polyarthritis closely resembling rheumatoid arthritis is also of common occurrence.

The effectiveness of regular injections of human IgG in preventing infections has increased the importance of early diagnosis. It is important to distinguish the Bruton type of agammaglobulinaemia, which requires life-long therapy, from *transient hypogammaglobulinaemia*. This latter condition presents similar clinical features and morphological changes in the lymphoid tissues, but is merely a delay, and not a permanent failure, of the capacity to produce immunoglobulins: it is familial, affects both sexes, and the defect disappears within the first three years of life. In most cases, severe immunoglobulin deficiency is limited to IgG, and normal levels of IgM and IgA in the serum may help to distinguish it from the Bruton type.

There are a number of less well-defined conditions which appear to fall within this group. In all of them, there is defective production of one or more classes of immunoglobulins, impairment of antibody production, and relatively normal delayed hypersensitivity responses. The evidence favouring a genetic predisposition, and a particular mode of genetic transmission, varies in the different types. In some forms, the immunological deficiency does not become manifest until adult life, and yet the disease tends to occur in families, and often exhibits a familial association with other immunological disturbances, e.g. hypergammaglobulinaemia and systemic lupus erythematosus. Some patients with such late-onset immunoglobulin deficiency also develop auto-immune diseases such as pernicious anaemia and connective tissue diseases, but without demonstrable auto-antibodies.

(2) Deficient delayed hypersensitivity responses. An example of this group is provided by the rare *Di George syndrome*, in which there is complete failure of development of the thymus, accompanied usually by absence of the parathyroids.

In those infants who survive the neonatal period, immunoglobulin production appears normal, although antibody responses, at least to some antigens, are impaired. The lymph nodes contain plasma cells and germinal centres, but the paracortical (thymic dependent) areas are deficient in small lymphocytes, and the number of circulating lymphocytes, although variable, is low in some cases. The condition may affect infants of both sexes, and there is no evidence for a genetic predisposition. Affected infants suffer from "*opportunistic*" infections, e.g. by *Pneumocystis carinii* and fungi (p. 154) and also from severe virus infections. Impairment of delayed hypersensitivity is demonstrable by failure to develop contact hypersensitivity to agents such as dinitrochlorobenzene (p. 110) and immunisation with live vaccines is liable to give rise to fatal generalised infections. The condition itself is a fatal one, but in a few instances life has been prolonged by transplantation of thymic tissue and bone marrow.

(3) Combined immunological deficiency. In *alymphocytic agammaglobulinaemia*, sometimes termed the *Swiss type of agammaglobulinaemia*, both the thymic-dependent and -independent immunity systems fail to develop. The thymus is hypoplastic and deficient in Hassall's corpuscles and small lymphocytes, the lymph nodes are extremely small and lacking in germinal centres, lymphocytes and plasma cells, and circulating lymphocytes are scanty. There is a near-absence of the three main classes of immunoglobulins from the serum, and both antibody production and delayed hypersensitivity are grossly defective. The condition is transmitted as an

E

autosomal recessive character, and affected infants show retarded growth, recurrent bacterial and virus infections, and response to antibiotics and chemotherapy is poor. Immunisation with living viruses is likely to prove fatal, and the condition usually results in death during the first or second year.

Secondary immunological deficiencies

These are conditions in which the immunity system and immunological responsiveness develop normally, but become defective as a result of injury to the lymphoid tissues by disease processes or immunosuppressive agents. Like the primary immunological deficiencies, the defect may affect mainly either antibody production or delayed hypersensitivity, or both types of response. In multiple myeloma and macroglobulinaemia (p. 440) antibody production is usually mainly affected, whereas in Hodgkin's disease, lepromatous leprosy, sarcoidosis and uraemia, delayed hypersensitivity is usually more severely depressed. In chronic lymphatic leukaemia, and also in patients with widespread lymphosarcoma, depression of both antibody production and delayed hypersensitivity is common. In all these conditions, there is involvement of the haemopoietic marrow and/or the lymphoid tissues, and replacement of these by the abnormal cells may account for the immunological defect, but the explanation may be more complex. For example, the rate of catabolism of immunoglobulins is increased in multiple myeloma, and in experimental mouse leukaemia immunological depression may precede the onset of leukaemia.

With the increasing use of immunosuppressive drugs—cortisone, azathioprine, cyclophosphamide, etc., and also radiotherapy, infections due to immunological deficiencies are becoming of greater importance, particularly as some of these agents may impair also the neutrophil polymorphs or macrophages, and the heavy immunosuppression sometimes necessary to prevent the rejection reaction is a common cause of fatal infections in the recipients of a renal transplant (p. 112).

CHAPTER 6

INFECTION:
HOST–PARASITE RELATIONSHIPS

By *infection* is meant the invasion of the tissues by living organisms. This must be distinguished from *contamination* which means the presence of organisms on the surfaces of the body, i.e. the skin and exposed mucous membranes, including those lining the gut and the upper respiratory tract. This distinction is also important in wounds. Infection may be caused by micro-organisms of many types and also by metazoan parasites.

Some difficulty arises over the distinction between contamination and infection as applied to the urinary and respiratory tracts, for bacteria may gain entrance to, and multiply within, the lumen of the bladder, and even extend up the ureters, without penetrating into the tissues; similarly they may extend down the bronchioles to the lung alveoli. Although such extension to these normally sterile parts of the body does not involve the penetration of the surface membrane, the micro-organisms have nevertheless broken through physiological barriers and their presence must be regarded as an infection. As a general rule, infection may thus be defined as the invasion by micro-organisms of parts of the body which are normally sterile.

For infection to occur, the micro-organisms must first make contact with the host, either directly with the surface of the body or by inhalation or ingestion, and must then proceed to penetrate into the tissues, and the factors concerned in this process of penetration provide the first major topic of this chapter. Following invasion, the microbes may be rapidly destroyed without causing obvious evidence of disease (inapparent infection) or they may multiply and produce clinical infection. Thirdly, virus infection, for example with herpes simplex, may persist for long periods without giving rise to disease. The factors determining which of these three possible courses will follow invasion form the second major topic of this chapter. The subject of infection is an enormous one, involving as it does a consideration of the host/parasite relationships which exist between man and numerous species of bacteria, viruses, rickettsiae, fungi, etc. The following account is limited to a brief outline of the subject.

It is necessary to define certain terms in common use in relation to infection. *Invasive capacity* indicates the capacity of a micro-organism to invade the tissues of the host, i.e. to establish an infection. *Pathogenicity* is the capacity to produce pathological changes in the host. A distinction is sometimes made between pathogenicity and *virulence*, but these terms are commonly used with the same meaning and both may be qualified to indicate various degrees of disease-producing capacity. *Commensal* is the term applied to an organism which is commonly present as a contaminant, e.g. on the skin or the pharyngeal mucosa of a particular species of host. In general, commensals are of low pathogenicity for a normal individual, although they may invade and cause disease under special circumstances. An example is provided by *Strep. viridans*, a normally harmless inhabitant of the mouth. Following extraction of teeth, it commonly appears in the blood but is eliminated rapidly without ill-effects. However, in individuals with abnormalities of the heart valves, it may settle and multiply in the abnormal cusps and cause the serious disease, subacute bacterial endocarditis.

Factors determining invasion

The skin and mucous membranes exposed to the environment are continuously contaminated by very many different types of micro-organisms present in expired droplets in the air, in dust particles, and in food and water. The skin and various mucous membranes on which these organisms may alight have properties which render them suitable for the survival and sometimes multiplication of certain organisms, but inhospitable to others. The requirements of a particular microbe for growth *in vitro* helps to explain its colonisation of particular parts of the surface of the body, but many of the factors determining such colonisation are still unknown, and indeed the predilection of certain bacteria for a particular host species is in some instances quite unexplained. There are, nevertheless, certain factors which are of great importance in limiting or preventing invasion by many types of organisms, and these must be considered briefly.

Barriers to invasion

(a) **Mechanical barriers.** The superficial keratinised layer of the epidermis is an excellent mechanical barrier to microbial invasion, and provided it is kept in a clean and dry state, direct invasion is extremely unlikely. Penetration may, however, occur when dirt is allowed to accumulate on the skin and particularly in moist warm areas subject to friction, such as the axillae and sub-mammary regions. In many skin diseases which result in exudation with loss or sogginess of the keratin layer, bacterial and fungal infections are common complications. The conjunctival, nasal, oral and gastro-intestinal mucosae, covered as they are by a film of mucous or serous secretion, also present a formidable barrier to most types of micro-organisms.

Mechanical injury to, or ulcerative lesions of, the skin and mucous membranes opens up pathways for bacterial invasion and are obviously important causes of infection, particularly when contaminated material is implanted below the surface. Burns are particularly liable to become heavily infected because the dead superficial tissue provides a good medium for streptococci, staphylococci, pyocyaneus and many other bacteria. Some parasitic organisms have evolved a life cycle in which they multiply in insect vectors and are introduced to man and other hosts by the insect bite. Examples include the protozoa which cause malaria, the metazoan filarial worms, and the virus of yellow fever, all of which are transmitted and injected by mosquitoes. *Pasteurella pestis*, the cause of bubonic plague (the Black Death), is transmitted by the flea of the black rat, and the rickettsiae which cause typhus by ticks, mites and lice. These organisms, themselves incapable of penetrating the skin barrier, have achieved a high degree of sophistication in their utilisation of biting insects as breeding grounds and vehicles and in some instances as "syringes". In the mouth, tooth extraction and tonsillectomy inevitably lead to bacterial infection, and tonsillectomy has been shown to predispose to invasion by the virus of poliomyelitis. The lesions resulting from certain vitamin deficiencies also impair the resistance to invasion. Thus in vitamin A deficiency the mucous membranes are affected, and in experimental animals the epithelium shows a remarkable change to squamous type. The lesions of the skin and mouth in scorbutic conditions, due to vitamin C deficiency, are also prone to infection.

(b) **Glandular secretions.** The secretions of glands opening onto the skin surface play an important role by maintaining the integrity of the layer, and also by providing an environment in which many types of bacteria cannot survive for long. The acidity of the sweat and the long-chain unsaturated fatty acids secreted by the sebaceous glands both exert a selective bactericidal effect, and consequently the bacterial flora of the skin surface tends to be rather constant: it has been shown that some types of pathogenic bacteria, when placed on the skin, are virtually all destroyed within an hour or two. The secretions of mucous membranes possess similar qualities. Lysozyme, an enzyme which digests polysaccharides of bacterial capsules, is present in high concentration in the lacrimal gland secretion and probably exerts an important protective effect in the conjunctival sac: it is secreted also by the salivary and nasal glands but in much smaller amounts. A modified form of IgA class of immunoglobulin is present in saliva, tears, intestinal contents, respiratory tract mucus, milk and urine (p. 79). Provided that IgA antibody has developed against a particular organism as a result of previous infection, it will be represented in these secretions. This is of importance in preventing invasion by certain viruses, for the virus may encounter the antibody in the surface mucus and be neutralised by it: its significance in relation to bacterial invasion is less certain, although there is evidence that union with IgA antibody may render bacteria more highly susceptible to the lytic action of lysozyme.

The acidity of the gastric juice is effective in killing most types of microbes ingested in food or water; but hypochlorhydria due to chronic gastritis is common, and minor illnesses and even emotional stresses can reduce temporarily the acidity of the juice. In general, those microbes which cause intestinal infections, such as the salmonellae and dysentery bacilli, are relatively acid-resistant. The parasitic amoeba *Entamoeba histolytica* produces cysts which resist the gastric juice and pass through the stomach before hatching out and invading the wall of the colon.

The normal acidity of the urine contributes to the defences of the urinary tract against infection. Also there appears to be a mechanism which eliminates bacteria in contact with the urinary tract epithelium, for it has been shown that when the mucosa of the rabbit's bladder is exposed and *Esch. coli* placed on its surface, the numbers of living bacteria diminish rapidly.

(c) Secretion currents. The continuous flow of tears over the surface of the conjunctiva has an important effect in the removal of contaminating bacteria, which are carried rapidly into the nasopharynx. In the nose and mouth also, the secretions covering the mucosa flow towards the pharynx and hence to the stomach, carrying with them residual food particles, bacteria, etc. The importance of the saliva is illustrated by the oral infections and severe dental caries which accompany loss of salivary secretion in Sjögren's syndrome (p. 477). The lacrimal secretion is also diminished, and conjunctival infections result. The importance of removal of contaminating bacteria by the saliva may explain the common occurrence of infection in the crypts of the tonsils and also in the periodontal sulci, for once bacteria gain entrance to these spaces, they are out of the main stream of salivary flow.

In the respiratory tract there is a continuous flow of mucus upwards over the surface of the bronchial and tracheal mucosa: inhaled particles are caught up and removed in this stream, and the air is almost sterile by the time it reaches the respiratory bronchioles. This defence mechanism is dependent on a normal production of mucous secretion and on the integrity of the cili-

ated respiratory epithelium. The virus of influenza parasitises the respiratory epithelium, interfering with its protective function; as a result, secondary bacterial infection invariably develops, and by extending into the alveoli may give rise to pneumonia. The integrity of the respiratory mucosa is also seriously impaired by chronic irritation, most commonly due to cigarette smoking but also to atmospheric pollution. This leads to metaplasia, the ciliated epithelium being replaced by goblet cells or squamous epithelium: there is increase in the amount of secretion, which also becomes more viscous, and this tends to stagnate and become infected.

The passage of intestinal contents is normally too slow to prevent the growth of contaminating pathogenic bacteria in its lumen, but if sufficient toxin is produced to injure and bring about an inflammatory reaction in the wall of the intestine, then increased peristalsis together with hypersecretion result in rapid and repeated evacuation of the gut and this helps to get rid of the offending bacteria.

The flow of urine is of importance in preventing growth and spread of any bacteria gaining entrance to the urinary tract by the urethra, and stagnation of urine resulting from urinary tract obstruction, particularly if partial and chronic, is complicated very commonly by infection.

(d) Bacterial commensals. In spite of the defence mechanisms described above, the skin, mouth, nasal cavity, conjunctival sac and intestines are all contaminated with bacteria of various types. The local environment provided by each of these various surfaces favours the survival of particular types of bacteria and thus each regional surface develops its own flora. Most of the commensals are non-pathogenic or of low pathogenicity, and they tend to prevent the establishment of other types of microbes, including pathogens, by competing for nutrients and by release of metabolic products which are toxic to other organisms. In normal circumstances the bacterial florae of the various surfaces are remarkably stable, but if they are disturbed, colonisation by pathogens may result: hence the common occurrence of fungal infections of the pharynx in patients on antibiotic therapy, and the overwhelming growth of resistant staphylococci in the intestines which may arise when the normal flora is depressed by broad-spectrum antibiotics.

(e) Phagocytes. There is evidence that phagocytic cells migrate onto the surface of various mucous membranes: for example neutrophil polymorphs pass through the thin epithelium lining the depths of the tonsillar crypts, and macrophages pass into the alveoli of the lungs. In both these sites the migrant cells have been shown to phagocytose particles on the surface of the mucosa and this may play a role in preventing invasion. It is possible, however, that the surface phagocytes may engulf living bacteria without killing them, and carry them back into the tissues. This has been suggested as of importance in aiding the invasion of the tonsils, lungs and intestine by *M. tuberculosis*.

Invasive capacity of micro-organisms

Micro-organisms vary greatly in their capacity to invade the host's defensive barriers. Some are virtually incapable of invasion and yet can produce disease. *Clostridium botulinum*, for example, is non-invasive to man—it grows in tinned or bottled foods which have been inadequately sterilised, and produces potent exotoxins which are absorbed from the gut. *Clostridium tetani* flourishes only in dead tissue, foreign material and exudate in wounds, and also produces serious toxic effects. *Vibrio cholerae* does not penetrate the basement membrane beneath the mucosal epithelium and yet produces a severe acute enteritis, and the corynebacteria of diphtheria remain superficially in the throat and produce a generalised toxaemia. Other organisms, and particularly some of the viruses, are very highly invasive and infect virtually all individuals who have not previously encountered or been immunised against them, e.g. the viruses of smallpox and poliomyelitis. A great many bacteria lie intermediate between these extremes in their invasive capacity. This applies to the more important pyogenic bacteria which are commonly present as contaminants in the nose or throat, or on the skin. Their presence carries a risk, but infection is by no means invariable.

In general, bacteria of high invasive capacity are also highly pathogenic, but there is little correlation between the invasive capacity and pathogenicity of viruses. For example, poliovirus invades readily but only a small proportion of infected individuals develops clinical disease, and non-pathogenic strains are administered orally to produce infection and immunity. Also

the protozoan *Toxoplasma gondii* is highly invasive and yet, apart from the lesions it causes in fetal life, it is of low pathogenicity.

Pathogenic effects of bacterial infection

Bacteria which have invaded the host tissues may be destroyed without causing clinically apparent disease, may produce a local inflammatory lesion, or may spread to other parts of the body and produce widespread lesions. The two major ways in which bacteria are known to produce pathological changes are, firstly, by the production of toxins, and secondly by promoting hypersensitivity reactions on the part of the host.

Bacterial toxins

These are of two main types, exotoxins and endotoxins.

Exotoxins are secreted by living bacteria: they are simple proteins, are often extremely potent, and vary considerably in their biological effects upon the host. They are antigenically specific and their biological activity is neutralised by union with antibody. Many pathogenic bacteria have been shown to produce a number of different exotoxins when cultured *in vitro*. Thus *Streptococcus pyogenes* and *Staphylococcus aureus*, two of the most important pyogenic bacteria, are capable of producing haemolysins, and hyaluronidases. *Strep. pyogenes* also produces a leukocidin which kills leukocytes, and *Staph. aureus* a coagulase which clots fibrinogen. Some exotoxins are injurious to virtually all types of host cell and their effects thus depend on their concentration and distribution. The diphtheria bacillus produces such a toxin and at the site of infection, usually the pharynx, it causes local tissue necrosis. Less florid but still severe cell injury is far more widespread and is reflected morphologically in fatty change of the parenchymal cells of the various organs: in severe cases, death may result from its effect upon the myocardium (Fig. 14.14, p. 307). The mechanism of injury by this particular toxin is known (p. 2): other toxins with a similar widespread effect are produced by many of the pathogenic Gram-positive bacteria but in most instances the mechanism of toxic action is not known. Some have enzymic activity, e.g.

phosphatases, proteases, lipases. Some bacteria produce toxins which act specifically on one type of tissue, e.g. the neurotoxins of *Cl. botulinum* interfere with the production of acetylcholine at cholinergic synapses in the peripheral nervous system, and cause a flaccid paralysis, while the neurotoxin of *Cl. tetani* has a contrasting effect on the synapses in the central nervous system, resulting in widespread tetanic muscular contractions in response to slight local stimuli.

Attempts to equate the pathogenic effects of a particular micro-organism with its toxins have encountered difficulties: not only are many toxins produced by a single strain of bacteria but different samples of a toxin, even in purified crystalline form, may have different biological properties. Also toxins vary greatly in their effects on hosts of different species, and experimental observations are not necessarily applicable to man. Finally, production or non-production of toxin in bacteria growing *in vitro* does not necessarily indicate a similar behaviour *in vivo*. It is a feature of exotoxins that their biological effects are neutralised by the corresponding antitoxin, and in some instances, e.g. diphtheria and tetanus, prior administration of the antitoxin or active immunisation by injection of *toxoid* (inactivated toxin which maintains its antigenicity) will protect animals against the effects of injection of the toxin and man against the disease. Thus in some instances, particular toxins have been incriminated beyond all reasonable doubt as the pathogenic agents responsible for the disease; in others, it seems most likely that toxins are responsible, but there remains the possibility that the bacteria may have other, at present unknown, pathogenic properties in addition to toxin production.

Endotoxins are structural elements of bacteria and are released only when the bacterium dies. To conform with clinical usage, the term "endotoxin" is restricted here to complex substances which contain phospholipid, polysaccharide and protein in their molecules, form part of the cell wall of Gram-negative bacteria, and have characteristic biological effects. The endotoxins produced by different Gram-negative bacteria are antigenically different but they all have the same biological effects and the active component is believed to reside in the lipid. Endotoxin is responsible for fever, intravascular conversion of fibrinogen to fibrin, vascular lesions and cellular necrosis in various organs. In small dosage it causes a neutrophil leukocytosis, in large amounts leukopenia. In severe Gram-negative bacterial infections, a state of shock develops with some or all of the above features and is termed "endotoxic shock" (p. 189). Because they produce fever, endotoxins are sometimes termed *pyrogens*. They are heat-stable and unless special precautions are taken are liable to contaminate apparatus and fluids to be used in parenteral therapy.

Hypersensitivity reactions to micro-organisms

Although specific immune responses to micro-organisms provide an essential defence mechanism against infections, they may lead also to tissue injury from hypersensitivity reactions, as described in Chapter 5. This is best known in relation to *Mycobacterium tuberculosis*, which has not been shown to produce toxins and can colonise cultures of macrophages without inducing obvious injury in them. If sensitised lymphocytes are added to the culture, macrophages which have ingested tubercle bacilli are rapidly destroyed. The lesions of tuberculosis appear to result mainly, if not entirely, from a delayed hypersensitivity reaction between sensitised lymphocytes and mycobacterial protein (p. 107). Without doubt the reaction is beneficial to the host in limiting the growth and spread of tubercle bacilli, but this occurs only at the expense of tissue injury. Another example of hypersensitivity in infection is provided by leprosy: in the lepromatous form of this disease the patient lacks delayed hypersensitivity to *M. leprae* and the lesions consist essentially of aggregates of macrophages containing enormous numbers of the bacteria. In patients who have developed delayed hypersensitivity to lepromin (an extract of lepromatous tissue) the lesions resemble those of tuberculosis, with necrosis and a granulomatous reaction, and they contain far fewer bacteria than in the lepromatous form of the disease. Delayed hypersensitivity develops in many other bacterial infections, for example in brucellosis, syphilis and typhoid fever, but it is probably less well developed in the acute pyogenic bacterial infections. It is of importance in fungal and viral infections and may contribute to the skin lesions in the acute virus exanthemata.

Other types of hypersensitivity also develop in bacterial infections. Anaphylactic (type I) reactions may occur in individuals genetically predisposed to produce IgE class of antibodies (p. 102). Arthus (type III) reactions are a possibility whenever IgG class antibody reacts with microbial antigens, and may contribute to the acute inflammatory reaction seen in many infections. However, antibodies tend to limit infection and thus reduce the associated acute inflammatory reaction and it is thus difficult to determine whether the Arthus reaction contributes significantly to the inflammatory response to infections. There is recent evidence that the severe form of dengue is due to reaction of viral antigen with circulating antibodies. Cytotoxic (Type II) hypersensitivity reactions may possibly result from microbial infections when the infecting micro-organism possesses antigenic similarity to a normal tissue constituent. A possible example is provided by rheumatic fever in which antibodies to *Strep. pyogenes* appear to react with constituents of heart muscle (p. 311).

The pathogenic effects of virus infections are considered on p. 131.

Defence mechanisms in infections

When micro-organisms have invaded the tissues, there are three major defensive reactions which tend to limit their multiplication and spread, and bring about their destruction: these are the inflammatory reaction, phagocytic activity, and specific immune responses.

The acute inflammatory reaction. The defensive role of this reaction has been considered in Chapter 2. Without doubt, it is of considerable importance, and those infections which are accompanied by acute inflammation at the site of invasion are more likely to remain localised than those in which invasion is accomplished without local injury or reaction. The pyogenic bacteria are a common cause of the former type of infection, while silent invasion is illustrated by *Treponema pallidum*, the cause of syphilis, which spreads widely through the body before the appearance of a local lesion at the site of entry. Other bacteria which may enter the body silently and spread widely include *Neisseria meningitidis*, a cause of acute meningitis, and brucellae, the cause of undulant fever. Many of the parasites transmitted by biting insects, such as the plasmodia which cause malaria, produce

generalised infection without a significant local reaction, and many viruses invade the body and produce viraemia without first producing local inflammation.

Chronic inflammatory change also plays a defensive role by surrounding the micro-organisms by a layer of granulation tissue which has been shown to be an effective barrier. In the more prolonged infections, such as tuberculosis, surviving micro-organisms may be effectively confined within a zone of dense fibrosis resulting from chronic inflammatory change.

Phagocytosis. A general account of the phagocytic process is given on p. 43, but some factors relating especially to phagocytosis of micro-organisms require consideration. Both neutrophil polymorphs and macrophages are capable of engulfing living micro-organisms and destroying them. This phagocytic activity depends partly upon the nature of the *surface coating of the microbe*, and in general is promoted by a protein covering. Thus smooth forms of bacteria, i.e. bacteria with a non-protein capsule, are not phagocytosed as readily as rough forms, which lack a non-protein capsule, and in testing the pathogenicity of bacteria grown in culture it is important to provide conditions conducive to capsule formation for that particular organism. A second important factor is *toxin production*: toxins are almost certainly responsible for positive chemotaxis which is, in turn, of importance in establishing contact between phagocytes and bacteria, and the toxins of many bacteria also have a stimulating effect on the production of neutrophil polymorphs in the bone marrow and their release into the blood (p. 124). A very high local concentration of toxin may, however, bring about injury to polymorphs and macrophages and inhibit their phagocytic activity. A third factor of importance in promoting phagocytosis is the *presence of cellular or tissue structures*. It appears that the phagocyte must first get the microbe "up against the wall" and accordingly phagocytosis occurs less readily in fluid unless, like pus, it is very rich in cells. Conversely, a fibrin coagulum aids phagocytosis.

Once they have been phagocytosed, living bacteria are likely to be destroyed, but this is no foregone conclusion, and many organisms not only survive, but may multiply within phagocytes, e.g. the tubercle and leprosy bacilli and the brucellae which cause undulant fever. Some protozoa, e.g. *Leishmania donovani* and *Histoplasma capsulatum*, also colonise phagocytes. These organisms are seen within macrophages rather than in the shorter-lived polymorphs, but phagocytosis of bacteria by polymorphs also is not necessarily bactericidal. In the case of pyogenic bacteria, there is commonly a high mortality rate among polymorphs which have ingested the bacteria. In spite of these bacterial triumphs, phagocytosis of microbes is commonly followed by their death. How this is effected is not yet known: it does not appear to be due directly to lysosomal enzymes, although these will digest the microbes once they have been killed (p. 44). In general, those bacteria which are less readily phagocytosed, e.g. smooth forms, tend also to resist destruction within the phagocyte. A factor of importance in promoting phagocytosis and in the destruction of phagocytosed micro-organisms is *the immune response*. Antibodies facilitate phagocytosis by acting as opsonins, and also by immobilising and agglutinating bacteria, rendering them easier prey to the phagocyte.

The immune response. In addition to its agglutinating and opsonic effects (p. 77), the union of IgG and IgM classes of antibody with micro-organisms is likely to be followed by fixation of complement, and this may result directly in the death of the organism or, failing this, have an additional opsonic effect and render the microbe more susceptible to destruction following phagocytosis. The development of delayed hypersensitivity also promotes destruction of bacteria for, as explained on page 106, encounter of sensitised lymphocytes (produced in the delayed hypersensitivity response) with the corresponding antigen is followed by release of a factor or factors with the following properties. (1) They are chemotactic to other lymphocytes; (2) they bring about vascular dilatation and exudation; (3) they render the macrophages mutually adhesive and immobile, and (4) they enhance the killing capacity of macrophages for ingested micro-organisms.

The complex inter-relationships between the defensive processes outlined above are of great interest and importance. For example, acute inflammation provides conditions favourable for emigration of leukocytes and phagocytic activity. It also promotes the transport of microbial antigens to the lymphoid tissues where they stimulate immune responses; acute inflammation also promotes contact of antibodies and sensitised cells with the infecting micro-organisms. The reaction of antibody or sensitised lymphocytes with micro-organisms or toxins can contribute to the inflammatory reaction (see above), while phagocytosis plays a role in the development of immune responses (p. 92).

A further mechanism of importance in the defence against viruses is the production of interferon (p. 132).

Diminished resistance to infection. There is a wide range of individual variation in the resistance to microbial invasion and infection among apparently normal individuals, and in most instances the explanation is not evident. There are also a number of disease states which impair the body's defences. Factors affecting the local resistance of the skin and mucous membranes to *invasion* have already been considered on pp. 118 *et seq*. Once invasion has occurred, the defence mechanisms may be depressed by a variety of conditions. For example, severe diminution in the production of neutrophil polymorphs in agranulocytosis (p. 396), or in various other diseases of the haemopoietic marrow, renders the patient highly susceptible to bacterial infections, while defects of polymorphs which impair their phagocytic and bactericidal functions (p. 396) have a similar effect. There are also many diseases which affect the capacity to develop specific immune responses against micro-organisms: these include the congenital immunological deficiency states (pp. 114–116) and also protein deficiency and various other diseases which involve the lymphoid tissues and interfere with their immunological functions. Patients with diabetes mellitus are unusually prone to bacterial infections, including staphylococcal lesions and tuberculosis. The explanation is not known, but lactic acid has been shown to be bactericidal to various bacteria *in vitro*, and it has been suggested that a similar effect is brought about *in vivo* by the relatively high concentration of lactic acid resulting from glycolytic activity of inflammatory cells. The impairment of glycolytic activity in uncontrolled diabetes may thus possibly result in reduced resistance to infection.

Two important reactions to infection are leukocytosis and fever, accounts of which are given below.

LEUKOCYTOSIS

Causes

Acute inflammatory lesions are commonly accompanied by an increase in the number of neutrophil polymorphs in the blood (Fig. 16.6, p. 396). This may be moderate, e.g. 10,000 per cubic mm., or may be in excess of 20,000. There is a corresponding rise in the *total* leukocyte count, although the proportion of neutrophil polymorphs does, of course, increase. In general the degree of leukocytosis correlates partly with the size of the acute inflammatory lesion and also with the intensity of polymorph emigration into the inflamed tissues. By far the most important cause of leukocytosis is bacterial infection, particularly when brought about by the pyogenic bacteria. In inflammatory reactions due to injury of tissue by physical agents, leukocytosis is not pronounced, and chemical agents vary in their capacity to induce it. Infection with virulent staphylococci, streptococci, pneumococci or coliform bacilli, etc. are all accompanied by a vigorous leukocytosis; other bacteria, e.g. *Clostridium welchii, Clostridium oedematiens*, cause severe acute inflammation but without intense leukocyte emigration, and leukocytosis is also less marked. In the acute inflammatory lesions of the intestine in typhoid and paratyphoid fever, polymorph emigration is virtually absent (Fig. 6.1), and the number of polymorphs in the blood usually falls to below the normal range (neutrophil leukopenia). There is a corresponding fall in the total leukocyte count, often to below 3,000 per cubic mm. The leukocytosis which occurs in pyogenic infections depends on the properties of the bacterial toxins, although it is not known whether they act directly or by stimulating endogenous mediators. Excessive toxaemia, even in infections which are usually pyogenic, may depress the bone marrow with consequent failure of leukocytosis, and even leukopenia. This is sometimes observed in pneumococcal pneumonia and is a bad prognostic sign. Injection of certain organic compounds produces a leukocytosis; for example, peptones, nucleoprotein, or breakdown products of DNA ("pentnucleotide") and it may be that the breakdown of neutrophil leukocytes themselves, as occurs on a large scale in pyogenic infections, stimulates leukocyte production. However, intravenous injection of bacterial proteins produces a leukocytosis, and the endotoxin of Gram-negative bacteria also has this effect if injected in small amounts. The "leukocytosis-promoting factor" of Menkin has been considered on p. 38.

Leukocytosis may develop within a few hours of the onset of a bacterial infection and is of diagnostic value. This early output of polymorphs is due to release of young cells lying in the sinusoids of the haemopoietic marrow.

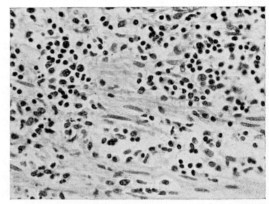

Fig. 6.1.—Inflammatory infiltration of the muscular coats of the bowel in typhoid fever, showing the mononuclear cells and absence of polymorphs. × 300.

Soon, however, there is an increased rate of formation of polymorphs in the marrow and the leukocytosis is thus maintained. The life of the neutrophil polymorph in the blood is estimated as about 3 days, and since there are approximately 5 litres of blood containing about 5,000 polymorphs per cubic mm., the normal daily production must be of the order of 7.5×10^{10}. In a suppurating infection, ten times this number may be lost daily for weeks or months in the pus discharging from an abscess, while at the same time the blood level may be maintained at 20,000 per cu. mm. or more. It is thus apparent that output of polymorphs is capable of enormous and sustained increase, and the process responsible for this is hyperplasia of the bone marrow, considered below.

A polymorphonuclear leukocytosis may result from causes other than inflammation and infection. It follows strenuous physical exertion, severe mental stress, and administration of glucocorticoids, corticotrophin or adrenalin.

After severe haemorrhage a moderate leukocytosis also occurs and is followed by a rise in the number of blood platelets.

Production of polymorphs

In the normal adult, production of the granulocyte or myeloid series of leukocytes is restricted to the haemopoietic marrow, where it occurs along with production of red cells (p. 387), platelets (p. 444) and monocytes (p. 399). The origin of blood lymphocytes is described in Chapter 4. All these cells probably originate from differentiation of the primitive haemopoietic stem cells, a brief account of which is necessary.

Haemopoietic stem cells appear first in the embryonic yolk sac and subsequently in the primitive blood and fetal liver: in the adult, this stem cell population is maintained in the haemopoietic marrow, and from it the supply of red cells, granulocytes and platelets (from megakaryocytes) is provided by proliferation and differentiation. Also stem cells pass into the blood and supply the thymus and probably other lymphoid tissues, where they differentiate into lymphoid cells.

Recent observations indicate that the primitive stem cell is pluripotent in being capable of giving rise to unipotent precursors of red cells, granulocytes, platelets and lymphocytes, and that the differentiation towards one or other of these lines is determined by the micro-environment of the tissue in which the stem cell settles and divides. These conclusions are drawn from experimental studies which indicate also that haemopoietic tissue may be likened to a large number of very small rooms, each of which represents a micro-environment capable of directing a stem cell settling within it into a particular line of differentiation. The nature of the cells which create the haemopoietic micro-environment is not known, but it is of interest that they are capable of withstanding 10,000r of X-irradiation and they must therefore be a remarkably stable (non-dividing) population.

Like other stem cell populations, the primitive haemopoietic cells are self-maintaining and it appears that their division gives rise not only to cells which differentiate, but also to undifferentiated stem cells. This must apply also to the stem cells for other labile cell populations, such

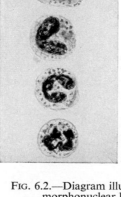

Myeloblast: non-granular, moderately basophil cytoplasm, oxidase negative, nucleus of finely meshed chromatin with two or more prominent nucleoli; about 10–18µ diameter.

Promyelocyte: appearance of coarse dark granules giving positive oxidase reaction, cytoplasm deeply basophilic; nucleoli still present but less conspicuous; about 12–18µ diameter.

Myelocytes: the early forms are still larger than promyelocytes, and the cytoplasm is less basophilic; coarse dark primitive granules are still present but are being replaced by the strongly oxidase-positive specific granulation which appears first in the area of less basophil cytoplasm opposite the nuclear indentation. The nucleus becomes progressively more condensed, and reniform. At this stage mitotic activity is at a maximum, and thereafter the daughter cells are reduced in size and maturation proceeds without further mitotic division; about 12–18µ diameter, becoming reduced as maturation proceeds.

Metamyelocytes: the coarse primitive granules are wholly replaced by the specific neutrophil granulation; the nucleus is more condensed and curved sometimes to a horseshoe shape; about 12–15µ diameter.

Polymorphonuclear leukocytes: the cells are further reduced in size, about 10–12µ, and the nucleus becomes horseshoe-shaped, and then segmented, the lobes being connected by a filament of chromatin. The older cells show further segmentation, and have 3 or 4 lobes.

Fig. 6.2.—Diagram illustrating formation of polymorphonuclear leukocytes. × 1000.

as epidermal and intestinal epithelium and spermatozoa.

Stages of myeloid (granulocyte) differentiation. The earliest recognisable granulocyte precursor is termed a myeloblast: small numbers of these are present in normal haemopoietic marrow and they divide to give rise to a population of cells which undergo successive multiplications and form the largest cell population in the marrow. This proliferation is accompanied by a continuous process of differentiation up to the granulocyte stage: representative stages are illustrated in Fig. 6.2. Throughout the process the ratio of cytoplasm to nucleus increases and after initial enlargement up to the early myelocyte

stage diminution in size is a feature of differentiation. In the primitive stages the nucleus is large, ovoid or indented, and the chromatin is finely distributed. Gradually the nucleus shrinks, becoming more deeply staining and eventually it becomes elongated giving the "band form", followed by division into lobes, the number of which increases during the life span of approximately 9 days of the polymorph in the blood. In preparations stained by a Romanowsky dye (e.g. Leishman's, Wright's or Jenner's stain) the cytoplasm of the myeloblast is moderately basophilic and has few or no granules; in the promyelocyte stage, basophilia is increased and a few unusually large lysosomal granules

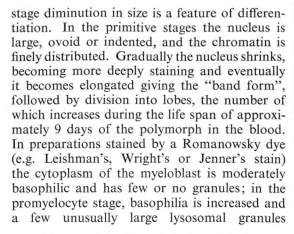

FIG. 6.3.—*Top left*. Normal haemopoietic bone marrow, showing the high proportion of fat cells, among which are foci of haemopoietic tissue. × 450.

FIG. 6.4.—*Bottom left*. Bone marrow after leukocytosis of moderate degree, showing distinct increase of the cellular marrow with diminution of the fat cells. × 450.

FIG. 6.5.—*Bottom right*. Bone marrow after long-standing leukocytosis. The fat cells have been replaced by a cellular tissue in which the great majority of the cells are myelocytes. × 450.

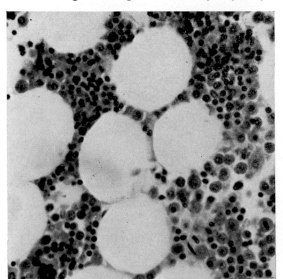

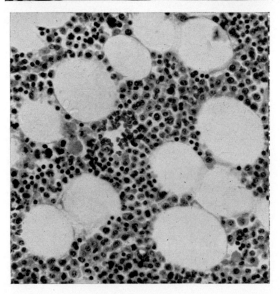

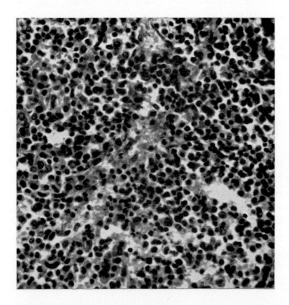

develop, of blue-reddish colour and giving a positive oxidase reaction (p. 433). In the myelocyte stage the cytoplasm loses most of its basophilia, becoming pale blue, and the large primitive lysosomal granules are gradually replaced by more numerous smaller specific granules, also lysosomal, which are intensely oxidase-positive. In the neutrophil myelocytes the granules are small and have a reddish or purple tint: in the eosinophil they are larger and bright orange, while in the basophil they are large and dark blue. These characteristic granules persist in the three types of mature granulocytes or polymorphs. In a neutrophil leukocytosis of recent origin there is an increased proportion of young cells and even myelocytes may appear in the blood.

Leukocytosis is brought about by hyperplasia, i.e. an increase in the number of cells in the haemopoietic marrow, and the proportion of myeloid cells and particularly of myelocytes is increased. This is termed a *leukoblastic reaction* and is analogous to the erythroblastic reaction in response to an increased requirement of red cells, e.g. after haemorrhage. The fat cells normally present in haemopoietic (red) marrow diminish in number as the cellularity increases (Figs. 6.3, 6.4, 6.5) and also foci of haemopoietic tissue appear in the yellow fatty marrow of the long bones, arising presumably from latent stem cells. These foci extend rapidly and in a severe infection, e.g. pneumococcal pneumonia, much of the yellow marrow in the shafts of the femur and other long bones may be replaced by red marrow, the change starting in the upper ends of the bones and extending downwards. All the cellular constituents of normal marrow are present in this newly formed haemopoietic tissue, but myelocytes and later forms predominate (Figs. 6.6, 6.7). The increased supply of neutrophil polymorphs is thus provided for. It is at the myelocyte stage that active proliferation occurs and this is why myelocytes predominate in the marrow, whereas myeloblasts are relatively few.

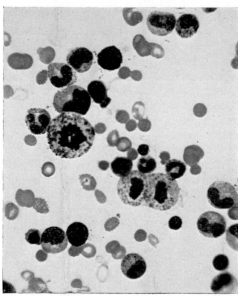

FIG. 6.6.—Film preparation from sternal marrow in leukoblastic reaction. Note granular myelocytes in mitosis and various stages of transition to polymorphonuclear leukocytes. × 600.

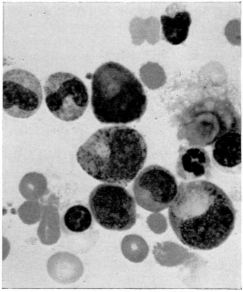

FIG. 6.7.—Film preparation from marrow showing finely granular myelocytes and transitions to polymorphonuclear leukocytes. × 1000.

FEVER

Elevation of the temperature above the normal—*pyrexia*—occurs in infections of various kinds, lesions of the nervous system, heat-stroke and after certain drugs. It is advisable, however, to restrict the term "fever" to the pyrexia which occurs in many infections.

Clinical manifestations. In an attack of fever, the clinical features vary according to whether the temperature is rising, steady, or falling. During the onset, while the internal temperature is rising, the patient feels cold and shivers, and sometimes a rigor occurs. The blood vessels and the smooth muscle of the skin are contracted, giving the appearance of pallor and "goose-flesh". Consequently the surface temperature falls, the patient feels cold, and there is diminished loss of heat. The involuntary contraction of the muscles in shivering and rigor contributes to the increased production of heat.

During the *fastigium* (while the temperature is raised and steady) the vessels of the skin are dilated, the face flushed, and there is a general feeling of heat and discomfort. Usually the skin is dry, though a considerable amount of moisture is still being lost by insensible sweating. In some fevers, however, and notably in rheumatic fever, there is much perspiration. The temperature may show only slight diurnal variation, as in pneumonia, or a distinct morning fall, as in typhoid fever, or it may have an irregular course.

Fall of temperature may be comparatively rapid, by *crisis*, as in untreated lobar pneumonia and is accompanied by sweating and increased loss of heat; or it may fall by *lysis*, i.e. over several days, as in typhoid fever.

Mode of production of pyrexia. Pyrexia is due to a disturbance of the normal balance of heat production and heat loss. Loss of heat results from the physical processes of conduction, radiation, and evaporation of moisture, and these depend mainly on the distribution of the blood and the secretion of sweat, which are controlled by the nervous system. Increased heat production is due to a rise in metabolism, to which the muscular work of shivering contributes. During the onset, when the patient feels cold, there is decrease in heat loss and increased production, causing a rise of temperature. During the fastigium the temperature of the skin

s raised; there is thus increased loss by radiation and conduction, which may be as much as 50 per cent above the normal in acute fevers such as typhoid, malaria, etc. The dryness of the skin is usually the result of both inhibition of the secretion of sweat and more rapid evaporation, but in some febrile states the loss of moisture by the skin may not be diminished, and may even be increased, resulting in still greater heat loss. This increased loss of heat while fever is maintained implies increased heat production, and this has been clearly established by studies on metabolism in fever. There is increase in the respiratory exchange, with other evidence of excessive metabolism, such as increased nitrogen excretion. Hard physical work in very hot climates, e.g. in troops on active service in the tropics, may bring about febrile inhibition of sweating, and this may so diminish heat loss that a serious state of hyperpyrexia rapidly develops. This occurs more readily in persons who are already dehydrated by loss of salt and water through previous excessive sweating and inadequate replacement, especially of salt. This is discussed more fully later (pp. 179 et seq.).

While increased heat production is an important factor in fever, it is not the whole explanation of the pyrexia. For example, much more heat may be produced by muscular exercise than occurs in fever, and in hyperthyroidism the basal metabolism may be 60 per cent or more above the normal, although there is no pyrexia. Accordingly, in addition to increased heat production in fever, there is a fault in the *temperature-regulating mechanism*, so that the loss of heat necessary to adjust the temperature within normal limits does not occur; this is probably the main factor in the rise of temperature. In fever the temperature control is unstable, and the temperature can be lowered artificially, e.g. by cold sponging or antipyretic drugs, far more readily than in health. It is as if the thermostat, represented by the heat-regulating centre in the hypothalamus, were set at a higher level and the metabolism is adjusted to maintain the raised level by increased heat production and often diminished sweating.

Pyrogens. Experimental work suggests that readjustment of the heat-regulating mechanism in fever is brought about by the action of pyrogens, and bacterial endotoxins appear particularly important examples. Their injection is followed after some hours by pyrexia and the features of shock noted on p. 189. The effective dose of purified endotoxin is very minute (0·1 µg. in man) and, if injection is repeated daily, tolerance is rapidly acquired. If bacterial pyrogens are incubated with whole blood or a suspension of polymorphonuclear leukocytes and the mixture is then injected intravenously the febrile response is almost immediate. This is interpreted as the result of interaction between the endotoxin and the leukocytes which liberate into the medium a heat-labile *endogenous pyrogen* to which tolerance is not acquired. Recent experimental evidence in lower animals and in man points to the action of this endogenous pyrogen on the hypothalamic centres as the intrinsic mechanism by which fever is produced probably in all infections.

Metabolism in fever. Excessive catabolism of protein leads to a great increase in the urinary excretion of urea, ammonia and other nitrogenous metabolites. Thus in typhoid fever the excess of nitrogen, sulphur and phosphorus excretion may sometimes represent a loss of over two kilograms of muscle in a week. Digestion and absorption are impaired and the old-fashioned "fever diet" is usually not sufficient to supply the necessary calories for a normal individual, much less a fevered patient. The carbohydrates in liver and muscle are soon used up and energy is provided by the breakdown of proteins and fats; the respiratory quotient usually falls and wasting occurs. Thus a state resembling starvation develops. Fats are catabolised in excess but incompletely and ketone bodies may appear in the urine. Urobilinogen may be present in the urine in excess, partly from increased red cell destruction, and partly from impaired liver function. After the temperature falls to normal the increased excretion of nitrogen may continue for a day or two, e.g. after lobar pneumonia, where it has been ascribed to the absorption and degradation of proteins present in the exudate.

The true nature and significance of the increased protein catabolism in fever are still not fully understood. High calorie diets, rich in protein and carbohydrate, diminish greatly or even prevent excessive catabolism of body protein in typhoid fever and the diminished excretion of creatinine and sulphur indicates that the catabolism of tissue protein is actually reduced. Cuthbertson has found that there is a marked increase of protein catabolism after injury, e.g. fractures, and that a high caloric protein-rich diet, while failing to maintain nitrogen equilibrium at the height of the process, does greatly diminish the breakdown of body protein. Whether it is wholly desirable to prevent this breakdown is uncertain as it may be an important source of amino-acids used in repair. It is now thought that a protein-rich diet is of the maximum benefit during convalescence.

The view that the increased temperature in fever represents a beneficial reactive process lacks proof, and there is no conclusive evidence that the heightened temperature stimulates the production of antibodies.

The symptoms of fever result from the increased temperature and from the action of toxins produced by the infecting organisms; both effects are accentuated by continued duration of the fever. Rise of temperature caused by exposure to a hot moist atmosphere alone leads to marked increase of the pulse-rate, a tendency to dyspnoea, general discomfort, headache, etc. A temperature of about 108°F (42°C) continued for some time causes coagulation of the protein in the nerve cells, but no doubt finer molecular change is brought about at a lower level. However, toxic action is the more important factor, and the earliest signs of structural damage to the cells of the body in fever, e.g. cloudy swelling, fatty change, etc. result mainly from toxic action. Neither these changes nor the clinical disturbances correlate well with the height of the temperature. Thus in many severe infections, toxaemia and general debility may be very marked when the temperature is little raised. However, pyrexia in itself becomes a formidable danger when it increases towards the level of *hyperpyrexia*, i.e. to more than 106°F (41°C).

Other causes of pyrexia. As already noted, abnormally high temperatures occur in conditions other than fever as above defined, and of these the two most important are heat-stroke and lesions of the nervous system. In all cases where the environmental temperature is abnormally high, the *regulating mechanism* may fail, and then there is a tendency for the resulting pyrexia to raise the production of heat and so the body temperature to a still higher level; this factor apparently plays an important part in hyperpyrexia. Owing to the efficiency of the regulating mechanism, the temperature of a normal individual may be little raised in a very hot atmosphere provided that it is dry, but regulation may fail when the atmosphere is moist. Thus a rise of the wet-bulb temperature to 88°F (31°C) elevates the temperature of a normal individual even at rest. Such a failure of regulation is an all-important feature in heat-stroke, as is seen amongst soldiers on the march, stokers, workers in mines, etc., and in its production a warm, moist and stagnant atmosphere, excess of clothing and severe muscular exercise are precipitating factors.

Excessive sweating leads to marked loss of salt, and the drinking of water without salt to replace that lost may lead to severe muscular cramp and even collapse. The increased temperature gives rise to further heat production with deficient regulation. In heat-stroke the temperature may rise to 108°F (42°C), while the pulse becomes rapid and feeble; there may be dyspnoea, delirium and convulsions, followed by death. In some cases symptoms of collapse or *heat exhaustion* are more prominent than the high fever, and are due mainly to salt depletion. After recovery from heat-stroke there may be symptoms of damage to the nervous system for some time. *Sunstroke*, in which again hyperpyrexia may develop, is probably merely a variety of heat-stroke (see p. 179).

Pyrexia and even hyperpyrexia are observed with certain *lesions of the central nervous system*, and result from damage to the heat-regulating centre, which is in the hypothalamus. Lesions occurring naturally, e.g. pontine haemorrhage and less commonly cortical lesions, may cause abnormally high temperature as does experimental puncture in the region of the basal ganglia. While the nervous mechanism concerned with heat loss by control of the cutaneous circulation and secretion of sweat is fairly well understood, little is known of the manner in which the nervous system brings about increased metabolism. The pyrexia resulting from puncture of the basal ganglia has been called *neurogenic*, and it appears to depend chiefly on excessive metabolism of carbohydrates, especially in the liver. Lusk has suggested that it has much the same relation to fever as "puncture glycosuria" (p. 902) has to true diabetes.

In some cases of Hodgkin's disease a remarkable relapsing pyrexia known as Pel-Ebstein fever is observed, and in certain tumours, and also in leukaemia, pyrexia occurs, quite apart from the presence of bacterial infection, probably from absorption of products of protein disintegration. Necrosis of tissue may lead to pyrexia; for example it is common in myocardial infarction and also after extensive tissue injury such as a fracture of a long bone. Pyrexia may be produced also by certain drugs.

CHAPTER 7

TYPES OF INFECTION

This chapter consists of a brief account of some of the more important types of infection. Infections in which the effects are dependent largely on their location, e.g. osteomyelitis, virus hepatitis, appendicitis, meningitis, are described in the appropriate regional chapters, and some of these later accounts should be read in conjunction with this chapter, which is restricted to a few illustrative examples of the different types of infection.

VIRUS INFECTIONS

Of all the pathogenic organisms which affect man, viruses show the most extreme degree of parasitism. In the extracellular state viruses are metabolically inert and depend absolutely on the metabolism of the host cell for their replication. Basically, all viruses consist of a protein shell or *capsid* which surrounds and protects a single molecule of nucleic acid—which may be either DNA or RNA. When a virus enters a susceptible host cell, the nucleic acid is released from the capsid and becomes functionally active: it re-directs the synthetic pathways of the host cell to manufacture components for new virus particles. This involves the replication of nucleic acid molecules and the production of proteins which include both the non-structural proteins (e.g. enzymes) necessary for viral replicative processes and also the structural proteins which become incorporated in the capsid of new virus particles.

Apart from those viruses which enter the host by the bite of an insect (e.g. yellow fever), or in the case of rabies virus by the bite of an animal, all parasitic viruses must enter the body by invading the surface epithelial cells of some part of the body. In many instances the site of initial infection is in the alimentary or respiratory tracts. In the case of some viruses the ability to invade and replicate in certain types of host cell appears to depend on the presence of receptor sites on the cell surface to which the protein coat of the virus can become attached.

In man, most virus infections are mild and are followed by complete recovery. Many infections are entirely symptomless and immunity to re-infection is acquired without serious disturbance at the time of primary infection. Although latent infection with virus may continue for months or occasionally even for years, viruses do not form a non-invasive flora in the way that some bacteria do. A few virus infections, such as smallpox, regularly cause serious disease and even viruses such as herpes simplex or the enteroviruses, which generally cause mild or symptomless infection, may occasionally give rise to severe disease in an unusually susceptible host. Viral infections, and especially respiratory virus infections, are extremely common in the community and are, in general, more frequent in childhood than in adult life.

Viruses are structurally simple parasites and do not produce disease by the elaboration of toxins as bacteria do. Lesions in viral infections are due to direct invasion of body tissues with subsequent cell damage due to the effect of viral replication in the host cells. In most clinically-apparent virus infections, replication of the virus is accompanied by death of the infected cell. Some viruses induce fusion between infected and adjacent non-infected cells, with the formation of multinucleated giant cells, e.g. the Warthin–Finkeldey cell of measles pneumonia (Fig. 15.31, p. 358). Such giant cells usually die, at least in tissue culture preparations, but their formation may be important in allowing virus to spread without entering the surrounding medium. There is increasing evidence that the immune response of the host may sometimes play an important role in causing lesions—for example in the development of bronchiolitis due to respiratory syncytial virus, which seems to be due largely to an immunological reaction in the lungs of the host. In arbovirus encephalitis, it has been postulated on the basis of some results of animal experiments that the lesions may be due to the cytotoxic effects of virus–antibody complexes rather than to the direct effect of the virus on the cells of the brain.

Unlike some bacterial infections, virus diseases are not usually accompanied by a polymorpho-nuclear leukocytosis, but a lymphocytosis is common. Most are associated with fever, and rash and lymphadenopathy are quite commonly seen. In the acute phase of virus infection a protein, *interferon*, can be detected in the blood and tissues. Interferon is released from cells in response to virus infection and when taken up by other cells makes them refractory to virus infection. Although the production of interferon is induced by virus, the protein itself is a species-specific cellular protein. It is not virus-specific in its antiviral effect but inhibits virtually all viruses. Interferon production is an important host defence mechanism against virus infection and is probably the major factor in bringing about recovery from acute virus infections. Although specific neutralising antibody is responsible for immunity to re-infection, it begins to appear in the blood stream only when the acute infection is subsiding. It is notable that infants with immunological deficiencies resulting in impairment of delayed hypersensitivity responses (p. 114 *et seq.*) are prone to develop chronic progressive vaccinia (vaccinia gangrenosa) following vaccination, and chronic infection with measles virus has also been reported.

Distribution of lesions in virus infections

In some instances, the main lesion is at the site of the initial infection. For example, the myxovirus responsible for influenza gives rise to a localised infection which spreads rapidly throughout the epithelial lining of the larger air passages of the respiratory tract. This results in epithelial necrosis of varying extent, and the cell injury and loss results in acute inflammatory oedema, which is the major clinical feature of influenza. The severity of the illness depends on the extent of epithelial necrosis, but secondary bacterial infection of the damaged mucosa is also of importance, especially in major epidemics. Influenza virus may enter the blood stream, but appears unable to replicate successfully in the cells of other tissues. Other examples of virus infections which remain localised, and produce lesions mostly at the site of initial infection, are molluscum contagiosum (p. 922) and the common cold.

In many other instances, the initial infection is usually clinically silent, but the virus invades various other tissues and organs and produces characteristic lesions in them. Thus in *smallpox*, the initial infection is probably in the respiratory tract. From there the virus spreads widely, invading the blood (viraemia) and many other tissues and organs. The characteristic vesicular lesions in the skin are due to invasion of the epidermal cells, and are one manifestation of the systemic infection. Suppuration of the skin lesions (pustulation) is due to secondary bacterial infection.

Because of the mode of virus spread in smallpox, the incubation period between initial infection and appearance of symptoms is about 12 days, and it may be even longer in some other exanthemas, e.g. measles and varicella (chickenpox). *Poliovirus* also spreads in a complex fashion within the body: following ingestion of the virus, there is an initial infection of the Peyer's patches in the small intestine. The virus then spreads to the regional lymph nodes, and in some instances produces viraemia. In a few individuals (e.g. about 1% of those infected with poliovirus type 1) the organism invades the anterior horn cells of the spinal cord (Figs. 20.35–20.37, pp. 640, 641), causing paralytic poliomyelitis. The intestinal infection is clinically silent, but it nevertheless results in the development of antibody in the blood, in the appearance of IgA antibody in the gastro-intestinal tract (p. 79), and confers immunity to subsequent infection with the same type of poliovirus.

Persistent virus infections are known to occur in man, e.g. with herpes simplex virus, which remains latent but becomes activated from time to time, e.g. during pneumonia or other febrile illness, to produce vesicles around the mouth. Varicella virus may also remain latent and then multiply within the cells of the dorsal root ganglia to produce an attack of zoster.

There is considerable interest at present in *slow virus* infections, which may be defined as virus diseases having a long incubation period, in some instances years, and a prolonged course. Such diseases have been demonstrated to occur in certain animals, e.g. Aleutian disease of the mink, and it seems very likely that *kuru* (p. 646) is an example in man. The agent of scrapie, a widespread chronic disease of sheep, is most unusual in its small size and remarkable resistance to heat and viricidal chemicals.

Active immunity can readily be produced by the administration of attenuated viruses, e.g. Sabin poliovirus vaccine, measles and yellow fever vaccines, and also—although somewhat less effectively—by inactivated viruses, e.g. influenza and rabies vaccines. Naturally-acquired immunity after virus infection is generally life-long and is due to the development in the blood of antibodies which neutralise the infectivity of viruses. However, in a few virus diseases, re-infections or repeated infections are common. This may be due to the existence of numerous serologically distinct strains of virus, e.g. the common cold, or to the virus undergoing antigenic variation, e.g. influenza. In the case of certain viruses, and especially herpes simplex and varicella zoster viruses, reactivation of virus in the tissues despite the presence of circulating antibody is not uncommon. The recurrences of infection are probably due to the ability of these viruses to remain latent within cells and to spread on re-activation directly through cell walls to infect neighbouring cells. The presence of antibodies in people who have experienced a virus infection can be demonstrated by various *in vitro* tests such as complement fixation, haemagglutination-inhibition and neutralisation tests.

ACUTE BACTERIAL INFECTIONS

These may be of several types, depending on the site of infection and the characteristics of the infecting bacteria.

Catarrhal infections

The term is applied to an inflammation of a mucous membrane accompanied by increased discharge of secretion. The surface epithelium is damaged and desquamates, and proliferation of the surviving cells in an attempt to repair the damage follows. When the cause is bacterial, the irritant may persist and bring about inflammatory changes in the mucous membrane. The secretion varies in different conditions, but there is an increased formation of mucus which may be tough and inspissated or dilute and watery. In nasal catarrh, the discharge may be very profuse, and another striking example is the acute catarrhal colitis of mild bacillary dysentery. In cholera (p. 517), a superficial infection of the colonic mucosa, there is little desquamation, but the causal organism, *Vibrio cholerae*, produces a toxin which renders the lining epithelium highly permeable to fluid, and there is a copious watery exudate, with excessive mucus secretion, into the lumen. In severe catarrh the secretion may be reddish, owing to the admixture of red cells. At first it is clear, but as leukocyte emigration is established, it becomes opaque and ultimately muco-purulent, with loosening or diminution of the tenacity of the mucus, apparently by the action of leukocytes. Single epithelial cells may be desquamated, but sometimes sheets of epithelium become detached, as in severe bronchitis (Fig. 7.1). The surviving cells proliferate; the young cells may in turn be desquamated, and the two processes of loss and repair may go on for a time. Ultimately complete repair may be effected. While such changes are occurring in the epithelium, the usual phenomena of inflammation are present in the underlying connective tissues. There is marked vascular engorgement with emigration of leukocytes, etc., and these cells pass through the basement membrane in increasing numbers and mingle with the secretion, which in consequence may be purulent.

Chronic catarrh. If the inflammation does not resolve completely, but passes into a chronic stage, proliferation of connective tissue cells with formation of new vessels forms a layer of vascular granulation tissue, which may cause swelling and unevenness of the mucosa. In chronic catarrh of the stomach, the epithelium in the upper portion of the glands may be repeatedly lost, and in the superficial part of the mucosa much granulation tissue may form.

Later, the fibrous connective tissue contracts, the mucous membrane becomes atrophic, and the epithelium degraded. In chronic catarrh, the dusts of glands may become occluded, with formation of small retention cysts, while in some

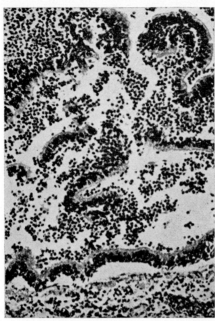

Fig. 7.1.—Wall of bronchus in acute inflammation, showing desquamation of epithelium and polymorphonuclear leukocytic infiltration. × 200.

situations, e.g. stomach and cervix uteri, small papillary outgrowths from the mucous membrane may develop. Clearly the efficient treatment of catarrh in the acute stage is of great importance, so that a return to normal as far as possible should be obtained and the later structural changes avoided.

Pseudo-membranous infections

These are infections, usually of a mucous membrane, in which the bacteria remain in the superficial tissues where they produce powerful exotoxins causing local necrosis, and fibrinous exudation from the underlying inflamed tissues. The dead epithelium becomes impregnated with fibrin, forming an opaque false membrane, which becomes detached when the infection subsides. Pseudo-membranous inflammation of the nasopharynx, throat, larynx or trachea is typical of diphtheria, caused by

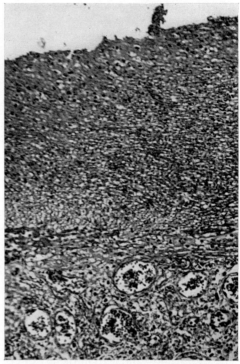

Fig. 7.2.—Diphtheria. The superficial part of the pharyngeal wall is shown. There is a thick pseudo-membrane, composed mainly of fibrin, on the surface, and congestion of the underlying connective tissue. × 100.

Corynebacterium diphtheriae (Fig. 7.2) and sometimes occurs also in infections with *Strep. pyogenes*: infection of the colonic mucosa with *Shigella shigae* produces a severe form of bacillary dysentery in which the lesion is of pseudo-membranous type. In both these instances there is also a severe systemic effect due to toxaemia.

Pyogenic infections

Acute infections caused by many bacteria have a marked tendency to progress to *suppuration*, i.e. destruction of tissue and production of an abscess. The term *pyogenic* (pus-producing) is applied to such lesions and to the bacteria which cause them. Such infections may remain localised, or may become generalised, the bacteria entering and spreading by the bloodstream and setting up a bacteraemia, septicaemia or pyaemia: these processes are described later.

Suppuration

Suppuration consists of the formation of *pus*, i.e. an accumulation of inflammatory exudate rich in neutrophil polymorphs, in a space resulting from destruction and digestion of tissue (Figs. 7.3, 7.4). Such an accumulation of pus is also termed an *abscess*, although pus can also

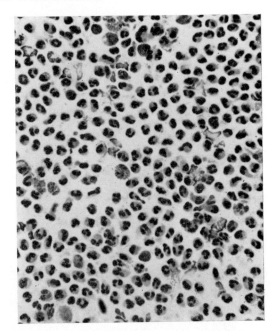

FIG. 7.4.—Smear of pus. Most of the cells are neutrophil polymorphs: some are undergoing autolysis. × 400.

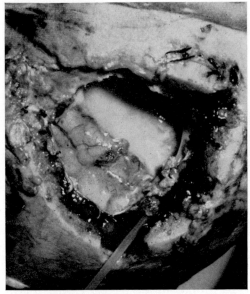

FIG. 7.3.—Abscess of brain. Part of the skull has been removed surgically and a cavity containing pus is seen in the brain. (Photographed at necropsy.)

collect in a natural body cavity, e.g. the pleura or peritoneum, without necrosis and digestion of tissue. While suppuration may be produced by chemical substances under experimental conditions, its natural occurrence is practically always due to bacterial infection.

Composition of pus. The opacity of pus is due to its content of cells; centrifugation separates it into an upper layer of clear yellow fluid, the *liquor puris*, and a lower creamy layer of cells. The fluid is essentially inflammatory exudate with, in addition, products of proteolytic digestion, e.g. proteoses and even amino-acids. Microscopically, most of the cells, called "pus cells", are seen to be neutrophil polymorphonuclear leukocytes. When the pus is recently formed many of these cells may show amoeboid movements on a warmed microscope stage, but when the pus is older most of the cells have died and show nuclear degeneration, etc. Some red cells are usually present in pus of recent origin,

and if numerous give it a pinkish tint. There are also macrophages in varying proportions (Fig. 2.12, p. 42). Some of the special cells of the tissue, showing various degrees of degeneration, may also be found. Fatty globules and cholesterol crystals may also be present in old pus.

Histological changes. Suppuration is brought about by two major changes which occur concurrently in the infected, inflamed tissue, viz. (a) a progressive emigration of polymorphonuclear leukocytes, which come to pack the tissue, and (b) a gradual destruction and disappearance of the tissue elements. The tissue cells are killed by bacterial toxins, and break down into fragments which are digested and melt away. The supporting connective tissue fibrils, capillaries, etc. are likewise digested and disappear. In suppuration there is thus an actual destruction of tissue, and a return to normal is no longer possible. With continuing accumulation of leukocytes, the tissue gradually becomes replaced by pus, in which the remains of the destroyed tissue are gradually digested. By contrast, in simple necrosis the dead tissue may persist for a long time.

Although the pyococci are most frequently responsible, suppuration may be produced by a great variety of organisms, the essential point being that they should be able to persist in the tissues and produce their toxic and chemotactic effects. Digestion or liquefaction of the tissues is due mainly to proteolytic enzymes produced by the leukocytes. Certain pyogenic organisms have a digestive action on proteins, but others, such as streptococci and pneumococci, which are scarcely less active in producing suppuration, have no such property. Digestive softening of the tissues by leukocytes follows on damage or actual necrosis due to bacterial toxins. Fibrin present in the exudate may also be digested by the polymorphs and disappear, as occurs also in resolution. Dense tissues may resist suppurative softening and a portion of dead tissue or *slough* then forms, and may persist for a considerable time (Fig. 7.5). This is well exemplified by a boil

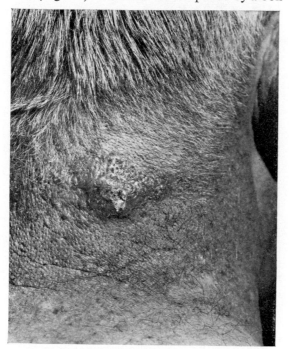

FIG. 7.5.—Furuncle ("boil") of back of neck. The centre of the lesion is necrotic, and is about to be sloughed off.

in the skin, the "core" of which consists of a necrotic portion of the cutis.

When suppuration ceases to spread, at the periphery of the abscess a reactive proliferation of the connective tissue cells with new formation of blood vessels forms a zone of granulation tissue around it (Fig. 7.6). The outer part becomes denser and a definite wall to the abscess is formed—the so-called "pyogenic membrane". If the abscess is small, the pus may be absorbed

and a small scar result. In larger abscesses, the pus may become inspissated and changed into granular debris; eventually deposition of calcium salts may convert this into a stone-like mass. In a chronic empyema, large calcareous plates may

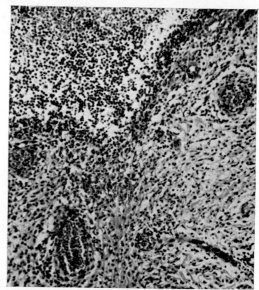

FIG. 7.6.—Wall of an abscess. The abscess cavity is seen at the top left. The wall consists of vascular connective tissue showing an inflammatory reaction. × 120.

thus be formed in the pleural cavity. Further, the longer an accumulation of pus lasts the greater will be the surrounding fibrous thickening, and accordingly any abscess cavity ought to be opened so that evacuation may allow the walls to come together and healing to occur with the minimum of fibrosis. When an abscess forms near a free surface, for example subcutaneously, the tension of the contents causes the suppuration to extend in the direction of the surface so that the overlying skin is involved. The abscess is then said to "point" and it may ultimately discharge its contents spontaneously.

Septicaemia, bacteraemia and pyaemia

When bacteria enter and multiply in the blood, the term *septicaemia* is applied. In certain acute bacterial infections in animals, for example anthrax in the guinea-pig, the organisms rapidly invade the blood stream from the site of inoculation and may be found on microscopic examination of the blood. In septicaemia in man, organisms are rarely so numerous as to be detectable by microscopy, though they may often be readily obtained by culture of the blood. They are more abundant in the capillaries of the internal organs than in the peripheral circulation, as judged by microscopic examination of the tissues after death, but the appearances are often exaggerated by bacterial growth *post mortem*. Where there is an absence of resistance the organisms actively multiply in the circulation and unless they are checked by intensive antibiotic therapy, are usually rapidly fatal, e.g. in virulent streptococcal and in meningococcal septicaemia, where death may result within a few hours. When the organisms represent merely an overflow from the tissues and do not multiply in the blood, the term *bacteraemia* is usually applied, and here their significance is not so grave. The outstanding examples of this are typhoid and paratyphoid fevers, in which organisms can usually be cultured from the blood early in the disease. In the course of the infection, even before the healing of the lesions, the organisms disappear from the circulation, as do the pneumococci in untreated lobar pneumonia at the time of the "crisis". In subacute bacterial endocarditis, organisms may be shed into the blood over weeks or months, but they do not multiply and their detection may require repeated blood culture. In certain conditions, including relapsing fever and malaria, proliferation of the causal organism in the blood is a characteristic feature and does not indicate an overwhelming or even serious infection.

In bacteraemia and septicaemia, there is always the risk that bacteria may settle in some part of the body and produce serious metastatic lesions, e.g. suppurative meningitis or arthritis in pneumococcal infections, or periostitis in typhoid fever. Sometimes, and especially in acute suppurative staphylococcal infections, the secondary lesions are in the form of multiple abscesses and the condition is then termed *pyaemia*. This results from bacteria becoming arrested in the capillaries of various organs and proliferating to produce small (pyaemic) abscesses (Fig. 7.7); they are likely to arise from blood dissemination of minute fragments of infected, suppurating thrombi which have escaped from veins involved in the primary focus of infection (p. 170). Serial section of pyaemic abscesses shows a central area of necrosis (Fig. 7.8), which may represent infarction brought about by septic embolism, but the toxic effects of proliferating bacteria may also be partly responsible.

Staphylococcal pyaemic abscesses occur especially in the lungs, brain, kidneys and myocardium. In addition to pyaemic abscesses, septic infarcts may develop in pyaemia as a result of arterial

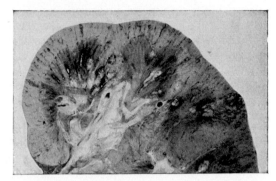

Fig. 7.7.—Pyaemia: kidney, showing multiple small abscesses which are seen as pale areas surrounded by dark haemorrhagic zones.

arrest of larger fragments of septic thrombus, and the abscesses which develop are relatively large: such lesions occur in the lungs in cases of septic thrombosis of systemic veins, and in various organs from the infected, crumbling vegetations on the heart valves in acute bacterial endocarditis.

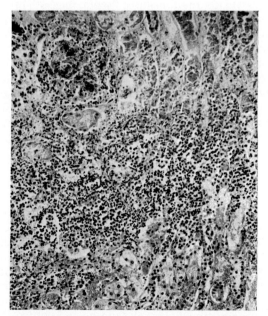

Fig. 7.8.—Septic infarct of kidney in a case of staphylococcal pyaemia. Infarcted tissue (above) is separated from congested living tissue (below) by a zone of suppuration. The dark patches in a glomerulus are masses of staphylococci, and have probably increased after death. × 50.

The common pyogenic bacteria

Pyogenic infections in man are most commonly caused by *Staphylococcus aureus* and *Streptococcus pyogenes*. The former is the usual cause of boils, carbuncles, and septic lesions of the fingers: the infection usually remains localised, although suppurating lymphadenitis may occur in the local nodes, and septicaemia and pyaemia (see below) are not rare. Some types of *Staph. aureus* are resistant to penicillin and sometimes to other antibiotics. Symptomless nasopharyngeal carriers of resistant types are commonly responsible for outbreaks of infection of surgical wounds, burns, etc., in hospital: phage typing has proved of great value in tracing the source of such outbreaks. Staphylococci are also a cause of pneumonia complicating influenza and other virus infections of the respiratory tract, and may produce a fulminating enteritis in patients receiving broad-spectrum antibiotics. The staphylococcal lesion shows the usual features of acute inflammation, and unless checked by antibiotic therapy frequently progresses to suppuration and discharges a thick creamy pus.

Strep. pyogenes commonly produces acute pharyngitis and tonsillitis, "septic fingers", otitis media and mastoiditis, also extensive inflammation of the subcutaneous connective tissues (*cellulitis*), and *erysipelas*, a spreading infection of the dermis producing a raised, red, painful lesion of the skin, usually of the face, with a well-defined margin. Before the introduction of antiseptics, *Strep. pyogenes* was a very common and important cause of fatal peritonitis or septicaemia, arising from infection of the genital tract following childbirth, and also of fatal septicaemia resulting from a minor injury, e.g. a finger prick sustained by the surgeon or pathologist dealing with a streptococcal infection.

The differences between infections due to staphylococci and streptococci are partly explicable by their toxins (p. 120). Staphylococcal infections show a greater tendency to remain localised, possibly due to the production of staphylocoagulase which clots fibrinogen, producing a deposit of fibrin which may help to limit spread of the organism and promote phagocytosis (p. 122). Streptococcal lesions tend to spread, possibly due to the production of hyaluronidase, which digests hyaluronic acid and thus liquefies the ground substance of connective tissues. They also produce fibrinolysins, and leukocidin which kills polymorphs.

Other pyogenic bacteria include *Strep. pneumoniae*, the common cause of lobar pneumonia, which may be complicated by metastatic blood-borne lesions, e.g. suppurating meningitis or arthritis; *Neisseria meningitidis* (meningococcus) which invades the nasopharynx, often silently, and produces a septicaemia or bacteraemia with the subsequent development of meningitis; *Neisseria gonorrhoeae* (gonococcus), transmitted by coitus and producing an acute urethritis, etc. The coliform bacilli normally present in the gut may produce ulcerating lesions of the intestines and also acute infection of the appendix, of the urinary tract, and of skin wounds. Another organism which is of low invasive capacity but may produce acute pyogenic infections of wounds and other skin lesions is *Pseudomonas aeruginosa*. The lesions produced by these various bacteria are described more fully in the various systematic chapters. Two rare infections, anthrax and glanders, deserve brief comment.

Anthrax

This epizootic disease of herbivorous animals is caused by a large Gram-positive spore-forming bacillus which is occasionally conveyed to man by animal contacts. Lesions occur in the skin from direct contact and are known as *malignant pustules*, and in the lungs or intestine from the inhalation or swallowing of the spores in dust from infected wool or hides, hence the name *wool-sorter's disease*.

Malignant pustule occurs by contamination of the exposed skin with infected animal products. A red painful papule forms and soon vesiculates; it is surrounded by a zone of intense congestion and inflammatory oedema, and central necrosis follows, resulting in a black crust (Fig. 7.9). Leukocytic emigration into the lesion is often inhibited by the combined action of a specific lethal factor together with a d-glutamic acid polypeptide and a lipoprotein. The regional lymph nodes are enlarged. In man, spread of infection to the blood stream occurs only rarely, but may result in a haemorrhagic meningitis (p. 626).

In wool-sorter's disease, the local lesion is usually in the lower trachea or large bronchi; it consists of a patch of haemorrhagic and ulcerated mucosa with intense oedema and involvement of the mediastinal lymph nodes, with haemorrhagic pleural and pericardial effusions.

Intestinal anthrax is rare in man, but ingestion is

the common mode of transmission in animals. The site of infection is usually in the upper small intestine and the lesions consist of one or more haemorrhagic foci with central necrosis and massive oedema; the mesenteric lymph nodes are involved and anthrax septicaemia may follow.

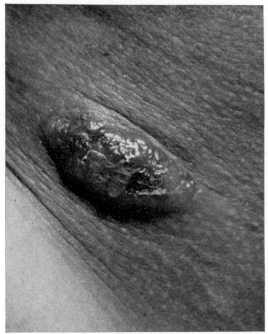

FIG. 7.9.—Anthrax pustule on skin of neck. × 1·5.

In anthrax septicaemia, death is due to the production of small amounts of a specific lethal factor or toxin but in experimental anthrax the total number of infecting organisms is so great that the cumulative effect suffices to produce death, apparently by circulatory failure from loss of blood volume (acute hypovolaemic shock, p. 189) owing to increase in local and general capillary permeability.

Glanders

This disease of equines due to *Actinobacillus mallei* is characterised by inflammatory thickenings and nodules in the nasal septum and upper respiratory passages, which tend to ulcerate. Infection in the horse occurs also through the skin and lymphangitis and suppurative enlargement of the lymph nodes result—the so-called farcy pipes and buds. In man direct infection of a scratch or abrasion by contaminated material leads to a local inflammatory reaction and spreading lymphangitis, the lesions being more acute than in the horse.

Gangrene

Definition. The term gangrene means digestion of dead tissue by saprophytic bacteria, i.e. bacteria which are incapable of invading and multiplying in living tissues. Many types of bacteria, often present in various combinations, may participate, and breakdown of tissue proteins, carbohydrates and fat may result in simple end-products: volatile bodies and gases may be formed, giving the foul odour of putrefaction, and the same changes are observed in putrefaction of meat, etc. Gas production may give rise to emphysematous crackling. The various changes in colour—dark-brown or greenish-brown, and sometimes almost black—are chiefly due to changes in haemoglobin, and are most pronounced when the dead tissue contains a lot of blood.

Gangrene may be either *primary* or *secondary*. In the former, tissue death is caused by the toxins of anaerobic bacteria which then invade the dead tissue and bring about digestive changes in it. In secondary gangrene, tissue death is produced by some other cause, e.g. cutting off the blood supply, and then saprophytic invasion and putrefaction follows.

Primary or gas gangrene. This is caused by a group of anaerobic sporulating bacteria, the *Clostridia*, of which the three most important are *Cl. welchii*, *Cl. oedematiens* and *Cl. septicum*. These organisms are normal intestinal inhabitants of man and animals; their spores are widespread, and are liable to contaminate wounds. Being anaerobic and saprophytic, they cannot multiply in living, oxygenated tissue, but they flourish in blood-soaked foreign material and dead tissue in lacerated wounds such as are caused by shrapnel and road accidents. Given such a favourable environment, the *Clostridia* produce exotoxins which diffuse into and kill the adjacent tissues and these in turn are invaded, so that the process spreads rapidly, particularly along the length of skeletal muscles (Fig. 7.10). Gas gangrene is most often due to *Cl. welchii*. Before the muscle and other tissues are killed, they become intensely oedematous, are extremely painful, and appear swollen and pink. Microscopically emigration of leukocytes is minimal. Among a number of toxins, *Cl. welchii* produces a lecithinase (α toxin) which, by its action on phospholipids, lyses cell and mitochondrial membranes, also hyaluronidase which liquefies ground substance. The action of α toxin on fat cells, with consequent release of fat, may be responsible for the occurrence of fat embolism. *Cl. welchii* ferments sugars, producing CO_2 which collects as bubbles in the dead tissues, rendering

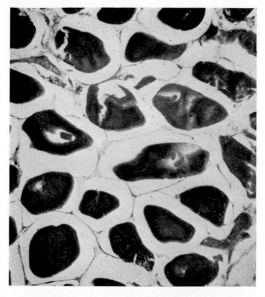

FIG. 7.10.—Gas gangrene of skeletal muscle. There is necrosis with loss of nuclei. × 250.

them crepitant on palpation. The subcutaneous tissue and skin are also affected, and the area involved, e.g. a limb, may burst open as a result of the swelling of oedema fluid and pressure of gas. The dead tissues are commonly invaded by a mixture of other organisms, which may play a major role in putrefaction. Gas gangrene may complicate intestinal lesions, e.g. appendicitis or strangulation of the gut (p. 527), clostridia being present in the intestine; it occurs also as a puerperal infection of the uterus from contamination via the perineum.

In addition to the rapidly spreading local lesion, gas gangrene is accompanied by acute haemolysis and a severe toxaemia which affects all the internal organs, and death results from peripheral vascular collapse. At necropsy, all the tissues may contain large numbers of clostridia, with extensive digestive changes.

If lacerated wounds are treated by early excision of the devitalised tissue, and toxic action is controlled by the use of antitoxic sera, clostridial infections are unlikely to establish themselves. Antibiotics have also contributed greatly to the prevention of gas gangrene by preventing the growth of clostridia.

Noma (*cancrum oris*) is a gangrenous condition which occasionally occurs in poorly nourished children, especially in kala azar and some other debilitating infections; it begins on the gum margin and spreads to the cheek, where an inflammatory patch of dusky red appearance forms and then becomes darker in colour and ultimately gangrenous. The original necrosis is caused by a characteristic fusiform bacillus (*Fusobacterium fusiforme*); the dead tissues then undergo putrefaction. Deficient intake of the vitamin B complex, especially of nicotinic acid, predisposes to the condition.

Secondary gangrene. Here death of the tissue is produced by deprivation of the blood supply or by necrotising chemicals, and putrefying bacteria then invade the dead part. This occurs wherever the necrosis involves the skin surface or a mucous membrane to which the necessary organisms have access, and two varieties are distinguished, namely dry and moist.

Moist gangrene occurs in the internal organs. When a portion of the bowel has had its blood supply cut off by strangulation, e.g. in a hernial sac, gangrene commonly follows. First there is interference with the venous return, and the consequent tissue swelling which results ultimately arrests blood flow; the part becomes haemorrhagic and then invasion of organisms brings about gangrenous softening. Moist gangrene occurs also in the appendix, pancreas, lungs, etc., and in infarction of the lower leg in an oedematous or obese individual, particularly in diabetics (see below). Gangrene of the fauces is a rare complication of diphtheria.

The occurrence of gangrene is favoured by any condition of depressed vitality. For example in diabetics, pneumonia is apt to be followed by gangrene of the lung. Occasionally the entrance of putrid fluids into the tissues may cause both necrosis and putrefaction. For instance, a cancer of the oesophagus may ulcerate into a bronchus and, by allowing access of contaminated food and secretions, may lead to gangrene of the lung.

Gangrene of the leg. Infarction of toes, a foot, or the lower leg is not uncommon as the result of arterial blockage (Fig. 13.27, p. 281), the collateral circulation being insufficient to keep the part alive. This occurs most often in old people (hence the term *senile gangrene*) and is caused by arterial thrombosis complicating advanced atheroma (p. 264), which tends to be marked in diabetes. It may occur also in early or middle adult life, due to thrombo-angiitis (p. 279), a disease which affects multiple arterial branches, especially in the lower limbs. Another occasional cause is the symmetrical spasmodic contraction of arteries in Raynaud's disease (p. 283).

If there is much subcutaneous fat, and particularly when the limb is oedematous, as in congestive heart failure, moist gangrene commonly supervenes in the infarcted tissues, with blebs of fluid in the skin, sometimes gas production, and rapid putrefaction: there is no sharp line of demarcation between dead and living tissue, and indeed gangrene may spread proximally beyond the tissues primarily affected. When infarction occurs in a non-oedematous leg, particularly when there is little subcutaneous fat and when gradual arterial occlusion has preceded the actual infarction, so-called *dry gangrene* is liable to ensue. The skin becomes cold and waxen, while the haemoglobin diffuses out along the veins and produces reddish-purple staining of the tissues, which then become brownish red and ultimately almost black, while the part becomes drier and shrinks, and *mummification* results.

Use of the term dry gangrene is controversial. Commonly, mummification occurs with little or no putrefaction. Saprophytic organisms are, however, usually present in small numbers, particularly in the dead tissues adjacent to the line of demarcation. If amputation is not performed, putrefaction becomes established at this site, and a process of slow putrefactive ulceration penetrates the soft tissues, ultimately down to the bone.

INFECTIVE GRANULOMAS

Under this heading may be included the numerous infections which give rise to chronic inflammation with a granulomatous reaction, i.e. production of granulation tissue which eventually progresses to fibrosis. The general features of chronic inflammation have been described on pp. 44–47, and a more detailed account of the production of granulation tissue is given on pp. 51–61. The following account gives the specific features of two most important chronic infections, tuberculosis and syphilis, and brief accounts of some other chronic infections. Because of its wide prevalence and tuberculous-like features, sarcoidosis is also included here, although there is no evidence that it is an infection.

Tuberculosis

Formerly one of the great killing diseases of temperate climates, tuberculosis is now much less common in Western Europe and North America. It is, however, prevalent in communities with a poor standard of living, and still ranks among the world's most important diseases. The disease illustrates well various basic features of bacterial infection, and in particular the importance of the reaction of the host in determining the nature of the lesions, and the spread of infection within the body. The causal organism, *Mycobacterium tuberculosis*, is an aerobic rod-shaped bacterium possessing a waxy capsule which renders it difficult to stain. Once the stain has penetrated the capsule, however, it is also difficult to remove, and the mycobacteria are sometimes referred to as acid- and alcohol-fast bacteria, since they resist decolourisation by various strengths of acids and by limited exposure to alcohol. *M. tuberculosis* grows slowly in culture; it is highly pathogenic for the guinea-pig, a feature which has been much used for its detection when present in small numbers in sputum, etc. In man, it gives rise to chronic disease but in certain circumstances can produce a much more acute and even overwhelming infection. In addition to *M. tuberculosis*, of which there are two major types causing human disease (see below), the mycobacteria include *M. leprae*, which causes leprosy, and there are also various ill-defined organisms, sometimes termed *anonymous or atypical mycobacteria*, which cause lesions in the lymph nodes, lungs and elsewhere.

Epidemiology

The two types of *M. tuberculosis* mainly responsible for disease in man are the human type, *M. tuberculosis hominis*, and the bovine type, *M. tuberculosis bovis*. The *human type* is the more important: infection with it is usually contracted by inhalation, and the initial, or primary, lesion is nearly always in the lungs. Patients with chronic pulmonary tuberculosis provide the reservoir of infection, and subjects with this condition commonly spread the disease by exhaling infected droplets and by coughing up infected sputum. The organism is resistant to drying and can survive for long periods in dust, inhalation of which is the usual method of contracting the disease. Infection of the tonsils or of the intestine can also occur from swallowing the human type of tubercle bacillus in contaminated dust, or the bovine type of bacillus in contaminated milk from cows with tuberculous mastitis.

Several factors are responsible for the declining incidence of tuberculosis in Western Europe and North America. Firstly, the rising standards of nutrition and housing: there is no doubt that under-nourishment predisposes to tuberculosis and impairs the resistance of the individual who has contracted the disease. Overcrowding and inadequate personal and domestic hygiene are also of importance in spreading the disease in the home and in public transport and meeting places, etc. The environment of a subject coughing up the organism is likely to be heavily contaminated, and spread within families is especially common, giving rise to both pulmonary and alimentary infections.

Since the 1939–45 war, the use of specific chemotherapeutic bactericidal agents has also helped to reduce the incidence of the disease by diminishing greatly the infectivity of patients with chronic pulmonary tuberculosis. Mass miniature radiography has revealed unsuspected cases of tuberculosis in the community, and protection against *M. tuberculosis* has been provided by means of BCG vaccination.

In countries where the disease is rife, infants and young children are particularly at risk, and in this country the mortality rate in children contracting the infection before the age of 3 years was formerly very high. Those who overcome the infection develop partial resistance to the organism, but may become re-infected and develop chronic pulmonary tuberculosis in adult life. The bacteria may survive for many years in dormant lesions, without clinical manifestations, and these may become active as a result of malnutrition, as in war or famine, as a complication of other debilitating diseases such as diabetes mellitus, or from administration of corticosteroids or other immunosuppressive agents. In Western Europe, a high proportion of "new" cases are middle- or old-aged, and have had dormant lesions for many years from the time when the disease was much commoner: childhood cases are now relatively uncommon.

The *bovine* type of *M. tuberculosis* causes mastitis in cattle, and is transmitted to man by consuming infected milk and milk products. Infection results usually by way of the gut or tonsils. In many countries, bovine infection in man has been eradicated by pasteurisation of milk, which kills the organism, and by tuberculin testing of cattle and elimination of infected cows.

Hypersensitivity and immunity

The immune response to the tubercle bacillus provides the classical example of delayed hypersensitivity, i.e. the production of specifically sensitised lymphocytes which are capable of reacting directly with antigenic protein of the mycobacterium. The mechanism of this type of response, and the state of hypersensitivity which results from it, have been described in Chapters 4 and 5 respectively. It is not understood why delayed hypersensitivity is the dominant type of immune response to *M. tuberculosis*, but it may be of significance that mycobacteria, living or dead, have a powerful enhancing effect on the immune response to antigens in general, and this forms the basis of their use in Freund's adjuvant (p. 83). Whatever the explanation of its adjuvant effect, infection with *M. tuberculosis* results, within two weeks or so, in the development of a high degree of delayed hypersensitivity to a protein fraction (tuberculoprotein) of the organism,* and thereafter the course of the infection and the features of the lesions are profoundly influenced by the hypersensitivity state.

---

* This state of hypersensitivity was demonstrated by Robert Koch (1891), using a crude preparation termed "old tuberculin". A more refined preparation is termed "purified protein derivative" (PPD).

Lymphocytes are produced which are specifically sensitised to tuberculoprotein, and their encounter with tuberculoprotein results in the release of the various factors described on p. 106. The results are both beneficial and harmful. *M. tuberculosis* has not been shown to produce any direct toxic effect, and can survive and multiply within macrophages in tissue culture without harm to the cultured cells. Indeed, it is likely that the tissue injury resulting from tuberculous infection is due mainly or entirely to the delayed hypersensitivity reaction against the bacteria. Nevertheless, without an immune response, multiplication of the organism would presumably continue unchecked. The delayed hypersensitivity reaction is therefore to be regarded as protective in reducing or eliminating the infection, but at the same time injurious to the tissues. Interpretation of the features of the lesions of tuberculosis in terms of delayed hypersensitivity is attempted in the account of the structural changes (below).

Tuberculin skin testing. This is carried out by intradermal injection of very small amounts of tuberculoprotein, as in the *Mantoux test*, or by applying tuberculoprotein to the skin in the *patch test*. In individuals who are, or have previously been, infected, a delayed inflammatory reaction develops, the features of which are described on p. 106. In some patients with very severe tuberculosis, the test is negative, presumably because the large amount of tuberculoprotein being released from the lesions has overwhelmed the state of hypersensitivity. Tuberculin skin tests give positive reactions in infections with both human and bovine types of *M. tuberculosis*, and with other types of mycobacteria. For this reason they may be positive in individuals infected with *Mycobacterium leprae*.

Immunisation against tuberculosis. Protective immunisation requires the induction of a state of delayed hypersensitivity to tuberculoprotein, and so far this can be reliably achieved only by injecting living mycobacteria. Attenuated strains of the bovine type, e.g. *bacille Calmette-Guérin* (BCG), or other non-human strains such as *M. tuberculosis muris* (the vole bacillus), are used for this purpose. Lesions result at the site of injection and in the draining lymph nodes, but these heal spontaneously and the attenuated bacteria are destroyed.

Structural changes

When a guinea-pig is inoculated with *M. tuberculosis* there is little reaction during the first day or so apart from local infiltration with neutrophil polymorphs, which soon disappear. During the next few days, macrophages migrate into the area and ingest the bacteria without bringing about their destruction. These very early stages of infection cannot, of course, be observed in man, but the subsequent changes are closely similar in man and the guinea-pig. After ten days or so, macrophages derived mainly from monocytes of the blood, but also from local histiocytes, aggregate in increasing numbers to form a minute nodule or *tubercle* (Fig. 7.11). These cells become swollen, oval or spindle-shaped, with foamy cytoplasm and a pale-staining elongated nucleus. It is likely that these altered macrophages, which are termed *endothelioid* or sometimes *epithelioid* cells, have been modified by humoral factors released by specifically sensitised lymphocytes (p. 106), rendering them immobile and mutually adhesive, and enhancing their capacity to destroy tubercle bacilli; this view would explain the aggregation of macrophages into tubercle follicles and also their protective role. Small lymphocytes accumulate around the margin of the nodule, which becomes visible to the naked eye about 3 weeks after the injection. In the central part of the lesion, multinucleated giant cells termed *Langhans' giant cells* are formed by coalescence or by nuclear division of endothelioid cells without cytoplasmic division: they have abundant foamy cytoplasm and commonly over a hundred nuclei arranged around the periphery (Figs. 7.11–7.13). At about the same time as the formation of giant cells, the endothelioid and giant cells in the central part of the tubercle undergo necrosis: the cells lose their outline and nuclear staining and become fused into a homogeneous or slightly granular material, which may also contain fibrin from vascular exudation. The tubercle thus comes to consist of a necrotic centre, surrounded by endothelioid and sometimes giant cells (Fig. 7.13), with a peripheral aggregation of small lymphocytes. The necrotic material is creamy-white, and resembles cream cheese in appearance and consistence—hence the terms *caseation* and *caseous material*.

Tubercles are avascular, but reticulin forms around their margins, and in a favourable case

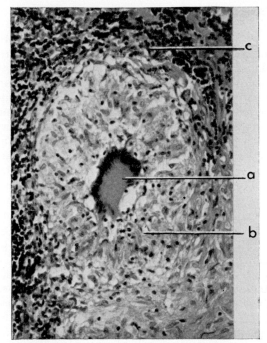

FIG. 7.11.—Tubercle follicle at early stage.

(*a*) Langhans' type giant cell; (*b*) endothelioid cells; (*c*) lymphocytes. × 250.

progresses to fibrous tissue. The central necrosis may be due in part to ischaemia, but probably the cell injury which results from the delayed hypersensitivity reaction of lymphocytes and macrophages with tuberculoprotein is an important factor. The further course of the infection depends on several factors, including the infecting dose and virulence of the organism, and also the degree of resistance of the host. What determines virulence in strains of *M. tuberculosis* is not understood, but the so-called virulent strains are those which are capable of relatively rapid multiplication *in vivo*. If the bacteria continue to multiply in the lesions, they may escape and gain a foothold in the surrounding tissues, with further tubercle formation. A cluster of tubercles may thus arise, and as these enlarge, they become confluent, and the central areas of caseous necrosis eventually unite to give a large caseous patch with tubercles around the periphery. Such lesions may reach several centimetres in diameter. When they arise in the lungs, they seldom reach this size without involving the wall of a bronchus, and the caseous material is then discharged, leaving a tuberculous cavity (Fig. 15.42, p. 364). In other tissues, and particularly in the kidneys and in lesions of bone extending into the surrounding soft tissues, caseous material may be invaded by neutrophil polymorphs, with resultant liquefaction ("tubercu-

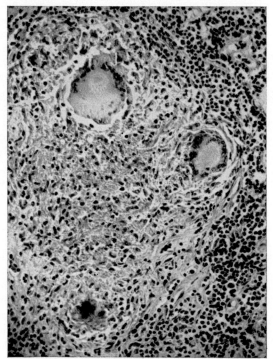

FIG. 7.12.—Tubercle nodule more fully formed with three giant cells.

Note peripheral aggregation of lymphocytes. × 150.

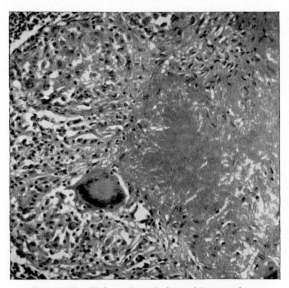

FIG. 7.13.—Tuberculous lesion with caseation.

On the left, there is cellular tissue with tubercle follicles and giant cells; on the right, caseation and loss of nuclear structure. × 150.

lous pus"). Such a lesion used to be called a *cold abscess*, because it is not accompanied by the acute inflammatory features of a pyogenic abscess. The softened caseous material may track through the tissues and may eventually reach a surface and discharge.

In certain situations, the lesions of tuberculosis may present features different from those described above. For example, rapid dissemination may occur by the air passages throughout the lung, giving a severe *bronchopneumonia*. Microscopy then shows extensive filling of the alveoli with large rounded macrophages containing fatty globules in their cytoplasm; these cells rapidly undergo necrosis, and the lesions enlarge with little or no attempt at healing. In the subarachnoid space, *M. tuberculosis* multiplies rapidly, and produces an exudative inflammatory lesion with deposition of fibrin, and accumulation of neutrophil polymorphs, macrophages and lymphocytes. Tubercles are usually poorly formed, and involvement of the walls of arteries and veins lying in the subarachnoid space may cause severe narrowing of their lumina by endarteritis (Fig. 20.25, p. 631) or occlusion by thrombosis. The lesions which result from infection of the pleural and peritoneal cavities are also commonly exudative, with a serous or serofibrinous exudate, and when the pericardium is involved the exudate may be rich in fibrin and is often haemorrhagic, presumably as a result of the mechanical effect of the heart beat.

Primary and reinfection tuberculosis

Infection of an individual who has not been previously infected or immunised gives rise to the *primary lesion* in the lung, tonsil or small intestine. This usually remains small, and commonly heals without becoming detectable. Early spread of bacteria to the regional lymph nodes is, however, the rule, and their rapid multiplication may occur in the affected nodes, i.e. at the root of the lung (Fig. 15.33, p. 360), in the neck or in the mesentery, depending on the site of the primary lesion. The combination of the primary lesion and enlarged, caseous regional lymph nodes is thus common—the *primary complex*.

Reinfection tuberculosis results from infection of an individual who has overcome a primary infection or been immunised by BCG. The reinfection lesion is usually in the apex of one or

other lung and may extend to give a large local lesion (Fig. 15.44, p. 365). There is usually little or no involvement of the local lymph nodes. Reinfection lesions occur also in the tonsils, small intestine, pharynx and skin, again without much involvement of the regional nodes, but these are relatively uncommon sites. Individuals with reinfection tuberculosis of the lungs may, however, develop lesions in the larynx, mouth and intestines as a result of endogenous infection by coughing up and swallowing sputum containing tubercle bacilli (Fig. 18.56, p. 518). These metastatic lesions resemble those of reinfection tuberculosis in spreading locally with minimal or no involvement of the local nodes.

The differences between primary and reinfection tuberculosis appear to depend mainly on the multiplication and spread of the bacilli in the early stages of the primary infection, i.e. before the development of delayed hypersensitivity.

The spread of infection within the body is discussed below, but more detailed accounts of the resulting lesions are given in the chapters on regional pathology, e.g. pulmonary tuberculosis, pp. 359 *et seq.*

Spread of infection

M. tuberculosis is very prone to spread by lymphatics and to produce lesions in lymph nodes. This occurs especially in the early stages of the primary infection, with resulting involvement of the draining lymph nodes and infection may spread from these to adjacent nodes or groups of nodes, e.g. in the mediastinum (Fig. 15.33, p. 360). In chronic (i.e. reinfection) tuberculosis, lymphatic spread is usually localised to the tissue immediately around the lesions, the draining lymph nodes seldom being severely involved. This limitation of lymphatic spread is probably attributable to the modified behaviour of macrophages which results from delayed hypersensitivity. There is experimental evidence that lymphatic spread results from ingestion and transport of *M. tuberculosis* by macrophages, and the lymphocytic factors which convert macrophages into "killer" cells and interfere with their mobility (p. 106) are likely to impede such spread.

Spread of *M. tuberculosis* also occurs by the blood stream. This is seen notably in *acute miliary tuberculosis*, in which large numbers of bacteria gain entrance to the circulation and give rise to innumerable tubercles in the various organs. The condition arises most commonly in primary tuberculosis and is due usually to chance involvement of a vein by the large caseating lymph node lesions of the primary complex—in most cases the pulmonary hilar nodes: the caseating process extends into the wall of an adjacent vein, usually one of the pulmonary veins, and caseous material containing large numbers of mycobacteria are then discharged into the circulation. The lesions which arise are particularly numerous in the lungs, liver, kidneys and spleen. They consist of tubercles of fairly uniform size, and without specific therapy death usually results from tuberculous meningitis after about a month, at which time the tubercles are of approx. 1–2 mm. diameter (Fig. 15.45, p. 366): they are rather poorly developed, often without giant cells, but with central necrosis (Fig. 7.14) and are termed *miliary tubercles* (latin *milium*— millet seed). In some instances, the bacteria escape into a systemic vein, either directly or by involvement of the thoracic duct, and as a result the number of miliary lesions in the lungs far exceeds those in other organs. When a relatively small number of tubercle bacilli gain entrance to the blood stream, few tubercles are produced in the various organs, and since the patient may survive much longer than is the case in untreated acute miliary tuberculosis, the lesions may become larger. One or more large metastatic lesions may also occur, for example in the bones, joints, kidneys, epididymes or fallopian tubes, and less

commonly in the brain. Although blood-borne lesions arise most commonly as a complication of the primary tuberculous complex, they may also occur in chronic pulmonary tuberculosis, particularly in advanced cases: haematogenous lesions are also observed when tuberculosis is complicated by other debilitating diseases, or as a result of corticosteroid or other immunosuppressive therapy.

Spread of tuberculous infection occurs also along hollow viscera and in body cavities. Spread by the air passages of the lungs is of great importance in pulmonary tuberculosis; mycobacteria coughed up in sputum may settle and give rise to lesions in the larynx and intestine. Spread may occur from the fallopian tubes to the endometrium, and from the kidney to the urinary tract, and dissemination may occur within the pleural, pericardial and peritoneal cavities and within the subarachnoid space and ventricles of the brain.

Healing of tuberculous lesions

The healing of tubercles or larger tuberculous lesions is dependent on the elimination or reduction in numbers of mycobacteria. Healing is brought about by formation of reticulin around the lesions, and by maturation of this into fibrous tissue. If caseation is slight or absent, as in early tubercles, the whole lesion may be gradually replaced by fibrous tissue, leaving a scar (Fig. 7.14), but extensive patches

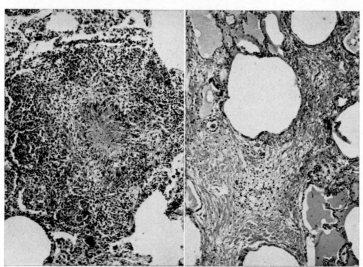

FIG. 7.14.—On the left is shown a miliary tubercle of lung with central caseation and acute exudate in the surrounding alveoli from a patient with untreated miliary tuberculosis; on the right a fibrous scar containing a few lymphocytes, the remains of a miliary tubercle after specific chemotherapy. × 72.

of caseation usually persist and become encapsulated in fibrous tissue. Slow, progressive deposition of calcium salts commonly occurs in the caseous material, which eventually may become stony hard and clearly visible in radiographs, and in some instances the calcified material may be replaced by bone, which may even develop spaces containing haemopoietic marrow (Figs. 15.34, 15.35, p. 361). The course of the disease depends on the balance between success of bacterial multiplication, with extension and caseation of the lesions, and success of the reactive processes in killing the bacteria, preventing their spread, and promoting a fibroblastic reaction.

The course and prognosis of tuberculosis have been radically changed by effective specific chemotherapy, which has also greatly modified the appearance of tuberculous lesions. When healing occurs "naturally", i.e. without specific chemotherapy, large caseous lesions become walled off first by cellular tubercles and then by new-formed fibrous tissue, which penetrates the outer zone of tubercles and finally encapsulates the central caseous mass. Dense fibrosis and calcification complete the process: there is little resolution. Treatment with streptomycin, which is bactericidal but does not readily penetrate into cells, hastens this process but its essential features remain as in "natural" healing, ending with much fibrosis and little resolution; thus miliary tubercles may heal, leaving small hyaline scars. The therapeutic combination of streptomycin, *p*-amino-salicylic acid (PAS) and isonicotinic acid hydrazide (INAH) is more effective, perhaps because the phagocytic cells are highly permeable to INAH, which acts specifically on tubercle bacilli in the actively growing phase. Combined therapy is accompanied successively by resolution of the surrounding exudative lesions, increased vascularity, and reversion of the endothelioid cells to foamy macrophages, formation of granulation tissue, absorption of necrotic and caseous material, and finally by healing with the production of minimal amounts of fibrous tissue. A notable result of combined treatment is the appearance of attempts at regeneration of the parenchymatous cells of the affected tissue, e.g. bronchiolar and alveolar epithelium. Combined therapy thus strikingly modifies the outcome; recent exudative lesions may clear up almost completely without residual effects and chronic caseous and fibrotic lesions

with excavation are transformed to smooth-walled cavities, at least partially relined by epithelium.

Syphilis

Historical note

It is generally believed that syphilis was introduced into Europe on the return of the Spanish sailors of Columbus from America and that by the end of 1494 it had spread throughout Spain and along the Mediterranean coast into Italy. Within a century it had become widespread throughout Europe, having been carried everywhere by the mercenary troops returning to their own countries after the Siege of Naples (1495). At this time syphilis was clearly recognised as a new disease and its manifestations became so well known that Shakespeare was able to give a remarkably accurate account of them in *Timon of Athens* (Act IV, Scene 3). If the above view of the introduction of syphilis to Europe is correct, this is, of course, an anachronism! Confirmation of the previous absence of syphilis from the Old World is afforded by the complete lack of evidence of the disease in skeletal remains dating back before 1494, whereas in Central America, bones found in ancient tombs bear clear indications of the disease.

Formerly common, syphilis is now relatively infrequent in the United Kingdom: recent reports show some increase, particularly among homosexuals, but the rise is much less than for gonorrhoea. Syphilis is an important *venereal disease*, i.e. it is usually contracted by coitus and the primary lesion is then on the genitals. Extragenital infections occur on the lip, tongue or breast and also on the fingers from handling infective lesions. The causal agent is a small motile spiral micro-organism or spirochaete, *Treponema pallidum*. Infection is usually by direct contact, the presence of a minute abrasion or crack in the skin apparently facilitating the entry of the organisms. The disease has a distinct incubation period, followed by a primary lesion and then a secondary, febrile stage with skin eruptions, and this may be followed by a tertiary stage, with localised lesions, and a late stage with disease of the central nervous system. It is convenient to give a general survey of the course of the untreated disease at this point. The special features of the individual lesions will be considered in the appropriate sections later.

F

"Stages" of syphilis

The primary sore. The *primary sore* or *hard chancre* (Fig. 7.15) appears usually on the external genitals, after an incubation period of 3–4 weeks, as a small, slowly growing papule of hard, almost cartilaginous consistence and pale coppery-red colour. The centre ulcerates and there may be some exudate which, in a skin lesion, is usually scanty and forms a crust. When the lesion is on a mucous surface and the part is not kept clean, there may be a lot of superficial necrosis and ulceration, and a great variety of organisms is

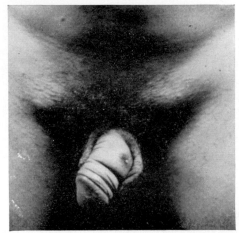

Fig. 7.16.—Primary chancre and bilateral inguinal bubo.

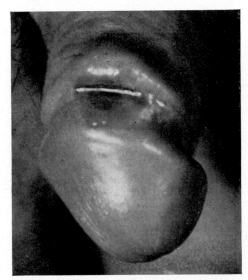

Fig. 7.15.—Primary chancre.

then present along with the spirochaetes. The ulcer persists for some weeks, but eventually resolves and heals. During this period the inguinal lymph nodes, usually on both sides, become somewhat enlarged and hard (bilateral inguinal "bubo"—Fig. 7.16). At this stage the organisms are abundant in the serous exudate from the primary sore, and the diagnosis can be made most readily by examination of the exudate by dark-ground illumination; if this fails they may be demonstrable in fluid withdrawn by puncture of the bubo. Dissemination of the organisms by the blood takes place before the appearance of the primary lesion, and syphilis is known to have been accidentally transmitted by transfusion of blood withdrawn before the primary lesion had appeared in the donor.

Secondary lesions appear at a variable interval, usually from 2–3 months after infection; the organisms are already distributed throughout the body and give rise to multiple symmetrical lesions of the skin and squamous mucous membranes as well as in the lymph nodes. In the former, eruptions of various kinds occur, at first *macular* and *papular* but even pustular (rupia), the palms of the hands and soles of the feet being important sites. Lesions of the hair follicles in the scalp lead to loss of the hair—*alopecia*. On the moist cutaneous and muco-cutaneous surfaces of the vulva, anus and perineum, flat raised papules develop—*condylomata lata*—and these are intensely infective: they must not be confused with *condylomata acuminata*, the so-called venereal warts. The buccal and pharyngeal mucosa shows *catarrhal patches*, white and shining owing to thickening of the keratinised layer, and these break down, giving "*snail-track ulcers*". General slight enlargement of lymph nodes is also common and is most easily detected in the superficial groups, the epitrochlear nodes and those along the posterior border of the sternomastoid being often conspicuous. The lesions are usually accompanied by systemic disturbances such as fever, anaemia and general malaise. After some months all these lesions disappear spontaneously and the patient may remain free from symptoms for some years.

Tertiary lesions appear irregularly, especially in the internal organs, and in the skin and mucous membranes, so that the lesions are asymmetrical and less numerous but are also larger than those of the primary and secondary stages, and lead to serious and permanent damage. Tertiary lesions rarely appear within the first few years, and sometimes only after many years. They are characterised by both diffuse chronic interstitial inflammation and the formation of masses of granulation tissue which may undergo central necrosis. This latter is known as *gummatous change* and such lesions are called *gummas*; they may occur in any site but chiefly in the liver, testes and bones, associated with much diffuse syphilitic granulation tissue. The central necrotic portion is dull yellowish, firm and rubbery; this is surrounded by a more translucent capsule of young connective tissue which has often a very irregular outline (Fig. 23.2, p. 818). Thus extensive destructive changes are brought about, e.g. in the nasal bones with loss of the bridge of the nose and perforation of the palate, ulceration and destruction of the larynx, creeping ulcers in the skin, etc.—indeed no organ or tissue is exempt from tertiary syphilis. Of especial importance are the cardio-vascular lesions, which formerly took a serious toll of life. All tertiary lesions tend to undergo healing, and much distortion of the organs and interference with function may result from scarring.

Neurosyphilis. Lastly, in a small proportion of cases there occur two important nervous diseases, *tabes dorsalis* and *general paralysis*. Since these develop usually only many years after infection they are sometimes called *quaternary* lesions; they are due to the actual presence of the spirochaetes in the central nervous system.

Serological diagnostic tests

Syphilis results in the development of antibody which may be detected in the patient's serum by a flocculation test (e.g. Kahn, Meinicke or Hinton tests) or by a complement-fixation test, the Wassermann reaction. An alcoholic extract of normal beef heart, termed *cardiolipin*, is generally used as antigen, although extracts of various animal and human tissues may be used. By the time the primary chancre has developed, these tests are positive in approximately 60 per cent of cases: in the secondary stage, they are invariably positive; thereafter the percentage of positives falls, and many cases of neurosyphilis are negative, although in some of these the cerebrospinal fluid may give a positive result. False-positive results occur in a number of conditions, including malaria, leprosy, glandular fever and systemic lupus erythematosus, and occasionally in apparently normal pregnancy. It has been shown recently that more than one antibody may develop in syphilis, and more reliable serological diagnosis is provided by immobilisation and immunofluorescence tests, using *Tr. pallidum* as antigen.

Microscopic appearances

A fully formed **chancre** consists of cellular granulation tissue extending close up to the base of the irregularly thickened and stretched epithelium. In the central parts the cells are densely packed in the connective tissue spaces (Fig. 7.17),

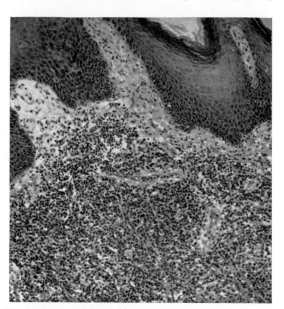

Fig. 7.17.—Section of primary chancre, showing extensive infiltration of the dermis with lymphocytes and plasma cells and some newly formed blood vessels. × 120.

and this gives rise to the typical hardness of the chancre. The tissue is very vascular and the small vessels are often surrounded by a sheath of pale and rather swollen cells accompanied by inflammatory infiltrate. Proliferation of the intimal cells and blocking of the lumen may be seen in the minute vessels, while larger twigs show endarteritis and periarteritis (Fig. 7.18). The interstices of the tissues are packed with cells: plasma cells very often predominate, but lymphocytes and some macrophages are also present. Polymorphonuclear leukocytes are absent or scanty except in the superficial parts when there is ulceration. Proliferation of the connective tissue cells and thickening of the stroma take place and increase the induration. After a time the reactive changes decline, the cells gradually diminish and only a little thickening of the fibrous stroma remains. As a rule there is little or no residual scarring, unless there has been much ulceration. The histological changes along the indurated lymphatics are essentially of the same nature. In the primary chancre there is little or no necrosis and giant cells are seldom present.

The lesions in the skin and mucous membranes in the **secondary stage** are essentially small areas of reaction around the spirochaetes distributed by the blood stream to the sub-epithelial connective tissue. The main changes are vascular engorgement and round-cell infiltration, the large number of plasma cells being a prominent feature (Fig. 7.19). Cellular infiltration occurs also around and into the hair follicles, and the hairs may fall out. All these disseminated lesions of the skin and mucous membranes usually subside naturally, i.e. without specific therapy.

The **gumma** of the **tertiary stage** is a cellular granulation tissue mass, but the central parts soon undergo necrosis, and accordingly it usually consists of yellowish necrotic material, surrounded by fibrous tissue. In course of time gummas have a great tendency to undergo absorption and shrinkage, and thus severe scarring results. In addition, chronic interstitial inflammation or fibrosis, often spreading extensively, is common, and this may be accompanied by foci of gummatous necrosis. Structurally a gumma resembles the primary sore, but differs in the early occurrence of necrosis (Fig. 7.20). This may be due in part to obliterative changes in the blood vessels, and possibly in part to the direct action of the spirochaetes, but these are so scanty that such an explanation is unsatisfactory and it seems more likely that the necrosis is chiefly due to a hypersensitivity reaction. In the necrotic areas the structural outlines may be preserved for a long time, the cells not having the same tendency to fuse into amorphous material as is seen in caseous tuberculosis. Giant cells may be present in the granulation tissue at the periphery, but they are usually smaller than in tuberculosis, and there are no well-formed follicles. Nevertheless the histo-

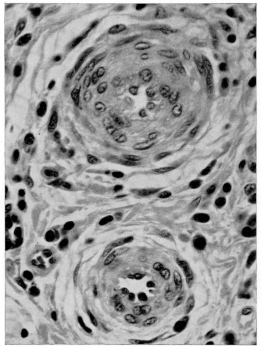

FIG. 7.18.—Section of chancre at late stage, showing obliterative changes in two arterioles. × about 450.

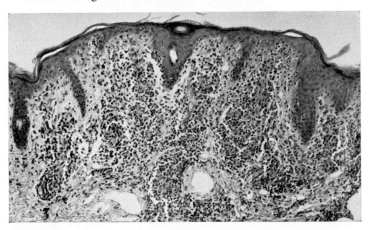

FIG. 7.19.—Papular syphilitic rash, showing abundant infiltration of the corium by lymphocytes and plasma cells. Note the hyperkeratosis. × 115.

logical diagnosis between the two diseases may be a matter of difficulty. The important *vascular lesions* of syphilis are described later: those in the larger arteries are due to the lodging of the

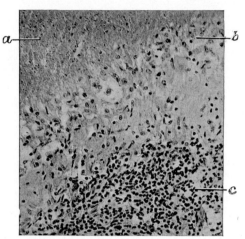

FIG. 7.20.—Part of gumma.

(*a*) Necrotic area with granules of chromatin. (*b*) Zone of connective tissue growth. (*c*) Infiltration with plasma cells and lymphocytes. × 200.

spirochaetes in the adventitial sheath, whence they extend into the media. Here, they give rise to cellular infiltrations like those described above, and some necrosis may follow.

Congenital syphilis

The first pregnancy after infection is likely to terminate prematurely with a stillborn macerated fetus, in the tissues of which spirochaetes are abundant. The parenchymatous organs show diffuse proliferation of connective tissue cells with minute foci of more severe reaction with necrosis—miliary gummas, and there is severe damage to the liver, lungs, pancreas, etc. (q.v.). In subsequent pregnancies the effects are progressively less severe. The next child may be born alive with the stigmata of congenital syphilis, namely a papular rash around mouth and nose, and on the buttocks, palms of hands, soles of feet. Disease of the nasal bones and mucosa leads to "snuffles" and interference with feeding. There is also syphilitic hepatitis with jaundice and splenomegaly, and lesions in the bones are common. Later a characteristic deformity appears in the incisor teeth, which are peg-shaped with notched edges (Hutchinson's teeth)

and there is also pitting of the first permanent molars. Still later, interstitial keratitis produces corneal opacity and blindness. Pregnancy has a curiously ameliorating effect on syphilitic lesions in the mother, who may appear healthy in spite of producing syphilitic offspring.

Actinomycosis

This disease is produced by organisms which are normal commensals in the mouth and gut, and only occasionally invade the tissues to produce infection. The actinomyces are branching bacteria which grow in the tissues to produce characteristic radiate colonies, sometimes visible macroscopically. In man, the micro-aerophilic *Actinomyces israelii* is the chief pathogen, but occasionally aerobic organisms—*Nocardia*—are involved, and also other species, which grow more diffusely. In bovines, in which actinomycosis is common, the lesions are localised and are large granulomatous masses which occur especially in and around the jaw. In man, the lesions are of a more suppurative type, and in about 50 per cent of cases are in the region of the mouth or jaws, the parasite gaining entrance commonly from a tooth socket; in 25 per cent the infection is in the appendix or caecal region, from which spread by the blood stream to the liver may occur; in about 15 per cent the initial lesion is in the lung and in 5 per cent it is subcutaneous. The lesion is usually a chronic suppurative one, with formation of multiple abscesses, each containing one or more colonies—the so-called honeycomb abscess (Fig. 19.29, p. 574). A fibrous tissue wall forms and is lined by granulation tissue which characteristically contains many foamy cells— macrophages laden with lipid—which give the lining of each abscess a yellowish colour. In the centre is pus containing actinomyces colonies (Fig. 7.21), which are sometimes visible by naked eye in the pus as small yellow or grey, gritty granules. Lesions in the face and neck, originating about the jaw, may produce much granulation tissue in which many small foci of suppuration persist and break down on the surface, resulting in multiple sinuses. The infection spreads directly through the tissues but does not usually involve the regional lymph nodes; if untreated it tends to invade the blood stream, giving rise to pyaemia with secondary abscesses in the liver, lungs and other organs.

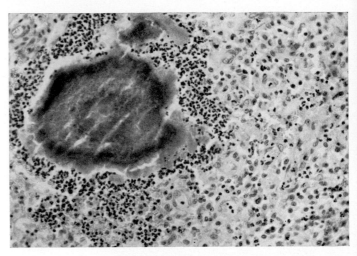

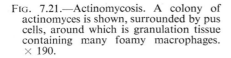

Fig. 7.21.—Actinomycosis. A colony of actinomyces is shown, surrounded by pus cells, around which is granulation tissue containing many foamy macrophages. × 190.

Leprosy

It is estimated there are throughout the world some 12–16 million people with leprosy. The disease was at one time not unusual in Great Britain, and in recent years it has again appeared among immigrants from countries in which it is still endemic. It is caused by an acid-fast bacillus, *Mycobacterium leprae*, but the exact mode of transmission is uncertain: it is not highly infectious and close contact is probably essential. The infection is often acquired in childhood. Unlike many other mycobacteria, *M. leprae* cannot be grown in artificial media, and so far has been cultured only *in vivo* in the mouse footpad. Experimental reproduction of the disease has been achieved by injection of infected material into mice with depressed immunological responses brought about by anti-lymphocyte serum (p. 87), or neonatal thymectomy followed by X-irradiation.

Two types of lesions are distinguished, the lepromatous and the tuberculoid, but less well defined types are also recognised. In the *tuberculoid type*, the lesions are granulomatous and undergo fibrosis and shrinkage; lepra bacilli are scanty. The organisms have a predilection for the cutaneous nerves, in which they multiply and spread, giving rise to multiple nodular thickenings, with destruction of nerve fibres and consequent anaesthesia, paresis, and trophic changes in the skin such as perforating ulcers.

In the *lepromatous type* the lesions consist of cellular aggregations of foamy macrophages, in which lepra bacilli are present in enormous numbers.

Skin testing with lepromin, a sterilised preparation of lepromatous lesions, gives a positive delayed hypersensitivity reaction resembling the tuberculin reaction in individuals with tuberculoid leprosy; the test is non-specific, being commonly positive in individuals who have never been infected. A later granulomatous reaction may develop, and becomes maximal in approximately 4 weeks: this also is not diagnostic of leprosy. The test is usually negative in lepromatous leprosy, and the significance of this is discussed on p. 121.

Sarcoidosis

This disease, which is of unknown causation, is characterised by multiple granulomatous lesions, and may affect lymph nodes, lungs, skin, eyes, salivary glands, liver and the bones, particularly of the hands and feet. It is of world-wide distribution, and is more common in Negroes than whites in the U.S.A., and in immigrants than natives in Great Britain. The highest reported incidence is in Sweden.

The disease most commonly gives rise to enlarged mediastinal and pulmonary hilar lymph nodes, often without symptoms, but sometimes accompanied by fever. Other groups of lymph nodes are often affected and minute lesions in the lungs may present an X-ray picture resembling that of miliary tuberculosis. Skin lesions of erythema nodosum are sometimes the earliest clinical feature, but sarcoid lesions may also occur in the skin. Microscopically, the lesions consist of tubercle-like follicles composed of endothelioid cells with occasional giant cells and scanty peripheral lymphocytes (Fig. 7.22 and Fig. 17.8, p. 460). The giant cells may contain curious star-shaped or conchoid inclusions (*asteroid* or *Schaumann bodies*). Unlike tuberculosis, the lesions do not undergo caseation although there may be a little central necrosis.

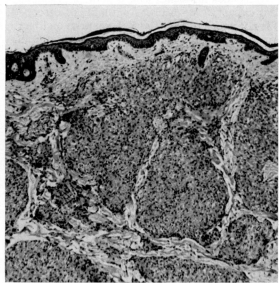

FIG. 7.22.—Sarcoidosis of skin. The lesions consist of aggregates of epithelioid cells with relatively few lymphocytes. In contrast to tuberculosis, there is little or no necrosis. × 80.

Intradermal injection of a sterile suspension prepared from sarcoid lesions (Kveim test) leads to the development of a lesion becoming maximal in about six weeks and having the histological features of sarcoidosis: the test is specific for sarcoidosis although recently, positive tests have been reported in Crohn's disease (p. 505). During the course of sarcoidosis, tuberculin tests are negative in most cases even when known to have been previously positive. The capacity to produce antibodies is not, however, impaired.

The course of the disease is unpredictable: it may be acute or chronic, and temporary or permanent remission may occur spontaneously. It can cause blindness by involving the uveal tract, and is occasionally fatal, usually as a result of fibrosis of the pulmonary lesions with consequent cor pulmonale (p. 369), or as a result of intercurrent infections. Hypercalcaemia may develop with consequent renal damage (p. 905). Some patients eventually develop frank tuberculosis with a positive tuberculin reaction.

Theories on the etiology of sarcoidosis include hypersensitivity to pine pollen, an atypical response to tubercle bacilli or other organisms, and a reaction to beryllium or other irritants. None of these explanations is entirely satisfactory.

Other granulomas

There are many other infections characterised by granulomatous lesions and caused by organisms of different kinds—bacteria, moulds, yeasts, dimorphic fungi and protozoa. The diagnosis of these infections rests as a rule on the identification of the parasite concerned. Some of these may be mentioned briefly.

Rhinoscleroma is an infection which produces nodular thickenings of the nose, pharynx and larynx. The lesions are essentially granulomatous and consist of numerous round cells, the cytoplasm of which contains many droplets which may fill the whole cell and push the nucleus to the side. Within these cells a bacillus, *Klebsiella rhinoscleromatis*, is present in large numbers. The disease is not uncommon in some European countries but rarely occurs in Great Britain.

Aspergillosis, most commonly produced by *Aspergillus fumigatus*, may occur as a chronic lung infection. However the effects of this particular fungus depend on whether or not the individual is hypersensitive (p. 368). The lesions are sometimes present in old tuberculous cavities or infarcts. They are often nodular with associated coagulative necrosis. In Northern Sudan a tumour-like granuloma may occur in the paranasal sinuses and orbit.

Histoplasmosis is most commonly caused by the dimorphic fungus *Histoplasma capsulatum* and produces a low-grade granuloma, usually of the larynx or lung, but occasionally more widespread and involving the reticulo-endothelial system: the degree of necrosis varies greatly. Judging by skin tests for delayed hypersensitivity, infection appears to be common in some countries, particularly the U.S.A.

Cryptococcosis is produced by the yeast *Cryptococcus neoformans*. Lesions may occur in lymph nodes and may simulate Hodgkin's disease, or in the lungs, simulating tuberculosis. A chronic granulomatous reaction is the rule, and multinucleated giant cells are common. The yeasts appear as round or ovoid bodies with a thick refractile capsule and occur both free and intracellularly. *Cryptococcus neoformans* infections are serious owing to the danger of spread to the central nervous system resulting in meningitis, which has a characteristically gelatinous character.

Sporotrichosis is caused by a dimorphic fungus, *Sporotrichum schenkii*. Diffuse granulomatous lesions develop, chiefly in the skin, with a tendency to suppuration. Occasionally lesions occur in the internal organs.

Delhi sore or **tropical ulcer** is an example of an ulcerating or granulomatous lesion produced by a protozoon, *Leishmania tropica*.

Lymphopathia venereum (lymphogranuloma inguinale) is a venereal infection in which the chief lesions are in the lymph nodes. It occurs especially where social conditions are poor, e.g. in large sea ports and in the tropics. The primary genital lesion is a small, superficial ulcer which often escapes notice. Swelling of the inguinal lymph nodes ("tropical bubo") becomes distinct from fifteen days to three weeks after exposure to infection and is accompanied by fever. Microscopically, the lymph nodes show a rather characteristic picture of multiple stellate abscesses containing polymorphonuclear leukocytes surrounded by a zone of endothelioid cells arranged in palisade fashion. The swellings become firm and tender and in white persons the skin over them assumes a reddish-violet tint. Adhesion of the nodes to the skin then occurs, and the abscesses discharge, producing multiple fistulae. In the female, owing to the lymph drainage of the cervix being to the nodes in the pelvis, the lesions are mainly in the latter and serious complications often follow: discharge into, and stricture of, the rectum may result, formation of fistulae and occasionally a condition of genital elephantiasis. Spread may occur to other groups of lymph nodes. The disease has been shown to be due to a member of the psittacosis group of virus-like organisms. Intradermal inoculation of the killed organisms (*Frei test*) produces an allergic reaction in sensitised individuals, with the appearance of an erythematous reaction at the site of inoculation. Complement fixation tests can also be used for diagnosis, a rising titre during the course of the illness being indicative of infection.

Granuloma inguinale. This is another granulomatous disease, quite distinct from that just described; it is not uncommon in tropical countries and North America. The lesions are in the cutaneous and subcutaneous tissues, and occur in and around the external genitals; chronic ulceration often follows. The characteristic feature is the presence in the granulation tissue of macrophages containing numerous small pleomorphic bacilli ("Donovan bodies"). Morphologically, this organism resembles a klebsiella, and it cross-reacts serologically with *Klebsiella rhinoscleromatis*.

Various other micro-organisms which cause granulomatous disease are of relatively low pathogenicity, and although they can cause lesions in otherwise apparently healthy individuals, are more prone to complicate diseases associated with depressed immune responses, such as the congenital immunological deficiencies (pp. 114–116), sarcoidosis, Hodgkin's disease and malignant neoplasms. Use of immunosuppressive or cytotoxic therapy, such as corticosteroids, azathioprine or actinomycin C, also predispose to such opportunistic infections, which include aspergillosis, cryptococcosis, systemic moniliasis, and pneumonia due to *Pneumocystis carinii*.

CHAPTER 8

DISTURBANCES OF THE CIRCULATION

Disturbances in the circulation, whether general or localised, are of major importance because of the dependence of tissues on the supply of oxygen and nutrients, and the removal of metabolites, by an adequate flow of blood.

A localised increase in blood flow—*hyperaemia*, is an essential feature of acute inflammation, but occurs also following temporary obstruction of the circulation. A general increase in circulatory rate results from impaired respiratory exchange in the lungs, or from congenital abnormalities of the heart or major blood vessels leading to a mixing of blood in the systemic and pulmonary circulations: it occurs also in anaemia and in conditions of increased metabolism, e.g. fever or hyperthyroidism. Local reduction in blood flow through an organ or tissue (*ischaemia*) can result from spasm or pathological obstruction of the supplying arteries and arterioles, from obliteration of the capillary bed, or from venous obstruction.

General reduction in blood flow results from failure of the heart to maintain its normal function, or from peripheral circulatory failure as seen in *shock*. This may be due to a fall in blood volume from various causes or to a general loss of capillary tone.

The *amount* of blood in any particular tissue is not necessarily indicative of the rate of blood flow. An excessive content of blood—*congestion*—may indicate increased flow, as in acute inflammation, but is observed also in association with reduced flow: for example there may be capillary congestion in association with arterial spasm, as in Raynaud's disease (see below). These various circulatory disturbances are considered in general outline in this chapter, together with an account of disturbances in the balance of the body's water and salt content, including the important condition *oedema*, i.e. accumulation of an excess of fluid in the tissues and serosal cavities.

ARTERIAL AND CAPILLARY HYPERAEMIA

The essential features of arterial and capillary hyperaemia have been discussed in connection with acute inflammation (pp. 33–34). An important point is that temporary deprivation of blood supply of a part by arterial occlusion is followed by active hyperaemia when the obstruction is released. This is of importance in bloodless operations, as the full degree of hyperaemia is not established till some time after the circulation has been restored, and thus bleeding may occur from the smaller blood vessels if they have not been ligated. If the ischaemic condition is prolonged irreversible damage may follow and the local capillaries become leaky so that great loss of plasma occurs into the damaged part; the blood in the vessels thus becomes inspissated and stasis and coagulation may result.

There are also conditions where the capillaries are dilated and the arteries contracted. When, for instance, the hands are exposed to cold, congestion is sometimes associated with blueness and coldness, due to impairment of the circulation by contraction of the arteries, while the capillaries are dilated and the blood within them is imperfectly oxygenated. There is neither arterial dilatation nor venous obstruction, and the congestion is apparently the direct effect of cold on the capillary walls. Local dilatation of capillaries alone, though increasing the amount of the blood in the part, will not increase the *rate* of blood flow. In fact capillary flow will be slowed because the capillary bed is so much wider than the sectional area of the corresponding arterioles.

Capillary dilatation in inflammation following various forms of injury, mechanical, chemical, thermal, etc., usually occurs within a few seconds, but when the skin is exposed to ultra-violet rays, the capillary dilatation does not occur till some hours afterwards, and then the capillaries may remain in a dilated state for days. The difference between heat rays and ultra-violet rays in this respect is noteworthy, and a delayed effect is also characteristic of X-rays. Capillary hyperaemia may thus be transitory or more persistent. If the capillary damage is more severe the flow of blood through the capillaries is interfered with and its rate diminished. The extreme degree of this is complete stoppage of the flow or *stasis* which may be reversible. A still more severe injury to the capillaries may cause necrosis of their walls with haemorrhage and thrombosis, and then restoration of the circulation is impossible. These different degrees of capillary injury are accompanied by increased permeability of the wall, leading to exudation, etc., and are of great importance in various pathological processes.

VENOUS CONGESTION OR PASSIVE HYPERAEMIA

Two varieties of this condition are recognised, namely *general venous congestion*, in which the whole venous system is affected. and *local venous congestion*, where excess of blood is present only in a limited area. Although the change is essentially the same in the two cases, the causal factors and results are different, and the two varieties are best described separately.

General venous congestion

This condition is of great importance in view of its frequency, and when it is long continued serious results follow from excess of blood in the venous system throughout the body. It may develop rapidly shortly before death, and at necropsy all the organs show venous engorgement; it may also be temporary and reversible. The essential factor in its production is diminished output of blood by the left ventricle, as will be explained below. The important form known as *chronic venous congestion* (CVC) is of long duration, is often permanent, and brings about important structural alterations. The cause of chronic venous congestion lies either in the *heart* or in the *lungs*, as these are the organs through which all the blood passes in each complete circulation. In the heart, lesions of the valves or myocardium, and in the lungs chronic bronchitis and emphysema or fibrosis, are the common causes.

All of these lesions impair the circulation through the heart or lungs: the mechanisms involved are described in the appropriate chapters, and the essential point is that they all lead to a diminution in the amount of blood passed into the aorta in a unit of time. This would lead to a fall in the arterial blood pressure if there were no compensating mechanism, because the pressure depends on the amount of blood passed into the aorta and on the peripheral resistance. But in the various conditions of diminished output mentioned, it is found that for a considerable time the blood pressure is maintained about the normal, and this is brought about by a tonic contraction of the arterioles and also by an increase in the blood volume. The amount of blood in the arterial system is thus diminished, while that in the veins is increased—in other words there is a general venous congestion. Later, however, the blood pressure may fall, the circulation then becomes embarrassed, and the heart ultimately fails.

Accumulation of blood in the venous system may be allowed by passive dilatation of the veins, and theoretically need not at first involve a rise of venous pressure. Later the resistance of the vessel wall to further dilatation may bring about an increase in the venous pressure. This can be detected by observing pulsation in the neck veins when the patient is sitting up or standing: normally the veins in the neck are partly collapsed, and do not pulsate, the blood pressure in them being slightly below atmospheric, but when the pressure rises markedly, they are distended in the lower part of the neck and pulsate at about the level where the blood is at atmospheric pressure. Increased venous pressure may also be measured directly by catheterisation. In general venous congestion the capillaries and veins contain an excess of slowly-flowing blood with a larger proportion of reduced haemoglobin than the normal; hence the oxygen supply to the tissues may be reduced and hypoxaemia and cyanosis result, and are followed by oedema and structural changes. With the exception of oedema, which is discussed on pp. 180–185, these effects are considered below.

Hypoxaemia

This term means deficiency of oxygen in the blood; it is applied to the various conditions in which the oxygen supply to the tissues is reduced: (*a*) due to lowered oxygen saturation of the arterial blood—*hypoxic type* (p. 346), or (*b*) to deficiency in the actual or available haemoglobin in the blood—*anaemic type* (p. 400), or (*c*) to decrease in the proportion of oxy-haemoglobin within the congested capillaries —the *congestive* or *stagnant type*. The oxygen available for the tissues is proportional to the concentration in the plasma, and this in turn depends on the amount of oxyhaemoglobin in the red cells. In normal arterial blood, for example, the amount of oxygen in solution is about 2 per cent of that combined with haemoglobin. As the oxygen in solution is used up by the tissues additional oxygen separates from the oxy-haemoglobin, and thus in the passively congested capillaries the degree of oxygen saturation of the haemoglobin is reduced below the normal; accordingly the amount of oxygen in solution is also reduced and thus the supply to the tissues is diminished. The normal degree of oxygen saturation of arterial blood is about 95 per cent while that of venous blood is about 65–75 per cent. In the congestive form of hypoxaemia the difference between the arterial and venous saturation is greater than the normal of 20–30 per cent, for the reasons stated. General chronic venous congestion due to cardiac disease may, however, exist without hypoxaemia. It is especially when cardiac compensation begins to fail, and the cardiac output is still more diminished, that the oxygen unsaturation of the venous blood becomes increased. Further, in the later stages of cardiac failure there are oedema and other changes in the lungs, and the aeration of the blood in the pulmonary capillaries is im-

paired. Thus the arterial saturation also may fall below the normal, that is, *hypoxic* hypoxaemia may be superadded, and then the degree of venous unsaturation becomes increased.

Longstanding congestive hypoxaemia interferes with cellular metabolism: it commonly causes fatty changes in the liver cells, and may be concerned in the production of oedema.

In cases of congenital heart disease, e.g. pulmonary stenosis with deficiency in the interventricular septum, not only may there be venous congestion but also there is admixture of the arterial and the venous currents. In such cases the arterial blood is not fully oxygenated and congestive failure may aggravate the consequent tissue hypoxia.

Cyanosis

This term is a descriptive one, indicating varying degrees of blueness or lividity of the skin and mucous membranes; it occurs in chronic venous congestion, resulting from an increased *amount* of reduced haemoglobin in the capillaries and small veins. Cyanosis depends also on the relative transparency of the skin and other tissues. In severe anaemias the *degree* of venous unsaturation may be much higher than in venous congestion and yet cyanosis may not be present because the amount of reduced haemoglobin is insufficient.

Causation. The chief conditions producing cyanosis are as follows: (*a*) Accumulation of blood in the capillaries with diminished rate of flow through them. This is seen in severe chronic venous congestion, as already described. It occurs also when a similar condition of capillary congestion and reduced flow is produced by exposure to cold. The initial reaction to cold is usually a general contraction of arterioles and capillaries, but after a time the capillaries become dilated from loss of tone, and cyanosis occurs. These two effects of cold are seen in intensified form, in the "local syncope" and "local asphyxia" of Raynaud's disease (p. 283). (*b*) Cyanosis may occur also, in proportion to the deficient oxygen saturation of the arterial and venous blood, in pulmonary disease with deficient aeration, e.g. in bronchitis and emphysema, pneumonia, pulmonary oedema, etc. Further, cyanosis tends to occur from this cause in individuals living at a high altitude, especially on exertion. But in extreme cyanosis there is usually a combination of the two factors (*a*) and (*b*). (*c*) Cyanosis is often a prominent feature in cases of congenital heart disease with admixture of the venous and arterial streams—"admixture cyanosis"—for example, in pulmonary stenosis with deficiency in the interventricular septum. In such cases, the haemoglobin concentration is above normal due to secondary polycythaemia (p. 390), and as it is largely in a reduced form within the capillaries the cyanosis is thereby intensified.

General venous congestion may exist for a long time without the occurrence of any *oedema* but ultimately this may appear, at first in the tissue round the ankles, and then steadily increase (p. 182).

Structural changes

When chronic venous congestion has persisted for some time, the organs are not only moderately swollen and purplish owing to excess of venous blood, but they become firmer in consistence, especially the kidneys and spleen, hence the term *cyanotic induration*. The induration appears to be due chiefly to thickening of the capillary walls in response to the state of overdistension. There is little increase in the interstitial tissue.

In the **lungs** (Fig. 8.1) red cells escape from time to time from the congested capillary walls and are taken up by macrophages (p. 44), within which their haemoglobin is broken down, and haemosiderin and other brown pigments are formed, and may be demonstrated *in vitro* by the Prussian blue reaction (p. 202). These macrophages may accumulate in the alveoli in considerable numbers, and they are often known as heart-failure cells, but the term is misleading as they are present when compensation is well established; in fact all that is necessary for their formation is an escape of red cells into the alveoli. Haemosiderin accumulates also in the interstitial tissue of the lungs and in the pleural membrane; the tracheobronchial lymph nodes are often only slightly pigmented. The lungs thus develop a brownish tinge and often feel firmer than normal (*brown induration*). In mitral stenosis, however, the lungs may show numerous dark brown spots due to massive aggregations of iron-containing macrophages around the

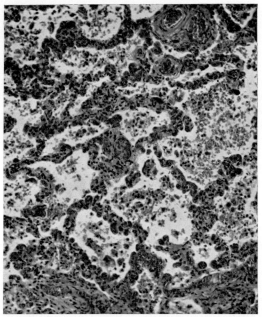

Fig. 8.1.—Lung in chronic venous congestion, showing thickening of alveolar walls and varicosity of capillaries; macrophages containing haemosiderin are lying free in alveoli. Note thickening of pulmonary arteriole. × 105.

terminal respiratory bronchioles, while the intervening alveoli are practically free from cells. This uneven distribution is probably due to macrophages taking up escaped red cells in the alveoli and then migrating to the interstitial tissue where they become arrested: the same distribution is seen after repeated injections of blood intratracheally in animals, and in man particles of inhaled coal-dust become similarly aggregated (p. 345). In CVC the aggregations of iron-containing cells may be sufficiently dense to be visible on X-ray examination and may be mistaken for miliary tubercles.

In the **liver**, congestion is most marked in the central parts of the lobules, where the liver cells undergo atrophy and ultimately disappear; the central zone is then constituted by the sinusoids and stroma (Fig. 8.2). At the same time fat may accumulate in the more peripheral surviving liver cells, and the lobules thus show dark red and yellow areas respectively, the term "nutmeg liver" being applied from the mottled appearance (Fig. 8.3). These atrophic and fatty changes are chiefly the results of hypoxaemia. Owing to the considerable loss of liver parenchyma in the central parts of the lobules, compensatory changes in the form of hypertrophy and hyper-

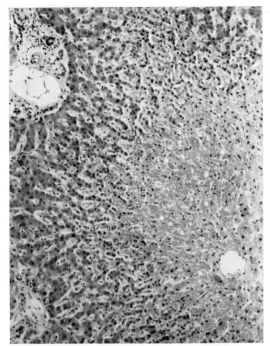

FIG. 8.2.—Liver in chronic venous congestion, showing centrilobular atrophy and disappearance of liver cells accompanied by dilatation of sinusoids (rt. side of figure). × 102.

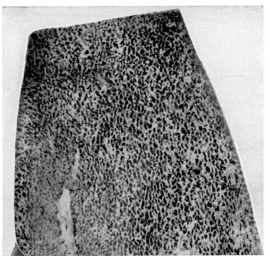

FIG. 8.3.—Liver in chronic venous congestion— "nutmeg liver".

Note the dark congested central parts of lobules, and pale periphery due to fatty change. (Natural size.)

plasia of surviving liver cells may follow. The pale hypertrophic areas may be small and regularly distributed (Fig. 8.4), or they may be larger and irregular. The changes are sometimes known as "*cardiac cirrhosis*", although they do not constitute a true cirrhosis (p. 569). Hypertrophic changes are seen only in longstanding cases and occur especially in young patients, in whom there have been several attacks of cardiac failure with subsequent recovery.

The **kidneys** are severely congested in most cases, the medulla especially being dark purplish (Fig. 8.5). The organs are firmer and more elastic than normal and the weight is slightly increased. In cases where passive congestion of the kidneys is marked, the urine is usually decreased in quantity and is highly concentrated; it often contains a small amount of albumin and a few red cells.

The **spleen** is moderately enlarged (up to 250 g.) and of firmer consistence so that it preserves its shape and on section shows a clean sharp edge. The cut surface is smooth and firm and the pulp is dark purple against which the paler Malpighian bodies and trabeculae stand out prominently. Histologically (Fig. 8.6) there is an

increased amount of blood in the red pulp, and dilatation of the venous sinuses with thickening of the fine reticular fibrils in their walls and of the connective tissue of the trabeculae, including the elastic tissue. More severe chronic congestion of the spleen, often with greater enlargement, occurs in portal venous hypertension (p. 452).

Local venous congestion

This results from mechanical interference with the return of blood from a part—by the forma-

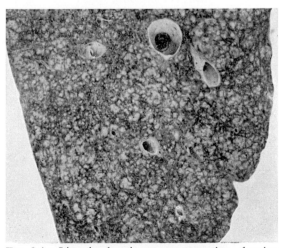

FIG. 8.4.—Liver in chronic venous congestion, showing numerous pale hypertrophic areas. × 1.

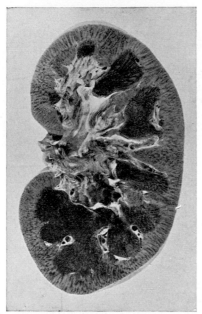

FIG. 8.5.—Kidney in chronic venous congestion, showing the intense vascular engorgement. × ⅔.

tion of a thrombus within a vein, or by pressure from outside, e.g. by a tumour or an aneurysm, or by the contraction of fibrous tissue. It may develop rapidly or slowly.

(*a*) If a vein is *rapidly obstructed*, e.g. by a thrombus or by a ligature, the local effect depends on the degree of anastomosis: if this is inadequate, venous congestion develops in the drainage area of the vein. Local swelling and lividity result, and, if the part is on the surface, also some fall in temperature. Owing to the increased filtration pressure there occurs an excessive transudation of fluid into the tissue

spaces. Experimental venous obstruction does not cause oedema in otherwise normal tissues, the excess of fluid being carried off by the lymphatics. In man, however, obstruction of a vein is often followed by oedema of the congested tissue, e.g. a leg. The relation of venous obstruction to oedema will be considered later. Red cells also may escape from the engorged capillaries, and there may even be gross *haemorrhage* and infarction. For example, when the superior longitudinal sinus is obstructed by thrombus, as occurs sometimes in severely debilitated children, the cortical veins of the brain become enormously dilated, and some of

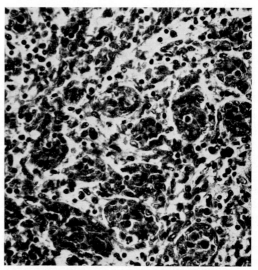

FIG. 8.6.—Chronic venous congestion of the spleen. The vascular sinuses are distended with blood, and the intervening medullary cords are relatively inconspicuous. × 250.

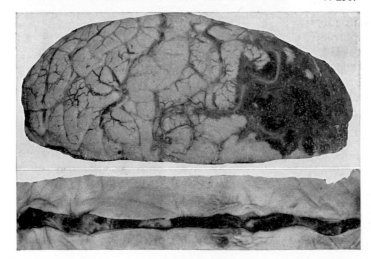

FIG.8.7.—Thrombosis of superior longitudinal sinus with resulting haemorrhage over frontal lobe of brain.

Note the greatly dilated and thrombosed cortical veins. The thrombosed sinus is shown below. × ⅔.

them may give way and cause irregular haemorrhage on the surface of the brain (Fig. 8.7). So also, obstruction of a branch of the splenic or renal vein may cause widespread haemorrhage in the area drained by it, the lesion resembling a haemorrhagic infarct produced by arterial obstruction. A similar result is seen when thrombosis of the mesenteric veins extends down into the small branches, diffuse haemorrhage and infarction then occurring in the related part of the bowel wall.

When a part of the intestine is impacted in a hernial sac, it often becomes distended by gas, and the pressure may then occlude the venous drainage: no collateral venous return is possible, and the gut is referred to as *strangulated*: it becomes engorged with blood, diffusely haemorrhagic, and finally necrotic and gangrenous. In most situations, however, when a vein is blocked, the blood is carried off from the part by the collateral veins and the circulation through it is maintained, though for a time at a decreased rate.

(*b*) *Chronic obstruction*, either complete or partial, and especially when it is slowly produced by compression of a vein, is accompanied by a marked enlargement of the collateral veins (Fig. 8.8). Thus obstruction of the superior vena cava, which may result from lung cancer extending into the mediastinum, is accompanied by great enlargement of the veins lying above the clavicle. This is not due simply to distension of the veins: the walls actually hypertrophy. In portal venous congestion, commonly due to cirrhosis of the liver, enlargement and varicosity develop in those veins which can pass blood from the congested portal system to the systemic venous system. One such group of veins runs longitu-

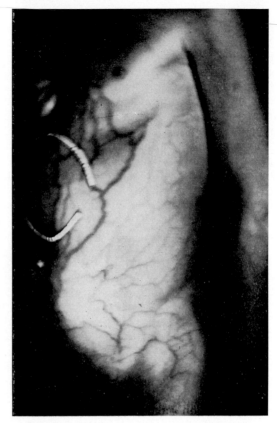

Fig. 8.8.—Enlargement of superficial collateral veins in obstruction of the inferior vena cava, shown up by infra-red photography.

dinally in the submucosa of the lower oesophagus; in their enlarged, engorged state, these veins are liable to rupture with serious or fatal bleeding into the oesophagus. Local oedema and ascites frequently result from chronic portal obstruction in cirrhosis (p. 572).

PETECHIAL HAEMORRHAGES

Examples of haemorrhage from large vessels by rupture as the result of injury or disease will be given later. We shall consider here first the multiple haemorrhages which may occur in various general conditions, and which are often minute capillary haemorrhages or *petechiae*. Observations on the circulation during life show that in inflammatory and other conditions, an escape of red cells may take place through transient breaches in the capillary walls, and this is called *diapedesis* to distinguish it from haemor-

rhage due to actual rupture of the wall, termed *rhexis*. Multiple petechiae are probably produced in the latter way in most cases, and the escape of blood is apparently the result of damage to the capillary endothelium. Such haemorrhages occur in two main groups of conditions: (*a*) in *acute infections* such as septicaemias, scarlet fever, yellow fever, etc., chiefly in the skin and serous surfaces, although bleeding may take place also from mucous membranes, e.g. in the stomach in yellow fever and in various septic conditions, without any gross breach of the mucosa to account for it. Multiple haemorrhages occur also in phosphorus poisoning. (*b*) various *blood diseases*—pernicious anaemia, leukaemia, purpura, scurvy, haemorrhagic disease of the newborn, etc. Here also, the haemorrhages are often multiple and there may be slight or more severe bleeding from mucous membranes.

In infections, haemorrhages are sometimes produced by the actual presence of organisms; for example, plugs of organisms are found in the capillaries in cases of meningococcal and pneumococcal septicaemia. In other cases, however, they are apparently due to endothelial damage by toxaemia. In anaemias and purpuric conditions, the occurrence of haemorrhage is often associated with diminution of the blood platelets and a prolongation of the bleeding time. Deficiency of vitamin K gives rise to a haemorrhagic tendency by lowering the prothrombin content of the blood. In scurvy the haemorrhagic tendency is due to vitamin C deficiency, which brings about some defect in the capillary endothelial cell junctions. In some cases the cause of spontaneous haemorrhages is imperfectly understood.

HAEMOSTASIS AND THROMBOSIS

The haemostatic and fibrinolytic mechanisms

The vital importance of keeping the blood fluid within an intact and patent vascular compartment following vascular injury is reflected in the complexity of the mechanisms which exist to this end. Continued blood loss from a leaking vessel is prevented by temporary vasoconstriction and the formation of a haemostatic plug. Initially, the haemostatic plug consists of platelets which rapidly accumulate at the site of vascular injury; the platelet plug is subsequently reinforced by fibrin formation. When the fibrin has served its function, it is removed by the fibrinolytic system, and more permanent repair processes of healing and fibrous tissue replacement then follow.

The haemostatic mechanism can be considered to function at two different levels: in response to an obvious major challenge such as a surgical incision or childbirth to seal off severed blood vessels, and also in every-day life to seal off the many tiny injuries to small blood vessels. The "spontaneous" haemarthroses of patients with a defect in the clotting mechanism, as in severe haemophilia, illustrate the need for effective haemostasis as a continuing physiological mechanism. The opposite effect, inappropriate or pathological thrombosis, is very common, and while there is often some predisposing cause, such as an abnormality of the wall of the blood vessel, or defective blood flow, it is to be regarded as a disturbance of the haemostatic mechanism.

The normal haemostatic mechanism

There are four components in the haemostatic mechanism: vascular contraction, platelets, the formation of fibrin (blood coagulation), and the fibrinolytic mechanism. Vascular constriction and normal platelet function are themselves not sufficient for physiological haemostasis. When a tooth is extracted from a patient with haemophilia, vascular constriction and the platelet component of haemostatis may prevent bleeding for a few hours after the extraction but unless the platelet haemostatic plug is reinforced by normal deposition of fibrin, haemostasis is only temporarily secured and bleeding, which may be very persistent, then occurs.

Platelet function. In normal blood, platelets circulate as single disc-like fragments of cytoplasm at a concentration of $1 \cdot 5 - 3 \times 10^5$ per cu. mm. In addition to providing a factor active in blood coagulation (platelet factor III), the platelets play a vital role in haemostasis. Following injury to the endothelium, they adhere initially to collagen in the connective tissue beneath the damaged endothelium. Contact with collagen provokes complex biochemical and morphological changes in the platelets (see Fig. 8.13). Adenosine diphosphate (ADP) is released from the platelets at the site of injury and causes further aggregation of platelets, leading to progressive occlusion of the vessel by a platelet mass. Simultaneously vascular injury initiates the process of blood coagulation which leads to thrombin production and fibrin formation. Thrombin, in addition to converting fibrinogen to fibrin, causes an explosive release of ADP, 5-hydroxytryptamine and other components from the platelets. These cause further platelet aggregation. The build-up of fibrin around the platelets is an essential step in the formation of an effective haemostatic thrombus.

Platelet function may be studied in various ways, e.g. by assessment of the percentage of platelets in a given sample which adhere to a standard column of glass beads through which the blood is passed, or the aggregation of platelets in plasma following the addition of aggregating substances such as ADP. These techniques have shown that there are a number of syndromes in which, although platelet counts are normal, platelet function is abnormal. Conditions with deficient platelet function include uraemia, the primary thrombocytopathies and hereditary haemorrhagic telangiectasia (p. 444): increased platelet adhesiveness and aggregation have been found in diseases associated with thrombo-embolic phenomena such as ischaemic heart disease, peripheral vascular disease and venous thrombosis. In the puerperium and following surgical operations, platelet adhesiveness is increased, the effect being maximal around the tenth post-operative day. This contributes to the post-operative thrombotic tendency.

Blood coagulation—extrinsic and intrinsic systems. When blood is withdrawn from the body by clean venepuncture and placed in a plain smooth glass test tube it will clot in five to ten minutes. However if the test tube contains an extract of minced tissue, the blood will clot in ten seconds. In this simple experiment the blood *alone* clots under the influence of a system which is derived from the components within the blood itself without any contribution from the tissues. This system is called the *intrinsic* or *blood thromboplastin system*. The more rapid clotting which occurs in the presence of tissue extract is described as clotting under the influence of the *extrinsic* or *tissue thromboplastin system*. The plasma components which contribute to the formation of fibrin by both the intrinsic and extrinsic systems are complex (Table 8.1).

The relationships between blood clot, the haemostatic plug and thrombus. When blood is placed in a test tube and allowed to clot, the cellular elements are randomly distributed throughout the fibrin network. However for-

Table 8.1.—International classification of the plasma coagulation factors (Roman numerals), together with their commonly-used names. The term "factor VI", formerly applied to an intermediate product, is no longer used.

Factor I	Fibrinogen
Factor II	Prothrombin
Factor III	Tissue factor
Factor IV	Calcium
Factor V	Proaccelerin
Factor VII	Proconvertin
Factor VIII	Antihaemophilic globulin
Factor IX	Plasma thromboplastin component or Christmas factor
Factor X	Stuart–Prower factor
Factor XI	Plasma thromboplastin antecedent
Factor XII	Hageman factor
Factor XIII	Fibrin stabilising factor or plasma transglutaminase

mation of a haemostatic plug or a thrombus takes place in flowing blood, and the cellular elements of the blood are not randomly deposited. In a haemostatic plug an occluding mass of platelets forms at the site of the leakage, and upon this is deposited fibrin which spreads into and reinforces the platelet plug. In a pathological thrombus a similar histological picture is seen with the white "head" of agglutinated platelets and numerous white cells, followed by a red "tail" consisting of fibrin and entrapped red cells (see p. 169).

Conversion of fibrinogen to fibrin. The conversion of fibrinogen to fibrin is brought about by the highly specific proteolytic enzyme thrombin, which splits off two small peptides from each fibrinogen molecule, converting it into fibrin monomer. Monomers of fibrin then polymerise to form a network of fibrin. In purified systems fibrin is soluble, but in the body it is converted to an insoluble form by the enzyme transglutaminase or fibrin stabilising factor (factor XIII) which is present in the plasma.

Conversion of prothrombin to thrombin. The ability of the body to keep the blood fluid and free of fibrin formation within the blood vessels is a remarkable phenomenon which suggests that no effective amount of thrombin can be in circulation. Blood coagulation occurs only when the thrombin is elaborated from its inert precursor prothrombin (factor II), under the influence of one or both of the two pathways already mentioned, the intrinsic or blood thromboplastin system and the extrinsic or tissue thromboplastin system.

In both the intrinsic and extrinsic pathways, the components probably do not react together simultaneously to produce their final "pro-thrombin converting principle", or thromboplastin; a sequence of reactions probably takes place in stepwise fashion in which one component acts as an enzyme and the other as a substrate. Two essentially similar series of sequential reactions, termed the "cascade" and "waterfall" sequences, have been suggested to explain the mechanism of blood coagulation (Fig. 8.9). This hypothesis is likely to be further modified as more information becomes available as the result of purification of known clotting factors. The intrinsic thromboplastin system is activated by contact of blood with a water-wettable surface which activates factor XII (Hageman factor). This reaction presumably occurs in response to relatively minor injuries. The extrinsic or tissue system is triggered *in vitro* by contact with tissue extract, and presumably operates in more severe injury.

Normal vascular endothelium appears to have an important role in maintaining the fluidity of the blood within the vascular compartment. In addition, plasma contains natural inhibitors of clotting, and activated clotting factors are removed by the liver and the reticulo-endothelial system. Not much is known about the inhibitors but it is probable that they are of great importance in limiting the activation of the clotting mechanism and reducing the risk of intravascular fibrin formation when coagulant substances enter the blood stream.

The fibrinolytic enzyme system

The fibrinolytic enzyme system has four main components: plasminogen, plasmin, activators and inhibitors. Plasminogen, a β-globulin of the plasma, is converted by activators to plasmin, a proteolytic enzyme which under suitable circumstances digests fibrin to give soluble products (Fig. 8.10). Plasminogen activators are widespread throughout the body, being present in almost all the tissues with the exception of liver and placenta. Activity is concentrated around blood vessels, particularly veins and venules. Plasminogen activator activity is also present in the blood plasma and is responsible for physiological fibrinolytic activity of plasma. It is also present in many body secretions, e.g. milk, tears, saliva, seminal fluid. Normal urine contains urokinase, a physiological plasminogen activator which may represent in part excreted plasma activator and may also be produced in part in the kidney. In normal plasma, fibrinolytic activity is low, but increased activity is found after exercise or emotional stress, and also following surgical operations and other trauma.

Normal plasma possesses both anti-activator and anti-plasmin activity. Platelets also show anti-plasmin activity.

The fibrinolytic enzyme system is probably in dynamic equilibrium with the blood clotting system, the two acting together to maintain an intact and patent vascular tree. According to this hypothesis the coagulation and fibrinolytic systems may both be continuously active, the

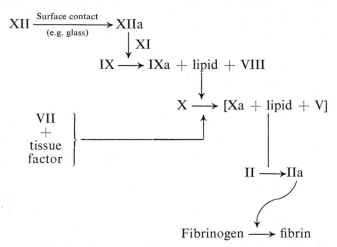

FIG. 8.9.—A simplified version of one current concept of the "cascade" reaction involved in coagulation. A series of reactions is involved in which inactive coagulation factors are converted to active forms, denoted by the letter "**a**" after the symbol for the factor.

former laying down fibrin where needed on the endothelium to seal any deficiencies which may occur, and the latter removing such deposits after they have served their haemostatic function.

Plasminogen (inactive plasma globulin)

Activators ⟶

Plasmin (proteolytic enzyme)

Fibrin ⟶ soluble products

Fig. 8.10.—The fibrinolytic enzyme system.

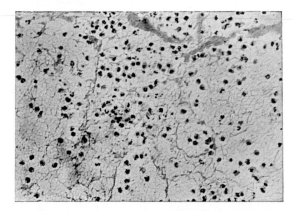

Fig. 8.11.—Red thrombus, showing a network of fibrin with leukocytes and numerous red cells between. × 250.

Thrombosis

Thrombosis is defined as the formation of a solid or semi-solid mass from the constituents of blood within the vascular system during life. As already explained, it differs from coagulation in that the latter occurs after death or in blood which has been withdrawn from the body.

Appearances and composition of thrombi

The composition of thrombi and thus their gross and microscopic appearances depend largely on their rate of formation and this in turn is determined mainly by the rate of the flow of blood from which they develop. As a general rule, thrombus forming in rapidly flowing blood, e.g. in an artery, consists mainly of aggregated platelets, with some fibrin; it enlarges slowly and is firm and pale, varying from greyish white to pale red, and is commonly called *pale thrombus*. By contrast, thrombus forming in stagnant blood, as for example in a blood vessel which has been occluded or constricted, consists of a network of fibrin in which are entrapped red cells, leukocytes and platelets (Fig. 8.11). It is called *red thrombus* and is formed by simple coagulation: like clot, it is soft and red and may retract from the vessel wall. Between these two extremes we have *mixed thrombi* which form in slowly flowing blood, usually in veins, and consist of alternating layers of platelet aggregates and red thrombus. The mixture may be intimate and only recognisable on microscopy: Fig. 8.12 shows such a thrombus in which the spaces between trabeculae of aggregated platelets are filled by a

fibrin network containing leukocytes and red cells. In other instances, veins may be filled with columns of red thrombus but with platelet aggregates at points of anastomosis. The formation of such thrombi is explained on p. 169. Except in recently formed thrombi, it is not easy to recognise aggregated platelets, for they soon lose their outlines, presenting microscopically a granular or structureless appearance. Immunofluorescence studies and electron microscopy (Fig. 8.13) have, however, facilitated their recognition.

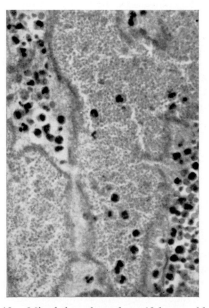

Fig. 8.12.—Mixed thrombus, about 12 hours old, showing dense masses of granular material, composed of fused platelets, with collections of leukocytes between. × 390.

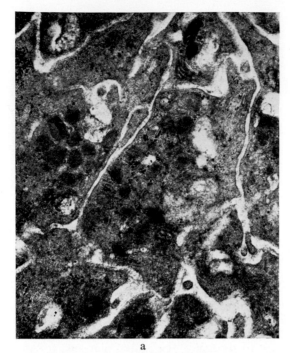 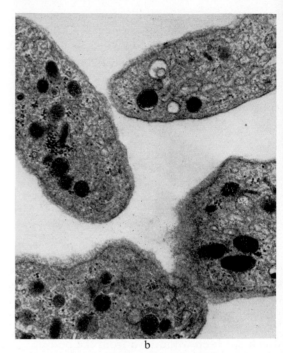

a   b

FIG. 8.13.—Electron micrograph of platelet thrombus (a), compared with free platelets (b). The platelets forming the thrombus fit closely together and are distorted, but can be readily recognised. × 28,000.

Factors predisposing to thrombosis

The three major predisposing factors are (a) local abnormalities of the vessel (or heart) wall; (b) slowing or disturbances in the flow of blood, and (c) changes in the composition of the blood. The parts played by these three factors in the formation of thrombi in the heart, arteries and veins are described below.

(a) Cardiac thrombosis. At necropsy, post-mortem clots are usually to be found in the chambers of the heart. They are soft and dark red with a glistening surface and are not firmly adherent to the endocardium. Occasionally the red cells settle before coagulation occurs and the upper (usually anterior) part of the clot is then yellow and gelatinous. Thrombi may form rapidly as the circulation is failing immediately before death. They are yellow or pinkish with a glistening surface and have a somewhat stringy appearance (Fig. 8.14). Such agonal thrombi originate at the apex of the ventricle to which they are attached and may extend through the valve orifice. They are composed mainly of fibrin, which separates out from the sluggishly moving blood before death, and may occur in either or both ventricles, although they are commoner in the right side of the heart. Quite apart from these terminal or post-mortem events, thrombi may form in any of the four chambers of the heart. In the atria, thrombosis is commonest in the appendices, especially that of the right atrium, in cases of heart failure with atrial dilatation. Stagnation of blood is probably the most important causal factor and this is accentuated by atrial fibrillation, which is very commonly complicated by thrombosis. Rarely small flattened globular thrombi form in either the atria or ventricles. They are pale, composed mainly of platelets and may show central softening. In mitral stenosis, a rounded thrombus may develop in the left atrium and lie free. It may exceed 3 cm. in diameter and is a rare cause of sudden obstruction of the circulation—the so-called "ball valve thrombus". The vegetations which form on the heart valves in certain diseases are essentially thrombi. In rheumatic fever the valve cusps are damaged along the line of apposition, and deposition of platelets results in the formation of minute pinkish-grey bead-like projections or vegetations (Fig. 8.15): in bacterial endocarditis the cusps are damaged by bacterial infection and not only platelets are deposited but also fibrin and interspersed leukocytes, and the important factors in its formation are the disturbances in blood flow caused by lack of pulsation in the dead muscle and also diffusion of factor III (tissue thromboplastin) from the dead tissue.

(b) Arterial thrombosis. Probably because of the rapid flow of blood, arterial thrombosis is uncommon in the absence of a local lesion of the vessel wall. In affluent communities, atheroma in arteries of various sizes is the commonest predisposing local lesion. In the aorta, atheroma is commonly severe and results in gross dis-

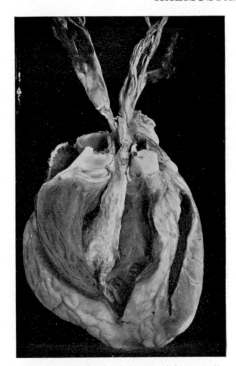

FIG. 8.14.—Agonal clot in right ventricle extending along the pulmonary artery in a case of pneumonia. × ½.

vegetations are consequently larger, softer, and more friable (Fig. 8.16). In the ventricles, mural thrombosis commonly occurs on the endocardium overlying an infarct (i.e. a patch of ischaemic necrosis of the heart wall—Fig. 8.17). Depending on the size of the infarct, the thrombus may be large or small. It forms a flat reddish plaque attached to the endocardium. Probably the

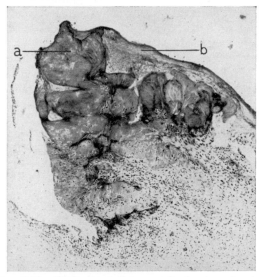

FIG. 8.15.—Early vegetation on mitral valve, showing surface deposit of hyaline material consisting of (*a*) fused platelets and (*b*) fibrin; early organisation is in progress. × 48.

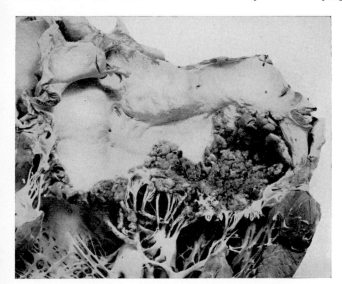

FIG. 8.16.—Numerous vegetations (thrombi) on atrial aspect of mitral valve, in a case of bacterial endocarditis. × ⅔.

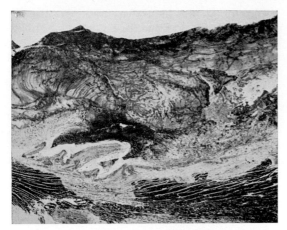

FIG. 8.17.—Mural thrombus in left ventricle (above), superimposed on a myocardial infarct (below).

tortion and unevenness of the wall, but because of the rapid flow of blood thrombosis is often not superadded. Sometimes, however, mural thrombi form over atheromatous plaques which have ulcerated or which have caused a local bulging of the aortic wall (Fig. 8.18). When blood is flowing smoothly in a normal vessel, the particulate elements are separated from the vascular endothelium by a layer of almost pure plasma, but atheromatous plaques, by causing irregularities of the wall, result in disturbed flow, and platelets can then impinge on the wall. This is possibly a predisposing factor to thrombosis, but the ulcerated plaque also brings the blood into contact with an abnormal surface on which platelet aggregation occurs. The irregularities also cause local disturbances in the rate of blood flow. When there is gross localised dilatation (aneurysm) of the wall of the heart, aorta or other arteries, stagnation and eddying of the blood usually result in some thrombosis. The thrombus may have a laminated appearance and may come to fill the aneurysmal sac (Fig. 8.19). Atheroma commonly gives rise to thrombosis in the arteries of the brain and heart. Because of

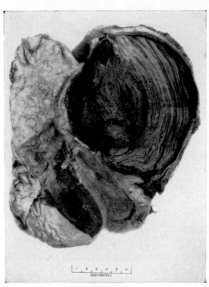

FIG. 8.19.—Aneurysm of aorta containing laminated thrombus.

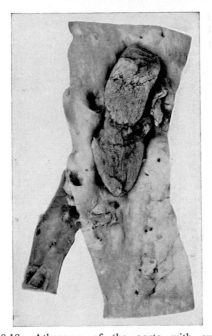

FIG. 8.18.—Atheroma of the aorta with extensive thrombus formation over the origin of superior mesenteric and other arteries. Infarction of intestine resulted.

their relatively small calibre, which is further reduced by the atheromatous plaques, thrombi readily occlude these vessels completely and ischaemic necrosis commonly results in the deprived tissues. This is described later in the section on infarction and also in the appropriate systematic chapters. Inflammatory lesions in the walls of arteries may also cause thrombosis: contributory factors may be irregularities of the wall, as in syphilitic aortitis, injury to the vascular endothelium, and release of tissue thromboplastin. In severe arterial hypertension, necrosis of the walls of small arteries and arterioles is commonly followed by thrombosis.

(c) **Venous thrombosis**. Because of the relatively slow flow of venous blood, veins are the commonest site of thrombosis. There may be a local predisposing factor, for example a patch of fibrous thickening in the wall, invasion or compression by tumour, and above all, inflammation of the wall of the vein due either to a phlebitis of unknown cause or to involvement in a pyogenic bacterial infection. Frequently, however, there is no demonstrable local predisposing lesion and thrombosis starts by platelet aggregation, usually within a small vein.

The structure of venous thrombi and the factors concerned in their formation are illustrated by thrombosis in the veins of the lower limbs, which is very common in elderly hospital patients, especially following a surgical operation. It is important because it is the usual cause of fatal pulmonary embolism. It starts in the relatively small veins in the calf muscles and may extend proximally as far as the femoral or iliac veins or rarely into the inferior vena cava (Fig. 8.20). The initial thrombus formed in the small calf veins occludes the lumen and for some distance proximal to the occlusion, blood flow is virtually arrested. This column of blood is rapidly converted into red thrombus as far as the next proximal venous tributary. Blood from this tributary continues to flow into the affected vessel and for a time arrests the formation of red thrombus. However, platelets in the moving column of blood coming from the tributary are deposited on the proximal end of the red thrombus, which thus becomes capped with more slowly formed pale platelet thrombus. This may eventually occlude the entrance of the tributary, again producing stagnation, and so red thrombus forms and extends proximally to the next tributary. So the process continues with thrombus extending into larger, more proximal veins. Once a tributary has been occluded, red thrombus also forms in the stagnant blood within it and so the thrombus in the main venous trunks comes to have branches extending into the tributaries. Leg vein thrombosis tends to occur especially in patients lying immobile in the supine position, and impairment of blood flow by pressure on the calves appears to be an important predisposing factor. It is particularly common after an abdominal operation, after childbirth, severe injury, myocardial infarction and in patients with congestive heart failure. Venous return from the lower part of the body is normally

aided by muscular movements of the legs and by the pumping action which ensues from use of the abdominal muscles and diaphragm in respiration, and in all the above conditions immobility of the legs interferes with the normal flow. To avoid the pain of abdominal movements, patients who have had an abdominal operation tend to use mainly the thoracic muscles for respiration, and this is a further factor in impairing venous return from the legs. Following operation, childbirth, or myocardial infarction, the platelets increase temporarily both in number and in adhesiveness and there is also a rise in the prothrombin level in the blood. These changes are maximal at about the tenth day, when thrombosis commonly occurs. The main factors predisposing to venous thrombosis in congestive heart failure are venous congestion, impaired venous flow and immobility. Another common site of thrombosis following operation, etc., is in the veins of the pelvis. This is seen especially after childbirth when the uterine blood flow diminishes considerably, predisposing to thrombosis in the hypertrophied uterine veins. Puerperal sepsis is also a predisposing factor in some cases. Pelvic venous thrombosis may also originate in haemorrhoids. Extension to large veins, including the internal and common iliacs, may complicate pelvic

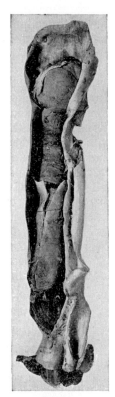

FIG. 8.20. — Large thrombus in inferior vena cava, with rounded projection at upper end. × $\frac{2}{5}$.

venous thrombosis and fatal pulmonary embolism may follow. It is partly to prevent venous thrombosis that patients are encouraged to leave their beds as soon as practicable after operation, childbirth, etc., and while bedridden to carry out muscular exercises and to practise abdominal respiration.

Venous thrombosis is also a common complication of malnutrition, severe debilitating infections and wasting diseases such as cancer. *Marantic thrombosis* occurs in severe debility in infants and young children. It commonly affects the superior longitudinal sinus and may give rise to haemorrhagic lesions in the cerebral cortex (Fig. 8.7). In patients with malignant tumours, and especially carcinoma of the pancreas, repeated episodes of thrombosis may occur in various veins and this may precede other symptoms.

(d) Capillary thrombosis. Thrombosis in capillaries and venules commonly occurs in severe acute inflammatory lesions. It is due partly to endothelial damage and partly to haemoconcentration, the thrombi being composed mainly of packed red cells.

There is no evidence that leukocytes play an important direct part in the formation of thrombi although they may be entrapped in considerable numbers in the fibrin network of rapidly formed thrombi. In cases of leukaemia, with huge numbers of circulating leukocytes, these cells may aggregate in masses and cause vascular obstruction.

The venom of certain snakes has a powerful thromboplastic effect and causes rapid and extensive coagulation of the blood. The thromboplastic factors in such venoms have been used as laboratory reagents in estimating the level of plasma prothrombin and also as local haemostatic agents as, for example, in haemorrhage following tooth extraction in haemophiliacs.

Sequels of thrombosis

Restoration of the vascular channel after thrombotic occlusion may occur by a combination of fibrinolysis and shrinkage of the thrombus. The fibrinolytic mechanism depends on the activation of plasminogen in the plasma and this may become very active when there has been large-scale intravascular coagulation such as may result from the entry of amniotic fluid into the maternal circulation. Veins thrombosed by venepuncture are usually restored to normal patency within a few weeks, and permanent occlusion only rarely follows. This mechanism is sometimes ineffective, and residual thrombus is then removed by the process of organisation (p. 60).

Venous thrombi may become infected with pyogenic organisms and undergo suppurative softening; fragments are then liable to be carried away by the blood stream, giving rise to pyaemia. In some instances, thrombosis is beneficial, for example when it occludes a vessel involved in an ulcerating lesion and thus precludes haemorrhage.

EMBOLISM

By embolism is meant the transference of abnormal material by the blood stream and its impaction in a vessel. The impacted material is called an *embolus*. In most cases it is a fragment of thrombus, occasionally material from an ulcerated atheromatous patch. A fragment of a tumour growing into a vein may form an embolus, and there may be embolism of the capillaries by bacteria, fat globules, air bubbles or collections of parenchymal cells. The site of embolism will, of course, depend on the source of the embolus. Thus embolism of the pulmonary arteries and their branches is secondary to thrombosis in the systemic veins or in the right side of the heart. Rarely, where there is a patent foramen ovale, an embolus may pass from the right side of the heart to the left atrium and thus be carried to the systemic circulation; such a condition is called *crossed* or *paradoxical embolism*. With this rare exception, emboli occurring in the systemic circulation are derived from thrombi formed in the left side of the heart, from vegetations on the aortic and mitral valves, and occasionally from thrombi or detached portions of atheromatous patches in the aorta or large arteries. Emboli carried from tributaries of the portal vein lodge, of course, in the portal branches in the liver.

Effects of embolism

Systemic emboli. The results are simply those of mechanical plugging and vary according to the site of the embolus, as described in pp. 173 et seq.

Pulmonary embolism is a specially important form resulting from the detachment of a thrombus in a large vein, usually in the lower limb. Such thrombi form in conditions which have already been described (p. 169) and in any of them pulmonary embolism may result. It is most common around the tenth day after operation, and may cause sudden death. The thrombus may become detached *en masse* and carried to the right side of the heart, causing a sudden blockage of the pulmonary trunk or one of its divisions, death usually occurring at once or after a short period of pulmonary distress. The thrombus is sometimes so long that it is found at necropsy coiled up like a snake in the right ventricle with one end extending along the pulmonary artery (Fig. 8.21); if smaller, it may be contained within the pulmonary artery or its branches. When the patient has lived some time after the embolism, a varying amount of haemorrhagic infarction may be present in the parts supplied by the blocked vessels. Infarction, however, is never co-extensive with the area of distribution, and sometimes there is none.

Septic emboli. With the widespread use of antibiotics, septic emboli, containing pyogenic bacteria, have become relatively uncommon. They may give rise to suppuration and this is the usual process by which multiple abscesses are produced in pyaemia. An infective embolus, when arrested in an artery, occasionally weakens the wall and gives rise to an aneurysm—*mycotic aneurysm* (p. 287). In various septicaemic and

pyaemic conditions, capillaries here and there may be plugged by organisms, most frequently pyococci, or by impaction of a small fragment of infected thrombus, the organisms then growing along the capillaries. The number of bacteria is also greatly increased by growth after death.

Embolism from tumours. This is of two kinds. One or a few cells of the tumour may enter the blood stream and impact in a capillary in some distant organ. In other instances there may be growth of a tumour into a large vein, and a larger fragment may become detached, carried by the blood, and impacted in a vessel, e.g. a branch of the pulmonary artery or of the portal vein. Both of these processes can result in metastatic tumours.

Fat embolism. Entrance of fat into the circulation results from laceration of veins surrounded by adipose tissue. It probably occurs after all fractures with displacement and injury of adipose tissue, of a fatty liver, and in Caisson disease (p. 661). In most instances the phenomenon is of no clinical importance but when the amount of fat entering the circulation is large, as in fractures of long bones, the *fat embolus syndrome* may develop within the following 3 days. The syndrome includes mental confusion, fever, dyspnoea, tachycardia, a petechial rash and sometimes cyanosis, haemoptysis, coma and death. It appears to be due largely to hypoxia resulting from pulmonary fat emboli complicated by oedema and haemorrhage. Fat may, however, pass through the lungs into the systematic circulation and cause emboli in the brain, giving rise to multiple small haemorrhages, in kidneys (Fig. 8.22), and in the skin. There may

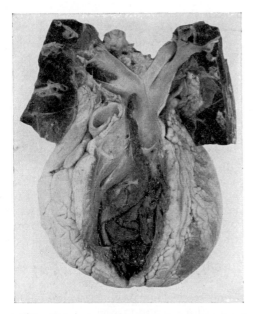

FIG. 8.21.—Pulmonary embolism; heart showing large cylindrical embolus in right ventricle extending up into right pulmonary artery. × ½.

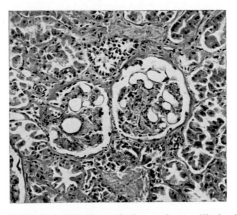

FIG. 8.22.—Fat embolism of glomerular capillaries in a case of caisson disease. The fat appears as unusually large clear globules. (A. C. L.) × 125.

also be thrombocytopenia. In patients who recover, there is usually no residual disability.

Air embolism. This occurs when air is aspirated into a severed vein, especially a large vein near the heart, but air may also enter the circulation in fatal amounts during blood transfusion if positive pressure is used without due care. The frequency and seriousness of the condition have probably been exaggerated. The air may produce effects in two ways. It may become mixed with the blood in the right ventricle, forming a frothy fluid, and thus may interfere with the proper emptying of the cavity, or the bubbles of air may become arrested in the pulmonary arterioles and lead to the mechanical effects of embolism. When air enters the circulation it is absorbed rapidly, and to produce serious results the sudden entrance of a considerable amount is necessary. Experiments have shown that rabbits are comparatively susceptible, while dogs can tolerate the entrance of large quantities without serious effects; man is said to occupy an intermediate position; less than 100 ml. has provoked alarming symptoms, but recovery has occurred after as much as 300 ml.

At necropsy, bubbles of gas may be found in the blood, due to the action of the *Clostridium welchii* after death, and this should not be mistaken for air embolism.

Parenchymal-cell embolism. In certain conditions special types of cells form emboli in the pulmonary vessels, for example the megakaryocytes of the bone marrow in severe infections, the syncytial cells from the placenta, and liver cells after laceration of the liver. Such cellular emboli are without serious effect, the cells in all probability disintegrating. By contrast, the entry of amniotic fluid into the maternal circulation during prolonged or obstructed labour may cause serious effects in two ways. Firstly, it may produce extensive and sometimes fatal embolism of the pulmonary circulation by fetal squames, vernix and meconium. Secondly, it may bring about both widespread intravascular fibrin formation and activation of the plasminogen fibrinolytic system, with the result that there is severe hypofibrinogenaemia, and dangerous post-partum haemorrhage commonly results.

LOCAL ISCHAEMIA

Complete arterial occlusion

The term ischaemic is applied to tissue in which the blood flow has ceased (complete ischaemia) or is abnormally low (partial ischaemia). Ischaemia localised to an organ, a part of the body, or a patch of tissue, is usually due to obstruction to arterial blood flow.

By far the commonest and most important causes of complete arterial occlusion are thrombosis and embolism; other causes include proliferative changes in the intima of small arteries, and also arterial spasm as in Raynaud's disease or ergot poisoning.

When an artery is obstructed the result depends on the extent of *collateral circulation*, i.e. alternative vascular routes by which blood can reach the deprived tissue. The arterial anastomoses in the limbs are such that blockage of any one artery does not usually result in severe ischaemia provided that the other arteries are not seriously diseased. Similarly, there are effective collateral arteries in the integument and muscles of the trunk. In the internal organs, however, the anatomical arrangement of many of the vessels does not allow a sufficient anastomic supply, and severe ischaemia follows arterial occlusion. When an artery of a limb is suddenly obstructed in a healthy subject, there is an immediate drop in the blood pressure beyond the obstruction, and the circulation is brought almost to a standstill; the arteries then contract and the part contains less blood than normally. Soon, however, the anastomotic arteries dilate and blood thus by-passes the obstruction to enter the vessels of the affected part, through which a flow of blood is gradually established and increased until ultimately it may approach normal. Thus in a healthy subject the femoral artery may be ligated without permanent damage resulting. The limb becomes cold and numb, and some time elapses before the pulse returns at the ankle; and it is much longer before complete muscular power is restored. The collateral vessels remain dilated and maintain the circulation, and in response to the sustained rise in blood flow there occurs a thickening of their walls, with increase of the muscular and elastic tissue corresponding with the enlarged lumen; in other words, the collateral vessels become permanently enlarged or hypertrophied. A good example is provided by the rare congenital condition of stenosis (*coarctation*) of the aorta beyond the arch, in which there occurs during development a great enlargement of vessels which link the arteries of the head and neck with those supplying the trunk and legs, the coarctation being thus by-passed.

The development of an efficient collateral circulation often depends on dilatation of healthy anastomotic arteries, and on a healthy heart. If, however, the collateral arteries are diseased, e.g. atheromatous, fibrosed or calcified, they are unlikely to dilate sufficiently to supply the necessary amount of blood to the ischaemic part, and a varying amount of necrosis will follow. In middle-aged or old people blockage of the main artery of a limb, or even of a large branch, may be followed by death of the tissues supplied by the obstructed vessel, the condition of "senile" gangrene resulting (p. 140). When there are multiple obstructions of limb arteries or spreading thrombosis, as in thrombo-angiitis obliterans (p. 279), serious results may follow and lead to gangrene even in young adults.

Infarction

Certain arteries of internal organs have imperfect anastomoses and their obstruction is always followed by serious results. Such arteries are called "end arteries", and they may have no anastomosis, e.g. the splenic artery, only capillary anastomosis, e.g. the branches of the renal artery, or arterial anastomosis, but insufficient to keep the part alive, e.g. the superior mesenteric artery. Obstruction of such vessels leads to ischaemia, usually sufficient to cause tissue necrosis, and sometimes congestion and haemorrhage in the affected tissue. The term *infarct* is applied to the altered area which has lost its blood supply, and use of the term implies that the tissue has undergone ischaemic necrosis. Infarcts are of two main types, *pale* or *anaemic*, and *red* or *haemorrhagic*. Pale infarcts occur in organs where there is little or no anastomosis, e.g. heart and kidneys; while in organs where there is some anastomosis, e.g. the intestine, or a double circulation, e.g. the lungs, red infarcts are found, blood passing from the marginal vessels into the damaged area. Infarction means literally a stuffing-in, and was originally applied to the haemorrhagic type, as the part appeared stuffed with blood. When pale infarcts were found to have a similar cause, the term was applied to them also.

Infarction is usually the result of acute occlusion of an artery by thrombosis or embolism. In the coronary arteries, atheroma with thrombosis is common, and is the usual cause of infarction of the myocardium: in the brain, thrombosis and embolism are both of importance, while in the lungs, kidneys and spleen embolism is a commoner cause than thrombosis.

Features of infarcts in various sites. In the kidneys, spleen and lungs, the vascular arrangements are such that most infarcts are roughly wedge- or cone-shaped, the apex lying most deeply, in the vicinity of the occluded artery, and the infarct enlarging as it extends peripherally, the base being visible as a necrotic area on the surface of the organ (Figs. 8.23, 8.24 and 8.26). The coronary arteries pass inwards from the epicardium, and accordingly myocardial infarcts involve especially the inner part of the wall, although commonly the whole thickness undergoes infarction.

In the **brain** a reduction in blood flow sufficiently severe to produce infarction is usually due to atheroma of the cerebral arteries or of major arteries in the neck that supply the brain, viz. the internal carotid and vertebral arteries. The artery may be occluded by thrombus formed on an atheromatous plaque but stenosis alone, by severely impairing blood flow through the artery, may cause ischaemic damage in the brain. Indeed cerebral infarction should be equated with a reduced cerebral blood flow rather than actual arterial occlusion as infarction may occur, even when the major neck arteries and the intracranial arteries are normal, as a result of a profound fall in cerebral blood flow due, for example, to cardiac arrest or an episode of severe hypotension. A not uncommon cause of occlusion of a cerebral artery is embolism. Even when a major cerebral artery is completely occluded, there is considerable variation in the size of the infarct, due partly to the severity and extent of the reduced blood flow and partly to the efficiency of the potential collateral circulation through arteries on the surface of the brain that link the major cerebral arterial territories, and through the circle of Willis. A cerebral

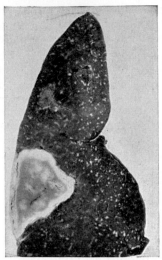

FIG. 8.23.—Pale infarct of spleen, showing process of decolorisation of the margin. × ⅔.

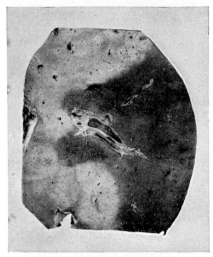

FIG. 8.25.—Atrophy and congestion of liver, due to plugging of branch of portal vein; thrombus is seen in the vein. × ⅔.

infarct may be pale or haemorrhagic (red) depending on whether or not some circulation becomes re-established through it. As the dead tissue soon breaks down and becomes soft, a cerebral infarct is often referred to as a *softening*. Thereafter, over a period of weeks or months, the necrotic tissue is gradually removed by phagocytes. The final result is a cystic shrunken area in the brain (see Figs. 20.18, 20.19, p. 624).

The central artery of the **retina** is an end-artery, and its obstruction causes retinal infarction, with loss of sight in the eye.

In the **heart**, obstruction of a coronary artery or a major branch gives rise to infarction of the ventricular myocardium; it is usually somewhat irregular in form, and is pale but with congestion and haemorrhage at the margin.

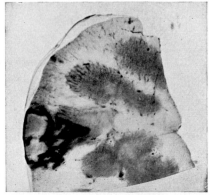

FIG. 8.24.—Infarct of kidney, showing pale necrotic centre with haemorrhagic margin. × ⅘.

The branches of the **pulmonary artery** have little anastomosis, but blood from the bronchial arteries provides a collateral circulation. Obstruction of a branch of a pulmonary artery does not invariably cause pulmonary infarction even when the occluded branch is a large one. This is due to the double blood supply. Pulmonary infarcts are haemorrhagic, the air spaces being filled with clotted blood (Figs. 8.26, 8.27). Experimentally-induced pulmonary emboli in otherwise healthy dogs do not usually cause infarction, and some general impairment of pulmonary blood flow is also required for infarction to result from the emboli, e.g. constriction of the pulmonary venous drainage. Similarly in man, impaired pulmonary blood flow, due to mitral stenosis, left ventricular heart failure or lung disease causing obliteration of pulmonary capillaries, predisposes to the development of infarction following pulmonary embolism. A rise in the pulmonary arterial pressure from the normal 18–25 mm. Hg. to 50 mm. or more is probably of importance, for it reduces the pressure difference between the bronchial and pulmonary arteries and prevents effective flow from the bronchial arteries into the pulmonary system of the ischaemic tissue beyond an embolus. Pulmonary infarcts are usually caused by emboli originating in the right atrial appendage of the heart or in a systemic vein. In pulmonary arterial hypertension, however, atheroma commonly develops in the pulmonary arteries and superadded thrombosis may then develop and lead to infarction.

Infarcts of the **spleen** are common and result usually from embolism. They are usually pale reddish at first, but soon become yellowish (Fig. 8.23); occasionally they are haemorrhagic. In the **kidneys**, infarcts seen at necropsy are

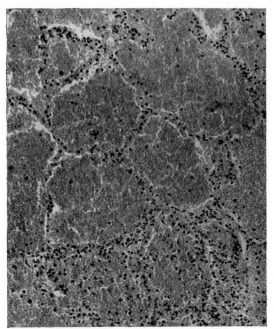

FIG. 8.27.—Haemorrhagic infarct of lung, showing alveoli filled with red cells. × 100.

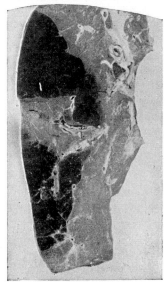

FIG. 8.26.—Two wedge-shaped haemorrhagic infarcts of lung. × ¾.

pale, with a deep red periphery due to congestion and haemorrhage. The pale portion involves chiefly the cortex, the affected part in the medulla being usually red and haemorrhagic (Fig. 8.24), but small infarcts may be haemorrhagic throughout. When an arterial branch in a kidney is blocked experimentally, the area supplied becomes at first swollen and red throughout owing to general congestion. Thereafter, the dying kidney cells take up water (p. 5), and their swelling expresses blood from the central part of the infarct, which thus becomes pale. At the periphery and in the medulla the hyperaemia and stasis persist, the nourishment of the capillary walls is impaired, and then haemorrhage occurs into the tissues. The fact that infarcts in the human kidney are usually pale is thus presumably due to the transitory nature of the early congested stage.

Blocking of the superior mesenteric artery produces a haemorrhagic infarct of the **intestine,** which is almost co-extensive with the distribution of the vessel (see below); death usually results unless the infarcted intestine is removed sur-

gically without undue delay. Obstruction of the inferior mesenteric artery, though the infarct is less complete, may likewise be fatal.

The sequence of events in the haemorrhagic infarct of the intestine, following obstruction of the superior mesenteric artery, has been studied experimentally in dogs. When this artery is ligated there is at first an arrest of the intestinal blood flow, accompanied by a contraction of the muscular coats of the intestine. The circulation is soon partially restored by blood flowing in from the arterial anastomoses, but without pulsation being present. The capillaries and small veins become engorged, but the flow through them is imperfect and irregular. Ultimately stasis occurs and there is diffuse haemorrhage into the wall of the intestine and its lumen. Correspondingly, the venous outflow becomes greatly diminished after the ligation; it then increases somewhat as the flow is re-established, and ultimately falls to a minimum. Complete deprivation of blood from 5–10 cm. of the bowel was found to lead to haemorrhagic infarction. Thus the collateral arterial supply may be able to fill the part with blood, but insufficient to maintain an adequate circulation.

In the **liver,** obstruction of a branch of the portal vein is not followed by infarction, owing to the supply of blood from the hepatic artery.

The obstruction does, however, reduce the blood flow sufficiently to cause atrophy and loss of hepatic parenchymal cells, and the sinusoids become widened and congested, giving an appearance resembling a red infarct (Fig. 8.25). Obstruction of the hepatic artery or of its branches may result in infarction of the liver (p. 545).

The susceptibility of tissues to ischaemia. The extent of infarction is usually less than that of the tissue supplied by the occluded artery, collateral circulation supplying the tissue at the periphery of the area. The extent of infarction may thus vary considerably, depending on whether the collateral arteries are healthy and capable of dilatation. Another factor of importance in determining the extent of the necrosis is the capacity of the tissue to withstand ischaemia. As a general rule, the parenchymal cells of the internal organs, which operate at a high metabolic rate, are relatively susceptible to ischaemia, whereas the supporting tissues—connective and fatty tissue and bone, are much less susceptible. The neurones of the central nervous system are perhaps the most susceptible cells of all, and cannot withstand deprivation of blood supply for more than a very few minutes. Glial cells are somewhat less demanding in their requirements, and accordingly at the margin of a brain infarct there is a zone of tissue exposed to partial ischaemia followed by restoration of the circulation by collaterals, in which the neurones have died while the glial cells persist and undergo reactive proliferation. Hepatic parenchymal cells are also highly susceptible to ischaemia and, as described above, thrombosis of a portal venous branch is commonly followed by atrophy and loss of liver cells with survival and dilatation of the sinusoids. The renal tubular epithelium has also a low resistance to ischaemia, and while in the central part of a recent renal infarct all the cells are dead, at the periphery there is a zone in which the glomeruli and intertubular capillaries have survived while the tubular epithelium has died.

Changes following infarction. Following occlusion of an end-artery, some time must elapse before morphological changes take place which afford recognition of tissue death, i.e. before the visible changes of infarction become apparent. The length of this interval depends on the type of tissue undergoing infarction and also upon the method of examination. In general, the changes are detectable first by electron microscopy; later they become apparent on light microscopy, and still later are visible on naked-eye examination. In examining necropsy tissues for the early changes of infarction, the interpretation of changes observed by electron- and light-microscopy is rendered difficult by post-mortem autolysis. The most reliable microscopic change is loss of cell nuclei, which undergo chromatolysis or karyorrhexis (p. 3). In most of the internal organs, infarcts remain solid and coagulative change occurs in the cytoplasm of the dead cells—*coagulative necrosis*: this is the usual sequel to tissue death in the kidneys, liver, myocardium, spleen and lungs. When there has been much exudation from the dying capillaries and venules, or actual escape of blood as in pulmonary infarction, coagulation of fibrin or blood contributes to the solidity and firmness of the infarct. Infarcts of the brain, however, usually undergo colliquative necrosis or softening, as described above, and softening occurs occasionally in infarcts of some other organs. For example, a myocardial infarct may undergo autolytic softening (*myomalacia cordis*), and this may be aggravated by the digestive enzymes of neutrophil polymorphs migrating into the dead tissue at the margin of the infarct (see below): rupture of the infarcted tissue may result, with escape of blood into the pericardium and fatal cardiac tamponade (p. 325). Central softening and liquefaction may occur also in a splenic infarct.

Tissue which has undergone coagulative necrosis remains recognisable microscopically for some days or even weeks. Cellular outline persists (Fig. 8.28), although the details of cytoplasmic structure are, of course, lost, and the dead cells have a refractile, homogeneous or hyaline appearance, well seen in myocardial infarction (Fig. 1.4, p. 4): the structural elements of blood vessels and stroma—collagen, reticulin and elastic fibres—persist for longer, and remain demonstrable by appropriate staining techniques.

At an early stage of infarction, products of dead cells at the periphery diffuse into the adjacent tissue and promote a mild acute inflammatory reaction, with exudation of fluid from the vessels and migration of neutrophil polymorphs into the peripheral dead tissue. This, together with ischaemia of their walls, accounts for the dilatation of the small vessels and

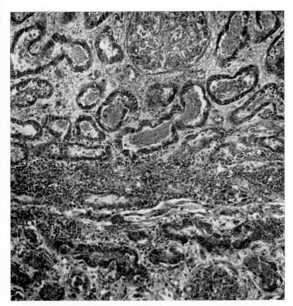

FIG. 8.28.—Infarction in kidney; the upper half shows the appearances of necrotic tissue. × 120.

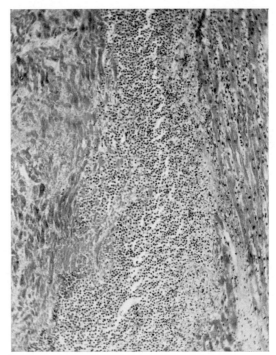

FIG. 8.29.—Septic infarct of heart. To the left, the dead heart muscle forms a slough, separated from the healthy myocardium on the right by a zone of polymorphonuclear leukocytes. × 85.

haemorrhage at the margin of the infarct. The acute reaction soon passes off, and the emigrated polymorphs die. The dead tissue stimulates a reaction similar to that around a foreign body: within a few days a zone of vascular granulation tissue forms around the infarct, and ultimately encloses it in a fibrous capsule. The dead tissue is gradually organised; macrophages migrate into and digest it from the periphery inwards, and they are accompanied by new capillary buds and fibroblasts, so that the granulomatous reaction progresses centrally, and as it matures into fibrous tissue the infarct is gradually converted to a scar. Extravasated red cells soon lose their outlines, and the pigment is slowly absorbed, although haemorrhagic infarcts, e.g. in the lungs, remain brown for a long time, and macrophages containing haemosiderin may long remain in and around the scar tissue. Loss of parenchymal cells and contraction of the fibrous tissue results in shrinkage; thus an old infarct of the myocardium presents the appearance of fibrosis and thinning of the ventricular wall (Fig. 14.8, p. 303). In solid organs, old scarred infarcts result in surface depressions, and when they are multiple, e.g. from repeated emboli in the branches of the renal arteries, the surfaces may be puckered and deformed by the scarring.

Septic infarcts. Multiple infarcts due to emboli containing pyogenic bacteria are an essential feature of pyaemia (p. 136) and thus a complication of acute bacterial endocarditis, acute osteomyelitis, carbuncle, etc. The bacteria may extend into, and multiply in, the dead tissue, and this results in an acute inflammatory reaction in the tissue around the margin of the infarct; thus the central dead tissue becomes surrounded by a ring of suppuration (Fig. 8.29). Occasionally, when putrefactive bacteria are present, the infarcts become gangrenous, for example in the lungs as a result of embolism from putrid thrombi in the pelvic veins in puerperal infection or in the transverse or sigmoid venous sinus in middle-ear infection.

The effects of infarction. The effects of infarction on function depend largely on the location and size of the infarct. In organs such as the kidneys, which have a large functional reserve, extensive or multiple infarctions of both kidneys are necessary to bring about any serious disturbance of function, and serious impairment of liver function also requires very extensive infarction. By contrast, single infarcts of the myocardium are commonly sufficiently large to reduce seriously the functional reserve of the heart, and cause heart failure; infarcts involving the conducting system of the heart may cause heart block, and occlusion of a coronary arterial branch not uncommonly causes death from ventricular fibrillation before infarction has become apparent. Infarcts of the brain are a major cause of serious dysfunction, and even a small one involving the internal capsule is followed by hemiplegia. As already explained, infarction of lung tissue tends to occur especially in association with embarrassment of the pulmonary circulation, and for this reason recent pulmonary infarcts are quite commonly observed at necropsy of patients dying of heart failure.

The effects of infarcts are considered more fully in the later, systematic chapters.

Partial arterial obstruction

Chronic narrowing of the lumen of arteries is very common, and is usually caused by atheroma (p. 264). It brings about the serious effect of ischaemic atrophy of specialised cells with accompanying overgrowth of fibrous tissue, for example in the myocardium and the kidneys. In the brain also, patchy loss of neurones and overgrowth of astrocytes is common, and owing to the prevalence of atheroma in the elderly, is an important cause of senile mental changes. Multiple or extensive atheromatous narrowing of the lumen is common in the arteries of the lower limbs, and the resulting chronic ischaemia brings about various trophic changes, and also limping, and cramp-like ischaemic pain, brought on by walking (*intermittent claudication*). Narrowing of the smallest arteries and arterioles —*arteriolosclerosis*—occurs commonly in the abdominal viscera and central nervous system as an ageing effect, and results particularly from arterial hypertension: it is usually most severe in the afferent arterioles of the glomeruli, where it brings about glomerular sclerosis. These regional changes are, however, more appropriately considered in relation to the various systems and organs.

DISTURBANCES OF WATER AND SALT BALANCE

Water and salt deficiency

The water content of the average male body, estimated by the deuterium method, is about 62 per cent, and that of the female about 52 per cent, the sex difference being accounted for by the higher fat content in females. A man weighing 70 kg. contains about 42 litres and this is distributed as 30 litres of *intracellular* water and 12 litres of *extracellular* water; the latter is subdivided into about 3 litres of *intravascular* fluid, the plasma, and about 9 litres of *interstitial* fluid which is distinguished from the intravascular and intracellular fluids by its very low protein content. The extracellular fluids contain practically all the sodium (except for that associated with collagen and that forming part of bone mineral), balanced chiefly by chloride and bicarbonate ions, whereas the intracellular fluid is almost devoid of sodium and chloride, its proteinate, sulphate and phosphate anions being balanced by potassium and magnesium. It is essential that the interstitial fluid should remain isotonic with the intravascular and intracellular fluids, and it contains a higher concentration of electrolytes which balances the colloid osmotic pressure of their proteins. Reductions in the water and salt content of the body are generally associated, but disproportionate depletion of either water or salt causes disturbances of the normal equilibrium which require different treatment. The continued daily loss by the lungs and by insensible perspiration of about half a litre of water without proportionate loss of salt must always be taken into account. Deficiency of water tends to cause hypertonicity of the extracellular fluids so that water is withdrawn from the cells, which thus share in *primary water depletion*. Conversely, in relative salt depletion the extracellular fluids tend to become hypotonic, but this effect is minimised partly by increased renal excretion of water and partly by diffusion of water from the interstitial fluid into the cells with maintenance of isotonicity. Thus in salt deficiency the extracellular fluids are reduced in volume, but the administration of water or glucose solution without salt is actually harmful as it merely dilutes further the extracellular fluids and increases the diffusion of water into cells. It is curious that whereas the need for water is normally indicated by thirst, in man there appears to be no urgent warning sensation when salt is lacking.

Deficiency in body water may be brought

about in various ways and in minor degrees is very common. In hospital patients it is seen most often as a result of insufficient intake owing to physical weakness, coma and pyrexia. The urine is reduced in volume (500 ml.) and is highly concentrated, the specific gravity rising to 1·040 or more. The plasma levels of Na^+, Cl^- and urea increase, probably as the result of diminished renal filtration, although the plasma volume is maintained relatively well by withdrawal of intracellular water and by active retention of Na^+ and excretion of K^- under the influence of the renin–angiotensin–aldosterone system (p. 185) which is stimulated by the diminished blood volume, the so-called reaction of dehydration. More severe water deprivation occurs under exceptional conditions, e.g. in men shipwrecked or lost in the desert, and then the deficiency of body water may ultimately reach over 12 per cent of body weight and amount to nearly 10 litres. Death is thought to be due to rise in the osmotic pressure of the cells. In children the ratio of body surface to weight is higher than in adults so that cutaneous losses of water are proportionately greater; also children cannot produce such a high concentration of urine as can adults. As a result, lack of fluid has a more severe effect in infants and young children than in adults.

Salt depletion is a commoner cause of serious effects than is water depletion, and also is more liable to remain unrecognised. Excessive loss of sodium chloride from the body occurs in various conditions and is commonly only one factor in complex fluid and electrolyte disturbances. Pure loss of salt results from excessive sweating when water is consumed freely, e.g. in the tropics or when working in a very hot atmosphere. It gives rise to a state of "heat exhaustion" which necessitates the administration of large amounts of salt as well as of water, the consumption of water alone being liable to produce severe cramps. Clinically, vomiting and diarrhoea are the most important causes of combined water and salt depletion: the former is complicated by alkalosis due to loss of H^+, and the latter by acidosis from loss of the alkaline secretions of the small intestine. If only water is restored the picture of pure salt depletion follows, with lowering of osmotic pressure of the extracellular fluid and so great a reduction in its amount, owing to renal excretion of water and to increased osmotic absorption by the tissue cells, that

G

peripheral circulatory collapse soon supervenes. Marriott states that the effects of this *secondary extracellular dehydration* are actually more serious than those of the disturbed acid–base balance which may develop from disproportionate loss of sodium or chloride ions, though the latter condition at one time received more attention. The symptoms of salt depletion when water is consumed freely include lassitude, weakness, giddiness, fainting attacks and cramps; also anorexia, nausea and vomiting occur and tend to aggravate the condition by establishing a vicious circle. Marked loss of weight and mental confusion may supervene. The plasma concentration of sodium, normally about 137–148 mEq/1, falls to 130–120 mEq/1 or less. The chloride and bicarbonate concentrations are also reduced *in toto* but their ratio varies with the presence of complicating acidosis or alkalosis. The blood is concentrated, with a rise in haemoglobin, haematocrit value and in plasma protein. The urine contains little or no sodium or chloride except when the salt depletion is due to renal loss, as in Addison's disease or diabetic ketosis. The blood urea rises, often to over 100 mg. per 100 ml., owing mainly to reduced renal blood flow and diminution in the volume of glomerular filtrate. These are common examples of pre-renal uraemia (p. 723).

Combined deficiency of water and salt is more common clinically than of either separately. Vomiting and diarrhoea are probably its most frequent cause. If water is ingested and retained, salt deficiency will predominate, as described above, but without fluid intake water loss exceeds salt loss. In such combined deficiency, the extracellular fluid therefore tends to become hypertonic and consequently fluid is withdrawn from the cells; this leads to thirst and oliguria in addition to the tendency to acute circulatory failure and other symptoms of salt depletion. The rise in blood urea often leads to the erroneous diagnosis of uraemia due to renal failure, but the administration of water and salt in adequate amounts may completely relieve the symptoms.

Regulation of the water content of the blood and urine is normally carried out by the kidneys, which in turn are controlled largely by the neurohypophysis through the action of the antidiuretic hormone on the renal tubular concentrating mechanism. The neurohypophysis is so highly sensitive to the osmotic influence of sodium chloride that an alteration of one per cent in the osmotic pressure of the arterial blood can bring about a tenfold variation in the excretion of water, and the osmotic pressure of the extracellular fluids is thereby regulated so as to maintain a practically constant state. Failure of this mechanism is seen in diabetes insipidus (p. 882), in which intense polyuria approaching maximum water excretion is constantly present. An analogous situation in respect of excessive salt excretion results from failure of the secretion of adequate amounts of aldosterone by the adrenal cortex, e.g. in Addison's disease, in which the cortex is largely destroyed. Uncontrolled sodium loss in the urine leads to fall of the plasma sodium to far below the level at which it normally ceases to be excreted. In consequence serious depletion of the body's store of sodium is brought about and this, if uncorrected, contributes greatly to the severe crises of Addison's disease and the tendency to acute circulatory collapse (p. 909). Other hormones also play minor parts in the regulation of water and salt excretion, e.g. ovarian hormones can cause a distinct retention of water, as is seen in the late phase of the menstrual cycle and in pregnancy.

The pathology of generalised oedema has to be viewed against this background of water and salt balance. Maintenance of osmotic equilibrium is more important for life and is therefore regulated more exactly than the total volume of fluid in the body or within any of its compartments. Most importance was formerly attached to the chloride anion, but it is now recognised that the sodium cation is even more significant in regulating the amount of body fluid in the extracellular compartment of the tissues, and that sodium is intimately concerned in the pathogenesis of oedema.

Water and salt retention: oedema

Oedema is an abnormal increase in the amount of interstitial fluid. It may be localised, e.g. in an organ, limb, etc., or more generalised. In generalised oedema there is usually accumulation of fluid also in the serous cavities (hydrothorax, ascites, etc.). When oedema affects the skin and subcutaneous tissues, swelling may be obvious, and momentary pressure will produce a depression ("pitting') which disappears in a few seconds as the oedema fluid returns to the tissue.

Control of interstitial fluid. It is generally accepted that the interchange of fluid between the capillaries and venules and the tissue spaces can be explained on a physical basis and that the distribution of fluid within and outside the vessels is regulated mainly by a balance of the two processes of filtration and osmosis. The intracapillary hydrostatic pressure tends to force fluid outwards into the tissue spaces, while the osmotic pressure of the colloids of the plasma tends to attract water and thus to induce its return from the tissue spaces into the capillaries and venules. The permeability of the capillary walls varies in different regions and also under different conditions of physiological activity in any one region, but the filtrate in all situations normally contains at least a small amount of protein, probably not exceeding 0·5 per cent in the more permeable areas such as the liver, and less than 0·1 per cent in the less permeable areas such as the limbs. In the normal exchange of interstitial fluid between vessels and tissue spaces most of the filtrate is returned to the circulation by the veins and only a small amount by the lymphatics, but the latter portion contains practically all the protein, so that the protein content of lymph is higher than that of the filtrate. The protein content of lymph therefore fluctuates widely, depending on the permeability of the capillaries in the area drained: for example, the hepatic lymph is very rich in protein (3–5 per cent).

The total exchange between the plasma and interstitial fluid is probably of the order of 7,000 litres of fluid daily, and presumably fluctuates widely in the varying states of the circulation to different parts. In the return of water and salt from the tissues to the blood stream, the chloride ion shift from plasma to red cells in de-oxygenated blood provides an additional force for the uptake of water and salt averaging 4 ml. per litre of venous blood. If the cardiac output is taken as about 7,500 litres per day the chloride shift alone would enable about 30 litres of fluid to be transferred from tissues to vessels and failure of this mechanism probably plays a part in the development of oedema in conditions of severe anaemia. The force provided by the chloride shift may also be concerned in the absorption of exudates and transudates and of physiological saline introduced subcutaneously. Further, this mechanism will automatically fluctuate in proportion to the physiological activity of the tissues. Any disturbance of the normal balance of these conditions will lead to increased or decreased passage of fluid in one or other direction as the case may be.

Water retention. It is important to an understanding of the problems of generalised oedema to realise that, regardless of the cause, this condition is accompanied by retention of water and cannot be regarded as a mere redistribution of the body fluids. There is always an increase in the extracellular fluids of the body and (in an adult) a rise of weight of about 5 kg. invariably precedes the appearance of clinically recognisable generalised oedema, a fact utilised in the attention paid to the weight during pregnancy. Indeed generalised oedema can be regarded as a method of disposing of excess fluid, which cannot be discharged by the usual channels, in order to regulate the blood volume. The body appears to tolerate badly an increase in the volume of the intravascular fluid; the excess is shunted into the interstitial spaces where its presence requires the simultaneous retention of a sufficient quantity of electrolytes, chiefly salt, to equalise the osmotic pressure of this fluid with that of the cells and of the plasma. The osmotic effect of the intracellular and plasma proteins is balanced by a higher concentration of electrolytes—chiefly salt—in the interstitial fluid. It is unlikely that increase of capillary permeability to macromolecules plays any major part in the common forms of generalised oedema, for the protein content of oedema fluid is not sufficiently high to support this possibility. Also, there is no gross fall in the blood volume, such as occurs in surgical shock where an increase in capillary permeability is believed to occur. In rare cases, cyclical oedema has been accompanied by shock, and it has been suggested that the oedema of hypothermia may be related to an increase of factors such as bradykinin, which increase capillary permeability.

Local oedema

Active hyperaemia: inflammatory oedema. Active hyperaemia occurs in acute inflammation, in which the exudation of protein-rich fluid from the capillaries and venules gives rise to inflammatory oedema: as indicated in Chapter 2, major factors in the production of inflammatory oedema are increased hydrostatic pressure in the small vessels, capillary and venular dilatation, and increased permeability. Another factor, the osmotic effect of metabolic products in the interstitial fluid, is probably of less importance.

Active hyperaemia of lesser degree occurs also under physiological conditions, for example in the skeletal muscles during exercise, in the gastro-intestinal tract during digestion, and in the skin as an important mechanism of heat loss. It has been shown experimentally that these physiological responses result in an increase in the volume and protein content of lymph draining from the hyperaemic tissues, indicating increased fluid and protein loss from the plasma. The increased flow of lymph removes the excess fluid, and active hyperaemia is not of importance in the production of oedema apart from its major role in the oedema of inflammation.

Oedema is a prominent feature of some types of hypersensitivity reactions, for example in hay fever, urticaria, the Arthus and delayed hypersensitivity reactions. These are all described in Chapter 5, and it is sufficient to state here that the oedema is of inflammatory nature, due to active hyperaemia and increased vascular permeability.

The term *angio-neurotic oedema* is applied to a heterogeneous group of conditions in which localised oedema results from increased permeability and dilatation of the capillaries and venules. It is usually acute and transient and may involve the larynx, skin, face, hands, stomach, intestines, external genitalia, etc; the factors determining localisation are obscure. In some cases attacks are induced by taking a particular food or encountering a particular foreign substance, and the oedema appears to be a local manifestation of anaphylaxis (p. 99). In other cases nervous disturbances are involved and localised oedema of the skin may occur in chronic nervous diseases, for example tabes dorsalis or syringomyelia, and also in hysteria.

Oedema may occur in severe cases of zoster (shingles) and is apparently a trophic effect due to inflammatory change in the posterior root ganglia. If the nerve lesion is unilateral, as it usually is, the oedema stops short in the midline of the body. A variety known as Quincke's disease often affects several members of the same family. In this condition the oedema occurs usually in the face or hands but may affect the larynx, and cause death from asphyxia. Oedema of the wall of the bowel with colicky pain has also been described. Recent work suggests that *hereditary angio oedema* is due to deficiency of a normal inhibitor to the first component of complement, with inappropriate activity of the complement system (pp. 103–104), leading to an inflammatory reaction.

Local venous congestion and oedema. In a healthy animal acute venous congestion produced by ligation of a large venous trunk does not usually lead to oedema, although there is an increased filtration of water and electrolytes owing to the heightened capillary pressure, and also an increase in the amount of protein leaving the vessels. Consequently a larger proportion of the tissue fluid is returned by the lymphatics and thus there is increased flow of lymph containing a lowered concentration, but increased amount, of protein. This increased flow along the lymphatics usually suffices to remove the excess transudate and consequently there is not sufficient accumulation of fluid in the tissue spaces to cause oedema. If, however, along with the ligation of the vein the vaso-motor nerves supplying the part are cut, the intracapillary pressure is still further increased and localised oedema follows, as the transudate is now too great to be carried away. Similarly, the application of an elastic band to a limb may merely produce venous congestion with increased lymph flow unless the band is tightened sufficiently to prevent the flow of lymph from the part, when oedema will result. These findings indicate that some other factor in addition to acute venous congestion is usually necessary for the production of oedema. In clinical cases, however, local venous congestion often lasts much longer than in the experimental animal, and this may possibly explain the common occurrence of oedema.

In acute venous obstruction there must be sufficient anastomotic drainage of venous blood to permit the circulation to continue; otherwise stasis, thrombosis and haemorrhagic infarction would follow as is seen in mesenteric venous thrombosis. After a time readjustment of the circulation occurs and arterial inflow diminishes. Persistent local venous obstruction is therefore not accompanied by any marked degree of chronic congestion of capillaries and venules, although the main venous anastomotic trunks remain dilated. This circulatory readjustment naturally leads to a reduction in the minute-volume of the circulation through the part, until in time the collateral circulation is fully able to deal with the normal flow. Until that stage is reached there must be a diminution in fluid exchange, which will have two consequences, both of which will tend to promote local oedema. Firstly, there is accumulation of local metabolites, which increases the osmotic pressure in the tissues, and secondly there is a reduction in the total chloride shift, which lessens the capacity to re-absorb water and salt from the interstitial tissue; the retention of fluid in the tissues thus brought about is likely to lead to local oedema.

The oedema of chronic lymphatic obstruction, e.g. that produced by cancer, fibrosis, tuberculosis, filariasis, etc. (p. 292), is usually of the non-pitting type, i.e. the swollen tissues do not yield readily to pressure. A characteristic feature of chronic lymphatic oedema is the tendency to elephantiasis with overgrowth of the connective tissue in the skin and subcutaneous tissue. This has generally been ascribed to an inflammatory reaction to the cancer, filarial infestation, etc., causing the lymphatic obstruction, but in some cases no such cause is obvious. Since the plasma protein normally present in the interstitial fluid is returned to the blood by the lymphatics, chronic lymphatic obstruction results in the accumulation of protein in the tissues while most of the water and electrolytes are taken up by the venules as usual. This accumulated protein may, either by providing nutrient or in some unknown way, be responsible for stimulating the connective tissue cells to increased production of collagen.

General oedema

Cardiac oedema is apt to develop at a late stage in cases of cardiac failure with long-standing general venous engorgement. It appears first in the most dependent parts of the body and gradually extends upwards. Thus it is usually noticed first round the ankles, and pitting may be elicited by pressure over the lower end of the tibia. When the condition is advanced, the limbs become greatly swollen, while the skin is tense and vesicles may form. Accumulation of fluid may occur also in the serous cavities.

As indicated above, increased transudation from congested, dilated capillaries is not sufficient to produce oedema, because the excess fluid is removed by the lymphatics. When, however, heart failure becomes severe, the diminution in cardiac output adversely affects renal function which depends upon normal renal blood flow (about one-fifth of the total cardiac output). There is evidence that the kidneys can compensate to some extent for reduced blood supply by increasing the proportion of fluid filtered off in the glomeruli; this is probably mediated by increased tone in the efferent arterioles. The volume of urine is reduced and it is highly concentrated, indicating that in spite of the undoubted reduction in the total glomerular filtrate, a considerable initial volume of filtrate must be formed and subjected to excessive tubular absorption. The mechanism of this excessive re-absorption is not fully understood, but the reduced renal blood flow may stimulate the juxta-glomerular cells to secrete excess of renin, and this in turn will enhance the secretion of aldosterone by the adrenal cortex, with consequent re-absorption of sodium by the renal tubules and a corresponding re-absorption of water. Direct evidence supporting such a mechanism has been provided in some, but not all cases of cardiac oedema (p. 186). The stimulus to this secondary aldosteronism has not yet been defined, as it occurs among different types of heart failure, both in low output and in high output types. The great increase in body weight confirms the enormous amount of fluid retained in the oedematous tissues in some cardiac cases, and the importance of water and salt retention is shown by the effect of diuretics in diminishing the oedema. Reduction in the intake of sodium chloride in the diet has sometimes a markedly diuretic effect, water being eliminated with preservation of the isotonic state of the oedema fluid.

Other factors may play a part in the genesis of cardiac oedema, e.g. the accumulation in the tissues of waste products which by their osmotic action will tend to attract more water from the blood; also the moderate fall in the concentration of plasma proteins, partly the result of dilution of the plasma. Possibly the diminished oxygenation may in time affect the capillary endothelium and increase its permeability, but this view is not supported by the protein content of the oedema fluid, which is usually about 0·5 per cent or less. We consider, however, that the fundamental cause of cardiac oedema lies in the faulty elimination of fluid consequent upon the deranged renal circulation. The distribution of the retained fluid in the tissues is determined by gravity because, with the reduction in cardiac power, the circulation is unable to absorb the tissue fluid and return it to the right heart against the hydrostatic pressure of the column of venous blood in the dependent parts. It is to be noted that in oedema generally, the distension of the tissue spaces with fluid will impair the tissue elasticity, so that tissue pressure will remain relatively low, and lymphatic drainage will not rise in proportion to the tissue distension. In failure of the left ventricle of the heart, venous congestion occurs mainly in the lungs so long as the right ventricle continues to beat forcibly: pulmonary oedema may then develop without generalised oedema (p. 297).

Renal oedema. Generalised oedema occurs in various diseases which affect the glomeruli, including some types of glomerulonephritis and also in acute renal failure due to injury to the renal tubules. The pathological changes in these conditions are described in Chapter 21. However, an understanding of the factors likely to be involved in the production of the various types of renal oedema depends not so much on a knowledge of the detailed structural changes but rather on the associated functional disturbances. Accordingly, renal diseases which give rise to oedema may be placed within three groups and these are considered below.

(1) Conditions in which all the glomeruli are affected, with reduction in renal blood flow and in glomerular filtration. This group is exemplified by *acute diffuse glomerulonephritis* and *rapidly progressive glomerulonephritis*. There is usually a rise in blood pressure and blood urea level, and production of a diminished amount of concentrated urine containing moderate amounts of protein. The oedema in these conditions is not influenced by gravity to the same extent as is cardiac oedema and is often noticed first in the loose connective tissues, e.g. of the eyelids and face: in ambulant patients, however, gravity is seen to have some effect. The protein content of the oedema fluid is usually less than 0·5 per cent and the oedema therefore cannot be attributed to increased capillary permeability. Also the proteinuria is usually only moderate and the loss does not result in any significant reduction in the levels of the plasma proteins. In our view oedema results from a failure of adequate excretion of salt and water and this is due to excessive re-absorption by the tubules. The factors responsible for this excessive re-absorption are not clearly defined. The renin–angio-

tensin–aldosterone system may be implicated, but even this is uncertain (p. 186).

(2) *The nephrotic syndrome.* In some renal diseases there is persistent and heavy loss of plasma proteins, particularly albumin, in the urine: when this exceeds about 10 g. daily, the plasma albumin level falls considerably and this is accompanied by generalised oedema which often becomes very severe. This condition is known as the nephrotic syndrome. As in other types of renal oedema, the distribution of the tissue fluid is not so dependent on gravity as in cardiac oedema. In patients with nephrotic syndrome, the blood pressure is often not raised and there is commonly no rise in the blood urea, indicating that renal blood flow and glomerular filtration rates are normal. The nephrotic syndrome may arise in a large number of conditions: in some it is regularly present, for example in *glomerulonephritis* of *minimal-change* and *membranous* types (q.v.). It is a common result of amyloid disease involving the glomeruli; it occasionally complicates other types of glomerulonephritis and the glomerular lesions of diabetes mellitus and various other diseases. In all these conditions, its development is dependent on excessive loss of plasma albumin into the glomerular filtrate.

Glomerular leakage of protein exhibits a molecular sieving effect, the amount of plasma albumin which escapes being disproportionately great because of its relatively small molecular size. Also because of its small size and its relatively high concentration in the plasma, albumin is the protein mainly responsible for the osmotic pressure of the plasma, and consequently, in states of severe hypoalbuminaemia, the amount of fluid leaving the capillaries and venules throughout the body greatly exceeds the amount drawn back into them by osmosis. Accordingly, the plasma volume tends to fall and this brings into play the renin–angiotensin–aldosterone mechanism which results in increased re-absorption of sodium and water from the renal tubules: this tends, in turn, to dilute the plasma protein still further and so transudation into the tissues remains excessive, a vicious circle is set up and continues to operate so long as gross albuminuria persists. As would be expected, the oedema fluid in the nephrotic syndrome has a very low protein content, and there is no evidence of general increased capillary permeability for macromolecules.

In experimental studies in which the levels of plasma proteins have been artificially lowered in dogs by plasmapheresis (removal of blood and returning the cells suspended in saline), oedema has not been found to develop unless physiological saline is administered by mouth. Since large amounts of salt and water taken by mouth can cause oedema, even in normal individuals, these findings do not provide strong support for the explanation given above for oedema in the nephrotic syndrome. Nevertheless, the importance of protein loss and hypoalbuminaemia is confirmed by the appearance of similar gross oedema in protein-losing enteropathy (p. 523) in which the kidneys are normal and there is gross loss of plasma protein into the gut. The participation of the renin–angiotensin–aldosterone mechanism is demonstrated by the very high plasma levels of aldosterone found in the nephrotic syndrome.

(3) In *acute tubular necrosis*, the acutely injured tubules lose their capacity for selective re-absorption and concentration of the glomerular filtrate. Consequently, most of the filtrate is re-absorbed and the small amount of urine produced approximates in its composition to a protein-free filtrate of plasma. There is retention of water and electrolytes and a progressive rise in blood urea. Apart from loss by sweating, vomiting, etc., most of the fluid taken by mouth is retained in the body and unless it is seriously restricted, gross oedema develops.

Acute tubular necrosis may result from shock or certain chemical poisons (p. 724). In some cases of acute renal failure following shock, the tubules show no convincing evidence of necrosis in a renal biopsy, and it has been suggested that hyperactivity of the renin–angiotensin–aldosterone system may be of importance in such cases.

In the various forms of renal disease which are complicated by arterial hypertension, cardiac failure is liable to develop with consequent generalised or pulmonary oedema.

Nutritional oedema

Generalised oedema may clearly be caused by malnutrition. Protein insufficiency seems to be the main factor, and the extreme example is termed kwashiorkor (p. 570). Examination of the blood shows a marked fall in glucose, lipids and proteins, the last being sometimes reduced to half the normal. It seems likely that fall in osmotic pressure of the plasma is the most important factor in the production of the oedema, but no strict parallelism has been found, some cases failing to become oedematous in spite of severe depletion of serum albumin, while others show gross oedema with plasma protein levels within normal limits; also the oedema may disappear before there is any significant rise in the colloid osmotic pressure of the plasma. Nutritional oedema is commonly associated with xerophthalmia, a condition in which opacity with ulceration of the cornea occurs, as a result of deficiency in fat-soluble vitamin A; possibly lack of the vitamin B complex is also concerned, and the wet form of beri-beri is perhaps related. A somewhat similar form of oedema has been observed in infants when there has been excess of carbohydrates in the diet with marked deficiency in other foodstuffs. In all such examples of nutritional oedema, the problem is a complex one, and the factors which we have mentioned may be concerned in varying proportions.

Oedema may occur in patients with chronic wasting diseases, e.g. cancer, tuberculosis, etc., and is due mainly to cardiac failure, although fall in the plasma proteins is a contributory factor in some cases.

Pulmonary oedema

The osmotic pressure of the plasma (25 mm. Hg.) is substantially greater than the normal hydrostatic pressure in the pulmonary capillaries (8–10 mm. Hg.). Consequently, the development of oedema of the lungs usually requires a considerable rise in the hydrostatic pressure. As elsewhere, this occurs, together with increased vascular permeability, in acute inflammatory lesions, and inflammatory oedema is pronounced in severe influenza and lobar pneumonia, etc.

Pulmonary oedema can be produced readily in healthy dogs by interfering with the flow of pulmonary venous blood, for example by compressing the left atrium or ventricle, or constricting the aorta. In man, it is produced similarly by left ventricular failure, as in some cases of myocardial infarction and in systemic hypertension. In this latter condition, acute pulmonary oedema ("cardiac asthma") comes on especially when the patient is lying down, probably due to improved venous return from the legs, and perhaps also to increase in the blood volume by re-absorption of oedema fluid from the legs, when recumbent. The attack is usually relieved by sitting up. Chronic pulmonary congestion, as for example in stenosis of the mitral valve, is not alone sufficient to produce pulmonary oedema in man. This is probably because reflex increase in tone of the pulmonary arterioles protects the pulmonary capillary bed from excessive rise in pressure. However, the situation is precarious, and pulmonary oedema is prone to result from physical exertion or other factors which increase the pulmonary blood flow. Chronic pulmonary oedema may occur as part of generalised renal oedema, particularly when there is, in addition, systemic hypertension, as in acute glomerulonephritis. Another important cause is overloading of the circulation by rapid transfusion of blood to patients with severe anaemia. Finally, pulmonary oedema results from certain experimental lesions of the nervous system, and occurs in man in conditions causing acute rise in intracranial pressure, most commonly in head injury or intracranial haemorrhage.

Apart from the above causes, oedema of the posterobasal parts of the lungs is a very common finding at necropsy, particularly in old people and where death is due to a toxic condition or has been preceded by coma. The oedema fluid is very prone to become infected by a mixture of bacteria, usually of low virulence, producing *hypostatic pneumonia* which, if untreated, is likely to be the immediate cause of death.

The renin–angiotensin–aldosterone system

Renin is an enzyme, stored and probably formed in the renal juxta-glomerular apparatus; it is present in high concentration in the cytoplasmic granules of cells of the wall of the terminal part of the afferent glomerular arterioles. The adjacent macula densa, a plaque of specialised epithelial lining cells in the wall of the distal convoluted tubule, is probably a sensory device, regulating the release of renin in response to changes in the composition of the fluid in the tubular lumen (Fig. 8.30).

Renin-substrate (angiotensinogen) is present in the α_2-globulin fraction of plasma and also in renal lymph.

The initial product of the action of renin on its substrate is an inactive decapeptide, angiotensin I. This is converted in the circulation (largely, it now appears, in the lungs) to the active octapeptide, angiotensin II. It remains uncertain whether or not conversion to angiotensin II can occur within the kidney, although the question is of considerable importance in considering the possible direct renal actions of angiotensin.

Renin is normally present in higher concentration in renal lymph than in renal venous plasma, but because of the much higher rate of renal plasma

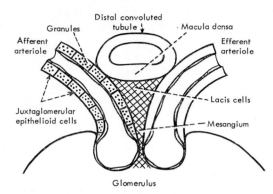

FIG. 8.30—Diagram of the juxta-glomerular apparatus.

flow, secretion into the renal vein is greater than that into lymph.

Effects of renin. Renin, by way of angiotensin, has three principal actions:—

(*a*) Aldosterone-stimulating.

(*b*) Pressor, mediated by peripheral vaso-constriction.

(*c*) A direct renal effect, modifying urinary output of water and electrolytes.

Other actions, which hitherto have been less fully studied, are the central stimulation of thirst, release of catecholamines and possibly release of kinins.

The relative dominance of the three principal actions mentioned above is much modified by the prevailing sodium status. Sodium deprivation, for example, enhances the aldosterone-stimulating effect, while minimising the pressor action, so that a marked rise in circulating renin, angiotensin II, and aldosterone occurs with little or no increase in arterial blood pressure.

The renal effects of administered angiotensin vary widely according to the dosage, the prevailing sodium status, arterial pressure, and species. At most doses which can safely be given to normal man, angiotensin reduces renal excretion of sodium and water, and this effect is enhanced by severe sodium depletion, as in untreated Addison's disease. By contrast, in hypertension, irrespective of etiology, and also in hepatic cirrhosis with ascites, angiotensin usually increases water and sodium loss.

Secondary hyperaldosteronism. The renin or angiotensin–aldosterone system is stimulated, and high circulating levels of all three components may be found, in sodium depletion, whether due to dietary sodium restriction, sodium-losing renal disease, diuretics or purgatives: haemorrhage produces a similar response. Because in these situations the increase in aldosterone is thought to be a consequence of a rise in renin, these are regarded as examples of "secondary" hyperaldosteronism.

Secondary hyperaldosteronism develops in some, but by no means all cases of untreated congestive heart failure, in hepatic cirrhosis with ascites, and in the nephrotic syndrome. It may seem paradoxical that patients with these oedematous states, with their retention of sodium and water, should react as though sodium deprived. The explanation lies probably in that the excess sodium is principally extra-vascular, and not therefore capable of recognition by the kidney. The kidney therefore responds as in sodium deprivation, hence plasma renin and angiotensin, and in consequence, aldosterone, are elevated.

Renal artery stenosis is another instance in which the kidney probably receives a stimulus to increased renin release which is inappropriate to the overall requirements of the body. The old belief that renal artery constriction, by leading to increased circulating renin and angiotensin, is simply and directly responsible for hypertension *via* the pressor effect of angiotensin (see p. 274) is now known to be a considerable oversimplification. It is clear, however, that in many cases of severe renal artery stenosis with hypertension, both renin and aldosterone are increased. A similar mechanism—possibly multiple intrarenal arterial stenoses—may be the cause of the secondary hyperaldosteronism which often accompanies the malignant phase of hypertension, irrespective of etiology. In advanced chronic renal disease with renal failure, occasionally such severe elevation of renin and aldosterone levels may occur that hypertension cannot be controlled until both diseased kidneys have been excised. This could well be an instance where sufficient angiotensin is circulating to have a direct pressor effect. It is noteworthy that the ability to secrete renin seems to be well-maintained even in the terminal stages of chronic renal disease.

Normal pregnancy is a special instance of secondary hyperaldosteronism in which an increase in renin-substrate seems of primary importance.

Other patterns of variation in circulating renin and aldosterone are readily predictable. Sodium loading, or the administration of sodium-retaining substances such as DOC, fluoro-cortisone, carbenoxolone, or liquorice, depress circulating renin and aldosterone.

Primary hyperaldosteronism. An adrenocortical adenoma secreting an excess of aldosterone will lead to the combination of renin suppression with elevated aldosterone. This is known as "*primary*" *hyperaldosteronism* (p. 912). The same combination will also be seen in any situation where excess aldosterone secretion is stimulated by mechanisms other than the renin–angiotensin system.

Hypoaldosteronism. In Addison's disease, the sodium deficiency stimulates marked secretion of renin, but aldosterone production remains deficient despite this stimulus, because the diseased adrenal cortex is unable to respond appropriately.

Direct effects of renin and angiotensin on the kidney. The renal actions of angiotensin, although undoubted, are difficult to study in isolation from the pressor and aldosterone-stimulating effects. It has been suggested that phylogenetically, renin and angiotensin may have appeared initially as components of a purely intrarenal sodium-conserving system, and that the peripheral pressor and aldosterone-stimulating actions evolved as subsequent refinements and modifications, perhaps made necessary by a terrestrial, as opposed to an aquatic or semi-aquatic, habitat. Much depends, in man, on whether or not conversion of the inactive decapeptide angiotensin I to the active octapeptide angiotensin II can occur within the kidney, a point which remains unresolved. If entry to the general circulation is necessary for this conversion, then the renal actions are likely to be subsidiary to the systemic effects. If intrarenal formation of angiotensin II can occur, then its renal actions could approach or exceed in importance its systemic effects.

In certain situations—for instance congestive heart failure—circulating renin appears to produce effects by acting directly on the kidneys, rather than by aldosterone-stimulation or peripheral vasoconstriction. For example, high circulating renin levels may be associated with uraemia, a marked fall in glomerular filtration rate, diminished total renal blood flow with relatively well-preserved filtration fraction, and reduced arterial pressure.

Many years ago Goormaghtigh suggested that a renal effect of renin might be responsible for the reduced renal blood flow and oliguria of acute renal failure (see p. 727); considerable circumstantial evidence now supports the hypothesis that several forms of acute renal failure may be the pathological extreme of the process outlined above in congestive heart failure. A wide variety of stimuli causing increases in renin secretion predispose to acute renal failure with or without renal tubular necrosis. These include cardiac failure, sodium depletion, pregnancy, haemorrhage, Addison's disease and renal artery occlusion. Conversely, sodium loading and renal denervation reduce renin levels and are thought to protect against acute renal failure. Moreover, it has recently been shown that two procedures not previously known to affect renin release—the administration of glycerol and the giving of the antibiotic cephaloridine—can each cause severe renal failure and tubular necrosis in experimental animals. Both procedures also cause very big increases in plasma renin concentration.

VARIATIONS IN BLOOD VOLUME

Hypovolaemia. When the volume of the blood is artificially decreased, homoeostatic mechanisms tend to restore the original volume. Following a moderate haemorrhage or artificial bleeding, the arterial pressure, after an initial fall, is restored nearly up to normal by contraction of the systemic arterioles and a sufficient arterial blood supply to the brain and heart is maintained. In severe haemorrhage, much of the arterial supply is diverted from other organs, e.g. the kidneys, which may be severely damaged by ischaemia if their blood supply is not quickly restored. Contraction of the arterioles leads to diminished flow through the capillaries and lowered pressure in them, and as the colloid osmotic pressure is thus less opposed, absorption of fluid from the tissues occurs and the blood volume is gradually restored. The rapidity with which this takes place varies in different animals and according to the state of the tissues. It occurs rapidly in rabbits, so that by the time an experimental bleeding has been performed, a considerable haemodilution has occurred, as shown by a fall in the red cell count and haemoglobin. In the dog the process is more gradual, and after the removal of about a quarter of the blood volume haemodilution is usually not completed for about 24 hours. In man, absorption of fluid from the tissues is rapid; for example, the removal of 500 ml. of blood from a healthy man is followed by restoration of the normal blood volume within a few hours. If, however, the loss amounts to 1,250 ml. the restoration of blood volume takes about 36 hours. The haemoglobin level is therefore not a good index of severe blood loss until about 30–36 hours later and it is then apt to be vitiated by other effects tending to produce haemoconcentration, e.g. shock, dehydration, etc.

Death from a severe haemorrhage is due to diminution in the volume of the blood, i.e. to loss of circulating fluid; loss of about half the blood volume may be fatal especially if the loss is rapid. When the blood volume is diminished, less blood reaches the heart, and the pressure can be maintained only by contraction of the arterioles. This means slower flow in the capillaries, and ultimately too little blood returns to the heart for the maintenance of the circulation. The importance of restoring the fluid part of the blood is thus evident. Saline injected intravenously is of only temporary value, as it passes rapidly out of the blood into the tissues and is also excreted in the urine. Similarly, restoration of blood volume is aided only slightly by the administration of fluid by the mouth or rectum. By far the most effective method is transfusion of a macromolecular solution which, by exerting an osmotic pressure, retains fluid in the vascular system. Blood, or failing that, plasma or dextran may be used. When haemorrhage is complicated by severe shock (p. 189), restoration of the blood volume becomes urgent, for hypoxia may bring about a condition of increased permeability of capillary walls, as a result of which fluid and proteins escape into the tissues and the blood volume cannot be restored ("irreversible shock").

Apart from haemorrhage, the blood volume can be reduced by loss of fluid in various conditions, for example by excessive vomiting, sweating, or by watery diarrhoea (p. 179). Diminution in blood volume may occur when there is an extensive escape of fluid into the tissues as a result of severe trauma and burns (see below).

Hypervolaemia. Increase of the blood volume occurs in normal pregnancy, and it may be artificially produced temporarily by the injection into the circulation of saline, plasma, whole blood, etc. The increased volume thus produced leads at first to a slight rise in venous and arterial blood pressure, and then to a vasomotor response, whereby dilatation of the arterioles results in increased rate of blood flow and increased pressure within the capillaries. In a given time more blood reaches the right side of the heart, and its contractions become more powerful, thus establishing a more rapid circulation of the blood. The increased pressure within the capillaries leads to more rapid filtration through the walls and the increased renal arteriolar pressure may inhibit the secretion of renin, with consequent loss by the kidneys of water and salt (p. 186). In these ways the increased volume returns to normal—rapidly after administration of saline, and more gradually in the case of plasma, since the additional protein persists, and exerts its osmotic effect, for some time. When the blood volume of an animal is increased by transfusion of blood, some reduction occurs in the plasma volume, and consequently there is an increase in the number of red cells per c.mm.; this condition of *polycythaemia* lasts for some weeks.

In pregnancy the plasma volume is augmented by 1·5 litres, but the volume of red cells by only 200 ml., resulting in a fall in the haematocrit from 42 per cent to 36 per cent. This latter fall can be largely prevented by the administration of iron. In congestive cardiac failure, too, the blood volume is substantially increased as a result of diminished renal excretion (p. 183). In polycythaemia vera there is an increase in the total red cell mass and in blood volume (p. 390).

Consideration of changes of blood volume are included also in the sections on oedema and electrolyte disturbances (pp. 178–185) and in the following account of shock.

SHOCK

Shock is a state of profound depression of the various functions of the body. It may be caused by many conditions, occurring singly and in combination. They include severe physical pain and unpleasant mental impressions, various injuries, particularly those of a crushing or lacerating nature, certain abdominal lesions such as perforation of the bowel, and surgical operations, particularly when anaesthesia is too light. Reduction in the blood volume either by haemorrhage or by exudation, as in burns, is a common cause. It is necessary to distinguish between the vaso-vagal attack (formerly, primary shock) which comes on immediately, and is often manifested by fainting, and true shock (formerly, secondary shock) which is more persistent and much more serious.

Vaso-vagal attack

This follows immediately on injury, physical or mental pain, or psychogenic stimuli. It is believed to be mediated by a vaso-vagal reaction, perhaps due to overaction of the carotid sinus reflex or to hypothalamic stimuli. The patient becomes pale and sweats, feels faint, often vomits and may lose consciousness. There may also be convulsions from cerebral hypoxia. The pulse is very slow and there is severe fall in blood pressure. Rapid recovery usually takes place.

True shock

In this condition there is a progressive inadequacy of the circulation until the normal exchange between the blood and tissue fluid is impaired. If it is severe and prolonged, general hypoxia causes the cell membranes to become incompetent, and intracellular enzymes are liberated. Refractory ("irreversible") shock occurs when the circulation cannot readily be restored, and cell structure and function are then likely to become irreversibly affected.

Clinically, the skin is pale, and the temperature is subnormal: the face is pinched and the eyes sunken. The patient may be restless or apathetic and drowsy. The pulse is weak, and, in contrast to the vaso-vagal attack, rapid, and the blood pressure is markedly lowered: the superficial vessels contain little blood, and bleeding from a wound is diminished. Respiration is rapid and shallow and may be irregular, and the volume of urine is low.

Although the factors initiating shock vary and may be present in combination, the following three main types may be distinguished.

1. Hypovolaemic shock. This results from diminution in the blood volume due either to severe haemorrhage or to exudation of plasma fluid as in burns and crush injuries. In severe injuries, both factors usually contribute. The condition tends to be aggravated by general anaesthesia and by exposure to cold.

Bleeding may occur externally or into the tissues, but it is usually accentuated by the marked transudation of plasma which results from trauma and gives rise to much of the local swelling. A badly bruised and swollen thigh may accommodate 1·5 litres of fluid derived from the circulating blood. The sequence of events is believed to be: reduction of blood volume → decreased venous return → decreased cardiac output → reduced arterial pressure (which through the carotid sinus reflex induces acceleration of the heart) → decreased blood flow to the organs with air hunger from hypoxaemia → reflex vaso-constriction with sweating from sympathetic over-activity. Thus at first the blood pressure may be sustained or occasionally even raised (hypertensive reaction), possibly due to the diversion of blood flow from the kidneys with consequent liberation of renin (p. 186). Later, however, the hypovolaemia results in failure of the heart to maintain the circulation and the blood pressure drops dramatically: this occurs in spite of sympathetic hyperactivity, and the blood stagnates in the venous system. Certain normal bodily constituents released at the site of injury, notably adenosine triphosphate, may participate in the genesis of shock and these are better described as *metabolic* rather than *toxic* factors. It seems clear that such tissue constituents play a part, albeit a minor one, in bringing about the essential changes of shock.

Hypovolaemic shock is aggravated by previous dehydration of the patient, e.g. by vomiting. Owing to the poor retention of fluids in the vessels, the infusion of physiological saline is useless, and the transfusion of whole blood in adequate amounts should be undertaken as soon as the need is apparent, as delay may permit the development of the refractory state. When haemoconcentration is marked, as in extensive superficial burns and in crush injuries, transfusion of plasma is indicated initially to reduce the viscosity of the blood, although blood transfusion is also usually desirable.

Since the vital organs in shock are suffering from inadequate circulation, it is not desirable to reduce this further by diverting blood to the skin by the application of excessive warmth, and experience in the treatment of air-raid and battle casualties showed that undue warming of the shocked patient might have undesirable results.

2. Cardiogenic shock. This is due to circulatory failure, resulting from an acute lesion of the heart. It is seen most commonly in myocardial infarction, but cardiac tamponade, pulmonary embolism or dissecting aortic aneurysm may sometimes be responsible. Reduction in cardiac output results in inadequate tissue perfusion.

3. Bacteraemic or endotoxic shock. This is associated with septicaemia due to Gram-negative bacteria and is probably brought about by endotoxin released from lysed bacteria (p. 121). It may develop in cases of peritonitis, biliary or urinary tract infections, and is recognised most frequently in elderly debilitated individuals. Predisposing factors include diabetes mellitus, cirrhosis of the liver and lymphoid neoplasia. The condition should be suspected when the state of shock is associated with fever, rigors, confusion or coma. In many cases antibiotics have already been administered and blood cultures are then usually negative. Impaired respiratory function is a constant and early feature and is associated with pulmonary collapse, oedema and sometimes pneumonia.

The mechanisms involved in endotoxic shock are still obscure. Endotoxin appears to act either directly or by inducing release of histamine, bradykinin and serotonin with consequent dilatation and increased permeability of the pulmonary capillaries and venules, and possibly loss of surfactant leading to collapse of the alveoli. These changes predispose to pulmonary infection. There is also evidence that endotoxin may result in lysis of circulating neutrophil polymorphs with release of their proteolytic and other enzymes. In some cases the condition is complicated by gross haemorrhage in the adrenals (p. 911) and by scattered small haemorrhages and necrosis in various other viscera and tissues.

Pathological changes. Death from shock is not readily diagnosable at necropsy. In addition to the responsible injury, heart lesion or infection, the viscera are usually congested and there may be pulmonary oedema or bronchopneumonia. One of the most reliable features is necrosis of the renal tubular epithelium (p. 723) but this is sometimes difficult to distinguish from postmortem change. In endotoxic shock, the special features noted above may also be present.

Shock associated with childbirth (*obstetric shock*) is usually due to a combination of painful and difficult labour, surgical manipulations and haemorrhage. In some instances activation of the clotting and fibrinolytic mechanisms results in afibrinogenaemia which aggravates the uterine haemorrhage, and at necropsy multiple microthrombi of fibrin are sometimes demonstrable in the small blood vessels (p. 443).

Anaphylactic shock is described in Chapter 5.

Burns

The pathology of burns is in certain respects closely related to that of shock. In burns, too, the factors of nervous disturbance, loss of fluid from the blood, and thus hypovolaemic shock, are involved. At a later stage local bacterial infection may develop and sometimes septicaemia. The area of skin is extensive in proportion to actual mass of tissue; it is very vascular and holds a high proportion of the extracellular fluid of the body. The effects of burning are of all grades of intensity from acute congestion and inflammatory oedema to actual charring of the tissues: surgeons describe burns as being of different "degrees" according to their depth. The area of skin affected is of greater immediate importance than the depth of the lesion and the effects are more serious in children than in adults. A vaso-vagal attack usually occurs almost immediately after the burn. There is a marked leukocytosis, and some hours later hypovolaemic shock develops, with fall in blood pressure, severe diminution in blood volume and a raised haematocrit. There is also marked retention of sodium and chloride. In the burned area many small vessels and capillaries are thrombosed but those lying more deeply are less severely damaged and take part in an acute inflammatory reaction, with gross inflammatory oedema and escape of exudate onto the surface. In consequence there is a fall in blood volume and loss of plasma proteins, varying in severity with the area of the burn. The onset of drowsiness and coma is due to inadequate perfusion of the brain and can be prevented by early correction of the hypovolaemia. If, however, treatment is delayed or inadequate, the circulation gradually fails, and delirium or drowsiness and finally coma precede death.

In a small proportion of cases, usually elderly subjects with extensive burns, a so-called *toxic stage* may develop on the 2nd or 3rd day, following partial recovery from hypovolaemia. The temperature rises, and the blood pressure again falls due to circulatory failure: pulse and respiration rates increase, and death may ensue. This stage is brought about by some unknown effect, the most likely explanation being the absorption of cell breakdown products from the burned area; removal of damaged tissue minimises this stage.

Bacterial infection of the burned area, and sometimes septicaemia, may arise after the first few days. Infection is likely to be serious, with severe toxaemia, especially in cases of deep burns. Before the widespread use of antibiotics, *Strep. pyogenes* infection was common, and often fatal. Today, in spite of antibiotics, deaths from severe burns are usually due to sepsis, and *Staph. aureus* and *Pseudomonas aeruginosa* are often the dominant bacteria in a mixed flora. Endotoxic shock (see above) may result from Gram-negative bacterial infection of the burned area.

The post-mortem changes are not characteristic: they are most marked when death has occurred late, and are chiefly degenerative changes in the liver with congestion and small haemorrhages in the viscera, notably in the adrenals, which commonly exhibit pronounced depletion of their cortical lipids. Acute ulceration of the duodenum (Curling's ulcer) occasionally occurs, especially in late deaths, but nothing definite has been established about its causation.

In cases where recovery takes place the usual processes of healing follow, but the extensive loss of skin often necessitates skin grafting. When the burn has been deep and healing has been slow, the fibrous tissue formed may be abundant and lead to scarring and deformity. The development of cancer of the skin in relation to the burn scar is sometimes seen many years later (Marjolin's ulcer).

BLOOD GROUPS AND BLOOD TRANSFUSION

The plasma (or serum) of one individual may contain iso-antibody which reacts with iso-antigens on the surface of the red cells of another. In carrying out transfusion it is essential to use red cells which are not thus affected by the plasma of the recipient, as otherwise the donated red cells may be destroyed rapidly and a serious or fatal transfusion reaction may result.

Haemolysis does not occur without agglutination, and the simplest test for compatibility is provided by mixing on a glass slide a drop of a suspension of the donor's red cells in saline or citrate-saline and a drop of the recipient's serum. The appearance of agglutination indicates gross incompatibility, and the blood must not be given. This simple *direct compatibility*, or *cross-matching test*, is not sufficiently precise for routine use, and is acceptable only when used in a life-saving emergency. Whenever possible, the blood group of the recipient should be known, and blood should be obtained from one or more donors of groups known to be compatible with the recipient. Blood grouping should include detection of the red cell iso-antigens within the ABO and Rh systems (see below). These are of most practical importance, but there are many others, and although the only natural iso-antibodies normally present are those of the ABO system, previous pregnancy or blood transfusion can result in the development of irregular iso-antibodies within the various other group systems. Accordingly, and also because of the possibility of clerical and technical errors in blood grouping, it is essential to carry out a direct cross-matching test, and this must whenever possible be carried out under more controlled conditions than the simple test described above: the donor's red cells and recipient's serum should be mixed in a tube and incubated at 37°C, and the cells should then be examined for agglutination, and also by the antiglobulin test (p. 80) which will detect incomplete (non-agglutinating) antibody of the IgG type (p. 78) in the recipient's serum. These procedures are essential to avoid the risk of a transfusion reaction due to any iso-antibody which may be present in the recipient's serum and which may react with the donated red cells. Also, by administering incompatible blood, e.g. Rh-positive to an Rh-negative patient, although there will not normally be Rh iso-antibody in the patient's serum, this may well develop as a result of the transfusion, and cause trouble in future transfusions or pregnancies (see below).

The ABO groups

The red cells and sera of different individuals can be classified into four main groups which interact as shown in the following table:—

Nomenclature, International	Iso-agglutinin Content of Serum	Red Cells of Group *				Average percentage Distribution in Great Britain †
		AB	A	B	O	
AB	Nil	−	−	−	−	3·0
A	anti-B	+	−	+	−	41·7
B	anti-A	+	+	−	−	8·6
O	anti-A and anti-B	+	+	+	−	46·7

* These four columns show the reaction of red cells of each of the four blood groups with serum from individuals of each blood group. + = agglutination; − = no agglutination.

† The distribution of the four groups varies throughout Great Britain, group O being more frequent in Scotland and group A less frequent; conversely A is more frequent in England and O less.

If sera of groups A and B are available one can determine the group to which any individual belongs. If the red cells are agglutinated by both sera the blood belongs to group AB, if agglutinated by group B serum alone the blood belongs to group A, if by group A serum alone to group B, and if by neither serum, it belongs to group O. Since the serum of group AB does not agglutinate the red cells of any of the groups an individual of group AB can receive the red cells of any other group and is thus a "universal recipient". The cells of an individual of group O are not agglutinated by the serum of any group; the red cells can be transfused into an individual of any group and such persons are known as "universal donors".

These results were originally elucidated by Landsteiner. They are due to the presence or absence of two iso-antigens, agglutinogens A and B, on the surface of the red cells of different individuals and to the invariable absence from each individual's serum of those agglutinating iso-antibodies of IgM class corresponding to the iso-antigens contained in his own red cells. The ABO groups are transmitted from parents to offspring in accordance with Mendelian principles, A and B being dominant over O; this fact is utilised in forensic work.

The Rh groups

In addition to the ABO group-substances there are many other antigens in the red cells, but most of these are rarely concerned in the use of blood for transfusion. Next in importance to the ABO system is the division of human cells into Rh-positive and Rh-negative. This was first achieved by Landsteiner and Wiener (1940) as a side-issue from experimental studies on the antigens of human and animal red cells. On testing human red cells with antisera prepared by injecting into rabbits and guinea-pigs the red cells of the monkey *Macacus rhesus*, they found that the cells of about 84 per cent of white persons are agglutinated by such anti-Rh sera; these persons are Rh-positive, whereas the 16 per cent of non-reactors are called Rh-negative. In contrast to the IgM agglutinins anti-A and anti-B, there are no anti-Rh agglutinins in normal human serum. The clinical importance of the Rh group lies in the danger of iso-immunisation, i.e. the tendency of Rh-negative recipients to develop anti-Rh antibodies, if Rh antigen is introduced parenterally. About 50 per cent of Rh-negative recipients transfused with Rh-positive blood respond by producing antibodies, and may in consequence suffer a severe reaction if subsequently transfused with Rh-positive blood of the same or compatible ABO group. Iso-immunisation may also be brought about in pregnancy. When the mother is Rh-negative and the fetus Rh-positive, fetal cells, which gain entrance to the mother's circulation shortly before or during labour or abortion, may stimulate the production of maternal Rh antibodies. These may be of either IgM or IgG class, or both. They rarely affect the pregnancy which has been responsible for their production, but in subsequent Rh-positive pregnancies Rh antibody of IgG class crosses the placenta and enters the fetal circulation where it may cause destruction of red cells (p. 102), the condition being known as haemolytic disease of the newborn (p. 412).

The Rh groups are inherited on Mendelian principles but are highly complex antigenically and full details are outside our scope. It is sufficient to say that each of the two Rh chromosomes carries at least three closely linked genes for each of which there is an allele. The six first recognised alleles each determine the presence of an antigen and the allelomorphic gene-pairs and the antigens they determine have been named Cc, Dd, Ee. Each of these antigens (except perhaps d) is known to exist in a number of slightly different forms which can be distinguished by certain antisera, and it has been found that genes present together in the same chromosome may exercise a combined effect to produce a compound antigen that differs from the sum of their separate effects. The relationship between the genes and the antigens they determine is certainly much more complex than was imagined a few years ago. The Rh group of the individual thus consists of the sum of the antigens represented on the two Rh chromosomes; the four types containing D are Rh-positive and the four types lacking D are Rh-negative. Individuals iso-immunised against an Rh antigen which they themselves lack produce immune iso-antibodies named according to the evoking antigen, e.g. anti-D, anti-C, etc. The number of genotypes which can be distinguished has been increased by the discovery that

Nomenclature		Rh-positive Types				Rh-negative Types			
British		cDe	CDe	cDE	CDE	cde	Cde	cdE	CdE
	American	R_0	R_1	R_2	R_z	r	R′	R″	R_y
Antisera									
anti-D	anti-Rh₀	+	+	+	+	−	−	−	−
anti-C	anti-rh′	−	+	−	+	−	+	−	+
anti-E	anti-rh″	−	−	+	+	−	−	+	+
anti-c	anti-hr′	+	−	+	−	+	−	+	−
*anti-d	anti-hr₀	−	−	−	−	+	+	+	+
anti-e	anti-hr″	+	+	−	−	+	+	−	−

* This type of antiserum has never been identified.

rare variants of the antigens are serologically recognisable; these are, however, relatively unimportant clinically on account of their rarity. The nomenclature and serological reactions of the commoner Rh types are given in the table on the opposite page.

The complexity of the Rh group is not yet fully known; certain red cell antigens have been found to be closely associated with the Rh factors but the exact relationships are still unsettled.

In addition to the ABO and Rh groups many other blood group systems are known, but like the Rh group natural iso-antibodies are absent, and the sera that detect these groups are ob-tained mostly from persons immunised by transfusion or by pregnancy. These groups only rarely bring about iso-immunisation. Neverthe-less the greatly increased use of blood transfusion necessitates their consideration and identification when a cross-matching test reveals an unexpected antibody. A satisfactory terminology has not yet been worked out; some are named after the person in whom they were first detected but the relationship of all the alleles is not yet clear. Some of these new antibodies have been recog-nised as the immunological response to the compound Rh antigens mentioned above.

CHAPTER 9

MISCELLANEOUS TISSUE DEGENERATIONS AND DEPOSITS

The degenerative changes which result from cellular injury, and the intracellular accumulation of lipids and glycogen resulting from certain disorders of metabolism, have been dealt with in Chapter 1. In the present chapter we describe a group of changes which, although heterogeneous, consist of either the accumulation in the tissues of various substances—amyloid material, mucus, pigmented compounds, calcium deposits and urates—or tissue degenerations which usually affect the stroma of supporting tissues, and are recognised by their microscopic appearances but are ill-defined chemically.

Amyloidosis

Amyloid is a predominantly extracellular fibrillar substance believed to be composed of a complex of protein and mucopolysaccharide: it is deposited in various tissues in a number of diseases. Extensive deposits are visible by naked eye, causing enlargement of the involved tissue and giving it a waxy appearance (Fig. 9.1). In sections stained by haematoxylin and eosin amyloid is seen as a homogeneous, pink, refractile material. Electron microscopy shows it to be composed of fibrils of 5–10 nm. in diameter (Fig. 9.2) which are frequently paired with a narrow gap between the pair. Some fibril pairs form a helix. Although immunoglobulins have been found in amyloid deposits, they are not essential constituents of amyloid.

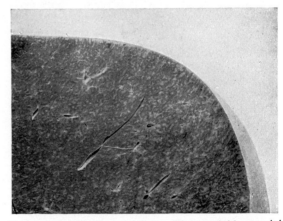

FIG. 9.1—Amyloidosis of liver. The amyloid material gives the organ a dark, homogeneous appearance. × 1.

Methods of demonstrating amyloid

The wide variety of methods currently used to demonstrate the presence of amyloid is an indication of their lack of specificity. Large deposits of amyloid are usually demonstrable by all the methods. If the amount of amyloid present is small, however, the results with each method vary from case to case and identification is correspondingly difficult; for this reason it is usual to use several methods, the best known of which are as follows.

(1) **Lugol's iodine.** Amyloid has a strong affinity for iodine (hence its name) and this forms the basis for a useful macroscopic test. When Lugol's iodine solution is poured over tissue, the amyloid is stained deep brown in contrast to the normal tissue which is only lightly stained. Congested tissues should first be rinsed free of excess blood as this obscures the test.

(2) **Congo red.** This stain may be used on gross specimens and sections for microscopy. Formerly the rate of disappearance from the serum of an intra-

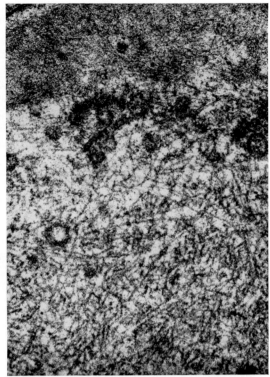

FIG. 9.2.—Electron micrograph of kidney showing amyl-oid deposition. The dense area above is glomerular capillary basement membrane; below, amyloid material is seen as a network of fibres of uniform diameter. × 50,000.

venously injected solution of congo red was used as a clinical test for amyloidosis but owing to lack of accuracy it was abandoned.

The staining by congo red is believed to be due to trapping of the dye in the gap between paired amyloid fibrils. In polarised light amyloid stained by congo red shows a green birefringence.

(3) Rosaniline dyes. These include gentian violet, methyl violet and crystal violet; they stain amyloid reddish while other tissue elements appear purple. This phenomenon of a dye reacting with a tissue constituent and undergoing a colour change is called *metachromasia*: it is believed that in this instance it is due to selective binding of impurities in the dyes by amyloid fibrils.

(4) Fluorescent dyes. Thioflavine-T binds to amyloid and its presence is demonstrated by fluor-escence microscopy (Fig. 9.3).

Classification

Amyloidosis is classified into *primary* and *secondary* types. The primary type occurs apart from any known predisposing cause. The secondary type occurs as a complication of certain diseases. Formerly, chronic infections, and especially chronic pyogenic osteitis, tuber-culosis, syphilis and bronchiectasis accounted

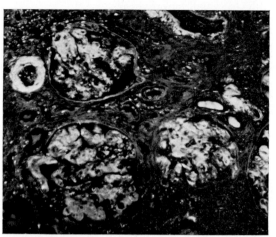

FIG. 9.3.—Amyloidosis of kidney, stained by thioflavine-T and photographed by ultraviolet light. Note fluores-cence of amyloid material in the glomerular capillaries and arterioles. × 100.

for most cases. One of the commonest causes today is rheumatoid arthritis in which careful examination of post-mortem tissues reveals amyloid in approximately 20 per cent of cases. It occurs also in 15 per cent of subjects with multiple myeloma and less commonly in Hodg-kin's disease and other neoplasms of the lym-phoid tissues.

Distribution and effects of amyloid

Organs severely affected by amyloid are en-larged, firm, and of increased specific gravity. The cut surface has a waxy, refractile appearance. In primary amyloidosis the organs and tissues are affected in the following order of frequency: heart, alimentary tract, tongue, skin, skeletal muscles, spleen, kidneys, liver and lungs. In secondary amyloidosis the liver, kidney, spleen and gut are most frequently affected. The microscopic distribution also reveals differences: in primary amyloidosis, deposition is in relation to collagen fibres, particularly in the adventitia of small veins, whereas the deposits of secondary amyloidosis are related to reticulin fibres, par-ticularly in the intima of arterioles. In both types, as the disease becomes more severe, deposits of amyloid are found in capillary and epithelial basement membranes.

Amyloid produces effects by pressure on adjacent cells and by interfering with the normal transfer of water and solutes across the walls of affected small blood vessels.

The **liver** is firm and elastic and may be palpable during life. The change usually begins in the sinusoids of the intermediate zones of the lobules: it may become very extensive and produce marked atrophy of the liver cells (Fig. 9.4). Even at an advanced stage, liver function is not usually severely impaired.

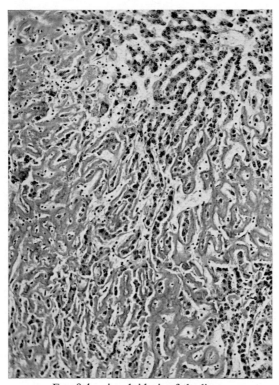

FIG. 9.4.—Amyloidosis of the liver.

The pale homogeneous amyloid substance occupies the mid-zone of the lobules. It extends along the walls of the sinusoids, enclosing the liver cells, which are undergoing atrophy. The zone around the central vein (top right) is least affected. × 110.

The **spleen** shows two distinct patterns of involvement. In one the Malpighian bodies are changed to translucent globules by amyloid deposition in their reticulum (Fig. 9.5); hence the term "sago spleen". In this form splenomegaly is not marked. In the diffuse form, the change affects reticulum of the red pulp, walls of venous sinuses, and many of the small arteries; the spleen may be palpable and weigh

up to 1 kg.; this variety is rare apart from tertiary syphilis.

Amyloidosis of the **kidneys** is particularly important because of its effect on renal function. Deposition occurs upon the basement membranes of the glomerular capillaries and of the tubules (Figs. 9.3 and 21.47, p. 720), in addition to involvement of the small blood vessels. Initially it causes polyuria, the urine being of low specific gravity and containing little or no albumin, but later oliguria and marked albuminuria develop. Nephrotic syndrome may result and the kidneys then show the enlargement, pallor and cortical lipid deposits typical of the syndrome (p. 705).

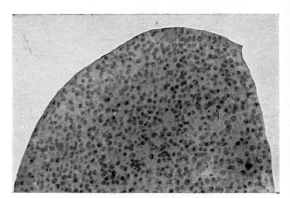

FIG. 9.5.—Amyloid spleen of "sago" type, i.e. affecting the Malpighian bodies.

Eventually many of the glomerular capillaries are obliterated, the kidneys become scarred and shrunken and chronic renal failure develops.

In the **stomach** and **intestines,** amyloid deposits may be widespread and this leads to atrophic changes in the mucosa. Diarrhoea may result from severe involvement of the gut, but even in its absence amyloid material is often demonstrable in rectal biopsy material, providing a useful diagnostic measure. Gingival biopsy is also useful, although less often diagnostic than rectal biopsy.

Deposits of amyloid may also be found in the adrenals, thyroid, lymph nodes and myocardium, especially of the right atrium. The nervous system is never affected (but see p. 653).

In primary amyloidosis, involvement of the myocardium may lead to heart failure, the cause of which may be obscure during life, and even at necropsy may only become apparent on microscopic examination.

Etiology

In spite of intensive investigation, the fundamental nature of amyloid production remains obscure. Amyloidosis may be induced in experimental animals by intensive immunisation and also by injections of casein. Cortisone accelerates the development of experimental amyloidosis, but it is not clear whether the high incidence in rheumatoid arthritis is partly due to the steroids used in its treatment. It has been shown that in animals sensitised lymphoid cells are associated with the deposition of amyloid fibrils but it is still uncertain which cells are responsible for the production of amyloid.

Genetically-determined amyloidosis. Several familial forms of amyloidosis have been described.

The best known are familial mediterranean fever and primary familial amyloidosis.

Familial mediterranean fever is principally found in Mediterranean Jews and Armenians and is inherited as an autosomal recessive factor. In its most typical form, recurrent fever is associated with pain in chest, abdomen, joints and skin; amyloidosis supervenes causing death by renal involvement, but affecting also the spleen lungs and liver. Variants of the disease are recognised in which the amyloidosis becomes apparent before the other features.

Primary familial amyloidosis. This is least rare in parts of Portugal and is inherited as an autosomal dominant. The disease presents in the 3rd and 4th decades with increasing leg weakness and loss of reflexes. Subsequently sphincteric disturbances and malabsorption from intestinal involvement lead to death within 10 years.

Hyaline and Fibrinoid

The term **hyaline** is used in a general descriptive manner to indicate a somewhat homogeneous or glassy, refractile appearance presented by various extracellular tissue elements or by the cytoplasm of cells; it does not indicate a specific substance. *Connective tissue hyaline* describes the homogeneous, usually eosinophilic appearance of collagen and background material in old dense connective tissue. It is seen also in lymph nodes in chronic inflammation, and is not uncommon in certain tumours, both in the stroma and in the walls of blood vessels. Hyaline change in arterioles is discussed below, under fibrinoid.

The term "hyaline" is also applied to thrombi. Fused and altered blood platelets and condensed fibrin may appear homogeneous and red cells may form so-called hyaline thrombi in capillaries. Droplets of homogeneous and somewhat refractile appearance described as hyaline are often a prominent feature in the renal tubular epithelium ("hyaline droplet change") where they are due to reabsorption of protein from the lumen of the tubule (Fig. 21.30, p. 705). Some of the plasma cells in chronic infective lesions commonly contain one or more rounded, brightly eosinophilic and refractile bodies in their cytoplasm: these are known as *Russell bodies*, and are seen by electron microscopy to lie in distensions of the cisternae of the endoplasmic reticulum. They are rich in immunoglobulin but contain also carbohydrate and are PAS-positive.

Other examples of hyaline cytoplasmic change are Crooke's change in the basophil cells in the pituitary in Cushing's syndrome (Fig. 24.2, p. 879), hyaline change in the liver cells in acute virus hepatitis (Fig. 19.13, p. 555) and "alcoholic hyaline" in the liver cells in some cases of cirrhosis (Fig. 19.22, p. 564). In these last two examples, the change represents severe cell injury.

Lastly, delicate transparent casts in the urine in nephritis are commonly known as *hyaline casts* (p. 685). These examples are sufficient to show how heterogeneous are the changes and substances commonly known as hyaline.

Fibrinoid change. This term is used to describe impregnation of tissues with homogeneous or granular, brightly eosinophilic material with staining properties suggestive of fibrin, e.g. bright red with the picro-Mallory method, and a gram-positive reaction. The occurrence of fibrinoid change was formerly regarded as indicating a particular type of disease process, and its occurrence in hypersensitivity reactions, e.g. of Arthus type (type III), led to the assumption that fibrinoid lesions were likely to have an immunological basis. Such conclusions are, however, unwarranted. In any exudative inflammatory lesions, fibrin is liable to be deposited in the inflamed tissues, e.g. in acute infections, and in the synovitis of rheumatoid arthritis. The change is also observed in infarcts, where it results from exudation through the walls of the ischaemic small vessels. Similarly in high blood pressure of rapid development (malignant hypertension) the walls of arterioles undergo necrosis and become impregnated with fibrin (Fig. 13.17, p. 273). In some fibrinoid lesions, the staining reactions are not sufficiently characteristic to indicate deposition of fibrin. Lendrum has demonstrated that plasma constituents may seep into the walls of small vessels and adjacent tissue elements and that, when recent, such lesions give the staining reactions of fibrin, but as they age their staining properties change, coming to resemble those of collagen. The deposits are then hyaline in appearance and are sometimes called *pseudo-collagen*. Such changes are seen in the arterioles in chronic arterial hypertension (p. 686) and in the glomeruli and renal tubules in old age and in diabetes (p. 719).

Fibrin is often not the only abnormal constituent in fibrinoid lesions. In some instances these are PAS-positive, indicating a carbohydrate component.

Fibrinoid change in systemic lupus erythematosus has been shown to contain DNA and immunoglobulins, and consists, at least in part, of DNA complexed with antibody (p. 814): in such complexes, the antibody appears to block the union of basic dyes with DNA, and basophilia is weak or absent.

Corpora amylacea. Under this term are included a number of rounded or oval hyaline structures, which may stain deeply with iodine, hence the name. They sometimes show concentric lamination and may undergo calcification. Such structures form in various situations and they cannot be regarded as all of the same nature. They are often a prominent feature within the acini of the prostate in the elderly; they occur also in the lungs, in old blood clots, and sometimes in tumours.

In the nervous system they are very common; e.g. in old age, in chronic degenerative lesions, and in the region of old infarcts and haemorrhages. They vary greatly in size, the smallest being spherical and homogeneous, and these usually stain deeply with haematoxylin. They appear to form simply by a deposition of organic material containing acid mucopolysaccharides in globular form in the intercellular spaces, but their exact composition is not known. They are of no importance except as a manifestation of the degenerative condition with which they are associated.

Mucoid Change

Under normal conditions mucin is produced both by the epithelial cells of mucous membranes, glands, ducts of glands, etc., and by connective tissue cells, notably in the tissues of the fetus; mucin produced in excess in pathological conditions is correspondingly of two main types—*epithelial mucin* and *connective tissue mucin*. The mucin in pathological states is not a single substance, but represents a group of muco- and glyco-proteins which have the common physical property of imparting high viscosity and sliminess to fluids, and which differ in their content of hexose and hexosamine. When treated with hydrochloric acid, the hexosamine is liberated and reduces Fehling's solution. Most mucins are precipitated by acetic acid and by alcohol, but the mucin of ovarian cysts is not precipitated by the former. Mucins are usually somewhat basophil, and often give a metachromatic reaction with toluidin blue, being stained a reddish purple; but variations in staining reaction are found as the pH is lowered, corresponding to variations in chemical constitution.

Increased formation of *epithelial mucin* is usually the result of increased secretion, as in catarrhal inflammation of mucous membranes. When a catarrhal inflammation has become chronic there is often an increase of mucin-forming cells; e.g. in chronic gastritis and chronic bronchitis. Cysts containing mucoid fluid may be formed by obstruction of ducts and retention of secretion. The constituent cells of the multilocular ovarian cystadenoma (p. 840) secrete much mucin. The cells of some carcinomas arising from mucin-forming epithelia produce mucin actively and also rapidly undergo degeneration to become lost in pools of inspissated mucin.

Mucin-forming connective tissue, usually called *myxomatous tissue*, is characterised by the presence between the cells of a clear matrix containing acid muco-polysaccharides, hyaluronic acid and chondroitin sulphate which give a strongly metachromatic staining reaction. The cells are stellate with branching processes and there are few collagen fibrils. Such tissue is a common constituent of some tumours (Fig. 12.6, p. 245), and intermediate stages between it and merely oedematous connective tissue are observed. Granulation tissue may sometimes present a myxoid appearance, apparently the result of chronic oedema and failure of maturation of the matrix. The term *myxoedema* is applied to the disease resulting from deficiency of the thyroid secretion: the connective tissue of the skin and elsewhere becomes swollen and gelatinous, owing to an increase of mucin in the connective tissue in the early stages of the disease, but later the amount may not be above normal. When the thyroid is removed experimentally in primates, the connective tissues become swollen and contain considerable excess of mucin.

Colloid change. The term "colloid" means glue-like, and may be applied to stiff translucent material. It is applied to the secretion of the thyroid, iodo-thyroglobulin, and when the thyroid becomes enlarged owing to the accumulation of intra-acinar secretion, the term *colloid goitre* is used. The term is also applied to the colloid cysts in the kidneys and the colloid casts in the tubules in chronic pyelo-nephritis. These casts are larger than the "hyaline" casts occurring in the more acute stage, and, unlike the latter, are readily stainable in sections, having an affinity chiefly for acid dyes.

Pigmentary Changes

Pigments are deposited in the tissues in many abnormal states, and may produce changes visible by naked eye or only on microscopy. Some are formed within the body—*endogenous* pigments; others enter the body from the outside—*exogenous* pigments. Of the former, the two main varieties are melanin and derivatives of haemoglobin.

(A) Endogenous pigmentation

(1) Melanin pigmentation

The melanins are iron-free sulphur-containing pigments varying in colour from pale yellow to deep brown. They are formed intracellularly from colourless precursors—melanogens—and are very stable substances, resistant to acids and many other reagents, but soluble in strong alkalis; they can be bleached by powerful oxidising agents such as potassium permanganate or hydrogen peroxide. They are related to the aromatic compounds, tyrosine, phenylalanine and tryptophane and may be formed from such substances by oxidation. On treating sections of skin with dihydroxyphenylalanine (dopa), "dopa-positive" cells in the epidermis oxidise this substance by means of an enzyme like tyrosinase and become blackened in consequence. The only cells in the skin which are "dopa-positive" *in vivo* are the *dendritic cells*, or *melanocytes*, which lie extended between the basal cells of the epidermis (Fig. 9.6); they are the only melanin-producing cells in the skin and after elaborating the pigment in the form of fine granules they transfer it by their processes into the basal epidermal cells and also into certain phagocytic cells (*melanophores*) in the dermis which may thus become heavily laden with coarse

pigment granules. Melanin granules possess the capacity to reduce certain silver salts, e.g. ammoniacal silver nitrate, with consequent deposition of metallic silver; melanin can thus be intensified in histological preparations, scanty or light-coloured

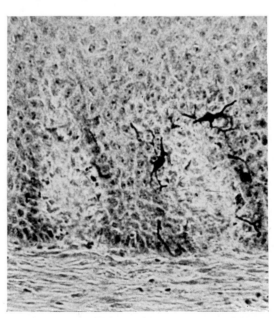

Fig. 9.6.—Dendritic cells (melanocytes) in the basal part of the epidermis. (Dopa reaction.) × 220.

granules being rendered conspicuous. This property is widely used histochemically. According to Masson, the dendritic cells are of neuro-ectodermal origin, being derived from the cells of the embryonic neural crest, as are also the melanocytes of the squamous mucous membranes, the meninges, choroid and adrenals. This view harmonises well with the evidence about the origin of the naevus cells of pigmented moles from neuro-ectodermal cells and also accords with the experimental work of Billingham and Medawar on the behaviour of melanocytes in skin autotransplants. This work seems to have rendered untenable the alternative view that melanocytes are modified basal epidermal cells. The Langerhans cells of the epidermis are now regarded as macrophages and may play a part in the control of keratinisation. Darkening of the skin on exposure to ultra-violet radiation is brought about first by migration of the melanin granules and subsequent darkening of their colour; later there is increased formation of pigment, apparently by the activity of the dendritic cells, which under further stimulation may increase in number.

In *Addison's disease*, which results from destruction of the adrenal cortex (p. 908), there occurs a general increase in melanin pigmentation of the skin, especially in areas exposed to light and in those normally pigmented. There may also be pigmentary deposition on the inner surface of the cheeks on a line corresponding to the junction of the teeth, and on the sides of the tongue, the position being apparently determined by irritation. In the skin the pigment is in the form of very fine brownish granules in the deeper layers of the rete Malpighii, and is present also as coarser granules, chiefly within macrophages in the underlying cutis, the appearance and distribution resembling those in the negro skin. The pigmentation in Addison's disease represents an increase of normal pigment, and occurs under the influence of the melanocyte-stimulating hormone of the pituitary (MSH) which is released in excess in the absence of adrenal inhibition (p. 877).

Chloasma is a condition observed principally during pregnancy, and occasionally in association with ovarian disease, in which pigmented patches occur in the skin of the face, and the pigmented parts, e.g. the nipples, may become darker under the influence of oestrogenic and melanocyte-stimulating hormones. A similar condition has been described in women taking oral contraceptives.

Leukoderma (*vitiligo*) denotes patchy depigmentation of skin and this may be accompanied by increase of pigment in the intervening areas. In the affected areas the dendritic cells are of abnormal structure and have lost their capacity to oxidise dopa to form pigment.

Irregular pigmentation of the skin is common in chronic arsenical poisoning and in neurofibromatosis. In haemochromatosis also, the colour of the skin is due partly to deposition of haemosiderin in the cutis, notably around the sweat glands (p. 204), but also to increase in melanin. A striking degree of melanotic pigmentation of the oral and labial mucosa occurs in association with familial multiple polyposis of the small intestine, especially the jejunum (Peutz-Jeghers syndrome): the disorder is transmitted as a Mendelian dominant. The control of pigment metabolism in the skin is obscure, but it is known to be affected by exposure to light, chronic irritation and increased vascularity, activity of endocrine glands including the adrenals, pituitary and ovaries, and nervous influences. Melanin pigment is formed in large amount in the melanotic tumours which arise from pigmented moles and warts of the skin or from the pigmented coats of the eye, and most analyses have been carried out on the pigment from such tumours. The urine of patients suffering from extensive melanotic tumours occasionally contains a melanogen which darkens on exposure to the oxygen of the air.

Melanosis coli. This is a rather uncommon condition characterised by varying degrees of brownish to black pigmentation of the mucosa of the colon, beginning in the caecum and ascending colon, and sometimes extending to the anus. The pigment is contained mainly in macrophages in the lamina propria; it is absent from the epithelial cells. The condition is commonest when there has been intestinal stasis or chronic obstruction, and it is now recognised to be the result of absorption of aromatic products from the gut. The condition is associated with the prolonged use of anthracene-derived purgatives, e.g. cascara, and the pigment consists of derivatives of anthraquinone combined with products of protein decomposition. The pigment resembles melanin in its reactions, but differs from it in being autofluorescent, weakly PAS-positive, and weakly sudanophilic. The cells containing pigment are dopa-negative.

Ochronosis. In this very rare condition, cartilages, capsules of joints and other soft tissues assume a dark brown or almost black colour, owing to pigment depositions. The pigment resembles melanin in some of its properties but does not reduce silver nitrate. In virtually all cases of ochronosis, alkaptonuria is present, a condition in which homogentisic acid (2,5-hydroxyphenylacetic acid) is excreted by the kidneys and causes the urine to blacken on standing owing to oxidation, especially in an alkaline medium. Homogentisic acid is formed from tyrosine and phenylalanine. Normally it is converted to malylacetoacetic acid by homogentisic acid oxidase in the liver and kidneys, but alcaptonurics lack this enzyme, and consequently homogentisic acid is not metabolised normally, but is oxidised into pigments and deposited in the tissues, producing ochronosis. The metabolic defect in alkaptonuria is inherited as an autosomal recessive character. In the early days of antiseptic surgery ochronosis occasionally followed the use of carbolic dressings for a long time, and the pigment is believed to be formed from the absorbed carbolic acid. This has been called *exogenous ochronosis.*

(2) Haematogenous pigmentation

The normal breakdown of haemoglobin from effete red cells takes place in macrophages of the reticulo-endothelial (RE) system. It begins with opening of the porphyrin ring system, the four pyrrole nuclei and globin now forming a long-chain molecule known as choleglobin. Next the globin and the iron are split off, the latter being re-used in haemoglobin synthesis (see below). The residual biliverdin pigment, consisting of the four pyrrole rings, is then reduced to bilirubin which is absorbed and carried by the plasma albumin to the liver cells. Here it is dissociated and the bilirubin, conjugated with glucuronic acid, is excreted in the bile. In pathological states involving red cell destruction, haemoglobin is broken down in the same way. The resulting pigments may be deposited in the tissues around local red cell destruction, e.g. following a haemorrhage, or in reticulo-endothelial organs when there is excessive destruction of circulating red cells. When haemorrhage occurs into the tissues the red cells become haemolysed, and their haemoglobin is released: much of it may be removed by the lymph and blood streams, to be taken up by RE cells elsewhere without local pigment deposition, but some haemoglobin is likely to be broken down locally in macrophages in and around the bruised tissues, and when the amount is great, there may be local deposition of *iron-containing* and *iron-free pigments.*

(a) Iron-free pigments. The chief of these is bilirubin, which occurs in the form of characteristic brown rhombic crystals (Fig. 9.7), though also as needles and granules. Experiments by Muir and Janet Niven showed clearly formation of bilirubin crystals within macrophages follow-

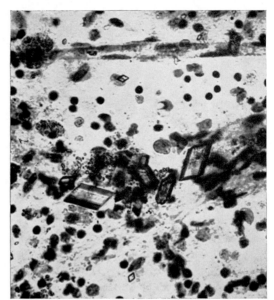

FIG. 9.7.—Bilirubin crystals and granular pigment, some of which is in phagocytes. × 500.
(From the wall of an old cerebral haemorrhage.)

ing ingestion of red cells (Figs. 9.8, 9.9). It may, however, be released from macrophages and come to lie free in the tissues around sites of haemorrhage. Crystals of bilirubin are thus commonly seen, both free and in macrophages, in the sites of old cerebral haemorrhages, thrombi, haemorrhagic infarcts, etc.

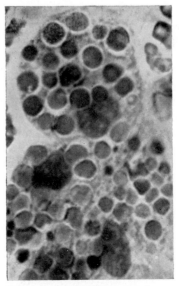

FIG. 9.8.—Two phagocytes from subcutaneous tissue of mouse containing numerous erythrocytes and some haemosiderin granules, 6 days after injection of erythrocytes. × 1500.

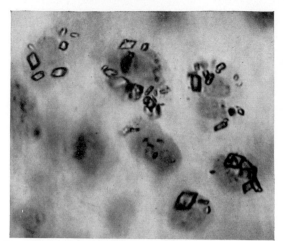

FIG. 9.9.—Intracellular formation of bilirubin crystals in macrophages of mouse, 16 days after injection of haemoglobin. × 1200.

From preparations by Dr. Janet S. F. Niven.

A rise in the level of bilirubin in the plasma results from increased breakdown of haemoglobin, or from failure of the liver cells to remove the normal amount of bilirubin from the blood and conjugate it with glucuronic acid. When the level exceeds 2–3 mg. per 100 ml. of plasma, jaundice appears, i.e. the skin and various other tissues become distinctly yellow. Jaundice *per se* causes little disability in adults unless severe and prolonged. In infants, however, the bilirubin shows a greater tendency to crystallise out in the tissues. Also, a rise of plasma bilirubin to over 15 mg. per 100 ml. in infants carries a risk of direct toxic injury to the brain (kernicterus—p. 605).

(b) Iron-containing pigments. Most of the iron in the body is in the haemoglobin of circulating red cells or stored in tissue cells, mainly in the liver, spleen and bone marrow. Haemoglobin released by normal red cell destruction is broken down in macrophages of the reticulo-endothelial system, particularly in the marrow and spleen. In these cells, iron may be detected histochemically by the prussian blue reaction. If relatively small amounts are present the cell cytoplasm is stained diffusely blue. When present in larger amounts the iron is in the form of granules of *haemosiderin*, a water-insoluble compound of unknown composition, which varies in its iron content and gives a strong prussian blue reaction (Fig. 9.10).* Intracellular iron is stored also

in the form of *ferritin*, a complex of the protein apoferritin and hydrous iron oxide. Ferritin is distributed throughout the cytoplasm and is never present in sufficient concentration to give a positive histochemical test for iron. It can, however, be detected by electron microscopy and also biochemically. The human liver normally contains 100–300 mg. of available iron, which is present in the liver cells mainly in the form of ferritin. Iron for haemoglobin production in the red cell precursors of the marrow is probably supplied by the local RE cells which derive their store from broken down haemoglobin, as mentioned above, and also by taking up iron from the

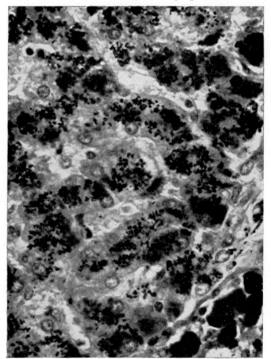

FIG. 9.10.—Granules of haemosiderin in liver cells, from a case of transfusional siderosis (prussian blue). × 500.

plasma. Plasma iron is carried in combination with a β-globulin, *transferrin*: it is derived from dietary iron absorbed from the gut and from exchange with ferritin-iron in the liver and RE cells. Plasma transport is thus essential in maintaining the normal equilibrium between the liver, spleen and marrow and also in distributing iron absorbed from the gut.

There is no physiological method of increasing the normal loss of iron in the bowel, urine, sweat

---

* On treating the tissue with potassium ferrocyanide and hydrochloric acid, any ferric iron present forms ferri-ferrocyanide which is bright blue.

and menstrual blood, and if excess iron enters the body, it is retained. Experimental studies have shown that iron is stored preferentially as ferritin, and haemosiderin is deposited within the liver cells, and probably also in RE cells, only when their concentration of ferritin is very high. For example, during iron overloading of rats, ferritin increases in liver cells to a maximum of over 30 times the normal before haemosiderin begins to appear in them. If the excess iron is then removed by repeated bleeding, iron is released from ferritin by the liver cells and passes to the plasma, but the high concentration of ferritin in the liver cells is maintained by transfer of haemosiderin iron to apoferritin and only when the liver cell haemosiderin is used up does the ferritin level fall.

When local haemorrhage occurs into tissues, as described above, there may be an accumulation of haemosiderin in local macrophages, first seen as a faint diffuse pigmentation of the cytoplasm but progressing to deposition of granules. Depending on the amount deposited and the state of the body's iron reserve, such local accumulations may remain for a long time or may be mobilised and passed to the plasma relatively quickly.

A general increase in red cell destruction, as in haemolytic anaemia, can occur from a large number of causes. In some types the red cells are phagocytosed by macrophages in the spleen, liver, marrow and elsewhere (*erythrophagocytosis*) and free haemoglobin is not then released into the plasma. In other forms of increased red cell destruction, the red cells undergo lysis while in circulation and haemoglobin is then released into the plasma. It is quickly bound to plasma α-globulins termed *haptoglobins* to form a relatively stable complex of molecular size 3×10^5. The amount of haptoglobin normally present in the plasma is enough to bind about 138 mg. of haemoglobin per 100 ml. plasma (representing lysis of about 27 ml. of blood) and release of haemoglobin up to this amount does not produce haemoglobinuria because none of the hapto-haemoglobin complex passes into the glomerular filtrate. When the concentration of haemoglobin in the plasma exceeds 150 mg. per 100 ml. (representing destruction of over 30 ml. of blood), some of the haemoglobin combines with plasma albumin to form methaemalbumin, which is slowly broken down and excreted later as coproporphyrin III by the liver, while the remainder

is rapidly excreted in the glomerular filtrate. When haemoglobinaemia is persistent or recurrent, the renal threshold for haemoglobin is lowered because the haptoglobin has been used up and its regeneration is slow; consequently haemoglobinuria occurs more readily.

When haemoglobin escapes into the glomerular filtrate, some of it is re-absorbed by the cells of the convoluted tubules, in which it is broken down with retention of haemosiderin. This may be observed within a few hours of initiating intravenous injections of haemoglobin into experimental animals: at first the tubular cells give a faint diffuse prussian blue reaction of iron, and within two days minute haemosiderin granules appear in them. In man, renal haemosiderosis (Fig. 9.11) is seen in marked degree in *paroxysmal haemoglobinuria* (p. 410) in which there is recurrent intravascular haemolysis and

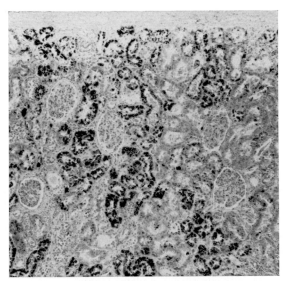

FIG. 9.11.—Kidney in paroxysmal nocturnal haemoglobinuria (prussian blue).

The cells of the convoluted tubules are filled with haemosiderin, the result of long-continued periodic haemoglobinuria. × 55.

so haemoglobinuria. As in the experimental injection of haemoglobin, there is eventual deposition of lesser amounts of haemosiderin in the liver and spleen. The abnormal red cells in pernicious anaemia (p. 417) undergo destruction at an increased rate in the blood, and although this is not sufficiently severe to result in detectable haemoglobinaemia, there may be heavy deposition of haemosiderin in the renal convoluted tubules (Fig. 16.30, p. 420). It was suggested by Muir (3rd ed.) that this might be due to a minimal degree of haemoglobinuria, and subsequent reports indicating that in untreated cases there is an absence of haptoglobin in the plasma lend weight to this possibility.

Accumulation of haemosiderin in organs, or *visceral siderosis*, is seen when there is excessive blood destruction, and can often be demonstrated macroscopically at necropsy by the prussian blue reaction or by ammonium sulphide which colours the haemosiderin black. It is a marked feature in chronic haemolytic anaemias and in pernicious anaemia in relapse, the liver and usually the kidneys and bone marrow giving a strong reaction. It is observed also where there has been much haemorrhage into the tissues, e.g. in purpuric diseases. Moreover, in some severe infections, notably those due to haemolytic streptococci and *Cl. welchii*, there may be sufficient acute haemolysis to produce marked haemoglobin staining of the intima of the large arteries and sufficient accumulation of iron to give a visible reaction.

Haemosiderosis can be produced experimentally by various haemolytic poisons such as toluenediamine, pyrogallic acid, arsenic hydride, and notably by haemolytic antiserum. Experiments by Muir and Shaw Dunn showed that iron derived from blood destruction, even when deposited in the liver and other organs as haemosiderin, is rapidly used again during regeneration of haemoglobin. This is also the case in pernicious anaemia, and adequate treatment by cyanocobalamin is followed by practically complete re-utilisation of the iron stored during the relapse phase. In cases of visceral siderosis the relative amount of iron in the various organs (liver, spleen, kidneys) varies greatly. This cannot be fully explained, but it would appear to depend very largely on the extent to which intravascular haemolysis and phagocytosis respectively are concerned in the process of blood destruction. The largest deposits of haemosiderin, however, occur in the disease known as haemochromatosis (see below). Sufficient haemosiderin to give a distinct iron reaction is a *normal* finding in the liver and spleen of infants up to the third month of life.

Haemochromatosis. This name was applied by v. Recklinghausen to a condition in which there is an extensive deposit of haemosiderin in the organs and tissues, without anaemia or increased red cell destruction. It appears to be an abnormality of iron metabolism leading to excessive absorption, and is considered by some to be genetically determined as either an autosomal recessive character or an autosomal dominant with incomplete penetrance. Along with the haemosiderin there is usually accumulation of the iron-free pigment *lipofuscin* in the smooth muscle of the intestine. However, the outstanding feature is the extensive deposition of haemosiderin, which reaches a degree not found in any other naturally occurring condition. The largest amount is present in the liver, but the haemosiderin concentration may be greater in the lymph nodes in the upper part of the abdomen. It is deposited in the skin, especially around the sweat glands, also in the pancreas, gastric glands, heart muscle, thyroid, etc.; in the kidneys and spleen it is very much less abundant. In the liver it is always accompanied by cirrhosis (p. 569). There is often also fibrosis and atrophy of the pancreas, and diabetes may result at a late stage. Commonly the skin is brown from excess melanin production (which is unexplained)—hence the term *bronzed diabetes*. Haemosiderin may also accumulate in the deeper part of the dermis and around the sweat glands in sufficient amounts to give the skin a characteristic leaden hue. Although the full picture of bronzed diabetes is rare, lesser grades of haemochromatosis are much commoner.

The causal factors in haemochromatosis are not understood. The large amount of iron that accumulates indicates a retention over a long period and indeed it is probable that there is excessive absorption of dietary iron from birth onwards. This may account for the observed increase in the level of plasma iron. The plasma transferrin level is not increased and may indeed be diminished owing to impaired production by the cirrhotic liver. Consequently the degree of iron saturation of the plasma transferrin is usually increased well above the normal 35 per cent, and this may favour its uptake by the liver cells and also by cells of the RE system. However, in haemochromatosis iron accumulates in the cells of the myocardium, gastric glands, pancreas, etc., which do not normally store iron. The nature of the relationship between iron storage, cirrhosis of the liver and pancreatic fibrosis in haemochromatosis is also not understood. Cirrhosis develops in adult life and if there is excessive absorption of iron from birth then there must be considerable accumulation in the liver and pancreas before the onset of cirrhosis and pancreatic fibrosis. However, these latter changes do not appear to be due directly to iron storage, for in patients with prolonged failure of red cell production (aplastic anaemia) who have been kept alive for years by very large numbers of blood transfusions, the amount of haemosiderin deposited in the liver and other tissues may equal or even exceed that commonly present in haemochromatosis (Fig. 9.10) and yet we have not observed the development of cirrhosis or pancreatic fibrosis in such cases. The distribution of the iron in the tissues following multiple transfusions is similar but not identical to that in haemochromatosis. In the Bantu people of South Africa, the dietary iron intake is very high because of the use of iron cooking pots: cirrhosis is common and may be associated with excessive iron uptake and storage, but the distribution of iron in the tissues is not the same as in haemochromatosis: for example, there is little in the gastric mucosa or choroid plexus and heavy deposition in the duodenum and upper jejunum. There is evidence that iron absorption from the gut is increased in some cases of cirrhosis and also in patients with chronic pancreatitis.

Malarial pigmentation. In malaria the parasites within the red cells produce from the haemoglobin a dark brown pigment, haematin, in the form of very minute granules, which accumulates within the parasites. It becomes free when the red cells are broken down, and is taken up by phagocytes and deposited in organs, especially the spleen and liver, where it remains practically unchanged for many years. Malarial pigment is not a melanin; it contains iron, though it reacts negatively with the ordinary prussian blue test. W. H. Brown showed that in its solubilities and spectroscopic properties it is essentially haematin, and it closely resembles the artefact pigment derived from formalin acting on blood. When there is much blood destruction, especially in severe cases of malaria, haemosiderin may be deposited in the organs in addition to the malarial pigment.

(3) Biliary pigmentation

Bile pigment consists mainly of bilirubin which has been taken up from the blood by the liver cells, conjugated with glucuronic acid, and secreted into the bile canaliculi (p. 590).

When bile is prevented by an obstruction of the major bile ducts from entering the intestine (*extrahepatic cholestasis*), the bile canaliculi gradually become distended with inspissated bile, which appears in histological sections as homogeneous, olive-green columns, with minute branches extending between individual liver cells (Fig. 19.25, p. 567). These appearances are seen also in obstruction of smaller bile ducts within the liver (*intrahepatic cholestasis*), as occurs in various acute and chronic diseases affecting the liver cells.

Failure to excrete conjugated bilirubin, due to extra- or intra-hepatic cholestasis, is the commonest cause of jaundice. The conjugated bilirubin is regurgitated from the liver cells into the blood. A rise of the plasma level of conjugated bilirubin to over 2 mg. per 100 ml. is associated with jaundice. Being relatively water-soluble, conjugated bilirubin does not show the same tendency as unconjugated bilirubin to become deposited in the tissues, nor does it cause brain injury. Another difference is that conjugated bilirubin passes into the glomerular filtrate and is excreted in the urine, which it renders dark. Some re-absorption occurs in the cells of the renal convoluted tubules, which may come to contain fine granules of conjugated bilirubin. Brown-green casts may also be seen in the lumina of the distal tubules.

(4) Lipofuscin: age pigment

In the later years of life a fine brownish-yellow pigment tends to appear in the heart muscle, smooth muscle, etc.; and in wasting diseases this accumulation of pigment is more marked. In some cases of malabsorption syndrome, for example due to coeliac disease, it is present in the smooth muscle of the small intestine and oesophagus, and in smaller amounts in that of the stomach and colon: experimental studies suggest that vitamin E deficiency may be responsible.

In the heart muscle the pigment accumulates in the central part of the cells around the poles of the nucleus, and when this is associated with wasting of the muscle, the term *brown atrophy* is applied. Similar pigment may occur in the liver cells, especially in the central parts of the lobules, in the cells of the testis, and in the nerve cells of the cortex of the brain. Heavy deposits of pigment in the cortical neurones is seen in senile insanity and allied conditions. The pigment must be distinguished from that which occurs normally in the pigmented neurons of the locus caeruleus and substantia nigra, which belongs to the melanin group. In brown atrophy the pigment is believed to be chiefly lipid, as it reduces perosmic acid and is usually coloured by the sudan stains. It is often called *lipofuscin*, but differs in its chemical and staining reactions in the various organs, some being fluorescent, doubly refracting or acid-fast in varying degree, e.g. *ceroid*, an acid-fast pigment found in the liver in certain forms of experimental cirrhosis. Electron microscopy suggests that age pigment consists of "indigestible" residues of lipid metabolism, lying in cytoplasmic vacuoles derived from lysosomes.

(B) Exogenous pigmentation

By inhalation. The most important exogenous pigments are those inhaled as dust particles and entering the body through the respiratory passages. A certain amount of coal dust and stone dust enters and accumulates in the lungs of all individuals living in urban conditions, but the accumulation becomes excessive in those exposed occupationally to an atmosphere rich in dust. The lungs may be infiltrated by foreign particles of various kinds—coal, carbon, silica, iron and other ores and various organic substances. The resulting pathological changes will be described later with the diseases of the lungs.

The entrance of such particles into the lungs is favoured by the presence of chronic bronchitis or other condition in which there is interference with the action of the ciliated epithelium, but even in a healthy animal, dust particles less than 5μ gain access to the pulmonary alveoli if the amount in the inspired air is great. The dust particles are quickly taken up by phagocytes in the pulmonary alveoli. Some of the phagocytes may be derived from flattened cells lining the alveoli, but these are supplemented by macrophages from the alveolar septa. Some of the phagocytes with the ingested particles are expelled via the bronchi; others enter the interstitial tissue of the lungs, and pass into the lymphatics to become arrested especially in the walls of the respiratory bronchioles and in the

lymphoid collections of the lungs. Many are carried to the hilar nodes and some also reach the pleura. The degree of irritation resulting depends on the nature of the particles. Large collections of carbonaceous particles may provoke little or no overgrowth of connective tissue—*anthracosis*—whereas fibrosis is very marked in the case of silica-containing stone dust, the condition of *silicosis* resulting (p. 372). The bronchial lymph nodes become pigmented and enlarged, the accumulation within their phagocytic cells being virtually permanent. Occasionally in anthracosis, a lymph node ruptures into a pulmonary vessel and pigment is distributed through the general circulation. It is then found in macrophages, especially in the spleen, where it may form small black areas visible to the naked eye, and also in the bone marrow and liver (Fig. 9.12). Some of the pigment which has accumulated in

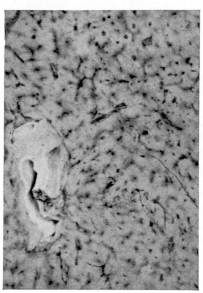

FIG. 9.12.—Anthracosis of liver, showing deposition of carbon pigment especially in and around the portal tracts. (Dr. J. F. Heggie.) × 1·5.

the lungs may be removed by phagocytes which appear in the sputum for a long time after removal of the individual from the dusty atmosphere.

By ingestion. The best example of pigmentation due to absorption from the alimentary canal is *argyria*, which results from the taking of silver preparations for therapeutic purposes for a long period. Silver forms an albuminate which is carried in the plasma to various tissues, and when it undergoes reduction minute brownish-grey granules are formed. These are present especially in the wall of the intestine, in the skin, liver and kidneys, where they occur especially in the basement membrane of the collecting tubules. The presence of the particles in the skin gives rise to a characteristic dusky appearance, which is practically permanent. In *chronic lead-poisoning* an albuminate is produced in a similar way, and around the teeth hydrogen sulphide reacts with it to produce the characteristic blue line on the gums.

Tattooing. In tattooing, fine particles such as india ink, ultramarine, cinnabar (mercuric sulphide), etc., introduced through the epidermis, are taken up by macrophages (p. 47) and lodge in small spaces or clefts in the connective tissue of the cutis. Some particles are carried also by the lymph stream to the regional lymph nodes and then are conveyed by phagocytes into the lymphoid tissue. Both at the site of introduction and in the lymph nodes the pigment persists for life.

Pathological Calcification

Pathological calcification of soft tissues occurs most commonly without any general disturbance of calcium metabolism: the level of plasma calcium is normal, and deposition is due to local changes in the affected tissue. This is termed *dystrophic calcification*. Less commonly, pathological calcification is a result of an increase in the level of ionic calcium in the plasma, and occurs in normal soft tissues: this is termed *metastatic calcification*.

In both dystrophic and metastatic calcification the deposits resemble in composition the minerals of bone, but show much greater variations in the proportions of calcium to magnesium and phosphate to carbonate.

Identification of calcium salts in tissues. Calcium salts have an affinity for haematoxylin, forming a lake with it, and the earliest sign of calcification is given by the appearance of hyaline or finely granular material of a deep violet tint. Later the calcium salts form irregular and somewhat refractile masses: they are, of course, readily soluble in weak acids, and small bubbles of carbon dioxide are released from the carbonates. When treated with diluted sulphuric acid, the characteristic crystals of calcium sulphate separate out. This occurs more readily when the sections are in 50 per cent alcohol, in which the solubility of the crystals is low. When calcium salts are treated with silver nitrate, yellow silver phosphate is formed, and this quickly undergoes reduction on exposure to light and turns black (von Kossa's method). Neither the affinity for haematoxylin nor von Kossa's method is specific for calcium. Silver nitrate is reduced by other substances, e.g. iron, and the reaction with haematoxylin is given by a substance formed before the deposition of calcium, and is positive after the tissue is decalcified. The best reagent is alizarin, the staining principle in madder, or its derivatives. Alizarin stains calcium salts red, but the reaction may not be given by very old deposits. When injected *intra vitam*, alizarin colours growing bone (but not fully formed bone) and also pathological deposits of calcium unless they are very old.

Calcification is often accompanied by deposit of iron compounds which give a prussian blue reaction. These may give a diffuse staining or may be granular.

Dystrophic calcification

This consists of the irregular deposition of calcium salts in altered or necrotic tissues and formed elements such as thrombi. Deposition is irregular and may be sufficiently heavy to render the part chalky or even stony hard.

Predisposing changes. The local changes which predispose to dystrophic calcification are as follows.

(1) *Hyaline change in fibrous tissue.* This occurs as an ageing change in arteries. Increase in calcium in hyalinised artery walls is usual, and it may be sufficient to convert the vessel to a rigid tube, as in Monckeberg's sclerosis (Fig. 13.19, p. 276). Calcification is also common in dense connective tissues, for example tendons, the dura mater, and the scarred heart valves following rheumatic endocarditis. It occurs in some tumours, for example in fibromas (Fig. 9.13) and in uterine myomas undergoing involution after the menopause. The "brain-sand" bodies of some meningiomas consist of concentrically arranged cells which undergo hyaline change followed by calcification.

(2) *Tissue death*, such as caseous patches in tuberculosis, the necrotic centre of a gumma, old infarcts and particularly fat necrosis (p. 859)

and the lipid-rich debris in atheromatous plaques all tend to become calcified, as do dead parasites (e.g. *Trichinella spiralis* and echinococcal cysts). Calcification of such dead tissue is a slow process, and occurs only when necrotic material persists for a long time without undergoing organisation.

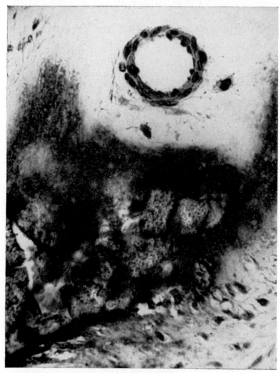

FIG. 9.13.—Area of calcification near a blood vessel in a fibroma.

Calcium is stained dark by haematoxylin, and the earliest change, in the form of a fine granular deposit, is seen at the margin. × 500.

(3) *Inspissated pus* and *organic material in ducts, etc.* A large collection of pus, unless discharged, eventually becomes inspissated, then calcified, and even ossified. Organic material accumulating in the ducts of salivary glands, or in the appendix, may become calcified, forming "stones" in these sites. Calcium deposition in the urinary tract, both as discrete stones and as soft, crumbling material, is caused by urinary infections, but stone formation occurs also as a result of increased calcium excretion (see below).

(4) *Thrombi.* Calcification occurs very commonly in old thrombi which have not undergone organisation: hard masses are thus formed in veins, e.g. in the legs, and show up on X-ray as *phleboliths.*

The chemical reactions involved in dystrophic calcification are not understood. Factors which may be involved include the following. (a) Local changes in pH of hyaline or necrotic tissue, etc.: calcium is deposited more readily from an alkaline medium. (b) Breakdown products of cells or tissue elements to provide a nucleus with an affinity for calcium salts. Release of phosphate from nucleoprotein breakdown is a possible example. The strong tendency for calcification of necrotic fatty tissue was formerly explained by the affinity of fatty acids for calcium, forming insoluble calcium soaps. This suggestion lacks supporting evidence, and in particular subcutaneous injection of fatty acids does not lead to calcification. (c) Local enzyme changes: the normal process of calcification of growing bone occurs in the presence of high local concentrations of alkaline phosphatase. In experimentally induced lesions, some correlation has been observed between high levels of alkaline phosphatase and deposition of calcium salts, but the correlation is not a very good one, and this is not a convincing factor in dystrophic calcification in man.

Calcinosis circumscripta. This is a condition in which irregular nodular dystrophic calcification occurs in the skin and subcutaneous tissues, especially of the fingers. The overlying skin becomes ulcerated and the chalky material is discharged or may be scraped out. This appears to consist chiefly of calcium carbonate, as shown by solution with effervescence in hydrochloric acid. Microscopically a mild chronic inflammatory reaction with giant cells surrounds the nodules. The causation of the lesion is obscure. The deposits are easily distinguished from gouty tophi by their dense opacity to X-rays and by histochemical tests.

Occasionally calcium deposition is more widespread, involving also muscles and tendons—this is known as **calcinosis universalis.**

Metastatic calcification

This occurs in the following conditions.

(1) Excessive absorption of calcium from the gut. This is seen most commonly in infants with hypervitaminosis D due to over-fortification of infant foods with vitamin D and calcium (p. 766). Similar experimental changes can be produced readily in the rat (Figs. 9.14, 9.15).

(2) Excessive mobilisation of calcium from the bones. This occurs in patients with widespread

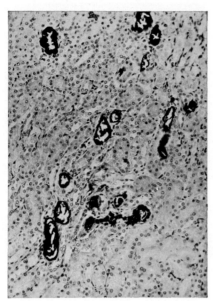 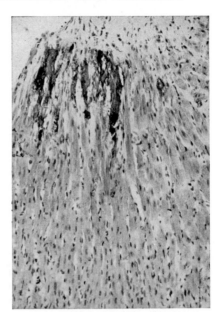

FIGS. 9.14 and 9.15.—Illustrations of hypervitaminosis D in rat. Calcium deposits stained dark.
Fig. 9.14, small calcified vessels in kidney; Fig. 9.15, calcified fibres of heart muscle.
From preparations kindly lent by Mr. J. R. M. Innes.

bone destruction, as for example in multiple myeloma or metastatic carcinoma. Prolonged immobilisation is also of importance, the bones undergoing disuse atrophy. Excessive mobilisation of bone calcium is also brought about by *primary hyperparathyroidism*, usually due to a parathyroid adenoma (p. 904), and by *secondary hyperparathyroidism* associated with parathyroid hyperplasia and resulting from chronic renal disease with retention of phosphate (p. 717).

Metastatic calcification occurs especially in the walls of arteries, the myocardium of the left side of the heart, the wall of the stomach, the kidneys and lungs. Apart from the arteries, these are otherwise rare sites of calcification, and it may be that, in the presence of a raised level of plasma ionic calcium, deposition is influenced by the local pH. Thus in the stomach, calcium deposition occurs around the acid-secreting glands where there is local alkalinity, and in the kidneys around the tubules, which produce ammonia.

Deposition of Uric Acid and Urates

Uric acid is formed as the final breakdown product of purine bases, and is thus derived from catabolism of nucleic acids. In the normal adult, the plasma level of monosodium urate is approximately 4–5 mg. per 100 ml., and levels above 6·5–7 mg. (depending on the method of assay) are pathological. The normal average daily excretion in the urine is 420 mg., and a smaller amount is excreted by the intestine. Renal clearance of uric acid is only 5–10 per cent of inulin clearance and is largely dependent on secretion by the distal tubular epithelium, since much of the uric acid in the glomerular filtrate is reabsorbed from the proximal tubules.

Hyperuricaemia is not uncommon, particularly in men over 40. It tends to be familial, but sporadic cases occur. The metabolic abnormalities concerned are not clearly understood. In some instances, increased production of uric acid results from a deficiency of the phosphoribosyl-transferase enzyme which is necessary for the re-utilisation of hypoxanthine for purine synthesis. This deficiency results in increased breakdown of hypoxanthine into uric acid. Other enzyme deficiencies with similar effect have been detected in some instances of hyperuricaemia. In others, there is a defect of unknown nature in renal excretion of uric acid. These defects account for at least some cases of *primary hyperuricaemia* in which nucleic acid breakdown is normal. *Secondary hyperuricaemia* results from increased nucleic acid breakdown, as in the myeloproliferative disorders (p. 435).

There is considerable variation in the effects of hyperuricaemia. In most instances, there are no associated pathological changes. In others there is deposition of uric acid or urate in the collecting tubules of the kidneys, seen macroscopically as brown-yellow streaking of the medulla: this may have little or no effect, or may be followed by formation of uric acid stones (p. 744). The most important complication of hyperuricaemia is *gout* (p. 799), in which crystals of sodium biurate are deposited in and around the joints, in the skin (Fig. 9.16) and elsewhere. It is always accompanied by hyperuricaemia, and yet the relatives of patients may have equally high levels of plasma uric acid without developing gout. As indicated above for hyperuricaemia in general, a number of individual abnormalities of purine metabolism can result in gout.

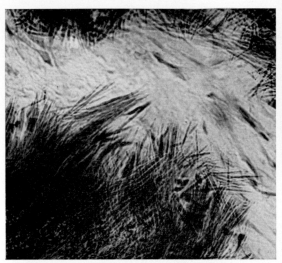

Fig. 9.16.—Section through gouty nodule of skin, showing deposit of needle-like crystals of sodium biurate. × 370.

CHAPTER 10

TUMOURS

I. ORIGIN, NATURE AND CAUSATION

Introduction. In previous chapters we have seen examples of cell proliferation and growth of tissues in the process of repair, in response to irritation, and as a hyperplastic process. Such growth is purposeful, and, up to a point, capable of explanation. In a tumour or *neoplasm*, however, the growth is not only excessive but apparently purposeless, progressing without regard to the surrounding tissues or the requirements of the individual as a whole. While forming a part of the body, a tumour and its cells seem to have become largely unresponsive to the factors which control the proliferation of non-neoplastic cells. Accordingly, tumours exhibit various degrees of uncontrolled growth and in some instances uncontrolled function, e.g. the production of hormones or enzymes. Such behaviour is commonly termed *autonomous*, but a tumour is, of course, parasitic on the host, and escape from host control factors is only relative.

Origin. Tumours show an extraordinary variety of structure, but the majority retain a resemblance to some normal tissue or cell type; occasionally the resemblance is to some precursor cell or tissue rather than to the fully differentiated adult type. These resemblances are attributable to the origin of all tumours from some normal cell or tissue, and the result of an abnormal and excessive proliferation of the cells derived from the previously normal structure. (The exact origin of some tumours is unknown or disputed, but this does not affect the general statement.) Most often, the origin can be traced to tissues in which there is active cell loss and replacement, and which are exposed to the various noxious agents in the environment (especially the skin and the epithelia of the alimentary and respiratory tracts). Many tumours do, however, originate from highly specialised cells such as those of the liver, thyroid, adrenal, cartilage or fat. The adult neurone is probably the only cell in the body incapable of giving rise to a tumour, and even here tumours derived from the precursor cells—neuroblasts—are not uncommon. The origin of a tumour in this respect is called its *histogenesis*, and provides the basis of a principal mode of classification—thus for instance nearly all tumours may be classified as *epithelial* or *connective tissue* tumours according to the cell of origin.

Behaviour

Tumours also differ greatly in behaviour. Some grow slowly, some fast: between one that hardly changes in size from year to year and one that can be seen to enlarge substantially within a week there are all gradations. They vary also in the mobility of their cells; in some (the *benign* tumours) the tumour cells are restricted to the site of origin and a single lump is formed, whereas in others (the *malignant* tumours*) the cells spread out from the primary site to invade the surrounding tissues—local malignancy—or are carried off in lymph or blood to form distant secondary deposits or *metastases*—full-blown malignancy. (For details of these processes see the later section on the spread of invasive tumours.) In addition, tumours vary in degree of *differentiation*: the well-differentiated growths closely resemble the tissue of origin, sometimes

---

* In this book *tumour* (or neoplasm) is used for all lesions of this type, benign or malignant. *Cancer* is used for all malignant tumours, regardless of their origin. *Carcinoma* is used only for malignant tumours of epithelium (see next chapter). Though purists often insist that cancer and carcinoma are the same word, it is quite obvious that "cancer research" for instance is not limited to epithelial tumours.

H

so much so that even with the naked eye the origin is obvious (as a lipoma, for instance, may be instantly recognisable as a lump of fatty tissue), whilst the *poorly differentiated* tumours diverge farther and farther from it, until they may consist of rapidly growing cells whose parent tissue is no longer recognisable. This loss of differentiation is known as *anaplasia*. These various features usually, but not always, run parallel: most benign tumours are well differentiated and grow slowly, most malignant tumours are poorly differentiated, grow rapidly and show numerous mitoses, both normal and abnormal (Fig. 10.1). Though benign tumours can be dangerous, especially if their site of origin leads them to press upon vital structures, the great majority of killing tumours are malignant. For this reason, the distinction between benign and malignant tumours is of outstanding practical importance, and the treatment received by the patient is greatly affected by it. The following table summarises the criteria of this

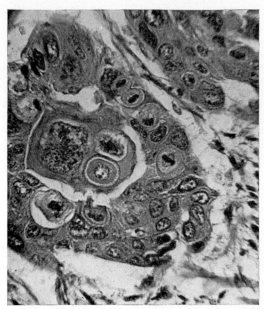

FIG. 10.1.—Section of squamous carcinoma, showing aberrant giant cells and numerous mitoses. × 400.

	Benign	Malignant
(a) *Evidence of rapid growth*		
Mitoses	Few and normal	Numerous and often abnormal
Nuclei	Little altered	Enlarged, often irregular (pleomorphic)
Nucleoli	Little altered	Usually large
Cytoplasmic basophilia	Slight	Marked
Haemorrhages and necrosis	Inconspicuous	Often extensive
(b) *Differentiation*		
Naked-eye resemblance to tissue of origin	Often close	Slight
Microscopic resemblance to tissue of origin	Usually very marked	Usually poor
(c) *Evidence of transgression of normal boundaries*		
Capsule intact	Frequent	Rare
Local invasion	Never	Very frequent
Metastases	Never	Frequent

distinction. In many cases, the transition from benign to malignant is so gradual that the crucial point is very difficult to recognise: indeed, one of

the principal functions of the pathologist in hospital is the application of his experience to prediction of the probable future behaviour of tumours, samples ("biopsies") of which are referred to him by clinicians. The behaviour of the innumerable different kinds of tumours of different organs varies greatly, and it is necessary to know these variations before one can apply the criteria of the table with safety to the individual case.

Examples of exceptions. *Rate of growth.* Some benign tumours (especially of the female genitalia, as myomas of the uterus and cystadenomas of the ovary) may grow very rapidly and reach a great size. Some malignant tumours—many rodent ulcers, some breast carcinomas and in particular argentaffinoma and "latent" carcinoma of the prostate—grow very slowly.

Differentiation. Some benign tumours (mucinous cystadenoma of the ovary, for example) look very unlike any tissue normally present at their site of origin. Some malignant tumours (some squamous carcinomas, for instance, and metastases of some well differentiated thyroid carcinomas) may closely resemble the parent tissue. Function is not always lost in malignant tumours: indeed, if one includes such basic functions as the production of keratin, mucin or melanin, its complete loss is exceptional. Among those tumours of the endocrine organs which secrete clinically important hormones malignancy is far from rare.

Invasion is perhaps the most nearly reliable criterion of malignancy, but it is often surprisingly difficult to assess in practice, especially where the normal structures are distorted by some other pathological process such as infection, metaplasia or congenital anomaly. A capsule may be absent in some benign tumours, such as papillomas, and present in some malignant tumours, including clear-cell carcinoma of kidney and some thyroid carcinomas.

Metastasis is another generally reliable criterion, but benign tumours and even normal tissue may sometimes become implanted at a distance as a result of trauma or surgical accident. Also some undoubted malignant tumours practically never metastasise: rodent ulcers are the best example, but intracranial tumours also fail to metastasise outside the cranio-spinal cavity. The placental trophoblast not only invades the uterus but is often carried to the lungs: and the fetus, incidentally, grows faster than any tumour.

Effects of tumours

These are various and many of them can be readily understood. The presence of a mass of growing tissue of whatever kind may lead to pressure effects on various important structures, e.g. on blood vessels (especially veins), nerves, tubes and organs, and the usual results will follow. This is true both of benign and of malignant tumours, but in addition the latter infiltrate and destroy such structures, and are especially liable to produce obstructive effects, e.g. stenosis of pylorus, intestine or bronchi. Compared with normal tissues, tumours have a reduced power of repair and a low resistance to bacterial invasion. Hence tumours of the skin or mucous membranes often become ulcerated, and extensive destruction follows. This is seen especially in malignant tumours, but in benign tumours also: a myoma in the cavity of the uterus, for example, may be extensively ulcerated. Ulceration often involves blood vessels, and thus serious and sometimes fatal haemorrhage may result. Highly cellular cancers in the stomach and elsewhere may be extensively invaded by bacteria and undergo sloughing, and there is no doubt that the absorption of bacterial toxins in such conditions plays a very important part in the production of the anaemia and wasting which are often such prominent features. The withdrawal of essential materials such as amino-acids from the metabolic pool by a massive or rapidly growing tumour is a further factor of

importance, e.g. tryptophan deficiency induced by argentaffinoma (p. 533). It has often been suggested that some more specific toxic effect is produced by tumours, but there is little evidence for this. Pyrexia can usually be ascribed to secondary bacterial invasion and in other cases may be due to absorption of products from dead and autolysed tissue. Many other effects of tumours will be exemplified in the accounts of individual organs.

Inappropriate hormone production and other special effects. There are a number of peculiar and specific effects produced by some tumours. Probably commonest of these is the production of anomalous hormones. Production of appropriate hormones by tumours of endocrine organs is to be expected. Production of the wrong hormone when it is one chemically related to the normal product, for example oestrogen by adrenal cortical tumours, or gastrin by pancreatic islet cell tumours, is rather more remarkable. But much more surprising is the lengthening list of hormones that have been shown to be produced by tumours of organs with no known relevant hormonal secretion— 5HT or ACTH by carcinoma of the bronchus, and insulin from fibrosarcoma for example. Such findings are by no means rare. Other hormones, as diverse as parathormone, antidiuretic hormone, TSH and erythropoietin have also been found. The tumours can be of many types, with bronchial carcinoma particularly often represented. There is some evidence that similarly inappropriate enzyme production would be found as often if looked for. These findings may be explained at least in part by the fact that the DNA in every normal cell in the body contains the whole genetic material of the individual, with the unwanted parts suppressed: these inappropriate hormone and enzyme productions may demonstrate simply that this suppression can sometimes be overcome during tumour growth.

There are a number of other apparently specific complications of tumours such as the pulmonary osteoarthropathy that sometimes accompanies intra-thoracic tumours (p. 772), the peripheral neuropathy and other neurological disorders complicating bronchial carcinoma (p. 382), thrombophlebitis migrans (p. 290) and acanthosis nigricans (p. 502). The mechanism of none of these is understood, yet the association with tumours is well-established.

The Causation of Tumours

This is an enormous and exceedingly difficult subject. An example will make this clearer than a great deal of explanation. If the back of a mouse is painted repeatedly with tar, a tumour will appear on the area in a few months. The cause (in one obvious sense of the word "cause") of *this* cancer is undoubtedly the tar. But the tumour will go on growing even if the painting with tar ceases. The tar has produced a change in the cells of the skin which causes them to grow and divide with abnormal speed, and they transmit this property to their progeny. The original cause is no longer relevant. The nature of the change in the cells of the skin which makes them continue to grow abnormally even in the absence of the original stimulus is the central mystery of cancer. What induces the cell to keep growing when the tar is no longer present? We know many differences between normal cells and tumour cells, but most if not all of them seem to be not the causes, but rather the consequences, of the change of behaviour. We do not even know if the change from normal cell to cancer cell is always of the same nature, or if there are several kinds of change which have similar biological effects.

Paradoxically, we know many causes for cancer, but not the Cause of Cancer. We know that many things, like tar, can produce tumours, but we do not know with certainty how any of them work. In the following section we shall review some of the more fruitful lines of enquiry and describe some of the key experiments of cancer research. In later sections we shall attempt a more complete survey of the known causes of cancer in man, and bring together the various threads into a review of some speculations on the nature of cancer.

Chemical carcinogens

In 1775 Percival Pott (of Pott's fracture and other eponyms) reported that London chimney sweeps developed cancer of the scrotum much more often than men in other occupations, and at a much earlier age (Fig. 10.2). (The capacity of the rugose skin of the scrotum to retain dust in the unbathed explains the localisation.) Other associations of skin cancer with occupations were discovered, the most important that by Volkmann (also a man of several eponyms) in 1874 affecting tar and mineral oil workers.

Experimental cancer. Many attempts were made to copy this process in experimental animals, with success finally in 1917 by Yamagiwa and Ichikawa, who produced cancers on the ears of rabbits by painting with tar over a prolonged period. It has recently been shown, ironically enough, that most of the lesions produced in rabbits in this way are not true cancers but examples of the reversible lesion called molluscum sebaceum (see Chapter 25): but this does not detract from the great significance of these experiments in stimulating experimental cancer research.

Very soon the much more susceptible mouse replaced the rabbit as the standard subject: the most active substances, when repeatedly painted on the back, will produce tumours in this animal in less than 3 months.

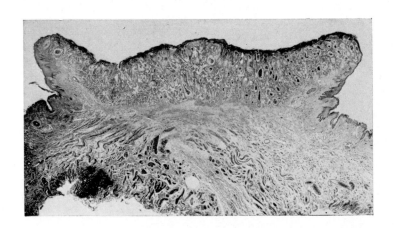

FIG. 10.2.—Chimney-sweeps' cancer of the scrotum. × 5.

A typical lesion showing the raised margins and infiltrating keratinising squamous carcinoma.

Carcinogens

Materials such as tar which produce tumours are called carcinogens. A search for the active constituents led Kennaway, Cook and Hieger in 1931 to the discovery of the first of the important group of *carcinogenic hydrocarbons* (Fig. 10.3). Of these *dibenzanthracene* was the first discovered: the other three are the most active of their type known. *Benzpyrene* occurs naturally in tar, soot and similar materials and is believed to be responsible for most of their activity. *Methylcholanthrene* is not a naturally occurring compound but is used very extensively for experimental purposes.

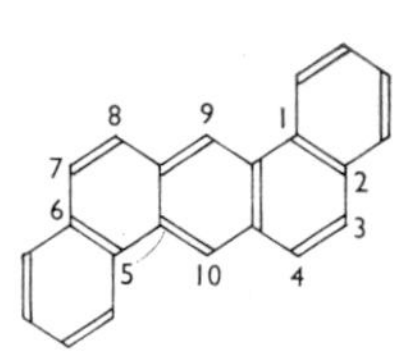

1 : 2, 5 : 6 dibenzanthracene 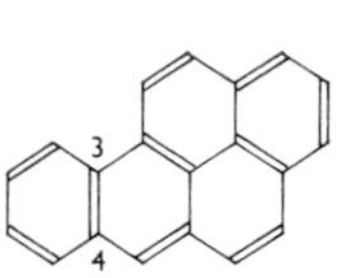   3 : 4 benzpyrene

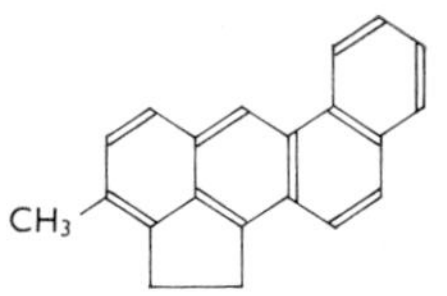

Methylcholanthrene 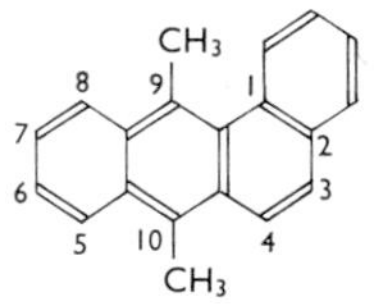   9 : 10 dimethyl
1 : 2 benzanthracene

FIG. 10.3.

Since their discovery an enormous amount of work has gone into the search for other chemical carcinogens, and some thousands of such substances are now known. It is natural to enquire whether the chemical structure of these compounds is related in any simple way to their carcinogenic activity, but although a great deal about the structure and the behaviour within the body of such compounds has been learned, remarkably little in the way of general principles has emerged. Experienced workers can often predict the probable activity of compounds closely related to known carcinogens, but they are sometimes wrong, and the only certain way to determine the activity of a compound is by animal experiment. Since a compound will often produce tumours in one animal and not in another, and since the effects of different ways of administering the compound are likely to be equally variable, the process of testing for car-

cinogenicity is a difficult one. The risk of inclusion of carcinogens among the great number of active chemicals constantly being released as new drugs, dyes, food additives, cosmetics, insecticides and the like is considerable.

Some compounds have special modes of action on particular organs, and a number of examples will be given in later sections. Of compounds with more general activity, the following, which include some of the simplest, must suffice:

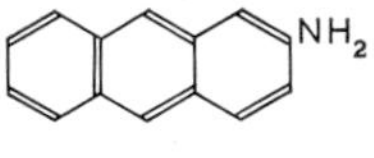

2-anthramine 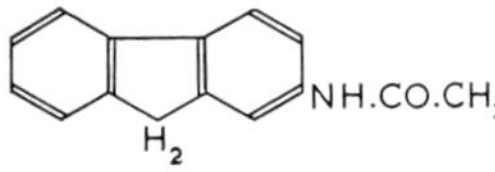   2-acetyl-aminofluorene

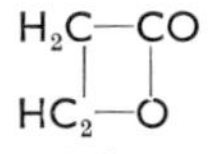

β-propiolactone   diazomethane

urethane

FIG. 10.4.

Only the first of these can be used to produce tumours in precisely the same way as benzpyrene, but most of the differences are readily explained by variations in the physical state of solubility of the compounds concerned. The effect of a readily soluble material such as urethane, which diffuses widely through the body, is likely to be different from that of a relatively insoluble material such as benzpyrene, which remains for some time at the site of application.

Bladder cancer in aniline dye and tyre workers. This is an interesting example of the way in which carcinogens can act on a single organ. It has long been known that workers in chemical factories making aniline dyes have a high incidence of cancer of the bladder. Analysis of the histories of the men affected showed that most had worked for a considerable time with 2-naphthylamine.

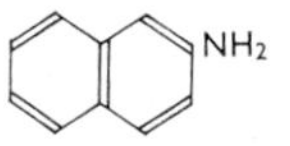

2-naphthylamine 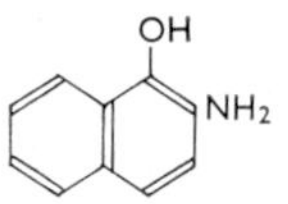   1-hydroxy-2-naphthylamine

FIG. 10.5.

Investigation of 2-naphthylamine, however, gave negative results at first. Under ordinary circumstances it is not carcinogenic, despite its resemblance to the carcinogenic 2-anthramine (see above). When fed to dogs for 5 years, however, it produced bladder tumours. It was then shown that dogs and man excrete the bulk of the compound in the form 1-hydroxy-2-naphthylamine, which *is* carcinogenic, when applied either to the bladder epithelium or to the skin. Because it is formed chiefly in the kidney, it affects the epithelium of the excretory tract almost exclusively. The normal processes of urine excretion and micturition mean that a relatively concentrated solution of any such material is held in contact with the bladder wall for substantial periods. Most experimental animals excrete the compound in some other form or forms (e.g. as a glucuronide) which is not carcinogenic. The reasons why only dogs and man are susceptible, and why only the urinary tract is affected, are thus obvious. In fact, the process is probably more complex, and 1-hydroxy-2-naphthylamine may not be the only or even perhaps the most important carcinogenic product, but nevertheless it provides a good example of a carcinogenic metabolite. A high incidence of bladder carcinoma in workers in tyre factories has been traced more recently to 2-naphthylamine, present as an impurity in 1-naphthylamine used as a rubber curing agent.

Apart from its value in eliminating an industrial disease, this work has important theoretical implications. It indicates one way in which species differences in susceptibility to carcinogens, or for that matter other noxious materials, can arise. It indicates also a way in which a material can circulate throughout all the body and yet act at only one point. And finally, as already mentioned, it shows that it is possible for a carcinogen to become active only after metabolism (just as fluoracetate is harmless until metabolised to the highly poisonous fluorocitrate, which blocks the Krebs cycle—Fig. 1.1, p. 3).

Benzidine (and probably a few other related aromatic amines) behaves in the same way as 2-naphthylamine. It also is a dye-stuff intermediary, and before this danger was discovered, had been used extensively in medical laboratories in testing for faecal occult blood.

Azo-dyes and liver cancer. Carcinogenesis in the liver has been much studied, partly because the liver is a convenient organ for biochemical analyses and the like, partly because geographical variations in incidence of primary liver cancer in man point strongly to the existence of carcinogens, presumably dietetic, whose identification might be of great practical value.

There are many liver carcinogens which are relatively non-specific in action. General carcinogens such as acetyl-amino-fluorene can produce liver cancers. Many liver poisons, such as carbon tetrachloride, are not directly carcinogenic, but in certain circumstances cause hepatic cirrhosis, which pre-disposes to the development of cancer of the liver. There are several with a more specific action, of which *Senecio* alkaloids and a fungal poison *aflatoxin* found in ground nuts damaged by *Aspergillus flavus* may prove important (p. 579), but the agents most studied are the *azo-dyes*.

(*a*)

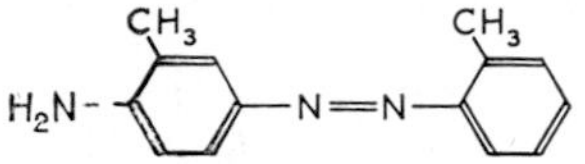

o-amino-azotoluene

(*b*)

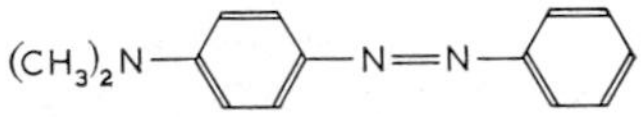

p-dimethylamino-azobenzene

Fig. 10.6.

Of these, *o*-amino-azotoluene was the first to be proved active, by Yoshida of Tokyo in 1931; *p*-dimethylamino-azobenzene ("butter yellow") is the most active. Fed to rats in large doses the dyes cause liver necrosis: with smaller doses immediate damage is relatively slight, but if the dosage is continued the liver shows progressive irregular hyperplasia and ultimately cancers (in 9 months or more).

Dyes of this type are banned from all foodstuffs, and rarely if ever have any opportunity of causing tumours in man: indeed their recognition has probably been valuable in emphasising the need for screening tests on all dyes or similar materials added to food. The lessons which can be drawn from experiments with these dyes are, however, numerous and important.

(*a*) *Continuity.* The transition from normality to malignancy is a continuous one, or more probably one with several successive stages, each of which seems to blend insensibly into its successor. This applies whether we consider the naked-eye appearance of the liver, the histology or the biochemistry. There is no sudden change from the normal to the malignant state.

(*b*) *Selection of resistant strain of cells.* The normal liver cell is damaged by the azo-dye, as shown by measuring oxygen uptake of liver slices exposed to a dilute solution of the dye. If the liver slices are taken from a rat which has been receiving the azo-dye by mouth for a few months, the depression of oxygen uptake produced by the dye *in vitro* is less than with a normal liver. With longer periods of feeding the depression becomes progressively less; when finally a tumour appears its oxygen consumption is found to have returned to normal. The liver cells appear to become progressively adapted to life in the presence of the azo-dye: very probably this occurs by the selection of resistant strains of cells, just as culture of bacteria in the presence of an antibiotic favours resistant strains of the organism.

(*c*) *Dye-binding.* The dye becomes bound to the proteins of normal liver cells. This dye-binding is reduced with time, and little or no binding occurs with tumour cells. We have here an indication of one reason for the selective effect of the dye on the liver, and a possible explanation for the progressive escape of liver cells from the effect of the dye indicated above.

(*d*) *Antigenic changes.* In normal liver cells it is possible to demonstrate antigens specific to the liver of the species concerned. Some of these are absent from hepatic cancer cells. There is evidence that the cells of chemically-induced tumours acquire new, tumour-specific antigens (p. 225).

(*e*) *Effect of malnutrition.* Production of tumours is much easier in rats on a poor diet. With butter-yellow it has been shown that most of this effect depends on a deficiency of riboflavin, which is required for a detoxification process which involves removal of one of the two terminal methyl groups. Since most geographical areas of high liver-cancer incidence in man are also areas of malnutrition, this may be important; it could well be that in such areas tumours result from exposure to some unrecognised substance which is detoxified, and so rendered harmless, in the well-nourished.

Radiation as a cause of cancer

Within 7 years of the discovery of X-rays, indiscriminate exposure was recognised as the cause of the numerous superficial cancers that appeared in the early workers. As late as the 1960s recurrences were still being seen, and few of the pioneers escaped unscathed. The early low-voltage machines produced "soft" X-rays with little penetration: the lesions were superficial skin cancers, mostly squamous carcinomas. Simple precautions soon all but eliminated these, but as the penetration of X-rays rose other deeper lesions were seen, and in the twenties and thirties of this century chronic myeloid leukaemia appeared as the main occupational risk in radiologists. With increasing knowledge, adequate protection seems to have almost removed this risk.

Both in man (whether by accident, occupational exposure, or as a hazard or an accepted risk of treatment) and in experimental animals, a wide variety of tumours can be produced by radiations of many sorts—not only by X-rays, but by α, β and γ rays and some at least of the many more recently recognised rays in the same categories; long-continued exposure to ultra-violet light is also effective. The differences in effect of these various forms of radiation are less than might be expected, and depend chiefly on the amount of energy absorbed on the passage of the rays through various tissues. Soft X-rays, α and β particles and ultra-violet light are all absorbed more or less completely on the surface and produce skin tumours: X-rays and γ-rays, penetrating deeply, can produce tumours in great variety, but a combination of the scattering power of bone with the sensitivity of marrow leads to an especially high incidence of leukaemia.

Tumours may arise in tissues affected by radiation necrosis (p. 27) or may occur where radiation injury appears to have been relatively slight.

The various radio-isotopes similarly produce effects which are related only to the amount or site of absorption of the radiation produced. Any radioactive dust inhaled into the lung is likely to produce lung cancers (see p. 379). Radio-iodine produces thyroid tumours experimentally because the thyroid is irradiated particularly heavily during the period when the isotope is held within the gland: external irradiation of the neck with X-rays can produce much the same effect.

Making due allowance for the effects of localisation, penetration and dosage, there is a remarkable similarity between the effects of irradiation and of chemical carcinogens. The tumours produced are the same, the intermediate "pre-malignant" changes seen in the tissue concerned are often closely similar, and the average time taken for a tumour to appear is similar. The latent period between application of a carcinogen and appearance of a tumour is much the same for a variety of active carcinogenic agents and a variety of tissues, but varies greatly with the species; in general the longer-lived the species, the longer the latent period. In man it is rarely less than five years and usually ten or more.

Xeroderma pigmentosum. This rare hereditary disease provides an unusual insight into the mechanism of action of one kind of radiation. Sufferers are intensely sensitive to sunlight, developing severe sunburn on slight exposure: they develop skin cancers on exposed sites at a very early age and usually die of them in their twenties. Exposure to UV light causes irreversible coupling of adjacent pyrimidine bases in the DNA chain: normally, an enzyme mechanism, acting after exposure has ceased, excises the coupled pairs and replaces them by normal bases, restoring the DNA chain to its original form. In xeroderma pigmentosa, the enzyme mechanism is absent and the DNA defect cannot be repaired. These defects presumably lead to the death of many of the affected cells, seen clinically as resembling acute "sunburn". Among the innumerable mutations which must arise, some presumably lead to tumour formation rather than cell death. It is particularly interesting to note that a radiation as apparently benign as sunlight can regularly produce in normal individuals nuclear damage which, if not repaired, is capable of giving rise to multiple tumours, and that only the existence of a highly specific enzymic repair mechanism prevents this happening to all of us.

Radiation treatment of tumours

It may seem illogical that we can both produce and treat cancer with the same radiations. In the one case, however, we use a moderate dose which will produce a statistically significant risk of cancer *in the future*: in the other we use a large dose which will destroy tissues *at once*. The occurrence of new tumours in tissues around the treated area, which necessarily receive some irradiation, is inevitable in some cases, but because the risk is usually not

great and always one for the relatively distant future, it can usually be accepted. Differences in susceptibility of tumours and normal tissues can be exploited in this form of treatment.

The injurious effects of ionising radiations on normal cells and tissues has been described in Chapter 1. The effects on tumours are mediated similarly, but in general, tumours are more sensitive to the immediate effects of irradiation than are normal tissues. As with normal tissues, the more rapidly growing tumours are usually the most susceptible. Slow-growing benign tumours are little if any more sensitive than the normal tissues from which they arise. There is usually a relation between susceptibility of tissue of origin and that of the tumour: the great sensitivity of lymphoid tissue and of gonadal epithelium is reflected in the often spectacular response to X-ray treatment of lymphosarcoma and seminoma. The complexities of the subject, however, are well illustrated by these two examples. Seminoma is remarkably sensitive, testicular teratoma, although also apparently arising from germinal epithelium, highly resistant even when anaplastic. Seminoma is often permanently cured: lymphosarcoma, whose immediate response may be as spectacular, nearly always recurs. There is, in fact, a difference between *radiosensitivity* and *radiocurability*. For many tumours, and especially for squamous carcinomas, it is approximately true that the least well differentiated are the most radiosensitive in terms of immediate response, but the better differentiated are the most radiocurable in terms of long-term prospects.

The effects of radiation on carcinomas may be dual—directly on the tumour cells, and indirectly through an inflammatory reaction and damage to the stroma. Inflammatory oedema with leukocytic emigration is followed by proliferation of fibroblasts and increased production of collagen fibres, which afterwards become dense and hyaline. An additional important effect is on the small vessels; many become thrombosed or are closed as a result of proliferative changes in their walls. The result is that the blood supply to the radiated part becomes very much diminished and in this way the nutrition of surviving cancer cells is reduced.

Viruses and tumours

Most squamous papillomas of the skin are due to virus infection and spread by contagion, and a virus is probably involved in the development of Burkitt's tumour (see below). The vast majority of human tumours, however, give no evidence of spread by infection or any other sign of relation to a virus or to any kind of parasite. Nevertheless, under the stimulus of the discovery of increasing numbers of viral tumours in animals, the view that viruses play a part in the etiology of tumours in man has long had its advocates, and this is supported by recent work on the subject.

Rous sarcoma. In 1911 Peyton Rous showed that, in contrast to most tumours of animals, a sarcoma of the domestic fowl could be transmitted (in this case to other fowls) by a cell-free filtrate. It has since been proved that this is due to an RNA virus related to the myxoviruses, which infects the cells of the host, causes them to multiply, and multiplies within them. The Rous sarcoma virus transforms normal cells into malignant cells within 48 hours, but for the replication of *infective* particles it requires the co-operative action of another virus to make the essential protein coat of the Rous virus particles. In its rapidity of action the Rous virus differs from all other fowl viruses including the common RNA virus of *fowl leukosis*, which is responsible for 10 per cent of deaths from disease in commercial poultry stock in this country. This latter virus is transmitted by the egg, and produces a leukaemia-lymphosarcoma-like disease with many variants (including for instance tumours of the kidney and bone), some of them due to distinct viral strains. The demonstration that fowl leukosis could be transmitted by a cell-free filtrate was made in 1908, before the Rous sarcoma, but the importance of this was not realised as leukaemia was not recognised as neoplastic at that time.

Shope papilloma. The relevance of a tumour of birds to human pathology is doubtful, but about 1930 certain mammalian tumours were shown to be viral in origin. Some of these were analogous to human warts, and of these the Shope papilloma is best known. Among the cottontail rabbits of Kentucky this is a common and harmless skin tumour which spreads by contagion, and can readily be transmitted by taking a cell-free filtrate of one of the warty growths, and rubbing it into the depilated skin of an uninfected rabbit. The warts appear within 21 days—a sharp contrast with the effect of a chemical carcinogen. The domestic rabbit (which is a different species) is not naturally affected, but rubbing in the cell-free filtrate produces a crop of warts. The warts differ in two major points from those in the cottontail, however: (*a*) filtrates are not infective (though the virus can be demonstrated by immunological methods); (*b*) many of the warts become malignant —which rarely happens in the cottontail—and the

virus often cannot be demonstrated by any method in the malignant cells.

Bittner milk factor. Breast cancer is commoner in some strains of mice than others, and experiments, designed originally to study the genetics of this, showed that pure lines of mice could be bred in which nearly all the breeding females died of breast cancer, while in other lines this was very rare. Crossing such lines, however, gave anomalous results. Few of the offspring of a high-cancer father and a low-cancer mother developed carcinoma: a high-cancer mother and a low-cancer father, on the other hand, invariably produced high-cancer offspring. The mother, in short, was the sole effective transmitter of the lesion. Such transmission suggests a non-genetic inheritance, and Bittner showed in 1940 that the essential element is the milk. Any suckling mouse that receives the milk of a high-cancer mother will be infected, and any mouse, even though it be born of a high-cancer mother, which receives milk only from low-cancer mothers, will escape. In the high-cancer strains all mice are infected in normal suckling, and the agent has been shown to be a virus shed in the milk.

In the males the virus has normally no effect. In the female, it has no outward effect for most of the life span, during which the normal number of litters will be produced and infected, but cancer will be induced late in life. By this time of course both mouse and its virus have reproduced sufficiently—an admirable example of host-parasite adaptation. The limitation of the tumour to the female depends on hormone levels. If a virus-infected male receives enough oestrogens to cause breast hyperplasia, breast cancer will follow: if a virus-infected female has her ovaries removed, she will not develop breast cancer.

Though breast cancer can be induced in non-infected mice by gross overstimulation with oestrogens or by suitable use of chemical carcinogens, most naturally occurring breast cancer in mice is viral in origin. Direct evidence for the existence of a human viral milk factor has recently been reported.

Polyoma virus. Many more tumour viruses have since been discovered, but one of the most interesting is the polyoma virus, discovered originally as a contaminant of a mouse leukaemia virus. It is a DNA virus that attacks the nucleus, and it is widespread among wild mice in many places, apparently causing them little trouble. When newborn mice are infected with it, however, it produces tumours remarkable for their variety, both sarcomas and carcinomas appearing in many organs. Moreover, newborn animals of other species—rats, rabbits, ferrets and hamsters—are susceptible. Sarcomas of the kidney are detectable in hamsters 4 days after infection, and death occurs in less than 2 weeks.

In the mouse it can produce cell destruction as well as proliferation, emphasising that the difference between the tumour viruses and the better-known ones which produce infectious disease (mostly cell-destructive) is less than might be supposed.

When polyoma virus is added to a culture of mouse cells, most of the infected cells are destroyed after the virus has multiplied within them, but a few become "transformed": these multiply rapidly and acquire other tumour-like characters, such as the tendency to grow irregularly, piled one on top of the other, instead of in an orderly monolayer ("loss of contact inhibition"). Transformed cells reimplanted into hamsters produce a sarcoma. In the transformed cell the virus can no longer be demonstrated. The virus can either multiply and destroy the cell, or can transform it, but not both. In the hamster, only transformation occurs: the virus can be propagated only in the mouse. As a corollary, the virus cannot be recovered from the actual tumours which it has produced in the hamster. This is an unusually clear-cut example of a remarkable phenomenon that occurs, with variations, in other virus tumours, for instance the Shope papilloma in the domestic rabbit, and even the Rous sarcoma at times. The virus seems to disappear and yet continues to produce its effects. Both in the induced tumours and in the transformed cells a new antigen can be demonstrated (p. 226), and immunization of hamsters with live polyoma virus protects them against transplantation of induced or transformed tumour cells.

Viruses and leukaemia. Since the demonstration by Gross in 1951 that mouse leukaemia could be transmitted by injecting cell-free extracts into newborn mice, several viruses have been shown to be capable of causing leukaemia in mice. They are all RNA viruses and, in general, produce leukaemia only in mice infected *in utero* or neonatally. Jarrett and his co-workers have demonstrated conclusively that naturally-occurring lymphoid neoplasms of domestic cats are caused by an RNA virus resembling those of mouse leukaemia. Infection with the cat virus is spread by contact, and oncogenesis can result from infection of adult cats. The virus can also infect and induce neoplasia in other species, including dogs, and replicates in cultures of human cells. The demonstration that the various neoplasms induced by the cat virus resemble lymphoid neoplasms and leukaemias of man, with the exception of Hodgkin's disease, is of the greatest interest. Very recent studies on childhood leukaemia support a similar virus etiology.

Burkitt's tumour. This interesting tumour is essentially a lymphosarcoma with a very curious distribution, both anatomical and geographical. In its most characteristic form it involves the jaw, but many other areas, including such unexpected organs as the ovary, may be involved. Response to small doses of cytotoxic drugs is often dramatic. It is chiefly though not entirely confined to children and to Africa: its distribution in Africa suggests that of an insect-borne disease so strongly that an infective cause for the tumour was proposed very soon after its discovery. Intensive search has so far failed to identify any causal virus with the unique relation to the tumour found in the animal work described above. The herpes virus, Epstein-Barr (EB) virus, has been shown to be associated with Burkitt's lymphoma, and most of the patients have high titre antibody to it. The presence of this virus and of chronic malaria have been suggested as causal factors. EB virus is also associated with infectious mononucleosis (p. 458).

Hormones in the causation of tumours

In general, any induced change of hormone level which causes prolonged hyperplasia of a target organ may cause tumours of the latter, but there are many exceptions. The following are the best known experimental situations.

Oestrogens can undoubtedly cause tumours; in susceptible strains of mice their administration in excess leads to an increased incidence of cancer of the breast in females and the appearance of cancer in males. Reduction of natural oestrogen levels by oophorectomy abolishes cancer of the breast in susceptible females. It might seem that the excessive proliferation of breast ducts induced by oestrogen, carried to excess, has been the actual cause of the cancer. But, as mentioned above, the oestrogens appear to act effectively only in the presence of the Bittner milk factor in mice. In virus-free mice (and in other species) the effect is much harder to demonstrate. In tissues other than the breast the position becomes somewhat anomalous. The most obvious oestrogen target organ, the endometrium, rarely develops tumours in treated animals, though connective-tissue tumours of the uterus are often produced. Oestrogen therapy in women rarely if ever produces endometrial carcinoma, though it often produces hyperplasia that can be mistaken for carcinoma: there is, however, some apparent association between endometrial carcinoma and the oestrogen-secreting granulosa-cell tumours of the ovary. Tumours can, however, be produced in organs not usually regarded as oestrogen-responsive, for example the kidney in the hamster, and the Leydig cells of the testis in the mouse.

These effects appear to depend only on the oestrogen-activity of the various compounds concerned, and not on their precise structure. A good deal has been made of the similarity between the basic ring structure of some of the carcinogenic hydrocarbons—especially methylcholanthrene which has oestrogenic activity in the rat—and the steroid hormones. This is more obvious if we re-draw the formula of methylcholanthrene (Fig. 10.7).

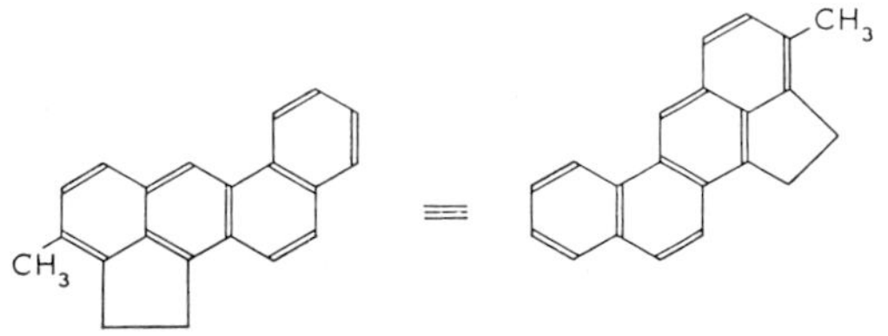

methylcholanthrene re-drawn as a steroid

Fig. 10.7.

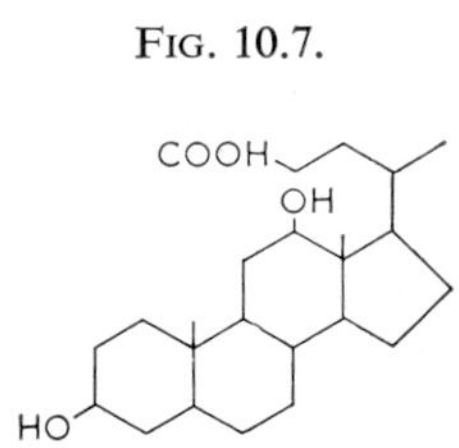

desoxycholic acid

Fig. 10.8.

Various hypothetical transformations of steroid components of bile (Fig. 10.8) and sebum have also been based on this resemblance, but there is no solid evidence for any of these attractive speculations.

Disturbances of the pituitary feed-back mechanism.

The following three examples, probably the most striking in the endocrine field, all depend on pituitary hormones.

(a) *FSH-induced ovarian granulosa-cell tumours.* The ovary is stimulated to various activities, including the secretion of oestrogens, by the follicle-stimulating hormone of the pituitary. A rise of oestrogen level in blood reaching the pituitary reduces the output of FSH, so that the system stabilises. Biskind removed the ovaries of rats and implanted pieces in the spleen. Oestrogen secreted by the grafts in this position passes into the portal blood, and so all of it is carried direct to the liver and is there inactivated by the normal hydroxylation process. Thus very little reaches the pituitary in active form, and FSH rises. This stimulates the grafts both to grow and to secrete oestrogen, but even the excessive oestrogen so produced is prevented from reaching the pituitary. Prolonged over-stimulation of the grafts leads finally to the appearance of granulosa-cell tumours. Although a fascinating experiment, this has no known relation to any situation occurring in man.

(b) *Thyroidectomy tumours of the pituitary.* The similar thyroid-pituitary feed-back, with thyroid-stimulating hormone increasing the secretion of thyroid hormone, and a rise of thyroid hormone lowering the secretion of TSH, can lead experimentally to tumours of either organ. If the thyroid is surgically excised or obliterated with radio-iodine, secretion of TSH is raised. In some strains of mice the TSH-secreting cells proliferate so actively under this stimulus that they give rise to malignant tumours of the pituitary. It is a point of special interest about these tumours that they can at first be transplanted only to other mice which have also lost their thyroids, but that after several passages they become less rigorous in their requirements and can be transplanted to normal mice. Again, there is no evidence of any comparable tumours occurring in man: patients with myxoedema, for instance, do not develop pituitary tumours.

(c) *TSH-induced thyroid carcinoma.* If the normal output of thyroid hormones is blocked by thiouracil or other goitrogenic drugs, TSH rises and stimulates thyroid proliferation. In rats, if this is continued for long enough, metastasising tumours may arise. Even after metastasis to the lungs, such tumours may regress if the goitrogen is stopped. This is a slow and uncertain way of producing thyroid cancers: the combination of a goitrogen with a chemical carcinogen (such as 2-acetyl-amino-fluorene) or with radio-iodine in doses insufficient to cause major damage to the gland, is much more effective than either alone.

This type of experimental tumour is less irrelevant to human cancer than the two preceding. Long-standing TSH-induced goitres, whether due to iodine deficiency or to one of the congenital defects of iodine metabolism, seem to carry a small but significant risk of development of cancer.

Hormone-dependent tumours. The pituitary and thyroid tumours just mentioned both may be "hormone-dependent" in the sense that they may regress if the hormonal stimulus that invoked them is removed. Related phenomena in man are few, but the following three carcinomas deserve mention (1) Most prostatic carcinomas are sufficiently dependent on a normal male hormonal environment to regress for long periods if oestrogens are given. (2) Some differentiated thyroid carcinomas are partially responsive to TSH, and their rate of growth and spread may be reduced or arrested by continued administration of thyroxin which suppresses secretion of TSH by the pituitary. (3) Some breast carcinomas regress under a variety of hormonal manipulations—treatment with male hormones or even oestrogens, oophorectomy, adrenalectomy, hypophysectomy. Application of these is largely empirical, and has not so far led to an increased understanding of the tumours concerned. Just as the hormone-dependent pituitary tumours become independent after serial transplantation, the tumours in man practically always ultimately resume growth, though with the thyroid and prostatic carcinomas the period of arrest and partial regression is often very long.

Co-carcinogens

These are substances which enhance the activity of carcinogens. The mode of action can best be understood by means of the following example. If methylcholanthrene dissolved in acetone at optimal strength is applied twice weekly to the skin on the back of mice, most of them will develop skin tumours within 3 months. If the solution is weakened progressively, a point is reached at which after a year of painting only a very few tumours have appeared. If to this weak solution of methylcholanthrene a 1 per cent solution of croton oil is added, the tumours appear within 3 months. The croton oil alone, no matter in what strength it is used, produces only a negligible number of tumours, but in 1 per cent solution it acts as a mild irritant and appears to enhance the action of the carcinogen: it is thus a *co-carcinogen*.

If, instead of mixing the two, they are applied one after the other, the nature of the effect is more clearly demonstrated. Instead of using a weak solution of methylcholanthrene, a strong solution can be applied for a short time, e.g. four times over a fortnight; this dose, applied alone, will give rise to only a few tumours after a long time. Croton oil applied in whatever strength and for however long *before* the methylcholanthrene, has no effect on the yield or rate of appearance of tumours. Applied *after* the methylcholanthrene, it leads to the appearance of numerous tumours after the usual 3 months. If a gap of some months is left after the brief exposure to methylcholanthrene, and painting with croton oil then begins, the tumours appear again after 3 further months.

It seems therefore that the carcinogen produces an irreversible change in the cells of the skin and that prolonged mild irritation by the croton oil converts the changed cells to frank neoplasia. Such a pair of substances are called *carcinogen* and *co-carcinogen*, or *initiating* and *promoting factors*. It must be supposed that most active carcinogens are mild irritants so that when applied in strong enough doses for a long time they act also as co-carcinogens. Urethane, however, for instance, produces no tumours of the skin at all unless combined with a co-carcinogen.

The practical importance of co-carcinogens is still doubtful. The high carcinogenicity of naturally occurring tars probably depends on their content of co-carcinogens as well as carcinogens. In particular, *the tar of cigarette smoke has an intense co-carcinogen activity* but is a relatively poor source of carcinogens and some of the relationships between lung cancer incidence and smoking probably depend on this (see p. 380).

Scars. Tumours do not ordinarily arise in a burn scar or surgical wound scar on a rabbit's skin. But if one paints a carcinogen evenly over an area which includes such a scar, the tumours appear first (and grow largest) around it. "Burn cancers" of man, or "brand cancers" of animals, occur almost always in areas exposed to excessive sunlight or similar carcinogenic stimulus. Scars thus seem to act as co-carcinogens. The paradox that chronic gastric ulcers are frequently complicated by cancers, but the almost exactly similar duodenal ulcers are totally free from them, is explicable on the view that the ulcer scar is acting as a co-carcinogen, but that in the duodenum no effective carcinogen is present with which it might co-operate.

If the term co-carcinogen is interpreted widely, some important examples can be brought within the concept. The *endocrine* stimuli that cause cancers often seem to be acting as co-carcinogens: the efficiency of the combination of 2-acetyl-amino-fluorene (or radioiodine) with raised TSH as a source of thyroid cancer suggests that since one factor is the carcinogen, the other is acting as a co-carcinogen.

Transplantation of tumours

Under appropriate conditions, pieces of a tumour growing in one animal can often be transplanted to another, and continue growing in the new host. The viral tumours we have discussed above can be transferred by a cell-free filtrate, and it is the cells of the new host which proliferate: but the transplants with which we are here concerned must contain live tumour cells, and it is the transplanted cells which proliferate, not those of the host. Transplanted carcinoma cells will, of course, induce growth of stromal cells in the host, but these stromal cells are not themselves neoplastic, merely a scaffolding for the tumours.

It is now clear that the major influence on the growth of tumour transplants is the same process of homotransplant immunity that affects transplantation of normal tissues (see p. 112). Tumours can practically always be transplanted (like normal tissues) elsewhere into the same animal, into monozygotic litter-mates, or into other members of a highly inbred strain. Since tumour cells possess the "transplant antigens" characteristic of the individual, tumour homotransplants are destroyed, just like homotransplants of normal tissue, by a rejection reaction.

Increase of transplantability. Some tumours are, however, more widely transplantable than the normal tissues from which they have arisen. Sometimes this is a characteristic of the original tumour, but it may arise only after the tumour has been maintained by serial transplantation through animals of the same pure line. Often the tumour will at first grow only in animals of nearly the same genetic constitution—litter-mates, or members of a closely related inbred strain. Later it may acquire the ability to grow in less closely related hosts, and ultimately in any animal of the same species: even, rarely, in other related species. The widening of the circle of transplantability has been said to occur, not as a gradual process, but as a series of well-defined steps.

On the whole the most readily transplantable tumours are malignant and poorly differentiated, and loss of transplant antigens by the tumour cells is probably a major factor. It is the heterogeneity of the cells of malignant tumours which renders difficult their complete destruction. No matter whether they are subjected to a transplantation reaction, a cytotoxic drug or radiotherapy, it is likely that some cells, because of their particular genome, will be more resistant than others.

Some strains of tumour have been maintained for hundreds of generations in this way and are used in laboratories all over the world. Many tons of tumour must have been derived in this way from a single original growth. They form convenient and reproducible if somewhat artificial sources of tumour tissue for experiments on cancer cell metabolism, the testing of anti-cancer drugs, and the like.

Tissue culture. Tumours can also be grown in tissue culture under conditions similar to those required by normal tissues. Most are at least as difficult to grow as normal tissues but some are less exacting. The tendency of normal cells maintained in tissue culture for many generations to undergo transformation which make them more like tumour cells complicates the picture. As with transplantable tumours, a relatively small number of easily propagable tumour cell strains have become useful and popular research tools: the best known is the HeLa cell strain, originally derived from a human uterine carcinoma, and now cultured in enormous quantities.

Age and heredity

Age. In both man and animals, tumours occur at all periods of life, but become commoner with advancing age. This is especially the case with carcinomas. Above the age of seventy the apparent incidence falls off, but this is due to the falling population at risk, and the true incidence at least of all the commoner carcinomas rises steeply throughout the later part of life. The actual rate often parallels approximately the sixth power of the age: thus for example the percentage incidence of most cancers at age 70 is 2–3 times that at age 60, and $70^6/60^6 = 2\cdot5$.

Among the less common tumours there are very many exceptions to the rule. Many kinds of sarcoma and the acute leukaemias are commoner in young subjects. Also some malignant tumours, for example nephroblastoma and neuroblastoma, usually occur in fetal life or early childhood.

The rising incidence of carcinomas with age may be due to the long time taken by carcinogens and co-carcinogens, perhaps encountered irregularly and in small doses, to bring about malignancy. There is, however, some evidence that the incidence of carcinoma in man, resulting from X-irradiation or industrial exposure to carcinogens, increases with the age during the period of exposure. Other evidence is conflicting, and tar cancer in mice occurs just as readily, and in as large a proportion of cases, in young as in old animals. When the tar painting is stopped before a growth has developed, malignancy, may appear later, as observed in man.

Heredity. There are considerable variations in the incidence of particular tumours, both spontaneous and carcinogen-induced. As exemplified by the Bittner milk factor, some of the most striking examples of this have proved to be due to pseudo-hereditary transmission of a virus. Apart from such cases, little is known of the mechanism of the variations in susceptibility. Similarly, there is a good deal of evidence for a minor role of heredity in many common human tumours. Cancer of the breast, for example, is about twice as common among relatives of patients with the disease as in the general population, and the same applies to carcinomas of oesophagus, uterus and prostate. In all such examples of familial aggregation of a disease it is necessary to consider the possibility of environmental factors, including virus infections, as an alternative to genetic predisposition.

A few rare tumours are clearly hereditary in origin. Polyposis coli and retinoblastoma are the classical examples: in both, at least most of those who inherit the gene concerned develop tumours without any additional stimuli. *Xeroderma pigmentosa* is another hereditary disease in which tumours of the skin arise as an inevitable consequence of exposure to UV light (p. 218). Beyond this, fully satisfactory examples are not easy to find. Intestinal polyposis of the Peutz-Jeghers type and neurofibromatosis are often familial, but more often apparently sporadic. Among conditions such as Lindau's syndrome and hereditary telangiectasis, of doubtful status as tumours, a familial incidence is commoner.

What makes the cancer cell multiply?

The preceding review of some of the known causes of cancer leaves us with the crucial questions unanswered. A few tentative conclusions can, however, be put forward.

(*a*) *A somatic mutation* is involved. This means no more than that a change has occurred in the cells of the tumour which can be transmitted to their descendants. The possible effects of a mutation in a somatic cell are limited. Germ cell mutation can of course give rise to changes in a later generation: and it is probable that somatic mutations in cells of the embryo can give rise to local defects. In the adult the fate of a mutation in a cell will depend on the effect of the mutation on the rate of multiplication of the cell. Unless it produces a clone of cells which multiply faster, or survive longer, than the surrounding cells, its presence will not be noticed. It follows therefore that *a tumour is almost the only kind of somatic mutation recognisable by ordinary methods.*

Such a mutation need not, of course, be a classical single-gene mutation. The same kind of inheritable change in a cell line may be produced by a chromosomal anomaly, or by the special kind of virus infection characteristic of tumour viruses (see above), and possibly in other ways.

(*b*) *Loss of specific features* is probably at least as important as *gain*. Malignancy at first sight seems a positive character, a new acquisition by the cell of the ability to do things (multiply rapidly, invade, metastasise, transplant out of its own pure line) that it could not do before. But some changes—dedifferentiation, loss of antigens, loss of hormone sensitivities— are clearly negative changes. Even active growth and invasion may be less positive characters than appear at first sight. Most normal cells—probably all that are capable of giving rise to tumours —migrate and multiply actively enough under the right conditions, such as following wounds or in tissue culture. They have the capacity both to grow when stimulated to do so and to stop when further growth is not required, i.e. they have brakes as well as accelerator: it is at least as likely that cancer cells have lost their brakes as that they have too powerful an accelerator.

The behaviour of epithelial cells in tissue culture is particularly significant here. Normal epithelial cells multiply and migrate to form a sheet, but once a continuous sheet has been formed, the cells within it cease growth as though contact with their neighbour inhibited further growth, which occurs only at the edges. Tumour cells grow at first no more rapidly, but they pile on top of each other indiscriminately without any of this contact inhibition. Part of the same difference is the tendency of normal epithelial cells to adhere closely to each other, whereas tumour cells lose such mutual adhesiveness.

(*c*) *Multiple stages* are usually involved. In most cases (excluding virus tumours) there is no sudden change, but a whole series of changes from normal to malignant tumour. This is obvious from the microscopic study of human material, but it also appears in such experimental situations as the induction of liver cancer in rats already described, where histological, biochemical and immunological changes all reflect a long process of transition. If a mutation is the basic process, there must be a series of mutations. The steep sixth-power rise with age in the incidence of many cancers has been interpreted mathematically as indicating that it depends on the concurrence of an average of seven independent events—which could be successive mutations.

(*d*) "*Survival of fittest*". Many experimental situations are most easily interpreted as the selective breeding out of cells which are more resistant to some noxious agent than are normal cells. From the first partly resistant strain, new and even more resistant strains are further selected, to be superseded in their turn. This does not explain why the selected cells should be cancerous, but it is clear that such a competitive atmosphere would favour the emergence of abnormally rapidly growing cells.

Conclusion. The cancer cell, then, is one with a modification which can be regarded as a somatic mutation: the type of mutation is probably very variable, but whatever its precise nature, the change must have two inescapable characters: (*a*) it must be transmitted to the descendants of the cell, and (*b*) it must give the cells some advantage in rate of growth or length of survival over the normal cells.

Most carcinogens, it must be assumed, increase the frequency of mutations within the tissue concerned, and in addition (either alone or aided by a co-carcinogen) increase the rate of turnover of cells so as to increase the chance of selection of a mutation with the essential features of malignancy. A virus tumour, however, short-circuits this process and supplies the mutation ready-made.

The role of viruses in human tumours

The section on virus tumours (p. 218) has demonstrated that in some species at least a large proportion of tumours are of virus origin. It is very difficult to prove that the same does not apply in man. Suppose, for instance, that cigarette smoke could produce bronchial cancer only if the bronchus was already infected with an appropriate virus? (It is known that at least one human respiratory virus can produce tumours in mouse cells.) One can only say that in this particular case there is no positive evidence for the intervention of the virus.

In some other types of human tumour there is indirect evidence suggesting the possibility of viral etiology (see previous and next sections). However, the carriage of "passenger" viruses by tumour cells, and the experimental demonstration that multiple factors (virus, X-ray, chemicals, etc.) may have additive effects in carcinogenesis, render the problem of human carcinogenesis a complex one.

The antigenicity of tumours

In the preceding sections, the emphasis has been on the causation of tumours. There are also various immunological aspects of neoplasia, one of the most interesting and potentially important of which is the antigenicity of experimentally-induced and human tumours.

Tumours in experimental animals

The possibility that tumours possess antigens not present in the normal cells of the host, raising the further possibility of the development of specific anti-tumour immunity, is an old idea. Early experimental work on the subject gave rise to false hopes, because what first appeared to be successful "vaccination" against tumours proved to be no more than homograft immunity, applicable to both tumours and normal tissues (p. 112). Further work on the subject in the 1930s and 1940s, using highly inbred strains of mice, gave disappointing results, and it is only since 1950 that evidence has accumulated to indicate that most tumours of inbred strains of mice, whether occurring naturally or induced experimentally, are antigenic to the host, and that it is possible to induce in the host some degree of resistance to the autologous and isologous tumour. Simple ligation of a tumour to induce ischaemic necrosis, or injection of small numbers of viable tumour cells or larger numbers of killed or irradiated tumour cells, are among the methods used to induce resistance to an oncogenic injection of tumour cells. It has become apparent from such procedures that resistance to tumours is by no means absolute, but that it may slow down the rate of growth of a tumour, increase the size of the minimal oncogenic dose of tumour cells, or diminish the number of tumours induced by transplantation to a group of mice.

Both chemically-induced and virus-induced tumours of mice have been shown to possess specific tumour antigens on the surface membrane of the tumour cells. Tumours induced by chemical carcinogens differ from one another in their tumour-specific antigens, and this has been observed even for two independent tumours induced in the same animal by the same carcinogen. By contrast, all tumours produced by a particular virus have common tumour-specific antigens, even when induced in animals of different species and arising in different tissues. These observations raise the possibility of an effective vaccine against tumours produced by a particular virus, but offer no such likelihood for tumours induced by chemical carcinogens.

The tumour-specific antigen for tumours induced by DNA viruses is virus-dependent, but differs from the antigens of the virus coat. Small oncogenic DNA viruses such as polyoma possess only enough DNA for the production of 6–8 different proteins, and since half or more of the total DNA is required to code for the constituents of the virus coat, very few viral factors remain to bring about changes in the host cell. Accordingly, any virus-induced cell change stands a good chance of being the one responsible for the difference between normal and tumour cells, i.e. the essential feature of neoplasia. The specific surface antigens of DNA-virus-induced tumour cells are thus of very great interest.

The major immunological defence against tumours is a delayed hypersensitivity reaction, injury to the tumour cells being mediated by specifically-sensitised small lymphocytes (p. 106). Circulating anti-tumour antibody, while capable of destroying tumour cells in the blood (e.g. leukaemia cells) or in body cavities (e.g. Ehrlich ascites tumour), and tumour cells in culture, has little or no inhibiting effect on the growth of tumours in the tissues. Indeed, anti-tumour antibody may have a stimulating effect on the tumour *in vivo*. This is known as *enhancement*, and may be due to a blocking effect, the antibody covering up the tumour antigen and interfering with the reaction of sensitised lymphocytes.

Human tumours

The cells of human tumours possess the individual's "transplant" iso-antigens (p. 112), and it is obviously important that these should not be confused with tumour-specific antigens. This danger does not arise when a patient is tested for an immune response against his own tumour, but it does complicate tests with homologous tumours, and also the use of antisera developed in animals against human tumour cells. However, some patients with certain types of tumour contain, in their serum, antibody which reacts specifically with their own tumour cells, and tumour-specific reactivity of lymphocytes has also been reported. In cases of melanoma, for instance, antibodies reactive with antigens on the surface membrane of the autologous tumour cells have been demonstrated by Lewis and other workers. These antibodies do not react with homologous melanoma cells; they are cytotoxic to autologous tumour cells in culture, and their presence appears to correlate with relatively slow advancement of the tumour and long survival. The situation is complicated by the occurrence of antibodies also to intracytoplasmic elements of the tumour cells, and these react with both autologous and homologous melanomas. Tumour-specific antibodies have also been reported in cases of osteosarcoma, chondrosarcoma and liposarcoma, and the occurrence of the same antibody in the serum of relatives and close contacts raises the possibility of viral oncogenesis. However, it is known from experimental work that viruses can colonise tumour cells and induce the development of cell-surface antigens without playing a causal role, and it is very difficult to exclude the possibility that such "passenger viruses" are responsible for tumour-specific antigens and antibodies in such cases.

The specific cytotoxicity of lymphocytes for autologous tumour cells has been reported in cases of melanoma, neuroblastoma, and carcinomas of bronchus, colon, breast, and urinary bladder. There is evidence also that, in cases of leukaemia, lymphocytes collected during a therapeutically-induced regression may react with the patient's (stored) leukaemic cells.

Evidence of immune reactions to human tumours. While the above findings indicate the occurrence of immune *responses* to tumours, in most cases there is no evidence that they play a protective role. Histological evidence of immune *reactions* to tumours is nevertheless provided by the common finding of lymphocytes and plasma cells both in and around early malignant tumours. The possibility that immune reactions do, in fact, occur in some malignant tumours, and that they may afford some protection, is suggested by reports claiming that lymphoid infiltration in carcinomas of the breast and stomach, seminoma and Hodgkin's disease, is associated with better than average prognosis.

Other indirect evidence of immunological protection against tumours comes from the reported high incidence of malignant tumours in individuals with congenital agammaglobulinaemia, and in patients treated by immunosuppressive drugs, for example following renal transplantation. Without doubt, there is a greatly increased incidence of reticulosarcoma in these cases, but this is a relatively rare and atypical tumour, and evidence that immunosuppression increases the incidence of the commoner forms of carcinoma is not yet convincing. There is thus little evidence to support Burnet's suggestion that the high incidence of cancers in old age is due to senile depression of the immunity system, which he regards as carrying out "immunological surveillance" for potentially neoplastic cells.

It has been shown that patients with Burkitt's tumour (p. 220) commonly have antibodies to virus-determined antigens of the tumour cells, and there is evidence also of immunological resistance to uterine choriocarcinoma (p. 260). These tumours are rare in most parts of the world, and their response to chemotherapy is much better than that for most other malignant tumours. Burkitt's tumour is likely to have a virus etiology and choriocarcinoma is really a neoplastic fetal transplant in the mother. Although of great interest, immunological findings in these two special tumours may not be of general relevance to resistance to the commoner human malignancies.

CHAPTER 11

TUMOURS

II. EPITHELIAL VARIETIES

After the introductory account of tumours in the last chapter, we turn for the next two chapters to the more practical questions of what kinds of tumour occur in man, what they look like and how they behave. There are many aspects of tumours that are best described as part of the pathology of the organs from which they are derived: these chapters are concerned with aspects of more general application, though they will be found to include also descriptions of a number of specialized tumours, sometimes because they illustrate some general principle, and sometimes for no better reason than that they are difficult to fit in elsewhere.

Classification

In the introduction to the previous chapter the distinction between *benign* and *malignant* tumours was discussed in some detail. We must now use the other chief mode of classification, the *histogenetic*, which is based on the tissue of origin. We may conveniently distinguish tumours of:

(a) epithelia;
(b) connective tissues (including muscle);
(c) blood vessels and lymphatics;
(d) the nervous system;
(e) the lympho-reticular and haemopoietic tissues;
(f) other tissues.

Of these, the epithelial tumours are overwhelmingly the commonest and are responsible for 90% of all cancer deaths in this country. This first chapter will be devoted to them alone.

General features of epithelial tumours

Epithelium has two essential characteristics which are carried over into its tumours.

(a) It forms continuous *sheets or masses* of cells of similar type, which adhere together without any intervening intercellular structures. This adherence of the cells into larger or smaller groups is retained as an indication of an epithelial origin even in tumours which have lost all the other distinctive features of epithelial cells.

(b) It requires a stroma of connective tissue and blood vessels for its support and nourishment. This is equally necessary for tumour epithelium, and all epithelial tumours appear to be able to stimulate the local connective tissues and blood vessels to proliferate and supply a stroma which surrounds and supports the epithelial cell groups. This "desmoplastic reaction", as it is called, varies in degree; it is often inadequate, so that much of the tumour dies from ischaemia, but it is sometimes excessive, so that the fibrous stroma becomes more conspicuous than the epithelium (scirrhous tumours, so-called). We know very little about the way in which the tumour cells can thus divert the normal connective tissue to their own ends, but it is clear that without such a capacity most epithelial tumours could not survive. As so often in cancer studies, the basic problem is a much wider one: the relationship between epithelium and connective tissue is established as a convenient form of organization in a large part of the animal kingdom, and we know little of its basic mechanism. The cancer cells are simply exploiting a normal process for their own ends.

The way in which an epithelium is organized naturally affects profoundly the structure of the tumours to which it gives rise, and this is especially marked in the case of the slow growing and well-differentiated benign tumours. Epithelia which cover surfaces generally give rise to *papillomas*; those which form glands give rise to *adenomas*, and the epithelia of solid organs give rise to solid tumours which, a little confusingly, are also called *adenomas*.

BENIGN EPITHELIAL TUMOURS

Papillomas

If one considers what will happen to a sheet of epithelium such as the epidermis when its cells have begun to multiply, it is clear that the first effect will be to thicken the layer. But since this is limited by the extent to which nutriments can diffuse from the underlying blood vessels, the tumour cells must soon spread in other directions. So long as the tumour is benign, they do not spread downwards into the underlying tissue, and so can only continue to spread sideways. To some extent this occurs by displacement of the surrounding normal epithelium, but, in addition and usually to a much greater extent, it occurs by expansion of the epithelium occupying the same spot. If one tries to visualize the epithelium as a sheet of cloth which is pinned down at the edges and then increased in area, it is obvious that it will be thrown into folds. If the increase is in one dimension only, the folds will be regular pleats, but since in a benign epithelial tumour it occurs in two dimensions simple folding cannot occur, and the result is an irregular mass of peaks and hollows. Where the epithelium is raised into peaks, a core of connective tissue is drawn into it (the "desmoplastic reaction" in effect) and the epithelium covering it remains well nourished and continues to grow. Since each peak is compressed by the other peaks around it, it can only grow upward, producing a higher peak which may finally become a long finger-like process. The resulting mass of "papillae" constitutes a papilloma.

If such a papilloma arises in a squamous epithelium the processes are naturally covered by squamous epithelium, thickened but otherwise not grossly abnormal. They are well seen in a papilloma of the skin, the commonest form of which is the virus-induced wart of children. (The name papilloma is derived from the prominence of dermal papillae in such tumours, well seen in Fig. 11.1. This is no longer regarded as an important characteristic, but the name has persisted).

The transitional epithelium of the urinary tract produces papillomas covered by transitional epithelium, in which the papillary processes are often exceptionally long and numerous (Figs. 11.2 and 11.3). This is probably not due to any special characteristic of the epithelium, but to

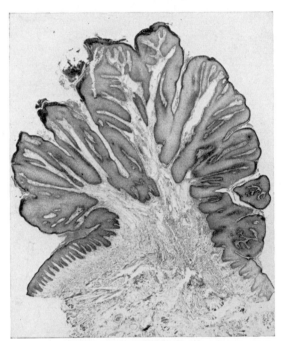

Fig. 11.1.—Papilloma of muco-cutaneous junction of lip, showing branching processes of connective tissue covered by stratified epithelium. × 10.

the environment provided by the bladder, in which the fronds of the papilloma float like seaweed in a sheltered bay: similar complexity is seen in the rare choroid plexus papillomas which float in the C.S.F.

While columnar epithelia can also give rise to papillomas (Fig. 11.4), the relation of these epithelia to glands tends to complicate the picture. Thus at the commonest site for such tumours, the large intestine, a papilloma (the so-called "villous papilloma") arises from the surface epithelium, and has very much the

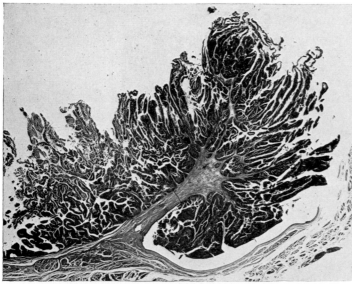

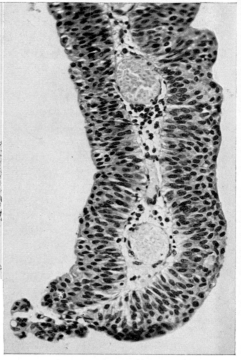

FIG. 11.2 (*above*).—Papilloma of bladder, showing stalk from which extend many delicate processes covered by epithelium. × 4.

FIG. 11.3 (*right*).—Papilloma of bladder.

Section of a process, showing the relation of transitional epithelium to the vascular core of connective tissue. × 200.

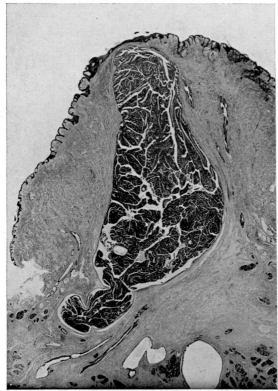

FIG. 11.4.—Intraduct papilloma filling a lactiferous sinus in the nipple. × 4.

structure one would expect (Fig. 11.5), but most tumours in this area tend to mimic the glandular structure of the crypts of the mucosa (the adenomatous polyps described below).

The papillary structure of papillomas is not usually obvious to the naked eye, though the educated naked eye may recognize it. In most skin papillomas it is hidden by the thick horny layer of keratin which develops on the surface, filling up the gaps between the fronds and producing a rough dry hard surface in which only an ill-defined cauliflower pattern gives a hint of the underlying structure. The result is a well defined little lump, usually round, always projecting above the surface (except when on the sole of the foot, where pressure flattens it) and at times slightly polypoid—i.e. having a slight neck between it and the skin level. In the case of bladder papillomas, the difficulties are of a different kind; the papillary projections (commonly called *fronds*) are narrow, and unless the excised tumour is submerged in fluid, they collapse against each other and leave nothing but a somewhat velvety surface to indicate their true nature. Seen *in situ* with a cystoscope, or examined with a lens under saline, the fronds will be obvious. The fronds are even harder to see in the soft velvety plaques of a villous papilloma

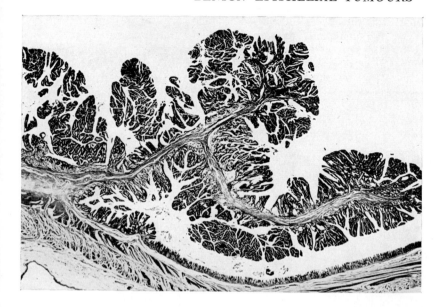

FIG. 11.5.—Villous papilloma of rectum. The tumour consists of a branching fibrous tissue core lined by epithelial processes composed of columnar cells. Note the continuity with rectal mucosa. × 3.

of the rectum, and a dissecting microscope may be necessary.

Adenomas

The simple tumours that arise from acinar glands and ducts vary a great deal in detail, but there is a basic pattern which can usually be recognized through all the variations. As the tumour cells multiply they arrange themselves into rounded packets, and in the centre of each of these packets there usually appears a lumen. Around the lumen the cells arrange themselves in a single regular layer (or sometimes two layers), and they assume a more or less columnar shape. The structure so formed has a fairly obvious resemblance to a gland acinus, and is usually called a tumour acinus. It may resemble quite closely the acini of the original gland from which it has been formed (as in the thyroid, for instance, or to a lesser extent the colon—Fig. 11.6) or it may look very different.

Though each tumour acinus looks like a gland acinus, it has no connection with ducts, so that anything that is secreted by the lining cells can only accumulate in the lumen. The endocrine glands dispose of their secretions directly into the blood, and probably for this reason tumours of endocrine glands retain their ability to produce their specialized products very much more often than those of the exocrine glands, and retain much closer histological resemblance to the parent tissue. It is altogether exceptional to see

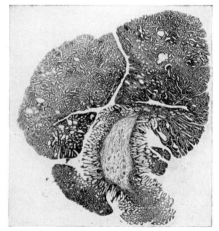

FIG. 11.6.—Polypoid adenoma (adenomatous polyp) of colon.

This growth was accompanied by a carcinoma (Fig. 11.11) and multiple polypi were present. × 6.

specialized secretory cells such as gastric parietal or peptic cells or pancreatic acinar cells in tumours: the acinic-cell tumour of the salivary glands is the only significant exception to this rule, and even it is a rarity. The rule does not apply to mucin-secreting cells, which commonly persist in adenomas, and even appear in situations (notably the ovary) where mucin-secreting cells are not found in the normal organ (Fig. 11.7). It will thus be clear that an adenoma of a gland, even though in general it retains a glandular appearance, will often have epithelium that is not easily recognized as derived from the particular gland of origin. Endocrine epithelium such as that of the thyroid may be little altered: some mucin-secreting epithelia such as that of the colonic mucosa may remain readily recognis-

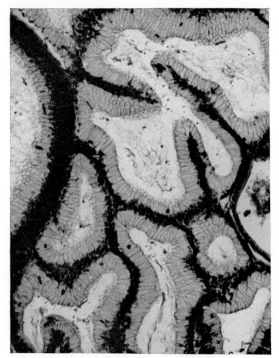

Fig. 11.7.—Cystic adenoma of ovary (mucinous cyst-adenoma), showing papilliform processes covered by tall mucin-forming epithelium. × 150.

able; and the same applies to the breast, the normal epithelium of which is not secreting for most of its life. But in most other cases transformation to a relatively nondescript simple or mucus-secreting columnar epithelium occurs.

In addition, the basic pattern of the acini in adenomas may be altered in two main ways:—

(a) The amount of secretion is usually small, but may be substantial (usually it is mucous, but there are some special exceptions, chiefly in thyroid and ovary). Since the adenoma has no organised duct system, the acini are distended with secretion, and the epithelium becomes stretched round it. At times the distension is so great that individual acini are large enough not merely to be seen with the naked eye, but to become cysts which may be larger than a football; they are full of secretion and the original epithelium usually persists as a single layer stretched over its surface. Such cyst-containing

adenomas, which are quite common in the ovaries, are called *cystadenomas*.

(b) The rate of multiplication of the cells may be a more pronounced feature than the production of secretion, and the cells tend to pile up round the central lumina, the acini becoming more and more solid: this feature often indicates the onset of malignancy. Sometimes, however, when there is enough secretion to distend the acini, and cells are well enough differentiated to retain the arrangement of a thin sheet, and yet still are multiplying, they behave like a surface epithelium and form papillomas which project into the lumina. Such a tumour is called a *papillary adenoma* or, if the lumina are large, a *papillary cystadenoma*. It might be expected that the pure cystadenomas, in which secretion is abundant and hence differentiation is good, are more benign than the papillary adenomas, in which proliferation is more prominent, and this is generally, although not always, true.

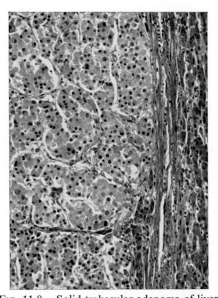

Fig. 11.8.—Solid trabecular adenoma of liver.

The cells are arranged in irregular columns and are demarcated from the compressed liver cells by a well-defined fibrous capsule. × 110.

To the naked eye the typical adenoma is a rounded lump, well defined, usually with a thin capsule of fibrous tissue and compressed normal gland. If lumina are small it appears solid when cut across, and is usually paler (because more cellular) and more homogeneous than the normal gland. If secretion is abundant it is obvious on section, and in a cystadenoma the bulk of the tumour consists of a mass of cysts full of mucus or other fluid; it may even sometimes form a single large cyst.

When an adenoma is formed from the glandular parts of a mucous membrane, as in the gut and most commonly the colon, it forms a very characteristic rounded nodule hanging upon a stalk formed by pulled-out normal mucosa, and is called an *adenomatous polyp*. (A "polyp" is a lump on the end of a stalk, without any commit-

ment as to the nature of the lump.) *Adenomas of solid organs* are not very common, but are seen mostly in the endocrine glands (adrenal, pituitary and parathyroid especially) and occasionally in the liver (Fig. 11.8). They consist of rounded well-defined solid lumps of tissue, usually encapsulated and very like that of the tissue of origin: an adrenal cortical adenoma, for instance, is usually a bright yellow lump hardly distinguishable except by its shape and size from the surrounding normal cortex.

MALIGNANT EPITHELIAL TUMOURS (CARCINOMAS)

The term *carcinoma* may be applied to any malignant tumour of epithelial origin. It may arise from one of the benign epithelial tumours just described, or arise directly from a non-neoplastic epithelium. In either case, it retains the two features already described as characteristic of epithelium and its tumours—the formation of sheets or masses of contiguous tumour cells, and the ability to excite a stromal reaction between and around the tumour cell masses. In addition, the epithelial element commonly retains some resemblance to the tissue of origin, though in poorly differentiated, and usually more malignant tumours, this may be tenuous.

The essential feature of a carcinoma is the presence of neoplastic epithelial cells which leave their proper site, migrate elsewhere to a greater or less distance, and there continue to multiply to form new masses of epithelium which displace and destroy the normal tissue of the area. The changes seen in the cells are those already described for malignant tumours in general in the previous chapter.

Naked-eye appearances

While there are many variations, it is possible to describe a typical carcinoma. It forms a firm lump, often irregularly nodular, its edge well defined in places and in others blending into the surrounding tissue (areas of invasion) so that it cannot be dissected out cleanly. On section it is predominantly whitish, as are most dense collections of young cells: there are often red patches of haemorrhage and, especially towards the centre, yellow areas of necrosis. Where the nodule lies on a surface it forms at first an

irregularly dome-shaped swelling. The centre of this swelling however has often a poor blood supply and has lost the original epithelium: it is exposed to trauma, infection and (in the case of lesions in the gut) digestive juices. It therefore often sloughs out, leaving a ragged ulcer. At the edges the tumour has a better blood supply and is partly protected by the original epithelium, and so survives: the ulcer therefore commonly retains a thick irregular raised edge which is responsible for the highly characteristic appearance of the ulcerated malignant tumour.

Varieties

There are many special types of carcinoma characteristic of particular sites, though the more highly malignant anaplastic ones all tend to look alike. Most malignant epithelial tumours can be included in the two great classes of squamous carcinoma and adenocarcinoma.

Squamous carcinoma

This is the characteristic malignant tumour of squamous epithelia, both epidermis and squamous mucosae. In addition there are some unexpected sites, where squamous carcinomas arise in organs containing no squamous epithelium: the most important of these is the bronchus, where squamous metaplasia of the bronchial epithelium is the probable cause, and similar metaplasia can account for less common sites such as the urinary tract and the gall bladder. Unstable squamo-columnar junctions such as the cervix are important also.

Histologically, most squamous carcinomas

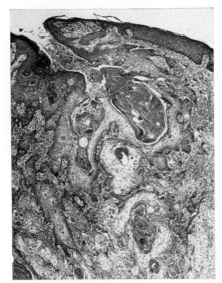

Fig. 11.9.—Squamous carcinoma of the tongue, showing keratinising squamous cell masses in continuity with the overlying epithelium and penetrating deeply to give rise to cell-nests. × 28.

are very readily recognizable. In early lesions, the downgrowth of the surface epithelium into the deeper tissues can be detected (Fig. 11.9). At the periphery, small masses and narrow columns of cells burrow into the surrounding tissues. Behind this margin, the invading cell groups have had time to enlarge and differentiate, becoming recognizable as prickle cells and usually forming keratin: the keratin forms rounded concentric nodules in the centre of the cell groups, a very characteristic appearance called "cell nests" or "epithelial pearls" (Fig. 11.10). The amount of keratin formed and the proportion of cells recognizable as prickle cells

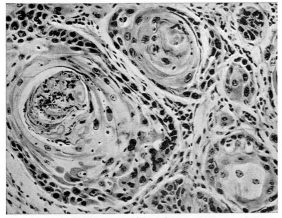

Fig. 11.10.—High-power view of squamous carcinoma, showing characteristic cell-nests. × 185.

both vary greatly: they are the best guides to degree of differentiation of the tumour, which, of course, affects its prognosis.

There are some variations from site to site— for instance, a squamous carcinoma of the bronchus or pharynx is usually less well differentiated than one of the lip or the skin. The site also naturally has a profound effect on the signs and symptoms produced by these tumours, and on their accessibility for treatment and hence on their prognosis.

Adenocarcinoma

This second group is a little less homogeneous than the last. Thus a histological section of an adenocarcinoma of the stomach can usually be distinguished from one of the colon with more confidence than a squamous carcinoma of the tongue from one of the bronchus. The grouping of adenocarcinomas together is, however, useful, for most of the malignant tumours of glands have a great deal in common with each other and with those that arise from all the ducts and surfaces lined by columnar epithelium. Important sites of origin include the stomach and colon, the pancreas, gall bladder and its ducts, breast and uterus; also the bronchi, which can produce both squamous and adenocarcinomas.

Histologically, almost everything that has been said of the adenomas applies to adenocarcinomas, with two differences.

(a) Instead of remaining localized, the tumour cells invade the surrounding tissues (Fig. 11.11).

(b) Differentiation is poorer (Fig. 11.12). In addition to all the general features of malignant tumours listed in the last chapter (p. 212), there is a marked tendency for acini to contain less secretion, to be lined not by one regular layer of epithelial cells but by a thick irregular layer, and in some tumours for most of the cell groups to form solid masses.

Several variations upon the basic pattern are common enough to be worth describing. Mixed and intermediate forms occur, and none of the following should be regarded as completely distinct entities.

(a) **Spheroidal-cell carcinoma,** (Fig. 11.13) an adenocarcinoma in which most of the cell masses are solid. This type of tumour is common in the breast, partly because of relatively poor differentiation, and perhaps partly because the gland is in a non-secretory state.

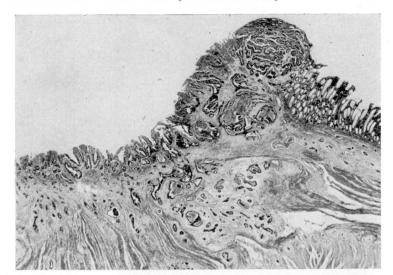

FIG. 11.11.—Adenocarcinoma of colon.

The rolled-over everted margin is seen, with abrupt transition from normal colonic mucosa; invasion of the lymphatics of the submucosa and muscular coat is advanced. × 11.

(b) **Cystadenocarcinoma,** in which cysts lined by columnar or cuboidal cells are prominent. This is common in the ovary and is seen occasionally in the pancreas and kidney.

(c) **Papillary adenocarcinoma,** in which papillary processes project into cysts. This is seen particularly in the thyroid, ovary and bile ducts.

(d) **Mucoid carcinoma.** An adenocarcinoma in which mucus secretion is unusually marked. The term should be used only when the whole tumour looks like a mass of jelly, and under the microscope most of the tumour cells float free in lakes of mucus (Fig. 11.14). The commonest site of origin is the stomach, but it occurs also fairly often in the colon and breast.

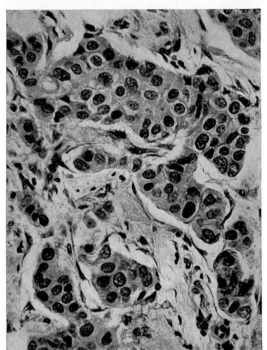

FIG. 11.13.—Spheroidal-cell carcinoma of breast infiltrating tissue spaces.

Note anaplasia of the cells. × 300.

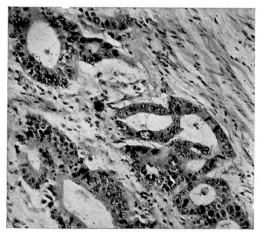

FIG. 11.12.—Adenocarcinoma of bowel invading the muscular coat.

Note the acinar arrangement of the cells with evidence of excessive proliferation in places. × 200.

Hard and soft carcinomas

Classification of carcinomas into the two following types depends on features of the stroma and not of the tumour cells. It is thus an essentially different mode of classification. For example both spheroidal-cell carcinoma and

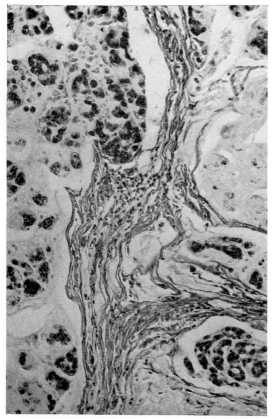

FIG. 11.14.—Mucoid carcinoma.

The degenerating carcinoma cells lie in large pools of mucin. × 65.

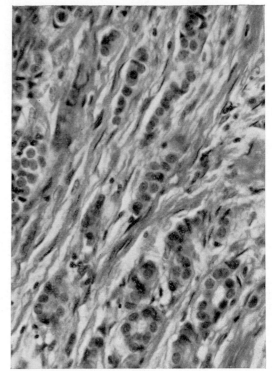

FIG. 11.15.—Scirrhous carcinoma of breast, showing tumour cells in tissue spaces with dense stroma between. × 240.

adenocarcinoma can be either scirrhous or encephaloid.

(1) **Scirrhous carcinoma** (Fig. 11.15) is a carcinoma in which there is an unusually marked fibrous reaction, so that the tumour cells are separated into small groups by dense fibrous tissue. Growth is often slow, but metastasis is not delayed by this reaction. It is common in the breast, and fairly common, in a rather special diffuse form (p. 500), in the stomach.

(2) **Encephaloid carcinoma** (Fig. 11.16). A carcinoma with minimal stromal reaction, so soft as to be brain-like in consistency, hence the name. The term is rarely used except for the occasional breast carcinoma that contrasts with the more usual scirrhous tumour of that site.

Special types of carcinoma

The names of some carcinomas reflect a striking appearance linked to a distinctive be-

haviour. Examples include clear-cell carcinoma of the kidney, trabecular carcinoma of the liver (Fig. 11.17), choriocarcinoma of the placenta, and rodent ulcer of the skin; these are highly distinctive lesions with very marked peculiarities of histogenesis as well as appearance and behaviour. They are described in the appropriate systematic chapters.

Spread of carcinoma

Local invasion

Local invasion by a carcinoma depends in part on the sheer expansive pressure of the mass of growing cells, but also on the active migration of motile tumour cells which penetrate the surrounding tissues and then multiply at the new site. Sometimes they appear to migrate as single cells: more often they appear to penetrate as columns of cells which extend by growth at the forward end. Such behaviour is unexplained, but, as we have indicated in the last chapter, it is possible that this is rather a loss of normal

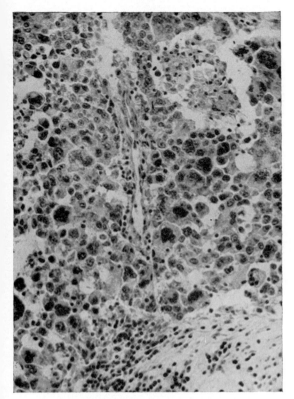

FIG. 11.16.—Encephaloid carcinoma of breast, showing a large mass of tumour cells with very little stroma. × 100.

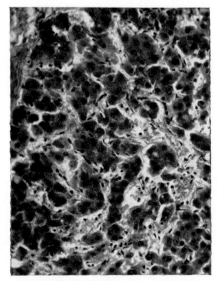

FIG. 11.17.—Carcinoma arising from liver cells, showing trabecular arrangement. × 150.

restraining forces than an assumption of new powers by the malignant cell.

Growth is easiest along the planes of loose connective tissue, and may be checked by dense structures such as thick fascia, the walls of large arteries, cartilage and compact bone. Structures such as glands and muscle, once penetrated, are rapidly destroyed, partly by pressure, partly by loss of blood supply. The carcinoma itself tends to outrun its blood supply, and necrosis of the tumour which ensues includes ischaemic destruction of any normal tissues which have been invaded. Unfortunately the growing edge of the tumour is hardly ever included in the necrosis.

Local invasion is important in the establishment of the primary tumour, and may of course result in damage to major structures nearby. Of greater significance from the point of view of the life of the patient in most cases is the appearance of *secondary deposits* or *metastases*—new areas of growth of the tumour at a distance from the primary tumour. These result from spread of tumour cells from the primary growth, usually by the lymphatics or blood vessels, as described below.

Lymph spread

This is one of the most characteristic features of carcinoma and is of prime importance from the surgical point of view. Cancer cells may enter the lymphatic vessels and be carried to the nodes at an early period, and they may also become arrested in their course and form small foci of growth which obstruct the lymphatics. In this way nodules are formed along the lines of the lymphatics, or the latter may be filled with proliferating cancer cells (Figs. 11.18, 11.19). The largest nodules, however, are those which form in and replace the lymph nodes. Early lymph node metastases usually lie in the peripheral sinus (Fig. 11.20). While the lymph nodes draining the region of the carcinoma are first, and usually most extensively involved, spread may take place in a direction contrary to normal lymph flow (Fig. 11.21) as a sequel to lymphatic obstruction.

Many of the secondary foci in the region of a carcinoma are of only microscopic size, and tissues may be unchanged in appearance though extensively involved. Accordingly it is impossible to assess the degree of secondary invasion by

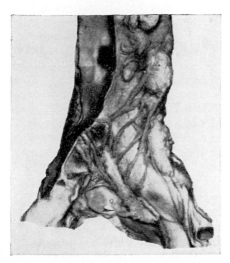

FIG. 11.18.—Carcinomatous invasion of lymph vessels
and nodes over lower end of aorta.

The lymphatics are seen as distinct cords. × ⅔.

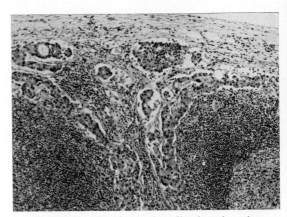

FIG. 11.20.—Carcinoma invading lymph node.

Carcinoma cells are seen in the lymph vessels in the capsule
of the node and in the peripheral lymph sinus, from which they
are extending into the medulla. × 66.

naked-eye examination alone (Fig. 11.22). The
presence of these minute collections of cancer
cells explains the so-called recurrence of cancer
after surgical removal. "Recurrence", in fact, is
not usually to be regarded as a fresh start or
recrudescence of the disease, but simply the
result of growth from cells which have been left
behind in the surrounding tissues. Such cells
may remain dormant, so that occasionally years
may elapse before a recognisable tumour re-
appears. True recrudescence of growth may,
however, occur in an area of pre-malignant
change (see below).

Blood spread

With most tumours, the effects of blood
spread are seen later than those of lymphatic
spread, though the wider dissemination makes
them usually of more serious consequence to the
patient. The small veins in and around the
primary tumour are the usual route of entry to
the circulation. Tumour cells are then carried
away to lodge in the next capillary bed that the
blood passes through, e.g. in the liver if the
primary tumour is in the portal drainage area
(Fig. 11.23), and in the lungs from tumours in
most other sites. Thence they may spread further,
from the liver to the lungs and from the lungs via
the systemic circulation to any part of the body
(Fig. 11.24). Blood-spread metastases in a solid
organ present a very characteristic picture of
multiple rounded nodules, varying in size but
with no single nodule conspicuously larger than

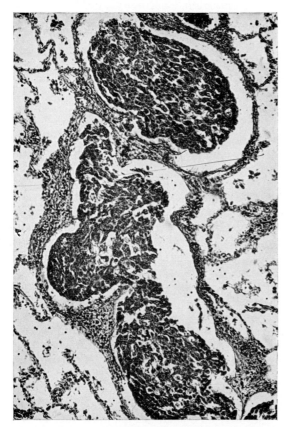

FIG. 11.19.—Lymphatic spread of carcinoma in
the lung. × 45.

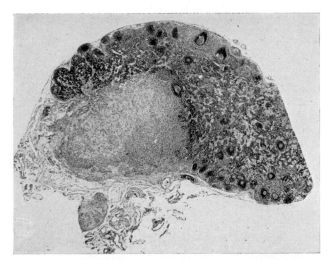

Fig. 11.21.—Retrograde invasion of lymph node by carcinoma.

The lymphatics at the hilum of the node are filled with cancer cells, which have spread into the node against the normal direction of lymph flow. × 7·5.

the rest, and scattered at random through the substance of the organ (Figs. 11.25 and 19.41, p. 581).

There are in practice many apparent anomalies in the distribution of metastases: some may be due to confusion between blood and lymph spread—there is for instance a strong case for considering the curious predilection of bronchial carcinoma to spread to the adrenals as a consequence of lymph spread rather than (as has been generally believed) blood spread. But even allowing for this, there must be great variations between capacities of different tissues to resist the growth of tumour cells arriving by the blood stream. It is highly probable that in most cases the great majority of cells leaving the primary

tumour by the veins fail to establish themselves.

In a painstaking necropsy study of a large number of cases of carcinoma arising in various sites, R. A. Willis gave the following incidences of metastases in various organs:—

liver	36%	brain	6%
lungs	29%	spleen	3%
bones	14%	skeletal muscles	1%
adrenals	9%	skin	1%

These incidences clearly do not correspond with blood flow, and so with the number of tumour cells likely to be arriving in the various organs. The liver and bone marrow are susceptible sites: the spleen and muscles resistant. There is experimental evidence for destruction of tumour

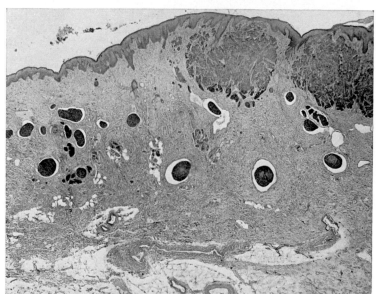

Fig. 11.22.—Squamous carcinoma of vulva, showing lymphatic permeation of the skin at the margin of the tumour. × 15.

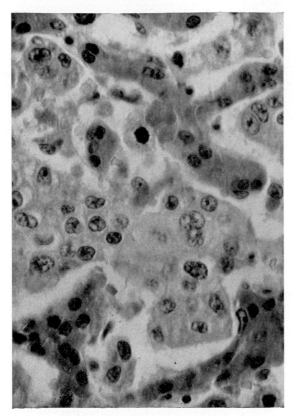

FIG. 11.23.—Secondary carcinoma in the liver.

Note masses of cancer cells in the sinusoids between the liver cells, without any formation of stroma. × about 200.

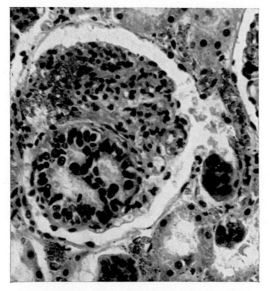

FIG. 11.24.—An embolus of carcinoma cells in a glomerulus, with extension into the tubule. × 150.

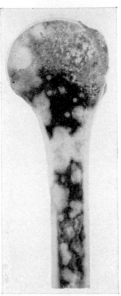

FIG. 11.25.—Multiple metastases in the humerus in a case of carcinoma of the breast. × ½.

cells by the spleen, but the nature of the defence mechanism is not known. The lung, which must receive by far the largest number of tumour cell emboli, provides an environment which is only moderately favourable to their growth. Cases of carcinoma in organs such as the kidney or thyroid often have multiple systemic metastases, for example in bone, with no obvious lung lesions: in such cases it can often be shown that there are minute microscopic foci in the lung where tumour cells have lodged in the pulmonary vessels, and, while failing to grow to any substantial extent at that site, have been able to launch further tumour emboli into the systemic circulation (Fig. 11.26).

Retrograde venous spread. One type of anomaly that has a special explanation is the localisation of metastases within the axial skeleton. Carcinoma of the prostate spreads early to the lumbar spine and pelvis, carcinoma of the breast to the thoracic vertebral bodies, and carcinoma of the nasopharynx to the cervical spine and the base of the skull. This is not attributable to direct or lymph spread but to spread by the blood. Yet blood spread in the usual fashion via the lungs should result in all parts of the vertebral column being equally affected, and this is not so. The explanation for the localised involvements of the spine appears to lie in the peculiarities of blood flow in the intra-vertebral venous plexus, in which differences of pressure above

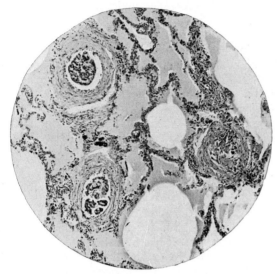

FIG. 11.26.—Section of lung from a case of prostatic carcinoma, showing two pulmonary arterioles containing tumour cells.

A third arteriole (to the right) has become obliterated, but at another level it also contained cancer cells. × 60.

and below the diaphragm often lead to reversal of flow: the effect of this is to draw blood at times into the vertebra from neighbouring organs, and this may carry malignant cells, which find a very favourable site for multiplication within the vertebral marrow.

Intracavitary spread

When carcinoma involves a body cavity, cancer cells may be liberated into the space and graft themselves on the surface to form new foci of growth. Any cavity can be involved, and the subarachnoid space, for example, is of some importance in the spread of intracranial tumours, but the serous cavities are especially important for carcinoma. Involvement of the peritoneum results most often from carcinomas arising in the stomach or the ovary, while the pleura and pericardium are most commonly invaded by carcinomas of breast or bronchus. In most cases there is an effusion of fluid into the sac concerned, and this may be bloodstained. Malignant cells are often present in such an effusion, but very often it is difficult to distinguish them with certainty from altered serosal cells. A special example of this form of spread is seen in transperitoneal metastasis to the ovary, usually before

the menopause and usually from a gastric carcinoma of the "signet-ring" type (p. 501): the ovaries may become very large, and have the characters first described by Krukenberg, who thought that such tumours originated in the ovaries (see p. 846).

Intra-epithelial and intracellular spread

Cancer cells may invade the epidermis, which is the only extensive epithelium in the body thick enough to withstand such invasion without disruption. Cells may spread for several centimetres in the epidermis without destroying it completely. Paget's disease of the nipple (p. 870) is the only common example involving carcinoma cells (the tumour being derived from the underlying breast): rarely this occurs in the epidermis at other sites, and something similar is seen in malignant melanoma of the skin (p. 946).

Carcinoma invading skeletal muscle may sometimes be seen under the microscope to be growing within the sarcolemma of muscle cells: this is the only known example of "intracellular" spread (Fig. 11.27).

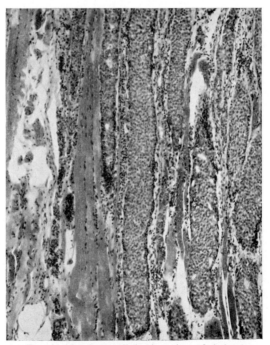

FIG. 11.27.—Intracellular invasion of skeletal muscle. × 60.

Premalignant lesions

These are conveniently considered here, as most such lesions involve epithelium, and are pre-carcinomatous.

A premalignant condition is one which can be recognized by either clinician or pathologist, and which indicates that the bearer has a substantially greater than the normal risk of developing a malignant tumour. The early stages of pre-malignant change (which presumably indicate the occurrence of the earlier mutations of a multistage conversion to malignancy) can often be recognized histologically. The signs include nuclear irregularity, increased mitotic activity, and abnormalities of differentiation, often combined with inflammatory infiltrates and stromal changes. The risk of such lesions becoming malignant can be established only in the light of experience of their behaviour in each particular site in which they occur. The following are examples of premalignant lesions.

(*a*) **Some benign tumours.** Probably all benign tumours carry some increased risk of malignancy, but in most it is very little more than that of the normal tissue, while in others it is high. There is little obvious logic about the differences. The villous papilloma of the rectum becomes malignant more often than the adenomatous polyp of the same site: similar tumours of the stomach carry a worse prognosis than either, while the uncommon similar tumours of the small intestine only very rarely become invasive.

Comparable anomalies could be quoted at other sites.

(*b*) **Certain chronic diseases.** Carcinoma may develop as a more or less common complication of some non-neoplastic diseases, such as cirrhosis of the liver, ulcerative colitis, asbestosis, and a variety of skin diseases.

(*c*) **Carcinoma-in-situ.** In the most extreme degrees of premalignant change in an epithelium, all the cytological changes of malignancy are seen in its cells, but the altered cells remain in the intact layer of epithelium and do not invade the underlying tissues. The name carcinoma-in-situ is often given to this lesion: it is not strictly accurate, as no carcinoma is present until invasion begins, but it is a vivid reminder of the need for action. It has been best studied in the cervix uteri, where its detection by the methods of exfoliative cytology is now widely practised in the prevention of invasive carcinoma at that site (p. 837). *Intraduct carcinoma* of the breast (p. 868) is an essentially similar lesion. The degree of risk of developing malignancy varies greatly with different lesions, and is often hard to determine with any exactness. In a few rare conditions, such as polyposis coli and xeroderma pigmentosa, it is practically 100%. In carcinoma-in-situ of the cervix, extensively studied but still controversial, it is also very high, though a period of twenty years may elapse between appearance of the lesion and the onset of invasive carcinoma. In most other lesions the risk appears to be much lower.

CHAPTER 12

TUMOURS

III. OTHER VARIETIES

There are far more kinds of non-epithelial tissue than epithelial, and equally there are far more kinds of non-epithelial tumour. As already indicated, however, the balance between this chapter and the last reflects the practical circumstance that the carcinomas greatly outweigh all other tumours in clinical importance. Nevertheless, even the tenth of cancer deaths that are due to non-epithelial tumours is a substantial number, and no-one can dismiss as unimportant a group that includes the lymphomas, gliomas, melanomas and bone sarcomas: they include also some benign tumours, such as the angioma and the myomas, which are common items of every doctor's experience even though they cause few deaths.

Though all the main types of non-epithelial tumours will be found mentioned here, detailed description will be given only of those varieties which are of such general distribution as not to be easily included under any one system. Length of description does not therefore always reflect importance.

TUMOURS OF THE MESODERMAL CONNECTIVE TISSUES

Nomenclature. In this group it is usual to name tumours by adding "-oma" to the appropriate stem for the benign lesion, and "-sarcoma" for the malignant—e.g. fibroma, fibrosarcoma; chondroma, chondrosarcoma.

Benign tumours. These are composed chiefly of fully developed tissues, such as are found in the adult body, e.g. fibrous tissue, cartilage, muscle. They are usually rounded or lobulated and well defined, being generally enclosed within a distinct fibrous capsule. They displace the surrounding tissues and produce atrophy by pressure, but they neither infiltrate tissues nor metastasise. Simple tumours are not infrequently multiple, but then each tumour represents an independent focus of growth. Blood vessels grow in relation to the tumour tissue, and are usually well formed, though the arteries are often deficient in muscle fibres. The well-formed fibrous tissue stroma of epithelial tumours is however altogether absent in most cases, the tumour relying for its support on the matrix produced by its own cells—though exceptions occur, for example the myomas.

Malignant tumours (sarcomas). In the corresponding malignant tumours, the activity of the cells is mainly proliferative, the tumour is more cellular, and although a certain amount of matrix is formed, this is imperfect and usually scanty. Sarcomas often form large masses, usually soft and with frequent haemorrhage and necrosis (Fig. 12.1). While these malignant tumours may appear to the surgeon to be encapsulated, diffuse destructive infiltration of the surrounding tissue occurs at the margin of most such masses so that wide excision rather than enucleation is required in their treatment. There is an extensive new formation of poorly formed blood vessels. Numerous capillaries, and larger channels composed of a single layer of endothelium, are supported by the cells of the tumour, while around the larger channels there is usually some fibrous tissue. Two results follow—(a) the cells of the tumour readily break through the vessel walls and are conveyed in the venous blood until arrested in the smaller vessels of lungs, liver, etc., and thus *metastases* may develop, and (b) *haemorrhages* are common. Spread by the

I

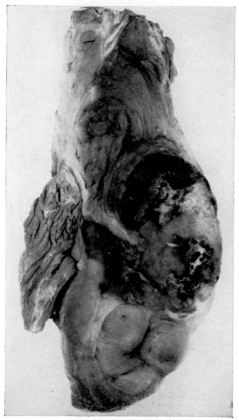

FIG. 12.1.—Spindle-cell sarcoma in intermuscular fascia of thigh, showing extensive haemorrhage and necrosis. × ½.

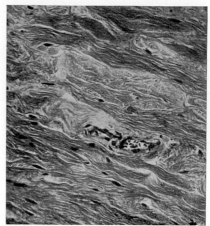

FIG. 12.2.—Hard fibroma, showing thick collagenous fibres with few cells. × 200.

lymphatic vessels is rare, except in the cases of synovial sarcomas and lymphosarcomas, but blood-borne metastases in the lungs are the usual cause of death.

Tumours of fibrous tissue

Although it is usual to regard these as the "typical" connective tissue tumours, they are in fact not very common and wholly typical benign fibromas are rare.

Fibroma. This is the name given to benign tumours of fibrous tissue. The cells of the tumour are fibrocytes; their nuclei are long and narrow and densely staining, the cytoplasm so scanty as to be hard to see, and mitoses are very rare. Bundles of dense collagen separate the cells, and the appearances, in short, may not be very different from that of fibrous tissue as seen in a thick fascia or a scar. A distinction is often made between *hard fibromas* with abundant collagen and scanty cells, and *soft fibromas*, with scantier collagen and more cells (Figs. 12.2 and 12.3): the latter are usually larger (Fig. 12.4) and more rapidly growing.

Fibromas are uncommon, but may occur in any type of connective tissue, and may be seen with varying degrees of rarity in most of the internal organs. Special varieties occur in the sheaths of nerves (neurofibroma, p. 679), skin (dermatofibroma, p. 947) and ovaries (p. 845) which have their own peculiarities of behaviour and which probably do not arise from ordinary fibroblasts.

Fibromatoses. There are a number of fibroma-like lesions which may cause considerable difficulties of diagnosis and which may not be true tumours. They include the following.

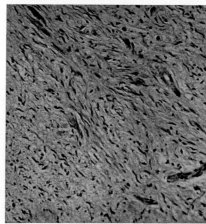

FIG. 12.3.—Soft fibroma, showing relatively cellular structure. × 200.

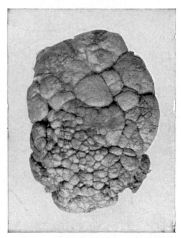

FIG. 12.4.—Lobulated soft fibroma removed from buttock. × $\frac{2}{3}$.

(*a*) *Desmoid tumour*, which is a curious lesion seen characteristically in the rectus abdominis muscle of multiparous women. It has the detailed histology of a fibroma, but is not encapsulated and infiltrates the surrounding muscle and destroys the muscle fibres (Fig. 12.5). It often recurs locally after excision, but never metastasises. Desmoids occur also in the thigh and shoulder, where they are difficult to eradicate and tend to recur, sometimes after many years.

(*b*) *Dupuytren's contracture.* This consists of a fibroma-like lesion, often quite cellular, involving the palmar fascia and producing flexion deformi-

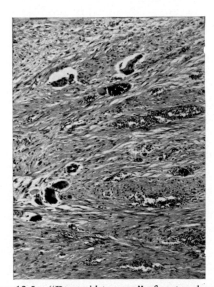

FIG. 12.5.—"Desmoid tumour" of rectus sheath.
Cellular fibrous tissue in which lie multinucleated giant cells derived from the destroyed muscle fibres. × 85.

ties of the fingers (see p. 804). A similar lesion of the plantar fascia (*plantar fibromatosis*) is often particularly cellular and sarcoma-like under the microscope: a similar penile lesion is termed *Peyronie's disease*. Two or even all three of these conditions may occur in one patient, and they are clearly related. Again, none of these ever metastasises.

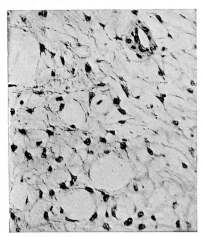

FIG. 12.6.—Myxoma of breast, showing branching cells in clear matrix. × 200.

(*c*) *Keloid.* Some people (Negroes more often than others) have a curious tendency to produce excessive masses of poorly cellular fibrous tissue, instead of the normal inconspicuous scars, after injury to the skin. They always cease growth after a time, and are clearly not tumours, but they are sometimes difficult to distinguish from hard fibromas.

Myxoma and mesenchymoma. The rare pure myxomas (Fig. 12.6) are translucent tumours, usually benign, composed of "myxoid" tissue, a kind of connective tissue with stellate cells widely separated by a mucoid ground substance with a high content of muco-polysaccharides, resembling that seen in the fetus and especially well in the umbilical cord. Tumours occur also in which similar tissue is mixed with other connective tissue elements (e.g. fat, giving a "myxo-lipoma"). Both mixed tumours of this kind and pure myxomas have a greater tendency to recurrence than most simple tumours. There is also a group in which a predominantly myxomatous tumour contains scattered elements of other mesenchymal tissue types, including muscle and cartilage. The name *mesenchymoma* is usually given to them, reflecting a belief, not necessarily well founded, that they represent a return to the capacity for multipotent differentiation of primitive mesenchyme. Those tumours, most often seen in the subcutaneous tissues of the trunk, rarely metastasise but have a high incidence of local recurrence. The "sarcoma botryoides" of children (p. 249) combines myxoid connective tissue with poorly formed muscle cells and sometimes other forms of mesenchymal tissue, but has a very different age and anatomical distribution and is much more malignant: it should not be confused with the mesenchymoma.

Fibrosarcomas. These tumours arise especially from fascia and subcutaneous tissues, but may occur almost anywhere in the body. Similar tumours arise from nerves, *neurofibrosarcomas* (Fig. 12.7). While most fibrosarcomas are clearly malignant from the start, some progress over a period of many years from an early stage in which they may be difficult to distinguish from a benign fibroma.

Fibrosarcomas differ greatly in their degree of differentiation. *Low grade fibrosarcomas* differ little from cellular fibromas: they are firm and fibrous, produce abundant collagen, and the cells differ little from normal fibroblasts. A moderately high rate of mitosis is often the only real evidence of malignancy. Such tumours are slow growing, are often cured by adequate local excision, and recurrences tend, at least at first, to remain localised. Tumours of intermediate

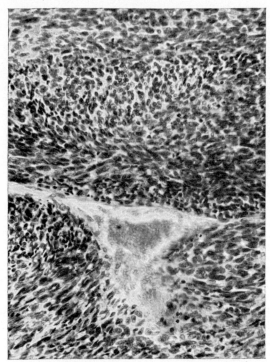

FIG. 12.8.—Spindle-cell sarcoma. × 250.

malignancy are often called "spindle-cell sarcoma" (Fig. 12.8). They are softer, more rapidly growing tumours in which the cells are still recognisably fibroblast-like and regularly arranged, but collagen is relatively inconspicuous: such tumours often metastasise and are usually ultimately fatal. From this type, transitions occur to the *pleomorphic sarcoma* (Fig. 12.9), a

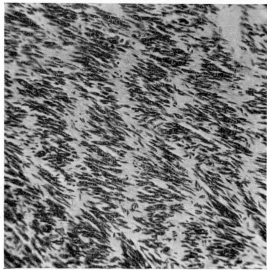

FIG. 12.7.—Neurofibrosarcoma arising in recurrent neurofibroma. × 190.

Note the very pronounced palisading of the nuclei.

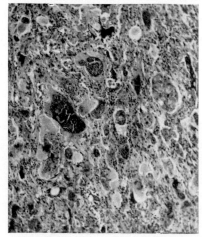

FIG. 12.9.—Pleomorphic sarcoma, showing great variation in the size of the cells.

Note the numerous enormous polyploid nuclei. × 85.

soft, rapidly growing tumour consisting of large irregular cells with large irregular nuclei, with little or no collagen and very little evidence of the tissue of origin; metastasis is usually rapid and prognosis poor. Obviously, in such tumours it may be impossible to say for certain what was the cell of origin, and indeed tumours with this kind of histology may arise from dedifferentiation of almost any kind of cell.

Fibrosarcomas, like most other sarcomas, may recur locally or metastasise by the blood stream, especially to the lungs, but hardly ever spread by the lymphatics.

The tumour cells of fibrosarcomas, unless very poorly differentiated, form enough collagen to produce an adequate stroma. As noted in the introductory section of this chapter, the blood vessels are often very poorly formed. Where this is very pronounced, the appearance under the microscope may be very striking, leading to their being called "telangiectatic sarcomas" (Fig. 12.10). Such tumours are extremely vascular and haemorrhage is especially common. The vascular change is however entirely secondary, and they must not be confused with true angiosarcomas.

Tumours of adipose tissue

Lipoma. This is a benign tumour of adipose tissue. It increases in size by proliferation of fibroblast-like cells which lie around the blood vessels and are typically sparse; subsequently, these cells become ballooned with fat. The common lipoma is a rounded, well-demarcated, subcutaneous mass. It sometimes reaches a considerable size, and may have blunt projections which pass into the tissues around. Multiple tumours may be present and occasionally they are symmetrical. They are commonest over the shoulders and buttocks, and occur also within the abdomen, especially in the perirenal fat but, like fibromas, they may arise almost anywhere in the body. Should the patient become emaciated, the fat in the tumour is not utilised—a good example of the failure of tumours to respond to the factors controlling the metabolism of normal tissues. In a lipoma there may be areas of fibrous, myxomatous or capillary angiomatous tissue—the tumour being then called a fibrolipoma, myxolipoma or angiolipoma respectively; occasionally there are areas of calcification.

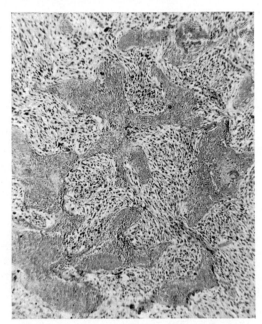

Fig. 12.10.—"Telangiectatic sarcoma" showing numerous thin-walled vessels. × 150.

In a rare variant the fat is finely divided in droplets within the cells, which thus closely resemble those of the brown hibernating-fat depots of rodents; this type of lipoma has been called "*hibernoma*" (Fig. 12.11).

Liposarcoma. This is rather uncommon. In the less malignant forms the tissue retains some naked-eye resemblance to fat and the microsco-

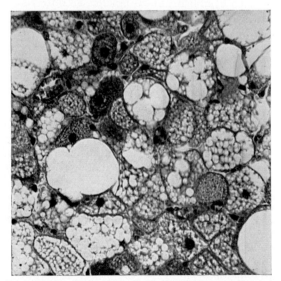

Fig. 12.11.—"Hibernoma" showing the characteristic appearances of the fat-laden cells, with central nuclei. × 400.

pic difference from lipoma may not be very striking at first sight. The fat cells vary in size; much more important, the scanty undifferentiated cells from which the benign lipoma arises are augmented to form broad bands of cellular connective tissue, with irregular nuclei, interspersed among the fat-containing cells. These well-differentiated liposarcomas are usually only prone to local recurrence. All transitions occur through myxoid liposarcomas to highly malignant, pleomorphic tumours in some of which gigantic lipoblasts may be seen (Fig. 12.12a). In others, however, the origin in fat cells may be

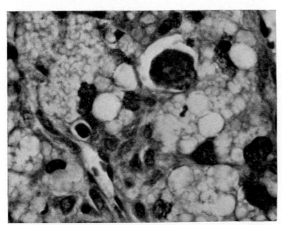

Fig. 12.12a.—Pleomorphic liposarcoma. In spite of gross pleomorphism, the cells contain globules of fat. Death resulted from metastasis. × 450.

hard to establish. Since normal adipose tissue has a lobulated architecture it is not surprising that liposarcomatous tumours show a somewhat lobular or alveolar architecture (Fig. 12.12b) and the cells may rarely be mistaken even for epithelium. Liposarcomas are commonest about the shoulders, in the perirenal fatty tissue, and in the intermuscular fasciae of the lower limbs, usually with an admixture of myxomatous tissue.

Alveolar soft tissue sarcoma. This rather uncommon variety of sarcoma arising in the soft tissues, usually of a limb. It is composed of large polygonal or round cells with coarsely granular cytoplasm, and arranged in a curiously alveolar pattern. In paraffin sections the appearances resemble those of liposarcoma or even carcinoma but the granules do not contain lipids, mucin, glycogen or other specifically stainable substance. Its origin and true nature are obscure, but some regard it as a variety of chemodectoma (p. 252).

Tumours arising in cartilage and bone

These are dealt with in detail in Chapter 22. The benign tumours of bone are a perplexingly various group, and their precise histogenesis is often obscure. The masses of cartilage called chondromas and the masses of bone called osteomas are developmental defects or hamartomas rather than true tumours. Osteosarcomas and, to a lesser extent, chondrosarcomas are among the commonest sarcomas. Osteosarcoma especially exemplifies many of the most charac-

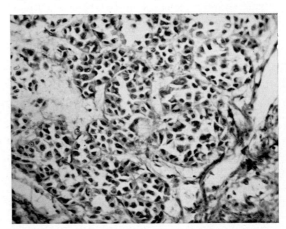

Fig. 12.12b.—Liposarcoma. The margin of the tumour, showing the pseudo-alveolar architecture. Elsewhere the cells contained much fat. × 210.

teristic features of sarcomas generally—a high incidence in childhood, a high mortality and a very low incidence of lymph-spread metastases combined with a high tendency to blood-borne metastases, especially in the lungs.

Fibrosarcomas may arise from bone. Conversely (though very rarely) bone-forming osteosarcomas sometimes arise from connective tissue elsewhere, and sometimes even from such organs as the breast, kidney, etc.

Bone and cartilage are sometimes seen in nonbony tumours. Both are common in teratomas. Cartilage, or something that looks very like it, is often seen in the parabuccal mixed tumours of the parotid and other glands. Bony metaplasia of the stroma of carcinomas is a rare but striking finding, least rare in man in large-bowel cancers, and not uncommon in breast tumours in bitches.

Tumours of muscle

Leiomyoma. There are two varieties of myoma, the leiomyoma, composed of smooth muscle fibres, and the rhabdomyoma of striped muscle. The latter is so rare that the term myoma without qualification is often used to signify leiomyoma.

The leiomyomas are composed of smooth muscle cells orientated in a more or less parallel manner within bundles, which are arranged in a whorled manner (Fig. 12.13). A small amount of

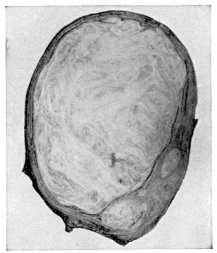

FIG. 12.13.—Transverse section of leiomyoma of the uterus, showing the characteristic whorled appearance. × ¾.

supporting connective tissue runs amongst the individual fibres, whilst broader bands separate the bundles. The proportion of fibrous tissue to muscle varies much in different specimens. The tumours are usually firm and rounded, and on section are pinkish with a characteristic whorled appearance due to the arrangement of the fibres (Fig. 12.14).

Leiomyomas of the *uterus* are among the commonest of tumours: their usually high content of fibrous tissue earns them their common name of "fibroids", though the muscle is the only true tumorous element and it is incorrect to call them fibromyomas. They are dealt with in more detail in Chapter 23. Of general interest is their tendency to cease growth or regress at the menopause.

Myomas are probably next most common in the muscular coat of the alimentary canal, though here most are too small to be found without

special search and few are large enough to cause trouble. They occur also in the skin, being remarkable here in that some are extremely painful on pressure; they appear rarely in other sites such as ovaries, prostate and bladder.

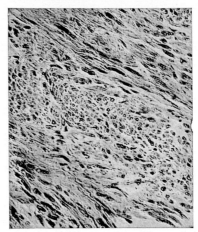

FIG. 12.14.—Leiomyoma.

The muscular bundles are seen in longitudinal and in transverse sections; the tumour is more cellular than usual. × 200.

Leiomyosarcomas occasionally arise from the same sites as leiomyomas, especially the uterus and the stomach. Most appear to be malignant from the first but some may arise by malignant progression in a benign myoma. The histological diagnosis of malignancy is usually easy on general cytological grounds, but the better differentiated tumours can be hard to distinguish from the more cellular benign tumours. It is a useful empirical rule, which cannot be extended to all other tumours, that a smooth muscle tumour in which mitoses can be found easily is liable to metastasise.

Rhabdomyosarcoma. In proportion to their bulk, the voluntary muscles are one of the rarest of sites for tumours of any kind, both primary and secondary: the reasons for this are not known. The rare tumours in which striped muscle fibres or their precursors are seen are nearly always malignant, and arise mostly in sites where no striped muscle is present normally. They are found most often in the genital tract, characteristically in the cervix or vaginal vault in young girls: probably next least rarely in the soft palate. Usually the tumours have a large myxoid element, and the muscle cells (though very characteristic when found) are often scanty and difficult to find, even with the help of special

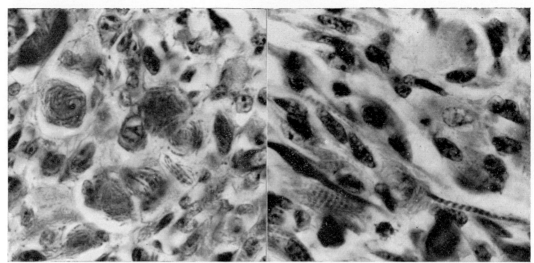

FIG. 12.15a.—Rhabdomyosarcoma showing coiled intracellular myofibrils.

FIG. 12.15b.—Strap-like cells showing characteristic cross-striation.

stains which accentuate their cross striations. Rounded or irregular cells with coiled myofibrils but without cross-striations are usually more readily apparent. (Fig. 12.15). When growing beneath a mucous membrane they often present with numerous blunt translucent processes— hence the name of *sarcoma botryoides* (grape-like sarcoma). These are highly malignant tumours: local recurrence after excision and blood-spread metastases are usual, and (unlike most sarcomas) lymph node metastases are common.

Rhabdomyosarcomas are also seen very rarely in the heart. Benign tumours, perhaps better regarded as hamartomas,* are seen there in children with epiloia (tuberous sclerosis): the lumps consist of swollen muscle cells packed with glycogen and some confusion has in the past existed between these findings and the cardiac lesions of glycogen storage disease.

TUMOURS OF BLOOD VESSELS AND LYMPHATICS

Haemangioma. A haemangioma consists of a mass of blood vessels, atypical or irregular in arrangement and size. A corresponding growth, lymphangioma, is composed of lymphatic vessels similarly altered; but, as this is rarer, the term angioma is often used as synonymous with haemangioma.

The majority of the lesions called angiomas are not true tumours, but hamartomas.* They are present at birth, even if not always visible, and their enlargement ceases with the growth of the patient. Most angiomas are well-defined masses of vascular tissue which *resemble* tumours sufficiently to justify their inclusion here. The two common varieties are as follows.

(*a*) *The capillary angiomas* consist of dense plexiform arrangements of vessels of capillary size (Fig. 12.16). They occur especially in the skin, where they form one of the two common types of *naevus*† or birthmark, but are also seen in the internal organs. Most are small, but larger lesions occur, e.g. the "port-wine stains" of the face, and these may contain vessels of larger size than capillaries. Capillary angiomas are usually well defined, and deep red or purple. The capillary vessels have a more prominent endo-

* *Hamartoma* is a convenient term for an ill-defined group of lesions on the borderline of true neoplasia. They are tumour-like lumps present at birth or appearing soon afterwards, growing with the patient and ceasing to grow when general body growth ceases. They can be best understood as a disorder of the relationships of normal tissues in a limited area, leading to a relative over-production of one element without any tendency to progressive growth beyond a definable point. Angiomas and pigmented naevi are the common forms, but there are many varieties. With some of them there is a tendency to later development of true tumour.

† A *naevus* (mole or birthmark) is a hamartoma of the skin made conspicuous by some definite colour difference from the surrounding normal area. Angiomas and pigmented naevi (p. 943) are the two common types.

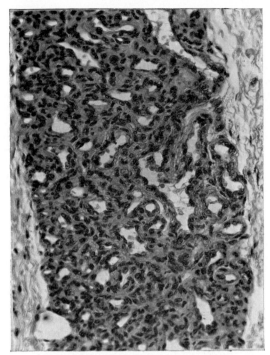

FIG. 12.16.—Capillary angioma showing well-formed capillaries with prominent endothelial lining. × 200.

Glomangioma (glomus tumour). This uncommon but interesting lesion apparently arises from the glomus bodies, small arteriovenous anastomoses with a coiled arteriole and abundant nerve supply which control blood flow and temperature, particularly in the fingers and toes. In its most characteristic form, the glomangioma is a small bluish nodule, usually near the end of a

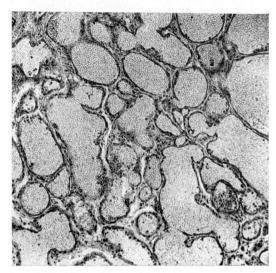

FIG. 12.17.—Cavernous angioma of subcutaneous tissue, showing large intercommunicating spaces filled with blood. × 80.

thelial lining than normal capillaries. Their stroma consists of well-formed collagen. There is no capsule, and outlying groups of capillaries in adjoining tissues often give a false appearance of invasion. The blood supply is usually clearly separated from that of the surrounding tissues, there being usually only one artery of supply.

(*b*) *Cavernous angiomas* are confined to the deeper tissues, being least rare in the liver. They consist of relatively large interconnecting sinus-like vascular spaces (Fig. 12.17). In the liver they form deep-purple well-defined masses, usually polygonal rather than round and not raised above the surface, signs of their lack of expansile growth.

Angiomas are often multiple, and are also an important component of several diseases with a strong hereditary element, e.g. hereditary haemorrhagic telangiectasia (p. 444) (multiple small angiomas in skin and mucosae with a strong tendency to haemorrhage), Lindau's disease (cerebellar and retinal angiomas with cysts of liver and pancreas) and Sturge-Weber syndrome (facial and meningeal angiomas).

A special form of angioma of the skin, the so-called sclerosing angioma, is dealt with later (p. 947).

finger, and extraordinarily tender to even light touch. On microscopic examination the tumour is found to consist of two kinds of tissue variously interblended (Fig. 12.18). The first is angiomatous, with spaces containing blood, lined by endothelium, and separated by connective tissue containing varying amounts of smooth muscle. The other is cellular, with rounded or cuboidal cells called "myoid", as transitions to smooth muscle fibres can be found. The growth contains numerous medullated and non-medullated nerve fibres and the pain is apparently due to distensile pressures of the blood-containing spaces, though the painfulness is not in proportion to the neural content. The origin of the growth seems to be distinctly related to trauma and it is doubtful if it should be regarded as a true neoplasm. A small dermal leiomyoma may likewise be painful and the two forms of growth may be related in origin. Glomangiomas have been described in deeper tissues, including the gut, but the characteristic pain occurs only with those in the limbs.

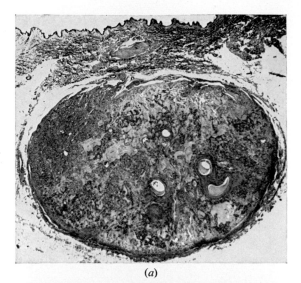

(a)

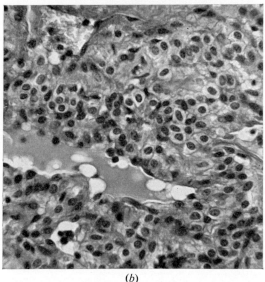

(b)

FIG. 12.18.—Glomangioma.

(a) Small subcutaneous encapsulated growth showing the coiled arteriole. × 8.

(b) The clear myoid cells surrounding a vascular space. × 350.

Chemodectoma. Because of their close anatomical relationship with blood vessels it is convenient to consider here the tumours arising from the chemoreceptor organs, viz. the carotid body, glomus jugulare, organ of Zuckerkandl and no doubt other less clearly defined structures such as the aortic bodies. These tumours have also been called non-chromaffin paragangliomas; they do not appear to produce any endocrine effects.

Chemodectomas are usually benign, but their anatomical sites may render complete surgical removal difficult. Thus carotid body tumours, which

are the commonest variety, closely embrace the bifurcation of the common carotid artery, and the glomus jugulare tumours involve the middle ear and present as recurrent bleeding aural polyps; they may also present intracranially. Microscopically the architectural pattern is similar to the normal structure and consists of many small masses of cells of variable size, sometimes enclosed in a boxlike framework of fine fibrous tissue (Fig. 12.19). The tumour cells are usually polygonal and may be spindle-shaped in places but aberrant types with hyperchromatic nuclei are not uncommon and do not indicate malignancy. The blood supply is very rich and of sinusoidal pattern.

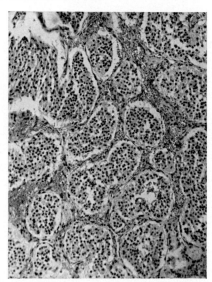

FIG. 12.19.—Chemodectoma of the carotid body, showing the characteristic boxlike pattern and highly vascular stroma. × 110.

Haemangioendothelioma: haemangiosarcoma. Occasionally tumours with the general histological features of capillary haemangiomas have formed numerous metastases. Fig. 12.20 is an example of this kind which originated in the breast (a not very rare site) and secondary growths developed in the orbit, lungs, liver, etc. Here one finds not only new formation of capillary channels but also active division of the endothelial cells to form solid processes which pass into and blend with the surrounding masses of cells and join with pre-existing capillaries. There was also growth within the small veins and pulmonary vessels of endothelial tufts, which appeared to distribute the tumour cells by the blood stream to give rise to metastases.

Tumours whose origin is traceable to the vascular endothelium and which forms both new capillaries and solid masses of cells, the two types being intimately blended, also occur in the intermuscular fascia of the limbs, and may extend much more

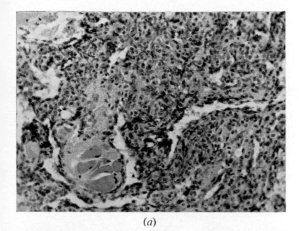

(a)

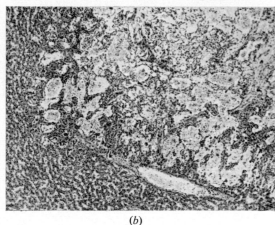

(b)

FIG. 12.20.—Haemangioendothelioma of the breast.

(a) Primary tumour, showing vascular channels and solid masses of endothelial cells. × 170.
(b) Metastasis in liver, showing wide vascular spaces lined by swollen endothelial cells which invade and replace the sinusoids, becoming continuous with them. × 45.

widely than is clinically apparent. Fig. 12.21 is from such a case; the tumour was in the upper arm and it ramified so extensively in the muscles that ultimately a fore-quarter amputation had to be performed.

Kaposi's disease: Idiopathic haemorrhagic sarcoma. This remarkable disorder is rare in Great Britain, we have seen less than 20 examples. It is less uncommon amongst the South African Bantu and in American Negroes, and is commonest in some well-defined areas of Central Africa, where it is much more frequent in males. The condition presents the syndrome of lymphoedema, multiple cutaneous tumours which later ulcerate, lymphadenopathy and ultimately visceral involvement. The skin tumours at first consist of lobulated masses of highly vascular and cellular tissue resembling granulation tissue deep within the corium and separated by fibrous trabeculae (Fig. 12.22). Later there is much haemorrhage in and around the lesions, the spindle cells and vascular

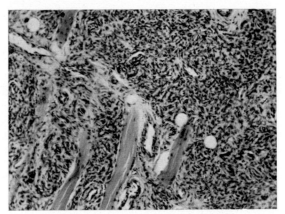

FIG. 12.21.—Haemangioendothelioma.

The tumour consists of solid cords of endothelial cells and poorly defined capillary channels, invading and destroying skeletal muscle. × 85.

sprouts increase progressively, mitoses are abundant, ulceration of superficial lesions occurs and the regional lymph nodes may be replaced by similar highly vascular spindle-celled tissue. Despite their tumour-like appearance many lesions ultimately heal, although the disease may progress elsewhere. However, in some cases at least (the proportion is

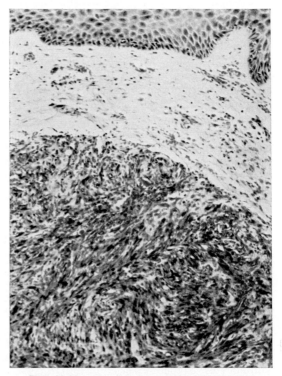

FIG. 12.22.—Kaposi's haemorrhagic sarcoma.

An early lesion showing the zone of fibrous tissue between the vascular spindle-celled tumour and the epidermis. × 130.

uncertain), the lesions become progressive in internal organs, especially the intestines. This occurs more frequently in Central African cases than in those in South Africa or elsewhere. The superficial lesions respond well to radiotherapy and chemotherapy.

It is uncertain whether this is a true neoplasm but in some cases it certainly behaves like one. Evidence from histochemistry and tissue culture indicates that the spindle cells are not fibroblasts and the lesion may be an angiosarcoma derived from lymphatic endothelium as the cells lack the enzymes characteristic of blood capillary endothelium.

Haemangiopericytoma. This also is a much disputed but probably genuine entity. The tumours are vascular, with uniform sheets of large pale cells around the vessels, the cells being separated from each other by a prominent reticulin network. They are usually malignant. The term should not be confused with "perithelioma", a term once mistakenly used to describe tumours, usually anaplastic carcinomas, in which the common tendency towards death of cells lying at a distance from blood vessels is exaggerated so that the surviving cells appear to form perivascular sheaths. The true haemangiopericytoma is believed to arise from pericytes, and the perivascular arrangement is not the result of pararterial ischaemic necrosis.

Lymphangioma. This may be composed of numerous lymphatic vessels—the *plexiform* lymphangioma—but more frequently it has a *cavernous* structure. Dilatation and diffuse growth of vessels may give rise to enlargement of a part, e.g. the tongue (*macroglossia*). In such lesions there is even less evidence than in haemangiomas of neoplastic growth, and the more diffuse lesions may be hard to distinguish from the effects of lymphatic obstruction, though in most cases it is clear from the anatomy that no such obstruction can be present, and a congenital malformation (or hamartoma) of the lymphatics is present. It is becoming increasingly common to describe such diffuse lesions as *localised lymphangiectasis* rather than lymphangioma. Lesions, whether diffuse or compact, are commonest in the skin and subcutaneous tissue. Each forms a somewhat ill-defined, doughy, or semi-fluctuant swelling, containing large, intercommunicating lymphatic spaces. The contents are a clear lymph, containing occasional lymphocytes. Sometimes bleeding into the spaces renders the diagnosis between haemangioma and lymphangioma difficult. Lymphangiomas occur

occasionally also in mucous membranes in the wall of the bowel (Fig. 12.23), in the tissues of the orbit and mesentery, and elsewhere.

In rare cases lymphangiomas of neck, retroperitoneum or mesentery undergo great dilatation, forming a multilocular ramifying cystic mass which may reach a large size. Occasionally a single cyst is formed, as in one form of *hygroma* of the neck or axilla. It may be distinguished from other cysts in this region by its endothelial lining.

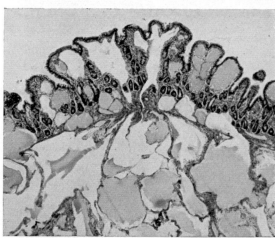

FIG. 12.23.—Cavernous lymphangioma of small intestine, showing intercommunicating spaces filled with clear lymph.

A cellular neoplasm designated *lymphangiosarcoma* has been described as arising in the lymphatics of the arm, following their obstruction by mastectomy and irradiation for mammary cancer. Very similar appearances may result from a slow and rather diffuse permeation of the lymphatics by carcinoma and it remains undecided whether the so-called lymphangiosarcoma secondary to chronic post-operative obstruction is a separate and distinct neoplasm.

"Endothelioma". This term was once used very freely for tumours of uncertain origin. The angiomas described above could be called vascular endotheliomas, but past misuse has led to the avoidance of this term. Meningiomas, formerly called fibro-endotheliomas, though possibly endothelial in origin, are no longer so described (see p. 667). Tumours of the serosal linings, which, though once suspect, have recently become more generally accepted as a genuine entity, are usually called *mesotheliomas*.

TUMOURS OF NEURO-ECTODERMAL ORIGIN

From the ectodermal cells of the neural tube and crest are derived the tumours of (*a*) the neuroglia, (*b*) nerve cells and their precursors, (*c*) nerve sheaths, (*d*) peripheral neuro-receptor organs, (*e*) the melanocytes, and possibly also of (*f*) the meninges. These tumours will be discussed in detail in connection with the nervous system (p. 669). It will suffice at this stage to mention very briefly a few types and their features.

Glioma. These tumours of the neuroglia occur commonly in the brain, but also rarely in the spinal cord. Because of their anatomical site and the pressure effects they may exercise on vital structures most gliomas in the end are likely to kill the patient, but even those of high cellularity and aberrant cellular structure do not metastasise outside the nervous system.

Gliomas may take origin from all types of neuroglia and may be firm, slow-growing, and rich in glial fibrils, but may nevertheless undergo central liquefaction. At the other extreme are highly pleomorphic rapidly growing cellular tumours in which necrosis and haemorrhage are conspicuous. A rapidly growing cellular tumour showing little or no pleomorphism occurs in the cerebellum of children—medulloblastoma (p. 674).

Neuroblastoma and ganglioneuroma. Neuroblastoma, also called sympathicoblastoma, is a highly cellular tumour which occurs chiefly in the adrenal medulla or in connection with the sympathetic chain elsewhere, usually arising in children. It consists of small round or oval cells with scanty cytoplasm, in places arranged in ball-like clusters which, on section, appear as rosettes. These tumours are highly malignant and metastasise widely, especially to the skull and other bones (p. 674).

Ganglioneuromas are rare tumours composed of mature ganglion cells and nerve fibres. They are found chiefly in relation to the sympathetic chain and adrenal medulla (p. 675). Clinically and histologically they behave as benign tumours except when they contain foci of neuroblasts.

Although strikingly different in appearance, it appears that these two tumours are benign and malignant variants of the same tumour. As a rare but striking event, neuroblastoma may undergo a form of self-cure by maturing into a ganglioneuroma.

MELANOCYTIC TUMOURS

The cells which form melanin are of neural crest origin and are called melanocytes (p. 199). The skin and the eye are their chief sites, and in both places they are important sources of tumours.

Skin tumours are dealt with fully in Chapter 25. The so-called *pigmented naevus* is very common. It is a benign lesion, probably better regarded as a hamartoma than a true tumour, formed by a mass of melanocytes ("naevus cells") which accumulate in the dermis as a result of excessive proliferation of melanocytes in their normal site in the basal layer. *Malignant melanomas* are much less common: they arise from epidermal melanocytes, often at the site of a pigmented naevus. They are highly malignant tumours on the whole, metastasising both to lymph nodes and by the blood: the unusually widespread black metastases commonly seen at necropsy may present a very striking picture.

Ocular melanomas. Malignant melanomas of the eye, though far from common, are the least rare of all intraocular malignant tumours. They may arise from any part of the uveal tract, but mostly from the choroid, where they form small buttons which push forward the retina causing detachment. They often grow extensively within the eyeball before penetrating the sclera to invade the orbit. They occur chiefly in the elderly, and are (like skin melanomas) much commoner in the white races. When metastasis occurs, it is almost entirely by blood-spread, with an unusually strong predilection for the liver. The tumour is notorious for the frequency with which a long interval (as much as twenty years) may elapse after excision of the eye with apparent cure, followed by discovery of a rapidly enlarging liver full of metastases (the big liver and glass-eye syndrome). Similar events can of course occur at times with other tumours (including skin melanomas). What the tumour cells are doing in the long latent intervals is largely a matter of speculation. A pure spindle-cell histology, production of reticulin, small size, origin in the anterior part of the uvea and an intact sclera are all factors making for a good prognosis in ocular melanomas: a small spindle-cell tumour arising in the iris can almost be regarded as benign.

Melanomas at other sites. Melanocytes spill over all the mucocutaneous junctions into the adjoining mucous membranes to varying distances and in varying numbers, and melanomas occur at the corresponding sites. They are least rare in the nose, but arise also in the mouth, conjunctiva, vagina and anus and even in such deeper sites as oesophagus and rectum. The presence of melanocytes in the meninges is also reflected in the rare occurrence of malignant melanomas, which are remarkable for their inability to metastasise outside the cranial cavity.

TUMOURS OF THE HAEMOPOIETIC, RETICULO-ENDOTHELIAL AND LYMPHOID TISSUES

Classification within this group is difficult, and it is only in the last two decades that some of its most important members—the leukaemias and Hodgkin's disease for instance—have become fully accepted as neoplastic. Nomenclature still tends to be anomalous and classification disputed. The principal varieties are described in Chapters 16 and 17 and only a few general points will be made here.

The characteristic cells of these tissues are far more mobile than those of most of the rest of the body. This is obviously true of the blood cells, lymphocytes, histiocytes and the like, but applies also to less prominently mobile cells—the blood cell precursors of the marrow, for example, appear in the blood in small numbers in various conditions of stress, and are capable of re-establishing themselves in the spleen and liver. None of these cells is tethered by being closely aggregated into a cell mass like epithelium, or by the formation of large amounts of extracellular matrix like most connective tissue cells. The tumours accordingly tend not to form a single mass, but to spread widely from the start: in most of them the spread is limited to a large extent to the regions which normally contain cells of the same type. This is particularly true of the better-differentiated tumours. For instance, in chronic myeloid leukaemia, a well-differentiated neoplasia of the granulocyte series, very large numbers of tumour cells appear in the blood from the start, but involvement of solid organs is usually limited to marrow, liver and spleen, i.e. to sites of leukopoiesis in fetal life. The poorly differentiated acute leukaemias on the other hand produce far fewer mobile cells in the blood (and sometimes none at all) and tend to a more destructive infiltration of the marrow and other organs. Similarly the better differentiated lymph node tumours characteristically cause widespread moderate enlargement of multiple lymph nodes and other lymphoid structures but often do not spread very much to non-lymphoid tissues, while the less well differentiated may cause large local masses and less discriminatory spread to other structures.

Any tissue which contains any of the cells belonging to the relevant categories (which means practically any tissue in the body) can give rise to tumours within this group, but the vast majority arise either in the bone marrow (leukaemias and myelomatosis) or the lymph nodes (lymphosarcoma, reticulosarcoma and the ill-defined group of "reticuloses" of which Hodgkin's disease is the best known). As will be obvious from what has been said above, a benign tumour in the ordinary sense of the word must be exceptional and may in fact be nonexistent. Localized nodules of abnormal lymphoid tissue are sometimes found, for example in the rectum and skin, and may be called "benign lymphoma" or "benign lymphocytoma" but it is doubtful whether these are tumours at all.

The immunological importance of these tissues is naturally reflected in their tumours. Immunological abnormalities are fairly commonly associated with some lymph node tumours, but the most striking example is production of immunoglobulin in large amounts by the neoplastic plasma cells of multiple myelomatosis.

Because of the proved viral origin of many animal leukaemias and lymphomas, the search for a similar cause in human material has been especially active; apart from the somewhat equivocal example of Burkitt's lymphoma, a viral etiology has not yet been established in man, though this now seems a very likely possibility, particularly in the leukaemias of childhood.

"MIXED" TUMOURS

A considerable number of tumours consist of two or more different kinds of tissue. The reasons for this are very diverse: the most important can be classified as follows:

(*a*) *"Collision" tumours* result when two different tumours arise close together and intermingle; presumably the juxtaposition may be a chance event, or the result of a single carcinogenic stimulus applied at one point and affecting several tissues.

(*b*) *Stromal changes in epithelial tumours.* The cartilaginous metaplasia of the stroma in mixed-salivary tumours, the bony metaplasia seen in a very few carcinomas of the colon, and the lymphoid stroma of some seminomas all produce the *appearance* of a mixed tumour, though only the epithelial element is truly neoplastic.

elements, which arise especially in uterus and bronchus, and more rarely in the stomach.

(*d*) *Tumours with variable differentiation.* This arises especially in carcinomas, parts of which are so poorly differentiated as to resemble sarcomas. It is almost certain that most so-called "carcinosarcomas", both human and experimental, are of this type (Fig. 12.24).

(*e*) *Truly mixed tumours* involving the co-ordinated neoplastic growth of two independent tissues are hard to find. The fibro-adenoma of the breast is the only completely acceptable example, though some connective tissue tumours, such as the angiolipoma, may qualify.

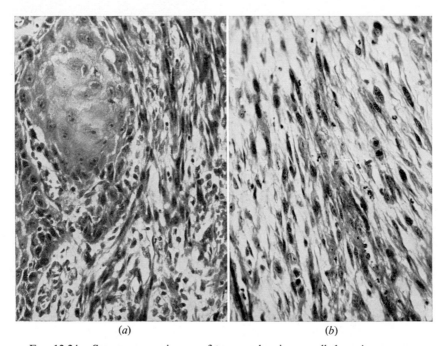

(*a*) (*b*)

Fig. 12.24.—Squamous carcinoma of tongue, showing so-called carcinosarcoma.
(*a*) On the left typical squamous carcinoma, showing continuity with spindle-shaped epithelial cells.
(*b*) On the right a purely spindle-cell area containing many mitoses. Transitions from (*a*) to (*b*) are readily found. × 200.

(*c*) *"Metaplastic" tumours.* Tumours arising from tissues which readily undergo metaplasia from one type to another often reflect this characteristic. Such are the "adeno-acanthomas", with mixed squamous and glandular

(*f*) *"Embryonal" tumours.* There is a group of tumours, mostly highly malignant, which arise usually in infancy and appear to be derived from immature tissue. Most of these (neuroblastoma, medulloblastoma, hepatoblastoma, for example) are not truly mixed, but the partial differentiation of some of the elements, while others continue to resemble primitive embryonal tissue, may give rise to appearances that simulate a mixed tumour.

One of the commonest of these tumours, the nephroblastoma (Wilms' tumour), consists of solid sarcoma-like masses of short spindle cells, amongst which some elements differentiate to tubules and occasionally glomerulus-like structures (Fig. 12.25). More discordant tissues such as cartilage and striped muscle are occasionally present, possibly representing a derivation of the tumour cells from the myotome at an earlier period in ontogeny (see also p. 740).

(*g*) *Teratomas.* These, the most extreme examples of mixed tumours, are dealt with in the following section.

It should be emphasized that the collection of these tumours together is not intended to indicate any special relation between them: they have, in fact, very little in common except the presence of more than one kind of tissue. Use of the term "mixed tumour" is somewhat arbitrary. It is most commonly applied to the salivary tumours, fibro-adenomas of the breast and teratomas, mentioned above.

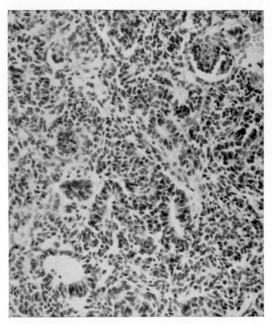

Fig. 12.25.—Nephroblastoma, showing cellular sarcoma-like tissue with transition to tubular and glomeruloid structures.

TERATOMA AND CHORIOCARCINOMA

Teratoma

A teratoma consists of a mass composed of various tissues, chaotically arranged and most characteristically including derivatives of all three germinal layers. They are not rare and are of practical importance. They are most common in the ovaries and testes, though they occur in other parts, such as the mediastinum, retroperitoneal tissues and pineal. They are usually single but occasionally more than one is present. There is great variation in naked-eye appearances, and cyst formation may be a notable feature, as in the common ovarian teratoma ("dermoid"). There is endless variety in the tissues and in their arrangement. Cartilage, bone, epidermis, glandular epithelium, hair, teeth, etc., are common components, but other specialised tissues such as liver, kidney, nervous, eye and haemopoietic are also represented (Figs. 12.26, 12.27), and sometimes there are structures resembling early embryos, with trophoblastic epithelium. There is, however, no evidence of the presence of the reproductive glands. While a teratoma may be of such a complicated constitu-

tion, there is no proper formation of organs, limbs, etc., and a very important fact is that there is no trace of a vertebral column and no metameric segmentation.

Because of their complicated structure, teratomas were formerly believed to arise from totipotent cells, i.e. from dislocated blastomeres. However, proliferation of a blastomere gives rise to an organised embryo, in contrast to the chaotic mixture of tissues in a teratoma. Another view is that teratomas are derived from the male or female germ cells. The frequency of teratomas in the gonads supports this possibility. Something of the nature of parthenogenetic development would have to be assumed, as is known to occur in amphibian ova under the influence of certain salt solutions. Bosaeus obtained striking results by stimulating frogs' ova to parthenogenetic development and then placing them in the internal tissues: tumour masses developed which he describes as having the structure of spontaneous teratomas. In cocks the intratesticular injection of solutions of zinc salts during the breeding season or after stimulation by pituitary gonadotrophin has led to the development of

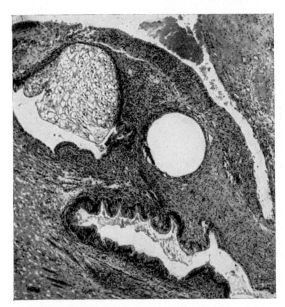

FIG. 12.26.—Section of ovarian teratoma.

Above there is a tube lined by squamous epithelium; and below, a space lined by columnar epithelium with smooth muscle around. × 60.

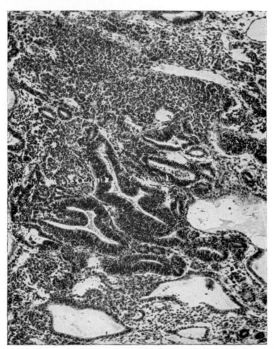

FIG. 12.27.—Section of testicular teratoma, showing solid cellular areas and spaces lined by epithelium of primitive neural type. × 60.

highly malignant complex teratomatous tumours closely resembling those in man (Bagg) but similar results do not appear to have been achieved in mammals.

Study of the sex chromatin has brought to light some evidence in favour of the parthenogenetic origin of teratomas. It has been found that all teratomas in women have female nuclei but about half of those in men have female nuclei, as would be expected if they arose by parthenogenetic development in the male gonad.

Many teratomas, especially in the ovary, are benign. Rarely, one element of such a teratoma may become malignant, and if metastases develop they contain only this one type of malignant tissue. Apart from those in the ovary, most teratomas, and especially those in the testis, are malignant from the start, and all of their elements are malignant.

Chorionic epithelium not uncommonly occurs in teratomas, apart from those in the ovary, and choriocarcinoma may develop and dominate the appearance and behaviour of the growth.

Monstrosities. When identical twins develop from a single fertilised ovum a variable amount of fusion may take place. This may be of limited extent as in so-called Siamese twins, or it may affect a considerable part of the body. Partial

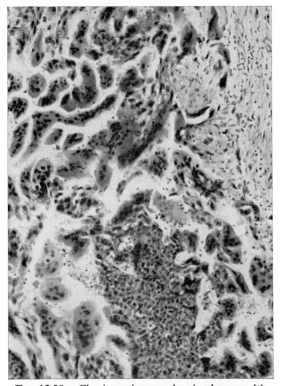

FIG. 12.28.—Choriocarcinoma, showing large multinucleated syncytia and Langhans' cells. × 250.

fusion of two germinal areas is often invoked. Then there are cases where one fetus is imperfectly represented and fused with the other, growing on it in parasite-like fashion or included within its abdominal cavity—*fetus in fetu*. Many sacral teratomas and epignathus probably belong to this group. All such abnormalities, which are extremely varied, are spoken of as monstrosities. They show wide deviations from the normal, but the formation of parts and the relations of the tissues to one another are well maintained: thus, organs may be doubled, and a limb, though abnormal in size or form, is still a limb. Monstrosities are now generally thought to be of a fundamentally different nature from teratomas and apparent transitions are almost certainly fallacious. A defect in the mechanism of the primary organisers at a very early stage of formation of the embryo may well be responsible for this type of abnormality.

Choriocarcinoma

This is mentioned here for convenience. It is not a teratoma although it may take origin from trophoblastic elements in a teratoma, and like teratoma it cannot readily be classified with any other group of tumours. Choriocarcinoma, in its usual uterine form, is a rare and highly malignant tumour originating from the trophoblast of the fetal placenta (Fig. 12.28): i.e. the cells are derived from the fetus and not from the mother. In spite of this, they invade the tissues of the mother like any ordinary malignant tumour. However, the existence of a homograft reaction on the part of the host probably accounts for the frequent occurrence of very extensive necrosis in the tumour and also for an unusually good response to chemotherapy. A more detailed description will be found on p. 853.

CYSTS

The term "cyst" properly means a space containing fluid and lined by endothelium or epithelium. Accordingly, cysts are not tumours and are included here only for convenience. Nearly all cysts arise by the abnormal dilatation of pre-existing tubules, ducts or cavities. A cyst may lose its cellular lining as a result of inflammatory or other change, and becomes lined by granulation or denser connective tissue. The term is, however, often applied in a somewhat loose way to other abnormal cavities containing fluid. For example, the term "apoplectic cyst" is applied to a space in the brain containing brownish fluid, which has resulted from haemorrhage. Some tumours e.g. gliomas, undergo softening in their interior, so that a collection of fluid is formed, and the term "cystic change" is often used even when no true cyst is formed.

The cysts peculiar to each organ will be described in the later chapters: we shall give here only a classification of their causes. The occurrence of true cysts in tumours—*cystic adenomas and teratomas*—has already been described. Apart from these, cysts fall naturally into two main groups, viz. (1) those due to congenital abnormalities, and (2) acquired cysts, i.e. those produced by lesions in post-natal life.

(1) Congenital cysts. These again fall into two main groups:

(a) Cysts may result from *abnormal development* of organs or parts of the body. Thus multiple cysts may arise in the kidneys from an error in development which disturbs the normal relationships of the tubules, and a similar condition occurs in the liver. Again, part of an epithelial surface may become detached or dislocated and come to form a cyst. In the skin the result of this is a space lined by epidermis and containing sebaceous material, degenerated epithelium, etc. Such a cyst is known as a *sequestration dermoid*, not to be confused with the teratomatous "dermoids" of the ovary (p. 842). Sequestration dermoid cysts occur most often in the middle line of the chest and neck and at the outer and inner angles of the orbit—in short, along the lines of closure of the embryonic fissures. Occasionally an epithelial-lined cyst may be found in the brain, and is apparently the result of dislocation of ependymal epithelium, and in the meninges one may rarely see cysts lined by a simple stratified squamous epithelium and filled with squames and cholesterol crystals, the so-called "pearly tumours" of Cruveilhier. Cysts occur in connection with the brain and spinal cord from an imperfect closure of the neural tube and its mesodermal envelope. Meningocele, encephalocele, and some forms of spina bifida belong to this group.

(b) Cysts may be due also to *non-closure of vestigial clefts, ducts or tubules*, which ought normally to become obliterated in the course of development. A cyst may form in this way from a branchial cleft or from the thyroglossal duct, urachus, vitelline duct, tunica vaginalis, etc.

Cysts of various embryological remnants are common in the internal genitalia of both sexes, though most are too small to be of any consequence.

(2) Acquired cysts. These are of several varieties, the three following being the most important:

(a) Cysts formed by retention of secretion produced by obstruction to the outflow—*retention cysts*. A single cyst, sometimes large, may be produced by the obstruction of the main duct, e.g. of a salivary gland or of a part of the pancreas. Obstruction of the orifice of a hair follicle gives rise to a cyst-like swelling filled chiefly with breaking-down keratin—the so-called sebaceous cyst, seen especially in the scalp. On the other hand, numerous small cysts may result from obstruction of small ducts, an occurrence which is not uncommon in fibrosing lesions of the kidney.

(b) Cysts may be formed from natural enclosed spaces, and are then called *distension and exudation cysts*. They occur in the thyroid from dilatation of the acini, and occasionally also in the pituitary: cystic dilatation of Graafian follicles in the ovaries is also common. Distension of spaces lined by mesothelium is also seen; for example, a bursa may enlarge to form a cystic swelling, and there is the common condition of hydrocele due to an accumulation of fluid in the tunica vaginalis.

Occasionally in the adult an *implantation cyst* occurs by the dislocation inwards of a portion of epidermis by injury. The epithelium grows and comes to line a space filled with degenerate epithelial squames (Fig. 12.29); rarely hair follicles are present in the wall. Implantation

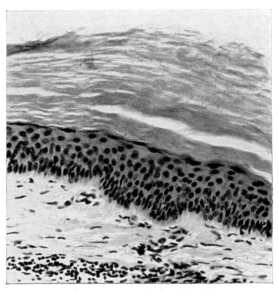

Fig. 12.29.—Section of implantation cyst in subcutaneous tissue, showing lining of stratified squamous epithelium and keratin in the lumen. × 200.

cysts may result also from wounds of the cornea.

(c) *Parasitic cysts.* These are cystic stages in the life cycle of cestode *parasites*. The most striking examples are the "hydatid" cysts produced by *Taenia echinococcus*, though small cysts may be produced in the brain and other parts by the cysticerci of *Taenia solium*.

CHAPTER 13

BLOOD VESSELS AND LYMPHATICS

ARTERIES

Introduction

Lesions of the arteries are very important because of their frequency and serious consequences. The commonest important disease is *atheroma*, which consists of prolonged, slow, patchy deposition of lipids with fibrosis of the intima of arteries of various sizes. The patchy thickening results in narrowing of the lumen with consequent chronic ischaemia of the various organs and tissues. Acute ischaemia can result from the occlusion of an artery by local thrombosis or embolism; these processes have been dealt with in Chapter 8, but it is important to emphasise here that arterial thrombosis is usually the result of disease of the artery wall, and atheroma is the commonest predisposing cause.

Another very common arterial change is termed *arteriosclerosis*. This is a diffuse change in the walls of arteries, in which the muscle and elastic tissue slowly diminish and are replaced by fibrous tissue, with the result that the arteries become more firm and rigid. These changes occur in various degrees with increasing age, but they are aggravated and accelerated by systemic hypertension in which the fibrous replacement is preceded, at least in some instances, by hypertrophy of muscle and elastic tissue. Arteriosclerosis alone is usually without serious consequences, but the accompanying changes in the arterioles—*arteriolosclerosis*—result in ischaemia, particularly of the kidneys. It should be mentioned that some writers apply the term arteriosclerosis to any condition causing increased firmness of the walls of arteries or arterioles: such usage, in which arteriosclerosis

would include atheroma, medial calcification (p. 276) and arteriolosclerosis, has led to considerable confusion between these conditions, and we prefer to restrict use of the term to the changes described above.

A very common and important condition which affects the arteries and arterioles is *systemic hypertension*. In most cases, the cause of the rise in blood pressure is not known, but it is likely that, in all instances, the rise is mediated by increased muscle tone in the arterioles. Prolonged hypertension, as mentioned above, leads to severe arteriosclerosis and arteriolosclerosis; it is by far the commonest cause of rupture of the cerebral arteries to produce haemorrhage into the brain, and is an important cause of heart failure.

Diseases of the arteries which bring about severe destruction of the muscle and elastic tissue, particularly of the media, may weaken the wall to such an extent that dilatation results, and if localised this is termed an *aneurysm*; rupture of the vessel wall may occur, with or without preceding dilatation. Severe weakening can result from various forms of *arteritis*, including that due to syphilis, but also from atheroma and from degenerative changes of unknown nature in the media. All three of these conditions can give rise to aortic aneurysm. Aneurysm formation and rupture may result also from developmental defects, as seen in the arteries at the base of the brain. Another effect of the various types of arteritis is to promote thrombosis, although atheroma is a much more important cause of this in certain arteries.

Effects of ageing. In the assessment of arterial lesions it must be considered to what extent the condition of the arteries can be attributed to the normal ageing process. In the arterial wall the normal adult has proportionately more fibrous tissue and less muscle than a child, and as

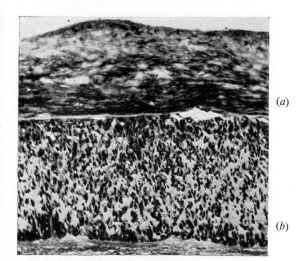

(a)

(b)

FIG. 13.1.—Longitudinal section of hypertrophied artery, showing hypertrophy of muscle in inner and middle coats.

The muscle fibres are stained darkly: *a*, longitudinal muscle fibres in intima; *b*, media. × 110.

the larger arteries become more fibrous and less elastic in later years they normally become less distensible and the lumina are dilated. As age advances there is also a progressive but histologically inapparent increase in the amount of calcium in the arterial wall. The alterations of arteries in ageing are sometimes intensified or accelerated by other arterial disease.

Adaptation and hypertrophy. The muscular and elastic nature of the arterial wall readily permits dilatation to provide an increased blood flow to the part supplied. If the requirement is more than temporary the lumen becomes persistently dilated and there is hypertrophy of the muscular and elastic tissue, e.g. the physiological hypertrophy of the uterine arteries during pregnancy. Analogous compensatory hypertrophy is seen in the walls of collateral vessels when a main artery is obstructed.

In persistent hypertension, a state in which the arterial blood pressure is abnormally raised, the tendency for the increased pressure to dilate and lengthen the arteries is partly prevented by compensatory hypertrophy of the circular muscle of the media and the intimal longitudinal muscle fibres which lie next to the internal elastic lamina

(Fig. 13.1). The vascular changes in hypertension are described in more detail on p. 270.

Endarteritis obliterans. Intimal thickening of arteries and arterioles occurs when well-vascularised concentric laminae of cellular connective tissue form in the intima and obliterate or narrow the arterial lumen. New elastic tissue is laid down independently of the internal elastic lamina and may appear as a layer under the endothelium or as a number of small new laminae at various points in the intima. This lesion is called *obliterative endarteritis* and is found near chronic peptic ulcers and tuberculous cavities (Fig. 13.2). In these circumstances it is beneficial in tending to prevent haemorrhage. It is due to external irritation, for similar lesions are seen in syphilis (the spirochaetes spread in the perivascular lymphatics),

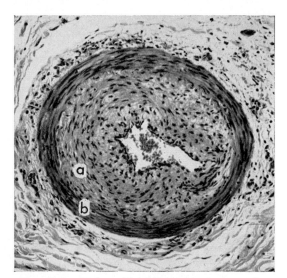

FIG. 13.2.—Endarteritis obliterans in the base of a chronic peptic ulcer.
a = intima, *b* = media

in tuberculous meningitis (Fig. 20.25, p. 631), and in silicosis. It is prominent also in small renal arteries in severe hypertension and in progressive systemic sclerosis.

When the functional requirements for blood flow through an artery are greatly reduced the lumen is narrowed by obliterative endarteritis which is the physiological mechanism of arterial involution. It occurs, for example, in the umbilical arteries and ductus arteriosus after birth and in the uterine and ovarian arteries after the menopause. The intimal fibrous tissue may be more collagenous and less cellular in these circumstances. Small renal arteries supplying an area destroyed by disease also show obliterative endarteritis.

Atheroma

Definition. The lesions of atheroma consist of patches of intimal thickening of the walls of arteries, due mainly to deposition of lipids and formation of fibrous tissue. The alternative term *atherosclerosis* (which literally means hard porridge) is inappropriate, particularly in Scotland, and its use has served merely to confuse the subject.

Naked-eye appearances. The early lesions are visible on the luminal surface of the walls of arteries as yellow patches, scarcely raised above the surface, and sometimes called *fatty streaks* or *patches*: they vary in diameter from 1 mm. up to several centimetres in the aorta and larger arteries. They are due to deposition of lipids in the intima (Fig. 13.3), and occur at all ages,

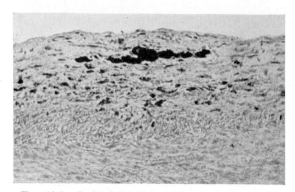

Fig. 13.3.—Intimal lipid deposit in the aorta of child aged 11, accidental death. × 115.

even in children who have died from injury or various other causes. At this stage, the changes may be reversible, but there is no proof of this. As the condition progresses, the patches enlarge and thicken by further deposition of lipid deep in the intima and by fibrosis more superficially adjacent to the lumen: the patches become distinctly raised and when viewed from the intimal surface they may appear yellow or white depending on the amount of fibrous tissue overlying the lipid deposits. In affluent communities, atheroma is often present in young adults and is

virtually always present in some degree in middle-aged and old people. In any one individual, the patches are at various stages of development, suggesting progressive formation.

Aorta. Atheroma occurs throughout the length of the aorta, but the abdominal aorta is usually most severely affected and patches often develop first around the origins of the intercostal and lumbar branches (Fig. 13.4): the plaques vary in size up to several centimetres diameter and may in places become confluent. If a sizeable plaque is cut across, lipid-rich paste-like

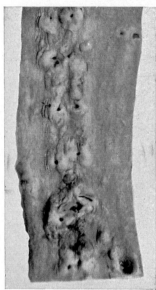

Fig. 13.4.—Atheroma of the aorta, showing irregular patches of thickening, especially round the orifices of the branches. × $\frac{2}{3}$.

material can be expressed from its deeper part, and fibrous thickening is seen as a white layer overlying this. The fibrous layer may break down, resulting in ulceration of the plaque, and mural thrombus is then likely to be deposited on the ulcerated surface; another common change is deposition of calcium salts which may convert the plaque to a hard brittle plate. Plaques showing ulceration, calcification or thrombus deposition are commonly referred to as *complicated atheroma*, and may produce great irregularity of the luminal surface of the aorta. Another important feature of aortic plaques is thinning of the overlying media, and in some instances extension of the plaque into the adjacent media: the wall is thus weakened and an aneurysm may result and even rupture (p. 285).

Other arteries. Atheroma occurs in arteries of all sizes down to approx. 2 mm. diam. and is seen occasionally in mild form in even smaller vessels. The features are similar to those seen in the aorta except that the plaques are necessarily smaller, often involve the whole circumference of the intima, and can cause all degrees of luminal narrowing down to virtual occlusion (Figs. 13.5, 13.6, 13.7). Atheroma tends to affect especially arteries supplying the heart, brain and abdominal viscera, and also the carotids and arteries of the lower limbs. There is considerable individual variation in its distri-

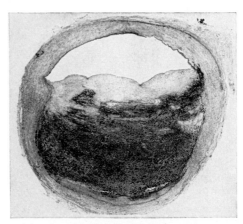

FIG. 13.6.—Severe atheroma of the superior mesenteric artery, causing marked reduction of the lumen.

Frozen section, stained with Scharlach R, showing the large amount of fatty material in the patch. × 10.

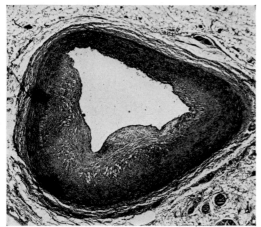

FIG. 13.5.—Coronary artery showing atheroma of moderate degree. The small spaces in the deeper part of the plaque represent lipid deposition. × 10.

bution, in some instances the aorta being mainly affected, in others the arteries at the base of the brain and/or the coronary arteries. The coronary arteries are often severely affected and are more often involved at a relatively early age than any other arteries. The cerebral arteries also are subject to severe atheroma, but this is found chiefly in elderly persons. For reasons which are unknown the renal arteries are seldom severely affected except in diabetics, in whom atheroma is often widespread and very severe.

In the smaller arteries, e.g. those of the brain, the patches are visible from both inner and outer aspects of the vessels, and their yellow opaque appearance contrasts with the reddish translucency of the normal parts of the vessel wall (Fig. 13.8). Thrombosis over a plaque in a small artery frequently causes occlusion and, as in the aorta, rupture of the fibrous layer may occur, with tracking of blood into the underlying lipid deposits.

Microscopic appearances. The early changes, consisting of fatty streaks or patches, are due to accumulation of lipids in proliferated spindle cells, shown by electron microscopy to be smooth muscle cells, lying in the intima (Fig. 13.9). Lipids also accumulate between cells deep in the intima, particularly in relation to elastic fibres and the internal elastic lamina. As the patch develops, thin laminae of connective tissue are found in the more superficial part of the intima and form the fibrous part of the lesion. Lipid-containing cells lie among the collagen

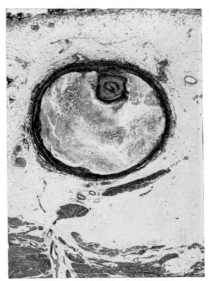

FIG. 13.7.—Extreme atheromatous narrowing of left coronary artery in a case of myxoedema.

The tiny residual lumen is closed by recent thrombosis. × 6·5.

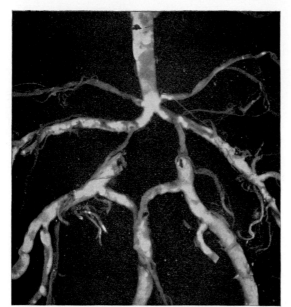

FIG. 13.8.—Circle of Willis and branches, showing marked patchy atheroma.

fibres in this region. Areas of necrosis then develop, converting the deep part of the patch into a structureless accumulation of lipids, tissue debris (Fig. 13.11) and sometimes altered blood, and the necrosis gradually extends into the overlying fibrous tissue. Calcium deposition may be visible microscopically. Infiltration of neutrophil leukocytes and other inflammatory cells is common, and lipid-laden macrophages—"foamy cells"—may appear around the lipid deposits,

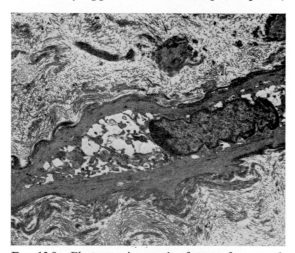

FIG. 13.9.—Electron micrograph of part of a smooth muscle cell in an atheromatous plaque. The cytoplasm is made up largely of myofibrils, and contains globules of fat, shown as light spaces. The fine fibres on either side of the cell are collagen. × 7500.

which usually contain crystals of cholesterol, represented in paraffin section by the typical elongated clefts (Fig. 13.10). The internal elastic lamina deep to the plaque usually fragments and lipid deposition, necrosis and fibrosis may then extend into the adjacent media. Quite apart from this, the media deep to the plaque becomes thinned and atrophic (Fig. 13.11).

Small blood vessels grow into the atheromatous patch from the adventitia of the affected vessel and sometimes also from the intimal surface. These may be the source of the haemorrhage which commonly occurs in the patch, although, as already stated, the overlying fibrous patch may be very thin and may rupture, allowing blood to track in from the lumen.

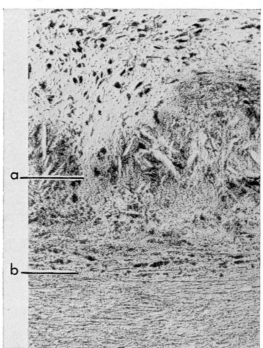

FIG. 13.10.—Advanced atheroma of the aorta, showing degenerate material in deeper part of intima.
The spindle-shaped spaces are due to collections of cholesterol crystals. *a*, intima; *b*, media. × 110.

Chemical analysis of the lipids of atheroma have shown that cholesterol esters and unesterified cholesterol, with smaller amounts of triglycerides and phospholipids, make up the bulk of the lipids within the plaques. Their composition closely resembles that of the low density lipoproteins of the plasma except in the most advanced lesions where there is a disproportionate increase in the quantity of unesterified cholesterol.

Effects

Large arteries. Uncomplicated atheroma of large arteries, such as the aorta, very often has no clinical effect because usually it does not substantially reduce the lumen or seriously weaken the wall. In advanced cases, however, there may be aneurysm formation in the abdominal aorta (p. 285). Thrombi which form on ulcerated

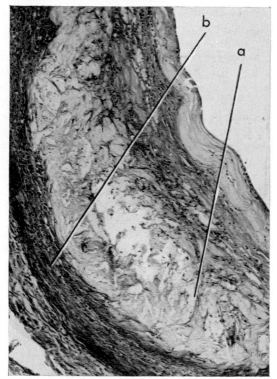

FIG. 13.11.—Atheroma of cerebral artery, showing great thickening of the intima with degeneration in its inner part.

a, degenerate material; *b*, atrophied media. × 110.

plaques in the aorta seldom cause complete occlusion, probably because the rapid flow prevents platelet aggregation. Occasionally, however, thrombus may extend to occlude the whole aortic lumen and when this occurs at the bifurcation it can result in gangrene of the legs unless adequate collateral circulation has developed. The patient may then experience merely coldness and weakness of the legs with muscle wasting and impotence but without ischaemic pain or gangrene (Leriche syndrome). Apart from occluding the aorta, thrombi and even atheromatous debris from ulcerated plaques may break away and form emboli in the arteries of the lower limbs and peripheral organs such as the kidneys.

Smaller arteries. By far the commonest important effects of atheroma are due to involvement of smaller arteries, the lumen of which may be progressively narrowed by an atheromatous patch, or suddenly occluded by superadded thrombosis (Fig. 13.7). These effects are well seen in the coronary arteries. Atheroma is the chief cause of ischaemic heart disease, the largest single cause of death in Europe and North America today (p. 300). Ischaemic brain damage is also very common and is usually the result of atheroma of the carotid, vertebral and basilar arteries and the vessels of the Circle of Willis (p. 623).

Peripheral arteries. Atheroma of the arteries of the legs often causes progressive diminution in blood supply. Eventually the collateral circulation becomes inadequate: relative muscle ischaemia can then be induced by the increased metabolic demands of exercise, which produces severe pain in the leg, relieved by rest. This is the clinical syndrome of *intermittent claudication.* In time ischaemia may be so severe as to cause gangrene, which usually starts in the toes and spreads proximally. Examination of legs amputated for gangrene usually shows narrowing or obliteration and calcification of the main arteries of the leg. Because atheroma is often widespread, patients with severe involvement of the arteries of the lower limbs frequently suffer also from ischaemic heart disease (p. 265). The arteries of the arms are rarely severely affected by atheroma.

Etiology

Many factors lead to the development of atheroma. Its patchy nature indicates that local factors are involved, and the siting of the earliest lesions at bends and branching points suggests that local stresses in the arterial wall or turbulence of blood flow are important initially.

A study of atheromatous lesions at different stages shows that the early change is deposition of fatty material in the intima and that the fibrous thickening occurs later, perhaps as a result of irritation due to the lipid or as a compensatory change when the vessel has been weakened; the general tendency to fibrosis with ageing may be a contributory factor.

The arterial intima has no vasa vasorum and is nourished by seepage of plasma through the endothelium. The "filtration theory" of atherogenesis explains the site of the early deposits by assuming that lipids filtered from the lumen are unable to penetrate the internal elastic lamina. If the lipids are not removed as quickly as they accumulate, atheromatous deposits will then occur. This explanation is supported by chemical analysis of the deposited lipids, which resemble those of the plasma lipoproteins. Duguid has revived the theory of Rokitansky (1852) that atheromatous lesions of the aorta and coronary arteries may result from small thrombi quite commonly found on the arterial lining; these are quickly incorporated in the intima by growth of endothelium over the surface and later they are converted into fibrous tissue with variable degrees of lipid accumulation in the deeper layers. Some intimal lesions probably do originate in this way. Fibrin and platelet constituents can be demonstrated by immunological methods within atheromatous plaques, findings which suggest that mural thrombosis contributes to their development. However, the thrombogenic theory of atherogenesis does not readily explain the gross accumulations of lipids which are such an important feature of atheroma, and it is probably not the whole explanation of the origin of the lesions.

The underlying cause of atheroma is not fully understood but it is clear that a number of factors determine the onset and distribution.

Age. Necropsy studies have shown that atheroma increases with advancing age except in extreme old age. This suggests that atheroma is a cumulative effect of causal factors operating usually over long periods. The somewhat reduced incidence of atheroma in very old people, and the great variations in severity in individuals within the same age group, however, indicate that the disease is not entirely dependent on age.

Sex. Atheroma is more severe in males than in females of the same age. Women do not usually develop it in severe degree until after the menopause, when it progresses as in men. This is believed to be related to the known effects of oestrogens on lipid metabolism, and explains why serious effects of atheroma generally occur earlier in men than women. Castration or the administration of oestrogens lower the serum cholesterol in males.

Local mechanical factors. Atheroma may develop in almost any artery but is more common and severe in certain situations; this indicates that local factors determine the site of formation. The distribution of lipid deposits around the orifices of arteries and in various smaller vessels which are poorly supported (e.g. the coronary, cerebral and splenic arteries) suggests the importance of local shearing strain, which may lead to loosening of the sub-endothelial connective tissue. This may explain the tendency for the disease to be most marked in the lowest part of the aorta.

Blood pressure. Atheroma is commonly found in the systemic arteries in patients with normal blood pressure but is intensified in patients with hypertension. The effect of hypertension is well shown in cases of coarctation of the aorta; in the segment proximal to the stenosis the blood pressure is raised and atheroma is more severe than in the distal segment where the blood pressure is low. In the pulmonary arteries atheroma develops early in patients with chronic pulmonary hypertension (e.g. with mitral stenosis).

Metabolic factors. Several facts suggest abnormal lipid metabolism is important in the genesis of atheroma. (1) The earliest recognisable atheromatous lesions are lipid in nature. (2) Atheroma is increased in severity in patients with hyperlipoproteinaemia (e.g. in diabetes mellitus, myxoedema, familial hypercholesterolaemia and xanthomatosis or the nephrotic syndrome). (3) Cachectic patients at necropsy have usually only mild atheroma. (4) Atheroma and its complications are more prevalent in wealthy societies than in undernourished communities. (5) Lesions closely resembling atheroma can be produced by the administration of large quantities of cholesterol to rabbits (which being herbivorous have a low blood cholesterol). Similar lesions are produced in dogs only when thyroid function is simultaneously reduced, as by the use of thiouracil.

The serum cholesterol level is related to severe atheroma and its complications. More elaborate physico-chemical investigations of lipid metabolism have been made in living subjects with a history of coronary artery occlusion, but there is no test applicable during life by which the severity (or presence) of uncomplicated atheroma can be established and the "normal" controls in many of these studies are likely to have atheroma even of severe degree; furthermore coronary occlusion usually results from thrombosis of an atheromatous vessel and any metabolic abnormality demonstrable in such studies may be more closely related to an *in vivo* thrombotic tendency or failure of fibrinolysis than to the atheromatous lesions themselves.

Studies on the mechanisms of lipid transport in the plasma show that this is effected by linkage of the cholesterol and phospholipid with α- and β-globulins, and that the resulting lipoproteins can be separated by chromatography and by the ultracentrifuge into a graded series depending on their lipid content and molecular size, the α-lipoproteins consisting of 35 per cent lipid and the β-lipoproteins about 75 per cent lipid. Quantitative differences in the proportions of the various factors and in the cholesterol-phospholipid ratio are found between men and women and between the subjects of coronary artery occlusion and normal persons. In atheroma, the proportion of plasma cholesterol carried on the β-lipoprotein is abnormally high. A diet rich in animal fat and cholesterol leads to distinctive changes in the lipoprotein pattern owing to increased transport of lipids by proteins of certain molecular sizes which normally form only a small fraction of the plasma lipoproteins. It has been claimed that the tendency to the formation of atheromatous deposits is associated with increase in this precise fraction of the lipoproteins (the "atherogenic" fraction) rather than with increase in the total plasma cholesterol, but this view is not generally accepted. Rabbits rendered atheromatous by cholesterol feeding develop marked elevation of the level of atherogenic lipoprotein in the plasma but less elevation of plasma phospholipid. Rabbits rendered diabetic by alloxan, and subsequently fed cholesterol, fail to develop atheroma, but this failure is perhaps due to absence of a rise in the atherogenic lipoproteins and to an equivalent rise in phospholipid so that the cholesterol-phospholipid ratio remains about normal.

In man it has been shown that the elevated cholesterol-phospholipid ratio and abnormal lipoprotein pattern can be modified towards the normal levels by the administration of certain hormones, especially oestrogens and thyroxin; but their usefulness is limited in practice by undesirable side-effects and the severity of the established lesions. The atherogenic lipoproteins and total cholesterol can also be reduced by diminishing the amount of animal and saturated fats in the diet, and by substituting unsaturated fats. It is not known whether this effect is mediated by the degree of unsaturation, by specific unsaturated acids, or by unsaponifiable fractions and unidentified sterols.

Smoking. There is a substantially greater mortality rate from coronary artery disease in cigarette smokers than in individuals who have never smoked or have given up smoking. The death rate correlates well with the number of cigarettes smoked. A factor of this sort may explain the increased death rate from ischaemic heart disease during the present century despite the lack of change in incidence of calcification of the coronary arteries as determined by necropsy.

Physical activity may be related to the incidence of complicated atheroma for it has been shown that people with sedentary occupations generally suffer more from coronary artery disease than those with strenuous jobs.

Psychological factors may be important by their effect on choice of occupation, smoking or eating habits or in some other way.

Systemic hypertension

Definition

Blood pressure usually increases with age but there is considerable individual variation in the increase, and recordings of the blood pressures in a general adult population show a wide range. Any definition of hypertension must therefore be arbitrary, and there is no general agreement on the level of blood pressure to be regarded as pathological. There is, however, good evidence, for example from insurance companies' statistics, of a general inverse relationship between the height of the blood pressure and the expectation of life.

Classification

In about 85 per cent of cases of hypertension the cause is not apparent and these patients are said to be suffering from *essential or idiopathic* hypertension. In the remaining 15 per cent hypertension is *secondary* to other disease processes: nearly always diseases of the kidneys are responsible ("*renal hypertension*") but occasional cases result from certain functioning adrenal tumours or as a feature of Cushing's syndrome (see Table 13.1). Coarctation of the aorta

Table 13.1. Classification of systemic hypertension

I. Essential { benign
             { malignant
II. Secondary { benign
              { malignant
  (*a*) of renal origin ("renal hypertension"), due to:
      chronic pyelonephritis
      glomerulonephritis
      diabetes
      polycystic disease of the kidneys
      renal amyloidosis
      connective tissue diseases, particularly poly-
          arteritis
      urinary tract obstruction (occasional cases)
      renal artery disease
      radiation nephritis
      some renal tumours
      some congenital diseases of kidney, possibly
          by predisposing to pyelonephritis
  (*b*) adrenal-mediated hypertension.
      Conn's syndrome (primary hyperaldosteron-
          ism)
      Cushing's syndrome
      phaeochromocytoma
  (*c*) coarctation of the aorta.

(p. 323) is accompanied by hypertension in the arteries arising proximal to the constriction. It is likely that, as diagnostic techniques improve, further causes of hypertension will be identified, and the proportion of patients with so-called essential hypertension will thus become smaller. Conn's syndrome (primary hyperaldosteronism, p. 912) is an example of a condition which has recently been distinguished from essential hypertension.

Regardless of the etiology, hypertension may be divided into *benign* and *malignant* types. In benign hypertension the rise of blood pressure is usually moderate, although sometimes marked. Many patients with benign hypertension lead active lives for many years with few or no symptoms, and may die of some independent disease. Frequently, however, it brings about disability and death from heart failure, and it increases the risk of myocardial infarction and cerebral vascular accidents.

Malignant hypertension is characterised by a very high blood pressure, by eye changes which include retinal haemorrhages, exudates and papilloedema, by rapidly progressive renal injury terminating in uraemia, and by hypertensive encephalopathy. The pathological hallmark of this state is fibrinoid necrosis of arterioles (see later). These special features appear to depend on the rapid development of a very high blood pressure. Unless treated, patients with malignant hypertension usually die within six months or so, but frequently the blood pressure can be reduced by anti-hypertensive drugs, and the outlook is then greatly improved.

Benign and malignant hypertension should not be regarded as independent conditions. Malignant hypertension supervenes in about 10 per cent of cases of benign essential hypertension and is commoner than this in patients with renal hypertension. Hence it is sometimes referred to as the *malignant* or *accelerated* phase of hypertension. However, it can also arise apparently *de novo*, i.e. without evidence of preceding benign hypertension.

Changes in the blood vessels

In addition to left ventricular hypertrophy (p. 298) changes develop in arterial vessels of all sizes as a result of hypertension. In the larger arteries, from the aorta down to vessels of about 1 mm. diameter, the changes are widespread, and are termed *hypertensive arteriosclerosis*. Changes in the vessels below this size, i.e. in the smallest arteries and arterioles, tend to affect especially the small vessels of the viscera, and in particular those of the kidneys. The changes occurring in the larger arteries are of the same nature in all types of hypertension, but those in the smaller vessels, particularly the arterioles, are different in benign and malignant types of hypertension, and require separate descriptions.

Large and medium sized arteries. The vascular changes in hypertension, uncomplicated by the arterial lesions common in the aged, are most readily studied in young patients with high blood pressure secondary to renal disease. *In the early stages* they consist mainly of hypertrophy of smooth muscle and elastic fibres. In the aorta, there is increase in both of these elements in the media. In muscular arteries the increase is mainly in the circular muscle of the media (Fig. 13.13) but also in the longitudinal muscle fibres of the intima; the internal elastic lamina becomes thickened, and very often new laminae

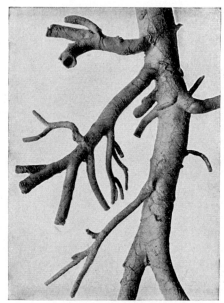

FIG. 13.12.—Aorta and arterial branches in hypertensive arteriosclerosis.

Note the relative enlargement of the branches and thickening of their walls. The patient (age 36) suffered from chronic glomerulonephritis. × ¼.

are formed towards the intima (Fig. 13.14). In *longstanding* hypertension, which is usually of benign essential type, these hypertrophic changes give way to fibrous replacement of muscle and the elastic tissue may break up and undergo partial absorption. The arterial walls are thickened and of increased rigidity, the lumina are dilated (Fig. 13.12) and the vessels are often elongated and tortuous. In the aorta, there is increase in the elastic and fibrous tissue of the

media. In the muscular arteries, the media is thickened and fibrosed with patchy loss of smooth muscle, and there may be fibrous thickening of the intima (Fig. 13.15). These changes are widespread, and vary in degree. They are without important effects, but in the brain they may be associated with formation of multiple micro-aneurysms of deep penetrating arteries, and rupture of these is the usual cause of cerebral haemorrhage (p. 288). Hypertension also increases the risk of rupture of the larger "berry" aneurysms which develop in the arteries at the base of the brain in some individuals (p. 287) resulting in subarachnoid haemorrhage.

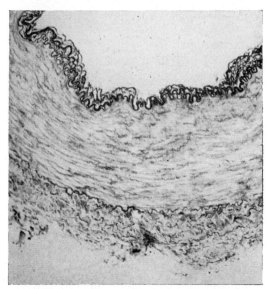

FIG. 13.14.—Another section of the same artery as in Fig. 13.13, showing increase of elastic tissue formed by splitting of the internal elastic lamina.

Elastic tissue stained black. × 110.

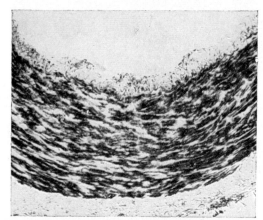

FIG. 13.13.—Section of hypertrophied radial artery, from a case of chronic glomerulonephritis in a young subject, showing hypertrophy of the media.

The muscle fibres appear black. × 100.

The arteriosclerotic changes described above are similar to those observed in normotensive elderly subjects (*senile arteriosclerosis*) but in the absence of hypertension they are usually less pronounced, and the media, although fibrosed, is often not thickened.

Atheroma tends to be particularly severe in individuals with chronic hypertension, and there is no doubt that prolonged elevation of the blood pressure aggravates this condition.

Hypertension thus results at first in hypertrophy of the arterial walls, with increase in muscle and elastic fibres, followed by arteriosclerosis and a tendency to severe atheroma.

The early hypertrophic changes are usually observed only in young hypertensive subjects: in older patients with chronic hypertension, arteriosclerosis and atheroma predominate.

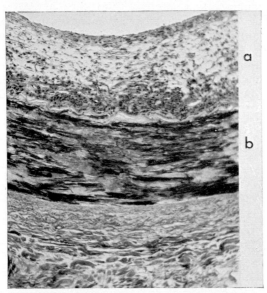

FIG. 13.15.—Medium-sized artery in arteriosclerosis.

a, thickened intima; *b*, media in which the muscle fibres stained dark are partly replaced by fibrous tissue. × 120.

Small arteries and arterioles. In arteries of 1 mm. diameter or less, and in the arterioles, the changes differ from those in the larger vessels, and they differ also in benign and malignant hypertension.

(*a*) *Benign hypertension.* The small arteries show the medial thickening seen in the larger vessels, but a more pronounced degree of intimal thickening, due to concentric increase in connective tissue; in the smallest arteries the intimal change predominates, and may result in narrowing of the lumen in contrast to the dilatation seen in the larger arteries.

The *arterioles* undergo *hyaline thickening* of their walls (*hyaline arteriolosclerosis*), which consists at first of patchy deposition of hyaline material, often beneath the endothelium, but sometimes more peripherally: the hyaline change gradually extends to involve the whole circumference, and when severe it replaces the normal structures of the wall apart from the endothelium. This change occurs also apart from hypertension, and is seen especially in old age. In both normotensive and hypertensive subjects it is observed most commonly in arterioles in the spleen, then in the afferent glomerular arterioles

of the kidneys (Fig. 13.16), and in the pancreas, liver and adrenal capsules. In all these sites, the change is appreciably commoner and usually more severe in hypertensives than in normotensive subjects of corresponding ages. Hyaline arteriolosclerosis is uncommon in the arterioles of the brain, gastro-intestinal tract, pituitary, thyroid, heart, skin and skeletal muscles (Smith, 1956).

When severe, hyaline arteriolosclerosis results in considerable narrowing of the arteriolar lumen. This has important effects upon the kidneys (p. 685). The nature of the change is not fully understood: initially, the hyaline material resembles fibrin in its staining properties, but later it stains like collagen. It also contains lipid material, and there is evidence that it may result from an exudative process in which plasma seeps into the arteriolar wall (p. 686). Apart from its occurrence as an ageing process and in hypertensive subjects, hyaline arteriolosclerosis is often severe and extensive in diabetes mellitus (p. 718).

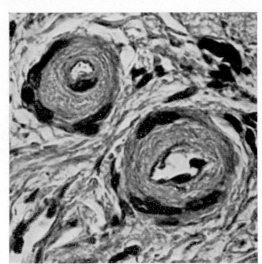

FIG. 13.16.—Hyaline arteriolosclerosis of afferent glomerular arteriole in chronic systemic hypertension. × 1500.

(*b*) *Malignant hypertension.* In this condition, the concentric fibrous thickening of the intima of the small arteries is often of extreme degree, particularly in the interlobular arteries of the kidneys (Fig. 21.10, p. 688). The arterioles are thickened and of hyaline appearance, as in benign hypertension, but the change is relatively acute, and consists of necrosis of the arteriolar wall, accompanied by permeation with plasma and deposition of fibrin (*fibrinoid necrosis*): pyknotic nuclei, neutrophil polymorphs and red cells can often be found in the necrotic wall. The lumen is considerably narrowed, and superadded thrombosis may complete its occlusion. These changes affect especially the viscera, and the arteriolar lesions may result in haemorrhages and in ischaemic necrosis (Fig. 13.17). Focal

The condition may be symptomless, and many cases come to light during routine medical examination for insurance or other purposes. Common symptoms include palpitations, audible pulsation in the head, headaches, attacks of dizziness particularly on stooping, and reduced exercise tolerance.

Approximately 60 per cent of deaths in

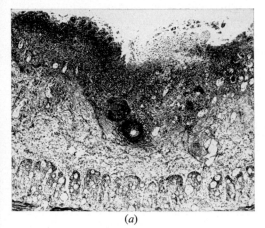

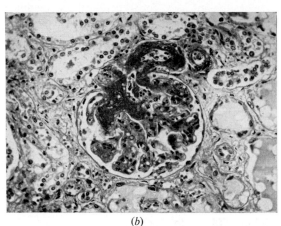

(a) (b)

FIG. 13.17.—Malignant hypertension.

(a) An arteriole in the submucosa of the colon shows fibrinoid necrosis and thrombosis. The overlying mucosa is ulcerated.
(b) The afferent arteriole and part of the glomerular capillary tuft are infiltrated with eosinophilic fibrinoid material.

fibrinoid necrosis may develop also in the small arteries.

In both benign and malignant hypertension, the changes in the small vessels in the kidneys bring about renal damage as described on pp. 685 to 689.

Course of benign and of malignant hypertension

Benign essential hypertension. As already stated, this is much the commonest type of hypertension. The blood pressure rises very gradually over a period of years, in most cases to moderately high levels, e.g. 180/110 mm. Hg but occasionally much higher. The increase nearly always starts before the age of 45 years, and individuals with a resting blood pressure consistently below 140/85 at this age are very unlikely to develop essential hypertension. The diastolic pressure is less subject to physiological variations than the systolic pressure, and a diastolic pressure persistently exceeding 90 mm. Hg is generally regarded as abnormal. However, the disease develops very slowly, and it may be some years before the rise in pressure clearly exceeds that which occurs normally with age.

patients with benign essential hypertension are from left ventricular or total heart failure (p. 296), and this is due to the increased work load thrown on the left ventricle and the commonly associated severe coronary atheroma. About 30 per cent of patients die from cerebral haemorrhage (p. 619), and the remainder from various causes unrelated to the hypertension. Although changes occur in the kidneys as a result of the vascular lesions, renal failure is uncommon in benign essential hypertension, although when heart failure develops, there is usually a moderate rise in the blood urea level. In those patients who progress from benign to malignant hypertension renal failure commonly supervenes.

Malignant essential hypertension. This develops in approximately 10 per cent of cases of benign essential hypertension. In those cases not preceded by benign hypertension, the onset is usually between 30 and 45 years. It can result in heart failure or cerebral haemorrhage, but without effective treatment *renal injury* is severe and usually causes death within a few months (p. 687).

Eye changes are another important feature in

malignant hypertension: lesions in the small arteries in the retina result in oedema, haemorrhages, infarcts and exudates, and blindness may ensue. Papilloedema, associated with cerebral oedema, is usually present. Hypertensive encephalopathy, characterised by epileptiform fits and transient paralysis is not uncommon, and is attributable to cerebral oedema, resulting from arterial spasm and focal cerebral ischaemia. This has been observed directly in rats with experimental hypertension and the fits have been shown to cease when the blood pressure is lowered and cerebral vasoconstriction ceases.

Secondary hypertension. Hypertension is a feature of chronic renal failure, and is more often of malignant type than is the case in essential hypertension. The superadded imposition of further renal injury from hypertensive vascular lesions, whether benign or malignant, aggravates and accelerates renal failure.

Etiology of hypertension

It is likely that increase in peripheral resistance is the basic causal factor in all cases of hypertension. In normal circumstances the peripheral resistance is controlled by the muscular tone in the arterioles throughout the body, and the major etiological problem is the elucidation of the factors which, by increasing arteriolar tone, bring about the various types of hypertension. The possibility that the structural changes of arteriolosclerosis initiate the hypertensive state is extremely unlikely, for such changes are sometimes absent, particularly in early cases, and moreover structural changes do not develop in arterioles which are protected from hypertension by occlusive changes in the larger arteries supplying them. For these reasons, it is widely accepted that the observed structural changes in the arteries and arterioles are the result of hypertension, and not the cause. It is likely, however, that structural changes in the arterioles and small arteries of the kidneys impair renal blood flow, and this may play a part in maintaining hypertension once the vascular changes have become pronounced.

Humoral vasoconstrictive factors. In patients with hypertension due to a phaeochromocytoma, the large amounts of catecholamines released by the tumour into the blood (see p. 917) are very likely to be the cause of the hypertension.

The vasoconstrictor substances renin and angiotensin (p. 185) may contribute to the increase of blood pressure in malignant hypertension secondary to renal disease, as plasma concentrations of these substances are increased in this state. By contrast, the levels of plasma renin in most patients with benign essential hypertension are quite normal, and in patients with Conn's syndrome (primary aldosteronism, p. 912) plasma renin concentration is actually reduced. It cannot be concluded from this that renin and angiotensin do not contribute to the increased blood pressure in these conditions, as sensitivity to the pressor effects of injected angiotensin is known to be increased in hypertensive patients, and thus the normal or subnormal amounts of angiotensin in the blood might conceivably raise the blood pressure to abnormal levels.

Search for other vasoactive substances in the blood of patients with hypertension has failed.

Renal hypertension. A firm experimental basis for renal hypertension was provided in 1934 by Goldblatt and his colleagues, who showed that partial clamping of the renal arteries produced hypertension in dogs. This has been confirmed repeatedly in several species and it has been shown that hypertension can be produced in the rat by partial clamping of the artery to one kidney. Vascular hypertensive changes have been produced by this method, and it is of interest that they do not affect the kidney which is protected by the clamp from hypertension. Experimental hypertension of short duration produced in this manner may be abolished by removing the clamp or excising the clamped kidney, but if the clamp has been left in place for some months, the hypertension persists in spite of these manipulations, because of arteriolar changes produced in the unclamped kidney.

Renal hypertension in man is similar in many ways to the experimental condition. The diseases which cause it are listed in the table on p. 270 and are described in Chapter 21: because of their relatively high incidence, chronic glomerulonephritis and chronic pyelonephritis are the most important ones. Release of excess renin from the abnormal kidney or kidneys may be an important factor in producing hypertension in such diseases. However high levels have usually been found only in malignant hypertension with underlying renal disease, and even in these the importance of renin is not fully established.

Secondary hyperaldosteronism in hypertension. In some cases of severe hypertension, particularly those with malignant hypertension and/or renal disease, secondary hyperaldosteronism develops. Plasma renin concentration is invariably increased and this leads to stimulation of aldosterone secretion which in turn produces potassium depletion (see p. 186). The condition is recognised usually by a decrease in the concentration of potassium, and often of sodium, in the plasma. It must be distinguished from primary hyperaldosteronism (Conn's syndrome) in which the hypertension and hypokalaemia are associated with *increased* sodium and *decreased* plasma renin concentration (see p. 912).

Neural factors in the pathogenesis of hypertension. The possibility that neural factors may play a role in primary hypertension deserves consideration. There is evidence that in both human and experimental hypertension the threshold of the vascular receptors is elevated, so that abnormally high pressures are necessary to initiate neurogenic anti-pressor reflexes. It may also be that variations in sensitivity to pressor agents, possibly genetically determined, are involved.

Pulmonary hypertension

The normal pressure in the pulmonary artery is 16–17 mm. Hg and this is raised in pulmonary hypertension to as much as 50–60 mm. Hg.

Etiology. Most cases of pulmonary hypertension are secondary to disease of the heart and lungs.

In *mitral stenosis* the pulmonary arterial pressure rises to elevate the left atrial pressure and force blood through the narrowed valve; a reflex constriction of small pulmonary arteries often develops in severe cases and although this diminishes the danger of pulmonary oedema resulting from very high pulmonary capillary pressure, it causes further marked increase in pulmonary arterial pressure. Less severe pulmonary hypertension is found when the mitral valve is incompetent.

Left ventricular failure, by leading to pulmonary venous congestion, causes mild pulmonary hypertension.

K

In *congenital heart disease* with septal defects, and in cases of patent ductus arteriosus, large amounts of blood may be shunted at high pressure from the systemic into the pulmonary circulation. If the volume passing through the lungs exceeds by three times the normal 5 litres/min., the pulmonary artery pressure rises to overcome the resistance of the congested pulmonary capillaries.

In *chronic lung disease* the pulmonary vascular bed is often much reduced. In emphysema this is due to loss of lung substance and alveolar capillary bed, and in fibrotic conditions such as silicosis, obliterative endarteritis is an additional factor. The hypertension is intensified by the high cardiac output required to compensate for poor pulmonary gas exchange; reflex spasm of small pulmonary arteries and arterioles, due to hypoxia or increased blood CO_2, leads to further increase in pulmonary arterial pressure, particularly during acute respiratory infections such as acute bronchitis in patients with chronic lung disease.

Much less frequently, pulmonary hypertension results from multiple small pulmonary emboli which are found in various stages of organisation. Obliterative pulmonary endarteritis has been described by Ayerza in the Argentine as a cause of pulmonary hypertension and severe cyanosis, but the cause is obscure and similar cases elsewhere have been attributed to syphilis or to massive thrombosis within the pulmonary arteries. Primary pulmonary hypertension analogous to, but not associated with, essential hypertension in the systemic circulation occurs, but is rare.

Vascular changes. In long-standing cases of severe pulmonary hypertension, the main pulmonary arteries dilate and develop atheroma which is otherwise rarely seen here. Superadded pulmonary thrombosis may occur, and the narrowing of the vessels further impairs the circulation. Nevertheless pulmonary infarction does not always occur in these cases.

In mitral stenosis there is thickening of the walls of pulmonary veins and marked muscular hypertrophy and fibrous intimal thickening in the medium and small pulmonary arteries. These changes are, for unknown reasons, more marked in the lower than in the upper lobes of the lung. Necrotic lesions of arterioles with fibrinous infiltration like those of malignant hypertension are sometimes seen in the small pulmonary arteries and arterioles and are probably hypertensive rather than inflammatory in origin. In cases due to congenital heart disease extreme fibro-elastic intimal thickening develops in the pulmonary arterioles, rendering irreversible the elevation of the pulmonary arterial pressure. It is clear that a state of *obliterative pulmonary arteriolitis* may be brought about by a variety of causes.

Effects. Pulmonary hypertension leads to compensatory hypertrophy of the right ventricle and failure of this chamber commonly causes death. In cases with left heart failure or mitral stenosis, pulmonary oedema may develop if the pulmonary capillary pressure so exceeds the plasma osmotic pressure that the lymphatics are unable to remove the transudate as quickly as it forms. This can occur acutely as a result of physical exertion in well-compensated cases where the tricuspid valve is not incompetent (see p. 315).

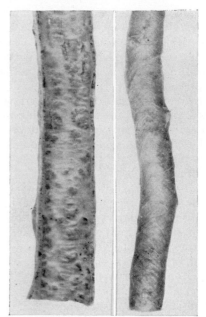

FIG. 13.18.—Calcification of media of iliac and femoral arteries, showing transverse markings caused by the calcified portions. × ⅘.

Calcification of the media (Mönckeberg's sclerosis)

Definition. This is a degenerative disease of unknown cause characterised by dystrophic calcification (p. 207) in the media, especially common in the major lower limb arteries in elderly people.

Naked-eye appearance. The affected vessels are generally dilated and show transverse bars of medial calcification due to deposition of calcium in the circular medial muscle fibres (Fig. 13.18). At a later stage the arteries may be converted into rigid tubes at places. There may be no noteworthy alteration of the intima though atheroma is sometimes present in addition.

Microscopic examination shows that the earliest change is hyaline degeneration of the muscle fibres and connective tissue, usually starting about the middle of the media (Fig. 13.19). Calcium salts are deposited first as fine granules, and continuous calcification follows. There may be little or no cellular reaction. Occasionally true bone may be formed in an area of calcification, and there may even be red marrow in the bone.

Etiology. This is essentially a senile change, an exaggeration of the natural increase of calcium salts in the arteries with age. It sometimes occurs earlier in arteriosclerotic vessels but in

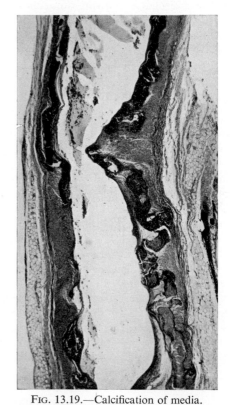

FIG. 13.19.—Calcification of media.

This calcification is indicated by the darkly staining areas. Note the marked irregularity of the lumen. × 14.

man is not intimately related to high blood pressure. A similar lesion has been produced in the aorta of rabbits by injections of adrenaline.

Effects. The radiological appearance is striking but the lumina of the arteries are seldom narrowed. Ischaemic effects, if present, are usually due to co-existing atheroma and its complications.

Syphilitic arteritis

Small arteries

Wherever syphilitic lesions occur there is intimal and adventitial fibrosis of small arteries associated with infiltration of lymphocytes and plasma cells (endarteritis and periarteritis). These changes are due to the presence of spirochaetes in the adventitia. In some cases the change is diffuse and a number of the vessels show general thickening, whilst in others it is of a patchy or nodular type.

Effects. Reduction of the arterial lumen due to endarteritis may contribute to necrosis in gummas. The essential change in syphilitic mesaortitis is probably involvement of the small nutrient vasa vasorum of the aortic media. Effects purely attributable to ischaemia are seen in the brain in tertiary syphilis (meningovascular syphilis) due to endarteritis obliterans of cortical vessels (Fig. 13.24) and this may be complicated by thrombosis leading to cerebral softening at an early age. Widespread obliteration of small pulmonary arteries, resulting in pulmonary hypertension, has been attributed to syphilis.

Syphilitic mesaortitis

This is a common manifestation of tertiary syphilis and an important cause of death in this disease. It occasionally occurs in congenital syphilis.

Naked-eye appearances can best be studied in untreated young subjects, in whom the disease occurs in the absence of other vascular lesions. The first visible lesions are greyish-white translucent areas of thickening in the intima, with little tendency to degenerate. Later they extend and fuse, forming areas with wavy or slightly wrinkled surface, whilst the intima in the parts between appears healthy (Fig. 13.20).

At places, contraction of the tissue may occur with formation of stellate scars. Localised depressions which are potential aneurysms may be seen. In older subjects, yellow patches of atheroma, which is often severe, may be associated with the syphilitic lesions. Occasionally, on cutting through the wall of the aorta, gummatous change may be seen extending inwards from the adventitia.

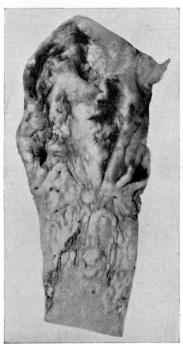

Fig. 13.20.—Extensive syphilitic disease of aortic arch, showing the thickened plaques and irregularity of the surface, also formation of aneurysmal depressions. ×½.
Note the sharp limitation of the disease below. The patient was aged 23.

The part of the arch immediately above the aortic valve is usually involved first and the aortic arch is by far the commonest and at times the only site of syphilitic lesions. They also occur at a lower level but are usually limited to the thoracic aorta.

Microscopic appearances. The earliest change is periarteritis and endarteritis of the vasa vasorum in the adventitia (Fig. 13.21). These changes then extend into the aortic media, in which foci of cellular infiltration appear (Fig. 13.22), with new formation of thin-walled vessels. This leads to breaks or windows in the elastic tissue and muscle of the media, best seen in a section stained to show the elastic fibres (Fig. 13.23). The elastic tissue is usually absorbed but

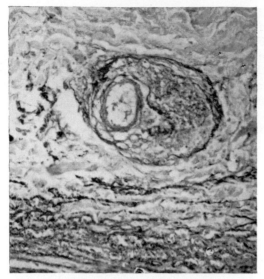

FIG. 13.21.—Section of adventitia in syphilitic disease of aorta, showing endarteritis and periarteritis of small arteriole, with fibrous thickening and extensive lymphocytic infiltration around. × 80.

gummatous necrosis may occur. Later, cellular infiltration is followed by formation of fibrous patches in the media in which no muscle or elastic tissue is present (Fig. 13.32).

In the intima overlying these medial lesions the connective tissue is increased and swollen and new vessels often extend from the media, usually without the cellular infiltration present

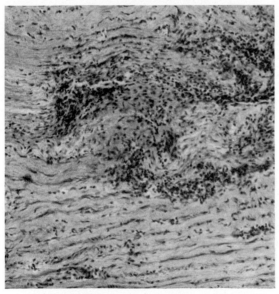

FIG. 13.22.—Section of syphilitic aorta, showing cellular accumulations around the small vessels in the media, with destruction of the laminae. × 160.

in the other coats. The intimal thickening is probably compensatory—secondary to the weakening of the media—and not part of the syphilitic lesion proper.

Effects. *Aneurysm* formation commonly results from syphilitic mesaortitis and is due to weakening of the vessel wall from loss of medial elastic and muscle tissue (p. 284).

Aortic incompetence. Syphilitic mesaortitis may spread to the aortic ring and cusps resulting in incompetence of the valve (p. 309). Dilatation of the valve ring due to loss of elastic tissue is another factor in the production of this valvular defect.

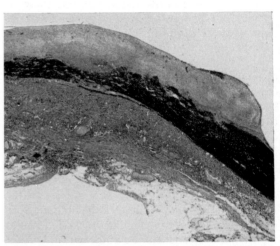

FIG. 13.23.—Syphilitic aortitis, showing the thick intimal patch overlying an area of irregular patchy destruction of the medial elastica. × 6.

Coronary artery narrowing due to involvement of their orifices by mesaortitis sometimes leads to myocardial ischaemia.

Embolism from thrombus formed on a syphilitic lesion is a rare complication.

Idiopathic aortitis in Africans

An inflammatory lesion affecting all parts of the aorta has been described in young Africans. There is infiltration of the adventitia and media with lymphocytes and plasma cells, and destruction of the elastic tissue, ending in dense collagenous fibrosis. The mouths of the renal arteries are often involved, resulting in unilateral or bilateral renal artery stenosis often leading in turn to hypertension. Micro-organisms have not been demonstrated and the etiology of the lesion is unknown.

Tuberculosis

Marked periarteritis and endarteritis sometimes occur in relation to tuberculous lesions. They are often a prominent feature in tuberculous meningitis, especially with late or inadequate treatment. These changes may lead to complete obstruction of the vessel and cerebral infarction. Occasionally, however, the wall of an artery adjacent to a cavity may be weakened before obliteration occurs and an aneurysm may form (p. 364).

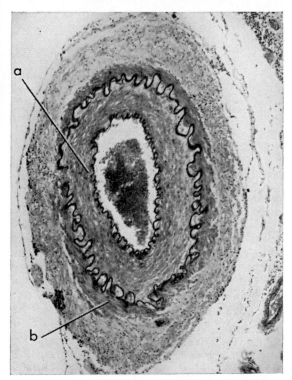

FIG. 13.24.—Syphilitic endarteritis and periarteritis in a cerebral artery.

The greatly thickened intima is seen between the elastic aminae, which appear black: *a*, intima; *b*, media. × 72.

Thrombo-angiitis obliterans (Buerger's disease)

Definition. A condition distinct from atheroma characterised by thrombosis and recanalisation of arteries and veins, and peripheral vascular insufficiency which predominantly affects the lower limbs of young men.

Etiology. The disease occurs almost exclusively in males and often starts before middle age, earlier than the period of arterial degeneration. It does not occur mainly amongst Jews as was at first supposed. The pathological features point to a specific etiology, but so far no organism of any kind has been found. Excessive cigarette smoking is almost universal amongst sufferers. Attacks of superficial migrating phlebitis often precede exacerbations of the arterial disease.

Pathological features. Legs amputated for gangrene have usually supplied the material for examination and consequently the late changes are best known. Usually many arteries are obliterated by thrombi which become completely organised and many are recanalised by comparatively wide vessels. The condition of the arterial walls varies greatly, but there is usually considerable fibrosis of the media and adventitia (Fig. 13.25), and an important feature is that the fibrosis involves the adjacent veins, nerves and muscle fibres. In some arteries there may be considerable endarteritis without thrombosis. A striking point is the occurrence in the intima and adjacent thrombus of cellular foci with giant cells; these are probably a reaction to damaged and fragmented elastic tissue. Similar changes may affect the accompanying veins—*thrombophlebitis migrans* (Fig. 13.26), which become filled with organised thrombus. It remains to be determined whether these changes usually follow an early, more acute stage consisting of infiltration of the arterial walls by polymorphonuclears and accumulation of these cells in the thrombi as suggested by Buerger, or whether the initial change is the formation of thrombi in the arterial lumen.

Clinical features. The symptoms are varied and depend on the degree of arterial obstruction. The earliest are pain, paraesthesia, and circulatory disturbances—local redness which disappears on elevating the limbs. On walking there is often cramp-like pain and inability to progress—"intermittent claudication"; this is a result of ischaemia of the calf muscles and occurs in other forms of arterial disease. Later, more severe trophic changes appear, including intractable ulceration, and gangrene which is apt to spread slowly (Fig. 13.27); amputation, sometimes repeated, is often necessary but the need for surgery may be minimised by therapy which improves the collateral circulation. In view of the widespread involvement of the arteries it has now been recognised that amputa-

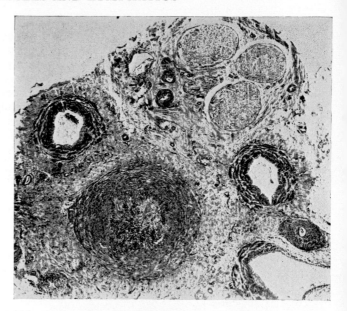

Fig. 13.25.—Thrombo-angiitis obliterans; posterior tibial artery with accompanying veins and nerves, showing occlusion of arterial lumen and fibrosis involving veins and nerves. × 32.

tion, if required, should be performed at a high level. The arms may also be involved and the disease sometimes causes Raynaud's syndrome in males.

Polyarteritis nodosa
(Periarteritis nodosa)

Definition. A focal but widespread arteritis with involvement of the media and a tendency to the production of aneurysms.

Etiology. This is a rare condition, more frequent in males than in females. No infective agent has been recognised in the lesions, but hypersensitivity to streptococci or drugs may be concerned, and also the Australia antigen (p. 558). Some observers have found a high incidence of antinuclear autoantibodies.

Pathological findings. The disease may be fairly acute and death is then usually caused by haemorrhage. The lesions are common on the visceral arteries, e.g. coronary arteries, pancreatic, renal, splenic, mesenteric, hepatic, etc., and also in muscle and subcutaneous tissue, and are indicated by the presence of nodules or patches of thickening along the course of the blood vessels. Aneurysms at various stages of formation may be comparatively numerous. On microscopic examination it is found

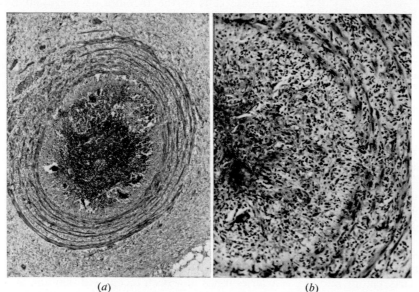

(a)   (b)

Fig. 13.26.—Thrombophlebitis migrans.

(a) A superficial vein is shown with early acute inflammatory infiltration of the wall, recent thrombosis and multiple giant-cell clusters in the intima. × 40.

(b) A more advanced stage of a similar lesion showing the abundant polymorphonuclear infiltrate and organisation of the occluding thrombus. × 170.

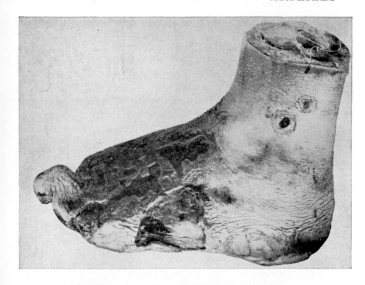

FIG. 13.27.—Foot from a case of thrombo-angiitis obliterans, showing ulcers and loss of toes from gangrene.

that in the affected parts there is an acute inflammatory lesion with extensive infiltration of neutrophil and eosinophil leukocytes in the adventitia. Along with this, there is fibrinoid necrosis in the adjacent media which rapidly spreads to involve the whole thickness of the wall (Fig. 13.28). Some compensatory proliferation may be found in the intima, but this is rarely marked. Stretching of the degenerate and necrotic tissue and formation of an aneurysm may follow.

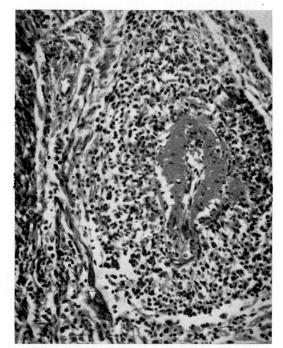

FIG. 13.28.—Acute polyarteritis nodosa. Small artery in kidney, showing inflammatory change. × 100.

More commonly, the disease runs a chronic course. The damage to the walls of the arteries is followed by reparative proliferation which compensates for the weakness and prevents aneurysm formation (Fig. 13.29). Nodular thickening of the arteries is the chief feature with dilatation, diminution or occlusion of the lumen. Such changes are met with mainly in the visceral arteries and vary greatly in distribution in different cases. The arteries of the kidneys and heart (Fig. 13.30) are most frequently affected and in these organs atrophy and fibrosis or infarction follow, according to the degree of obstruction. In the kidneys considerable surface irregularity may result owing to areas of local shrinkage (Fig. 13.31) and recovery may be followed by hypertension, which is sometimes severe. When the coronaries are affected nodular thickenings may be present on the branches on the surface of the heart.

Clinical features. The illness is often severe and accompanied by fever and a very high ESR. Abdominal or chest pain due to visceral or cardiac ischaemia is common and peripheral neuropathy may be present. Renal failure or hypertension may occur. There may be necrotic and granulomatous lesions of nose ("malignant" granuloma of nose) or lung (Wegener's granulomatosis), the latter often associated with symptoms of asthma and eosinophilia in the peripheral blood. It may be possible to confirm the diagnosis by biopsy of painful subcutaneous or muscular lesions.

A microangiopathic form of polyarteritis nodosa affects small arteries in the kidneys and elsewhere, and gives rise to uraemia, often without hypertension: the renal lesions (p. 710) include focal and rapidly progressive glomerulonephritis. In some cases, the renal changes are accompanied by features of Wegener's granulomatosis.

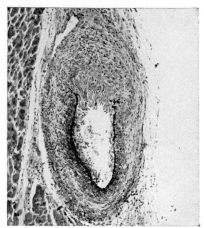

FIG. 13.29.—Polyarteritis nodosa of less acute type affecting branch of coronary artery of heart. Note eccentric character and rupture of elastic lamina. × 50. (Dr. Janet Niven.)

Localised polyarteritis, indistinguishable microscopically from that described above, is sometimes found in skin, gall bladder and appendix and has an excellent prognosis. Inflammatory lesions of small arteries and veins of the skin occur in erythema nodosum, erythema induratum and nodular vasculitis (p. 931), but these conditions are quite distinct from polyarteritis nodosa.

Other forms of arteritis

Rheumatic arteritis. Lesions similar to those found in the heart are produced by rheumatism in the walls of large arteries. In the aorta they commence in the adventitia and consist of an infiltration of the tissues with lymphocytes and plasma cells. There may be foci of histiocytes, and typical Aschoff bodies with characteristic cells (p. 311) may form. The cellular

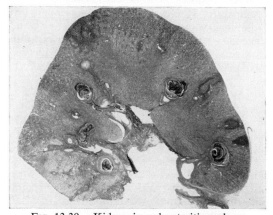

FIG. 13.30.—Kidney in polyarteritis nodosa.
Note the multiple aneurysms, partly filled with thrombus and the multiple infarcts. × $\frac{4}{3}$.

infiltration may spread into the media and lead to absorption of elastic tissue, but this rarely extends beyond the outer third of the media. Such lesions do not weaken the wall sufficiently to produce aneurysms. Syphilitic aortitis (p. 277) has similar features.

In the smaller arteries, rheumatic lesions of varying distribution have been found, especially in the visceral branches. They are acute and may be accompanied by necrosis of the media as well as by leukocyte infiltration; they thus resemble the lesions of polyarteritis nodosa but thrombosis and aneurysm have not been found. Further work is required to establish the relation of rheumatism to disease of the smaller arteries. There is no known clinical relationship, but the occurrence of focal lesions in the subcutaneous tissues and elsewhere illustrates the systemic nature of rheumatic disease.

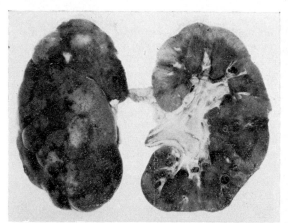

FIG. 13.31.—Kidneys in polyarteritis nodosa, showing multiple depressed scars from older lesions and some small infarcts and aneurysms from more recent acute lesions. × $\frac{1}{2}$.

Aortitis in ankylosing spondylitis. Unexplained lesions of the aortic valve and ascending aorta, identical in appearance to syphilitic arteritis but without serological evidence of syphilis, sometimes develop in males with ankylosing spondylitis.

Temporal arteritis (*giant-cell arteritis*). This is a subacute inflammatory disease affecting especially the temporal arteries in elderly people. It is associated with severe headache, fever and other general symptoms and sometimes results in blindness. Post-mortem examination has shown that the lesions are not limited to the temporal vessels but may occur also in the aorta and visceral arteries. The essential lesion is a subacute inflammation of the adventitia, spreading into the media where it is associated with foci of necrosis; a granulomatous replacement of the media follows and partial destruction of the elastica is seen, followed by new formation of elastic laminae. Giant cells may form and a poorly defined follicular architecture may result. The intima becomes concentrically thickened and in the smaller arteries thrombosis and organisation commonly follow. The lesions may be histologically similar to those of thrombo-angiitis obliterans, but the age and sex incidence are different, and the disease is usually self-limited.

Takayashu's disease

This is a rare condition, first reported from Japan, in which the aorta and the large arteries arising from the aortic arch are affected by an arteritis involving the whole thickness of the wall and resembling temporal arteritis. Intimal thickening, sometimes with superadded thrombosis, severely narrows or occludes the subclavian, carotid and innominate arteries (hence the term *pulseless disease*), with resulting ischaemia of the head and arms. The disease affects mainly young women, and the etiology is unknown. Occasional cases with vascular occlusions suggestive of Takayashu's arteriopathy are encountered in Britain. The patients are usually older, and may be of either sex. These cases are attributable to severe atheroma or syphilitic arteritis of the major arteries.

Thrombotic microangiopathy (thrombotic thrombocytopenic purpura)

This is characterised by the deposition of homogeneous eosinophilic material, at least some of which is fibrin, in the intima and lumen of visceral arterioles, without an associated inflammatory reaction. It sometimes accompanies, and may belong to, the group of connective tissue diseases. Further details are given on p. 416.

Raynaud's disease

Nomenclature. The name Raynaud's disease has been applied to a variety of conditions in which there is excessive vasomotor response to cold. It is now thought desirable to subdivide these conditions and to use the following arbitrary nomenclature—Raynaud's phenomenon, Raynaud's disease (primary or secondary).

Raynaud's phenomenon affects the extremities, usually the fingers, but occasionally also the ears, tip of the nose and the toes. It is provoked by cold, and consists of attacks of local ischaemia with intense pallor or cyanosis (p. 157), coldness and disturbance of sensation; the patient suffers from "dead fingers". Pallor is due to spasm of all the vessels of the affected part. Cyanosis, or lividity, may be accompanied by swelling, and is due to continued arterial contraction, while the capillaries and veins are dilated from loss of tone and filled with blood from which the oxygen has been largely dissociated. In Raynaud's phenomenon the circulation through the hands is normal between attacks; these can be generally terminated by warming even after the condition has existed for many years, and the structure of the digital vessels remains normal (Lewis). There are no trophic changes.

The disorder is familial, predominantly affects women, develops in early adult life, and is an exaggeration of the normal reactions to cold; the prognosis is excellent.

Raynaud's disease consists of attacks resembling Raynaud's phenomenon but accompanied by trophic changes. The tips of the digits develop atrophy of the skin with blisters, minor infections and finally progressive necrosis and ulceration of the fingertips, the changes usually being symmetrical. Studies on the digital circulation by angiography have shown that there is some degree of permanent arterial obstruction and this may be due either to intimal fibrous thickening or to thrombosis and imperfect recanalisation. Secondary Raynaud's disease results from the use of vibrating tools. It occurs also in scleroderma and the other connective tissue diseases (p. 812); in a paralysed limb following poliomyelitis; as a stage in the symptomatology of obliterative arterial disease; in certain forms of paroxysmal haemoglobinuria as a result of cold agglutinins acting on the red cells in the digital circulation; in chronic ergot poisoning. In a few cases no underlying cause is found and these are described as primary Raynaud's disease.

Aneurysms

Definition. An aneurysm is a local enlargement of the lumen of an artery.

Classification. A *true* aneurysm is formed by slow dilatation of an artery and is enclosed within the stretched vessel wall, or, when this is no longer recognisable, the surrounding connective tissue. A *false* aneurysm is produced by rupture of the vessel, the blood being enclosed from the start by the surrounding tissues. After a time the two forms come to be closely similar in structure.

A *diffuse* or *fusiform* aneurysm involves the whole circumference of the wall symmetrically whereas the *saccular* type is an asymmetrical bulge communicating with the artery through an aperture which does not involve the whole circumference. These terms may not be applicable to advanced lesions which are often very irregular in form.

In a *dissecting aneurysm* the space containing the blood is actually in the wall of the artery, usually the aorta. The essential cause of the condition is some lesion of the media, which allows blood from the lumen to dissect the media into two layers. Other varieties of aneurysm are mentioned briefly on p. 288.

Formation. The force which expands an aneurysm is the blood pressure, but for an aneurysm to form there must be an arterial lesion which weakens the media locally. Stretching usually results in further weakening, so that once an aneurysm has started it tends to expand and commonly ruptures. Occasionally thrombus forms in thick layers which fill the whole sac.

Syphilitic aneurysm

This usually occurs between the ages of 40–50, when tertiary syphilis is most common and the individual is still able to indulge in strenuous physical activity. Large aortic aneurysms were previously due in most instances to syphilis, but are now rare as a result of successful treatment in the primary and secondary stages of the disease. The commonest site is the aortic arch, because it is the part most frequently affected by syphilitic mesaortitis (p. 277); next come the thoracic and the abdominal aorta, and then the main branches from the arch. The disease

extends from outside the vessel, starting in the adventitia and passing inwards around the vasa vasorum. The lesion, having reached the media, leads to destruction of the elastic tissue and muscle fibres, and thus to local weakness (Fig. 13.32). In addition to a large saccular, fusiform or irregular aneurysm it is common to find small depressions or aneurysms in various stages of formation, along with the stellate scars and intimal thickening characteristic of syphilitic mesaortitis. As an aneurysm forms, the elastic tissue and muscle of the artery wall soon degenerate and the sac comes to be composed of layers of fibrous tissue, on which laminated thrombus forms. Blood infiltrates the wall of the aneurysm and may ooze for some distance into the tissues around; accordingly the limits of the aneurysm are badly defined.

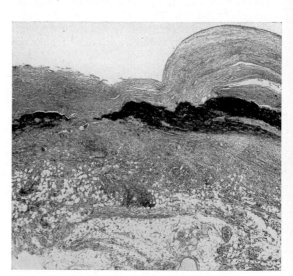

Fig. 13.32.—Section of syphilitic aorta, showing interruption and destruction of the elastic tissue of the media, which is stained black; aneurysmal dilatation occurs through such weak areas. × 15.

Effects. *Pressure* on surrounding structures leads to the syndrome of superior mediastinal compression; the great veins may be displaced and undergo thrombosis, resulting in congestion of the head and neck and the opening up of collateral channels. Implication of the oesophagus may cause dysphagia, whilst pressure on a bronchus leads to narrowing and retention pneumonia may occur. Aneurysms of the transverse part of the aortic arch may compress and stretch the left recurrent laryngeal nerve and cause paralysis of the left vocal cord. Rigid structures such as the bodies of vertebrae may be eroded and the bare bone come to form part of the wall of the sac; the intervertebral discs offer greater resistance to absorption and persist longer.

Rupture of an aneurysm may occur into practically any tube or cavity in its neighbour-

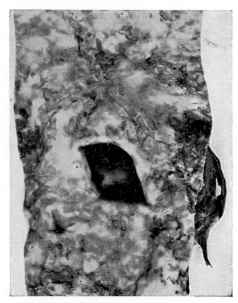

Fig. 13.33.—Abdominal aorta, showing orifice of aneurysm. × ⅔.

The intima of the aorta is affected by both atheroma and syphilitic disease.

hood, and occasionally takes place externally through the chest wall. The commonest site of rupture is into the trachea or a bronchus, but the sac may burst into the pleura or lung substance, the pericardium, the oesophagus, a large vein, or even into an atrium, the pulmonary artery or the right ventricle. Fatal rupture may be preceded by oozing of blood for some time; this is often clinically recognisable in the case of the respiratory passages. Rupture of an abdominal aortic aneurysm gives rise to a large mass of retroperitoneal clot in which the kidneys may be buried, and the onset is often marked by symptoms like those of an acute surgical emergency.

Embolism from thrombus within an aneurysm is uncommon.

Cardiac hypertrophy and dilatation occur only when the syphilitic mesaortitis affects the aortic valve and results in aortic incompetence. Other wise aortic aneurysms, even very large ones, do not affect the heart as there is no interference with cardiac output.

Atheromatous aneurysm

In Great Britain atheroma is now by far the most common cause of aortic aneurysm, due to the decline of syphilis and the concurrent increase in atheroma, a remarkable change from the position 50 years ago. Atheromatous aneurysms are found in an older age group than syphilitic aneurysms. They may be saccular, fusiform or, rarely, dissecting and they usually rupture while still quite small. The aneurysm forms as a result of penetration of the media by ulceration of necrotic atheromatous patches or damage from calcified plaques impinging on the media. The microscopic changes seen at the edges are those of atheroma, sometimes with a marked leukocytic reaction around the fatty debris, and there may be some lymphocytic infiltration round the vasa vasorum in the adventitia and media. Atheromatous aneurysms

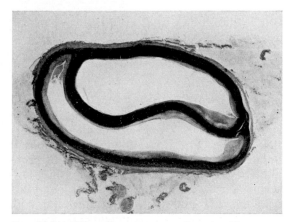

Fig. 13.34.—Dissecting aneurysm of aorta. Transverse section of the thoracic aorta, showing the double channel. × 3.

occur mainly in the presence of very severe atheroma and affect especially the abdominal aorta or its branches.

Effects. Death is usually due to rupture with retroperitoneal haemorrhage but in some cases thrombosis of the aorta or its branches takes place, producing ischaemia in legs, kidneys, etc. Pressure effects are not conspicuous.

Dissecting aneurysm

This is much less common than true aneurysm of the aorta. In most cases it results from incomplete rupture of the aorta (Fig. 13.36) due to degenerative and cystic changes in the media, the elastica and muscle being replaced by a metachromatic mucoid substance—Erdheim's medial degeneration—(Figs. 13.35*a* and *b*).

longitudinally; the intima is able to slide to and fro on the media because of the mucoid degeneration and ultimately it ruptures. The outer parts of the media and adventitia are not usually severed, but are widely infiltrated with blood, and dissecting aneurysm is thus produced. In proximal ruptures, blood commonly passes backwards and within a few hours bursts into the pericardial sac and causes death acutely from

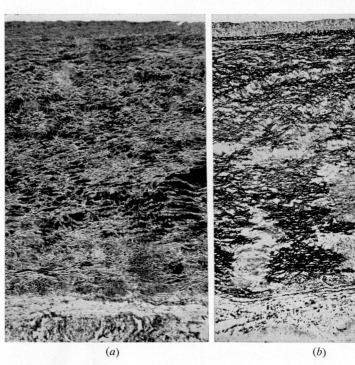

Fig. 13.35.—Cystic mucoid degeneration of aorta.

(*a*) The degenerate mucoid matrix is stained specifically and appears black;
(*b*) the elastic tissue is stained specifically, and is seen to show numerous gaps. × 45.

From a case of spontaneous rupture of the aorta in a woman of 24 years.

(*a*)   (*b*)

Sometimes there are small areas of necrosis with softening (*medionecrosis*) but in our experience this is rare. The cause of these conditions is unknown. Atheroma rarely, and syphilis probably never, causes dissecting aneurysm. Dissecting aneurysm is commonest in the later years of adult life and high blood pressure with hypertrophy of the heart is present in the majority of such cases. Dissecting aneurysms are found also in younger subjects and Figs. 13.35 (*a*) and (*b*) are from a woman aged 24.

The commonest site for rupture is shortly above the aortic cusps (Fig. 13.36); next in frequency is a point just distal to the insertion of the ductus arteriosus. The tear is usually transverse like a cut, and it may extend around almost the entire circumference. Rupture is probably brought about by the frictional tractive effect of blood flow during systole pushing the intima

cardiac tamponade; intra-pericardial rupture may be preceded by signs of coronary occlusion from pressure upon these vessels at their origin. In other cases the blood strips open the media distally between the outer and middle thirds and passes along the wall of the thoracic, and even the abdominal aorta, finally rupturing into the retroperitoneal tissues. Occasionally the blood bursts back into the lumen of the aorta or iliac vessels at a lower level, and when this happens the blood may flow through a new channel from the aperture of entry to the point of re-entry in the lower abdominal aorta and the patient may survive for some time (Fig. 13.34). Occasionally a dissecting aneurysm remains localised (Fig. 13.37).

Marfan's syndrome. In this inherited disorder, dissecting aneurysm of the aorta or fusiform aneurysm with incompetence of the aortic valve is associated with long tapering fingers (arachnodactyly) and other skeletal abnormalities, subluxation of the lens and other anomalies of the eye and ear. There may be multiple healed internal aortic tears, and the histological changes in the aorta resemble those of Erdheim's medial degeneration.

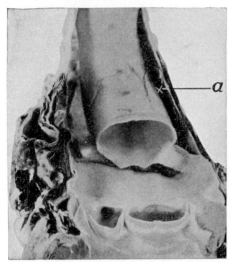

Fig. 13.36.—Rupture of aorta with acute dissecting aneurysm.

There is a transverse rupture above the aortic valve and the blood has separated intima and inner part of media almost as a complete tube. *a* points to dissecting aneurysm in which some blood is still present. × ⅔.

Other causes of aortic rupture. Apart from aneurysm, rupture of the aorta may result from damage to its wall from outside, as by the perforation of an impacted fishbone or other sharp foreign body in the oesophagus; also from very severe injury such as crushing of the chest. In children traumatic rupture can occur without fracture of the ribs. Carcinoma of bronchus or oesophagus may invade the aortic wall and cause fatal haemorrhage.

Infective aneurysm
(Mycotic aneurysm)

These may occur at the beginning of the aorta as the result of *direct extension* of organisms from vegetations in bacterial endocarditis, mainly the staphylococcal type (Fig. 14.31). The organisms settle on the intima, an infective thrombus forms, invasion and weakening of the wall follow, and an *acute aneurysm* is produced, which may rupture; occasionally multiple aneurysms are present. In smaller arteries infective aneurysms result from lodgment of small infected emboli in the vasa

vasorum, rather than from the presence of an infected embolus in the lumen of the artery. Inflammatory softening of the arterial wall results. They may occur in a limb or viscus, and the effects are similar to those seen in the *non-infective* aneurysms of polyarteritis nodosa where the vessel is weakened by inflammation due probably to a hypersensitivity reaction. Infected emboli in the lumen of an artery may give rise to acute inflammatory softening with rupture, e.g. in the cerebral haemorrhage of staphylococcal pyaemia.

A mycotic aneurysm is sometimes seen in the wall of a tuberculous pulmonary cavity, instead of the usual occlusion of the vessel by endarteritis obliterans or thrombosis.

Cerebral aneurysms

Aneurysms of the circle of Willis and its branches occur at all ages and appear to be due mainly to congenital weakness of the arterial wall. Evidence of this is destroyed when the aneurysm forms but a deficiency in the medial muscle, especially in the acute angle between large branches, is demonstrable in other arteries

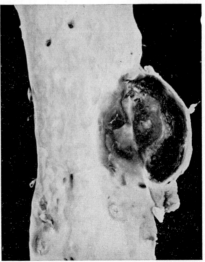

Fig. 13.37.—Localised chronic dissecting aneurysm; the space in the media is filled with dense thrombus. × 1.

at the base of the brain and similar deficiencies are sometimes found in apparently normal brains. An inherent defect in the elastica has not been demonstrated, but when dilatation starts the elastica probably soon degenerates. These aneurysms are often known as *congenital*, but only the defect is congenital. The aneurysms usually occur singly and are often about 5 mm. in diameter though they may be considerably

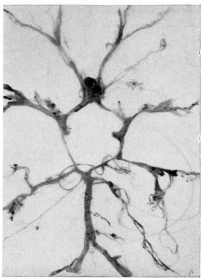

FIG. 13.38.—Circle of Willis, showing small aneurysm on the anterior communicating artery.

larger. The commonest site is at the origin of the middle cerebral followed by the anterior communicating artery (Fig. 13.38), but they may arise practically anywhere on the circle of Willis and major branches. Rupture of these aneurysms is the principal cause of spontaneous subarachnoid haemorrhage, but in many cases the sac is buried in the cortex and they bleed into the brain. Accordingly aneurysm should be suspected in the examination of any cerebral haemorrhage in an unusual situation. Not uncommonly, these aneurysms become partly or completely occluded by thrombus (Fig. 13.39). Occasionally aneurysms of the larger cerebral arteries are due to atheroma.

Micro-aneurysms. The occurrence of multiple micro-aneurysms on the small cerebral arterial twigs in hypertensive subjects was described over a century ago, but they are difficult to find without special techniques, and only recently has their common occurrence been reaffirmed. In a painstaking study, Cole and Yates (1967) using a micro-angiographic necropsy technique reported the occurrence of multiple (usually 15–25) aneurysms of up to 2 mm. diam., occurring mainly on arteries of less than 250 μ diameter. They were detected in over

50 per cent of hypertensives over 50 years of age, and the incidence increased with age: in normotensives, the incidence was low and aneurysms were found in only a few subjects over 65 years old. The aneurysms were most numerous in and around the basal ganglia, and occurred usually at or near branchings of the striate arteries: they were found also in the sub-cortical white matter and in the mid-brain and cerebellum.

The aneurysms may be saccular or fusiform, and the adjacent artery and wall of the sac show hyaline thickening of the intima, sometimes with fibrinoid change: the internal elastic lamina is usually absent from, or fragmented in, the wall of the sac, and muscle is usually absent. Thrombus, sometimes organised, may fill the sac, and there is often evidence of old or recent leakage of blood into the surrounding tissues.

Cole and Yates detected micro-aneurysms in 18 of 20 hypertensives dying from cerebral haemorrhage, and they provide evidence which suggests strongly that rupture of such aneurysms is the usual cause of cerebral haemorrhage in hypersensitive subjects (p. 619).

Other forms of aneurysm

Traumatic aneurysm may be produced by injury to the vessel wall by a stab or bullet wound, or by a spicule of fractured bone. A localised haematoma forms and later a layer of granulation tissue develops

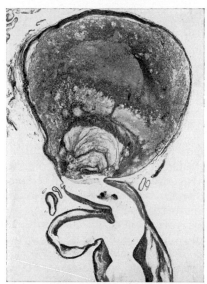

FIG. 13.39.—Aneurysm of circle of Willis, almost completely filled with thrombus. × 6.

around the blood producing a remarkably well-defined wall.

If a vein and adjacent artery are both injured, the arterial blood flows into the vein; if a blood-filled sac develops between artery and vein this is known as an *arterio-venous aneurysm*. Blood flow between a large artery and vein may seriously disturb the circulation and high output cardiac failure (p. 296) may quickly follow.

A *cirsoid* or *racemose aneurysm* is a form of arterio-venous fistula which appears as a pulsatile swelling consisting of tortuous and dilated arteries and veins with multiple intercommunications. The commonest site is the scalp, and atrophy of the underlying bone may be produced. The condition is sometimes of congenital origin, but more often is the result of a blow on the head; some of the allegedly congenital cases are probably the result of birth injury. Similarly a carotid-cavernous sinus aneurysm resulting from fracture of the skull base gives rise to great engorgement of the orbital veins and oedema of the orbit and conjunctiva.

DISEASES OF VEINS

Compensatory enlargement of the veins takes place, as in the arterial system, when an increased collateral flow is produced by obstruction in a large vein. As in the case of arteries, the dilatation is followed by hypertrophy of the various elements in the wall of the vessels. Veins are, of course, not exposed to the marked variations of blood pressure which occur in arteries, but when they are subject to chronic over-distension, compensatory changes occur in their walls. There is little or no hyperplasia of the muscle, but considerable increase of the elastic tissue occurs. At a later stage, this undergoes degeneration, whilst the fibrous tissue becomes thickened and hyaline. Localised patches of thickening in the intima of veins are not uncommon, but the fatty changes which are so prominent a feature of atheroma are rare.

Acute thrombophlebitis

A distinction is sometimes made between *thrombophlebitis*, by which is meant a primary inflammatory condition of the vein, with secondary thrombosis, and *phlebo-thrombosis*, in which a bland thrombosis of the vein occurs with, at most, mild preceding inflammatory change. In many instances, however, the distinction is more theoretical than practical because the presence of thrombus in the lumen of the vein sets up reactive changes so that the distinction between mild thrombophlebitis and phlebothrombosis may no longer be possible. It is, however, of value to distinguish between venous thrombosis due to acute pyogenic inflammation in the vein wall associated with abundant micro-organisms, which is liable to by followed by pyaemia, and milder conditions where the effects are chiefly those of local mechanical occlusion and of bland embolism.

Pyogenic thrombophlebitis is produced by extension of organisms from a septic focus outside. This was formerly common in the veins of the diploë and dural sinuses in middle-ear disease, in the uterine veins in puerperal sepsis, in the veins of the bone marrow in suppurative osteomyelitis, and occasionally in the pulmonary veins in cases of bronchiectasis. When a large vein such as the lateral or sigmoid dural sinus is involved the wall becomes intensely inflamed and infiltrated with pus, while secondary implication of the intima by inflammatory exudate leads to thrombosis. The thrombus formed is at first of the ordinary type, but it may be invaded by organisms so that purulent or even putrefactive softening may follow and lead to pyaemia; this may, however, be prevented by occlusion of the lumen beyond the site of infection by simple uninfected thrombus.

In the condition known as *pylephlebitis suppurativa* the inflammatory process starts in a small tributary of the portal vein and leads to progressive ascending thrombosis and suppuration, from which multiple abscesses in the liver may result.

Thrombophlebitis may also appear as a complication of conditions in which there is a bacteraemia, notably typhoid fever, and it is presumed that organisms circulating in the blood settle in the intima and produce an acute endophlebitis with secondary thrombosis.

It is uncertain whether post-operative and puerperal thrombophlebitis are in this category or whether venous stasis and changes in the blood are more important. The much higher incidence of such lesions in the veins of the leg suggests that infection plays at most a subordinate part in the etiology of these conditions.

Thrombophlebitis migrans is a conspicuous feature of many cases of Buerger's disease (p. 279) but it is also seen in association with carcinoma. It is a particularly common complication of carcinoma of the pancreas, but occurs also in association with carcinomas of breast, stomach, bronchi, etc.; it is then usually accompanied by vegetations on the mitral and aortic cusps. Thrombophlebitis migrans may be the presenting sign before the underlying malignancy has been recognised and may be associated with multiple deep-vein thromboses.

Tropical thrombophlebitis. Fisher in Northern Rhodesia described a variety of acute phlebitis occurring in adults, both European and Bantu, accompanied by fever, muscular spasm and pain and tenderness along the course of the veins, the femoral being most frequently affected. The disease runs a self-limited course, but in about 10 per cent of cases proves fatal from involvement of visceral veins. It is probable that this form of *primary tropical phlebitis* is the underlying cause of "Serenje leg", a fairly common disorder in Africa characterised by chronic oedema. Bacteriological studies failed to demonstrate micro-organisms of any kind. Lendrum described the histological appearances as a peculiar type of inflammatory reaction characterised by gross interruption of the vein wall by new capillaries with many polymorphs and macrophages, some of which contained phloxinophil inclusion bodies of unknown nature. Thrombosis is secondary to the lesion of the vein wall.

Chronic phlebitis

Chronic inflammatory processes may spread to the walls of the veins and lead to reactive thickening; in fact, the minute veins are affected in this way in all chronic inflammatory conditions. Chronic phlebitis is seen in syphilitic lesions, in the smaller venous branches, both in the primary and later stages and in association with syphilitic periarteritis (p. 149). Chronic phlebitis of obscure origin is occasionally observed in the large vessels, for example, in the portal vein, and may lead to thrombosis; after some time it may be impossible to say whether the changes present in the vein wall are primary in nature or secondary to the thrombosis.

Endophlebitis of the hepatic veins is the basis of the veno-occlusive disease of Jamaica and certain other tropical regions (see p. 544) and involvement of the hepatic ostia with thrombosis gives rise to the Budd–Chiari syndrome (p. 544).

Tuberculous invasion of veins, which is of great importance in relation to acute miliary tuberculosis (p. 146), is seen in two forms. In one, infection apparently takes place from the blood. Single or multiple foci form on the intima (Fig. 13.40) or the lesion may appear as a raised yellowish patch of considerable extent and thickness; when it ulcerates, numerous bacilli pass

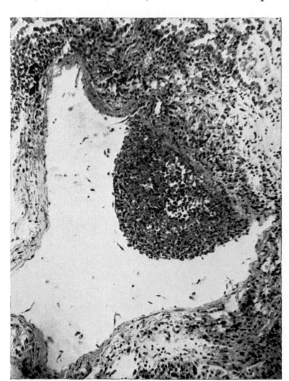

Fig. 13.40.—Pulmonary vein showing intimal tuberculous lesion. × 190.

into the blood stream, acute miliary tuberculosis resulting. This lesion has been found most frequently in the veins of the lungs, but occasionally elsewhere. More commonly blood infection develops when a caseous mass, usually in a hilar lymph node, invades and destroys the wall of the vein, and, on its erosion, a similar result follows.

Veins are often invaded by *malignant tumours*, from which the growth may extend in the lumen for some distance into the inferior vena cava. This is sometimes a prominent feature in cases of clear-cell carcinoma of the kidney; the tumour growth is often attended by thrombosis.

Varicosity, i.e. dilatation and tortuosity, may affect a group of veins diffusely or in the form of saccular dilatation. Varicose veins arise from chronic continuous or recurrent increase in the pressure of the blood within them, and this results mainly either from (a) the effects of gravity, e.g. in the leg veins, sometimes aggravated by compression proximally, or (b) when a major vein is obstructed leading to increased pressure in collateral veins.

The former class is represented by varicosity of the saphenous system of the legs, notably the long saphenous vein. The condition is much commoner in women and there is a distinct hereditary predisposition. Prolonged standing upright without much muscular movement causes marked rise in pressure and distension of the long saphenous vein. This leads to incompetence of valves and failure to maintain the flow of blood towards the heart. Any constricting band around the upper part of the leg or thigh, if worn habitually, increases the risk of developing varicose veins. Venous stasis in the legs, due to the pressure of the gravid uterus on the iliac veins, often results in the development of varicose veins. Without doubt pregnancy is a predisposing cause, perhaps accounting for the higher incidence in women than men, although obesity is also a predisposing factor. The increased column of blood, giving greater hydrostatic pressure, further increases the dilatation. The venous valves and the muscle and elastic tissue ultimately atrophy somewhat irregularly so that thinning of the wall and pouchlike dilatations occur; finally the wall comes to be composed chiefly of fibrous tissue.

The nutrition of the skin over varicose veins of the legs may be impaired. The skin becomes eczematous and pigmented, and chronic indolent ulceration often follows. Haemorrhage from the dilated veins may be severe, but is easily stopped by raising the leg with the patient lying flat. Thrombosis is also apt to follow. Organisation of the thrombus is generally imperfect and calcification may result.

Varicocele is another common example of "gravitational" varicosity, in the pampiniform plexus of veins around the spermatic cord: it is commoner on the left side than on the right and various ingenious explanations have been suggested for this.

The second category of varicose veins is best exemplified by chronic obstruction to the portal venous blood flow (due most commonly to cirrhosis or schistosomiasis of the liver), in which the vessels which form anastomoses between the portal and systemic venous systems become varicose (p. 543): the most important ones are those running longitudinally in the oesophageal and gastric submucosa (Fig. 18.20, p. 486), for they may rupture and bleed profusely. While it is true that haemorrhoids ("piles")—varicosity of the communicating veins between the haemorrhoidal venous plexuses in the rectal wall—are a complication of portal obstruction, they are also extremely common in otherwise healthy individuals. Obstruction of the inferior vena cava brings about dilatation of the veins of the abdominal wall, establishing a collateral circulation through the upper thoracic veins. Obstruction of the superior vena cava may occur in cases of bronchial carcinoma and leads to severe dusky cyanosis of the head, neck and arms, sometimes accompanied by pitting oedema of the hands.

DISEASES OF LYMPHATIC VESSELS

The lymphatic vessels form a closed system separated by an endothelial layer from the tissue spaces. The separation, however, is very easily broken. Not only do organisms, leukocytes and tumour cells readily pass into the lymphatic vessels; also red cells which escape from the capillaries by diapedesis may be present in considerable number in the lymphatics draining an inflamed area. The lymphatic vessels thus afford an easy means of communication between the tissues and lymph nodes. Involvement of the lymph nodes in this way occurs in two main conditions, namely infections and tumours, especially carcinoma. In both the extension may be due to transport of the organism or tumour cell by the lymph stream, *i.e.* to metastasis in the strict sense. There may also be progressive involvement of the lymphatic vessels by the disease. In infections this may involve either acute or chronic lymphangitis, whilst in tumours the growth of the cells within the lymphatics leads to lymphatic permeation.

Acute lymphangitis. In the course of the spread of organisms along the lymphatics, inflammatory changes may be set up in the walls. This is seen, for instance, in streptococcal infection of wounds, in erysipelas and in suppurating lesions. Along the lymphatics of the part, redness, swelling and tenderness are present, these indicating the spread of the inflammatory condition. Spreading lymphangitis is an important feature in puerperal sepsis and septic abortion and may be followed by suppuration in the loose connective tissue around the uterus. In other cases of bacterial infection, the organisms are carried by the lymphatic vessels without settling in their walls. Inflammation of the axillary lymph nodes may result in this way from an infected wound on the hand, without the occurrence of spreading lymphangitis. A similar striking example is seen in plague, where even at the site of infection there is usually no inflammatory reaction, the first lesion appearing in the related lymph nodes.

Chronic lymphangitis occurs in a variety of conditions; it may follow repeated acute attacks of erysipelas, and is an important feature in many types of chronic interstitial inflammation. A striking example of non-infective lymphangitis is seen in silicosis of the lungs, where fine stone particles which have reached the lymphatics from the alveoli are carried in various directions and lead to fibrosis of the pulmonary tissue (p. 372). In various chronic infections the spread of organisms by the lymphatics is of great importance. In *tuberculosis*, a disease which in the early stages may be regarded as essentially one of the lymphatic system, the organisms may be carried to lymph nodes without causing lesions on their way. They may however settle in the walls of the lymphatic vessels and give rise to tubercles which thus come to form rows along the vessels. In tuberculous ulceration of the intestine, small tubercles may be found along the lymphatics passing from the floor of the ulcer (Fig. 18.56, p. 518), and also in the mesenteric lymphatics. The thoracic duct may become involved by spread of bacilli along the lymph stream and ulceration of these lesions may set free a large number of tubercle bacilli into the circulation to set up acute miliary tuberculosis (p. 146).

In *syphilis* also, chronic lymphangitis is a prominent feature in connection with the primary lesion, and induration spreading along the lymphatics leads to the characteristic bubo in the regional lymph nodes. The chronic inflammatory change is due to the spread of the treponemata by the lymph stream, and is characterised by proliferation of the lining endothelium as well as of the connective tissue cells in the walls of the vessels. The organism of syphilis has a predilection for perivascular lymphatics, and the serious results caused in the aorta by this mode of spread have already been described (p. 277).

Lymphatic obstruction, lymphoedema. Chronic obstruction of lymphatics may give rise to interstitial accumulation of lymph (lymphoedema). When this is prolonged there is proliferation of connective tissue in the lymphoedematous area, resulting in a firm, non-pitting oedema. The most striking examples are seen in *filariasis*, in which obstruction of major lymphatics, together with recurrent inflammation in the affected region, may lead to gross thickening of the tissues known as *elephantiasis*: the lower limbs and sometimes the male external genitalia may be involved (see below). In this country, lymphatic obstruction was formerly not uncommon as a result of recurrent erysipelas, in which scarring and obstruction of multiple small lymphatics may lead to lymphoedema. Nowadays, extensive carcinomatous permeation of lymphatics is a more common cause, but surgical removal of lymphatics or destruction of lymphatics by radiotherapy can cause lymphoedema. This is sometimes seen following radical mastectomy and radiotherapy for breast cancer, where the ipselateral arm may be sufficiently deprived of its lymphatic drainage to develop gross lymphoedema without carcinomatous involvement of lymphatics. Several instances of tumour growth resembling haemangiosarcoma have been observed in the lymphangiomatous arm. It is not clear whether they are true sarcomas, or metastatic breast carcinoma, the appearance of which is modified by the lymphoedematous environment.

Filarial disease. The term *Filaria sanguinis hominis* is applied in a general way to the embryos of at least four species of filaria found in the tissues of the human subject, which are distinguishable by morphological and other characters. Microfilariae may appear only periodically in the blood, for example, at night— *Microfilaria nocturna*, during the day—*Microfilaria diurna*, or at all times—*Microfilaria perstans*. The most important of these filariae is the filaria *Wuchereria bancrofti*, the embryo of which is the *Microfilaria nocturna*. We shall give a brief account of this parasite and the important effects produced by it.

Wuchereria bancrofti. The parasite is widespread in tropical and sub-tropical countries, and more than a quarter of certain populations may be infested (Manson). The adult worms, male and female, are thin filiform organisms, little thicker than coarse hairs; they are whitish and show wriggling movements. The female is about three inches in length, whilst the male is shorter, thinner, and has a spirally

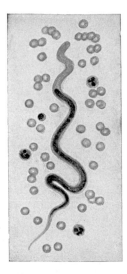

FIG. 13.41.—*Microfilaria nocturna* (embryo of *Wuchereria bancrofti*) in human blood. × 300.

twisted tail. Within the thoracic duct or in large lymphatic vessels, in the pelvis or groins, several worms often occur together coiled up in a bunch. The females are viviparous and produce microfilariae, which pass by the lymphatics to the blood stream, where they are readily found on microscopic examination. The microfilariae, about 0·3 mm. in length and about 8 μ in thickness (Fig. 13.41), are each enclosed in a loose sheath within which the little worm may be seen to move backwards and forwards. The microfilariae, which apparently do no harm, appear in the blood in the evening, and they can be easily detected microscopically by means of their movements. During the daytime they disappear from the peripheral circulation; some think that they collect in the blood vessels of the lungs, but others believe that they are quickly

destroyed, and that their periodicity is due to daily discharge of larvae by female worms in the lymphatics. The intermediate host is a female mosquito, usually of the *Culex* genus, which becomes infected by swallowing blood containing the microfilariae. Within the stomach they escape from their sheaths and pass to the muscles of the insect. Within these they undergo further development, and thereafter pass to the labium, where they are in a position to gain access to the human tissues when the insect bites.

In man the chief effects are produced by the masses of the adult worms in the lymphatics which have a twofold effect, namely, (*a*) the causation of obstruction and (*b*) the production of a certain amount of irritation and damage to the walls of the lymphatics, which often results in their permanent closure. When the thoracic duct is obstructed, it dilates below, and there is also a great varicose enlargement of the lymphatics drained by it, which may form large masses in the abdominal cavity. The anastomoses with the lymphatics, especially of the abdominal wall, become varicose. Thus the scrotum may become greatly swollen and swellings may form in the groins. These lesions are, however, only the outlying manifestations of the general lymphatic varicosity. The dilated lymphatics contain chyle which is passing off by the collateral channels, and when rupture occurs a milky fluid escapes, containing fatty globules, red cells in varying number, and sometimes microfilariae. When rupture takes place into the peritoneal cavity *chylous ascites* is produced; when it occurs in the kidneys or bladder *chyluria* results.

Another important result of filarial infection is the production of a form of elephantiasis— *elephantiasis Arabum*—which is of common occurrence in filarial regions. The condition usually starts with an attack of erysipelatoid inflammation and lymphangitis, and is intensified by subsequent attacks. The skin and subcutaneous tissues undergo marked thickening and swelling and become indurated, irregularly folded or nodular. In more than 90 per cent of cases, a lower limb is affected; less commonly the scrotum, breast, or an upper limb, are involved. The leg may slowly reach an enormous size, while a scrotal tumour may weigh 15 kg. or more. According to Manson, elephantiasis occurs when the lymphatic vessels become completely obstructed because the ova of the parasite are set free instead of the living embryos. Since the ova are broader than the living microfilariae, they could more readily cause obstruction and irritation. Thickening of connective tissue results also from attacks of secondary bacterial infection. As a rule microfilariae are not found in the blood in cases of elephantiasis. Manson considered this to be due to complete obstruction of the lymphatics, or to the actual death of the female parasites.

CHAPTER 14

THE HEART

Introduction

Disease of the heart now causes more deaths in Western countries than disease of any other organ, amounting to more than a third of all deaths in Great Britain according to the Registrar General's Statistical Review for 1969. Atheroma and thrombosis of the coronary arteries account for most of these deaths by causing ischaemic heart disease in its various forms. The other frequent causes of cardiac disease are congenital abnormality, rheumatic fever and its sequelae, hypertension in the systemic or pulmonary circulations, thyrotoxicosis and anaemia.

The work of the heart. Assuming that at rest the stroke volume of the heart is 66 ml. and the rate 72 beats per minute, the left ventricle has a minute volume of about 5 litres, and a daily output of 7,200 litres (about 7½ tons). The normal heart has great reserve power, and this can be substantially increased by physical training. During exertion, there is a greater venous return to the heart with consequent increase in diastolic filling and stretching of the muscle fibres; the response is a more vigorous contraction (Starling's law) and the blood pressure is raised. The rate of contraction also increases during exertion and these two factors together can raise the minute volume to above seven times that of the resting state.

This physiological performance can be maintained only if the myocardium is intrinsically healthy, if the valves function efficiently and if the conducting system of the heart co-ordinates contraction of the chambers properly.

CARDIAC FAILURE
Congestive cardiac failure. Cardiac decompensation.

Definition. Cardiac failure is that state in which the myocardium fails to maintain a circulation adequate for the needs of the body despite an adequate venous filling pressure.

Physiology. If the power of ventricular contraction is inadequate to expel the volume of blood received, stretching of the fibres goes beyond the point of increased energy of contraction and there is retention of residual blood. The dilated heart acts at a disadvantage because in order to bring about a given pressure within the larger cavity the contracting myocardium has to achieve a greater tension than is required in a smaller cavity. Excessive dilatation of the cavities is the essential physical condition underlying cardiac failure; emptying is incomplete, the venous pressure rises ("backwards failure"), cardiac output falls, and tissue anoxia occurs ("forwards failure").

Etiology. Cardiac failure may be due to:

(1) *Weakness of the myocardium*, e.g. as a result of myocardial ischaemia, rheumatic myocarditis, the toxic effects of diphtheria, isolated myocarditis and the myocardiopathies.

(2) *Intrinsic mechanical defects* of the heart with which the myocardium is no longer able to cope, e.g. stenosed or incompetent valves due to rheumatism, syphilis or congenital abnormalities. The dilatation of failure itself causes stretching of the valvular orifices with *secondary* (*functional*) incompetence of the mitral and tricuspid valves. Even a moderate augmentation of stroke volume increases substantially the total daily work required, and the reserve power of the heart is consequently reduced; if the left ventricle has to expel an additional 20 ml. to compensate for a diastolic aortic leak, then

the *additional* daily output will be over two tons.

(3) *Extrinsic conditions*, arising outwith the heart which increase the demands on the myocardium. Of these, systemic and pulmonary hypertension are common; in order to avert cardiac failure the ventricles have then to maintain a normal cardiac output against increased peripheral or pulmonary arteriolar resistance. In thyrotoxicosis, pulmonary emphysema, beri-beri, anaemia, arteriovenous aneurysm and Paget's disease of bone persistently high cardiac output is required to meet the oxygen and other requirements of the body and in these conditions cardiac failure frequently occurs when the cardiac output has fallen but is still greater than that required by the normal individual ("high output failure").

(4) *Disorders of cardiac rhythm* occur frequently in the presence of cardiac disease (Fig. 14.1) and occasionally in the absence of demonstrable lesions. Although minor irregularities such as sinus arrhythmia and occasional extrasystoles do not significantly impair cardiac function, severe tachycardia so shortens the time for diastolic filling of the ventricles and diastolic flow in the coronary arteries that the efficiency of the heart is substantially decreased; this happens in atrial fibrillation and flutter and the paroxysmal tachycardias. The bradycardia seen in complete heart block (about 30 beats a minute) causes a marked fall in cardiac output.

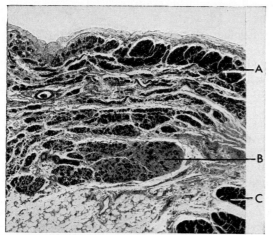

FIG. 14.1.—Section of atrio-ventricular node in a case of ischaemic heart disease with heart block and Stokes-Adams syndrome.

A. Atrial muscle.
B. Fibrosed A.V. node.
C. Ventricular muscle.

(5) *Coincidence of multiple factors*. Each of the above etiological groups may independently produce cardiac failure, but various factors often operate simultaneously. For example, a patient with mitral stenosis and myocardial fibrosis due to previous rheumatic fever may have only impaired exercise tolerance (i.e. diminished cardiac reserve) without evidence of cardiac failure at rest; with the onset of atrial fibrillation cardiac failure at rest may develop. An individual with systemic hypertension may develop cardiac failure as a result of occlusion of a minor coronary artery which would go virtually unnoticed but for the hypertension, or cardiac failure may be precipitated by an attack of pneumonia in a person with pulmonary hypertension due to emphysema.

Manifestations of cardiac failure. In the mildest form of cardiac failure, cardiac function is adequate for the needs of the body at rest, and failure becomes apparent as undue breathlessness on exertion; this is attributable to congestion of the lungs which stimulates respiratory reflexes. In more severe forms of cardiac failure, cardiac output is inadequate even at rest and structural changes in various organs result. The nature of the changes depends on the duration of the cardiac failure, and on which ventricle predominantly fails.

Acute cardiac failure is due to conditions of sudden onset, e.g. coronary artery occlusion, pulmonary embolism, acute infections, the hypertension of acute glomerulonephritis, the development of an arrhythmia, or rupture of a chamber or valve cusp. If death occurs rapidly the organs behind the failing ventricle show acute venous congestion and no compensatory changes are found in the heart except in cases where there has already been a cardiac lesion.

Chronic cardiac failure may follow acute cardiac failure if death or recovery does not occur rapidly. In cardiac disease of gradual onset, e.g. acquired valvular lesions, chronic failure is particularly common. At death the changes of generalised chronic venous congestion (see p. 156) are found, and the heart, in addition to the features of the causative lesion and the dilatation of failure, shows compensatory enlargement of the chambers. These are described below (p. 298).

Left ventricular failure is the cause of 60 per cent of deaths in essential hypertension, and is a common cause of death in myocardial infarction, a condition which mainly affects the left ventricle. It is usually the cause of death in patients with disease of the aortic valve. The clinical and pathological manifestations are predominantly pulmonary, for in the presence of an efficient right ventricle, congestion is confined to the pulmonary circulation in which an excessive volume of blood accumulates. Severe breathlessness, cyanosis and pulmonary oedema are the outstanding clinical features and there may be no evidence of right ventricular failure though some congestion of the neck veins is usual. Paroxysmal nocturnal attacks of dyspnoea ("cardiac asthma") are common in hypertensives and are due to acute left ventricular failure following a rise in pulmonary blood volume perhaps from resorption of peripheral oedema fluid when the patient is recumbent at night. At necropsy there is dilatation of the left ventricle and functional mitral incompetence: acute or chronic venous congestion of the lungs is found with pulmonary oedema and froth in the bronchi.

Right ventricular failure in its most acute form is found in cases of massive pulmonary embolism. The more chronic forms are found in patients with pulmonary hypertension due to lung disease (e.g. extensive pulmonary fibrosis, emphysema, etc.) and to mitral stenosis. In pure right ventricular failure pulmonary congestion is absent and the predominant findings are those of the causal disease, dilatation of the right ventricle with secondary tricuspid incompetence, distension of the great veins, well seen in the root of the neck, and acute or chronic venous congestion of the liver, spleen and kidneys. Oedema, ascites and pleural effusions are conspicuous in untreated advanced cases. Right ventricular failure also occurs in mitral stenosis, but in this condition chronic venous congestion with or without pulmonary oedema is found in the lungs owing to the rise in pulmonary venous pressure required to force enough blood through the mitral valve during diastole.

Total heart failure combines the features of left and right ventricular failure and is found not only in diseases which cause diffuse myocardial damage (e.g. extensive infarcts, myocarditis) but also in states requiring a persistently high cardiac output (thyrotoxicosis, etc.). In addition when there is left ventricular failure the strain imposed on the right side of the heart by the raised pulmonary pressure sooner or later leads to right ventricular failure.

Anoxic phenomena. When left ventricular output falls suddenly and markedly, the cerebral blood supply is so diminished that the patient loses consciousness. This may be momentary, as in a vaso-vagal attack (p. 188), or it may be rapidly fatal when due to occlusion of a main coronary artery, massive pulmonary embolism or rupture of a cardiac chamber. When the condition is reversible, e.g. during an attack of complete heart block, transient loss of consciousness may occur (Stokes-Adams attack); similar attacks occur in patients with incompetence of the aortic valve. In chronic cardiac failure oxygen deficiency in the tissues is less marked and is seen clinically in the form of cyanosis, sometimes accompanied by mental confusion. Pathologically, the effects of stagnation anoxia are best seen in tissues such as liver where fatty change and atrophy of liver cells are usually present in association with venous congestion. A compensatory increase in red cells (polycythaemia) may occur due to anoxia.

Cardiac oedema is dealt with on pp. 182, 183.

Thrombo-embolic phenomena. Patients with cardiac failure are prone to form thrombus in the leg veins as a result of muscular inactivity associated with bed rest, and in the auricles, especially when there is atrial fibrillation causing anoxia and slowing of the circulation. Many patients die or are disabled when these thrombi are lodged as pulmonary or systemic emboli resulting in infarction of lungs or other important organs (particularly brain, small intestine and main limb vessels).

Peripheral circulatory failure (Shock)

This is fundamentally different from cardiac failure, for it is the result of inadequate venous return to the heart. It is brought about (*a*) by lowering of the blood volume by haemorrhage and loss of plasma as in trauma or burns, (*b*) by severe dehydration in the crises of Addison's disease and diabetic coma or (*c*), from loss of tone of the arterioles with diversion of blood from the vital organs into the muscles, etc. In profound toxaemia, e.g. general peritonitis, diphtheria of the *gravis* type, a somewhat similar state may be observed and multiple

factors are concerned in its genesis, e.g. myocardial damage, peripheral arteriolar dilatation
and faulty cellular metabolism resulting from
toxic action. The subject is dealt with on
pp. 188–190.

Compensatory enlargement of the heart

When extra work is imposed on the myocardium as a result of a chronic disease (e.g. a
valvular lesion or hypertension) compensatory
changes gradually occur in the walls of the
affected chambers which enable these chambers
to deal more effectively with the increased work
of maintaining the circulation. The compensatory changes take the form of muscular hypertrophy of the wall, and in some cases dilatation
of the affected chambers; these changes are
often conspicuous clinical and pathological
features in patients with heart disease, and are of
great diagnostic value. When compensation is
effective there is, of course, enlargement of the
heart without evidence of cardiac failure; when
cardiac failure develops the dilatation of failure
is superimposed on these changes.

Compensatory hypertrophy of the myocardium is limited because the capillary blood (and
therefore oxygen) supply to hypertrophied
myocardial fibres is not proportionately increased; hypertrophy of fibres beyond a certain
diameter is therefore ineffective for lack of
adequate blood supply and cardiac failure then
readily results; for the same reason, hypertrophied myocardium is always unduly susceptible to local or general anoxia.

Manifestations of cardiac hypertrophy. In left
ventricular hypertrophy the weight of the heart
is increased above the normal 300–350 g., the
thickness of solid muscle at the thickest part of
the left ventricle exceeds 13 mm. and the
columnae carneae and papillary muscles are also
enlarged (Fig. 14.2). Hypertrophy of the right
ventricle alone seldom markedly increases the
total heart weight and is usually assessed visually
because of the difficulty of measuring the thickness of the right ventricle. For greater accuracy,
the right ventricular muscle can be dissected
from the rest of the heart and weighed. The
hypertrophy is due wholly to increase in the
average length and thickness of the myocardial
fibres.

Etiology of left ventricular hypertrophy. The

common causes of marked left ventricular
hypertrophy are (1) systemic hypertension
(essential, or secondary to renal disease, coarctation of the aorta, and certain endocrine
tumours), (2) stenosis of the aortic valve, (3)
compensatory dilatation of the left ventricle (in
aortic or mitral incompetence), (4) persistently
high cardiac output (thyrotoxicosis, anaemia,
arterio-venous fistula and Paget's disease of
bone). Mild and focal left ventricular hypertrophy is found in the absence of hypertension
or valvular lesions in certain patients with healed
myocardial infarcts, and is presumably compensatory for the loss of muscle. Various cardio-
myopathies (p. 305) are a less usual cause of
hypertrophy.

Etiology of right ventricular hypertrophy.
Most examples of right ventricular hypertrophy
are found in patients with pulmonary hypertension. The common causes are (1) chronic
lung disease, especially emphysema and widespread pulmonary fibrosis, (2) stenosis and/or
incompetence of the mitral valve, (3) congenital
heart disease with large shunts of blood from
one side of the heart to the other, and also in
cases of stenosis of the pulmonary valve, (4)
frequently right ventricular hypertrophy without obvious cause occurs in patients with massive
left ventricular hypertrophy. This may be
secondary to the raised pulmonary arterial

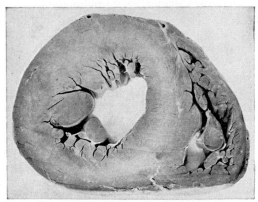

Fig. 14.2.—Transverse section of heart near apex in a
case of hypertension.

Note great hypertrophy of wall of left ventricle. $\times \frac{1}{2}$.

pressure associated with left ventricular failure;
some cases have been attributed to the hypertrophied interventricular septum distorting the
lumen of the right ventricle. Rarer causes of
right ventricular hypertrophy include disease of
the pulmonary arteries such as the presence of

multiple small emboli, pulmonary artery thrombosis and pulmonary arteriolitis (syphilitic or idiopathic). Patients with kyphoscoliosis and thoracic cage deformity have, for reasons not yet clearly defined, pulmonary hypertension and right ventricular hypertrophy but the severe reduction in total lung volume is probably the chief factor.

Clinical features. On clinical and radiological examination, the external measurements of a hypertrophied chamber may not be much increased unless there is co-existent dilatation. Characteristic electrocardiographic changes are found especially with hypertrophy of only one ventricle.

Compensatory dilatation. When a chamber of the heart is habitually overfilled during diastole because of incompetent valves, but continues to empty normally during systole, that chamber undergoes compensatory dilatation and this permits the chamber to maintain the required net forward stroke output.

Manifestations. The volume of the chamber is increased and the external size of the heart is substantially enlarged. Compensatory dilatation is accompanied by hypertrophy of the myocardium but this may not be obvious because of the increased diameter of the chamber.

Etiology. Compensatory dilatation of the left ventricle is associated with incompetence of the aortic or mitral valves or both, and to a lesser extent in patients with persistently high cardiac output (e.g. in thyrotoxicosis).

Clinical features. This condition can be recognised as enlargement of the external outline of the heart in the absence of signs of cardiac failure.

ISCHAEMIC HEART DISEASE

Classification

It is convenient to classify ischaemic heart disease under two headings.

(*a*) Chronic coronary insufficiency, associated with the clinical syndrome of angina pectoris.

(*b*) Coronary occlusion and myocardial infarction.

Coronary insufficiency

Diminished blood flow through the coronary arteries is associated with the clinical syndrome of *angina pectoris*, a paroxysmal substernal pain which may radiate to the shoulders and arms and which is usually precipitated by exertion, cold or emotion and relieved by rest and vasodilator drugs such as nitroglycerin. Anginal pain is of short duration, lasting no longer than a few minutes, but may be agonising while it lasts.

Etiology and structural changes. The primary factor in nearly all cases is narrowing of the coronary arteries. Atheroma is usually responsible, but syphilitic aortitis may also cause coronary insufficiency by constricting the mouths of the coronary arteries. A minority of cases are caused by inadequate filling of the coronary arteries because of regurgitation or stenosis at the aortic valve or sometimes by severe mitral valve stenosis. In most cases myocardial hypertrophy secondary to hypertension or valvular disease is a predisposing cause, the increased amount of muscle exaggerating the inadequacy of the diseased coronary arteries. *Coronary atheroma* shows the usual features of atheroma in other arteries (p. 264). There is patchy fibrous thickening of the intima with accumulation of lipid debris (Fig. 14.3). Calcification is usually

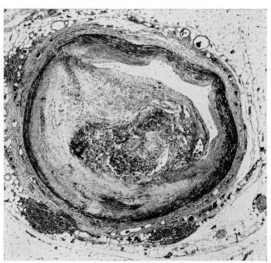

Fig. 14.3.—Coronary artery severely narrowed by atheroma.

Note the collection of degenerate fatty material in the depths of the intima, into which haemorrhage has occurred. × 17.

present, and confluent calcified patches of atheroma may convert lengths of the vessel into a rigid tube which cannot be cut with a knife; it is then very difficult to examine satisfactorily without decalcification. Atheroma affects all the main branches of the coronary arteries but the earliest and most severe lesions often develop in the first 2–3 cm. of the left coronary artery or in its anterior descending branch. Even small distal

organised thrombus (Mitchell and Schwartz, 1965). These workers raise some doubt as to the parts played respectively by chronic ischaemia and by acute thrombotic occlusion in the production of these patchy myocardial lesions.

Clinical Course. In general, chronic coronary insufficiency can be expected to shorten life, although there are wide variations in the clinical course and some patients survive for more than

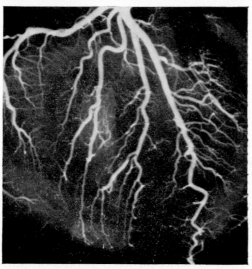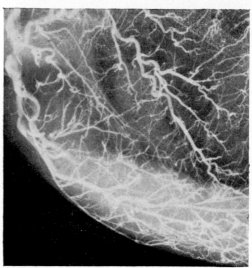

Fig. 14.4.—Angiograms of the coronary arteries, prepared after death. The enlargement of small intramural arteries to form an extensive anastomosis in occlusion of the major coronary arteries is shown on the right. Normal heart on left. (Mr. I. McA. Ledingham.)

epicardial branches may be narrowed, although branches that have penetrated into the myocardium are usually free of atheroma. At necropsy, occlusion of one or more major coronary vessels by organised thrombus can often be demonstrated. Extensive anastomoses commonly develop, as indicated by postmortem angiograms (Fig. 14.4). In most cases of angina pectoris, at the time of death there is myocardial scarring or recent myocardial infarction, but myocardial lesions are not invariably present.

Chronic coronary insufficiency may account for the finding of areas in which the myocardium is partly replaced by scar tissue, but in which some myocardial fibres persist (Figs. 14.10, 14.11), particularly around blood vessels. The difficulty in drawing conclusions as to the pathogenesis of such lesions arises from the frequency with which there is not only severe coronary narrowing due to atheroma, but also blocking of one or more vessels by

20 years. Many such patients die suddenly and unexpectedly; in some this is due to sudden occlusion of a coronary artery by thrombus, but in about half the cases no recent occlusion can be demonstrated. Death in these cases is assumed to be due to the sudden onset of ventricular fibrillation, and this has been confirmed in patients being monitored by electrocardiography at the time of death.

Myocardial infarction

Myocardial infarction is the commonest cause of death in many parts of the world today. Approximately 33 per cent of males and 25 per cent of females coming to necropsy in this department have evidence of old or recent myocardial infarction and mortality statistics for England and Wales and especially for Scotland suggest that the death rate from this disease is still increasing.

Etiology. By far the commonest cause of myocardial infarction is atheroma of the coronary arteries *with superimposed thrombosis.* There is some disagreement in the literature about the incidence of coronary thrombosis in myocardial infarction but our own studies have demonstrated that in patients who die shortly after the development of an infarct, recent occlusive thrombosis is usually present and also that this is commonly related to ulceration of an atheromatous plaque (Fig. 14.5). A study of the

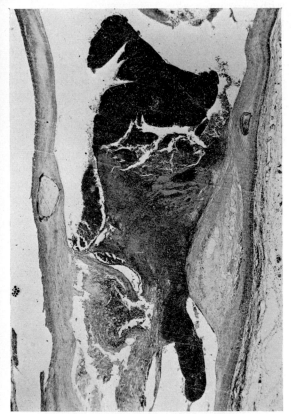

Fig. 14.5.—Coronary artery in longitudinal section, showing an ulcerated atheromatous plaque (left, lower) with occlusion of lumen by thrombus. × 15.

epidemiology of myocardial infarction indicates that many factors contribute to coronary thrombosis. The most significant etiological associations are with hyperlipidaemia, hypertension and cigarette smoking. The disease is commoner in males but its incidence increases in females after the menopause (p. 268). There is also some evidence to suggest that genetic predisposition, physical inactivity, psychological stress, soft drinking water and climatic conditions also play a part. On the evidence available it seems likely that dietary factors, particularly a high intake of saturated animal fat, are of fundamental importance.

Infrequent causes of myocardial infarction. Embolism of the coronary artery is a much less common cause of myocardial infarction. Emboli may originate from vegetations on the mitral or aortic valves in bacterial endocarditis or from thrombus in the left ventricle or auricular appendage. Myocardial infarction can result also from coronary artery involvement in syphilitic aortitis, Buerger's disease (p. 279) or polyarteritis nodosa (p. 280).

Clinical course. The onset of myocardial infarction is signalled by the appearance, often abruptly, of severe persistent chest pain. Many patients already suffer from angina pectoris and they often recognise that the pain is different, being continuous for some hours and failing to respond to rest and nitroglycerin. With the onset the patient may experience profound weakness and breathlessness, and there is usually evidence of peripheral circulatory failure with hypotension, cyanosis and a cold clammy skin. Fever, leukocytosis and a raised erythrocyte sedimentation rate are commonly observed within the first 24 hours. Certain tissue enzymes are released by the dead heart muscle, with a consequent rise in blood levels, which is of diagnostic value. The plasma concentration of glutamic oxaloacetic transaminase, for example, rises within 6 to 12 hours, and reaches a peak within 2 or 3 days. Characteristic abnormalities of the electrocardiogram are often demonstrable, but by no means always. The prognosis depends on the site and extent of the infarct and the age of the patient. Approximately 25 per cent of cases are fatal, mostly within the first few days after vascular occlusion, and sometimes instantaneously. Death is most commonly caused by ventricular fibrillation, cardiac failure or secondary embolic disease (see below).

Structural changes. Thrombosis of the interventricular branch of the left coronary artery is particularly common and usually causes an infarct involving the anterior wall of the left ventricle together with the apex and anterior part of the interventricular septum and the adjacent part of the anterior wall of the right ventricle. Occlusion of the right main coronary artery is somewhat less frequent and a proportion of such cases develop an infarct of the posterior wall of the *left* ventricle and the adjacent part of the interventricular septum. Occlusion of the circumflex branch of the left coronary artery can cause infarction of the lateral wall of the left ventricle. The site and extent of infarction do not, however, depend entirely on which vessel is occluded by thrombus. For example, in some cases the left coronary artery or its anterior descending branch has been grossly narrowed by atheroma, and the anterior wall of the heart is supplied mainly by the posterior descending and

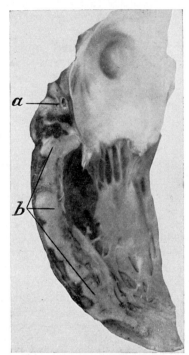

FIG. 14.6.—Recent infarction of myocardium.

The ventricular wall shows an extensive pale infarct (*b*) bordered by a zone of congestion and haemorrhage. Above, the occluded coronary artery is shown (*a*). × ¾.

other branches of the *right* coronary artery. Occlusion of the right coronary or its posterior descending branch by thrombosis may, in these circumstances, result in an infarct of the anterior wall. Effects such as this probably explain, at least in part, why some writers have reported a relatively low incidence of coronary thrombosis in patients with myocardial infarction.

The detection of thrombus in coronary vessels narrowed by atheroma is not always easy. If the arteries are opened lengthwise with scissors, a small thrombus may be displaced and disrupted by the point of the blade, and its presence thus obscured. A more satisfactory method of examining the vessels is by

transverse section at close intervals. The presence of extensive and grossly calcified atheromatous lesions prevents satisfactory naked-eye examination of the affected parts of the vessels at necropsy, and decalcification is first necessary.

Infarction may involve the whole thickness of the myocardium, or it may be confined to the inner part of the wall. Occasionally infarction extends round the whole left ventricle, involving mainly the deeper, subendocardial muscle. These so-called *global infarcts* occur in subjects with an unusually rich vascular plexus in the inner myocardium. It appears that this increased anastomotic plexus is a compensatory change which has resulted from atheromatous narrowing of larger coronary vessels. In spite of the richness of the plexus, the blood supply of the inner myocardium appears precarious. Fall of pressure in the plexus, following thrombosis in a major vessel, results in this characteristic distribution of infarction.

Although ischaemic death of myocardium results within a few minutes of loss of blood supply, the visible changes of infarction in the dead muscle do not appear for 8 hours or so.

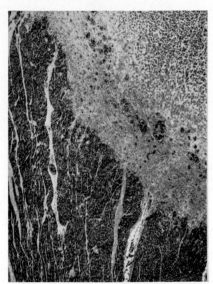

FIG. 14.7.—Infarct of myocardium of 12 days' duration.

The necrotic heart muscle (upper right) is separated from the surviving muscle by a zone of cellular and vascular granulation tissue. × 30. (See also Fig. 13.7.)

Accordingly, in patients who die suddenly at the time of coronary occlusion, or within the next few hours, acute changes in the myocardium are not observed by naked-eye or ordinary light microscopy. The dead muscle undergoes co-agulative change and after a few days appears as a dull yellow area surrounded by a zone of congestion and haemorrhage (Fig. 14.6). When the infarct extends to the outer surface of the myocardium, the pericardial surface is often covered by a layer of fibrinous exudate with marginal haemorrhages. On the inner aspect, the endocardium and a thin layer of adjacent myocardium remain alive, nourished by blood from the lumen, but in patients surviving for some weeks or even months, depending on the size of the infarct, and eventually a pale fibrous scar remains (Fig. 14.8). Occlusive thrombus in the coronary arteries also undergoes organisa-tion with some degree of recanalisation (Fig. 14.9), and anastomoses may increase from enlargement of small intramural arteries.

As already stated, it is sometimes not possible to determine whether myocardial fibrosis has resulted from infarction or chronic ischaemia (Figs. 14.10, 14.11).

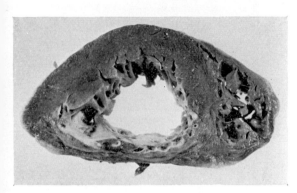

FIG. 14.8.—Old infarct, represented by a pale patch of thinning and fibrous scarring of the posterior wall (below) of the left ventricle.

several days this does not prevent thrombosis on the endocardial lining (see below).

Under the microscope the infarcted muscle shows the usual features of necrosis (Fig. 14.7). The necrotic muscle is invaded by polymorpho-nuclear leukocytes and, after a few days, diges-tion by macrophages and organisation can be seen at the margins. Gradually, the dead muscle is replaced by fibrous tissue, the process taking

Complications

(a) **Arrhythmias.** Death from myocardial infarction most frequently results from arrhythm-ias, particularly ventricular fibrillation. Healed infarcts may also be associated with cardiac arrhythmias and are the chief cause of heart block.

(b) **Cardiac failure.** Extensive infarction of left ventricular muscle can cause acute or chronic heart failure (p. 295), and this may develop at any time after infarction.

(c) **Mural thrombosis.** Following acute myo-cardial infarction, release of tissue throm-boplastin from the damaged muscle and localised eddying of blood leads to thrombosis in the ventricular chambers. This thrombus is a potential source of emboli. In time mural thrombus becomes organised.

(d) **Venous thrombosis.** Presumably because of reduced blood flow, systemic venous thrombosis is an important complication of myocardial infarction and tends to occur especially in the veins of the legs. Detachment of this thrombus is

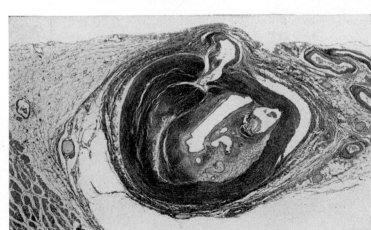

FIG. 14.9.—Coronary artery recanalised after occlusion by thrombus. There was extensive healed myocardial infarction. × 25.

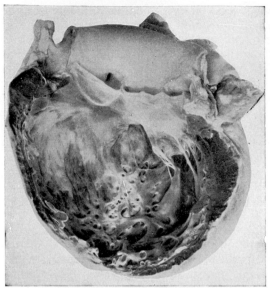

Fig. 14.10.—Extensive fibrosis of left ventricle with marked thinning at places; secondary to disease of left coronary artery. × ½.

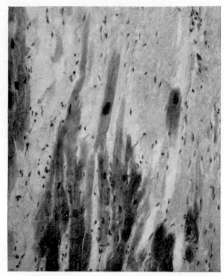

Fig. 14.11.—Myocardial fibrosis.
The surviving muscle fibres are hypertrophied. × 80.

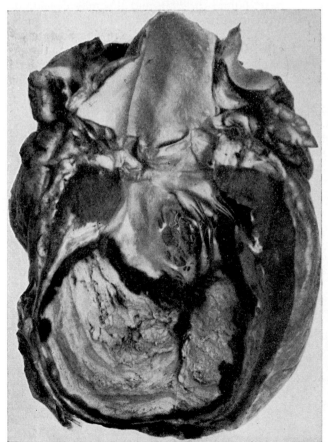

Fig. 14.12.—Aneurysm of the left ventricle following myocardial fibrosis.

The greater part of the ventricular cavity is filled with laminated thrombus. Note the white scar tissue forming the ventricular wall and the overlying peri-cardial adhesions. × ⅔.

common and consequently pulmonary embolism and infarction are not infrequently a cause of death in this disease.

(e) Rupture of the left ventricle due to myocardial softening (*myomalacia cordis*) causes 10 per cent of all deaths from myocardial infarction. It generally occurs 4 to 14 days after infarction, when autolysis of the infarct is active, and especially when leukocytic invasion is marked but repair just commencing. Rupture leads to sudden death from massive haemopericardium. When the interventricular septum is involved in infarction, it may rupture, leading to sudden onset of severe cardiac failure and a loud heart murmur. Rupture of a papillary muscle in the left ventricle may also occur, leading to incompetence of the mitral valve, with a loud murmur and intractible pulmonary oedema. Persistence of hypertension and physical activity after infarction predisposes to cardiac rupture.

(f) Cardiac aneurysm. In rare instances the fibrosed wall of a healed infarct of the left ventricle may stretch to form a cardiac aneurysm. As with other aneurysms, laminated thrombus tends to form in the cavity (Fig. 14.12).

(g) Angina pectoris. Whenever myocardial infarction has occurred, there is likely to be adjacent myocardium which, although not infarcted, is ischaemic (and is presumably the source of the prolonged pain associated with infarction). As anastomotic channels dilate and enlarge, the blood supply to such areas of partial ischaemia will improve. However, in some patients angina pectoris dates from a myocardial infarction, and it is apparent that thrombosis of a major coronary vessel may render areas of myocardium chronically ischaemic. In some instances, angina is cured by myocardial infarction, presumably because an area of myocardium which was previously clinically ischaemic has been included in the infarct and destroyed.

(h) Recurrence of infarction. Because atheroma is generally extensive, individuals who have had a myocardial infarct are prone to recurrence.

MISCELLANEOUS "DEGENERATIVE" CONDITIONS OF THE MYOCARDIUM

Fatty change of the myocardium (p. 17) is an expression of impaired metabolism of the heart muscle most frequently seen in severe prolonged anaemia. *Adiposity of the heart* is a deposition of fat in the epicardium which extends between cardiac muscle fibres (Fig. 1.18, p. 18). It affects the right ventricle especially and is usually but not always associated with general obesity. Very rarely cardiac function is impaired by this deposition of adipose tissue. *Brown atrophy* (p. 27) is not related to the occurrence of cardiac failure. *Primary amyloid disease* (p. 195) commonly affects the heart and is a rare cause of cardiac failure. The clinical picture may be similar to that of idiopathic cardiomyopathy, and diagnosis may be difficult both clinically and at necropsy, unless the possibility of amyloidosis is kept in mind. *Segmentation and fragmentation of the myocardium* indicate conditions in which the heart muscle cells either separate from one another at the intercalated discs or show irregular tearing. These changes have been observed in cases of violent death. It is supposed that these conditions result from irregular contraction at the time of death, although the possibility that they are artefactual cannot be excluded.

Cardiomyopathy

Cardiomyopathy is a convenient term for the classification of a very heterogeneous and ill-defined group of chronic myocardial disorders which are neither frankly degenerative nor inflammatory in nature. In most the etiology is obscure.

The main pathological finding is cardiac dilatation and there is usually myocardial hypertrophy sometimes focal but commonly generalised; no obvious underlying condition such as a valvular lesion, hypertension, shunt or coronary arterial occlusion is present. There is little if any evidence of inflammation apart from fibrosis which is often marked, especially in the subendocardial layer where it gives a "sugar icing" appearance to the lining of the cardiac chambers. Mural thrombus may also be present. In addition to replacement fibrosis and hypertrophy of myocardial fibres microscopy may reveal focal necrosis of cardiac muscle. Clinically the lesion may present as cardiac failure, arrhythmia, unexplained cardiac enlargement or sudden death, and sometimes the patient has a disease known to be associated with cardiomyopathy.

Etiology. Numerous hereditary forms are

recognised, particularly those associated with dystrophy of the skeletal muscles, Friedreich's ataxia or with glycogen storage disease of the Pompe type (p. 21), but in none of these is the precise mechanism of production of the myocardial lesion understood. In many cases cardiomyopathy is an unexplained and isolated finding, perhaps the aftermath of an attack of myocarditis. Thiamine deficiency is sometimes responsible and some cases have been associated with alcoholism. Cardiomyopathy may complicate pregnancy and the puerperium.

Endomyocardial fibrosis is a cardiomyopathy of unknown etiology found mainly in tropical Africa where it is one of the common forms of heart disease. It is also found in many other parts of the world. In the absence of significantly narrowed coronary arteries there is dense fibrosis of the endocardium affecting usually the apex and posterior walls of one or both ventricles. Sometimes the fibrosis partially obliterates the ventricular cavity and, by enveloping the posterior papillary muscles and chordae tendineae, distorts the posterior cusps of the mitral and tricuspid valves with resulting incompetence. Mural thrombus overlying the fibrotic endocardium is common though embolism seldom occurs. The fibrosis is dense and acellular on the surface but more loose with some inflammatory reaction in the deeper layers. Fibrous tissue bands may spread through the inner third of the myocardial wall and there may be atrophy of myocardial fibres with loss of sarcoplasm. Bacterial endocarditis is recorded in about 10% of fatal cases.

Endocardial fibro-elastosis. Though not strictly a cardiomyopathy as described above, this rare disorder, mainly of infants, is similar in that it is characterised by a thick smooth layer of collagenous and elastic tissue between the endocardial and muscular layers. Involvement of the left ventricle, which may be hypertrophied, is most common. Cases have been attributed to fetal endocarditis, to anoxia due to origin of the left coronary artery from the pulmonary trunk, and to hypoplasia of the left ventricle associated with premature closure of the foramen ovale.

INFLAMMATORY LESIONS OF THE HEART

Myocarditis

The term myocarditis is used loosely to cover various lesions of diverse nature in some of which micro-organisms are present in the myocardium while others are due to the action of toxins or to the interaction of the tissues with other bacterial products in ways not yet clearly understood. The subject is difficult because of the impossibility of confirming myocarditis in suspected cases which recover, and the poor correlation between pathological lesions in the myocardium and clinical evidence of heart disease. The possibility of serious metabolic disorder with no structural change in the myocardium, and the difficulty of interpreting the results of bacteriological cultures of necropsy material further complicate the subject.

Toxic myocarditis commonly occurs in diphtheria. Similar appearances, presumed to be toxic in origin, may be seen in pneumococcal pneumonia, typhoid fever, influenza and in other infective diseases.

Naked-eye appearances. The lesions do not usually produce any recognisable change, al-

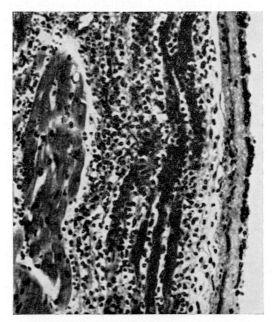

Fig. 14.13.—Inflammatory change round sub-endocardial branch of atrio-ventricular bundle in a case of diphtheria.

Note cellular infiltration round necrotic fibres. × 225. (Professor A. C. Lendrum.)

though sometimes the myocardium shows pale areas which suggest the existence of the condition; rarely there may be extensive mural thrombus between the columnae carneae of the left ventricle overlying damaged areas.

Microscopically there is a parenchymatous lesion with numerous small foci of coagulative necrosis in the muscle. The affected fibres appear swollen and glassy, with loss of striations and nuclei, and around them there is infiltration, mostly of mononuclears and lymphocytes, but polymorphonuclear cells also may be present. In some cases of diphtheria a lesion of this kind, with heavy leukocytic infiltration, is found in the atrio-ventricular bundle, and causes heart-block (Fig. 14.13). The necrotic fibres afterwards undergo absorption, whilst the supporting cells in the areas of infiltration proliferate, and small fibrous patches ultimately result (Fig. 14.14). The nature of the infection cannot be deduced from the appearances of the cardiac lesions.

Clinically toxic myocarditis is recognised by the onset of cardiac arrhythmia or acute cardiac failure in a patient with diphtheria, pneumonia, or other "toxic" illness. It may cause sudden

death. Peripheral circulatory failure may also be present in severe cases. The site of action of diphtheria toxin has already been discussed (p. 2).

Suppurative myocarditis is due to direct extension of pyogenic organisms from an adjacent valve in bacterial endocarditis, or to infection by way of the blood stream. In acute pyogenic infections, especially those due to staphylococci, e.g. acute osteomyelitis, the myocardium is often affected by cocci settling in the walls of the capillaries, rather than by

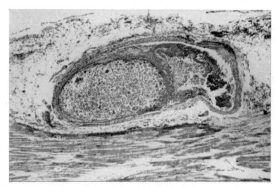

Fig. 14.15.—Septic embolus in coronary artery in acute bacterial endocarditis. × 36.

embolism in the ordinary sense. Similar lesions occur when a suspension of staphylococci is injected into the vein of a rabbit, the heart muscle being affected probably next to the kidneys in order of frequency. This distribution can be explained, at least in part, by the greater flow of blood through these organs.

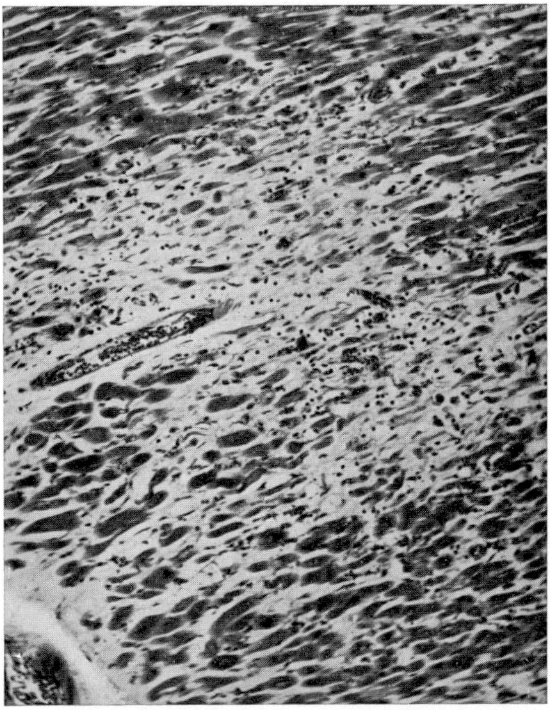

Naked-eye appearances. In cases of acute bacterial endocarditis the vegetations on the valves may infect the adjacent endocardium to give rise to haemorrhagic areas with crumbling surface vegetations; the organisms then invade the muscle substance and form an abscess, which sometimes leads to rupture of the heart or perforation of the interventricular septum.

In cases of pyaemia, infective emboli often lodge in branches of the coronary arteries (Fig. 14.15) and cause small abscesses, especially in the posterior wall of the left ventricle near the base; their presence at necropsy is indicated by small haemorrhages in the epicardium, which should always be incised to show any underlying areas of necrosis and suppuration.

The papillary muscles also are a common site of suppurative foci. Such abscesses occur especially in fatal infections, but occasionally small

Fig. 14.14.—Heart muscle in diphtheria, showing degeneration and disappearance of muscle fibres with focal cellular infiltration. × 115.

L

abscesses may be absorbed and scars left, especially in cases successfully treated by antibiotics and chemotherapy. Larger abscesses, usually haemorrhagic, are sometimes produced by grosser septic infarction.

Microscopy shows suppuration, and when the abscesses are pyaemic there may be recognisable myocardial infarction (Fig. 14.16). In various streptococcal infections, small inflammatory foci with many polymorphs may be present, and it is likely that in many instances these do not go on to suppuration but undergo healing with fibrosis, especially in treated cases.

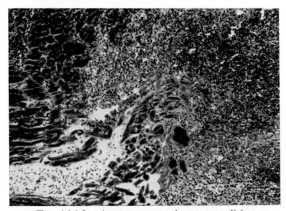

FIG. 14.16.—Acute suppurative myocarditis.
To the left of the field necrotic muscle fibres in process of digestion; in centre, clumps of staphylococci; to the right a collection of pus. × 85.

Myocarditis due to virus infection. An acute myocarditis occurs in the newborn and in young infants due to Coxsackie B virus, the infection being conveyed from the mother to the fetus *in utero*. The myocardium shows widespread damage to the muscle fibres with abundant macrophages, lymphocytes, plasma cells and eosinophils in the interstitial tissue. Coxsackie myocarditis may occur also in adults.

Isolated myocarditis. Various forms of subacute and chronic myocarditis without concomitant endocarditis or pericarditis have been described, and although the appearances resemble those in Coxsackie infection in the newborn, nothing is known of their causes or relationships. In one variety, known as interstitial myocarditis (Fiedler's myocarditis), the heart is dilated and hypertrophied and mural thrombi are common. Yellowish-white foci of necrosis may be visible and microscopically these show conspicuous infiltration of the interstitial tissue around the necrotic muscle fibres

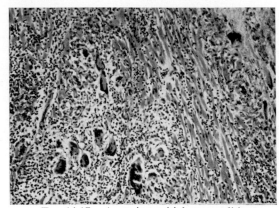

FIG. 14.17.—Acute interstitial myocarditis.
The heart muscle fibres are replaced by a granulomatous reaction, in which there are many giant cells derived from the muscle fibres. × 85. (Professor T. Symington.)

with macrophages, lymphocytes, plasma cells, eosinophils and multinucleated giant cells, apparently derived from the damaged muscle fibres. Fig. 14.17 is from a boy aged 14 who died suddenly after a brief illness.

Clinically the disease presents with cardiac arrhythmia, chest pain and embolic phenomena, progressing in a few weeks or months to cardiac failure without obvious cause.

Sarcoidosis may involve the heart, granulomata developing in the myocardium. The endocardium and pericardium are not usually involved.

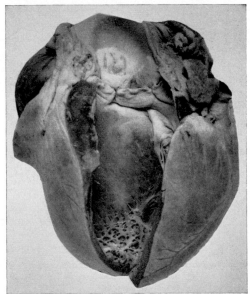

FIG. 14.18.—Chronic syphilis of aortic valve and aorta. Note the ventricular dilatation resulting from aortic incompetence and myocardial ischaemia. × ½.

Syphilis, formerly a frequent cause of serious heart disease, is now uncommon. It may affect the heart in four ways. *Incompetence of the aortic valve* is the commonest form and is due to involvement of the cusps or the valve ring as a result of extension of syphilitic mesaortitis. The cusps are elongated and pendulous but do not become adherent or calcify (Fig. 14.18). The mitral valve is not affected by syphilis but secondary incompetence may result from left ventricular dilatation. The effects on the chambers of the heart are similar to those resulting from any other variety of aortic incompetence (see p. 316).

Myocardial ischaemia may follow narrowing of the orifices of the coronary arteries by intimal fibrous plaques formed over areas of mesaortitis or by cicatricial contraction of healing lesions. This results in diffuse myocardial fibrosis and angina pectoris, but myocardial infarction is rare. Death is often sudden.

Gumma of the heart is very rare. It forms a tumour-like mass in the wall of a ventricle or in the interatrial septum where it may cause heart-block. It is found in both congenital and acquired forms of the disease (Fig. 14.19).

Interstitial myocarditis occurs in congenital syphilis and spirochaetes are often numerous, occurring in clumps throughout the cardiac muscle; there is a variable amount of fibrous tissue proliferation around them. In the adult, syphilitic myocarditis can be proved only by demonstration of the spirochaetes. The great majority of cases of myocardial fibrosis in adults are the result of ischaemic heart disease of which syphilis, by narrowing the coronary ostia, is a possible but now uncommon cause.

Tuberculosis sometimes causes pericarditis (p. 324) but seldom involves the myocardium even in miliary cases. Vegetations, tuberculous from the beginning or secondarily infected by tubercle bacilli, have occasionally been described.

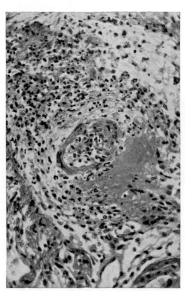

Fig. 14.19.—Miliary gumma of heart of child.

In the centre of field there is a small thrombosed arteriole and below it an area of necrosis. × 200. (Professor J. W. S. Blacklock.)

Rheumatic heart disease

Rheumatic fever
(Acute rheumatism)

This is an inflammatory disorder of the connective tissues, affecting especially the heart in the young and the joints in adults, and with a marked tendency to recur.

Age incidence. In about 50 per cent of cases the first attack develops during the second decade; of the remainder about one half occur earlier, usually between the fifth and tenth year. The primary attack occurs only rarely after the age of 30 years. Onset in childhood or adolescence is especially likely to result in a severe general affection of the heart—pancarditis—whereas if the primary attack is postponed until adult life joint manifestations are more prominent.

Etiology. Most attacks of rheumatic fever occur 2–4 weeks after infection of the throat by β-haemolytic streptococci of Lancefield group A. There is no doubt that such throat infection is a major etiological factor since prolonged administration of antistreptococcal drugs such as penicillin to patients who have had an attack of rheumatic fever greatly reduces the incidence of further attacks of this notably recurrent disease. Presumably the high incidence of rheumatic fever in the lower social classes is due to increased likelihood of streptococcal infection.

It is far from clear how preceding infection of the throat leads to the cardiac and other lesions of rheumatic fever. The 2–4 weeks delay in onset speaks against a direct infection of the heart, etc., or a direct effect of exotoxin. Streptococci have not been demonstrated convincingly in the cardiac lesions, and the failure of antibiotics to prevent the disease when first administered during the interval between the sore throat and the onset of rheumatic fever is not in keeping with simple spread of infection.

There are considerable grounds for believing that the lesions of acute rheumatism may have an immunological background. Compared with those who make an uncomplicated recovery from streptococcal sore throat, patients who develop rheumatic fever have unusually high antibody levels against various streptococcal antigens (including antistreptolysin O (ASO) titre, which is widely used as a diagnostic aid). The serum of many patients contains auto-antibody which reacts *in vitro* with antigen present in myocardial fibres, and becomes fixed to the patient's myocardial fibres *in vivo*. It is of particular interest that Kaplan has shown that certain antigens are shared by some types of group A streptococci and by myocardial fibres. A simple explanation of the pathogenesis of rheumatic myocarditis is that throat infection by streptococci leads in certain susceptible individuals to strong immunity against various streptococcal antigens; if, among these, the antibody response is directed towards the antigen shared by streptococcus and myocardium, an immunological cross reaction with myocardium takes place with fixation of antibody and complement and this leads to cytotoxic effects on the myocardial fibres. The real explanation is likely to be more complex since the above does not take into account the occurrence of rheumatic fever following infection by streptococci which do not contain the cardiac antigen, nor does it explain the typical lesion, the Aschoff body (see below)

which does not contain fixed immunoglobulin and is widely regarded as a lesion of connective tissue rather than one centred around myocardial fibres. Furthermore some unexplained factor must render the cardiac tissues abnormally permeable to permit the union of antibody and complement with cardiac muscle sarcoplasm *in vivo*.

Naked-eye appearances. Death may occur in the first attack of acute rheumatism or in an early recrudescence and at this stage is due to myocarditis and acute myocardial failure. This is often precipitated by the onset of pericarditis and pleurisy, which are not only indications of a severe carditis but further increase the load on

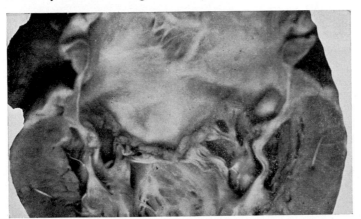

Fig. 14.20.—Acute rheumatic endocarditis of mitral valve, showing small vegetations along lines of contact. × 1.

the heart especially if there is much effusion. The weight of the heart may be increased by oedema and inflammatory infiltration and in cases of longer duration there may be some hypertrophy. Small, pale, focal lesions are often just visible in the heart wall, especially behind the posterior mitral cusp (Fig. 14.20).

An acute endocarditis usually accompanies the myocarditis, but plays little part in causing death in the acute disease. The endocarditis affects mainly the valves, and small thrombi referred to as vegetations are formed, first as minute rounded bodies of greyish or pinkish-grey translucent appearance along the lines of contact of the cusps (Fig. 14.20). Thus, in the aortic valve, they are found on the ventricular aspect of the cusps a short distance from the free margins, and in the mitral on the atrial aspect. The definite relationship of the vegetations to the lines of contact of the valve segments is clear evidence that the pressure along these lines on closure of the valves is a determining factor in the deposition of the vegetations.

It acts as a slight trauma on the surface endothelium altered by subjacent inflammatory oedema; the resulting lesion leads to the deposition of platelet thrombi. This factor has greater effect on the left side of the heart where the blood pressure is higher, and vegetations predominate on the valves of the left side. The mitral valve is more commonly affected than the aortic, the tricuspid being rarely and the pulmonary valve very rarely involved. The vegetations later enlarge and may extend on to the mural endocardium; for example, from the mitral valve they may spread over the atrial aspect of the curtains to the lining of the atrium, especially on the posterior aspect. In

collagen bundles surrounded by a zone of histiocytes and leukocytes (Fig. 14.21(*a*)). It often contains one or more giant cells (Fig. 14.22), though these are relatively small and contain only a few nuclei or a convoluted nucleus. The leukocytes are mainly lymphocytes and monocytes, though a few polymorphonuclears also occur. At a later stage the Aschoff bodies become fibrous (Fig. 14.21(*b*)). There also occur more diffuse polymorphonuclear and lymphocytic infiltrations along the connective tissue planes, and the formation of nodules is often associated with an inflammatory oedema. Bacteria are not demonstrable in these lesions.

Aschoff bodies are more common in the left

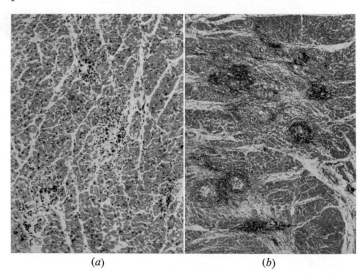

FIG. 14.21.—Rheumatic myocarditis.

(*a*) Acute stage, showing many Aschoff bodies. × 68.
(*b*) Later stage, showing early fibrosis around the Aschoff bodies. (Masson's trichrome stain.) × 40.

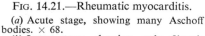

(*a*)   (*b*)

cases with a history of previous acute rheumatism, patches of white fibrous tissue with ill-defined margins may be present all over the lining of the heart. In early fatal cases the lungs are congested, sometimes brownish and of firm rubbery consistence, with hyaline membranes in the alveolar ducts (Fig. 15.13, p. 340). These appearances, previously thought to indicate a specific rheumatic pneumonia, appear to be merely the result of fairly acutely developing left heart failure and are met with sometimes in acute left heart failure from other causes.

Microscopic appearances. The cardiac lesion of acute rheumatism is a *pancarditis*, i.e. lesions occur in myocardium, endocardium and pericardium.

Myocardium. The characteristic lesion of acute rheumatic fever is the Aschoff body which, when fully developed, shows hyaline necrosis of

side of the heart both in atrium and ventricle. They are especially abundant beneath the endocardium of the left atrium just above the posterior mitral cusp; in long-standing cases this area becomes notably thickened, roughened and fibrous. The clinical effects of rheumatic fever indicate extensive myocardial damage and this may be a result of the fixation, *in vivo*, of antibody and complement to the myocardial fibres, as shown by Kaplan (p. 310), who reported also that such fixation correlates with marked eosinophilia and refractility of the fibres.

Endocardium. The whole of the endocardium may show innumerable focal lesions and a certain amount of diffuse inflammatory oedema and cellular infiltration, continuous with similar changes in the subjacent myocardium particularly over the chordae and papillary muscles.

At an early stage the connective tissue of the

valves shows inflammatory oedema, most marked in the subendothelial layer, where there may be localised swellings almost like vesicles. The condition is a general valvulitis (Fig. 14.23) upon which secondary changes are superimposed rapidly owing to the mechanical stresses to which the valves are subjected in the cardiac cycle. The inflammatory oedema is soon fol-

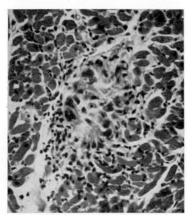

FIG. 14.22.—Aschoff body in child's heart, showing characteristic cells surrounding a focus of necrosis. × 180.

lowed by proliferation of fibrocytes and sometimes by the formation of poorly defined Aschoff bodies, especially near the base of the valve segments, and there is also an ingrowth of capillaries into the valve cusps which normally are avascular in man. The vegetations are composed chiefly of blood platelets and fibrin (Fig. 8.15, p. 167), and possibly also exudate from the inflamed valve. At a later stage organisation takes place from the valve and also fibrous thickening, and often calcification, of the valve cusps, and these may result in serious deformity.

Pericardium. Fibrinous pericarditis is common in rheumatic fever, giving rise to pain and a friction rub, and later undergoing organisation with resulting adhesions.

Clinical features. Marked variation occurs in the clinical features of rheumatic fever at different ages. In typical adult cases there is a transient febrile migrating polyarthritis which may be mild or very severe, affects the large joints mainly and leaves no deformity (p. 792). In children, early evidence of cardiac involvement includes tachycardia, disorders of conduction and dilatation of the heart with the murmurs of secondary valvular incompetence and, at a later stage, signs of pericarditis. The

vegetations on the valves have no clinical effect in acute rheumatic fever for they do not impair valvular function or give rise to emboli. Other features which may be seen are *chorea*—a mild encephalitis with degeneration of nerve cells of the basal ganglia which leads to involuntary movements—various skin rashes of which *erythema marginatum* is most common, and subcutaneous nodules consisting of areas of fibrinoid necrosis surrounded by a granulomatous reaction. The fever and arthritis usually respond dramatically to treatment with salicylates. There is a marked tendency for the disease to return after successive attacks of tonsillitis.

Laboratory findings. There is no specific test for rheumatic fever but a raised erythrocyte sedimentation rate, anaemia, slight leukocytosis and high titres of streptococcal antibodies are commonly present. C-reactive protein appears in the serum at an early stage but this reaction is not specific for acute rheumatic fever.

Subclinical rheumatic fever. Latent rheumatic fever is important for it may lead to chronic rheumatic carditis in later life. In a surprisingly

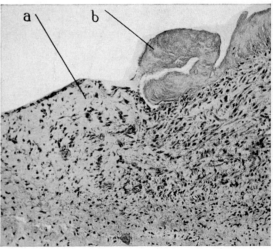

FIG. 14.23.—Section of mitral valve in early acute rheumatic endocarditis, showing (*b*) a small vegetation with commencing organisation. To the left side there is a patch of oedematous swelling (*a*) such as apparently precedes the deposition of platelets. × 60. (Professor A. C. Lendrum.)

large number of cases, examination of atrial biopsies taken at operation for mitral stenosis in carefully selected patients with no clinical evidence of active rheumatism shows the presence of Aschoff bodies in the subendocardial tissues (Fig. 14.24). Aschoff bodies are generally accepted as an indication of active rheumatism and it is clear that a very chronic smouldering form of the disease frequently leads to the serious valvular lesions encountered in the later stages.

Chronic rheumatic heart disease

Chronic rheumatic heart disease is a common sequel to acute rheumatic fever and is characterised mainly by chronic endocarditis in which overgrowth of connective tissue and its subsequent contraction leads to valvular deformities. Compensatory dilatation and hypertrophy of the chambers are found depending on the nature of the valvular lesions. In many cases Aschoff bodies are present together with minute foci of myocardial fibrosis representing healed Aschoff

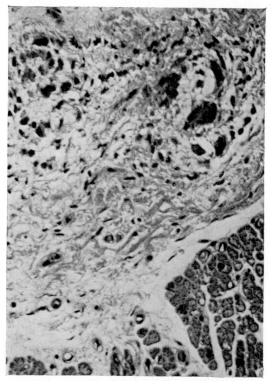

FIG. 14.24.—Aschoff bodies in the endocardium of the left atrial appendage, removed during operation for mitral stenosis. × 250.

bodies. Pericardial adhesions are common but these impede cardiac action only when the fibrous thickening is unusually severe and especially when the pericardium is adherent to other mediastinal structures.

Mechanism of production of lesions. The lesions represent a healing stage of acute rheumatic endocarditis and fibrosis results in all the sites previously inflamed in the acute stage. Thus the valves affected are the mitral, aortic and tricuspid in that order of frequency, and the chordae tendineae are much thickened and shortened. Fusion of the cusps along their contiguous edges by organisation of vegetations and fibrosis leads to narrowing or *stenosis* of the aperture. The chronic inflammatory process leads to thickening and retraction of the valve cusps which prevents efficient closure; valvular *incompetence* thus results. Both effects are frequently present. Subendocardial or myocardial Aschoff bodies or fresh vegetations on the valve cusps and atrial wall are fairly common and indicate recurrent rheumatic activity.

Effects

(1) *Cardiac failure* is common, mainly as a result of the mechanical problems created by stenosed and incompetent valves. These are considered in detail below.

(2) *Thrombi* frequently form in the atrial appendages especially in patients with mitral or tricuspid stenosis and atrial fibrillation, and may cause emboli with serious clinical consequences. A rare occurrence of interest is the formation in the left atrium of a so-called ball thrombus which lies free in the cavity and which may reach several centimetres in diameter.

(3) *Angina pectoris* occurs when the cardiac output is so reduced that coronary blood flow to the hypertrophied myocardium is inadequate.

(4) *Cardiac arrhythmias*, especially atrial fibrillation, are a common consequence and may be due to myocardial and subendocardial scar tissue.

(5) *Subacute bacterial endocarditis* is particularly prone to develop on valves even slightly damaged by rheumatic fever.

Mitral stenosis. Adhesion of the mitral cusps is very common, and the resulting stenosis may become very severe (Fig. 14.25). The orifice sometimes measures 5 mm. or less in diameter, and as the area is proportional to the square of the diameter, the reduction is extreme. (The mitral orifice usually measures 25–30 mm. in diameter.) The cusps may be adherent along the commissures, and form a thin fibrous diaphragm

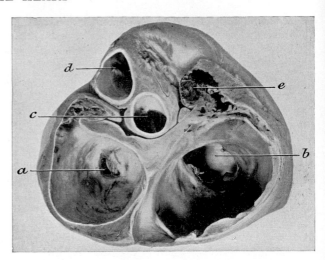

FIG. 14.25.—Horizontal section through atria in a
case of mitral and tricuspid stenosis, as seen
from above.

a, mitral valve, severely stenosed; *b*, tricuspid valve,
moderately stenosed; *c*, aorta; *d*, pulmonary artery;
e, right atrial appendage containing thrombus. × ½.

which is pliable and mobile; closure of the orifice
during ventricular systole can then be adequately
brought about by the constriction of the annulus
fibrosus, approximation of the nodular ridge,
and ballooning of the cusps towards the atrium.
In such cases a pure stenosis results and
operation for its relief may be remarkably
successful; unfortunately there is a marked
tendency to redevelop stenosis following operation. In other cases, in the later stages, the
segments are much shortened, thickened and
rigid, as well as fused at the commissures, and a
dense fibrous diaphragm with a slit-like aperture
results—the "buttonhole" mitral. There may be
marked thickening and shortening of the
chordae tendineae, and also fibrous induration of
the apices of the papillary muscles so that the
valve comes to form a funnel-shaped structure
with a small oval aperture. Calcification of the

cusps and valve ring may be present. The
endocardium of the left atrium is thickened and
opaque in most cases.

Effects of mitral stenosis. The left ventricle
can receive a normal volume in the diastolic
interval only if the blood is propelled more
forcibly through the narrowed mitral orifice;
commonly, it gets less blood than normally, can
easily pass it on and therefore does not undergo
hypertrophy; indeed it is often slightly atrophied.
The left atrium hypertrophies and it readily
dilates, sometimes to gigantic dimensions (500
ml. in place of the normal 30–40 ml.). Blood is
retained within the pulmonary veins and the
intra-pulmonary blood pressure is raised. The
work of driving the blood into the pulmonary
artery against the raised intrapulmonary pressure falls upon the right ventricle, which undergoes great hypertrophy (Fig. 14.26), until the

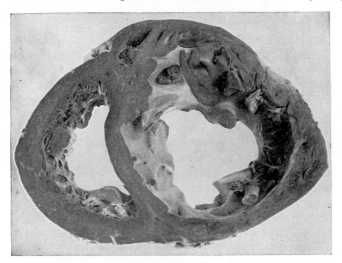

FIG. 14.26.—Transverse section of the ventricles
in a case of mitral stenosis, showing the
comparatively small left ventricle and the
greatly enlarged and hypertrophied right
ventricle (on the right). × ⅔.

pressure in the pulmonary veins is enough, in conjunction with atrial systole, to fill the left ventricle adequately during diastole. The stroke volume of the left ventricle may thus be normal —or very nearly so—even in quite severe mitral stenosis, and the patient may be very little incapacitated at rest. This is an extremely dangerous position, because if the tricuspid valve is competent then the relatively healthy and powerful right ventricle may in response to physical exercise raise the pulmonary capillary pressure to levels which produce pulmonary oedema.

Why pulmonary oedema does not develop more often is not completely known. The pulmonary capillary bed is partly protected by spasm and endarteritis of the pulmonary arterioles and the pulmonary lymphatics must remove enormous amounts of transuded fluid. In patients with mitral stenosis and tricuspid incompetence, any severe rise of pulmonary artery pressure is prevented by regurgitation into the easily distensible systemic venous system *via* the right side of the heart; this has the effect of decompressing the pulmonary circuit and bringing on right heart failure (p. 297), which is the common mode of death in mitral stenosis.

The passive hyperaemia of the lungs in mitral stenosis cannot be alleviated by any compensatory process. The lungs pass into the state of brown induration (p. 158) and there is often slight haemoptysis, to be distinguished from the more severe haemoptysis which results from pulmonary infarction when the heart is failing. The pulmonary arteries and arterioles develop marked hypertrophy of the muscular tissue of the media and some degree of fibrous thickening of the intima. Occasionally acute necrotising arteriolitis develops, very similar to that seen in systemic malignant hypertension. As a result of pulmonary hypertension there may be marked pulmonary artery atheroma. In mitral stenosis the heart as a whole comes to have a quadrangular form and the enlarged right ventricle constitutes the apex. The weight of the heart is not greatly increased. Mitral stenosis usually gives rise to a distinct murmur over the precordium and sometimes to a palpable thrill during atrial systole.

Rheumatic mitral incompetence often accompanies stenosis but may occur in its absence. Rigidity of the cusps due to fibrous thickening

or calcification favours the development of incompetence which depends not only on the size of the orifice but also on its consistence and configuration. If the stenosed orifice is small, and if the opening is directed posteriorly, the inward movement of the ventricular wall and papillary muscles and the tensing of the chordae in systole may completely close the orifice so that regurgitation is absent. Conversely, excessive shortening of the anterior cusp directs the valve orifice towards the ventricular outflow so that during systole these mechanisms cannot close the orifice and regurgitation then occurs. When the orifice is large and the cusps shortened, thickened and deformed, closure in systole fails and again regurgitation results.

In Great Britain nearly all cases of clinically significant chronic endocarditis of the mitral valve are attributable to rheumatism. In many cases there is a history of previous rheumatic fever. In other cases with no known history of rheumatism the appearance of the valvular lesion, the occurrence of endocardial fibrosis in the posterior wall of the left atrium and the finding of subendocardial or myocardial Aschoff bodies on microscopic examination point to rheumatic origin. This is supported by the known tendency of rheumatic fever to remain clinically latent. Secondary mitral incompetence associated with dilatation of the left ventricle due to heart failure is often due to causes other than rheumatism.

Effects of mitral incompetence. Mitral incompetence results in compensatory dilatation and hypertrophy of the left ventricle by means of which normal cardiac output is maintained. From the outset the left atrium is dilated and the pulmonary circulation congested. Increased work is thrown on the right ventricle which also becomes hypertrophied. The subsequent effects are similar to those occurring in mitral stenosis. Mitral incompetence is associated with an apical systolic murmur.

Rheumatic aortic stenosis is less common than mitral stenosis, probably because the cusps are forcibly thrown apart at ventricular systole. The segments are adherent at their adjacent margins and the aperture is triangular and considerably reduced (Fig. 14.27). Obstruction is the chief result but there is usually some incompetence of the valve.

Effects of aortic stenosis. Aortic stenosis produces pure hypertrophy of the left ventricle;

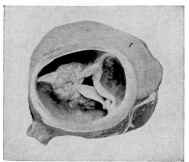

Fig. 14.27.—Chronic endocarditis of aortic orifice with severe stenosis and secondary calcification. × 1.

where there is significant incompetence, there is a certain amount of dilatation of the cavity as well, which becomes lengthened and more pointed. Later, the hypertrophied muscle may fail and then dilatation is the prominent feature. The passage of the blood during systole through the narrow aortic orifice gives rise to a loud ventricular systolic murmur audible over the base of the heart, and a systolic thrill. The pulse pressure is characteristically low.

Rheumatic aortic incompetence is often associated with stenosis and occurs when the margins of the segments are thickened and shortened or tacked down at their extremities so that the cusps can no longer come into apposition. Pure aortic incompetence in an adult is suggestive of syphilitic aortitis.

Effects of aortic incompetence. Aortic incompetence produces, from the outset, enlargement of the cavity of the left ventricle, accompanied by hypertrophy of the wall. The internal length of the cavity may reach 12 cm. or more (normal 8–9 cm.) resulting in twice the normal capacity. This indicates a very gross leakage. Thick white collagenous patches often develop on the mural endocardium beneath the incompetent valve and are known as "jet lesions", being attributed to forceful reflux of blood during diastole. So long as the mitral valve is competent the effects of the aortic lesion may

not extend backwards to the lungs and venous system; but as the enlargement of the left ventricle progresses, and especially as the muscle fails, the muscular ring round the mitral orifice becomes stretched and secondary mitral incompetence results; the effects of the latter lesion then become superadded. Incompetence of the mitral from rheumatic endocarditis may be present as a concomitant lesion, and such a combination causes most striking enlargement of the heart—the so-called *cor bovinum*, which may weigh 1 kg. or more. The pulse in aortic incompetence is characteristic. There is a large systolic wave owing to the increased output by the left ventricle, and this is followed by a rapid fall. The pulse has a bounding and collapsing character—the so-called "water-hammer pulse". A ventricular diastolic murmur, corresponding with the regurgitation, is usually audible over the base of the heart. There is a well-recognised tendency to sudden death in cases of aortic incompetence. It is probable that inadequate diastolic filling of the coronary vessels, due to lack of proper closure of the valve curtains, is responsible.

Rheumatic tricuspid stenosis is less common than mitral stenosis and is usually less marked (Fig. 14.25). It occurs most frequently when the right ventricular pressure is increased due to established mitral stenosis.

Tricuspid incompetence, most often secondary to cardiac failure, produces enlargement of both right atrium and right ventricle, while tricuspid stenosis affects mainly the atrium.

Effects of valvular lesions on right side of heart. Tricuspid stenosis restricts right ventricular output and this diminishes the likelihood of developing pulmonary oedema from the mitral stenosis which is almost invariably present. Pulmonary stenosis causes hypertrophy of the right ventricle. It is very rare, but occurs as a congenital abnormality, or in the carcinoid syndrome (Fig. 14.32, also p. 532).

Bacterial Endocarditis

Subacute bacterial endocarditis

Definition. An infection of the endocardium with bacteria of low virulence characterised by the formation of large crumbling vegetations usually on a pre-existing cardiac lesion, by bacteraemia and toxaemia and by multiple

embolic episodes over a period of months or years.

Etiology. Most cases are produced by non-haemolytic streptococci of the type classified as *Streptococcus viridans*; these are by no means uniform in their biological characters. In a small proportion of cases, *Staphylococcus albus* or organisms of the *Haemophilus* group have been isolated, notably *H. para-influenzae*. Infection probably takes place chiefly from the mouth, more rarely from the naso-pharynx, especially after minor operations. Firm biting on teeth affected by apical abscesses, dental extraction or tonsillectomy can lead to a temporary bacteraemia. The organisms tend to settle on previously damaged or abnormal valves, the result of previous rheumatic infection or a congenital abnormality, e.g. a bicuspid aortic valve. The roughened surfaces of the abnormal endocardium tend to attract platelet deposition, and bacteria in the blood stream, like other finely divided particulate matter, become attached to platelets and are deposited with them. Subacute bacterial endocarditis is often superimposed on still active rheumatic lesions.

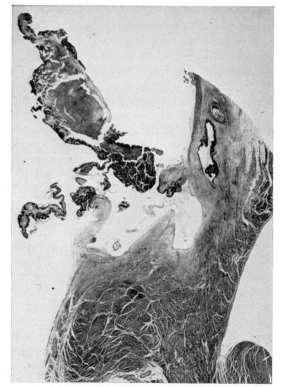

FIG. 14.28.—Subacute bacterial endocarditis of aortic valve, showing friable crumbling vegetations on the aortic cusp and adjacent aortic wall. × 4.

Bacterial endocarditis may occur in a patent ductus arteriosus and healing follows surgical closure in suitable cases.

Naked-eye appearances. *The heart* usually shows evidence of chronic rheumatic endo-

carditis or a congenital abnormality of a valve upon which are vegetations that are larger, softer and more crumbling than in the rheumatic form (Figs. 14.28, 14.29). In 40 per cent the mitral valve alone is affected, in 11 per cent the aortic and in 36 per cent both valves are

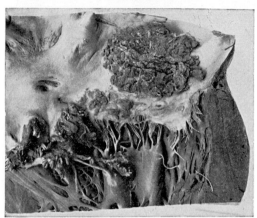

FIG. 14.29.—Bacterial endocarditis of mitral orifice.
The valve seen from atrial aspect shows crumbling and ulcerating vegetations extending to wall of atrium. × ⅔.

involved. The vegetations tend to spread on the endocardial surface and very frequently develop on the wall of the left atrium just above the posterior mitral cusp which frequently is the site of previous rheumatic lesions (Fig. 14.29). Possibly this results from retrograde propulsion of blood against the wall in this situation due to mitral incompetence. The lesions are not usually so destructive as in acute bacterial endocarditis, but give rise to emboli, both large and small, and infarcts are common in internal organs.

Other organs. The skin often has a *café-au-lait* colour and clubbing of the fingers is usual. Large emboli cause infarction in various organs but the infarcts seldom suppurate, probably owing to the high content of streptococcal antibodies which develop in the blood in the course of the prolonged infection. Petechiae found in the skin, beneath the nails and in the conjunctiva and retina, may be due to embolism (Fig. 14.30). The renal complications are described on p. 710. They include focal glomerulonephritis, which is common in cases of some months duration and is responsible for haematuria; also diffuse glomerulonephritis which may bring about renal failure. As a rule the spleen is enlarged, sometimes markedly so.

Microscopic appearances. The vegetations consist of fibrin, platelets and polymorphs togcthcr with masses of organisms and foci of calcification. The underlying cusp is vascular, oedematous and necrotic and macrophages, some multinucleated, often form a palisade round the necrotic areas.

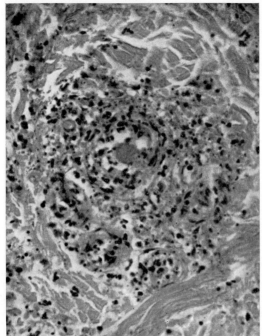

FIG. 14.30.—Section through haemorrhagic spot in dermis in subacute bacterial endocarditis. Note small thrombosed and degenerate arteriole surrounded by leukocytes—the result of infective embolism. × 160.

The myocardium, though grossly normal, often shows microscopic areas of infarction and inflammation.

Clinical features. Subacute bacterial endocarditis is relatively uncommon but is clinically important since it is often responsive to antibiotics though almost invariably fatal in a few months if left untreated. The clinical features leading one to suspect the diagnosis are an irregular fever accompanied by splenomegaly and haematuria, associated with small and large emboli in a patient with rheumatic or congenital heart disease. Cardiac failure is uncommon in the early stage of the disease. Non-haemolytic streptococci released from the vegetations can usually be obtained in blood cultures, especially during bouts of fever, but sometimes the result is negative because of the low virulence of the organisms and the marked antibody response, and cultures have to be repeated. The organisms in the inert substance of the vegetations are not destroyed by circulating antibody; they continue to grow and to be discharged into the blood stream from time to time.

Healed subacute bacterial endocarditis following antibiotic treatment leaves fibrosis and distortion of the valve cusps which are sometimes also calcified. The valvular defects and the minute myocardial scars often lead to cardiac failure later.

Rickettsial endocarditis complicating Q fever may present a clinical and morbid anatomical picture virtually identical with that of subacute bacterial endocarditis; this infection should be suspected when blood cultures are persistently negative.

Acute bacterial endocarditis

Definition. An infection of the endocardium by virulent pyogenic bacteria associated with the formation of large crumbling vegetations and severe damage to cardiac valves, septicaemia or pyaemia. Acute and subacute bacterial endocarditis are not, however, clearly demarcated by their morbid anatomy, and a distinction is based chiefly on the clinical course and on the finding of the responsible micro-organism.

Etiology. The disease is usually produced by pyogenic organisms, most frequently *Streptococcus haemolyticus*, the *Strep. pneumoniae* and *Staphylococcus aureus*. In Great Britain it is only occasionally due to other organisms. Infection of the valves is in most cases secondary to some other lesion caused by one of these organisms; it thus occurs in septic conditions, osteomyelitis, pneumonia, etc. Occasionally, however, the path of infection is obscure. Virulent organisms can attack previously healthy valves, as is shown by experimental work, but a pre-existing lesion may sometimes be found.

Pathological appearances. The vegetations are large and tend to break down; and the valve cusps may be largely covered by crumbling masses (Fig. 14.31), which consist of layers of fibrin in which are buried clumps of bacteria, resting upon a zone of leukocytes, macrophages and granulation tissue. The substance of the cusps may be softened and eaten away; or, especially in the aortic valve, rupture may take place, leading to severe incompetence. Aneurysm of a cusp is common, the organisms causing a softening of one side of the curtain, so that the thin tissue is stretched by the blood pressure and forms an aneurysmal bulging. An aneurysm or rupture of a valve is sometimes obscured by vegetations. Aneurysms of the aortic segments bulge downwards into the ventricle, due to the diastolic pressure. An aneurysm of the mitral valve bulges towards the atrium as the stretching occurs during the ventricular systole. The vegetations may spread also to the chordae tendineae which may soften and rupture. Infection may extend to the intima at the commencement of the aorta and an acute mycotic aneurysm may be formed (Fig. 14.31). The organisms may also pass directly into the substance of the heart wall, and lead to ulceration or to abscess formation. This occurs especially in infections with staphylococci and haemolytic streptococci. The valves most often affected are those on the left side of the heart. Affection of the tricuspid is not uncommon, but vegetations on the pulmonary valve are rare.

The lesions are more often localised to one part of a valve or are more irregularly disposed than in the other forms of endocarditis; for example, there may be massive vegetations at the junction of two aortic cusps, the rest of the valve being free.

The most severe and rapidly progressive examples of acute bacterial endocarditis are due to the *Staphylococcus pyogenes* and the *Streptococcus haemolyticus*. Staphylococcal endocarditis, which is now the more common, tends to produce valvular destruction, and to extend into the myocardium. It causes secondary abscesses in various organs more frequently than any of the other bacteria. *Pneumococcal endocarditis*, which is usually preceded by acute pneumonia, is characterised by massive, soft, greenish vegetations. It is one of the few infections that may affect the pulmonic and tricuspid valves.

Embolism is common and the resulting infarcts may undergo suppuration; multiple small abscesses may also be present in organs without gross infarction.

The clinical features of acute bacterial endocarditis are those of septicaemia or pyaemia in the course of which signs of acute cardiac involvement appear. Rupture of a valve cusp may be followed by the development of a very loud coarse murmur.

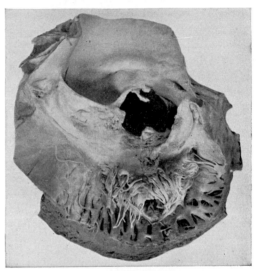

Fig. 14.31.—Chronic rheumatic and superimposed acute bacterial endocarditis of aortic valve, with ulceration and formation of acute aneurysm at beginning of aorta. × ½.

Other valvular lesions

Syphilitic aortic incompetence is described on p. 309.

Calcific aortic stenosis. Sclerosis, calcification and adhesion of the aortic cusps are sometimes found in elderly patients in the absence of mitral disease, and in spite of the distinct stenosis there may be little enlargement of the ventricle. The lesion itself is indistinguishable from chronic rheumatic endocarditis of the aortic valve (Fig. 14.27) and some writers attribute the lesion to this cause, but the absence of other signs of rheumatic heart disease and the advanced age of the patients suggest a degenerative lesion analogous to calcification of the arteries, which is a common accompaniment.

Degenerative changes of mitral valve. Yellowish patches of thickening and degeneration similar in structure to atheroma are fairly common in the mitral valve and may be attended by fibrosis and calcification, especially at the base of the cusps. The chordae tendineae are not affected and there is seldom any effect on cardiac function.

Endomyocardial fibrosis (see p. 306) frequently involves the chordae tendineae and posterior cusps of the mitral and tricuspid valves, causing severe mitral or tricuspid incompetence. The aortic and pulmonic valves are not affected.

Valvular lesions in carcinoid syndrome. Patients with secondary carcinoid tumours in the liver may develop stenosis of the pulmonary and, less often, the tricuspid valves. The cusps show marked fibrous thickening, have a rolled edge and are adherent along the lines of the commissures. Fibrosis may extend over the adjacent endocardium both in the right ventricle and in the wall of the right atrium (Fig. 14.32). Only trivial lesions are found in the left side of the heart, probably because of the amine oxidase enzymes in the lungs (p. 533).

Libman-Sacks endocarditis occurs in many patients with systemic lupus erythematosus. The vegetations are similar in appearance and consistency to those of acute rheumatism but are larger and are found on unusual sites such as the ventricular aspect of the mitral valves. Embolism and functional impairment of the valve does not occur.

Terminal endocarditis. A few vegetations on the mitral and aortic cusps are sometimes found in cases where death has occurred from wasting diseases, especially carcinoma. The vegetations are usually patchy and soft and consist of fibrin and platelets but no bacteria. There is sometimes an associated peripheral neuritis.

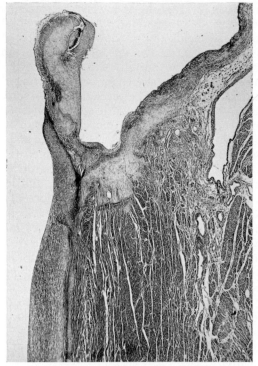

FIG. 14.32.—Pulmonary valve in carcinoid syndrome showing great fibrous thickening of the cusp and of the subendocardial connective tissue. × 12.

CONGENITAL ABNORMALITIES

Introduction

Little is known of the causation of congenital abnormalities, but the part played by rubella infection of the mother in the first three months of pregnancy is well established. About 10–20 per cent of the infants show serious abnormalities, of which heart disease constitutes about 50 per cent.

The most important congenital abnormalities of the heart result from defects or variations in the formation of the septa in the primitive heart. For details the student must consult a work on embryology and the classical studies of Maude Abbott and Helen Taussig, but it may be recalled that the heart at an early stage of development consists essentially of three chambers or parts, an atrial, a ventricular, and the aortic bulb; division of each of these into two takes place separately. Of special importance in this connection is the relation of the ventricular septum to the division of the distal portion of the bulb into two, which division results in the formation of the beginning of the aorta and of the

pulmonary artery. The ventricular septum grows upwards from the apex, with a curved margin resulting from the growing folds on the anterior and posterior walls, until ultimately there is a relatively small aperture at the base. The bulb, on its part, undergoes division into two nearly equal parts by the formation of longitudinal folds in its wall, which meet, and the two vessels formed undergo a certain amount of rotation in conformity with that of the ventricles. The septum of the bulb ultimately fuses with the up-growing ventricular septum, the last portion to close being represented by the *pars membranacea*. Important abnormalities occur in connection with the growth of these two septa. It is to be borne in mind that the position of the semilunar valve does not exactly correspond with the junction of the primitive ventricle and the aortic bulb. This is especially the case on the right side, where the lower part of the bulb becomes the upper part of the right ventricle or conus, and, as we shall see, this part is sometimes abnormally narrow.

While some of the anomalies are incompatible

with extra-uterine life, in many the circulatory dynamics are such that the patients may survive birth for varying periods of time. With the diagnostic methods of cardiac catheterisation and angiocardiography, successful surgical cure or alleviation of many of the conditions can be effected. It is convenient to divide the anomalies into those which produce *cyanosis* of the patient and those which do not. The cyanosis is produced by admixture of a relatively large amount of reduced haemoglobin, from the systemic venous return, with the oxygenated blood leaving the heart, i.e. a venous-arterial shunt exists. The resulting unsaturation of the arterial blood leaving the heart leads to an increase in the number of red corpuscles per c.mm. of blood, i.e. there is a *compensatory* or *secondary polycythaemia.* Cyanosis is then prominent. Later, when changes in the lung vessels occur and the heart begins to fail there may be added to this *admixture type of cyanosis* an element of faulty oxygenation of the blood by the lungs.

Cyanotic group

Malformations in connection with the aortic bulb.—Pulmonary and aortic stenosis. The commonest of these result from an unequal division of the bulb, and most frequently the septum is pushed to the right, so that the aorta is abnormally large and arises partly from the right ventricle, there being usually a defect in the ventricular septum at the same time (Fig. 14.33). The result is pulmonary stenosis or obstruction, in the wide sense of the term, but the condition of the pulmonary artery varies. Sometimes the pulmonary artery is small, the division of the bulb being markedly unequal and occasionally the small pulmonary artery is even obliterated or atretic. In other cases the narrowing is mainly at the valve, the cusps sometimes being partly fused to form a thickened diaphragm with an aperture of varying size. A third abnormality occasionally met with is a narrowing of the part of the right ventricle below the valve, that is, the part which is derived from the bulb. All these abnormalities interfere with the flow of blood into the pulmonary artery, and lead to a varying degree of hypertrophy of the right ventricle. Part of the blood from the right ventricle passes through the aperture in the interventricular septum and then into the aorta, and after birth the ductus arteriosus usually remains open and the lungs receive part of their blood supply through it. The foramen ovale also remains open and may be of considerable size.

The commonest anomaly of this group and one which is amenable to surgery is the *tetrad of Fallot.* In this there is obstruction in the outflow tract of the right ventricle, usually from stenosis of the pul-

monary valve but the obstruction may be in the infundibular portion of the right ventricle. This results in right ventricular hypertrophy and the pressure in this chamber is raised so that some of the reduced blood in the chamber is shunted through a high interventricular septal defect into the aorta, which, in addition to receiving the oxygenated blood from the left ventricle, partially overrides the septal defect and is thus in communication with the cavity of the right ventricle. In other words the aorta is dextraposed. All degrees of severity exist in the stenosis of the right ventricular outflow, the size of the septal defect and the dextraposition of the aortic root. In extreme cases the pulmonary orifice and artery may be atretic and blood reaches the lungs

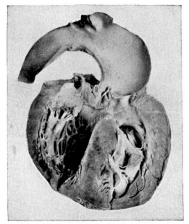

Fig. 14.33.—Pulmonary stenosis due to unequal division of the aortic bulb. × ⅔.

from the aorta through a patent ductus arteriosus. Obviously such cases will die when the ductus closes.

In about 25 per cent of cases of Fallot's tetrad, there is a right aortic arch.

Eisenmenger's complex. In this there is a strong resemblance in the gross morphology of the heart to that just described but there is no obstruction to the outflow from the right ventricle. The pressure gradients across the high interventricular septal defect are such that little right-to-left shunting of blood, and hence little cyanosis, occurs at first. Later, with the onset of pulmonary hypertension and changes in the pulmonary vessels, overt cyanosis occurs, partly from admixture cyanosis and partly from faulty oxygenation of the blood by the lungs.

Transposition of the great vessels. A curious anomaly results when the aortic bulb does not undergo the normal spiral twisting necessary to bring its septum into relationship with the interventricular septum. The pulmonary artery, instead of rotating forward and to the right, passes in the other direction, and the result is that the aorta rises from the right ventricle and the pulmonary artery from the left. While such a condition alone is incompatible with extra-uterine life, it may sometimes be compensated, for a time, by persistence of the ductus arteriosus, patent foramen ovale or a defect of the interatrial or interventricular septum; often these defects are present in combination. In this condition, the chief difficulty is not the volume of blood reaching the lungs but how effective is the mechanism allowing oxygenated blood to reach the systemic circulation. Hence the greater the volume of the shunt, the better the admixture of arterial blood to venous blood and the less marked is the cyanosis.

Truncus arteriosus. In this the arrangement of the heart and emergent arteries resembles that met with in elasmobranch fishes in that the aorta and the pulmonary arteries arise from a common stem vessel. The pulmonary arteries may be replaced by enlarged bronchials. The truncus arises from both ventricles, overriding a ventricular septal defect. Sometimes the septum may be missing so that a single ventricular cavity exists. Defects of the interatrial septum are also common.

Single ventricle with a rudimentary outlet chamber. This latter lies in the position of the normal conus of the right ventricle, and communicates with the main ventricular cavity which receives blood from both atria. One or both great vessels may arise from the rudimentary chamber; most often the pulmonary artery arises thus, with the aorta coming off the single ventricle. The interatrial septum may or may not develop normally, resulting in cor binatrium triloculare or cor biloculare respectively.

Tricuspid atresia. This is associated with defective development of the right ventricle which in extreme cases is virtually absent. Blood passes from the right to the left atrium through a defect in the septum between these two cavities. The pulmonary artery is small, arising from the underdeveloped right ventricle. In some cases the vessel is atretic or occupies an abnormal position. Usually blood reaches the lungs from the aorta by a patent ductus arteriosus.

Aortic atresia. In this rare condition the aortic orifice is hypoplastic, the ascending aorta hypoplastic or atretic and the left ventricle poorly developed or absent. Circulation of blood is maintained by shunting of oxygenated blood from the left atrium into the right atrium and thence to the right ventricle and pulmonary artery. From this the aorta is filled *via* a patent ductus arteriosus.

Pure pulmonary stenosis. Here the course of the circulation is essentially normal except for possible patency of the interatrial septum. The lesion is either a stenosis of the pulmonary valve or of the infundibulum of the right ventricle. The right ventricular myocardium is hypertrophied in order to force the blood to the lungs past the obstruction. If the interatrial septum is intact, cyanosis need not be present; if there is interatrial communication a right-to-left shunt may be established and cyanosis will then result.

Anomalies of the venous return. These may involve the systemic or the pulmonary veins. In the former the superior vena cava and/or the inferior cava may open into the left atrium, thus shunting reduced systemic venous blood into the arterial side of the systemic circulation. If, on the other hand, some of the pulmonary veins open into the right atrium the result will be merely that an excessive amount of oxygenated blood is pumped around the pulmonary circulation and cyanosis will not occur.

Acyanotic group

Aortic valve stenosis and subaortic stenosis. Apart from these localised abnormalities, the heart is normal. Another isolated abnormality here is bicuspid aortic valve, which may later become the site of bacterial endocarditis.

Patent ductus arteriosus. While it will be appreciated from the foregoing description that this may coexist with many other anomalies, patency of the ductus may be the only abnormality present and closure by surgery restores the patient to complete normality. Failure to close the ductus leads eventually to heart failure or the development of bacterial endocarditis or endarteritis at the site of the ductus. In a few cases there is associated pulmonary hypertension and in some the direction of blood flow in the ductus may be reversed so that unoxygenated blood passes from the pulmonary artery into the ductus and aorta distal to the ductus, usually immediately beyond the origin of the left subclavian artery. Such a patient may thus have a cyanotic tinge in the nailbeds of the toes but not in those of the hands.

Interatrial septal defect. This is one of the commonest congenital malformations of the heart. Such defects, even when of considerable degree, appear to have little effect on the circulation. They may occasionally be the means of allowing a portion of thrombus from a vein to pass from the right atrium into the left, in which case *crossed* or *paradoxical embolism* results. While probe patency of the foramen ovale is not uncommon in normal hearts (25 per cent approximately), the important malformations are of three main types, persistent ostium primum, ostium secundum and persistent atrio-ventricularis communis. In this latter condition, there is often fusion of the tricuspid and mitral valves to form a common atrio-ventricular valve. Lutembacher's disease consists of an interatrial septal defect with mitral stenosis.

Interventricular septal defect. A high septal defect is frequently part of another congenital anomaly, e.g. tetrad of Fallot, but an isolated high interventricular septal defect is not uncommon. Maladie de Roger is the name sometimes applied to an isolated perforation of the interventricular septum; the size and location of the aperture varies.

Anomalies of the aortic arch. As shown by Blalock, these are common in association with tetrad of Fallot, but as isolated anomalies they rarely cause symptoms. When, however, a vascular ring is formed around the trachea and oesophagus by a right aortic arch and left descending aorta together with a persistent ductus arteriosus or ligamentum arteriosum or from an anomalous left subclavian artery, pressure effects mainly on the trachea may result. A double aortic arch may give similar symptoms.

Coarctation (stenosis) of the aorta. Slight narrowing of the aorta between the left subclavian artery and the orifice of the ductus arteriosus, i.e. in the interval where the two main streams of the fetal circulation cross, is not very uncommon. The stenosis is rarely marked, but it may be severe and all degrees of narrowing up to complete atresia of the aorta at this point have been recorded. In such a condition an extensive collateral system from the carotids and subclavians links the aorta above and below the narrowed segment. The pulses in the lower limbs are poor as compared with those of the upper. Hypertension develops and death is likely to ensue from cardiac failure, cerebral haemorrhage or

less commonly from local complications associated with the coarcted site, e.g. aneurysm or rupture of the aorta. Coarctation of the aorta may be associated with other congenital abnormalities, but frequently it is the only abnormality present and, moreover, it is one that can be cured by surgery. The condition is distinctly commoner in the male sex.

Ebstein's disease. In this condition there is downward displacement of the tricuspid valve so that the upper part of the right ventricle comes to be a functional part of the right atrium. The course of the circulation is normal.

Other abnormalities of the valves. Sometimes there is excess or deficiency in the number of the segments of the semilunar valves; occasionally there are four segments, usually somewhat unequal in size, but, as a rule, there is no interference with the efficiency of the valve. Occasionally, on the other hand, only two segments are present, and this abnormality is more frequently met with at the aortic valve. One segment is, as a rule, somewhat larger than the other and often shows evidence of fusion of two segments; the competence of the valve may not be interfered with. Such valves have a tendency to become subsequently the seat of bacterial endocarditis (p. 317). Very rarely cases have been recorded in which two mitral valves have been present.

DISEASES OF THE PERICARDIUM

Pericarditis

Definition. Pericarditis refers to a group of inflammatory diseases of the pericardium of varied etiology; some are frankly infective, others result from chronic disturbances of metabolism and the infective origin is less conspicuous.

Classification. Pericarditis may be classified according to its cause and may be acute or chronic. Acute cases are usually fibrinous and are divided into those with effusion (which may be serous, haemorrhagic or purulent), and those without. Some chronic cases are classified according to their effects on cardiac function (e.g. chronic constrictive pericarditis).

Etiology. *Pyogenic infection.* Acute pericarditis may be the result of invasion by organisms from a lesion in the vicinity, e.g. empyema, suppuration in the mediastinum, or from some ulcerating growth, e.g. of the oesophagus. In most cases, however, infection is by the blood stream in the course of septicaemias. The suppurative type is produced chiefly by pneumococci, streptococci and staphylococci; and infection by the last may be secondary to small abscesses in the heart wall.

Tuberculosis. The pericardium and heart are relatively immune in cases of acute miliary tuberculosis; but tuberculous pericarditis is not uncommon, due to spread of infection along lymphatics from caseous upper mediastinal lymph nodes.

Non-infective types. A sterile pericarditis commonly occurs in the later stages of an acute attack of rheumatic fever and may gravely impair the heart's action. In uraemia due to subacute or chronic nephritis, pericarditis is a common terminal event, and appears to be due to metabolic disturbances rather than infection. Acute fibrinous pericarditis usually accompanies myocardial infarction and is often more extensive than the infarct; it is probably due to release of active vasodilator polypeptides from the products of autolysis, causing increased capillary permeability and fibrinous exudation. Pericarditis is a feature of polyserositis (Pick's disease, Concato's disease, p. 540), in which great thickening of the subserous fibrous tissue occurs.

Naked-eye appearances. *Fibrinous pericarditis* is found in rheumatism, uraemia, myocardial infarcts and some infective cases. The exudate usually appears first posteriorly round the large vessels at the base of the heart as an opaque, dull and roughened layer, and when it becomes abundant it forms a rough covering to the heart with irregular projections, giving rise to the so-called "bread and butter" appearance. *Pericardial effusion* up to or over a litre is usually accompanied by fibrinous pericarditis. The effusion may be serous in rheumatic fever or myocardial infection, haemorrhagic in tuberculosis, uraemia, myocardial infarction and metastatic tumours, and purulent following invasion by pyogenic bacteria. A variety of chronic pericarditis with massive effusion is occasionally seen in which none of the above etiological factors appears to be implicated.

Chronic pericarditis. The ordinary sequel to pericarditis is organisation of the exudate, and adhesions ultimately form with partial or complete obliteration of the pericardial sac. Sometimes, especially in rheumatic cases, there may be repeated attacks, and great thickening of the pericardium may result. Adherent pericardium may contribute to the need for cardiac hypertrophy.

Slightly thickened patches of opaque and whitish appearance in the epicardium are known as "milk spots". They occur especially over the anterior surface of the right ventricle and the apex of the left ventricle, and occasionally a large area of opacity is present. They are common in hypertrophied hearts and occasionally fibrous adhesions are present over an area of thickening. Milk spots are of no clinical significance.

Tuberculous pericarditis. At an early stage the disease may appear like an ordinary fibrinous pericarditis and its real nature may be discovered only on microscopic examination. In other cases caseation may occur in the exudate and this is usually followed by much thickening of the layers of the pericardium (Fig. 14.34), and later sometimes by calcification. In certain cases at an early stage there is an abundant exudate, both fibrinous and fluid, and it may contain a considerable admixture of blood. Ultimately the sac may be enormously distended. Tubercle bacilli may be present in very large numbers in the exudate.

Chronic constrictive pericarditis denotes a condition of dense fibrous adhesions around the heart, usually commencing in childhood with a febrile illness and pericarditis clinically resembling rheumatism. Pericardial effusion is often followed by pleural effusion and later by absorption and healing with very dense fibrous tissue and sometimes calcification. The effect is to constrict the chambers of the heart and the caval openings, which interferes with diastolic filling; a marked rise of venous pressure occurs and cardiac failure ultimately ensues. It is now accepted that the majority of cases are of tuberculous origin. Surgical resection of the visceral and parietal layers of the pericardium gives relief of symptoms in about one-third of the cases.

Effects of pericarditis. Many examples of pericarditis are not recognised during life. In acute pericarditis there may be pain in the chest or neck, and pericardial friction. Signs of pericardial effusion include enlargement of the "heart" on percussion and radiologically with a feeble apex beat in the normal position. Chronic constrictive pericarditis may be associated with

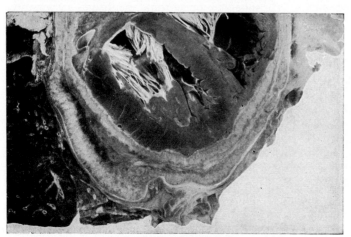

Fig. 14.34.—Tuberculous pericarditis in a child, with obliteration of pericardial sac and caseous change between the layers— shown on section. (J. W. S. B.)

systolic retraction of the chest wall and with increased venous pressure and ascites due to interference with filling of the heart; the pulse pressure is low and decreases on inspiration (pulsus paradoxus).

Pericardial haemorrhage

Haemorrhage into the pericardial sac, giving rise to *haemopericardium,* may be due to rupture of the heart itself following infarction, to rupture of a saccular (syphilitic) aneurysm, to rupture of the aorta (p. 286) caused by an acute dissecting aneurysm which strips open the aortic wall to the base of the heart, or to a stab wound involving the heart or a large vessel. When the bleeding takes place rapidly, the pressure of the accumulated blood interferes with the diastolic filling of the chambers. The output of blood from the left ventricle is greatly diminished, the blood pressure rapidly falls and death from heart failure results—this is known as *cardiac tamponade.*

Multiple minute haemorrhages occur into the layers of the pericardium in the various purpuric conditions. They are sometimes a prominent feature also in cases of death by suffocation.

TUMOURS OF THE HEART AND PERICARDIUM

Primary tumours are of rare occurrence in the heart wall. *Fibroma, myxoma, lipoma,* and *lymphangioma* are occasionally encountered, especially in the left atrium, the commonest being a myxomatous mass of considerable size projecting into the cavity from the margin of the foramen ovale: it is uncertain whether this is a true tumour or an organised thrombus of unusual appearance. *Haemangioma* is another rare growth; we have seen one of considerable size at the upper margin of the right ventricle. *Rhabdomyoma* of congenital origin occurs especially in the ventricles as multiple rounded nodules of pale and somewhat translucent tissue. It consists of large branching cells in which striped fibrils are found; the cells have a somewhat vacuolated appearance and contain much glycogen. In a number of cases, the tumour has been associated with multiple discrete gliomatous growths in the cerebral hemispheres—tuberous sclerosis (p. 666); in some cases there have been also malformations of the kidneys and liver, and adenoma sebaceum on the face (Bourneville's disease).

Metastatic growths in the heart and pericardium are less uncommon than is generally realised, occurring in about 10 per cent of all fatal malignancies, secondary melanotic tumours being disproportionately numerous in relation to their total incidence. In this Department, primary carcinoma of the bronchi has been found to present cardiac metastases more frequently than any other neoplasm (31 per cent of cases); no doubt the proximity of the primary growth is a factor in this high incidence, as direct extension readily occurs to the base of the heart and pericardium. There is, of course, an element of selection in the cases studied at necropsy, as those with bronchial carcinoma more commonly die in hospital. The presence of tumour growth in the pericardium is usually attended by inflammatory changes, often accompanied by haemorrhagic exudate.

CHAPTER 15

RESPIRATORY SYSTEM

Introduction

The majority of diseases of the respiratory system are initially acute or chronic inflammations, and by far the commonest cause is infection, sometimes bacterial, but often primarily due to viruses. The respiratory tract affords a direct pathway from the external air to the interior of the alveoli and there is continuity of mucous membrane along which infection may spread from the nose and mouth to the finest air passages. Normally the defensive mechanisms of ciliary action and leukocytic activity prevent organisms from gaining access to the lungs, and accordingly the alveoli and the minute bronchi are practically sterile. At what level this bacterium-free state is reached cannot be definitely stated, and no doubt it varies from time to time. Certain viruses have, however, the important pathogenic action of damaging the ciliary mechanism and inhibiting leukocytic emigration; accordingly the resistance of the respiratory mucosa to bacterial invasion is lowered and thus bacterial growth may extend farther downwards and set up inflammatory change. The most striking example of this type of bacterial invasion is seen in influenza, where organisms of many kinds may invade the air passages in succession to the causal virus; but the same principle holds also in the pulmonary complications of fevers, e.g. measles.

In other cases, *specific pathogenic bacteria* may gain entrance through the inspired air, for example tubercle bacilli, virulent pneumococci, plague bacilli, etc., and the possible role of diminished resistance in leading to infection may not be evident. Lesions, initially inflammatory, may lead to other changes; for example, chronic bronchitis, often complicated by emphysema, may cause important circulatory disturbance. Bacterial infection of the lungs may occur more rarely by way of the blood stream.

The *effects* of pulmonary lesions are of two kinds, namely, (*a*) toxaemia, as in infections elsewhere; (*b*) those due to interference with the functions of the lungs and the flow of blood through them. It is important to have in view these two main effects, though not infrequently both are concerned.

(*a*) The bacterial infections vary in course and character. Some are primary diseases, whilst others are secondary and often terminal phenomena occurring in other infections, notably the specific fevers. In untreated lobar pneumonia, the disease behaves as a specific fever, the temperature running a definite course and terminating usually by crisis; in contrast the course and fever in bronchopneumonia are irregular. The tuberculous infections are more prolonged and cause irregular fever and wasting.

(*b*) Extensive lesions such as oedema, collapse, pneumonic consolidation or fibrosis, may interfere with the oxygenation of the blood and moreover hypoxia may readily bring about pulmonary oedema and thus set up a vicious circle. In affected parts of the lungs blood will be circulating in the walls of alveoli which do not contain air, or in which there is impaired circulation of the air. For example, in rapid shallow respiration, as in lobar pneumonia, expansion of the lungs is not general and in places there is little movement of the air. The result of such conditions is that the blood returning from the lungs and passed on into the arterial system is not saturated with oxygen, in other words, there is a certain degree of hypoxia. Further, if at the same time, there is diminished output of blood from the heart, then venous congestion results with excess of blood in the capillaries and diminished rate of flow through them. Thus a stagnant or *congestive hypoxaemia* may be produced. Both types of anoxaemia may be present, and it is in such circumstances that cyanosis becomes marked. Certain permanent lesions in the lungs, notably vesicular emphysema and fibrosis (silicosis, etc.), diminish the total sectional area of the pulmonary capillaries and thus bring about obstruction to the blood flow. Hypertrophy of the right side of the heart and general venous congestion thus result, and death is then brought about by heart failure with its accompanying oedema, etc.

Many acute infections of the upper respiratory tract are attributable to viruses, many types of which have been isolated from clinically similar infections. The virus enters the upper respiratory passages and leads to acute catarrh with watery secretion. It also lowers the resistance of the mucosa of the air passages to secondary growth of various pyogenic bacteria and to their extension down the bronchial tree. Since bacterial growth itself is responsible for purulent

secretion it is not possible to distinguish the effects of the virus *per se* from those of the bacteria.

The variety and number of viruses concerned in human respiratory disease is now so large that it may be useful at this stage to summarise the present situation with regard to their classification and their relationship to clinical syndromes. This is done in an admittedly over-simplified form in Tables 15.1 and 15.2.

Table 15.2. Viruses Associated with Acute Respiratory Syndromes

Syndrome	Common Causes
Epidemic influenza	Influenza A, B
Sore throat	Adenoviruses
Common cold	Rhinoviruses Para-influenza Respiratory syncytial virus Some enteroviruses
Feverish cold	Para-influenza
Croup	Para-influenza 1,2,3
Bronchiolitis of infancy	Respiratory syncytial virus
Pneumonia	Respiratory syncytial virus (in infants) (also psittacosis, Q fever and primary atypical pneumonia—not true viruses: *q.v.*)

(modified from Stark, 1969)

Table 15.1. Respiratory Viruses

Classification	Virus	No. of Serotypes
Adenoviruses	Adenovirus	31
Myxoviruses	Influenza	A, B and C (and subtypes)
Paramyxoviruses	{Para-influenza {Resp. syncytial	4 1
Enteroviruses	Coxsackie Echo	30 34
Rhinoviruses	Rhinovirus	70+

(modified from Tyrrell, 1968)

NOSE, NASAL SINUSES AND NASOPHARYNX

Inflammatory conditions

Acute rhinitis is the common inflammatory disorder of the nasal mucosa. The familiar clinical form, the common cold (acute coryza), is caused by any one of a group of RNA rhinoviruses or sometimes by para-influenza virus and may be followed closely by secondary bacterial infection. The rhinoviruses concerned form a group of over 70 antigenically distinct strains which probably accounts for the short-lived immunity following the common cold. The specific infectious fevers, such as measles,

are often preceded by acute rhinitis. Nasal diphtheria is another cause, but is now a rarity in this country (see p. 330).

Another common clinical disorder is *hay fever*, or *acute allergic* or *atopic rhinitis* which occurs as a result of sensitisation to certain pollens, such as the pollen of Timothy grass, or to house dust, animal dandruff, feathers or other specific allergens (p. 99). Atopic hypersensitivity is also a factor in some cases of nasal polyposis.

Acute sinusitis is generally a complication of acute infection of the nose, less commonly of dental sepsis. Gram-positive cocci such as

Strep. pyogenes, Strep. pneumoniae or *Staph. aureus* are the usual causal organisms.

Acute nasopharyngitis usually accompanies either acute rhinitis or acute tonsillitis in which *Strep. pyogenes* is the common pathogen. The histopathology of acute inflammation of the nose, sinuses and nasopharynx is similar. There is hyperaemia and oedema of the mucosa, and the mucosal glands are hyperactive. Until the development of secondary bacterial infection, neutrophil polymorphs are generally sparse in both the mucosa and the exudate, but thereafter increasing numbers of neutrophils migrate through the mucosa and the exudate becomes mucopurulent in character. There is a variable degree of loss of the superficial ciliated epithelium. In atopic inflammation, oedema of the submucosa is a prominent feature, giving rise to polypoid thickening of the mucosa. The mucosal glands are often enlarged and distended and the oedematous stroma is characteristically infiltrated by numerous eosinophil polymorphs.

Chronic rhinitis, sinusitis and **nasopharyngitis** may follow an acute inflammatory episode which has failed to resolve. Inadequate drainage of the sinuses, nasal obstruction due to polypi, or enlargement of the nasopharyngeal lymphoid tissue (adenoids), may be underlying factors.

Nasal polypi. Chronic inflammation of the nose may lead to polypoid thickening of the mucosa. Polyps are rounded or elongated masses commonly arising from the region of the middle turbinate. They are often bilateral, a point of distinction from nasal tumours. Nasal polypi are usually gelatinous in consistency with a smooth shiny surface. Their microscopic structure consists of a core of loose oedematous connective tissue containing occasional submucous glands and covered by normal ciliated respiratory type of epithelium (Fig. 15.1). Lymphocytes, plasma cells and eosinophils infiltrate the submucosa to a variable degree. Polypi in which eosinophils predominate in the inflammatory infiltrate are considered to have an atopic basis.

Chronic granulomatous rhinitis. In contrast to acute infection, specific forms of chronic infection of the nose are rare in this country. Chronic granulomas may be due to tuberculosis, tertiary syphilis, leprosy, scleroma (*Klebsiella rhinoscleromatis*) or fungal infections such as aspergillosis or rhinosporidiosis.

Two rare forms of necrotising granuloma of uncertain nature occur in the upper respiratory tract. In one form, *Wegener's granuloma*, a necrotising lesion with giant cells develops usually in the nose or the maxillary sinus, followed by necrotic lesions in the lung and associated with disseminated polyarteritic lesions, particularly in the lungs and kidneys. The other, *malignant granuloma of the nose*, or *midline lethal granuloma*, presents as an ulcerated lesion which spreads progressively to erode the soft tissues and bones around the nose. Histologically the lesion consists of proliferating lymphocytes and histiocytes, and closely mimics a lymphoid neoplasm.

Tumours

Benign. The common benign lesions of the nose are haemangioma of the septum and squamous papilloma of the vestibule. A much less common tumour is the *juvenile angiofibroma* which usually occurs in the nasopharynx but occasionally presents as a nasal polypoid lesion. It occurs almost exclusively in males, presenting in childhood and tending to become quiescent by the end of the second decade. It is an enlarging vascular tumour which may cause

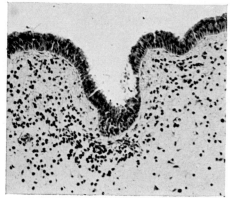

FIG. 15.1.—Section through the margin of a nasal polyp, showing the respiratory epithelial lining and the loose oedematous stroma infiltrated with chronic inflammatory cells. × 100.

bone erosion and destruction by pressure atrophy. The histological structure consists of numerous small vascular spaces set in poorly cellular fibrous tissue. The histogenesis of the lesion is uncertain and like haemangiomas, it may be a hamartoma of the nasal erectile tissue rather than a true neoplasm.

Malignant. The commonest malignant tumour of the nose and nasal sinuses is squamous carcinoma but anaplastic carcinoma and adeno-carcinoma also occur. The so-called lympho-epithelioma of the nasopharynx is now generally accepted as a highly anaplastic carcinoma admixed with the normal non-neoplastic lymphoid tissue of the region (see also p. 475). Naso-pharyngeal carcinoma, usually squamous, often poorly differentiated or of lympho-epithelio-matous type is particularly common in China, Malaysia, Indonesia and East Africa. There is some evidence that the anaplastic forms of this tumour are associated with the same virus as Burkitt's lymphoma (p. 220). Adenocarcinoma of the nose and nasal sinuses, especially the ethmoid, has been found to be unduly frequent in woodworkers in the furniture industry and following radium ingestion (p. 759). In both instances the latent period may be 40 years or more.

A group of transitional cell tumours of the nose is of particular interest; commonly they present as a papilloma with a tendency to recurrence but no other features of malignancy. Transitional cell carcinoma also occurs.

Sarcoma, including reticulum cell sarcoma and lymphosarcoma, is much less common than carcinoma. The nose or the pharynx are rarely the site of a solitary extra-skeletal deposit of myeloma (plasmacytoma).

LARYNX AND TRACHEA

Acute inflammations of these structures are of two main types, viz. (*a*) catarrhal and (*b*) croupous or pseudo-membranous.

(A) *Acute catarrhal inflammation* is common, and although exposure to cold, irritating vapours, etc. may be predisposing factors, it is mainly due to the action of viruses and of bacteria which extend from the mouth and fauces. The bacteria chiefly concerned are *Strep. pneumoniae*, *Strep. pyogenes* and *Neisseria catarrhalis*; and further extension of such organisms may produce bronchitis. Acute fevers and debility favour the occurrence of acute catarrh; it is accordingly specially common in measles, influenza, typhoid, etc. The naked-eye and microscopic appearances correspond with those seen in catarrhal inflammation in other parts. An acute catarrh may subside and the tissues return to normal, or it may pass into the chronic stage.

Chronic catarrh may occur without any very acute onset and is not uncommon in combined excessive smoking and consumption of alcohol. It is accompanied by leukocytic infiltration, new formation of blood vessels in the mucous membrane, and fibrosis. Sometimes there is distinct thickening and opacity of the epithelium; in the larynx, this may be a marked feature, and then the term *pachydermia* is applied. The mucous glands are swollen and give the surface a granular aspect, and occasionally chronic catarrh is accompanied by the formation of small papilliform projections.

(B) *Pseudomembranous inflammation* may, for practical purposes, be distinguished as "diphtheritic" (caused by *C. diphtheriae*) and "non-diphtheritic"; the latter may be associated with *Strep. pyogenes*, *Staph. aureus* or *Strep. pneumoniae*, following infection with para-influenza virus. Severe lesions of this type have been designated *laryngo-tracheo-bronchitis*, and are characterised by epithelial necrosis and the formation of an extensive fibrinous membrane in the trachea (Fig. 15.2) and main bronchi and by marked oedema of the subglottic area, resulting in stridor. In a minority of cases

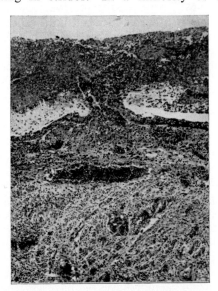

FIG. 15.2.—Acute laryngo-tracheo-bronchitis.
Showing fibrinous exudate, patchy necrosis of the mucosa and much congestion and inflammatory infiltration. × 57.

Haemophilus influenzae is the secondary invader, with severe sore throat, fever, tender lymph nodes and great swelling of the epiglottis. In most cases of laryngo-tracheo-bronchitis the danger of laryngeal obstruction is greater than that of toxaemia or sepsis, but bronchopneumonia and lung abscess are recognised complications and interstitial emphysema is not uncommon. Pseudomembranous inflammation may result also from the action of corrosive substances or from the inhalation of irritating gases, notably ammonia.

Diphtheria is an acute inflammation which affects most frequently the fauces, soft palate and tonsils (see p. 480), but may also attack the nose, or the larynx and trachea. The local lesions are characterised by the formation on the affected surface of a false membrane composed of fibrin, leukocytes and necrotic epithelium. In the larynx and trachea the epithelium is columnar; the coagulated exudate rests on the basement membrane from which it separates easily and is coughed up. Over the vocal cords, however, where the mucosa consists of squamous epithelium, the membrane is firmly adherent. When it is coughed up from the trachea it may remain attached to the vocal cords and may then impact in the larynx and cause death from suffocation.

In nasal diphtheria the infection is often unilateral and the child may appear to have a "cold in the head" with discharge from one nostril. This type is often overlooked until other toxic manifestations appear, e.g. palatal paralysis, myocardial damage; sometimes its nature is recognised only on the occurrence of secondary cases.

In *typhoid fever*, swelling and ulceration of the lymphoid tissue, analogous to that in the intestines, sometimes occurs (p. 514); typhoid bacilli have been recovered from such lesions. The catarrh so common in typhoid is, however, more often produced by other organisms. Occasionally ulceration involves the perichondrium of the laryngeal cartilage and necrosis; suppuration of the cartilage may follow. In *smallpox*, in addition to catarrhal or membranous inflammation, nodular inflammatory foci, similar to those in the skin, may form in the larynx and especially in the trachea. They are accompanied by intense congestion and haemorrhages but have less tendency to necrosis than those in the skin; sometimes, however, they break down and form ulcers.

Oedema glottidis. This term is intended to designate an acute inflammatory oedema of the loose tissues of the upper part of the larynx and not of the vocal cords. The aryepiglottic folds and the tissues around the epiglottis become greatly swollen and tense (Fig. 15.3). The false cords also are affected. The lesion is important, as the swelling may lead to obstruction and death by suffocation, but after death the tissues become less swollen and tense than they were during life. Oedema of the loose tissues mentioned may occur in cardiac and renal disease, but rarely to such an extent as to cause serious results; the severe type occurs as a complication of other lesions of the larynx, e.g. diphtheria, or the deep-seated ulceration and perichondritis seen in tuberculosis, syphilis, and sometimes in typhoid. It may result also from erysipelas or from the spread of inflammation from tonsillitis and suppurative conditions in the neighbourhood, and in conditions of agranulocytic angina (p. 396). Oedema glottidis is caused also by the trauma following impaction of a foreign body in the larynx or by endotracheal intubation, and may be produced by irritating gases, scalding fluids, etc. It occurs in *angioneurotic oedema* (p. 181) and in some cases this form has proved fatal. In some of the above conditions infection of the tissues by pyogenic organisms may lead to diffuse suppuration.

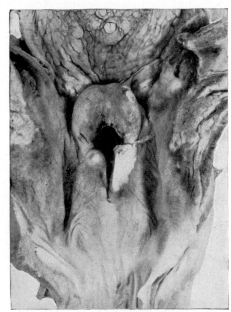

FIG. 15.3.—Oedema glottidis, showing great swelling of tissues around orifice of larynx.

Chronic inflammation

Two important *chronic infective lesions* of the larynx, although rare nowadays in this country, are tuberculosis and syphilis.

Tuberculosis. In most cases tuberculosis of the larynx is secondary to tuberculosis of the lungs, the disease being the result of direct infection by bacilli in the sputum. The bacilli enter the mucosa and give rise to tubercles which then become eroded and form small ulcers which

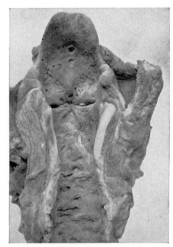

FIG. 15.4.—Tuberculous disease of larynx, showing ulceration of vocal cords and also small ulcers above and below them.

tend to spread. Any part of the larynx, or less commonly the trachea, may be affected but the disease usually starts first and is most marked in the arytenoid region and on the vocal cords (Fig. 15.4). Occasionally, small papilliform excrescences form at the margins of the tuberculous ulcers, and epithelial hyperplasia may be mistaken for carcinoma. The disease may spread deeply and involve the perichondrium of the arytenoid cartilages, there being chronic thickening with caseation and ulceration from which portions of dead cartilage may be separated and discharged. These various changes are often accompanied by great pain and considerable inflammatory swelling; sometimes oedema glottidis is superadded.

Lupus of the larynx, although also tuberculous, is quite a different condition from that just described. Mostly it occurs secondarily to lupus of the nasopharynx, occasionally to lupus of the face. The commonest site is the epiglottis, also the aryepiglottic folds, whilst it is unusual for

the vocal cords to be involved. Small pale reddish nodules form, which spread and slowly ulcerate. Healing occurs in some places whilst superficial ulceration extends in others, and much cicatricial contraction may result. Lupus in the larynx is an indolent lesion, which differs markedly from the ordinary form of tuberculosis clinically in that there is none of the severe pain of the latter nor is there usually much secondary inflammatory change.

Syphilis. In the secondary stage, catarrh of the larynx, mucous patches and superficial erosions may be present. The most important effects, however, are in the tertiary stage. The lesions usually start in the submucosa of the larynx or trachea, or in the perichondrium as a diffuse but irregular thickening and stiffening which often leads to immobility of the cartilages. Gummatous change follows: the epiglottis and affected cartilages may be extensively ulcerated and the latter may become necrosed and separated. Almost a distinguishing feature of syphilitic disease, however, is the tendency to secondary fibrosis and its contraction leading to stenosis and deformity of the larynx (Fig. 15.5). The upper part of the trachea may also be involved and narrowed, but the commonest site in the trachea is at the bifurcation, where ulceration with secondary scarring can cause stenosis of a main bronchus. These lesions are all much rarer nowadays.

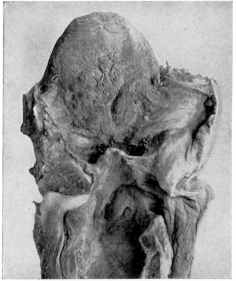

FIG. 15.5.—Chronic syphilitic laryngitis, showing extensive destructive change with irregular fibrosis and contraction.

Tumours

Benign. Papilloma and fibroma are most frequent, the former being the commoner; angioma, myxoma, and lipoma are described but they are very rare. Small inflammatory polypi are common and may contain amyloid or show mucoid degeneration. They may simulate neoplasm. *Papilloma* occurs usually on the vocal cords and especially at the commissure; it is generally single in the adult, but in children below the age of five may be multiple and arise anywhere within the larynx. Those in the sub-glottic region are especially liable to plug the larynx. Papillomas in children are mostly of viral origin and they regress spontaneously at puberty, sometimes with astonishing rapidity. In the adult, when a papilloma is removed, there is sometimes recurrence and malignant change may rarely develop. The *fibroma* is usually a small hemispherical growth, rounded and occasionally pedunculated. Like the papilloma, it is common on the vocal cords, and both are apt to occur in singers and others who use their voices a lot.

Granular-cell myoblastoma (p. 473) sometimes arises in the larynx, and the irregular hyperplasia of the covering squamous epithelium may closely mimic squamous carcinoma (Fig. 18.3, p. 473). Recognition of the characteristic granular cells beneath the irregular squamous epithelium is vitally important. It usually behaves as a benign tumour.

Malignant. Carcinoma is the commonest malignant tumour of the larynx and is of highest incidence in men over 50 years of age. An association with pipe smoking has been postulated. In most cases it is a squamous carcinoma with little or no formation of cell-nests. When the tumour is on the true or false vocal cords it is usually less invasive, and the prognosis after removal is better, than when it arises in the upper part of the larynx or in the subglottic region. Carcinoma of a vocal cord appears first as a small indurated patch (Fig. 15.6), sometimes with a papillary surface; in the latter case diagnosis will be unsatisfactory if only a superficial part is removed for microscopic examination. A carcinoma of the larynx infiltrates and destroys the surrounding parts by ulceration. This may be accompanied by septic infection, from which the discharge passes down the bronchi into the lungs and causes suppurative or gangrenous change.

Sarcoma is much less common. Various histological types are seen, the commonest being the spindle-cell sarcoma; lymphosarcoma and chondrosarcoma also have been described and we have seen an example structurally resembling giant-cell tumour of bone.

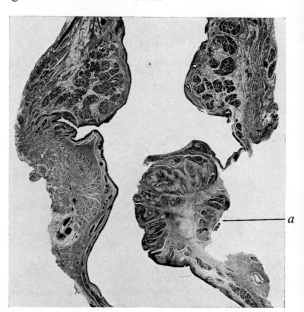

Fig. 15.6.—Squamous carcinoma of the larynx, affecting the vocal cord.

A coronal section through the soft tissues of the larynx shows the right vocal cord region swollen and replaced by hyperplastic keratinising squamous epithelium and in the centre an infiltrating squamous carcinoma. × 4.

a—lymphatic invasion of the deep tissues.

THE BRONCHI

Inflammatory changes (bronchitis)

This may be considered conveniently under the two headings of *acute* and *chronic bronchitis.* The common acute bronchitis of the adult affects the large and medium-sized bronchi. It is usually mild, but is the cause of much disability when it aggravates an established chronic bronchitis especially in aged or debilitated subjects. Acute bronchiolitis, however, is a much more serious lesion owing to its tendency to spread and lead to pneumonia.

It is comparatively rare in the healthy adult, if we except cases of influenza, as the organisms do not readily extend so low in the bronchial tree; but it is common in children and in old people. It will be described below in connection with bronchopneumonia.

Acute bronchitis

Classification. Acute bronchitis affecting the larger tubes is usually of three varieties, viz. (*a*) catarrhal, (*b*) fibrinous or membranous and (*c*) putrid bronchitis.

Etiology. In acute catarrhal bronchitis at the present time the most important bacterium is probably *Haemophilus influenzae*, but pneumococci are also concerned especially in acute exacerbations of a chronic lesion. It is probable that bacterial growth is often favoured by damage to the respiratory epithelium and its ciliary mechanism by the action of the many viruses that attack the respiratory tract, e.g. influenza and para-influenza. Sometimes acute bronchitis is an early symptom in typhoid fever. Recovery from acute bronchitis is usually complete but catarrh may persist for some time and may become chronic after repeated acute attacks.

Structural changes. In *acute catarrhal bronchitis* the changes are those of a simple catarrhal inflammation in which there is congestion and leukocytic infiltration of the bronchial mucosa accompanied by outpouring of mucus. The secretion may be scanty and tough, abundant and more serous, sometimes bloodstained and in the later stages it becomes mucopurulent. There may be considerable desquamation of the columnar ciliated epithelium. *Staphylococcus aureus* infection causes a severe purulent bronchitis in infants.

Fibrinous bronchitis is occasionally seen in diphtheria as a downward extension from the trachea. It may be produced by the para-influenza viruses and by streptococci, staphylococci and other organisms; in severe influenza there may be fibrinous exudate in the bronchi, but usually it is scanty. In chronic membranous bronchitis abundant exudate forms on the surface of the bronchial mucosa, and large casts of the bronchi may be expectorated. The condition is rare and its etiology is unknown.

Putrid bronchitis occurs as a result of decomposition of the secretions by putrefactive bacteria when there is stagnation in dilated bronchi or in bronchiectatic cavities. It is also associated with gangrene of the lung set up by the inhalation of infected fluids during narcosis or coma and it is a common result of ulceration of malignant growths into the trachea or bronchi. During life the sputum is abundant and fetid.

Chronic bronchitis

This may follow repeated acute attacks but in about half the cases it develops insidiously without a clinically recognisable acute stage.

Clinical features. The most constant finding is increased secretion by the bronchial mucosa and glands of abundant clear tenacious mucus which is expectorated by frequent coughing. During exacerbations the secretion becomes mucopurulent and opaque. It is important to distinguish between the opacity due to pus cells and that due to eosinophils in large numbers as may occur in asthma, which is often associated with chronic bronchitis.

Epidemiology. Chronic bronchitis and its complications have a high morbidity and mortality; in Great Britain they far exceed that of all other countries, especially between 45 and 65 years of age. The male death rate is about five times that of females. Heavy cigarette smoking, poor housing conditions and occupation are important factors, but the greatly increased prevalence of the disease in highly industrialised areas points to atmospheric pollution, especially by sulphur dioxide and other components of the lethal aerosol called smog, as an important factor in its pathogenesis. Bronchitis is one of the principal causes of loss of working time amongst older men in industry.

Structural changes. Chronic catarrh is followed by changes in the mucous membrane that prevent a complete return to normal. The columnar ciliated epithelium of the smaller bronchi and the cubical epithelium of the bronchioles are partly replaced by numerous goblet cells (Fig. 15.7) and the bronchial mucous glands are much hypertrophied (Fig. 15.8). Later there is marked thickening of the basement membrane and overgrowth of vascular fibrous tissue so that the bronchial mucosa is thickened and irregularly congested, the surface being uneven and granular beneath the abundant mucopurulcnt sccrction. This has been termed the *hypertrophic stage.* The bronchial tubes are often somewhat dilated, notably in the intervals between the cartilaginous rings, so that both the transverse markings and the longitudinal

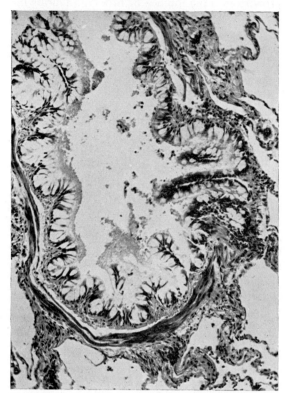

Fig. 15.7.—Chronic bronchitis. A small bronchus showing replacement of the columnar ciliated epithelium by mucin-secreting goblet-cells. × 115.
Section kindly loaned by Professor Lynne Reid.

folds are more distinct. The bronchial epithelium may be represented merely by a few pyramidal cells on the surface of the thickened basement membrane, but much of this shedding of the epithelium is a post-mortem artefact. In the so-called *atrophic stage* there is general thinning of the mucous membrane with atrophy of the glands and other structures. Chronic bronchitis is very frequently associated with emphysema of the lungs.

Asthma (bronchial asthma)

Asthma is a condition characterised by widespread bronchial obstruction due to muscular spasm and plugging by thick mucus. The obstruction varies in intensity from time to time, or is intermittent, and is completely reversible spontaneously or by therapy. When used alone, the term *asthma* is usually regarded as synonymous with bronchial asthma; it should not be confused with the so-called *cardiac asthma* which is unrelated, and due to acute pulmonary oedema in patients with left ventricular failure (p. 297).

Clinical features. Asthmatic patients usually suffer from acute attacks characterised by a feeling of tightness in the chest, difficulty in breathing, and particularly in exhaling, which is accompanied by loud wheezing, and often coughing which during the attack tends to be non-productive. As the attack subsides, thick viscid sputum is coughed up which contains eosinophil leukocytes. An attack may last from a few minutes to days and may vary in severity from mild dyspnoea with wheezing to severe respiratory distress. During attacks, the lungs become distended with air—acute vesicular emphysema, but in uncomplicated asthma residual lung injury and right ventricular hypertrophy develop only after a very long time, if at all.

Etiology and classification. Bronchial asthma

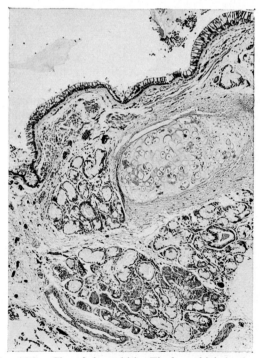

Fig. 15.8.—Chronic bronchitis. The bronchial glands are enlarged, extending between and behind the cartilaginous plates. × 40.

may be classified into *extrinsic* and *intrinsic* types. *Extrinsic asthma* usually starts in childhood or early adult life and may be preceded by infantile eczema or hypersensitivity to foodstuffs in childhood. It is due to *atopic* (type I) *hypersensitivity* (p. 99) to one or more extrinsic antigenic substances ("allergens") and inhalation of the offending allergen brings on an attack within a few minutes. As already explained (p. 101), such hypersensitivity occurs in individuals who have a genetically-determined predisposition to develop reaginic antibodies of IgE class, and skin tests or provocative inhalation tests with the allergen(s) responsible typically produce an immediate (type I) reaction. The allergens commonly responsible include various pollens, animal danders, house dust, and various fungi.

An interesting and important development is the finding that the most important allergen in house dust is provided by house mites, and particularly *Dermatophagoides pteronyssinus* (Fig. 15.9) which infests mattresses and lives on human

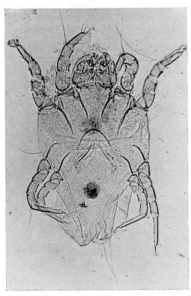

Fig. 15.9.—The house mite, *Dermatophagoides pteronyssinus.* × 300.

squames: this mite is commonly found in house dust, and inhaled excreta or fragments of the mite produce an asthmatic reaction in sensitised individuals. The prognosis in extrinsic asthma is good, although deaths may result from overmedication or from sudden withdrawal of corticosteroids.

Intrinsic asthma usually develops later in adult life in subjects without an individual or family history of previous atopic diseases: in contrast to extrinsic asthma, skin tests or provocative inhalation tests fail to reveal a responsible allergen. Nasal polypi are common, and microscopic examination of the polyps shows infiltration with eosinophil polymorphs. The prognosis is less good than in extrinsic asthma. Patients tend to develop drug hypersensitivity, particularly to aspirin and penicillin, and administration of these drugs may then be followed by a generalised atopic reaction which is sometimes fatal; palliative therapy tends to become ineffective, although corticosteroids are beneficial.

In both extrinsic and intrinsic asthma, there is commonly a blood eosinophil leukocytosis of 700–1000/c.mm., and an eosinophil infiltration of the bronchi. Intrinsic asthma is commonly associated with chronic bronchitis, and it has been suggested that atopic hypersensitivity develops to allergens provided by bacteria in the infected bronchi, although this has seldom been established. Psychological factors are of importance in asthma, and in many patients the attacks are more likely to occur during periods of anxiety or emotional disturbance.

Structural changes. During an attack of asthma, there is acute bronchial obstruction due partly to plugging of the bronchi by tough gelatinous mucus secreted by the bronchial glands. As a result, breathing is difficult and acute generalised emphysema develops. The bronchial and bronchiolar smooth muscle becomes hypertrophic and there is oedema and eosinophil polymorphonuclear infiltration of the submucosa of the bronchi: these latter features do not extend to the bronchioles, and chronic vesicular emphysema does not usually develop unless chronic bronchitis supervenes.

The endogenous pharmacological mediators of asthma have already been considered (p. 101), and the pulmonary diseases due to an Arthus-like reaction, or to atopic and Arthus-like reactions together, are described on pp. 376–7.

Bronchiectasis

Definition and classification. Bronchiectasis means a dilatation of the bronchi, which may be generalised or localised, and may result in the formation of multiple large spaces or cavities.

Bronchiectasis is said to be *cylindrical* or *digitate* when the bronchi are affected in most of their length; this is most pronounced in the lower lobes and may present as an almost generalised dilatation of the tubes.

In *saccular bronchiectasis* the dilatation is more localised and of greater degree; less frequently the dilatation is *fusiform*.

Congenital bronchiectasis results from agenesis of pulmonary alveolar tissue and atelectasis of large portions of a lobe or lobes.

The affected lobe is small and shrunken and dilated bronchi form cyst-like spaces which extend almost to the pleural surface, there being virtually no trace of lung substance between them.

Structural changes. In chronic bronchitis the transverse markings of the bronchial lining are often increased and depressions are present between the ridges; from this condition all degrees are seen up to the generalised dilatation of fully established cylindrical bronchiectasis.

Saccular bronchiectasis is, however, usually due to fibrosis of the surrounding lung tissue with obliteration and destruction of the smaller bronchi and bronchioles (Fig. 15.10). The dilated sacs so clearly displayed in a bronchogram appear to be the expanded terminations of the first few branches of the segmental bronchi. The lining of the bronchiectatic spaces resembles an irregularly swollen and vascular bronchial musosa and is often much congested. For a time the cavities are almost dry but later secretion accumulates and becomes purulent, and ulceration of the wall occurs.

Bilateral saccular bronchiectasis is seen in the upper lobes in the more fibrotic varieties of chronic tuberculosis, where the fundamentally tuberculous nature of the lesion may be difficult to prove; such cases are now rather less common. Apart from tuberculous infection saccular bronchiectasis is usually unilateral and is commonest in the lower lobes of the lung, especially in the left posterior basal segment.

In chronic bronchiectasis there is usually considerable enlargement of the bronchopulmonary anastomoses so that the bronchial blood flow is substantially increased, and this may be a factor in raising pulmonary arterial pressure and increasing the degree of cor pulmonale that results.

On *microscopic examination*, an epithelial lining may be present to a varying extent, the cells being columnar, rounded or flattened, and occurring in a single layer or in several layers; sometimes there is metaplasia to the stratified squamous type. In specimens removed surgically at an early stage, the walls of the larger affected bronchi often show surprisingly good preservation of their structural elements, the chief change being dilatation of the lumen, with collapse and obliteration of their terminal divisions and fibrosis of the lung tissue. In the later stages the epithelium disappears, the surface is formed by a thinned basement membrane beneath which

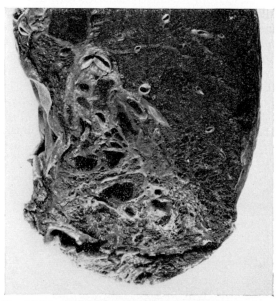

FIG. 15.10.—Bronchiectasis. The lower part of the lung is shown, with gross bronchial dilatation, destruction of lung tissue and fibrosis in the lower lobe. × ⅔.

there is granulation tissue. The blood vessels are numerous and greatly dilated. Deeper ulceration also may be present. The various structures of the bronchial wall—muscle, elastic tissue, glands—become atrophied and may disappear; this is the usual state found in necropsy specimens.

Effects. Ultimately an abundant purulent secretion accumulates within the bronchiectatic cavities and this tends to stagnate and undergo decomposition because in the absence of air-containing pulmonary alveoli distal to the affected bronchi an effective expulsive cough cannot be made. Accordingly, patients suffering from bronchiectasis often have a very abundant and foul-smelling sputum. Organisms may extend from the bronchiectatic cavities, either by the air passages or by direct ulceration, to the alveolar tissue; pneumonia with abscess formation may result and occasionally gangrene. In such conditions the wall of a vein may become involved, septic thrombosis may follow, and this may in turn give rise to embolism, pyaemia, and multiple secondary abscesses in the brain. The abundant putrid secretion from the bronchi may lead to infection of the nasal sinuses and further complications.

Causation. In the production of saccular bronchiectasis three main factors are concerned: (*a*) loss of aerated lung substance so that the force of the inspired air is exerted on the bronchial walls alone, (*b*) weakening of the supporting tissue of the bronchial wall caused by inflammatory changes, and (*c*) contraction of fibrous bands connecting the bronchial walls with the fibrosed and adherent pleura. In long-established cases these factors are variously combined and usually all three are present, but it is important to ascertain which is of primary importance in the pathogenesis of the condition.

Bronchiectasis is usually a sequel to bronchiolitis and bronchopneumonia in childhood with partial collapse and imperfect resolution; it may also follow congenital atelectasis of a portion of the lung. The bronchopneumonia may be primary or it may complicate whooping cough or measles; in adults, influenza may have similar effects. In the study of some early examples obtained from children by lobectomy Macfarlane and Sommerville found that the bronchi are ensheathed in hyperplastic lymphoid tissue, which causes narrowing of the lumen (Fig. 15.11). The condition closely resembles that seen in certain virus infections of the lung in cattle ("cuffing pneumonia"), and in most of these cases evidence of the presence of one of the adenoviruses has been obtained, either by isolation of the virus or by means of serological tests. Infection by adenoviruses may prove to be important in the etiology of this variety of bronchiectasis in children, to which the name *follicular bronchiectasis* has been applied.

There has been much uncertainty about the relative parts played by infection with consequent weakening of the bronchial walls and by collapse with subsequent fibrosis. Radiological investigations clearly indicate that any major degree of collapse with negative intrapleural pressure is followed almost at once by dilatation of the bronchi supplying the collapsed zone; this dilatation may subsequently disappear when the lung becomes re-expanded. Permanent collapse is, however, followed by fibrosis and the bronchi remain dilated. The evidence of X-ray examinations indicates that this state is commoner than had been supposed and that it may exist for long periods without the clinical symptomatology associated with bronchiectasis. The dilated bronchi are relatively dry, and if lobectomy is performed at this stage remarkably little structural change in the larger bronchial walls may be seen. Infection, with destruction of the special-

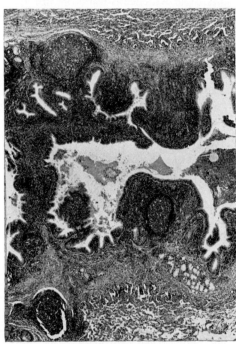

FIG. 15.11.—Juvenile bronchiectasis associated with adenovirus infection.

A bronchus showing the massive lymphoid infiltration of the submucosa and marked irregularity and narrowing of lumen. (Dr. Peter Macfarlane.) × 21.

ised elements and consequent weakening of the wall, cannot therefore be the primary change in these cases, and it is probable that pulmonary collapse is the all-important initial causal lesion. No doubt bronchial dilatation is hastened by the forced inspiration which follows the act of coughing, and the cough, being unproductive from the lack of air in the lung beyond the affected bronchi, tends to be frequently repeated. A vicious circle is thus set up, the effects of which become more severe when the accumulation of infected secretions has produced inflammatory damage to the bronchial walls with the loss of the cartilage, muscle and elastic tissue. In other cases collapse is by no means complete and persistent infection of the bronchial walls with damage to the deeper structures plays the more important part. Ogilvie, in a detailed study of 35 lobectomy specimens, found extensive collapse in 21 and only scanty collapse in 10, all of which showed well-marked damage to the bronchial walls. Nevertheless damage to the bronchial wall was slight in only two of the 21 collapsed specimens and in more than half there was severe destruction of the specialised elements. The evidence is therefore not yet clear as to the importance to be attached to collapse on the one hand and to inflammatory damage on the other in the pathogenesis of bronchiectasis. Certainly in those with persistent infection, repeated attacks of localised pneumonia may occur in subsequent years, resulting in dense fibrous adhesions between lung and parietal pleura. The third factor, viz. contraction of fibrous bands connecting bronchi with pleura, may then operate in increasing still further the bronchial dilatation, and especially in producing the sacculated condition, but this factor is regarded as of less importance.

Undoubtedly the bronchopneumonias of childhood are the most important antecedent to bronchiectasis, but any extensive pulmonary fibrosis may have this effect. In chronic pulmonary tuberculosis with fibrotic change, bronchiectatic cavities are common in association with tuberculous cavities, and they also occur in silicosis and fibrotic conditions generally. In congenital syphilitic pneumonia with diffuse fibrosis, generalised bronchiectasis may be present. In infants of a few months suffering from fibrocystic disease of the pancreas, the trachea and bronchi are lined by tough mucoid secretion which soon becomes purulent; bronchopneumonia follows, and if the infant survives, bronchiectasis is a common sequel.

Honeycomb lung: bronchiolectasis. This name has been applied to an acquired form of cystic disease of the lung brought about by post-inflammatory obliteration of bronchioles and their associated air passages and alveoli. The spaces arise by dilatation of neighbouring unaffected bronchioles and the walls of the spaces incorporate the fibrosed and obliterated lung substance. The condition is usually patchy affecting only one lobe or part of a lobe and it may be found in association with coal-miners' pneumoconiosis, and with the healing of various granulomatous lesions such as sarcoidosis, berylliosis, tuberculosis and other forms of bronchopneumonia. It also occurs in association with a

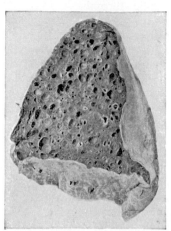

FIG. 15.12.—Honeycomb lung. Portions of child's lung, showing bronchiolectasis and emphysema (associated with histiocytosis). × ¾.

widespread histiocytosis of the lungs in children (Fig. 15.12), usually as part of a generalised histiocytic infiltration of the reticulo-endothelial system of unknown etiology (*Letterer–Siwe disease*, p. 455).

Bronchial obstruction

Various degrees of obstruction may occur up to complete closure and either large or small bronchi may be affected, the causation being different in the two cases. Obstruction of a large bronchus is most frequently produced by primary carcinoma infiltrating the wall and growing into the lumen, or by pressure of massively enlarged hilar nodes. Cicatricial contraction from a syphilitic lesion at the tracheal bifurcation, and pressure on a main bronchus by a syphilitic aneurysm of the aortic arch, both formerly common, are now exceedingly rare. A foreign body lodged in a large bronchus may obstruct it completely, whereupon the air in the related part of the lung is absorbed rapidly and pulmonary collapse follows. Usually, however, obstruction is partial at first, oedema fluid and secretions then accumulate, and this results in a degree of bronchial dilatation. Bacterial growth in the part beyond the obstruction is the most important result and this sets up a purulent bronchitis which by further extension may bring about suppurative bronchopneumonia. This is the usual sequence of events when a major bronchus is invaded by tumour growth or otherwise progressively obstructed. Obstruction of individual small bronchi does not lead to collapse of the segment of lung supplied, because collateral ventilation from adjacent lobules, through the pores of Kohn and the canals of Lambert connecting bronchioles to distal air passages, supplies enough air to expand the obstructed segment; indeed it is more likely to become emphysematous. Obstruction of bronchioles is usually produced by inflammatory exudate, e.g. purulent plugs in bronchopneumonia, or by fibrinous exudate, but narrowing of the lumen by hyperplastic lymphoid tissue in the bronchial wall is also a cause. In bronchial asthma the obstruc-

tion is due to the spasmodic contraction of the walls of the bronchioles, aided by the presence of tough secretion. If the obstruction is such that air can be sucked in and cannot be expelled, as may occur in bronchiolitis and in asthma, then acute emphysema, inspiratory in origin, may result in the area supplied by the obstructed bronchioles. Such a condition may be recovered from when the obstruction is removed, but when bronchiolitis is repeated and failure to resolve results in organisation and fibrosis, structural changes result and emphysema of centrilobular type may supervene.

Tumours of the bronchi are considered later along with tumours of the lungs and pleurae (p. 379).

THE LUNGS

Circulatory Disturbances

Many of the chief facts with regard to these have been given in Chapter 8, but certain details deserve mention.

Chronic venous congestion. Chronic excess of blood in the pulmonary vessels is produced by any lesion of the left side of the heart which leads to deficient output of the blood into the aorta (p. 156), but it is seen in most marked degree in cases of mitral stenosis; and, in this condition it cannot be overcome by any adjusting mechanism. In fact, the more powerfully the right ventricle contracts, the greater would be the distension of the pulmonary capillaries but for the reflex pulmonary arteriolar constriction that develops, especially in the lower lobes, and this may be followed by marked intimal fibrous thickening. In mitral stenosis when the pulmonary arterial pressure is high, oedema of the interlobular septa precedes incipient pulmonary oedema and may be detected radiologically by the appearance of horizontal parallel lines in the costophrenic angles (*Kerley's B lines*). In a typical example of long-standing venous congestion, the lung tissue feels coarser and tougher than normally, and it has a brownish red tint—hence the term "brown induration" applied to the condition. Blood scraped from the surface also may show a brownish tint. The microscopic appearances, etc., have already been described

(p. 158). It is noteworthy that the lingula usually contains much less haemosiderin than other parts.

With regard to *acute congestion* of the lungs—often used as a descriptive clinical term—we know nothing definite beyond the fact that it occurs in the earlier stage of acute inflammation, e.g. lobar pneumonia.

Hypostatic congestion and oedema. Some hypostatic congestion is always present in the lungs *post mortem*, even when death has occurred suddenly in a healthy individual, as from injury; the blood accumulates in the dependent parts and some serous fluid escapes into the alveoli. But in cases where dying has been gradual, and notably in those in coma, hypostatic congestion and oedema become much more marked.

Pulmonary oedema. Sometimes a large proportion of the posterior parts of the lungs may be airless and waterlogged, and when the tissue is squeezed, a large quantity of more-or-less frothy serous fluid, with little admixture of blood, escapes. Pulmonary oedema is, however, most severe in cases of nephritis with general oedema, and also sometimes in cardiac disease; here it may result from relative failure of the left side of the heart, as may occur in hypertension, and also after physical exertion in

M

mitral stenosis when the tricuspid valve is competent. Experimental production of pulmonary oedema has already been discussed (p. 185).

Uraemic lung. This term is used to describe a chronic form of pulmonary oedema long known to radiologists on account of the butterfly-shaped shadow that results from severe chronic oedema extending outwards from the hilum of both lungs. The lungs are voluminous and rubbery and on section exude, under pressure, a frothy fluid. Microscopically the reluctance of the oedema fluid to drain out of the cut surface is seen to be due to a fine fibrin network in the alveoli, and well marked hyaline membranes may be formed. In longstanding cases organisation of the exudate may take place here and there.

Hyaline membrane disease. In the newborn, especially in premature infants delivered by Caesarean section, the respiratory bronchioles and alveolar ducts may become filled with a protein-rich fluid which condenses into a fibrinous membrane over the mouths of the air sacs and alveoli. The origin of this lesion is uncertain, but inadequate opening of the pulmonary vascular bed and deficient formation of the lipoprotein lining film ("surfactant") that normally lowers the surface tension of the alveoli are thought to be concerned. Continued breathing for some time is essential for the formation of the membranes and previous inhalation of liquor amnii may assist in the conversion of fibrinogen to fibrin. Affected infants develop a severe metabolic and respiratory acidosis which, if uncorrected, may prove fatal. The condition is also known clinically as *respiratory distress syndrome of the newborn*.

Apart from neonates, hyaline membranes are found in children dying of acute rheumatic carditis (Fig. 15.13) and occasionally in adults dying of influenza, acute left ventricular failure, or the uraemic lung syndrome.

Pulmonary embolism. The pulmonary artery or one of its large branches may be plugged by an embolus, the source of which is usually a thrombus in a peripheral vein or in the right side of the heart; but we have also seen fatal embolism produced by a large mass of crumbling vegetations from the tricuspid valve. Sudden death may result from pulmonary embolism, and this appears to be brought about by an abrupt diminution of the blood supply to the left side of the heart, fatal syncope resulting; and in our experience there is usually a history of the occurrence of pallor rather than of cyanosis. The conditions giving rise to pulmonary embolism and the results are dealt with on pp. 169–170. The typical *haemorrhagic infarcts* are seen in chronic cardiac disease, with chronic venous congestion of the lungs, and it would appear that in such conditions the collateral supply from the bronchial arteries is sufficient to distend the vessels with blood, but not to maintain the circulation; diffuse haemorrhage thus occurs. Though the commonest cause of such infarcts is embolism, often arising from a thrombus in the veins of the legs or right atrium, infarction may also result from thrombosis in branches of the pulmonary arteries, especially when they are affected by atheroma. Occasionally a massive thrombus may form on an atheromatous patch in a large vessel and we have seen such a thrombus over-riding the bifurcation of the main pulmonary artery and producing so extreme a degree of narrowing of the lumen that severe pulmonary hypertension resulted. Old pulmonary infarcts are rarely found, as the conditions which lead to infarction are usually followed by death within a short time. The old infarcts, which are composed of brownish necrotic and haemorrhagic tissue, shrink and become surrounded by fibrous tissue.

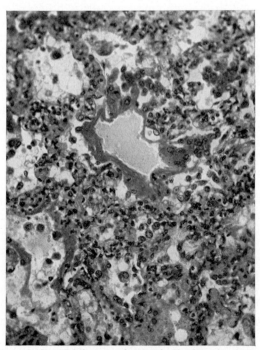

Fig. 15.13.—Hyaline membranes in the lung in cardiac failure from acute rheumatic carditis. × 220.

If organisms are present in the embolus which causes infarction, suppuration commences at the periphery, so that the infarct becomes surrounded by a pale zone of softening, and ultimately an abscess may result. The infection may be by organisms of mild virulence giving rise merely to localised pleurisy without any suppurative softening in the infarct.

Pulmonary alveolar proteinosis. This name has been applied to an uncommon condition of unknown etiology occurring at all ages, in which all the distal air spaces of the lung over wide areas are filled with fluid rich in protein and lipids. In places the fluid appears homogeneous but in most parts it is coarsely granular and contains more deeply staining lumps and numerous needle-shaped clefts in which lie doubly-refractile lipid crystals (Fig. 15.14). A few macrophages containing sudanophil material are present but there is virtually no inflammatory reaction except in those areas affected by terminal infection. The disease is characterised by chronic progressive dyspnoea with cough and spit.

Idiopathic pulmonary haemosiderosis (Ceelen's disease). This is a rare and obscure condition arising in children and young adults, characterised by repeated haemoptyses, anaemia of iron-deficiency type and pulmonary mottling on X-ray examination owing to the large amount of iron in the abundant alveolar phagocytes and saturating

the elastic and reticular stroma of the lung. The etiology is unknown. Occasionally it is associated terminally with acute glomerulonephritis (see Goodpasture's syndrome, p. 711).

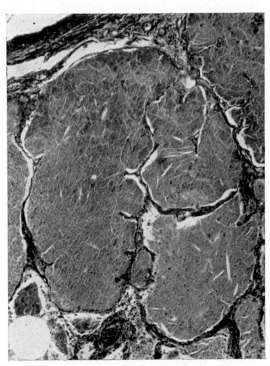

Fig. 15.14.—Pulmonary alveolar proteinosis. The alveoli and ducts are filled with a protein-rich fluid in which many needle-shaped clefts are seen. × 65.

Emphysema

Definition. Emphysema means the presence of bullae or abnormal spaces containing air. In the lung these may be derived from the respiratory bronchioles and alveoli—*vesicular emphysema*, or may be in the connective tissue framework of the lung—*interstitial emphysema*. The latter is due to escape of air into the connective tissue framework of the lung as a result of trauma of some kind and will be considered later. The clinically important form of vesicular emphysema is defined as "a condition of the lung characterised by increase beyond the normal in the size of the air spaces distal to the terminal bronchiole either from dilatation or from destruction of their walls". When the abnormal air spaces are greater than 1 cm. diam. they are termed *bullae*. A relatively unimportant variety is that known as *atrophic* emphysema, which occurs in old age and in wasting diseases.

Vesicular emphysema

In all cases of emphysema, the lungs should be examined after fixation in the expanded position, e.g. by running fixative into the bronchi. The study of normal and diseased lung has also been advanced by two additional techniques. First, the preparation of sections of approximately 300 μ thickness of gelatin-embedded whole lungs: the sections may be mounted on paper and preserved as dry specimens. Secondly, barium sulphate impregnation of slices of fixed lung tissue which allows the relationships of the abnormal air spaces and their connections to be assessed in three dimensions with the dissecting microscope (Figs. 15.15–15.17).

Classification. Vesicular emphysema occurs in *acute* and *chronic* forms. The further classification of the latter is based on its distribution within the pulmonary lobules, a brief description of which is appropriate. When the lung is fixed in the inflated position, the cut surface shows hexagonal areas of parenchyma, some 1 or 2 cm. across, delineated by fibrous septa (Fig. 15.15). Each hexagonal area is a section of a lobule; each lobule consists of 3–5 terminal bronchioles which radiate from the centre of the lobule,

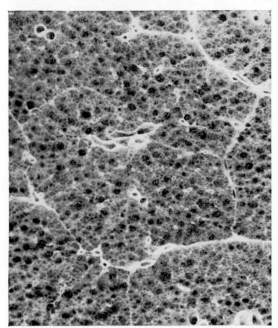

Fig. 15.15.—Normal adult lung. Note the hexagonal lobule in the centre of the field with the terminal bronchioles in its centre. (Barium sulphate impregnation.) × 4.

accompanied by pulmonary arterial twigs, and further subdivide into respiratory bronchioles from which arise the alveolar ducts and alveoli. The parenchyma supplied by one terminal bronchiole is termed an *acinus*, so that a lobule contains 3–5 acini.

Chronic vesicular emphysema is subdivided into the following three types:

(*a*) *Panacinar* (*panlobular*) *emphysema*, in which all the air spaces of the lobule distal to the terminal bronchiole are dilated (see diagram).

(*b*) *Centrilobular emphysema*, in which the abnormal air spaces are derived initially from the respiratory bronchioles, and are clustered in the centres of the lobules. Centrilobular emphysema is further classified into *destructive* and *distensive* types. The former is associated with chronic

bronchitis and bronchiolitis, and the respiratory bronchioles are destroyed leaving a punched-out hole in the centre of the lobule. Distensive emphysema is usually associated with injury to the respiratory bronchioles by inert dust, e.g. coal dust. The dilated respiratory bronchioles persist and are seen clustered together in the centres of the lobule, often around a focus of dust aggregation; it is also called *focal* or *perifocal* dust emphysema and is the main feature of *simple coal miner's pneumoconiosis.*

(*c*) The third type of chronic vesicular

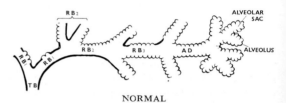

NORMAL

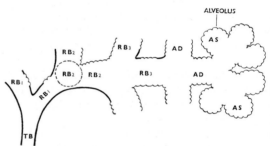

PANACINAR EMPHYSEMA

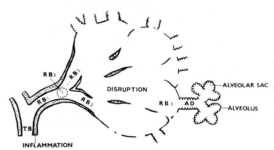

DESTRUCTIVE CENTRILOBULAR EMPHYSEMA

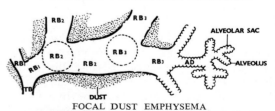

FOCAL DUST EMPHYSEMA

Diagram illustrating the anatomy of the terminal bronchial tree and lung lobules in relation to emphysema. T.B. = terminal bronchiole; R.B. = respiratory bronchioles of 1st, 2nd and 3rd order; A.D. = alveolar duct.

(*diagrams kindly provided by Professor A. G. Heppleston*)

emphysema is *irregular* or *scar emphysema* in which the spaces are localised around scars, e.g. healed tuberculous lesions or silicotic nodules, and results from traction on the adjacent lung tissue by the contracting scar, and compensatory over-inflation. Large bullae may be formed in this way and if these are near the lung surface they may rupture and give rise to pneumothorax (p. 378).

Although each of these forms of chronic vesicular emphysema may occur alone, they frequently co-exist in the lungs of city dwellers.

Acute vesicular emphysema

This is usually of panacinar type. It is sometimes seen as an agonal phenomenon, when, owing to the swelling of the bronchial mucosa or the presence of secretion in the bronchial tubes, air cannot be expelled from the lungs though it is sucked into the lung by strong inspiratory effort. The lungs thus become over-distended and voluminous and there may be also actual rupture of the air vesicles. It was a prominent feature in death from chlorine gas in the war of 1914–18. Acute emphysema occurs in a similar way during an attack of asthma, the bronchial obstruction in this case being caused by contraction of the muscular coat of the bronchioles, aided by tough secretion. If attacks recur in association with chronic bronchitis, the permanent changes of chronic emphysema may develop. This is, however, not invariable; sometimes dilatation of only the terminal bronchioles occurs, without involvement of the alveolar ducts and alveoli.

Acute emphysema frequently occurs *locally* around areas of collapse, such as are produced by obstruction of the bronchioles in acute bronchiolitis and bronchopneumonia. A ring of dilated air spaces can often be seen around the collapsed part, and microscopic examination shows that the affected respiratory bronchioles are overstretched, and the dilated alveoli have a rounded or oval form. Sometimes over a considerable area collapsed lobules alternate with overdistended tissue. Such emphysema is often termed *compensatory*, and is regarded as the result of the overdistension during inspiration, secondary to the adjacent collapse. No doubt that is the case, but during the course of plugging of the minute bronchioles, there will often be a stage at which air can be sucked in and not expelled, just as in acute panacinar emphysema.

When recovery takes place, acute emphysema in great measure disappears, as the collapsed areas re-expand.

Chronic vesicular emphysema

Clinical features. It is extraordinarily difficult to correlate the pathological findings in emphysema with the clinical state of the patient during life. Typically the patient is a middle-aged male who has suffered from chronic bronchitis for years and who now has some degree of dyspnoea on exertion; this is the only constant sign. The chest is said usually to be barrel-shaped, with a wide sub-costal angle, a degree of kyphosis and impaired expansion; the accessory muscles are used in respiration, the lungs are hyper-resonant, breath sounds are impaired, the cardiac dullness is reduced and the liver and diaphragm are displaced downwards. The vital capacity is much reduced and the volume of residual air is increased.

Eventually exertional dyspnoea may prevent the patient from working and finally he may become an asthenic, chair-bound, respiratory cripple, depending on his accessory muscles for ventilation. Hypoxia and CO_2 retention develop early in some patients and may be associated with cyanosis, polycythaemia, mental deterioration and right ventricular failure. An abrupt deterioration in respiratory function may result from afebrile inflammatory episodes or from a spontaneous pneumothorax. There is an increased incidence of peptic ulcer in emphysematous patients, and perforation may have an atypical clinical presentation.

Panacinar (panlobular) emphysema. *Macroscopically*, the lungs appear very voluminous but are not larger than normal lungs in full expansion; the anterior surface of the heart is covered and the diaphragm pressed downwards. The emphysematous tissue is distended and raised above the surface, thus rounding off the sharp margins of the lung. It is paler than the rest of the lung as less carbon pigment is present; it contains little blood and usually it pits on pressure, owing to lack of elasticity. It has a soft, downy, almost non-crepitant feeling to the touch, and air may be passed along by gentle pressure from one part to another, owing to disruption of the alveolar walls. On section, the essential feature is the enlargement of air spaces throughout the whole of the lobule (Fig. 15.16), and

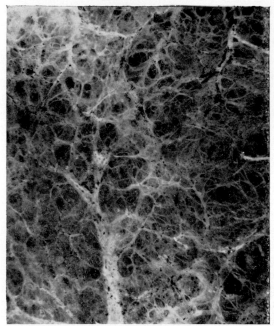

FIG. 15.16.—Severe panacinar emphysema. Note the fine fibrous strands which are the surviving remnants of the alveoli. An interlobular septum is present in the centre of the field, therefore this illustration shows the periphery of two lobules. (Barium sulphate impregnation.) × 8.

spaces of all sizes may be present up to large bullae, from the walls of which the remains of vessels in the ruptured pulmonary tissue project. Emphysema is most marked at the apices and along the margins, especially the anterior borders, but in extreme cases practically the whole of the lung substance may be affected, though the condition is always slight on the posterior aspect. This severe degree of emphysema inevitably results in respiratory insufficiency and cor pulmonale.

Microscopic examination confirms that the condition develops from dilatation of the respiratory bronchioles, alveolar ducts and alveoli, and that the larger spaces are formed by destructive coalescence of adjacent air sacs.

The pathogenesis of generalised panacinar emphysema is not fully understood and writers on the subject are not in agreement about the degree of bronchiolar involvement with narrowing that may be present. Although chronic bronchitis very often accompanies panacinar emphysema, it is not always present, and the etiology remains obscure.

Destructive centrilobular emphysema. *Naked-eye appearances.* In this form of emphysema also

the lungs are voluminous but the dilated air spaces at an early stage occupy the centre of the lobules and each peripheral zone is relatively unaffected; the changes are more pronounced in the upper lobes than elsewhere. As the condition develops the spaces enlarge, occupy more of the lobule and often coalesce (Fig. 15.17). The changes of chronic bronchitis and of bronchiolitis are invariably present. Centrilobular emphysema is commonly associated with some degree of diffuse panacinar emphysema.

Microscopic examination. The bronchi and bronchioles are somewhat dilated down to the bronchiole supplying the primary lobule; in nearly half the cases the supplying bronchiole shows no noteworthy narrowing but in all cases the bronchiolar walls show chronic inflammatory changes, with fibrosis and loss of muscle fibres resulting from organisation of previous acute inflammatory exudate. These chronic inflamma-

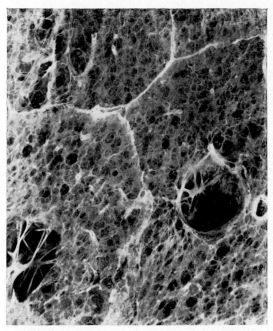

FIG. 15.17.—Early destructive centrilobular emphysema. Note the punched out centrilobular spaces containing fibrous strands and blood vessels and the relatively normal parenchyma at the periphery of the lobules. (Barium sulphate impregnation.) × 6.

tory and fibrotic changes extend to the respiratory bronchioles and the large air spaces of centrilobular emphysema are in the first place the dilated respiratory bronchioles. Finally the walls may rupture and adjacent dilated air spaces become confluent, thus forming the larger bullae which are traversed by the fibrous remnants of respiratory bronchiolar walls containing blood vessels. At this stage most of the lobules may be involved and the centrilobular origin of the condition is recognisable only in the less severely affected parts of the lungs.

Distensive centrilobular or **focal dust emphysema.** This form of emphysema is responsible for most of the disability from dyspnoea in the *simple pneumoconiosis* of the coal miner and those exposed to other non-fibrogenic dusts. The finer inhaled particles penetrate to the terminal air passages and alveoli from which they are removed by macrophages. These dust-laden phagocytes accumulate in and around the walls of the respiratory bronchioles, especially those of the second order and the smooth muscle fibres within their walls undergo atrophy. The respiratory bronchiole dilates under inspiratory pressure and the presence of the dense mass of dust cells associated with the dilated respiratory bronchioles produces on transverse section the stellate foci of dust aggregation and perifocal emphysema, so characteristic of simple pneumoconiosis (Figs. 15.18 and 15.49, p. 370). There is little actual tissue destruction and cor pulmonale

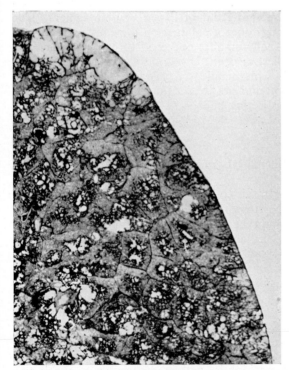

FIG. 15.18.—Centrilobular (focal dust) emphysema in coal-worker's pneumoconiosis. × 1.

may be very slight unless chronic bronchitis and bronchiolitis are also present, when destructive centrilobular emphysema, with its more serious effects, will be superimposed.

Causation of chronic vesicular emphysema. Irrespective of the nature and site of the damage done to the lungs, the initial force which expands the damaged portions into emphysematous spaces is the atmospheric pressure of the inspired air. On purely physical and mathematical principles the force required to distend an elastic sphere is inversely proportional to the radius and therefore becomes progressively less as the sphere enlarges. A vicious circle is initiated as soon as a weakness develops in the air passages and continuing dilatation and destruction is inevitable, particularly if the emphysematous lung is subject to the powerful inspiratory effort of the coughing which is associated with chronic bronchitis. In destructive centrilobular emphysema associated with chronic bronchitis, the essential lesion is post-inflammatory weakening of the terminal and respiratory bronchioles and this is the most likely cause of the dilatation. It also seems probable that in the initial phase there is proximal bronchiolar narrowing (fibrosing bronchiolitis) which prevents the escape of inspired air and leads to increased pressure in the distal bronchioles and alveolar ducts. Such narrowing is recognised in only half of the cases examined, but it should be noted that the technical procedure of fixing and inflating the lungs prior to examination might dilate air passages which were narrowed in life. As the process continues, destruction of the surrounding parenchyma leaves the surviving bronchioles unsupported and kinking of these air passages and loss of elastic recoil leads to further air trapping.

In focal dust emphysema the selective localisation of the dust accumulation in and around the walls of the second respiratory bronchiole leads to rigidity and loss of the unstriped muscle so that the affected segments are progressively dilated under the pressure of inspired air.

In advanced panlobular emphysema, air trapping and damage become progressive once there is insufficient surrounding parenchyma to keep open the terminal bronchioles in the expiratory phase, but the initial process of panlobular dilatation is more difficult to explain. This form of emphysema is not always associated with chronic bronchiolitis and speculations as to its etiology include the possibility that there is a primary, genetically determined bronchiolar atrophy or that the atrophy is ischaemic and results from obliterative endarteritis of either pulmonary or bronchial blood vessels.

Functional effects. Emphysematous air spaces not only replace functioning lung tissue, but also have serious effects on the flow of air into and out of the lung. Air is trapped by increased airways resistance and diminished force of elastic recoil, so that the volume of air which can be removed by forced expiration is decreased and lung function studies invariably reveal a diminished vital capacity: the clinical term *obstructive airways disease* is therefore appropriate. The presence of abnormal air spaces increases the residual volume and total capacity of the lung, but this serves no useful purpose and the net effect is irregular mixing and distribution of inspired and residual air which in turn leads to inefficient gas exchange. The increased muscular effort required to hyperventilate the lungs against airways resistance leads to wasteful oxygen consumption and adds to the retention of carbon dioxide. Thus blood gas analysis reveals a fall in the oxygen saturation of the pulmonary venous blood from the normal 96 per cent to 90 per cent or less—hypoxic hypoxaemia—and this may be associated with a secondary polycythaemia. Poor ventilation of well-perfused areas of lung also leads to CO_2 retention and respiratory acidosis which is compensated by a raised plasma bicarbonate—a compensated respiratory acidosis. In some patients the respiratory centre becomes insensitive to the increased plasma CO_2 and respiratory control depends on the stimulus of a depressed oxygen saturation; if such individuals are given oxygen therapeutically, the reduced stimulus to the respiratory centre can produce a disastrous apnoea. In spite of the destruction of many alveolar walls and capillaries the pulmonary blood flow is maintained for a time by compensatory hypertrophy of the right ventricle (*cor pulmonale*, i.e. right ventricular hypertrophy resulting from lung disease). There is also evidence that hypoxia can bring about constriction of the pulmonary arterioles, thus increasing the resistance to blood flow. The systolic pressure within the pulmonary arteries is raised from the normal level of 18–25 mm. Hg to about 60 mm. Hg and in consequence there is often considerable atheroma in these vessels. Cardiac

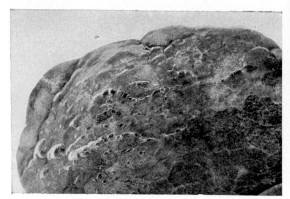

Fig. 15.19.—Interstitial emphysema of apex of lung, showing numerous small air bubbles along the lines of interlobular lymphatics. (J. W. S. B.)

catheterisation has revealed that the cardiac output is high and is accompanied by a marked rise in venous pressure. Polycythaemia is sometimes found but is rarely severe.

Atrophic or senile emphysema. This is common in old age, but it is caused also by conditions of malnutrition, e.g. the cachexia of malignant disease, and was often a feature in chronic untreated pernicious anaemia. The changes are simple atrophy of the alveolar walls and confluence of air vesicles, the result not of overstretching, but of imperfect nourishment. The lungs do not enlarge; on the contrary, they are usually smaller and tend to collapse when the chest is opened *post mortem*. The emphysema is widespread as a rule; the affected tissue is soft and silky to the touch and there are no large projecting bullae. Atrophic emphysema usually does not lead to hypertrophy of the right heart.

Interstitial emphysema

In this condition the air is in the lymphatics of the supporting tissue of the lungs, and spreads along them. For its occurrence some laceration of the lung substance is necessary, either (*a*) *overdistension* of the air vesicles, such as is present in severe coughing and in dyspnoea with forced inspiration, or (*b*) *traumatic laceration* of the lung tissue by a fractured rib or by a perforating wound. Interstitial emphysema, due to rupture of the alveolar walls from over-distension, is much commoner in children than in adults, and occurs in such conditions as whooping-cough, bronchiolitis, and in diphtheria of the larynx and trachea. The alveolar walls give way as the result of over-expansion during forced inspiration, and air in the form of small bead-like collections or blebs extends along the lines of junction of the interlobular septa with the pleura, thus producing a sort of reticulated appearance on the pleural surfaces (Fig. 15.19). When the air is abundant, it passes by the lymphatics to the root of the lungs, and in exceptional cases it may extend even to the tissues at the root of the neck and lead to subcutaneous emphysema. Occasionally in interstitial emphysema a bleb may rupture and give rise to pneumothorax (p. 378). In traumatic emphysema the air follows a similar course, and here again there may be extension to the chest wall. We have seen interstitial emphysema as the result of severe injury to the body where there has been no fracture of ribs or wound of the lungs.

Collapse of Lung Tissue

Atelectasis and collapse. A distinction is usually drawn between these two conditions, the former being *congenital* and the latter *acquired*. The congenital lesion is really due to non-expansion of the lung tissue, and the term *atelectasis* is properly applied; sometimes it is used loosely but erroneously to indicate all forms of collapse. In poorly nourished infants the lungs may fail to expand fully at birth, due to muscular weakness and consequent feeble inspiratory movement. Mucus and amniotic fluid causing obstruction in the bronchi bring about failure of expansion of parts of the lung tissue by inspiration, and may lead to collapse of parts which formerly contained air. These are more frequent in the lower lobes, are usually superficial in position and somewhat depressed below the surface; owing to the non-oxygenation of the blood in the capillaries they are usually of dark purplish colour. Apart from these conditions, the two commonest causes of collapse are (a) *direct pressure* on the lung substance from without, and (b) *bronchial obstruction*, with resulting absorption of air in the corresponding area of lung tissue. With regard to the former, a lung may undergo collapse from accumulation of fluid in a pleural cavity, for example, as the result of serous effusion, haemorrhage or empyema. In the last-mentioned condition, the collapse is sometimes very great, and the lung becomes very small and lies posteriorly against the side of the vertebral column. When the exudate on the pleural surface becomes organised, and a "pyogenic membrane" has formed, the lung is incapable of expansion to its former size, and may ultimately be enclosed by a fibrous layer. It is therefore important to drain the pleural cavity and obtain re-expansion of the lung before this happens. Collapse of a part of the lung may be produced also by direct pressure of an aneurysm or neoplasm. The relation of *bronchial obstruction* to collapse has already been considered.

In a collapsed area, the walls of the alveoli are approximated, and their capillaries are usually dilated. Owing to lack of movement of air the haemoglobin of the blood in the capillaries of the collapsed area is largely in a reduced state—hence the purple colour on naked-eye examination. When the collapse has lasted for some time, the alveolar epithelium forms a prominent lining of cubical cells. Later it tends to desquamate, progressive fibrosis follows, and permanently prevents expansion and return to normal. Such areas of collapse and fibrosis are very often accompanied by bronchiectasis.

Acute massive collapse. This condition is seen most frequently after operations, especially those on the upper abdomen and after open wounds of the chest. It may occur in strong and well-nourished patients and has no relation to shock. The onset is comparatively sudden, usually within one or two days after operation, and is characterised by pain in the chest, dyspnoea, cyanosis and a certain degree of pyrexia. The collapse may affect a large portion of a lung, usually the right, and is commonest in the lower lobe. The chest wall is indrawn and more or less motionless and the heart is displaced to the affected side, as is well seen on X-ray examination. The condition usually passes off within a day or two, sometimes quite rapidly. The view generally held is that it is the result of obstruction of large bronchi by tough mucus, this being probably aided by weak and shallow respiration. Natural relief of the condition is sometimes preceded by the expectoration of much tenacious mucus. It has been shown experimentally that massive collapse can be produced by bronchial obstruction and rapid re-expansion of the lung occurs when the obstruction is removed. However, the mode of production of massive collapse is not fully understood. On the supposition that shallow respiration during anaesthesia is a factor, carbon dioxide has been administered to stimulate the respiratory centre; collapse, however, cannot be entirely prevented in this way.

Acute Inflammatory Conditions

In conformity with general pathological terminology it might be expected that inflammation of the lungs would be called "pneumonitis" or "pulmonitis", but it is customary instead to use the term "pneumonia", a direct transcription of that used by the ancient Greek physicians. In its usual connotation it implies the presence of solidification of the lung substance. Recently the term "pneumonitis" has been introduced to designate certain inflammatory states of the lungs in which consolidation is not a feature clinically, but the term has not yet gained general acceptance.

Classification. The acute inflammatory conditions of the lungs are most conveniently classified according to the mode in which the infection spreads.

(A) In one variety the inflammation starts at one place and then spreads by direct continuity, involving the various structures in its course and leading to extensive consolidation of the lung substance—*lobar pneumonia*.

(B) In another type the infection is disseminated by means of the air passages, inflammation of the minute bronchi preceding that of the pulmonary tissue. The resulting lesion is aptly termed a *bronchopneumonia*. It is also called *lobular* on account of its distribution, in contrast with lobar.

(C) Organisms may be carried by the blood stream and arrested in the pulmonary vessels, and thus give rise to inflammatory foci, which are often suppurative. The term *embolic pneumonia* may be applied. It occurs as a complication in other infections.

(D) Lastly, the accumulation of secretions in the posterior parts of the lungs may supply a medium for the growth of organisms, which set up inflammatory changes. To this variety, in which the distribution is influenced by gravity, the term *hypostatic pneumonia* is given.

Acute lobar pneumonia

Since the widespread use of antibiotic therapy, the full-blown picture of lobar pneumonia is not often seen in this country. It is, however, a classic example clinically of a specific bacterial infection and pathologically of acute inflammation.

Etiology. In the majority of cases, lobar pneumonia is caused by *Strep. pneumoniae*, of which four types have been distinguished by their serological and other features. The typing of pneumococci is of importance in epidemiology, but since the advent of the sulphonamide drugs and penicillin, etc., typing is no longer so important clinically. Types I and II are responsible for most cases of typical acute pneumonia. Type III, *Pneumococcus mucosus*, is relatively uncommon, but causes the most severe form of pneumonia. It produces a mucoid exudate as is seen also in the comparatively small proportion of cases caused by *Klebsiella pneumoniae*. Type IV includes a large number of strains which are serologically distinct; it is often called "group IV" for this reason. Pneumococci of this group are often present in the normal nasopharynx and the pneumonia caused by them is relatively mild.

Natural history. Lobar pneumonia starts usually at the base or about the hilum and then spreads directly, leading to a progressive consolidation of the lung tissue. Ultimately almost the whole of the lung may be involved. The essential factor is a rapid and diffuse spread of pneumococci throughout the pulmonary tissue and the organisms are found in the interstitial tissue, as well as in the contents of the air vesicles. It spreads rapidly by continuity, and resolves rapidly when immunity is established with the appearance in the blood of antibodies. When these reach a certain level, bacterial multiplication ceases and the crisis occurs. In some cases the crisis fails to occur, bacterial growth with inflammatory change continues, and suppuration in the lung tissue follows (see below). Less frequently the disease begins in the apex—"apical pneumonia". The disease is usually one-sided, but occasionally it affects both lungs—double pneumonia; and when this is the case, the consolidation in one lung is more extensive than in the other, and is usually at a somewhat later stage. Lobar pneumonia is more common on the right than on the left side. The disease occurs most frequently in adult life and is comparatively uncommon in children, in whom bronchopneumonia is the common pneumonic type; this suggests that there may be an element of hypersensitivity to the pneumococcus in the pathogenesis of the lesions.

Clinical features. Untreated lobar pneumonia forms the best example of a bacterial infection running a definite course of 6 or 7 days like a specific fever and terminating by crisis. The onset is sudden, with a rigor and pain in the side, and the inflammatory changes in the lung are accompanied by rapid and shallow respiration, the rise in the respiratory rate being disproportionate to that of the pulse rate.

Throughout the stage of fever there is usually a well-marked polymorphonuclear *leukocytosis* of 25–30,000 cells per c.mm., which rapidly falls at the time of crisis or with successful treatment, being followed often by a percentage increase of mononuclears. The presence of leukocytosis indicates that the cellular defence of the body is satisfactory, and it is a favourable sign; but it does not signify that the patient will recover, as death may occur from various causes—heart failure, etc. The absence of a marked leukocytosis, or its disappearance before the crisis, indicates a severe toxic action on, or lack of response of, the bone marrow and is therefore of grave significance. Diminution of leukocytosis is, however, a common result of antibiotic therapy.

In some cases of pneumonia the degree of oxygen saturation of the arterial blood is normal or practically so. This is remarkable in view of the fact that the alveoli of one or more lobes are out of action, and one would expect that the blood from them would return to the heart in a non-oxygenated state and thus *hypoxic hypoxaemia* would result. The explanation may be that the circulation of blood through the consolidated parts is much reduced. Some flow must, of course, be present, since serious ischaemic effects do not occur, and the antibodies reach the bacteria. The whole matter is puzzling and requires further investigation. In other cases of pneumonia, however, anoxic anoxaemia is present, and at the same time there may be deficient output of blood from the heart and thus accumulation of blood in the venous system with accompanying *congestive hypoxaemia* (p. 157). In such circumstances the amount of oxygen unsaturation of the venous blood may be very high and cyanosis may be present. When the latter is marked the prognosis is usually grave.

Structural changes. The lesion is essentially a spreading inflammation with abundant fibrinous exudation, which leads to consolidation. The inflammation progresses till the time of crisis; it then stops and thereafter undergoes resolution in favourable cases, and the lung may return to a practically normal condition. In other cases, however, there follow various complications (see below). It has been customary to describe the stages of the process under the headings of (1) *acute congestion*, (2) *red hepatisation*, (3) *grey hepatisation*, and (4) *resolution*. The first mentioned is simply a necessary stage in every acute inflammatory condition.

In *red hepatisation* a portion of the lung, one lobe or more, has become consolidated or "hepatised", that is, liver-like in its consistence. The affected tissue feels solid, and on section is red and mottled by the presence of carbon pigment and the pale connective tissue of the lung. The cut surface is comparatively dry, smooth or slightly granular. This appearance is due to filling of the alveoli with fine strands of fibrinous exudate, feebly translucent when fresh, through which the intensely congested alveolar walls can be seen. Overlying the area of lung affected, the earlier stages of acute pleurisy are present, the pleura being intensely congested, often showing minute haemorrhages, and covered with a variable amount of dense fibrinous exudate. Fibrinous plugs may be present in the minute bronchi, and occasionally may extend into those of larger size, whilst the pleural layers between the affected lobes may be greatly swollen and glued together by fibrinous exudate. All these changes are the results of the direct spread of the pneumococci through the pulmonary tissue.

Grey hepatisation results from even more complete consolidation, and the lung tissue feels denser and heavier. The cut surface is, on the whole, pale; there is a greyish or pinkish-grey background, against which the carbon pigment of the lung stands out prominently, the appearance being aptly compared to that of grey granite (Fig. 15.20). The pleurisy is more marked than in the stage of red hepatisation, and the fibrinous exudate is sometimes very abundant.

Resolution. At the time of crisis most of the pneumococci are rapidly killed, the process of consolidation ceases to spread, and in favourable cases the process of resolution begins. During this period the fibrinous exudate in the alveoli is gradually liquefied, the consolidation becomes less dense, and when the lung tissue is pressed, a certain amount of fluid exudes from the surface. The process of softening or digestion of the fibrin progresses until the fibrin has completely disappeared, and thereafter the fluid within the alveoli gradually is absorbed and replaced by air. The process of resolution is usually to be seen at various stages in different parts. The liquefied exudate undergoes absorption by the lymphatics, though possibly in part by the blood vessels: a portion is expectorated, but as a rule the amount discharged in this way is comparatively small.

The absorption of the fibrin on the *pleural surface* is relatively slow, and organisation

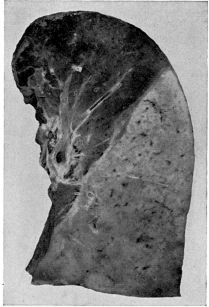

Fig. 15.20.—Acute lobar pneumonia with grey hepatisation in lower lobe, red hepatisation in part of upper lobe. × ¼.

usually occurs, giving rise to fibrous adhesions between the layers of the pleura. This is apparently due to the exudate on the pleura being denser and more abundant than in the alveoli. It is also less thoroughly permeated by leuko-

cytes and is farther removed from blood vessels.

The microscopic appearances need only be described briefly as they are essentially those of a typical acute inflammation. In the early stage of red hepatisation a delicate fibrinous reticulum

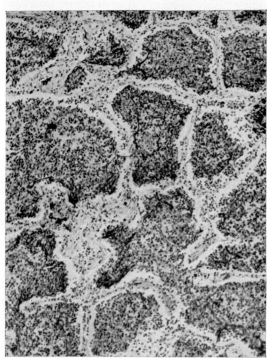

Fig. 15.21.—Lobar pneumonia in stage of red hepatisation, showing general consolidation with abundant network of fibrin in the alveoli, which appears dark. (Stained by Weigert's fibrin method.) × 60.

fills the alveoli (Fig. 15.21), and also fibrin extends as strands through the pores of Kohn between adjacent alveoli. Fibrin is present also in the septa, and the minute bronchioles may sometimes contain fibrinous plugs. Within the alveoli a number of polymorphonuclear leukocytes and of red cells, which have escaped by diapedesis, are present in the fibrinous reticulum. Some of the cells of the alveolar epithelium, which have become swollen and desquamated, may be seen lying free (Fig. 15.22). The alveolar capillaries are at first markedly congested. In the stage of grey hepatisation, the fibrin has contracted from the walls and forms more condensed, and often somewhat granular, masses within the alveoli. There is marked increase in the number of polymorphonuclear leukocytes and the alveoli appear packed with them. Some show signs of degeneration and many of the red cells have undergone lysis

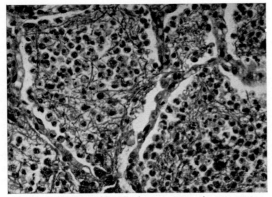

FIG. 15.22.—Lobar pneumonia.

The early exudate showing the fibrin network and many polymorphonuclear leukocytes. × 235.

and disappeared. The lung tissue has also become less congested. During the stage of resolution the fibrin becomes still more granular or amorphous in appearance, and seems to be melting away by a process of peripheral digestion. Along with the disappearance of the fibrin there occurs a gradual diminution in the number of leukocytes, these being carried off chiefly by the lymphatics, whilst there may be a considerable proliferation of the lining epithelium. Ultimately the fluid contents and the remaining cells in the alveoli are absorbed, the epithelial lining of the alveoli is restored and the condition returns to normal. The lymph nodes draining the affected lung are markedly enlarged, and when resolution is going on, the sinuses are greatly distended, and contain macrophages actively engulfing whole cells and detritus which have been removed from the lung.

Complications. Whilst resolution is the normal

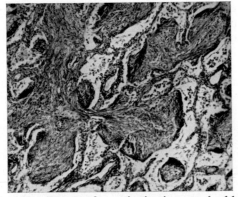

FIG. 15.23.—Process of organisation in unresolved lobar pneumonia, showing new formation of fibrous tissue and ingrowth into fibrinous masses within the alveoli. × 80.

termination of lobar pneumonia, it may fail, and we have to consider now some less favourable results or complications which may follow.

Organisation of exudate and fibrosis. We have already pointed out the difference between the fate of the exudate in the alveoli and that on the pleural surface. In some cases, however, digestion of the fibrin in the alveoli and absorption do not take place, and then a process of organisation occurs from the alveolar walls. In such cases one usually finds that leukocytes within the alveoli are scanty, whereas the fibrinous plugs are dense and hyaline in appearance (Fig. 15.23).

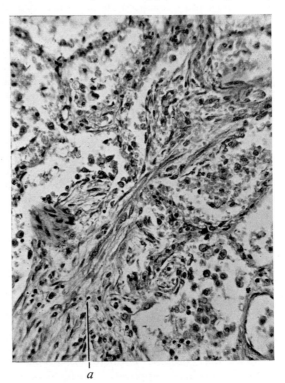

a

FIG. 15.24.—Organisation of alveolar exudate in lung.

The alveolar exudate is replaced by a cellular vascular fibrous tissue. Note the fibroblasts passing from one alveolus to another through the pore of Kohn; also the destruction of the alveolar wall at *a*, with preservation of the alveolar walls elsewhere. × 390.

Probably deficiency of leukocytes is of greater importance. In the cases in question there is proliferation of the connective tissue cells of the alveolar walls, and this is accompanied by a formation of new capillary buds and their growth into the alveoli often from only a single point in the wall (Fig. 15.24). The later stages are the usual ones of devascularisation and diffuse fibrosis with contraction. However, diffuse pulmonary fibrosis rarely results with antibiotic therapy.

Suppuration. Failure of resolution from continued multiplication of the pneumococci may be followed by *suppurative softening*. There is advanced grey hepatisation and the lung appears comparatively bloodless, but, in addition, there is softening of the pneumonic tissue. The alveoli are filled with enormous numbers of polymorphonuclear leukocytes, while in affected parts the fibrinous exudate has entirely disappeared and the walls of the alveoli are undergoing digestion, so that ill-defined areas of suppuration or more localised abscesses are formed by their confluence. This process may be seen in cases where death has occurred about the eighth day without crisis or resolution, and results from persistent multiplication of the pneumococci. Occasionally abscesses become chronic and may perforate into the pleural cavity. Suppurative change is more likely to occur in diabetics and alcoholics.

Gangrene of the lung (p. 356). This is a rare complication and is due to the secondary invasion of the affected lung by putrefactive organisms. It is observed sometimes in diabetic patients, in alcoholics, and in others whose powers of resistance are markedly diminished; it occurs also sometimes in the pneumonia following influenza. In the great majority of cases it is rapidly fatal.

Other complications. In addition to the various results in the lung, pneumococcal infection may ensue in other parts. Sometimes the pneumococci extend to the pericardial sac and set up *pericarditis*, and this takes place more frequently when the pneumonia is on the left side. The exudate may become purulent. *Empyema* (p. 378) is another complication, which occurs, however, more frequently in children than in adults. In cases of pneumonia, the pneumococci pass into the blood stream, and in severe cases may be present in considerable number, so that various degrees of septicaemia result. The organisms may then settle in different parts of the body and give rise to inflammatory change. The leptomeninges are sometimes invaded, and the resulting lesion found *post mortem* varies from an intense congestion to a *meningitis* with abundant greenish-yellow and semi-purulent exudate. Another complication is infection of the heart valves, and the *bacterial endocarditis* which results is characterised by the formation of large crumbling vegetations. Acute *arthritis* occasionally occurs as a sequel to pneumonia.

Bronchopneumonia

Classification. This condition is characterised by spread of infection from the terminal bronchioles to the alveoli; there are several varieties, which include:

(A) *Simple (non-suppurative) bronchopneumonia*, a condition in which there is pneumonic consolidation of lobular or patchy type, and in which, as in lobar pneumonia, resolution may follow.

(B) *Suppurative or septic bronchopneumonia*, where the consolidation is followed by suppuration and the formation of groups of abscesses, which may become confluent. This occurs frequently behind bronchial obstruction and the term *retention pneumonia* may then be suitably applied.

(C) *Tuberculous bronchopneumonia*. This is a condition in which the tubercle bacilli become disseminated by the air passages and in which the pneumonic change is succeeded by caseation (p. 362).

While in the first type resolution may occur, in the second and third types this is not possible, as there is actual destruction of lung tissue.

Simple bronchopneumonia—non-suppurative

Epidemiology and etiology. This is a common and serious complication of whooping-cough and measles. It occurs, however, apart from these diseases, and is frequently fatal, especially in poorly nourished children. In infants under one year bronchiolitis is due chiefly to respiratory syncytial virus, and if bacterial infection is superadded it is commonly due to penicillin-resistant *Staphylococcus aureus* which the infant probably picked up in the Maternity Hospital during the neonatal period.

The bronchial mucosa of the adult has much greater resistance to bacterial invasion than that of the child, and in the healthy adult it is comparatively rare for a descending infection to extend to the alveoli and cause bronchopneumonia. In old age, however, the liability to bronchopneumonia again occurs. When the resistance is lowered by other infections, especially by viruses, bronchopneumonia is not uncommon in the adult; the outstanding example of this is seen in *influenza*, where bronchopneumonia is the chief pulmonary complication. Further, it may be caused by the inhalation of irritating gases. Simple bronchopneumonia is usually caused by *Strep. pneumoniae*, and there are comparatively few cases in which this organism is not present. It may be produced by other organisms, such as *H. influenzae*, *Staph. aureus*, *Esch. coli*, *Pseudomonas pyocyanea* and *Strep. pyogenes*, the complicating organism varying in different localities and in different epidemics. *Staph. aureus* and *Esch. coli* are of particular importance in hospital-acquired and post-operative pneumonia. The diphtheria bacillus and typhoid bacillus may be involved in the respective diseases along with the pneumococcus or other organisms.

In considering the causal organisms of simple bronchopneumonia the importance of virus infections of the respiratory tract as a predisposing factor cannot be overemphasised.

Structural changes. In all cases the initial lesion is an acute inflammation of the terminal and respiratory bronchioles (that is, a *bronchiolitis*—Fig. 15.25), which become plugged with purulent exudate extending to the alveolar ducts and alveoli. In young children some alveoli become collapsed by absorption of the contained air because collateral ventilation is not yet fully established. These alveoli appear as purple depressed areas of the lung: they are surrounded by a ring of alveoli showing compensatory emphysema and clearly visible on the pleural surface. The occurrence of collapsed areas has been rather overemphasised and in most parts the inflammation spreads to the alveoli without previous collapse.

In the stage of acute bronchiolitis there is little change to be seen on naked-eye examination. The lung tissue is usually congested, and when it is squeezed small purulent drops exude from the minute bronchi. Areas of collapse are usually small but may be much larger if a major bronchus is obstructed by mucus and inflammatory exudate. Bronchopneumonia usually involves both lungs, though one may be much more affected than the other. The change tends to occur earlier and to be more advanced in the lower lobes and in the posterior parts of the lung, but there are exceptions to this. The implication of the lung tissue is shown by the

appearance of numerous patches of consolidation which can be felt to be almost airless. Their size and colour vary. At first they are minute and tend to be red and often they can be felt more readily than seen; later they become larger, paler, and are almost grey. They are arranged in groups and their margins are somewhat ill-defined; they may be interspersed amongst the

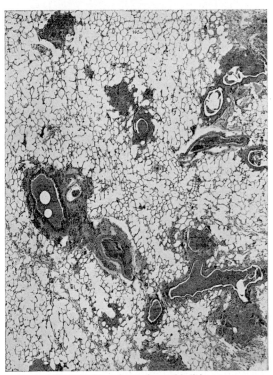

FIG. 15.25.—Acute bronchiolitis.
The bronchioles are filled with inflammatory exudate, which in a few places is seen to extend into the alveolar ducts and alveoli. × 10.

collapsed parts, as already explained. As the condition advances, the pneumonic areas enlarge and become confluent (Fig. 15.26), and sometimes a considerable proportion of the lung may be consolidated. Occasionally the consolidation may be almost as complete as in lobar pneumonia, but the consolidated areas have always a patchy appearance, some parts being paler than others. Moreover, in the less affected parts, the lobular distribution can be quite easily recognised. Pleurisy is usually present over the affected lung; there may be little more than a dimming of the surface, or there may be a distinct fibrinous exudation.

Microscopic examination at an early stage of the disease shows that most of the terminal bronchioles are plugged with an exudate (Fig. 15.25) containing numerous polymorphonuclear leukocytes along with red cells and desquamated epithelial cells, and sometimes sheets of detached

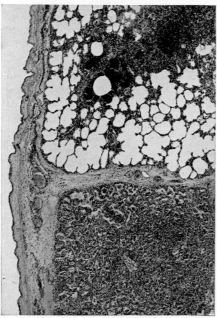

Fig. 15.26.—Early and advanced bronchopneumonia.

The upper lobe shows early bronchopneumonic consolidation with compensatory emphysema; the lower lobe shows confluent consolidation. × 30.

epithelium may be seen. In relation to the distribution of a bronchiole there is a collection of consolidated alveoli, and at places it can be seen that the exudate in the bronchioles is continuous through the alveolar ducts with that in the alveoli; this is, of course, an indication of the direct distal extension of the inflammatory process (Fig. 15.25). Spread of the inflammatory process, however, takes place also directly through the bronchial wall, which is swollen and extensively invaded by leukocytes (peribronchiolitis), and usually surrounded by a ring of consolidated alveoli (Fig. 15.27). The inflammatory process here is fairly severe, and these alveoli may contain fibrinous plugs (Fig. 15.29). While in a consolidated patch near a bronchiole most of the cells are polymorphonuclear leukocytes, at the margins where the reaction is less intense the alveoli may contain numerous macrophages which have come from the alveolar walls. In the intervening parts of the lung many of the alveoli may be over-distended with air (Fig. 15.26).

Cellular infiltration of the bronchial walls and interstitial tissue is often a marked feature of bronchopneumonia, but it varies in extent from case to case. It is especially prominent in cases due to *Strep. pyogenes*.

Results of bronchopneumonia. When recovery takes place, as in lobar pneumonia, resolution with absorption of the inflammatory exudate may occur; but in bronchopneumonia this is more protracted without a distinct crisis, because bacterial growth does not cease abruptly. Moreover, the lung tissue often does not return completely to normal, but undergoes organisation. Peribronchiolitis may be followed by fibrosis, sometimes nodular, sometimes more diffuse. Fibrosis may later lead to bronchiectasis, or patches of honeycomb lung. There is no doubt that failure of resolution of bronchiolitis and bronchopneumonia is an important factor in causing destructive centrilobular emphysema at a later stage. Suppuration may sometimes occur in the consolidated areas, but this is not common if we except cases of aspiration pneumonia (p. 355). Empyema is an uncommon complication nowadays.

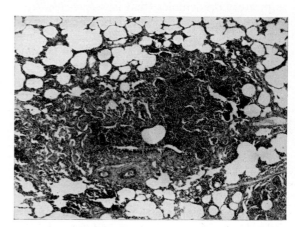

Fig. 15.27.—Bronchopneumonia, showing acute bronchiolitis with consolidation of surrounding alveoli. × 60.

Suppurative bronchopneumonia

This is produced as a rule by the entrance of fluids containing various pyogenic organisms into the small bronchi. It may complicate surgical operations about the mouth or throat, and it occurs also when the bronchi become partially or completely obstructed, e.g. by tumour, so that secretions are retained and form a suitable medium for the growth of organisms. In neoplastic obstruction of a main bronchus the consolidation resulting from this infection may be lobar in distribution; later multiple abscesses may develop (Fig. 15.61, p. 380). Repeated attacks of pneumonia and failure of complete resolution are now regarded as so suspicious of bronchial carcinoma as to demand full diagnostic investigation. Occasionally septic bronchopneumonia results from the presence of an *aspirated foreign body* in the trachea or in a main bronchus, especially in children. Bronchopneumonia of similar type occurs in cases of *immersion in contaminated water*, a common sequel of this being suppuration and sometimes gangrene. Another cause

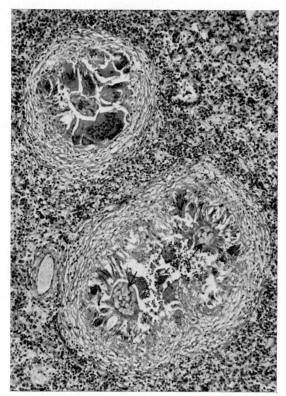

Fig. 15.28.—Aspiration bronchopneumonia, showing inhaled lentil-starch grains (arrows), with granulomatous foreign-body giant-cell reaction. × 72.

is *inhalation of vomited material*, e.g. following alcoholic intoxication or anaesthesia.

In suppurative bronchopneumonia the consolidation occurs in patches which run together, and these afterwards undergo suppurative softening. A portion of the lung may thus come to be riddled with small abscesses, whilst a considerable amount of general pneumonic consolidation may be found between. The abscesses form most frequently in the substance of the lower lobes, though they may reach the surface and infect the pleura. In contrast, pyaemic abscesses are situated chiefly under the pleura.

Lipid pneumonia

This variety of aspiration pneumonia results from the inhalation of oil instilled into the nose as medicated drops, but infants and children may aspirate cod liver oil given by mouth. There may be considerable accumulation of oil in the posterior and basal parts of the lungs especially on the right side. Liquid paraffin produces little more than a macrophage response in the alveoli, vegetable oils are a little more irritant, but oils of animal origin containing much unsaturated fat may evoke a severe inflammatory and fibroblastic response and give rise to areas of firm granulomatous pneumonic consolidation.

Haematogenous pneumonia

In various *pyaemic conditions* resulting from septic invasion of peripheral veins, abscesses varying in size and number may occur in the lungs. Such abscesses were frequent in the days when surgical pyaemia was rife, but they are now much less common, and are seen mainly in such conditions as septic thrombosis of the cerebral sinuses and suppurative thrombosis of the uterine and other veins in puerperal conditions. They are wedge-shaped suppurating infarcts. Occasionally infective emboli may be derived also from ulcerative endocarditis of the tricuspid valve. In acute pyogenic infections, e.g. suppurative periostitis and osteomyelitis, there may be groups of small, often haemorrhagic abscesses in the lungs. In some very acute cases, especially those caused by the *Staphylococcus aureus*, the lesions may appear as numerous small haemorrhagic areas without any actual suppuration. In the haemorrhagic areas staphylococci may be found in enormous numbers, as plugs within the capillaries and also outside. This condition is often rapidly fatal, and at necropsy the lesions may be confined to the lungs and inconspicuous.

Pneumonic conditions may occasionally be

produced by other organisms carried by the blood stream, for example in meningococcal septicaemia; and it is possible that pneumococci sometimes reach the lungs in this way from lesions elsewhere. In typhoid fever, the bacilli may be carried to the lungs by the blood, and may there take part along with pneumococci or other organisms in causing pneumonia. In plague two types of infection occur. In the bubonic type, secondary invasion of the lungs may take place by the blood stream, whereas in the pneumonic type infection is by inhalation. The resulting pneumonia is usually accompanied by much haemorrhage and oedema, and sometimes by necrosis; the bacilli are present in large numbers.

Hypostatic pneumonia

This results from accumulation in the posterior parts of the lung of secretions which serve as a nutrient medium for pneumococci and other organisms. Infection is most often due to organisms of low virulence growing under specially favourable conditions. Hypostatic pneumonia is very common in cases of coma and also in weakly and bedridden subjects. It is frequently a terminal phenomenon in such patients. All degrees exist from a congested and oedematous condition of the lungs to true consolidation. The consolidation is most marked in the posterior parts of the lungs and gradually fades off in front, merging into oedema; it is never so complete or so well-defined as in lobar pneumonia. The microscopic appearances vary much in different cases, and also in different parts of the lungs in the same case. In some, there is chiefly catarrh, with oedema and a varying amount of haemorrhage, whilst in others the alveoli may be largely occupied by leukocytes, and occasionally even fibrin may be present. The pleura may be normal, or there may be fibrinous or serous pleurisy.

Gangrene

This condition, which is uncommon nowadays, is the result of the entrance of putrefactive organisms into the lung by one of two routes, the bronchi or the blood stream. Infection by the bronchial route may occur in various conditions, for example in cases of ulcerating carcinoma of the tongue or larynx where the putrefactive material is aspirated and from carcinoma of the oesophagus which has invaded the trachea. Gangrene occasionally complicates lobar pneumonia or bronchopneumonia. In addition to various bacteria, coarse spirochaetes and fusiform bacilli may be present, such as are common in lesions of the mouth or throat.

Influenza

Epidemiology. Influenza occurs endemically in this country, but about every three years it assumes epidemic form, and about every forty years a major epidemic or worldwide pandemic appears as in the great pandemic of 1918, when a large percentage of the world's population of all ages was affected. Influenza is an acute virus infection of which two chief strains, A and B, have been distinguished, but there are other serological variants, the occurrence of which renders the problem of protective immunisation very difficult and complicated. Infection is probably spread by droplets and infected secretions reaching the respiratory tract of susceptible subjects.

Structural changes. The lesions of the respiratory passages in influenza merit special notice because of their variable and sometimes serious nature. Commonly the whole tract is invaded, and an outstanding feature is the implication of the terminal bronchioles to a degree which is not observed in any other disease in adults. It has been shown by the fluorescent antibody technique that influenza virus attacks not only the bronchial epithelium but also the lining of lung alveoli. The trachea and large bronchi usually show signs of intense inflammation, which may be accompanied by haemorrhage and occasionally in very severe types also by some superficial necrosis of the mucosa and fibrinous exudate. There is leukopenia, sometimes severe, and neutrophil polymorphs are absent from the lesion. In the majority of cases, the disease progresses no further, but during epidemics when the virulence of the virus may have become enhanced, extension of the disease to the bronchioles and lung parenchyma becomes increasingly frequent.

When bronchiolitis occurs, there is intense inflammation in the alveoli around the walls of the bronchioles, often accompanied by fibrinous exudate and haemorrhages (Fig. 15.29). Exten-

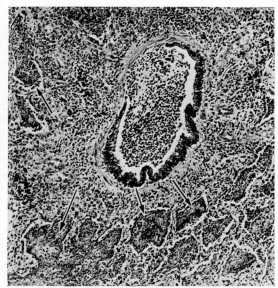

FIG. 15.29.—Influenzal bronchopneumonia, showing acute bronchiolitis and peribronchiolitis.

Note the fibrinous exudate in the air vesicles around bronchiole (e.g. arrows). × 60.

sion of the inflammation occurs also by way of the alveolar ducts to the alveoli beyond, i.e. an early bronchopneumonia is present. The walls of the bronchioles also show marked interstitial inflammation—peribronchiolitis; in fact this is a prominent feature in influenza and is of importance as it often leads to permanent fibrosis.

In susceptible experimental animals influenza virus may produce consolidation of the lung without superimposed bacterial infection, and during epidemics when the virulence of the virus is enhanced, this may happen also in man. But the lowering of the resistance of the respiratory tract to secondary bacterial invasion is a striking and characteristic feature and the development of pneumonia is usually associated with the presence of *Haemophilus influenzae, Strep. pneumoniae, Strep. pyogenes* or *Staph. aureus.* Haemophilus organisms are usually present in the exudate in the bronchi, and may be seen invading their walls, but the infection is commonly mixed. *Staph. aureus* gives rise to an especially severe and often fatal pneumonia. The areas of consolidation vary greatly in size; sometimes they are massive and confluent and may exhibit patches of necrosis (Fig. 15.30). Severe influenzal pneumonia is characterised by a peculiar violaceous cyanosis, a grave prognostic sign. Pleurisy is usually present, especially when the condition is advanced. In uncomplicated influenza there is no polymorph leukocytosis, and later the paucity of these cells in the pneumonic lesions, even in the presence of pyogenic micro-organisms, suggests a pronounced depression of the marrow. No doubt this increases the tendency to incomplete resolution.

Complications. Occasionally pneumonia of lobar distribution may be superadded and may prove fatal before there is much consolidation, the fatal parenchymal lesion consisting of dilatation of alveolar ducts and outpouring of fluid leading to the formation of hyaline membranes on their walls and in the alveoli. Such lesions are produced by the virus of influenza rather than by secondary bacterial invasion. We have seen also cases where there was a very intense inflam-

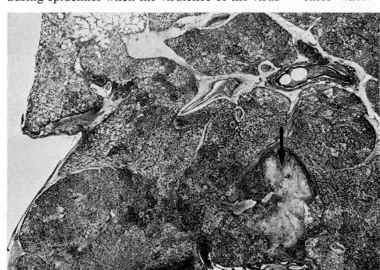

FIG. 15.30.—Influenzal bronchopneumonia.

There is widespread consolidation, in places confluent, and an area of necrosis of the lung tissue is seen (arrow). (From a child who died of epidemic influenza.) × 9.

matory oedema with haemorrhage, but comparatively little consolidation, and where *Strep. pyogenes* was abundant in the fluid exudate. Infection of the influenzal lung by *Staph. aureus* may lead to widespread patchy necrosis and haemorrhage, the lesions resembling multiple septic infarcts; this complication is one of the most serious and has a high fatality rate. It was the chief cause of death in Great Britain in the 1957 pandemic. The patchy pneumonic consolidation is occasionally followed by suppuration, usually in multiple foci, and the organisms may reach the pleura and give rise to an empyema. Sometimes abscesses are chronic and lead to much local fibrosis. Apart from suppuration, however, interstitial fibrosis is a comparatively common sequel of influenzal pneumonia. In fact in some cases at an early stage acute interstitial inflammation is a marked lesion, and this is followed by increase of the connective tissue. Organisation of the exudate in the bronchioles may occur and lead to their obliteration with permanent collapse and fibrosis of the lung tissue beyond. Some small bronchi, probably as a result of damage to their muscle, undergo dilatation and thus permanent bronchiectasis may result. Occasionally in the acute stages of influenza, septicaemia due to pneumococci or streptococci may appear and prove rapidly fatal, as was seen in the severe epidemic in 1918. Death may be caused by the severity of the pulmonary lesions or by septicaemia and while bronchopneumonia may resolve, recovery is often prolonged, with some residual fibrosis.

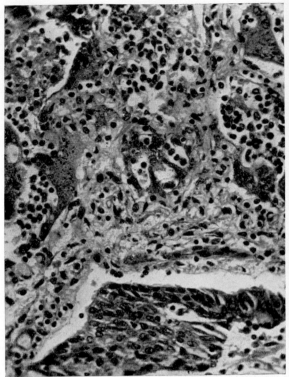

Fig. 15.31.—Giant-cell pneumonia in measles. Note the marked hyperplasia of the bronchiolar epithelium and the numerous giant cells in the alveoli with acidophil cytoplasmic inclusions. × 240.

Other types of pneumonia

Giant-cell pneumonia. In cases of measles dying early in the disease the epithelium of the bronchioles may be hyperplastic and contain intracytoplasmic inclusion bodies (Fig. 15.31). The alveoli may show many giant cells derived from the lining epithelium by fusion, and they, too, contain inclusion bodies. There is good evidence that this form of giant-cell pneumonia is due to the measles virus, and that it represents an altered immune response to the virus, in which the titre of serum antibody remains low or nil. In cases developing a secondary bacterial pneumonia the characteristic changes are lost.

Psittacosis and Ornithosis. Infection with various species of micro-organisms of the genus *Miyagawanella* (sometimes termed *Bedsonia*) is very common in various species of birds, and can be transmitted to man. When contracted from members of the parrot family, including budgerigars, the condition is termed *psittacosis*, while *ornithosis* is used for infection spread to man from birds of other families.

The organisms were formerly classed as viruses because of their small size and their intracellular growth: however, they contain both RNA and DNA, a bacterial type of cell wall, and they are susceptible to antibiotics, particularly tetracycline: they are now classed with the *Rickettsiae*. Similar organisms are responsible for lymphogranuloma inguinale and trachoma (p. 154).

The disease in man is a generalised infection, but the most characteristic feature is a patchy pneumonia. It resembles grossly influenzal bronchopneumonia, and there is a leukopenia and the cellular infiltrate is largely of mononuclear cell type, as in virus pneumonias. There may also be capillary thromboses.

Ornithosis may be contracted from turkeys in N. Africa, from fulmar petrels in the Faroes, and the pigeons in Trafalgar Square have been shown to harbour *Miyagawanella*, although of a type of low virulence to man. Antibodies occur in the serum of bird-handlers who give no history suggestive of the disease.

Primary atypical pneumonia. This form of pneumonia is poorly defined. Some cases are caused by *Rickettsia burnetii*—Q fever, but the majority are associated with Eaton's agent, a member of the pleuro-pneumonia (PPLO) group, now classified as *Mycoplasma pneumoniae*, which has been demonstrated within the bronchial epithelium by the fluorescent antibody technique (p. 80). The lesions consist of a low-grade inflammation of focal character centred on the bronchioles, the walls of which are thickened by interstitial mononuclear infiltration, while the lumina contain mucopurulent material. In some alveoli there is fibrinous exudate tending to undergo organisation, in others oedema and haemorrhage. The morbid anatomy resembles that of influenzal pneumonia; polymorphs are scanty in the lesions but a mild leukocytosis may be found. The onset is usually gradual and the mortality is low but resolution is often somewhat delayed. A remarkable feature of the disease is the appearance in the patient's serum of agglutinins against *Streptococcus MG* and of cold haemagglutinins for red cells, which reach a peak about 21 days after onset but fall rapidly thereafter.

Pneumocystis carinii **pneumonia.** Premature and weakly infants may develop an atypical pneumonia of insidious onset, with trivial physical signs but massive patchy consolidation which accentuates the lobular pattern of the lungs. The alveoli are filled with a rather acellular non-fibrinous exudate of characteristically honeycomb appearance (Fig. 15.32), within which are small intensely staining granules thought by some to be a protozoal parasite,

Pneumocystis carinii, but by others to be a saccharomycete. Sometimes the interstitial tissue of the lung is extensively infiltrated with plasma cells but in a substantial proportion this feature has been absent, particularly in cases attributable to congenital immunodeficiencies. The disease occurs also as an "opportunistic infection" in patients with an immunological deficiency due to neoplasia of the reticulo-endothelial system or to the administration of cytotoxic or immunosuppressive drugs as in renal allotransplantation (p. 154).

Fungal diseases of the lungs are dealt with on p. 368. It should be noted that various fungi give rise to "opportunistic infections", including bronchopneumonia.

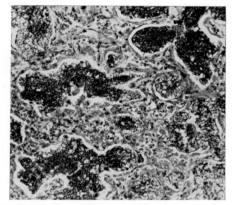

Fig. 15.32.—Pneumocystis pneumonia. × 160
(Dr. T. Bird.)

Chronic Infections

Tuberculosis

General considerations

The general features of tuberculosis have already been described (pp. 141–7), and it has been pointed out that the causal organism, *Mycobacterium tuberculosis*, has not been shown to produce any agent which is significantly toxic to normal cells and tissues. A remarkable feature about tuberculous infection is the high degree of delayed hypersensitivity to tuberculoprotein which accompanies it. Very likely the delayed hypersensitivity reaction between host cells and mycobacteria or their products is responsible for most if not all of the structural changes of tuberculosis. The basic features of delayed hypersensitivity reactions, a knowledge of which is essential to the full understanding of this account, have been given on pp. 106–9.

In this country, the lungs are more often

affected by tuberculosis than any other organ, partly because inhalation is now the commonest mode of infection, but also because lung tissue provides a favourable environment for growth of the organism.

Pulmonary tuberculous lesions present a wide diversity of appearance and behaviour. In communities with a high infection rate, tuberculosis is usually contracted during infancy and childhood, and the resulting primary lesions may either heal or prove fatal. Subsequent infection may occur in adult life, giving rise to *re-infection tuberculosis*, which may either heal or produce chronic pulmonary disease. In communities with a low rate of tuberculous infection, lesions of the primary type may occur in adults, and it is thus no longer appropriate to refer to primary and re-infection tuberculosis as the childhood and adult types respectively.

Broadly speaking, the morbidity and mortality

rates of tuberculosis reflect the general health of the community. Overcrowding, malnutrition and poor hygiene all predispose to a high rate of the disease. The course of pulmonary tuberculosis varies greatly. The most favourable outcome is healing of the lesion at an early stage. Failing this, the disease may become chronic; spontaneous arrest may occur at any stage, but equally the infection may flare up, become relatively acute and severe, and cause death from extensive lung lesions or generalised

infection in childhood has continued to fall, and is now very low.

Primary pulmonary tuberculosis

The early primary lesion is now seldom available for histological examination. However, when tuberculosis was much commoner in this and other European countries, primary infection was frequently observed as an incidental post-

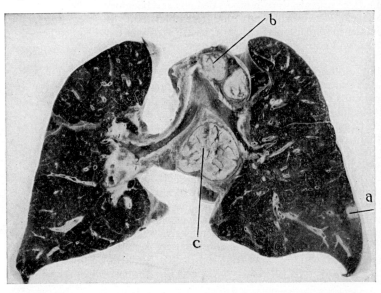

FIG. 15.33.—Lung of child with (*a*) primary lesion in right lower lobe, and (*b*) and (*c*) enlarged caseous tracheobronchial nodes in relation to the lesion. (J. W. S. B.)

dissemination. The factors determining these courses have already been considered on pp. 141–7. Briefly, factors predisposing to an unfavourable course are a heavy infecting dose of *M. tuberculosis*, infection at an early age, i.e. in infancy or early childhood, malnutrition, or chronic debilitating disease.

In this country, as elsewhere in W. Europe and in N. America, the general conditions of living have improved so greatly during the last century that the incidence and mortality rates of tuberculosis are now low. In particular, childhood infections are greatly diminished. In the city of Glasgow, for example, the rate of positive reactors to tuberculin skin tests carried out on 13-year-old school children had by 1953 fallen to 40 per cent, and by 1964 to 16·5 per cent, indicating a decreasing rate of primary infection in childhood. Subsequently, the percentage of positive reactors has increased as a result of mass BCG immunisation in infancy, but there is every reason to believe that the rate of natural

mortem finding in children dying from various other causes. The primary lesion, also termed the *Ghon focus*, is usually single; it consists of a caseating nodule of 1 cm. or so diameter, but sometimes larger, and situated close beneath the pleural surface in any part of any of the lobes (Figs. 15.33, 15.34). Microscopic examination of the early Ghon focus shows central caseation and peripheral tubercles; the lesion enlarges by spread of mycobacteria, which are taken up and carried by macrophages, so that tubercles form in the adjacent lung tissue, replacing alveolar walls and filling air spaces, and as they enlarge these peripheral tubercles become incorporated in the central caseous area.

In most instances, the primary infection is overcome, the Ghon focus undergoing healing: if small, it may be completely replaced by fibrous tissue, but if larger, the caseous centre usually persists and is converted into a hard calcified nodule, often partly ossified (Fig. 15.35), enclosed in fibrous tissue: such a healed lesion is readily visible on X-rays. Very commonly, lymphatic spread of *M. tuberculosis* takes place in the primary infection; tubercles are frequently seen along the line of the lymphatics between the Ghon focus and the hilar lymph nodes, and

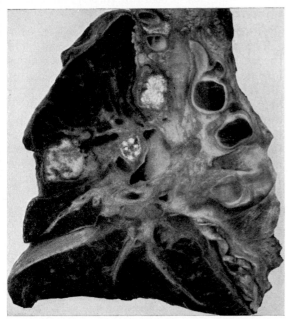

FIG. 15.34.—Primary lung focus of tuberculosis, showing well marked calcification of the sub-pleural lesion and of the tracheo-bronchial lymph nodes. × 1.

both the tracheobronchial and adjacent mediastinal nodes become extensively involved (Fig. 15.33). Tubercles are found in large numbers in these nodes and undergo caseation and coalesce, finally converting the nodes into large caseous masses with marginal tubercle follicles. The combination of the Ghon focus and tuberculous lymphadenitis is termed the *primary complex*. At this stage, healing is also the usual outcome, and, like the Ghon focus, the affected lymph nodes eventually may become heavily calcified (Fig. 15.34), but are rarely ossified.

Healing of the primary lesion with a favourable outcome is not invariable and, depending on the various factors which have already been stated above, the disease may progress to *tuberculous bronchopneumonia*, or to *blood-borne spread* (pp. 366–7) which gives rise to innumerable disseminated lesions in various organs (generalised miliary tuberculosis), to smaller numbers of disseminated foci, or to one or two *metastatic foci*.

Acute tuberculous bronchopneumonia can

develop from the primary infection by aspiration of infected caseous material throughout the bronchial tree, either from the Ghon focus or, more commonly, from caseous lymph nodes at the hilum or in the mediastinum (Fig. 15.36). In the former case, the Ghon focus continues to enlarge until eventually it incorporates a bronchus in the caseous process. Caseous material is then discharged into the lumen from which it may be aspirated through adjacent and more distant parts of the bronchial tree. Bronchial dissemination results similarly when a caseating lesion in the hilar or mediastinal lymph nodes ulcerates into a major bronchus. The resulting tuberculous bronchopneumonia is relatively acute, and usually affects both lungs, although one is often involved to a greater extent than the other. The lung tissue is studded with numerous small pneumonic patches, which are arranged in groups or clusters round the terminal bronchi. These patches are yellowish in the centre and are comparatively firm. Large consolidated

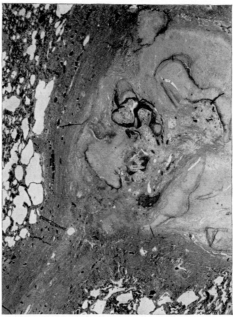

FIG. 15.35.—Healed Ghon focus, showing dense fibrous encapsulation, calcification and central ossification. × 15.

areas may be formed by their confluence. Microscopic examination of the lesions shows caseation of a small central bronchus and of the adjacent lung tissue (Fig. 15.37). Further out, inflammatory reaction with fibrinous exudation is seen within the alveoli, with numerous rounded macrophages, which often contain fatty globules. The tubercle bacilli, after reaching a bronchiole, thus produce bronchopneumonic consolidation followed by caseation.

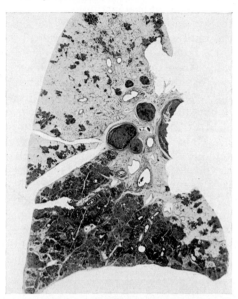

FIG. 15.36.—Tuberculous bronchopneumonia in a child. One of the caseous hilar lymph nodes has eroded a bronchus, leading to tuberculous bronchopneumonia, mainly in the lower lobe. × ⅘.

There may be considerable fibrinous exudate in and around the lesions, which advance too rapidly for tubercle formation or the development of granulation or fibrous tissue. As the condition progresses, the lesions may become confluent in the lower parts of the lungs, where they are most numerous. The enlarging caseous patches may also soften and discharge into bronchi, with dissemination of more mycobacteria and aggravation of the condition. The cavities resulting from discharge of caseous material have ragged caseating walls without surrounding fibrosis, and in these respects they contrast to the smooth fibrous walls of chronic tuberculous cavities (p. 364). Tuberculous bronchopneumonia with cavity formation is termed *acute phthisis*. Tuberculous pleurisy usually develops in tuberculous bronchopneumonia, and in acute phthisis a small cavity opening into a bronchus may rupture also into the pleura, resulting in pneumothorax.

Extensive tuberculous bronchopneumonia is associated with fever, severe debility and rapid weight loss. Unless treated early and effectively, it is rapidly fatal.

As stated below, acute tuberculous bronchopneumonia can occur also in patients with re-infection pulmonary tuberculosis (Fig. 15.38).

Re-infection (post-primary or chronic) pulmonary tuberculosis

The individual who has experienced and successfully overcome a primary tuberculous infection, or who has been immunised against *M. tuberculosis*, has developed a partial resistance, and should re-infection occur, the resulting disease is quite different from the primary infection. By far the commonest site of the re-infection lesion is the apex of the lung, or rather a short distance below the extreme apex (Fig. 15.39), the right lung being the more frequently affected: the predilection for the apical region may be attributable to the relatively low venous pressure there, and the rarity of the development of pulmonary tuberculosis in patients with mitral stenosis, despite the former frequency of both conditions, suggests that venous congestion is protective against pulmonary tuberculosis. It is of interest that, in four-legged mammals, the lesion is not at the apex, but in the parts of the

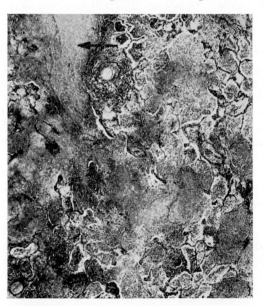

FIG. 15.37.—Section of lung in acute tuberculous bronchopneumonia.

A terminal bronchiole (arrow) is seen opening into its ducts and alveoli, the walls of which are identified by the persisting elastic tissue. The bronchiole and alveoli show diffuse caseation. × 26.

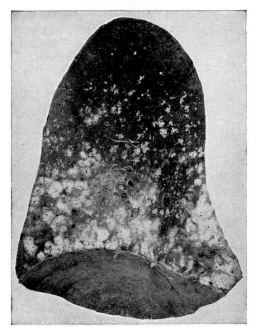

FIG. 15.38.—Tuberculous bronchopneumonia. Note the particularly severe involvement of the lower part of the lobe. This arose in an adult with re-infection tuberculosis in the upper lobes (not shown in photograph).

lungs which are uppermost in the standing posture. The point is of some interest, for sub-apical predilection in man suggests that tubercle bacilli inhaled into other parts of the lungs are destroyed or rejected, and it is noteworthy that in some cases, lesions develop sub-apically in both lungs.

Structural changes. The re-infection lesion results from *M. tuberculosis* gaining a foothold and proliferating, probably in the wall of a bronchiole or of an alveolus. The usual re-action takes place, with formation of tubercle

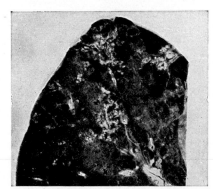

FIG. 15.39.—Chronic tuberculosis of apex of lung. Note the collections of grey tubercles without cavity formation. × $\frac{4}{5}$.

follicles, and the lesion enlarges by formation of new tubercles at the margin and in the adjacent lung tissue. The infection spreads by the lymphatics, but, as a result of the previous primary infection a state of delayed hypersensitivity exists from the onset, and this may explain why lymphatic spread is not usually extensive (p. 145), tubercles appearing mainly in the lung tissue below the sub-apical lesion, and in the peribronchial fibrous tissue. The hilar lymph nodes are not affected, or only slightly involved with development of a few

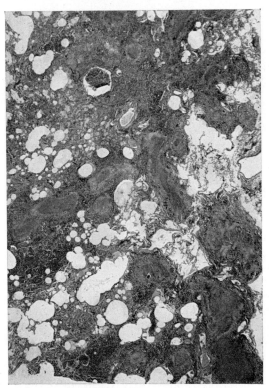

FIG. 15.40.—Chronic pulmonary tuberculosis, showing well-developed conglomerate tubercles.

tubercles in them. The developing reinfection lesion thus comes to consist of a cluster of follicles which, as they enlarge and caseate, tend to become confluent, producing one or more larger lesions. Because of the partial state of immunity which exists, progress of the lesions is slow, the tubercles are well-developed (Fig. 15.41) and there is conspicuous formation of fibrous tissue at their periphery (Fig. 15.40). The caseous material is yellowish, or sometimes greyish due to inclusion of carbon pigment, which is often abundant in the fibrous tissue. If healing does not now occur, some of the nodules will spread to involve the wall of a bronchus in caseous necrosis and blockage of the lumen follows. The lesion may become encapsulated by fibrous tissue or the caseous material may be slowly discharged along the bronchus leaving a small cavity (Fig. 15.42). Spread by the bronchi then occurs, but provided that the number of mycobacteria

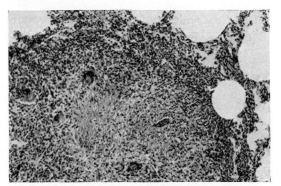

Fig. 15.41.—Chronic pulmonary tuberculosis, showing a nodule composed of several follicles, sharply demarcated from the surrounding tissue. × 90.

discharged remains small and resistance is maintained, development of new tubercles is slow and, like lymphatic spread, occurs mainly in the adjacent part of the lung, i.e. a localised form of tuberculous bronchopneumonia. The resulting tubercles are well-formed and are distinguishable from the lesions arising by lymphatic spread mainly by their lobular or segmental distribution. Bronchial spread to the upper parts of other lobes, and to the other lung, may, however, occur, and chronic pulmonary tuberculosis is frequently bilateral.

Variations and complications. Cavitation, as described above, may occur in a number of lesions, the condition then being termed *chronic phthisis* (chronic pulmonary tuberculosis with cavitation) (Fig. 15.43). The cavities may coalesce and can become very large. Even with cavitation, the tuberculous lesions usually enlarge slowly; they are accompanied by considerable overgrowth of fibrous tissue, not only around the cavities (Fig. 15.44), but also in a diffusely spreading manner. In this way, the lung shrinks and bronchiectasis may be superadded. In fact, bronchiectatic cavities with a red vascular lining are often found along with tuberculous cavities whose walls are covered with caseous material. Ultimately, a cavity may

become very large, and may occupy a considerable portion of the upper lobe. The walls of the chronic cavities are somewhat irregular and contain raised bands, which represent obliterated blood vessels and other structures which have more resistance than the rest of the tissue. In very chronic cases the lining of cavities may be comparatively smooth, but there is usually adherent caseous material, or there may be debris with sometimes an admixture of blood. The contents of the cavities have as a rule no putrid odour, and the organisms present along with the tubercle bacilli are chiefly pyogenic cocci; they aid the ulcerative process, while their toxins play a part in increasing the cachexia. The pulmonary vessels usually become obliterated by endarteritis before the ulcerative process reaches their lumina, but if not, the wall of an artery may be weakened when the vessel still contains blood, and an aneurysm may result. A pulmonary aneurysm may be 5–15 mm. in diameter and give rise to serious, sometimes fatal haemorrhage by its rupture.

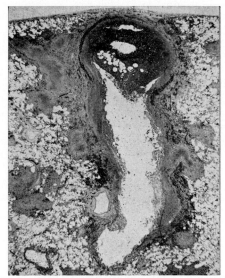

Fig. 15.42.—Chronic phthisis, showing the formation of a cavity by discharge of caseous material into a peripheral bronchus. × 4.

In some cases, the spread of the disease is so slow and is accompanied by so much fibrosis, that the tuberculous nature of the lesion may largely be obscured. The disease then appears as a chronic fibrosis with much pigmentation, cavity formation and also bronchiectasis. This type of tuberculosis is seen also in coal miners as *progressive massive fibrosis*, in which the cavities continue to enlarge without tubercle formation (p. 371).

If at any time there should occur a rapid diffusion of large numbers of bacilli by the air passages, as may happen when a caseous focus suddenly discharges into a bronchus, the patient's resistance may be overcome and acute rapidly spreading tuberculous bronchopneumonia supervene. It is not uncommon to find the latter in the lower parts of the lungs, whilst chronic cavity formation is present in the upper lobes. Such an event is prone to occur if the patient with chronic phthisis is debilitated by intercurrent disease, e.g. influenza, diabetes, etc., or by overwork and unfavourable environmental conditions.

In patients dying from chronic pulmonary tuberculosis, and particularly when there has been breakdown of resistance with extensive bronchopneumonia, blood dissemination with acute miliary tuberculosis may occur, but this is much less common than in primary tuberculosis in young children.

In phthisis, both acute and chronic, *tuberculous ulcers* often develop in the intestines from infection by bacilli in swallowed sputum. Tuberculosis of the larynx (p. 331), likewise produced by direct infection from the sputum, is

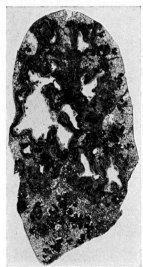

FIG. 15.43.—Apex of lung showing multiple chronic tuberculous cavities with fibrous walls. × ½.

a serious and not infrequent complication. *Secondary amyloidosis* is common (p. 195).

Clinical features. During the development of tuberculous lesions in the lungs, bloodstained sputum or more frank haemoptysis is not uncommon; in fact, it is often the earliest sign of the disease. It is apparently due to erosion of some of the smaller vessels, and is to be distinguished from the larger, sometimes fatal haemorrhage from

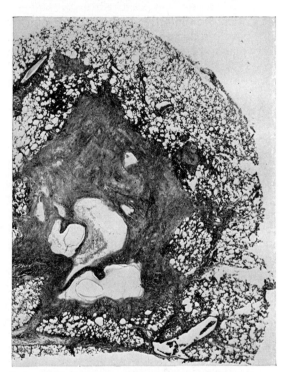

FIG. 15.44.—Apical reinfection tuberculosis in an adolescent. Two small cavities are surrounded by dense fibrosis; at the periphery are a few chronic tubercles. × 3·5.

an artery or aneurysm within a cavity in the later stage of the disease (p. 287). Another frequent early manifestation of pulmonary tuberculosis is serous effusion into a pleural sac.

Chronic pulmonary tuberculosis may progress to an advanced stage with little or no clinical illness, but more commonly it is accompanied by cough, haemoptysis, loss of appetite and weight, and low-grade fever. When advanced, it gives rise to severe emaciation, night sweats, some secondary anaemia and irregular fever. These features are often attributable in part to secondary pyogenic infection of tuberculous cavities, although the delayed hypersensitivity reaction to the tubercle bacilli is, without doubt, an important factor in their production.

The effects of specific chemotherapy. The above account of pulmonary tuberculosis refers essentially to the disease as it occurs when unmodified by chemotherapy. We have previously (p. 147) described the changes brought about in tuberculous lesions in general by streptomycin alone and in combination with *p*-amino-salicylic acid and isoniazid. In pulmonary tuberculosis combined therapy is imperative in order to render the patient non-infective and to reduce quickly the risk of producing antibiotic-resistant strains. If adequately carried out in the early stages of the apical lesion, chemotherapy leads to rapid resolution and healing with minimal fibrosis. In excavated lesions the caseous lining disappears and is replaced by a layer of vascular granulation tissue which in turn is converted to a thin smooth fibrous layer over which an epithelial lining may ultimately grow leaving a persistent cavity which may or may not openly communicate with a bronchus. The epithelial lining is rarely complete except in very small lesions. Small fibrocaseous lesions may be almost completely absorbed or, if larger, may become hyalinised and acellular with a thin fibrous capsule. In favourable cases even actively caseating bronchopneumonic lesions may cease to progress, the caseous material becoming liquefied and absorbed or discharged, and the cavities, walled off by granulation tissue which eventually becomes fibrosed, are re-lined to some extent by epithelium. A notable feature is the lack of the dense fibrosis which characterises healing under natural conditions, and healing of open cavities, i.e. with a persistent residual lumen, is a common result of modern therapy which can then be completed by surgical resection. Patches of active disease may however persist for long periods and tubercle bacilli may be isolated from such resected cavities despite long-continued chemotherapy so that it is advisable to consider the disease process to be arrested rather than cured by specific therapy. The naked-eye appearance of the treated lesions is therefore a rather unreliable guide to the bacteriological state.

Haematogenous tuberculosis

(a) **Generalised miliary tuberculosis.** The pulmonary lesions of this condition are part of an acute generalised tuberculosis, which occurs when a considerable number of mycobacteria gain entrace to the blood stream. The ways by which this is brought about have already been considered (p. 146). In miliary tuberculosis the

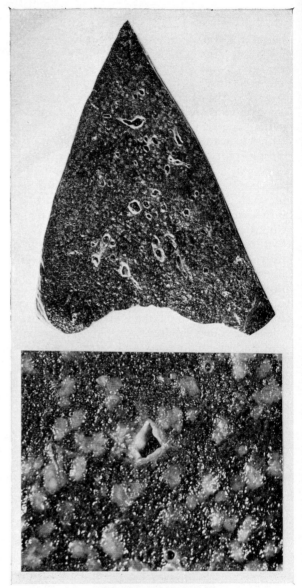

FIG. 15.45.—Acute miliary tuberculosis of lung. Above, lower lobe, $\times \frac{3}{4}$; below, part of same specimen. $\times 5$.

lesions in the lungs are usually more numerous than in any other organ. The lesions are scattered equally in both lungs and are usually numerous small greyish tubercles (Fig. 15.45), though sometimes they are larger and yellowish. They may be so small as to be invisible to the naked eye or may be 1–3 mm. in diameter. They are often more numerous and rather larger in the upper lobes than in the lower.

Microscopically, the lesion is found to consist

of minute tubercles in the interstitial tissue of the lungs, i.e. in the peribronchial connective tissue and septa (Fig. 15.46), and also in the alveolar walls. Each tubercle starts from a capillary and the proliferation is primarily interstitial, but it is soon followed by consolidation in a ring of air vesicles. Necrosis then occurs in the centre of the areas. In very acute cases the tubercle follicles are poorly formed and giant cells are virtually absent; occasionally the lesion is less acute, and the nodules are less numerous, larger, with yellow caseous centres, and are clearly derived from the fusion of several typical

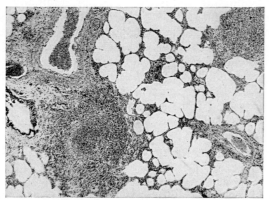

FIG. 15.46.—Section of lung in acute miliary tuberculosis, showing two small well-circumscribed nodules. × 40.

follicles with giant cells. Such a condition presumably results when a smaller number of mycobacteria gain access to the blood stream. In acute miliary tuberculosis, there is no breaking down of the lesions, and *M. tuberculosis* is rarely found in the sputum.

The prognosis in miliary tuberculosis has been greatly improved with the advent of specific therapy, the lesions readily undergoing healing with minimal fibrosis (p. 146).

(b) Localised metastatic tuberculosis. In tuberculous infections, a few tubercle bacilli sometimes gain access to the blood stream and are carried to distant parts, where they give rise to local lesions in the bones, kidney, epididymis, fallopian tube, or various other organs. Secondary tuberculosis in the lung may also be produced in this way, but the lesions cannot readily be distinguished from those resulting from inhalation and local spread.

The pleurae in pulmonary tuberculosis

In tuberculosis of the lungs the pleural cavities are affected in various ways. At a very early stage of localised lung disease tubercles may form in the visceral pleura, and this may be followed by an extensive effusion into the affected pleural sac. Tuberculosis is a frequent cause of the apparently idiopathic pleurisy of young adults. The fluid is usually clear and the cells in it are scanty and mainly lymphocytes. A large proportion of desquamated mesothelial cells, as is seen in the centrifuged deposit of the serous transudate of cardiac failure, strongly contra-indicates tuberculosis. In many cases tubercle bacilli cannot be found. Sometimes the exudate is serofibrinous and there may be some admixture of blood. The lesion usually resolves and the fluid is absorbed, leaving only scanty adhesions to mark its previous existence.

In chronic tuberculous lung lesions there is thickening and adhesion of the overlying pleural layers, and in longstanding cases this may be marked. Owing to such adhesions, perforation of an underlying cavity into the pleural sac is uncommon; but in acute phthisis a necrotic patch in the lung may rapidly involve the pleura and cause pneumothorax, which is usually accompanied by inflammation and suppuration—pyopneumothorax. Apart from actual perforation, pyogenic organisms occasionally invade the pleural cavity and give rise to an empyema. Occasionally tubercle bacilli gain access to the cavity from a tuberculous rib or vertebra, and there may then be fibrinous exudation, followed by an eruption of tubercles of considerable size on both layers. Great thickening of the pleural layers may result, with a collection of caseous material between them—that is, chronic tuberculous pleurisy, which may be followed by calcification (Fig. 15.47).

Sarcoidosis

The lungs are a common site of sarcoidosis. Lesions resembling miliary tubercles are widely scattered throughout both lungs, and produce on radiological examination a typical "snow-storm" appearance. There is usually also bilateral hilar lymphadenopathy. Often these lesions regress spontaneously, but they may undergo fibrosis and much destruction of lung

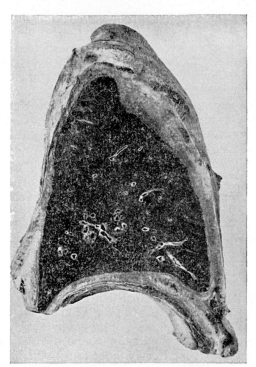

Fig. 15.47.—Chronic tuberculous pleurisy, showing enormous thickening of pleural layers with caseous material between. × $\frac{3}{5}$.

tissue, especially in the upper lobes, may follow, producing the appearances of "honeycomb lung". Other aspects of sarcoidosis and the microscopic features of the sarcoid granuloma have already been considered (p. 152).

Syphilis

In *congenital* syphilis, an interstitial pneumonia occurs mainly in the peribronchial and perivascular regions, but it may involve large areas, so that practically the whole pulmonary tissue is affected. The lungs are pale and tough and contain comparatively little air; the term *pneumonia alba* has been applied. The alveoli are small and lined by a cubical type of epithelium, whilst the small bronchi undergo dilatation. The diffuse nature of these lesions is related to the large number of treponemata in the pulmonary tissue. Gummas also may be present, and occasionally these reach a considerable size.

In *acquired* syphilis, gummas in the lungs are rare.

Fungal infections

Pulmonary aspergillosis

The spores of *Aspergillus fumigatus* are widespread in the environment, and the organism is commonly found in sputum cultures. It gives rise to three more or less distinct types of lung disease in man. *Firstly*, atopic subjects may develop reaginic antibody to antigenic constituents of *Aspergillus*, and as a result suffer from attacks of bronchial asthma on heavy exposure to the spores. *Secondly*, on exposure to *Aspergillus* some patients with asthma develop also precipitating antibodies, and in addition to asthma suffer from attacks resembling "farmer's lung", with ill-defined pulmonary consolidation, fever, and often blood eosinophilia (p. 376). Such attacks are probably due to an Arthus-type reaction in which *Aspergillus* spores are inhaled and the antigens react with precipitating antibody: it appears that this condition is triggered off by an atopic reaction to *Aspergillus*, and skin tests show a biphasic result, an immediate (atopic) reaction being followed by an Arthus-type reaction.

Thirdly, *A. fumigatus* can colonise tuberculous or bronchiectatic cavities in the lung, producing a rounded mass of fungus (*mycetoma*) with a characteristic X-ray appearance. There are usually high serum levels of precipitins to various *Aspergillus* antigens, but unless there is also atopic hypersensitivity skin tests are usually negative.

Candidiasis

Candida albicans is a yeast-like fungus and is a normal commensal in the throat and nasopharynx, where it can give rise to the lesion of *thrush* (p. 471). It is also commonly present in the bronchi in chronic bronchitis and bronchiectasis, and in tuberculous cavities in the lungs. While commonly regarded as saprophytic in these latter situations, it can probably induce reaginic antibodies and cause asthma in atopic individuals. It may also assume more direct pathogenicity, producing bronchopneumonia and rarely pyaemic candidiasis, in patients with debilitating diseases or an immunological deficiency.

Pulmonary fibrosis

This is characterised by an overgrowth of the connective tissue of the lungs, especially in the situations where it is normally most abundant, namely, around the bronchi and blood vessels, along the interlobular septa, and in the deep layers of the pleura. In the fibrosis following organisation, the alveoli become compressed and many of them entirely disappear (Fig. 15.23, p. 351), while at places the epithelial cells lining them become cubical, resembling the cells in the fetal lung. Pulmonary fibrosis if extensive usually leads to obstruction to the pulmonary circulation. Thus hypertrophy of the right side of the heart often results and may be followed by cardiac failure (cor pulmonale).

Varieties and causation. Pulmonary fibrosis may result from organisation of an acute inflammation, or be chronic from the outset.

With regard to the first variety, it has already been described how in acute lobar pneumonia organisation of the exudate occasionally follows, and thus areas of diffuse fibrosis may result (p. 351). A corresponding change is sometimes seen as a sequel to ordinary bronchopneumonia, the fibrosis being usually patchy and sometimes accompanied by bronchial dilatation or centrilobular emphysema; in the influenzal type a considerable degree of fibrosis may result.

Primary chronic pulmonary fibrosis is usually due to either *inhalation of irritating particles* (pneumoconiosis), or *chronic infections, especially tuberculosis.* Two special conditions, however, deserve brief description.

Hamman–Rich syndrome. This is a severe but patchy chronic interstitial fibrosis of the lung in which progressive thickening of the alveolar walls develops from an acute oedematous and inflammatory stage without the organisation of intra-alveolar exudate. The appearance is thus quite different from that in organised pneumonia. The cause is unknown but some attribute it to a hypersensitivity reaction, others assign it to the so-called "connective tissue diseases" (p. 812). The disorder is characterised by dyspnoea as a result of severe deficiency in gaseous interchange in the lung.

Paraquat poisoning. A number of cases of acute lung disease has been observed recently to follow ingestion of paraquat (1,1'-dimethyl-4,4'-bipyridylium dichloride), which is widely used as a weed killer. Within two days, there may be severe ulceration of the mouth, and acute renal failure may develop from tubular injury: renal function usually returns, although sometimes haemodialysis is required. After several days, progressive respiratory embarrassment develops. Biopsy shows fibroblastic proliferation in the alveolar walls, and electron-microscopy suggests that this follows damage and loss of the alveolar epithelial lining. Fibroblastic reaction rapidly obliterates the alveolar spaces, and death commonly results from impaired respiratory exchange.

Pneumoconioses or Dust Diseases

These are produced by inorganic or organic particles of various kinds.

Inorganic dusts

The commonest of these are coal and stone dust; also dust in potteries and pigment factories, iron particles, etc. Lesions produced in this way were formerly frequent, but under improved hygienic conditions in industry some have become much rarer.

Classification. The principal varieties are:
1. *Anthracosis* or coal-worker's lung; 2. *Silicosis* or stone-mason's lung, also found in sandblasters and in workers in the abrasive soap industry; 3. *Asbestosis* due to inhalation of asbestos dust; 4. *Siderosis* in knife grinders, etc. and in workers in haematite mines, due to a mixture of iron and stonedust.

The general disposal of inhaled particles. The entrance of particles of dust into the alveoli is favoured by any abnormal condition of the bronchial mucosa, but it has been found that even when healthy animals are exposed to an atmosphere containing much dust, the finer particles (about 5 μ or less) gain access to the alveoli in a short time whereas coarse particles are deposited on the bronchial mucosa, from which they are swept upwards entangled in mucus, by the action of cilia. The alveolar particles are then taken up by phagocytic cells (Fig. 15.48) and are carried into the lymphatics of the lung, where they become widely distributed. They tend to accumulate in certain situations, for example, in the walls of the respiratory bronchioles, along the peribronchial lymphatics and at the junctions of the interlobular septa and the pleura. In the various positions where they are arrested they give rise to reactive changes, which vary according to the nature of the particles. The nature of the phagocytes in the lung alveoli has already been considered (p. 158).

Anthracosis

In all town dwellers there is accumulation of carbon particles in varying degree, but in coal-workers this is excessive: the whole lymphatic system of the lungs becomes impregnated and the lungs come to be almost uniformly

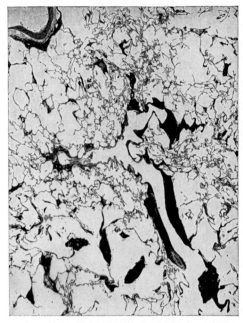

Fig. 15.49.—Coal-worker's pneumoconiosis. Focal dust emphysema showing the localisation of dust accumulation in the walls of the second order of respiratory bronchioles. × 7.

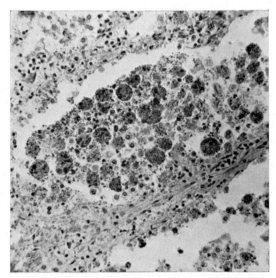

Fig. 15.48.—Silicosis, early active stage of development, showing accumulation of dust within phagocytic cells in lung alveoli. × 190.

black. The effects of anthracosis are now recognised to be more serious than was formerly believed. The work of the M.R.C. Pneumoconiosis Research Unit has made it clear that the liability of coal-miners in different mines to pneumoconiosis is directly proportional to the concentration of air-borne dust rather than to qualitative differences in its composition. The important work of Gough and his associates in Cardiff showed that the lesions of anthracosis are at first essentially focal. Inhaled coal dust tends to accumulate within phagocytes, especially at the divisions of the respiratory bronchioles and adjacent alveoli and the smooth muscle of the bronchiole atrophies; delicate fibrosis follows. Later the lesions become condensed and shrunken, acquiring a somewhat stellate outline (Fig. 15.51). This probably corresponds

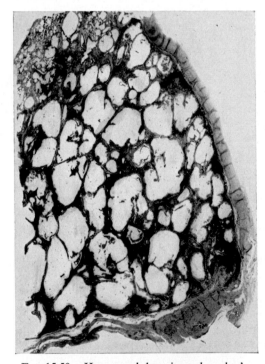

Fig. 15.50.—Honeycomb lung in coal-worker's pneumoconiosis. × 1.

to the radiological stage of "dust reticulation". The respiratory bronchioles, especially of the second order, become progressively dilated and the spaces thus formed constitute a very characteristic *focal dust emphysema* (Fig. 15.49), which has already been described (p. 345).

derived from dilated respiratory bronchioles. The changes may produce a "honeycomb lung" appearance (Fig. 15.50). Chronic bronchitis and constriction of a large bronchus by massive fibrosis (see below) may be contributory causes. Micro-incineration shows that the lesions of dust

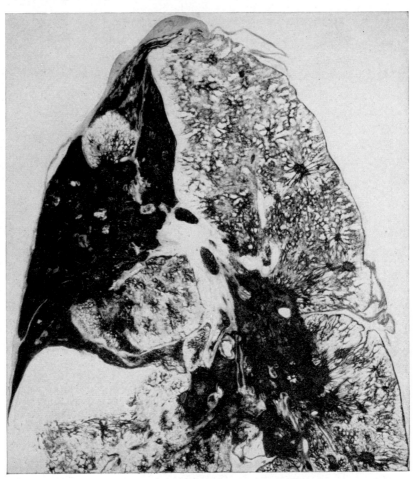

FIG. 15.51.—Coal-miner's lung, showing severe anthracosis.

Note the discrete lesions with focal emphysema, and also the areas of gross fibrosis and pigmentation. $\times \frac{7}{10}$. From a whole lung section kindly lent by Professor Gough.

It later becomes almost confluent, but in many cases remarkably little obstruction to the pulmonary circulation is brought about unless there are concurrent chronic bronchitis and bronchiolitis which induce destructive centrilobular emphysema. Thus despite the considerable disability, the disease often does not appreciably shorten life. The resultant deficient respiratory exchange, characteristic of severe emphysema (see p. 346), leads to great disability from dyspnoea. In some instances, large areas of lung tissue may be completely destroyed and replaced by large spaces lined by fibrous walls and possibly

N

reticulation usually contain a considerable amount of silica, but the response of the tissues to a mixture of finely divided coal and silicious dust is greatly modified from that brought about by silica alone, perhaps because much of the silicious dust is inhaled in the more complex and less harmful forms.

A further change in some cases is the development of progressive massive fibrosis of the lungs, especially in the upper lobes (Fig. 15.51), and these lesions may undergo central softening and cavitation. Progressive massive fibrosis is not due to excessive amounts of silica along with coal dust as the proportions do not differ from those found in simple pneumoconiosis and we have observed a precisely similar lesion in a carbon-electrode maker in whose lungs silica was present in minimal amount. Accordingly, it is now generally accepted that the additional factor is in most cases the concomitant presence of tuberculous infection, and virulent tubercle bacilli

sive fibrosis. They are surrounded by a zone of inflammatory reaction with polymorphs and macrophages and the whole lesion bears some resemblance to caseous tuberculosis but tubercle bacilli are absent. The condition is regarded as rheumatoid nodules in the lung aggravated and modified by the simultaneous reaction to dust.

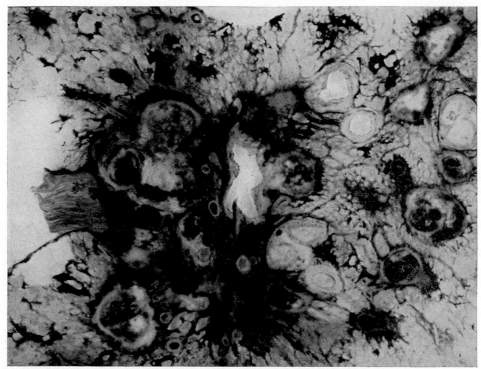

FIG. 15.52.—Caplan's syndrome, "rheumatoid" nodules in the lung of a coal-miner who had suffered from rheumatoid arthritis.
Note the concentric lamination of the nodules.

have been isolated from the central cavity of such lesions in cases with minimum silica content. It seems probable that the action of coal dust in some way mitigates the effects of silica and tubercle bacilli, both locally and generally. The initial dust reticulation and focal emphysema, however, appear to depend more upon the mechanical accumulation of a sufficiently large amount of foreign particles than on their chemical composition.

Caplan's syndrome. Miners suffering from rheumatoid arthritis develop multiple discrete rounded nodules in the lungs, larger than ordinary dust foci and of more rapid progression (Fig. 15.52). These nodules show concentric layers of paler necrotic collagen and darker dusty material and they may fuse into larger masses resembling progressive mas-

Silicosis

Conditions of occurrence. This is a more serious disease than anthracosis. In Great Britain it occurs in stone-masons, sand-blasters and workers in the abrasive-soap industry where the very finely divided particles and perhaps also the effect of alkali lead to a rapidly fatal form of the disease. The use of power-driven abrasive tools to dress sandstone or clean the surface of sandstone buildings is more dangerous than simple hand-tools, for they produce a much finer dust. Wet processes for drilling or abrading silicious stone may greatly reduce the risk, but face masks are of little use unless they remove particles of less than 3 μ.

Structural changes. The stone particles have a

markedly irritating effect and may give rise to much fibrosis. The layers of the pleura are usually adherent and thickened, and on the surface of the lung there are often scattered grey firm nodules. These occur especially at the junctions of the interlobular septa and the pleura, and when cut into may be gritty to the touch. Similar nodules are present throughout the lung and larger fibrous masses may be formed by their confluence, especially in the upper lobes. The lesions are surrounded by a variable degree of diffuse fibrosis of the lung and of the hilar lymph nodes. Some bronchiectasis may occur, and there may be ulceration of the nodules into the bronchi, with formation of cavities. The lung tissue is dark greyish and as a rule there is also a considerable amount of carbon pigment. Tuberculous lesions of various kinds are often present in addition.

Microscopic examination shows that the nodules are composed of very dense connective tissue arranged in a laminated fashion, and between the fibres there are collections of stone particles which are usually very minute, angular, and greyish-brown; their appearances, however, vary according to the nature of the stone. Most of the particles are doubly refracting and are

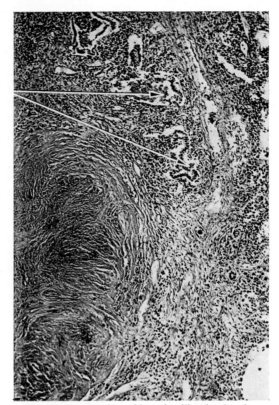

FIG. 15.54.—Section of lung in silicosis, showing characteristic laminated fibrous nodule.

The compressed alveoli at the margin (arrows) are lined by cubical epithelium. × 100.

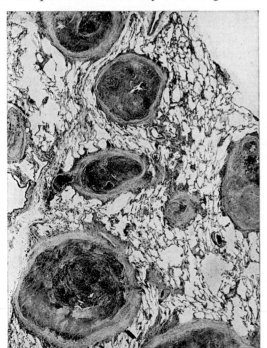

FIG. 15.53.—Fibrotic nodules in lung in silicosis.
Note dense laminated connective tissue. The nodules are unusually well circumscribed. × 7.

thus readily distinguished by the polarising microscope. The nodules are cellular at the periphery, while the central parts become hyalinised (Figs. 15.53, 15.54). In silicosis the walls of the small arteries are usually hyaline and endarteritic and the narrowed lumina may be occluded by organised thrombus. These arterial lesions may produce central necrosis in the related nodules.

Clinical effects. Silicosis leads to serious results in two ways. (*a*) In the first place, owing to the great fibrosis and destruction or replacement of the alveolar tissue, the vascular area is diminished and, accordingly, there is not only obstruction to the circulation, but also hypoxia, resulting in cor pulmonale (p. 346). The right side of the heart undergoes hypertrophy, and this may be followed by dilatation, with congestive heart-failure and oedema. (*b*) The other serious result is tuberculosis. Silicosis renders the lungs very susceptible to invasion by the tubercle bacillus, more than 50 per cent of cases being affected, and the lungs may then be extensively involved by both types of disease. A fibrocaseous lesion is specially common amongst gold miners in the Transvaal. The silicotic nodules are radiologically opaque and X-ray examination reveals both the nodules and the more diffuse lesions.

The pathogenesis of silicosis. The action of silica is characterised by two main features, viz. (*a*) the extensiveness of the resulting fibrosis, as contrasted with that in other pneumoconioses, and (*b*) the susceptibility to tuberculosis. It has long been known that the action of the stone particles on the tissues is not the result of their physical properties merely as foreign material, but is due to the slow formation of silicic acid which diffuses around the particles and, after polymerisation to colloidal silica, becomes fixed to the cytoplasm of the cells. Colloidal silica is a powerful cell poison (p. 11), leading to fibrosis which later becomes hyaline. The hyalinised silicotic lesions, however, contain only about 40 per cent of collagen, the remainder consisting of globulins, polysaccharides and lipids, the composition resembling that of amyloid. Accordingly it is now thought that silica may not merely have a toxic action on tissues but that it may combine with tissue proteins to produce a conjugated antigen, the silicotic lesions resulting at least in part from immunological processes. It has been shown experimentally that colloidal silica breaks down the defence of the tissues against tubercle bacilli, and tuberculosis, if present, tends to become extensive. In this way, the increased susceptibility of silicotic lungs to tuberculous infection is brought about, and the essential features of silicosis are explained. The production of experimental silicosis can be prevented by the repeated inhalation of metallic aluminium powder. This action depends chiefly on the formation of a gelatinous aluminium hydroxide which covers the quartz particles with an insoluble and impermeable coating. It remains to be seen to what extent this result may have practical application in the prevention of silicosis in man.

The nature of the silicious materials concerned in the production of silicosis is still a subject of enquiry, but it is generally agreed that *crystalline silica* (SiO_2) is chiefly responsible, especially in the form of quartz; tridymite and cristobalite are even more toxic but give rise to a diffuse interstitial fibrosis without nodularity. The size of the inhaled particles is important, and those in the range 1–3 μ in diameter have been shown to be the most intensely fibrogenic. Many of the complex silicates present play little or no part in the production of silicosis; indeed some exercise a protective influence by delaying the formation of colloidal silicic acid on which the harmful effects largely depend. Sericite, felspar, hornblende and kaolin are compound silicates found in many rocks and some are also used in certain industrial processes; their fibrogenic action after inhalation is minimal (King).

Asbestosis

Asbestos is a fibrous silicate, the silica being combined chiefly with magnesium and iron; it is much used in industry and the carding and spinning of the fibres produces a very dusty atmosphere, from the inhalation of which a serious form of interstitial fibrosis arises among workers in asbestos factories.

Structural changes. Small fibres, 50–200 μ in length, are inhaled into the respiratory bronchioles from which, aided by respiratory movements, they gain entrance to the alveoli by piercing their walls. There they give rise to a well-marked macrophage reaction with numerous giant cells, and colloidal silica is liberated. As the impacted fibres cannot be transported along the lymphatics, nodular reaction is absent and fibrosis of the lungs of a diffuse type results (Fig. 15.55). This is usually most marked in the lower lobes, diminishing in intensity in an upward direction; it is often accompanied by much pleural thickening. In a chest X-ray the lesion presents a striated rather than a nodular appearance.

Pleural plaques. Sharply demarcated plaques of fibrous tissue are seen on the pleural surfaces in some individuals who have been exposed to asbestos dust, with or without developing pulmonary asbestosis. The common sites are the diaphragmatic pleura and the posterior intercostal pleura. The lesions consist of acellular collagen and they may become calcified and radio-opaque.

Microscopy of the lung reveals areas of fibrosis in which the alveolar structure has disappeared, and other areas alongside in which the alveoli show an advancing fibrosis of their walls along with a varying amount of inflammatory change in the alveolar spaces. Peribronchial fibrosis is often specially marked. Scattered in the fibrous tissue and also within the alveoli, one finds the so-called "asbestos bodies", which are of great importance in the diagnosis of the disease. They are thin and of considerable length, often clubbed or bulging at the extremities and transversely fissured or notched along their length. They are brownish-yellow and contain stainable iron. The bodies represent asbestos filaments coated with some protein deposit from the tissues (Figs. 15.56, 15.57), the curious

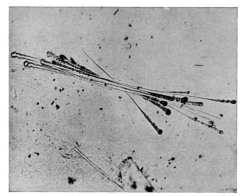

FIG. 15.56.—Asbestos bodies in sputum from case of asbestosis.

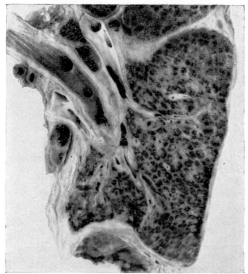

FIG. 15.55.—Pulmonary asbestosis showing massive fibrosis and shrinkage of the lower lobe. × ¾.

ringed structure being probably due to the effects of respiratory movements on the process of deposition. In the lung tissue they are often arranged in radiating clumps, though there are also irregular fragments, and they are accompanied by deposition of much carbon pigment. They have also been found to appear in the lungs of guinea-pigs within two or three months after artificial exposure to the dust. Asbestos bodies have been found in the sputum of persons exposed to asbestos dust without there being any evidence of a pulmonary lesion; similarly, small numbers of asbestos bodies can be demonstrated at necropsy in the lungs of about 40 per cent of city dwellers. Their presence thus indicates that there has been exposure. The presence of the bodies in clumps has, however, another significance, for these form only in the pulmonary lesions, and their presence in the

sputum probably indicates breaking down of the tissues, either as a result of tuberculosis or suppurative change.

There is a distinct tendency for tuberculosis to occur in asbestosis, though the incidence of the disease is not as high as in silicosis. There is also an increased liability to bronchial carcinoma, greatly in excess of that in silicosis or anthracosis. More recently a relationship has been demonstrated between exposure to asbestos dust,

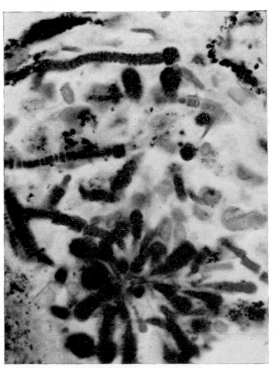

FIG. 15.57.—A characteristically radiating clump of asbestos bodies within the lung and many single knobbed and ringed bodies. × 600.

although not necessarily asbestosis, and the rare tumour *malignant mesothelioma* of the pleura or peritoneum.

Asbestosis, when well established, is a very serious disease, and leads to death more rapidly than silicosis. However, dust control measures have greatly reduced the incidence of severe disease.

Other inorganic dust diseases

Pulmonary siderosis. This may be due either to iron or steel dust, or oxide of iron (haematite). The former variety has now practically disappeared as a result of precautions adopted in industry, but the latter is encountered in workers in haematite mines and occurs in this country. The haematite lung is rusty brown and may be extensively fibrosed. The fibrous tissue is in coarse bands or is diffuse, but with localised denser areas. The fibrosis is coarser than in asbestosis and less nodular than in silicosis. In fact, it resembles that in the progressive massive fibrosis of coal workers, and like it is probably due to associated tuberculous infection. Microscopically the haematite pigment consists of brownish-yellow granules, which are abundant throughout the fibrous tissue. Most of the pigment is free and does not give the prussian blue reaction, but a considerable amount contained within cells reacts positively. The iron is absorbed from the lungs, probably in a colloidal state, and carried to other parts of the body, so that a varying amount of siderosis of the reticulo-endothelial system may result. Haematite lungs contain a large amount of silica and this no doubt plays an important part in leading to the fibrous changes, and for this reason the condition is called silico-siderosis. As in silicosis, there is a marked tendency to frank tuberculosis, and 15 per cent of fatal cases have also developed carcinoma of the lung, chiefly in relation to the areas of scar tissue.

A considerable degree of nodular siderosis of the lungs is observed in electric-arc welders, who inhale fumes consisting largely of iron oxide. The lesions do not appear to progress beyond the stage of nodulation and in spite of marked changes visible on X-ray examination disability is usually slight.

Cadmium fumes, from ore-smelting or from over-heating of cadmium-plated articles, can give rise to an acute fatal chemical pneumonia, with gross oedema and formation of hyaline membranes and a remarkable proliferation of the alveolar lining epithelium. In chronic cases it gives rise to centrilobular destructive emphysema.

Aluminium, despite its use in the prophylaxis of silicosis, can cause a form of pneumoconiosis, first observed in the German aircraft industry. In Great Britain cases have been detected amongst men using very finely divided aluminium in the fireworks industry. The lungs show a diffuse fibrosis of rather characteristic pattern, accompanied by emphysema (Fig. 15.58).

Certain other metallic dusts encountered in industry may be very harmful, and when inhaled as fine dust or fumes may also cause an acute chemical pneumonia. Manganese, osmium, vanadium and

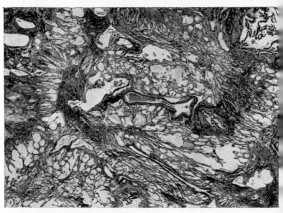

FIG. 15.58.—Pulmonary fibrosis and paraseptal emphysema from inhalation of aluminium. (Section kindly loaned by Dr. Manning.) × 12.

especially beryllium, extensively used in the manufacture of fluorescent lighting tubes, all may have this effect. Beryllium also gives rise to remarkable granulomatous lesions resembling sarcoidosis not only in the lungs but also in the skin and internal organs.

Organic dusts

Farmer's lung

This disease results from inhaling the spores of micro-organisms growing in mouldy hay. *Micropolyspora faeni* is usually responsible, and enormous numbers of its spores, which are of approx. 1 µ diameter, are released from hay stored without adequate drying, so that the farm worker handling such hay in an enclosed space may inhale a million or so spores per minute, and many of these reach the alveoli. In sensitised subjects, the features of the illness depend on the frequency of inhaling the spores. When this occurs at long intervals, i.e. of one or more weeks, an acute illness develops 6–9 hours following exposure, and is characterised by fever, malaise, and persistent dry cough. X-ray shows diffuse pulmonary infiltrations, and biopsy has revealed inflammatory changes in the alveoli with polymorph infiltration, for which the term "extrinsic allergic alveolitis" has been suggested; in some instances granulomas develop resembling those of sarcoidosis, and these also may be discernible by X-ray. The illness usually subsides after a few days; in severe cases, glucocorticoids are beneficial. With more frequent exposure to mouldy hay at short intervals, a more insidious alveolar reaction occurs, with malaise, general ill health and weight loss: pulmonary fibrosis may eventually result.

The occurrence of this disease has been shown to be related to the presence of high serum levels of precipitating antibodies to antigens of *Micropolyspora faeni*, and the condition is due to an Arthus-like (type III) reaction (p. 104), in the alveolar walls, between *Micropolyspora* antigens and precipitating antibodies. Skin tests have not proved helpful in making the diagnosis, and most patients do not have a history of atopy. The disease is not uncommon, particularly in areas where a wet climate interferes with the adequate drying of hay before storage.

Other diseases resembling farmer's lung

Inhalation of dusts in various occupations can lead to an alveolar reaction resembling that of farmer's lung, and due to Arthus-like reactions between precipitating antibodies and antigens in the inhaled dust. In some of these conditions, there is evidence that atopic (type I) hypersensitivity is necessary to promote the Arthus (type III) reaction. Examples are as follows.

Bird-fancier's lung results from inhaling dust from bird cages, pigeon lofts, etc. As in farmer's lung, intermittent exposure is followed by an acute febrile condition and more regular exposure leads to chronic ill-health and in some instances to pulmonary fibrosis. Precipitins to various antigenic constituents of bird droppings and to bird serum proteins are usually detectable, but are found also in the serum of some exposed individuals without illness. The disease is associated with a biphasic (atopic and Arthus-type) reaction to skin tests, and it appears that the Arthus-type of reaction is triggered off by atopy.

Other conditions in this group include *bagassosis*, due to inhalation of moulds from sugar cane bagasse, *flour-miller's disease* from antigens of wheat or the wheat weevil, *mushroom-picker's lung* from thermophilic actinomycetes; and possibly *byssinosis*, a disease resulting from inhalation of dust of the cotton plant. Patients with diabetes insipidus may also develop true asthma and a farmer's-lung type of lesion from inhaling bovine or porcine pituitary "snuff". Precipitating antibodies which react with both foreign and human pituitary extracts are detectable in the serum.

THE PLEURAE

A number of lesions of the pleurae have been described incidentally, earlier in the chapter, but others have to be added.

Hydrothorax is the term applied to the common effusion of serous fluid into the pleural cavities in cardiac and renal cases; it is a simple transudate and both pleural cavities are generally affected. It may also be produced by tumours, or other lesions at the root of the lung which interfere with the lymph flow. The presence of fibrous adhesions will prevent the accumulation, and when these are on one side, the corresponding lung is usually more oedematous than the other.

Haemothorax, i.e. a collection of blood in a pleural cavity, is usually the result either of trauma, e.g. a perforating wound of the lung or fracture of ribs with displacement, or rupture of an aneurysm. The pleural cavity may be distended with blood and coagulum, and the lung is compressed. The association of haemorrhage with pleurisy will be referred to below.

Acute pleurisy

Sources of infection. Pleurisy is caused usually by spread of micro-organisms from a local lesion, although it can result also from blood spread. It is most commonly a complication of pulmonary infection, e.g. lobar or bronchopneumonia, lung abscess, or tuberculosis. It may result also by extension from pericarditis and from abdominal lesions, especially subphrenic abscess, or from ruptured oesophagus and mediastinitis.

Acute pleurisy may result from carcinomatous involvement of the pleura, without superadded infection, and it may occur also in rheumatic fever and in uraemia.

Naked-eye appearances. The exudate in pleurisy varies greatly in character. It may be chiefly fibrinous, serofibrinous, purulent, haemorrhagic, or even gangrenous. The appearances depend mainly on the organisms present. Thus pleurisy occurring in rheumatic fever or due to *Strep. pneumoniae* is usually fibrinous or sero-fibrinous, though the exudate caused by the latter organism sometimes becomes purulent (*empyema*). In streptococcal and staphylococcal infections, the exudate is usually purulent, whilst in the gangrenous type a great variety of organisms, both aerobic and anaerobic, may be present. As in the pericardium, a haemorrhagic effusion is seen in invasion of the cavity by malignant tumours, and occasionally in scurvy.

The results vary according to the nature of the exudate. Serous and, to a certain extent, fibrinous exudate may undergo absorption, but in the latter, a process of organisation is usually involved, and this will be in proportion to the amount and density of the fibrin. When suppuration has occurred the pus tends to increase in amount and sometimes forms an enormous *empyema*, the lung becoming collapsed against the side of the vertebral column. A layer of granulation tissue then forms on the pleural surfaces, and this is followed by fibrosis in the subserous layers, which is apt to extend into the collapsed lung. These changes prevent the proper expansion of the lung, and hence it is of great importance that empyema should be evacuated without undue delay. If the empyema is small, its contents may be absorbed or changed into inspissated material; great pleural thickening, sometimes followed by calcification, is apt to occur.

Pleural fibrosis

This condition, often with pleural adhesions, and sometimes with obliteration of the cavity, may follow acute pleurisy, or may be the result of chronic pulmonary lesions such as silicosis and tuberculosis, as already described. The presence of some pleural adhesions is common after middle adult life.

Pneumothorax

This condition is produced by the entrance of air or gas into the pleural cavity and is usually the result of some breach of continuity of the lung substance. Spontaneous pneumothorax may occur suddenly in an apparently healthy individual probably from the rupture of an emphysematous bulla. The air usually undergoes rapid absorption without any untoward effects. Similarly air may gain entrance from the rupture of an interstitial emphysematous bulla in whooping-cough. Recurrent pneumothorax of unknown cause may occur in apparently healthy young adults. Pneumothorax may also be the result of injury, e.g. a punctured wound of the chest, or laceration of the lung from a fractured rib. In such conditions there may be no bacterial infection of the pleura, and if healing of the wound in the lung occurs, the air in the pleura is rapidly absorbed. Sometimes the opening into the pleura is small and admits the entrance but not the exit of respired air; great distension of the pleural cavity with much displacement of the heart may result—*tension pneumothorax*.

Pneumothorax may occur secondarily to abscesses of the lung, and to acute caseating tuberculosis. It can result also from rupture or ulcerating cancer of the oesophagus. In these conditions the pleural cavity becomes infected with pyogenic and sometimes with putrefactive organisms; suppuration follows, the condition being then called *pyopneumothorax*. Unless adhesions are present, the lung collapses and the changes described above in connection with empyema may follow.

TUMOURS OF THE BRONCHI, LUNGS AND PLEURAE

Benign tumours

In the *trachea, bronchi* and *lungs*, benign tumours such as fibroma, leiomyoma and chondroma have been described, but they are all very rare. *Bronchial adenoma* is less rare, forming under 10 per cent of bronchial neoplasms; it occurs mostly in young persons and is about equally distributed between the sexes. This tumour is of clinical importance because it usually projects into the lumen as a pedunculated mass which causes partial obstruction (Fig. 15.59), with bronchiectasis and sometimes haemoptysis. Extension through the bronchial wall is the rule, so that the intra-luminal portion is the smaller part of the growth; endoscopic resection is therefore not practicable. In our own series, most bronchial adenomas have been solid trabecular growths not unlike "carcinoid" tumours of the intestine (Fig. 15.60). Although they rarely give the argentaffin reaction some produce the carcinoid syndrome (p. 532) and 5-hydroxytryptamine may be excreted in the urine along with 5-hydroxy-indole-acetic acid. In some adenomas a more glandular architecture is found; in others more proximally situated, a cylindromatous structure resembling that of salivary and mucous gland tumours is seen, but these are less common (Fig. 18.13, p. 478). It is not always easy to make the diagnosis from fragments removed endoscopically, and the benign nature of such tumours is not certain, for they are prone to repeated local recurrence and may rarely metastasise.

Malignant tumours

Bronchial carcinoma

General features, age and sex incidence. This is by far the commonest primary tumour of the lungs and bronchi. It usually takes origin from one of the main bronchi at the hilum of the lung, less frequently from a more peripheral bronchus. It may also arise from the lung alveoli, but this cannot be distinguished with certainty. Bronchial carcinoma is more often found on the right side, and in our necropsy reports the incidence in males is about four times that in females. The incidence of cancer of the lung has

undergone a striking increase, indeed it is now one of the commonest forms of malignancy. The magnitude of the increase is best assessed from the returns of the Registrar-General for England and Wales, which show a rise in the number of deaths registered as due to cancer of the lung from 6,500 in 1944, 16,000 in 1955 and over 30,000 in 1969.

Etiology. Bronchial carcinoma has no definite relation to common chronic conditions such as

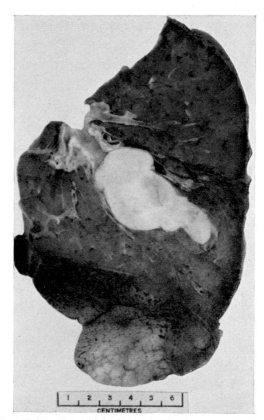

Fig. 15.59.—Bronchial adenoma. The tumour projects as a polyp into the bronchus.

tuberculosis but the greater frequency in males suggests some external environmental factor. The first recognised industrial lung cancer was that occurring amongst the workers in the Schneeberg cobalt mines in Saxony. It is almost certain that radioactive substances were concerned; these tumours were almost exclusively of oat-celled and anaplastic squamous types. Workers in the chromate industry also have an abnormally high death rate from cancer of the respiratory tract; this is true also of workers in nickel refining, of workers with asbestos, and of haematite miners. These industrial hazards, however, have little bearing on the rising incidence of lung cancer reported from most countries. Long-continued exposure of the respiratory tract to carcinogenic agents is a most important causal factor of bronchial carcinoma. Two sources of smoke are important in this respect, atmospheric pollution and tobacco. Statistical evidence shows that bronchial carcinoma is more common in towns than in rural districts and that its incidence is closely correlated with

bronchial carcinoma occurs mainly in cigarette smokers, and the risk appears to increase proportionately to the consumption of cigarettes. This conclusion, first indicated by retrospective studies, has been confirmed in a prospective study of the causes of death of medical practitioners. It has been clearly established (*a*) that the victims of bronchial carcinoma include a marked excess of heavy smokers and also (*b*) that in some areas in this country, the habitual smoking of 25 cigarettes or more per day over a period of years is associated with a 12 per cent risk of dying from bronchial

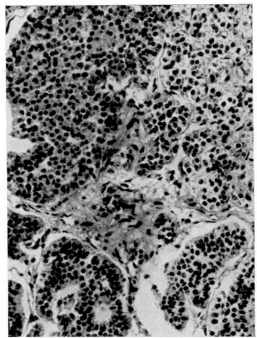

FIG. 15.60.—Bronchial adenoma of the carcinoid type. × 230.

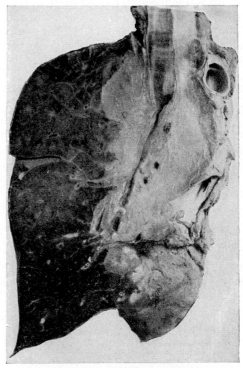

FIG. 15.61.—Primary carcinoma of bronchus, oat-cell type, showing marked bronchial obstruction.

Note the extensive consolidation in adjacent parts of the upper and lower lobes; the lower and inner part of the lower lobe is the site of multiple abscesses, resulting from retention pneumonia. × ⅖.

the degree of atmospheric pollution. It is commonest in large towns with an atmosphere heavily polluted by industrial and domestic smoke and by the fumes from internal combustion engines. The carcinogenic agents liberated in the combustion of coal include benzpyrene and arsenic and the concentration of the former in the air of large towns (up to 5 μg. per 100 cubic metres of air) is such that under normal weather conditions about 0·5 μg. may be inhaled in 12 hours. The amount is greater in winter than in summer and may be increased almost tenfold in foggy weather.

There is also good statistical evidence that

carcinoma. The mode of action of cigarette smoke is uncertain; there is about 1 μg. of 3 : 4 benzpyrene in the smoke of 100 cigarettes. It is by no means certain that benzpyrene is the only carcinogen involved, and it may be more important that the tar from cigarette smoke has been found to be a powerful co-carcinogen. Accordingly it may be that the correlation of the incidence of bronchial carcinoma with smoking represents the summation of the effects of a number of different substances, including carcinogens and co-carcinogens.

Naked-eye appearances. Bronchial carcinoma presents a variety of appearances depending upon the site of origin, the extent of local spread and the degree of bronchial obstruction produced (Fig. 15.61).

Hilar type. In the commonest type the tumour forms a massive growth surrounding the main bronchus to the lung or to one lobe; the bronchial mucosa is ulcerated or may be merely roughened and nodular, while secondary extension by lymphatics produces further nodules in the mucosa towards the bifurcation of the trachea. The growth narrows markedly the lumen of the affected bronchus, producing obstruction. Retention of secretions then occurs, and is followed by infection with consequent septic bronchopneumonia and abscess formation; occasionally gangrene ensues, resulting in production of ragged cavities in the lung. The tumour soon spreads by the lymphatics giving rise to massive secondaries in the mediastinal nodes which are often so incorporated with the bronchial mass as to be indistinguishable separately (Fig. 15.61). Extension upwards into the lymph nodes of the neck is often seen. Retrograde spread also occurs along the peribronchial and perivascular lymphatics so that even the smaller bronchi and vessels may be ensheathed by whitish collars of tumour. Invasion of the pericardial sac occurs by direct extension along the lymphatics around the walls of the pulmonary veins, and the carcinoma may compress and occlude the superior vena cava causing marked cyanosis. The tumours form bulky cellular masses in which necrosis is often widespread and pressure effects within the mediastinum give rise to severe dyspnoea.

Peripheral type. Less frequently the tumour originates from a peripheral bronchus, and sometimes apparently arises in such a small bronchus that the exact site of origin is uncertain. Some writers claim to recognise a form arising in the pulmonary alveoli. However, the histological appearances are deceptive and both carcinomas of unequivocally bronchial origin and metastatic tumours may use the alveolar walls as a convenient stroma and thus simulate an alveolar origin. Alveolar tumours are usually, but not invariably, mucus-secreting adenocarcinomas and they may produce consolidation of large areas of the lung resembling pneumonia, the cut surface presenting a greyish, rather mucoid appearance. A variant of this neoplasm appears to arise in the respiratory bronchioles and may spread by way of the air passages producing a rather characteristic type of pulmonary invasion, to which the name *pulmonary alveolar adenomatosis* has been applied (Fig. 15.62).

The spread of lung cancer. The early and widespread invasion of the lymphatics has been emphasised and this may involve the pleura, forming a thick ensheathment of the surfaces or take the form of multiple discrete nodules.

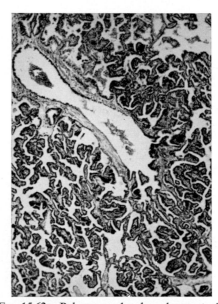

Fig. 15.62.—Pulmonary alveolar adenomatosis.

Showing the papillary architecture and the relation to the terminal bronchiole. × 42.

Pleurisy with effusion, often haemorrhagic in character, is common. When the growth is at the apex of the lung, extension to the adjacent thoracic cage may involve the lower cords of the brachial plexus and the sympathetic chain, so that pain and sensory disturbances together with signs of sympathetic palsy may occur—*Pancoast's syndrome.* Owing to the peripheral situation of the lung cancer, symptoms and signs referable to the lung may appear only late in the disease.

Metastases. The liver and adrenals are nearly always involved sooner or later. Onuigbo, working in this Department, has shown that the spread of lung cancer is predominantly to the ipsilateral side and this distribution indicates the lymphatics rather than the arterial blood stream as the usual route of metastases. Sometimes spread occurs to the lymph nodes of the neck, axilla or even groin, before the primary tumour presents localising signs. This ipsilateral spread is particularly true of the adrenals, which are a very common site of secondary deposits. The kidneys, with a larger arterial supply, are much

primary bronchial carcinoma. Metastases in the bones are common, the thoracic vertebrae being especially frequently involved, possibly by the retrograde venous route. Bronchial carcinoma may also be associated with very widespread secondaries in the internal organs, especially the liver, while the primary tumour remains small and clinically silent.

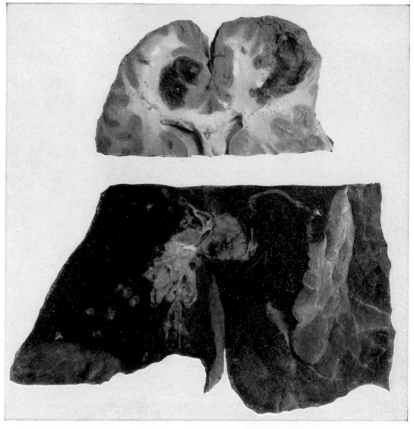

FIG. 15.63.—Primary bronchial carcinoma of oat-cell type causing multiple cerebral metastases while the primary was still small and undeclared clinically. × ½.

less often involved and the contrast to the localisation of blood-borne metastatic abscesses in staphylococcal pyaemia is very striking.

Ipsilateral spread predominates also in certain other organs, such as liver and kidneys, but in the liver the appearances may be rendered difficult of interpretation by subsequent widespread dissemination within the organ (tertiary spread). There is a special tendency to the formation of secondary tumours in the brain (Fig. 15.63), a phenomenon of particular importance because it may overshadow the primary bronchial growth clinically. In fact surgical exploration of a cerebral neoplasm should always be preceded by a careful survey of the lungs to exclude

Associated clinical phenomena. Bronchial carcinoma is sometimes associated with widespread neuropathy and myopathy not related to direct effects of secondary deposits (p. 665). Cushing's syndrome with adrenal cortical hyperplasia occurs too frequently for the association to be fortuitous: it has been shown to be due to secretion of ACTH by the tumour (p. 912), which is almost always of the oat-cell type. Other rare systemic effects of bronchial carcinoma are the carcinoid syndrome, hypercalcaemia, hyponatraemia, encephalopathies and neuropathies, and gynaecomastia. Migrating phlebitis and gross lymphoedema may also occur and may cause the initial symptoms.

Hypertrophic pulmonary osteo-arthropathy is also associated with bronchial carcinoma (p. 772).

Histological types of carcinoma. Microscopically bronchial carcinomas fall into three main groups, the oat-cell, the squamous and the mucus-secreting adenocarcinoma, but the structure may be mixed owing to the appearance of

Squamous carcinomas form an increasingly high proportion of bronchial cancers, and especially in cases subjected to surgical excision. Some are frankly squamous, of dense creamy-opaque appearance (Fig. 15.66) and with typical cell nests. More commonly they are anaplastic, with very little keratinisation and are largely spheroidal celled. Squamous carcinoma

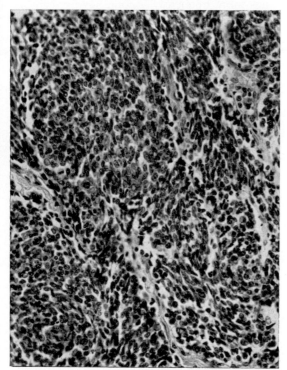

Fig. 15.64.—Oat-cell carcinoma of bronchus showing many very short spindle cells. Others cells appear round in transverse section. × 115.

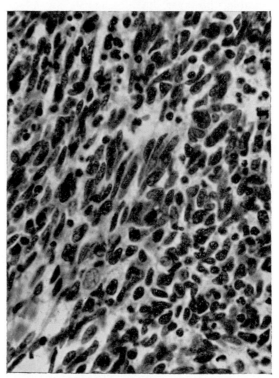

Fig. 15.65.—Oat-cell carcinoma; a vertebral metastasis. × 450.

small lumina in the oat-celled type, or to some degree of squamous metaplasia in the adenocarcinomas.

Oat-cell carcinoma. Many of the hilar growths belong to the so-called "oat-cell" type, i.e. they consist of very short spindle cells which may appear oval or round depending upon the plane of section (Figs. 15.64, 15.65), but are loosely arranged in alveoli. These tumours were formerly confused with lymphosarcomas, but are now recognised as of epithelial origin, the prototype being the cells of the deepest layer of the bronchial epithelium. In places they may be arranged around the small vessels and stroma in palisade fashion and thus present a columnar appearance, or small lumina devoid of mucus secretion may develop.

arises from bronchial epithelium which has undergone squamous metaplasia (Fig. 15.67), and such areas are frequently seen in the bronchial lining with or without bronchiectasis. Blood-borne metastases and secondary spread to the hilar lymph nodes usually occur later in squamous than in oat-cell carcinomas. This behaviour renders squamous cancer the more favourable type of tumour for radical excision. Keratinising squamous, anaplastic squamous, polygonal-cell and oat-cell tumours comprise about 75 per cent of bronchial cancers and these types are responsible for the major part of the greatly increased incidence of the disease, and for the striking difference in the sex incidence.

Adenocarcinoma is the least common of the

main types, and is composed of cubical or columnar cells which are usually mucus-secreting in places; sometimes the tumour has a distinctly papillary architecture, or it may be more scirrhous. Adenocarcinomas form about 25 per cent of primary lung cancers, and of these a substantially higher proportion arise in the more peripheral intrapulmonary sites. It is not possible, however, to distinguish an adeno-carcinoma from the other types merely by its site and naked-eye appearance. In striking contrast to the other types, adenocarcinoma is about equally distributed between the sexes.

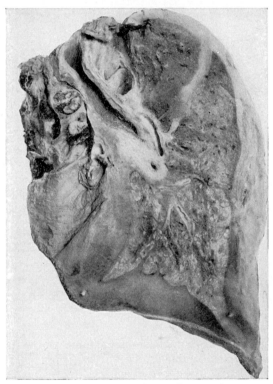

Fig. 15.66.—Primary bronchial carcinoma of squamous type. The lung is greatly collapsed, and there is widespread lymphatic permeation, with great pleural thickening. × 2/5.

Other primary malignant lung tumours

Primary *sarcoma* and *haemangio-endothelioma* are occasionally encountered in the lungs, but are rare. The latter may be simulated by a form of vascular malformation leading to an arterio-venous shunt. Any form of malignant growth in the lungs may give rise to haemoptysis, and this is sometimes an early symptom.

Secondary tumours in the lung

These are fairly frequent among *sarcomas* of all kinds. The metastases occur chiefly by the blood stream, and the tumours in the lung are usually multiple discrete rounded masses. The spread of *carcinoma* to the lungs may take place by the blood stream, but we believe that the lungs more frequently become involved by way of the lymphatics. For example, in cases of breast carcinoma, the cells may spread to the pleural lymphatics and thence to the lungs, while in cases of abdominal carcinoma there may be a

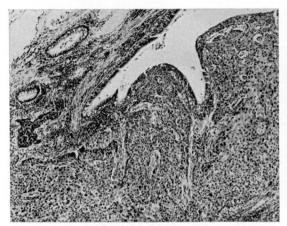

Fig. 15.67.—Squamous carcinoma of bronchus.
The normal columnar ciliated lining is seen at one side, but elsewhere has undergone metaplasia to squamous type and is continuous with masses of squamous carcinoma below. × 44.

spread to the hilar lymph nodes, and from there extension into the lungs may follow. When the lymphatics of the lungs become involved, the tumour may be diffuse and produce only minute nodules. The pleural lymphatics may, for example, appear as whitish threads outlining the lobules, and we have seen cases where the lungs contained very numerous nodules, no larger than tubercles and in some instances scarcely palpable. Blood-borne metastases may form large rounded masses, the so-called "cannon-ball" secondaries, often seen with renal carcinoma, and with testicular tumours. *Lymphosarcoma*, involving the bronchial lymph nodes, either primarily or secondarily, has a great tendency to extend along the peribronchial lymphatics, forming sometimes an encasing sheath to the bronchi and also irregular masses of tumour. It is, however, relatively rare: many of the cases formerly described were really examples of oat-cell carcinoma. The appearance and distribution accordingly resemble this form of cancer, but the tissue tends to be somewhat more cellular with an even greater tendency to necrosis.

Pleura

In the pleura, various benign mesodermal tumours have been described, but are all rare. There is, however, a form of pleural fibroma which may become large and is then usually accompanied by osteo-arthropathy. Some writers regard this as a benign form of pleural mesothelioma. Neurofibroma, sometimes containing ganglionic or neuroblastic elements, is occasionally seen on the posterior wall subpleurally, near the thoracic inlet. *Primary* malignant tumours are also rare, and of these the most characteristic is the so-called *mesothelioma* of the pleura. There has been much interest in this tumour in recent years since an association with exposure to asbestos dust was first described in South Africa. The relationship has been confirmed in the United Kingdom, particularly in the shipbuilding and insulating industries. There

has usually been a history of light exposure to asbestos dust a long time ago. Mesothelioma tends to involve the whole surface, and the pleural layers may be fused and changed into a thick, white, neoplastic mass encasing the lung. In other cases there are nodules in both layers and inflammatory exudate between; extension may take place to the pericardium and also along the lymphatics into the interior of the lung. Such tumours present a widely variable structure with either carcinomatous or sarcomatous features or a mixture of the two. The carcinomatous pattern usually consists of tubular and papillary structures in a loose stroma, or of solid alveolar tumour; the sarcomatous pattern is spindle-celled. The origin of the tumour is usually ascribed to the covering mesothelium of the pleura. Such primary pleural neoplasms are rare and many alleged examples are in fact secondary to an undetected carcinoma in the lung, stomach or elsewhere; sometimes papillary renal carcinoma invades the pleura in such a fashion while the initial growth is still small. The occurrence of *secondaries*, particularly carcinoma, is common. As in the pericardium, malignancy is often accompanied by fibrinous or haemorrhagic pleural exudate.

CHAPTER 16

THE BLOOD AND BONE MARROW

Introduction

Abnormalities of the blood most commonly result from diseases which do not have their origin in a primary disorder of the tissues of the haemopoietic system. This is especially so when the abnormalities are of a chemical nature involving the blood plasma, but it is also true when the cellular elements are affected. An obvious example of this is the leukocytosis which accompanies pyogenic infections, but the changes in the blood secondary to other diseases may be very complex and their connection with the primary disease so little apparent that the blood changes may be mistakenly regarded as a primary abnormality. Thus severe anaemia is observed in some forms of renal failure, while the reverse condition, polycythaemia, may sometimes result from renal abnormalities of a different kind (p. 390).

The body possesses a remarkable regulating mechanism whereby the state of the blood is kept constant. Blood volume, specific gravity, chemical content, number of erythrocytes and leukocytes, varieties of leukocytes, etc., each has an average value within a narrow range of normal limits, and if in conditions of health any one of these is artificially altered a rapid return to normal follows. Deviations from normal in either the cells or the plasma are of great importance, and can often be used in diagnosis. We shall consider here the changes in the cells, while the main chemical changes will be dealt with in connection with the diseases of the various organs concerned in their production.

Essential data. In disease of the haemopoietic tissues, examination of the blood is essential and should include at least the following estimations: the haemoglobin content, the packed red cell volume by centrifuging in a haematocrit, and the red cell count, for from these are derived the *absolute values*, described below, which are of great importance in the differential diagnosis and management of anaemia: also the total number of white cells and examination of a stained blood film by which the morphology of the cellular elements may be assessed. In certain cases further examinations are required, e.g. differential count of the white cells, the percentage and number of reticulocytes, the serum bilirubin, enumeration of the blood platelets, etc., while in many cases marrow biopsy by sternal puncture yields decisive information.

The *haemoglobin* is expressed preferably in grams per 100 ml. whole blood (in males, 13·5–18; in females, 11·5–16·5).

Variations in haemoglobin content. Confusion arises from the use of different scales when haemoglobin concentrations are expressed as percentages. This does not occur when the haemoglobin is expressed in grams per 100 ml. and a British Standard (B.S. 3985: 1966) has been specified for a solution of cyanmethaemoglobin to be used for haemoglobinometry. Nevertheless, the clinical convenience of a percentage scale is great and the modified Haldane standard of 100 per cent = 14·6 g. haemoglobin per 100 ml. blood is in practice satisfactory for this purpose.

The *packed cell volume*, or *haematocrit* value, is expressed as the percentage of whole blood occupied by the red cells: the normal range is 40–54% for men and 35–47% for women.

While it is customary to refer to the percentage of the various white cells in the differential count, the *absolute number* of each variety should be calculated from the total, for it is only from this figure that a true estimate of the number present is obtained.

The absolute values

The *mean corpuscular haemoglobin concentration* (*MCHC*) gives precise information on the *degree of saturation* of the red cells with haemoglobin and therefore indicates unequivocally whether inadequate formation of haemoglobin is a factor in the development of the anaemia, e.g. in iron-deficiency states. It is given by the formula:

$$\frac{\text{grams of haemoglobin per 100 ml.}}{\text{packed-cell volume per 100 ml.}} \times 100$$

and is thus expressed as a percentage (normal 32–36, average 34).

The *mean corpuscular volume* (*MCV*) (normal 76–96 cμ, average 86 cμ) is given in cubic microns by the formula:

$$\frac{\text{volume of red cells in ml. per litre}}{\text{number of red cells in millions per c.mm.}}$$

This gives an indication of the volume and therefore the size of the red cells.

The *mean corpuscular haemoglobin* (*MCH*) is given in picograms by the formula:

$$\frac{\text{grams of haemoglobin per 100 ml.} \times 10}{\text{number of red cells per million per c.mm.}}$$

(Normal = 27–32 pg. per cell)

This indicates the average *amount* of haemoglobin per red cell.

The main purpose in determining the absolute values is in the classification of states of anaemia (i.e. reductions in the haemoglobin concentration of the blood), depending on the average size of the red cells and their degree of haemoglobin saturation. The terms used in such classification depend upon the appearances of the red cells in a stained blood film, and the three main groups are as follows:

Type of anaemia	*Absolute values*		
	MCV	MCHC	MCH
(1) Normochromic normocytic	normal	normal	normal
(2) Hypochromic microcytic	low	low	low
(3) Normochromic macrocytic	high	normal	high

The absolute values are more reliable than the microscopic apperances of the red cells in making this classification, on which diagnosis and therapy usually depend.

The marrow is the all-important tissue in supplying the formed elements of the blood; it is the source of the erythrocytes, granular leukocytes and platelets. All these are in a sense end-products; there is no multiplication of them in the blood stream, though, as described below, both erythrocytes and leukocytes undergo a process of maturation after having entered the blood.

The development of the cells of the blood

The development of the granular leukocytes from primitive precursors has already been outlined (p. 125). The red cells likewise arise from primitive cells in the marrow and proceed through a series of stages to the ultimate non-nucleated erythrocyte. In the peripheral circulation the mature granular cells survive only a relatively short period (2–3 days) as compared with the red cells (100–120 days) and in normal marrow leukoblasts outnumber erythroblasts, in fact the normal leuko-erythrogenic ratio is about 3:1, suggesting that the red cells mature more quickly than the white. When hyperplasia of the marrow occurs this ratio is usually disturbed, e.g. in an active erythroblastic reaction it may be less than 1:1 whereas in a leukoblastic reaction it may be 10:1. In actively proliferating marrow there are primitive cells whose developmental potentiality is not yet revealed by their morphology and these elements are called haemocytoblasts. Normally, differentiation proceeds so rapidly that such indeterminate cells are scanty and the great majority of the early progenitor cells are quite distinctly recognisable as belonging to either the red or white cell series. Only in abnormal conditions, when differentiation is for some reason slowed down or the intermediate cells are being rapidly destroyed, are such primitive undifferentiated cells readily found. The red and white cells arise from a common stem cell (p. 125). The findings of the abnormal 22(Ph') chromosome* in the red cell and megakaryocyte series as well as in the granular cells in chronic myeloid leukaemia (p. 436) provides stong support for this view, which is now widely accepted.

In adult life the primitive stem cells destined to erythroid differentiation normally pass through successive stages known as haemoctyoblast → basophil pronormoblast → polychromatophilic normoblast → reticulocyte → normal red cell. This is known as normoblastic proli-

---

* Formerly classified as No. 21.

feration and the typical stages are depicted in Fig. 16.1, but there are, of course, innumerable gradations as the cells mature from one stage to the next. In the course of maturation from haemocytoblast to red cell there is: (1) progressive diminution in cell size; (2) progressive reduction of nuclear size with condensation of the chromatin, culminating in pyknosis and ultimate disintegration or extrusion; (3) progressive loss of the basophil substance (RNA) of the cytoplasm and concurrent development of haemoglobin.

In early fetal life the first red cells to become filled with haemoglobin are very much larger and were called by Ehrlich *megaloblasts*. By the fourth month of fetal life megaloblastic haemo-

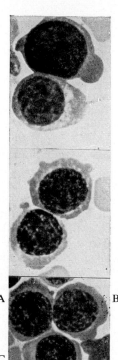

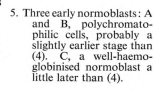

1. Haemocytoblast with finely dispersed chromatin and basophil cytoplasm.

2. Pronormoblast: basophil cytoplasm, early condensation of nuclear chromatin.

3. Early normoblast with basophil cytoplasm and coarse well-marked condensation of the nuclear chromatin.

4. A slightly later normoblast with commencing haemoglobinisation.

5. Three early normoblasts: A and B, polychromatophilic cells, probably a slightly earlier stage than (4). C, a well-haemoglobinised normoblast a little later than (4).

6. Late normoblast showing marked nuclear condensation.

7. Late normoblasts showing early pyknosis and more haemoglobinisation.

8. Late normoblasts—the lower showing complete pyknosis. The cytoplasm in a Leishman-stained film would still be polychromatophilic.

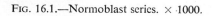
FIG. 16.1.—Normoblast series. × 1000.

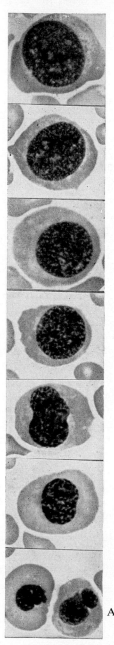

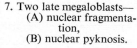

1. Haemocytoblast: note the basophil cytoplasm and evenly dispersed nuclear chromatin containing several nucleoli.

2. Promegaloblast: nucleoli persist, nuclear chromatin shows commencing fine reticular condensation, cytoplasm basophilic. Note contrast to the coarse aggregation of nuclear chromatin in the normoblast series.

3. Early megaloblast: nuclear chromatin is finely reticulate, cytoplasm shows diminished basophilia and early haemoglobinisation.

4. Polychromatophilic megaloblast with haemoglobinisation in advance of nuclear maturation.

5. Later polychromatophilic megaloblast.

6. Late megaloblast with some nuclear condensation.

7. Two late megaloblasts—
    (A) nuclear fragmentation,
    (B) nuclear pyknosis.

FIG. 16.2.—Megaloblast series. × 1000.

poiesis is replaced by the normoblastic type, but for a considerable time the red cells are larger than in adult life (macrocytes). There is no conclusive evidence that the change in the character of fetal blood formation is related to the effects of vitamin B_{12} or of folic acid, but in post-natal life deficiency in the supply of B_{12} or of folic acid, however brought about, leads to abnormal erythropoiesis which resembles superficially that of the fetus, and is therefore termed megaloblastic. Development then proceeds from haemocytoblast to promegaloblast and then successively through basophilic and polychromatophilic megaloblasts to reticulocytes and macrocytes. These stages are depicted in Fig. 16.2.

The feature of megaloblastic erythropoiesis is that the maturation processes do not proceed synchronously. Lack of vitamin B_{12} or folic acid slows the mitotic rate and interferes with nuclear maturation and reduction in cell size, both of which proceed more slowly than usual, while haemoglobinisation proceeds at a more normal rate. This results in the appearance of haemoglobin in cells which, judged by their large size and large finely reticulated nuclei, are very immature, i.e. are at the stage of development where normally the cytoplasm would be basophilic and lacking in haemoglobin. As they mature the cytoplasm becomes more fully haemoglobinised and the nucleus becomes smaller and consequently more dense. These large nucleated cells of various degrees of maturity are known as *haemoglobinised megaloblasts*. Megaloblastic

marrow rapidly becomes transformed into normoblastic marrow when the deficiency in vitamin B_{12} or in folic acid is rectified.

The normal development of the red cells thus requires an adequate supply of vitamin B_{12}, folic acid, and all the other components essential for the formation of haemoglobin; namely iron, vitamin C, thyroxine and protein to furnish amino-acids for globin synthesis. The iron required to replace the haemoglobin destroyed by the daily loss of senescent red cells is made good largely by re-utilisation of the iron from the broken-down haemoglobin, and the balance required is provided by absorption from the diet and by the iron reserves.

Extramedullary haemopoiesis. When the bone marrow has been destroyed by tumour or by fibrous transformation or osteosclerosis (p. 429) there is often extensive formation of marrow in the spleen and liver and great splenomegaly may result—*extramedullary haemopoiesis* (p. 453). It occurs more readily in infants, for example in the liver, spleen and the pelves of the kidneys, but it is also found in the adult within bone formed by metaplasia in various sites (p. 147) and it is noteworthy that the new tissue exhibits erythroblastic as well as leukoblastic formation. Extramedullary haemopoiesis is often associated with the presence of primitive red and white cells in the peripheral blood (*leuko-erythroblastosis*) possibly indicating that in the newly-formed marrow there is imperfect control over the entry of cells into the circulation.

THE RED CELLS

Erythropoiesis, its magnitude and control. In the course of 1 hour 10,000 million red cells are destroyed and replaced, resulting in the synthesis of 300 mg. globin and 12·5 mg. haem. The normal stimulus to red cell production is provided by the hormone erythropoietin, secreted in response to the diminished oxygen carrying capacity of the blood brought about by the physiological destruction of 1% of the total red cells per day. The juxtaglomerular apparatus in the kidney is regarded as the chief source of this hormone, which acts as a proliferative stimulus to the erythropoietic stem cells in the bone marrow.

Variations in number. The normal number of red cells varies between 4·5 and 6·5 millions per

c.mm. in the male and is slightly less in the female. There is a natural diurnal variation of about 10 per cent and the normal fluctuations in the state of hydration of the patient, or prolonged venous constriction of the arm before collection of a venous sample, can readily cause alterations in the count. While decrease is the usual effect of disease, there are certain conditions where an increase occurs. In the first place, the number may be increased simply by the withdrawal of fluid from the blood; this is known as *haemoconcentration* and may result from profuse perspiration or severe diarrhoea, e.g. in cholera, or from increased capillary permeability as in extensive burns. It is most easily assessed by estimating the packed cell volume in the haematocrit. In such cases there is no alteration in the total red cell mass, but simply an increased concentration; the red cell count soon returns to normal by addition of fluid when recovery takes place. In people living at a high altitude, a true increase in the total red cell mass takes place (*secondary polycythaemia*). The red cell count may rise to $7-8 \times 10^6$ at an altitude of about 4,000 metres, and the increase of the total amount of the haemoglobin in the blood is proportionate. The condition is a compensatory one, brought about by the diminished oxygen tension in the atmosphere.

Compensatory or secondary polycythaemia occurs also in chronic diseases of the heart and lungs which interfere with adequate oxygenation of the blood. It is seen, for example, in those forms of congenital heart disease which result in admixture of oxygenated and de-oxygenated blood, the red cell count sometimes exceeding 7×10^6/c.mm. In adults, a lesser degree of polycythaemia may occur in chronic bronchitis and emphysema, or pulmonary fibrosis—conditions which reduce pulmonary blood flow or impair gaseous diffusion in the lungs. Secondary polycythaemia is also observed as a rare association of certain renal lesions such as cysts, hydronephrosis and neoplasms which secrete erythropoietin, including some renal carcinomas and some hepatic tumours. This association has also been suggested to explain the occasional occurrence of polycythaemia in patients who have uterine fibroids or a cerebellar haemangioblastoma, the surgical removal of which corrects the red cell count. In these latter cases excessive erythropoietin activity has not been demonstrated in either the tumour tissue or the patient's blood but as the methods for detecting this are crude, the matter cannot be regarded as settled. In secondary polycythaemia marrow hyperplasia is slight.

In *primary polycythaemia* with splenomegaly (*polycythaemia vera*) there is an increase in the total red cell mass, the blood volume being increased and the red cell count raised, e.g. 8×10^6 per c.mm. The nature of the marrow stimulus here is unknown. The polycythaemia, usually accompanied by an increase in the white cells and platelets also, is due to overproduction of red cells by the marrow, which is grossly hyperplastic, and the disease is included in the group of myeloproliferative disorders (p. 437).

Decrease in the number of red cells per c.mm. is very common. The term "anaemia" includes all conditions where there is a diminution in the percentage of haemoglobin; the two conditions are usually associated, but there may be considerable anaemia with little or even no diminution in the number of red cells. The most severe reductions in the red cell count occur in the so-called primary anaemias; for example, in pernicious anaemia the number of red cells may fall to 5×10^5 per c.mm.

Changes in size and shape. Anaemia is frequently associated with variations in the size of the erythrocytes—*anisocytosis*—and irregularities in form—*poikilocytosis*. Abnormally large red cells, termed *megalocytes* or *macrocytes* (see p. 388–9), are numerous in pernicious anaemia and some related anaemias; in air-dried films they may measure 10–12 μ in diameter, (p. 417). Although undersized cells also are present in pernicious anaemia, the *average size* of the red cells is usually greater than the normal, and the anaemia is thus termed *macrocytic*. The typical macrocytes in pernicious anaemia appear well coloured, as the MCHC is normal. Abnormally small red cells, or *microcytes*, occur in all forms of anaemia, but in certain types they preponderate so that the average size of the cells is diminished; the anaemia is then called *microcytic*.

Erythrocytes of irregular shape and usually small, known as *poikilocytes*, may occur in any severe anaemia (Fig. 16.23). Their number is not in proportion to the severity of the anaemia, and while their presence is of no absolute diagnostic importance they are usually a striking feature in pernicious anaemia and may appear even before the anaemia is pronounced. They occur also in other anaemias. For example, in certain disorders of small blood vessels, e.g. microangiopathic haemolytic anaemia and malignant hypertension (p. 416), triangular, helmet-shaped or *burr cells* may be numerous in the circulation. The term *irregularly contracted red cell* has now become popular to describe these poikilocytes, which are believed to result from mechanical damage in the abnormal vessels. They are frequently found along with obvious red cell fragments (*schistocytes*).

Another pathological variation is that the erythrocytes may be thicker than normal while their diameter is reduced and their volume is unchanged. They thus tend towards a globular shape and the term *spherocytosis* is applied. Characteristically this is associated with haemolytic anaemia and acholuric jaundice (p. 406). Other morphological abnormalities are associated with inborn abnormalities of haemoglobin structure, e.g. (*a*) the sickle form assumed by de-oxygenated cells containing Hb-S (p. 408), (*b*) the abnormally thin cells which sometimes have a central area of thickening (*target cells*) found in thalassaemia and other haemoglobinopathies (p. 409). In *hereditary elliptocytosis* the majority of the erythrocytes are oval, but in most instances this is a harmless trait; occasionally a mild haemolytic anaemia is present. The

The normal haemoglobins. The globular protein globin is composed of two pairs of coiled polypeptide chains. To each chain a haem group containing an atom of iron is attached, the whole forming a molecule of haemoglobin. The amino-acid sequence in the polypeptide chains determines the type of haemoglobin. Four different polypeptide chains occur normally and have been named α, β, γ, δ. The normal haemoglobins they form consist of two pairs of chains which may be represented as in Fig. 16.3.

Haemoglobinopathies result from abnormalities in the synthesis of the globin fraction due to *gene mutation*, the haem groups being normal. Usually these mutations cause an abnormality in the amino-acid sequence of a peptide chain so that an abnormal

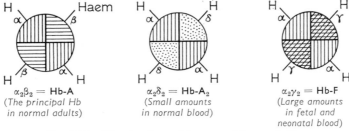

$\alpha_2\beta_2$ = Hb-A
(*The principal Hb in normal adults*)

$\alpha_2\delta_2$ = Hb-A$_2$
(*Small amounts in normal blood*)

$\alpha_2\gamma_2$ = Hb-F
(*Large amounts in fetal and neonatal blood*)

FIG. 16.3.—The structure of the normal haemoglobins.

genes for the trait appear to be carried on the same chromosome pair as those for the Rh blood group. (Non-hereditary elliptocytosis occasionally occurs in association with myelofibrosis.)

Variations in haemoglobin content. Reduction in the amount of circulating haemoglobin constitutes anaemia; this may be the result either of diminution in the numbers of circulating red cells or of the amount of haemoglobin within them or of both. For example, in pernicious anaemia, reduction in the numbers of red cells is the cause of the anaemia; the increase in size of the individual cells does not compensate for this. In the hypochromic anaemias of iron-deficiency states, on the other hand, the anaemia is due chiefly to reduction in the haemoglobin content of the cells, as a result both of lowered concentration and reduced size of cells (but some diminution in cell numbers is also present); accordingly the MCHC is lowered, e.g. to 25 per cent or less, and the MCH is also low. When the MCHC is greatly reduced, the cells in films show red staining only at the periphery, giving the so-called ring-staining, but there are so many possible artefacts that this criterion, unless gross, is quite unreliable and should not be used as an indication of the haemoglobin content of the cells.

haemoglobin, e.g. Hb-S (see p. 408), is produced. In classical (β-chain) thalassaemia, however, a common form of haemoglobinopathy, no abnormal haemoglobin is present as the mutation affects not the chemical composition of the peptides but their *rate of synthesis*, which is reduced.

Of the *abnormal* haemoglobins the best known are those designated S, C, D and E where the β chain contains an abnormal amino-acid sequence. By 1970 over a hundred variants had been recognised. The effect on the blood of a haemoglobinopathy, however caused, is interference with the synthesis of haemoglobin so that the marrow output falls and anaemia results. The cells have a reduced survival time in the circulation and the anaemia therefore is partly due to increased blood destruction. These defects in haemoglobin formation are hereditary and are especially marked in the homozygote while the heterozygote may even be asymptomatic (see p. 409).

Haemoglobins differ in their electrophoretic mobility, solubility, resistance to alkali denaturation, and these features, together with chromatography, are used in their identification. Thus fetal haemoglobin (Hb-F) has long been known to differ from adult haemoglobin (Hb-A) in these respects and its resistance to alkali-denaturation provides a method of estimation. Hb-F begins to be replaced by Hb-A before birth and the latter, together with Hb-A$_2$, accounts for over 99 per cent of the haemoglobin normally present by the end of infancy. In the adult less than 0·4 per cent of Hb-F is found normally but increases occur not only in the haemoglobinopathies but in other blood disorders such as pernicious anaemia and chronic myeloid leukaemia.

Polychromasia and reticulocytes. If a film of normal blood is stained with a Romanowsky stain (a combination of a basic and an acid dye such as Leishman's stain or Giemsa's or Wright's stain), practically all the erythrocytes are purely eosinophilic (*normochromic*). In certain conditions, however, in addition to the eosinophilia a proportion of the erythrocytes show a slight bluish-violet tint (basophilia) and the term *polychromasia* or *polychromatophilia* is applied to this double staining. These are young cells, which have recently lost their nuclei, but still retain some of the basophilic RNA which is abundant in the early erythroblast and is concerned in haemoglobin synthesis. Such cells become numerous when there is increased output from the bone marrow, for example, after haemorrhage, haemolysis, or in response to treatment. As they mature in the circulation the polychromasia gradually disappears and they become normochromic. The young erythrocytes tend on the whole to be slightly larger than those thoroughly mature.

By supravital staining with certain dyes, cresyl blue being most frequently used, any basophil substance remaining in the erythrocytes is precipitated or condensed within the cells as a sharply stained skein or reticulum, hence such corpuscles are called *reticulocytes*. When the basophil substance is abundant it can be recognised both as polychromatic staining and as reticulum, but when scanty, only as the latter. Accordingly enumeration of young corpuscles as reticulocytes is the easier and more exact method. The reticulum has nothing whatever to do with remains of the nucleus, and it is not visible within the cells by dark-ground or phase-contrast illumination until it has been precipitated by the action of the supravital basic dye (Fig. 16.4). Reticulocytes are normally present in a proportion of less than 1 per cent in males, but may occur up to 2 per cent in females after menstrual loss. Reticulocytosis in response to specific therapy, e.g. vitamin B_{12} in pernicious anaemia, provides valuable confirmation of the diagnosis. In all exact work the total number of reticulocytes per c.mm. should be calculated because their estimation as a percentage introduces the

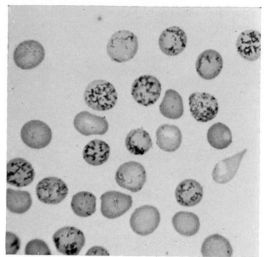

FIG. 16.4.—Blood film in haemolytic anaemia, showing numerous reticulocytes containing various amounts of reticulum. Supravital staining with cresyl blue. × 1000.

fluctuating figure of the red cell count which makes comparison of percentage figures meaningless.

Red cell inclusions. In *punctate basophilia* (Fig. 16.5), films stained by Leishman's stain show some red cells studded with minute basophilic granules. Punctate basophilia occurs especially in anaemias produced by toxic substances and when scanty can be most easily demonstrated in smears from the buffy coat. In chronic lead poisoning without anaemia its presence is sometimes of value in diagnosis, although a much less sensitive indication

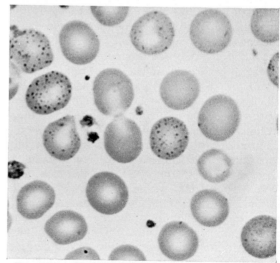

FIG. 16.5.—Blood film showing punctate basophilia. × 1250.

than lead or porphyrin estimations (p. 415). It occurs also in pernicious anaemia and may be produced experimentally by various haemolytic poisons. Punctate basophilia may be associated with polychromatophilia in the same red cell. It would seem that punctate basophilia is an abnormality produced in most cases by toxic action on the erythroblasts; as these show the condition as well as the erythrocytes. It results from clumping of RNA in the cell cytoplasm.

Pappenheimer bodies are small deeply basophilic granules, usually solitary and less than 1 μ, which give a positive Prussian blue reaction. Red cells containing them (siderocytes) appear most abundantly in the peripheral blood of adults after splenectomy but are present in some erythroblasts in normal marrow (sideroblasts).

Howell–Jolly bodies are granules of nuclear chromatin, 1–2 μ or more in diameter (Fig. 16.24), but which, if very small, resemble Pappenheimer bodies; they are, however, *iron-negative*. They are most common in the red cells in macrocytic anaemias but are found also in a variety of other blood diseases or following splenectomy in normal individuals.

Heinz bodies, composed of granules of denatured haemoglobin, appear in wet unstained preparations as irregularly-shaped, highly refractile granules, which often aggregate or coalesce under the red cell membrane. Not visible in Romanowsky-stained films, they are readily demonstrated in supravital methyl violet preparations (Fig. 16.15, p. 408). Also by using brilliant cresyl blue they are easily seen, though less well stained than reticulocytes. They are associated with the presence of methaemoglobin, and the blood in consequence tends to be brownish. Solitary very small Heinz bodies can be found in the peripheral blood of normal people if the spleen has been removed, is atrophied, or is congenitally absent. They are numerous in many forms of drug-induced haemolytic anaemia (p. 415) and in cases of "unstable haemoglobin" disease (p. 408) following splenectomy. It is believed that a normal function of the spleen is to remove intracellular inclusions as the erythrocytes pass from the red pulp into the sinusoids. This is known as the "pitting" function of the spleen (p. 448), and accounts for the appearance of the Heinz bodies in the peripheral blood in some diseases only after splenectomy.

The red cell inclusions of *malaria* are described on p. 414.

Presence of erythroblasts. The term *erythroblast* is used throughout to mean nucleated red blood cells of all types; normally in the adult they are present only in the marrow, but they appear in the blood in a variety of conditions.

Normoblasts are about the size of an ordinary red cell or a little larger, and have a single spherical nucleus which is condensed and thus stains very deeply. The nucleus shows a coarse network of deeply staining chromatin, or it may appear very dense and practically homogeneous in the pyknotic nuclei of the more mature erythroblasts (Fig. 16.1). The nucleus may be fragmented into two or more rounded pyknotic portions. A few normoblasts appear in the blood in various types of anaemia; the rapid appearance of a large number usually indicates specially active red cell regeneration.

Megaloblasts, as their name indicates, are larger; the nucleus is fairly large, is usually of less mature character, stains less deeply than the nucleus of a normoblast, and shows a somewhat granular or reticular structure (Fig. 16.27); in later forms it may be fragmented or pyknotic. The cytoplasm of megaloblasts often gives a polychromatophilic reaction of varying depth, and may show punctate basophilia; Howell–Jolly bodies are frequently present. In pernicious anaemia the presence of megaloblasts is an important feature, and at least a few are to be found as a rule, especially if smears of the buffy coat are examined; they are encountered similarly in the other types of macrocytic anaemia referred to later (p. 422). Although they are often associated with a few normoblasts their presence is certain proof of a profoundly abnormal type of haemopoiesis in the marrow. In anaemias in children, megaloblasts appear much more frequently in the circulating blood than they do in adults.

The presence of erythroblasts in the circulation does not always indicate special regenerative activity on the part of the bone marrow. In myeloid leukaemia, for example, erythroblasts of all types may be present in the blood, sometimes in large numbers along with other primitive cells. When the bones are extensively invaded by malignant tumour, erythroblasts may be present in the blood, and this may be due simply to disturbance of the marrow by the tumour, or to the premature escape of cells from sites of extramedullary haemopoiesis (p. 430). Again, in some very severe infections erythroblasts may appear in the blood, often accompanied by a few myelocytes.

Variations in the osmotic fragility of the erythrocytes. When red cells are placed in a hypotonic salt solution they become swollen and finally rupture, the haemoglobin diffusing out. With normal blood, the first trace of lysis is usually seen in a concentration of 0·42–0·46 per cent of sodium chloride; initial lysis occurring below 0·4 or above 0·5 per cent may be taken as abnormal, indicating diminished or increased fragility respectively; in some cases the abnormality may be detected only by careful quantitative methods. There is a close parallel between the thickness/diameter ratio of red cells and their osmotic fragility; increase of the ratio, as in the globular cells of hereditary spherocytosis, conferring increased fragility and conversely the reduced ratio of the thin cells in thalassaemia and other haemoglobinopathies conferring reduced fragility.

The *mechanical* fragility of erythrocytes (susceptibility to trauma) is much increased in certain states associated with cold agglutinins, and sometimes in lead poisoning.

Erythrocyte sedimentation rate. This is determined by placing the blood, to which anticoagulant has been added, in an upright calibrated tube and observing the rate of sedimentation of the red cells, as indicated by the length of the column of plasma after a given period of time. The range of normality depends on the details of technique, and is greater for women than men. Abnormal variations are chiefly in the direction of increased rapidity of sedimentation and are associated with increased concentration of plasma proteins, especially the globulins. The test has no specific value but has been found useful as an aid to detection of organic disease in the absence of physical signs, and notably as a prognostic aid in a particular condition, e.g. in tuberculosis or rheumatoid arthritis in which approximation of the rate to normal is taken as a favourable sign.

THE LEUKOCYTES

Introduction

The three classes of leukocytes in the blood—polymorphs (granulocytes), monocytes and lymphocytes—differ in their precursor cells, their morphology, and in their function. The three types of polymorphs—neutrophil, eosinophil and basophil—originate in the bone marrow (p. 126). The neutrophil polymorphs, as already explained in Chapter 2, are concerned in inflammatory reactions, and their chief function is the phagocytosis and digestion of micro-organisms and other foreign materials, damaged tissue elements and dead cells. The monocytes of the blood are also phagocytic, and provide most of the macrophages at sites of inflammation; they belong to the reticulo-endothelial system, and originate from precursor cells in the reticulo-endothelial tissues, including the haemopoietic marrow. Disturbance of the functions of neutrophil polymorphs and monocytes, with consequent tissue injury, is a feature of certain types of hypersensitivity reaction (Chapter 5). The eosinophil polymorphs increase in the blood, and appear in the lesions, of patients with atopic hypersensitivity (p. 102) although their physiological role, like that of the basophil polymorphs, is largely unknown. The origins of lymphocytes and their essential functions in immune responses have been considered in Chapter 4.

Increase or decrease in the numbers of the leukocytes in disease can affect any or all of the different types; increase in the total number of leukocytes above 11,000 per c.mm. is termed *leukocytosis*, while diminution below 4,000 per c.mm. is termed *leukopenia*: to determine the *absolute numbers* of different types of leukocytes, it is necessary to determine the total number and also the proportion of different types by performing a *differential count* on a stained film. The normal range of numbers of the leukocytes in adults is given in Table 16.1.

Table 16.1.—The Normal Numbers of Leukocytes

	No. per c.mm. blood
Polymorphs	
neutrophil	2,500–7,500
eosinophil	40–440
basophil	0–100
Lymphocytes	1,500–3,500
Monocytes	200–800
Total	4,000–11,000

Changes in the Leukocytes in Disease States

Neutrophil polymorphs

Neutrophil[1] leukocytosis. An account of neutrophil leukocytosis, and the accompanying myeloid hyperplasia of the haemopoietic marrow, is given on pp. 124–7. The commonest cause is bacterial infection, which should always be suspected in a neutrophil leukocytosis of over 20,000 per c.mm., and may cause an increase to 50,000 per c.mm. Moderate rises may accompany tissue necrosis without infection, such as myocardial infarction, and occur within a few hours after a large haemorrhage, passing off within a day or two; acute haemolysis is also accompanied by a neutrophil leukocytosis, and drug reactions, e.g. to steroids, sometimes promote a leukocytosis.

Increased production of neutrophil polymorphs in the circumstances given above is a controlled response to a stimulus, and may be regarded as a physiological reaction on the part of the myelopoietic marrow. By contrast, the neutrophil leukocytosis which occurs in myeloid leukaemia and in some of the other myeloproliferative disorders (p. 429) is not a controlled response to a known stimulus, but is of neoplastic nature.

In any acute neutrophil leukocytosis, the proportion of young neutrophils in the blood increases (Fig. 16.6), and some myelocytes or metamyelocytes may be found. This was made use of in the *Arneth* and *Cooke–Ponder* counts, in which the proportions of cells judged, by their nuclear configuration, to be of different ages or degrees of maturity, was used to give an indication of the duration of the leukocytosis. These methods, which have been largely abandoned, are based on the increasing degree of nuclear segmentation as the neutrophil ages. Another change is diminution in the amount of alkaline phosphatase. In megaloblastic anaemias, there is a "shift to the right" in the Arneth count, etc., i.e. an increase in the proportion of cells with hypersegmented nuclei, but simple observation of the unusually large hypersegmented neutrophils (macropolycytes, p. 418) is adequate to establish this feature.

Toxic granulation. In severe infections and toxic states the young polymorphonuclear leukocytes entering the circulation may show morphological evidence of damage; their cytoplasm contains deeply staining granules showing abnormal variations in size, and giving a poor oxidase reaction, and their nuclei fail to undergo the normal degrees of segmentation. It is likely that there is impairment of the functional capacity of such cells, which are termed *staff cells*, and their presence is indicative of severe toxaemia. Cell injury of greater degree results in failure of production of polymorphs, and leukopenia is thus a grave sign when associated with severe infection by pyogenic bacteria.

Neutrophil leukopenia (neutropenia). The term leukopenia means diminution in the number of circulating leukocytes below the normal limit of 4000 per c.mm.; as the neutrophil polymorphs constitute so high a proportion of the leukocytes, it is for practical purposes synonymous with neutropenia. It occurs both as an isolated haematological feature and also as part of a reduction of all cell types in the blood (pancytopenia).

Neutropenia has already been mentioned in typhoid fever and virus infections. It may occur also in overwhelmingly severe infections by bacteria of a type which usually promote a leukocytosis, for example in pneumococcal pneumonia in alcoholics, and absence of leukocytosis or leukopenia are then of grave significance. Leukopenia is caused by certain toxic chemicals which depress leukopoiesis, and in various blood diseases as part of a general failure of haemopoiesis and pancytopenia. In anaphylactic shock (p. 99) marked leukopenia may develop very rapidly, due apparently to aggregation of leukocytes in the capillaries of the lungs and other internal organs, and bacteraemic (endotoxic) shock (p. 189) may also be accompanied by leukopenia.

Since leukopenia usually represents a deficiency of granular leukocytes, it may be called *agranulocytosis*, but this term is generally restricted to the specially severe form, with consequent infections, described overleaf.

---

[1] The term "neutrophil" was originally applied by Ehrlich in view of the reactions given by certain mixed stains. With the eosin-containing stains now ordinarily used a faintly acidophil reaction is given by the granules of the neutrophil leukocytes, though the colour is not quite of the same tint as that of the granules of the eosinophil leukocytes, the granules of which are also much coarser.

Agranulocytosis: malignant neutropenia. In this formerly common condition there is a marked neutropenia. The erythrocytes and the platelets are not usually affected. It is especially associated with a severe acute inflammation of the fauces and gums, which may be accompanied by intense lymphadenitis and be followed by gangrene—*agranulocytic angina*. This condition occurs more commonly in women than in men, and has a high mortality, but subacute and relapsing or cyclical cases are also encountered. Examination of the marrow has shown in most cases an almost complete absence of polymor-

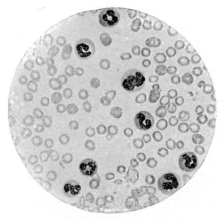

FIG. 16.6.—Blood film: neutrophil leukocytosis. × 400.

phonuclears and sometimes also a great diminution of myelocytes. As a rule myeloblasts are readily found, but sometimes even they are unduly scanty.

The abnormally low leukocyte count precedes the severe infection of the throat or other region, and a very important fact is that in most cases the condition has followed the administration of various drugs. A large number of different drugs have now been implicated, including barbiturates, sulphonamides, dinitrophenol, gold, sanacrysin. Amidopyrine and related compounds were formerly often responsible and their use has been largely discontinued. Thiouracil, used in the treatment of hyperthyroidism, gives rise to various degrees of agranulocytosis in about 2 per cent of cases. In large dose, many compounds may depress the marrow, but agranulocytosis is more often the result of the development of hypersensitivity to a particular compound, subsequent administration of even a small dose then inducing the condition. It may not always be

possible to trace the offending sensitising drug, but it is now regarded as improbable that the disease ever occurs spontaneously. The drug appears to become attached in some way to the proteins of the leukocytes and thus gives rise to a new complex or conjugate with antigenic properties. The resulting antibodies, in the presence of the conjugated antigen (i.e. when a further dose of the drug has been administered), react with the drug-modified leukocytes and their more mature precursors in the marrow, leading to their destruction either by the cytotoxic action of complement or by phagocytosis. With so many new synthetic drugs introduced into therapeutics the danger of sensitisation must constantly be borne in mind, and it is noteworthy that the haemopoietic system is often the first to show evidence of unwelcome toxicity by the occurrence of neutropenia, thrombocytopenia or anaemia, or a combination of these results, viz. pancytopenia. Not only the mature elements, but also the earlier precursors may be affected, although as a rule less severely; consequently there is a *relative deficiency* of later forms in the marrow, and so the appearances of maturation arrest may be simulated. When the granular leukocytes are greatly diminished as part of a general failure of the marrow, e.g. in aplastic anaemia or advanced myeloid leukaemia, similar acute infections are apt to follow: this may be called *symptomatic agranulocytosis*.

The presence of myelocytes. The appearance of these cells in the blood has an important clinical significance. In addition to myeloid leukaemia, where their presence in large numbers along with myeloblasts is a prominent feature, they are found occasionally in pernicious anaemia in small numbers. In the anaemia accompanying secondary carcinoma of the bone marrow and in myelofibrosis, myelocytes may be found in relatively large numbers, as may also nucleated red cells (p. 429), and the term leukoerythroblastosis is then applied. A few myelocytes may be found also in some very severe infections.

Functional deficiency of neutrophil polymorphs. The protective function of neutrophils against micro-organisms is essential to life and health. Infections result not only from agranulocytosis, in which the number of neutrophils is greatly reduced, but also in a group of uncommon conditions in which the neutrophils are functionally defective. In some of these conditions, the abnormality appears to be intrinsic. Thus in *chronic granulomatous disease of childhood* the neutrophils have been shown to have an enzyme defect and as a result they lack the capacity to destroy phagocytosed bacteria. The disease is transmitted by a gene defect on the X chromosome, and so, like haemophilia, affects males; female carriers have been shown histochemically to have in their blood a mixture of normal and defective neutrophils, which supports the Lyonisation hypothesis.* From early childhood, affected males suffer from protracted infections, with extensive abscess formation and granulation, even from bacteria of low pathogenicity.

Another example is the *Chediak–Higashi syndrome*, in which there is an abnormality of lysosomes affecting many types of cell, including the neutrophil polymorphs. The abnormal lysosomes enclose and digest portions of the cytoplasm, giving rise to large cytoplasmic inclusions visible in the neutrophils by light microscopy. The condition is transmitted as an autosomal recessive character and gives rise to recurrent infections: other variable features include leukopenia, defective pigmentation, neuropathies, lymph-node enlargement and hepato-splenomegaly, and malignant reticuloses commonly supervene. There are several other conditions, all rare, in this group, and others in which impaired neutrophil function is attributable to deficiency of a factor normally present in the plasma.

Pelger anomaly. This is a genetically-determined morphological curiosity of the nuclei of the granulocytes, which fail to become fully segmented as they mature, two lobes being the maximum. The abnormality is transmitted as a Mendelian dominant factor, and the heterozygous condition has an incidence of the order of 1 in 10,000: it is apparently not associated with susceptibility to infections or other harmful effects. A similar abnormality occurs in rabbits and dogs, where the homozygous condition is accompanied by skeletal and other deformities incompatible with life. The homozygous condition is unknown in man.

Eosinophil leukocytes

Eosinophil leukocytosis resembles neutrophil leukocytosis in being evoked by certain stimuli which act by increasing the cellular output of the marrow. Just as neutrophil leukocytosis occurs in pyogenic infections, so eosinophil leukocytosis is observed in these conditions which are characterised by infiltration of the tissues with eosinophils. The factors responsible for this local and general increase in eosinophils are not understood. It occurs in the following conditions.

(*a*) In certain chronic skin diseases, such as dermatitis herpetiformis, urticaria, psoriasis, etc., eosinophilia of moderate degree is usually present. An increase of eosinophils often observed in scarlet fever probably belongs to the same category.

(*b*) In infestation with certain animal parasites, e.g. ankylostoma, filariae, trichina spiralis, bilharzia, echinococcus, the increase is often very marked; this is especially the case with nematodes, the eosinophils in ankylostomiasis sometimes reaching 3000 per c.mm. or 40 per cent of the total (Fig. 16.7). The examination of the

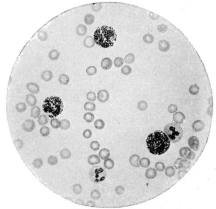

Fig. 16.7.—Eosinophil leukocytosis in ankylostomiasis; three eosinophil and two neutrophil leukocytes are shown. × 400.

blood in such cases has accordingly diagnostic importance.

(*c*) In atopic hypersensitivity reactions (p. 99) such as asthma and hay fever, eosinophilia is usually present, and is related to the local emigration of eosinophils in the tissues. It is possible that eosinophilia in skin diseases is, in part at least, also due to hypersensitivity, and also the eosinophilia of polyarteritis nodosa. The functions of the eosinophil leukocyte, and the part they play in the conditions noted above, are unknown, in spite of much experimental investigation. There is, however, some evidence sug-

* This postulates that the inactive X chromosome represented by the sex chromatin of females' cells, can be *either* of the X chromosomes, selection being random in each individual cell.

gesting that they may antagonise the phlogistic effects of histamine.

Further, in some cases of malignant disease involving the bone marrow, a considerable degree of eosinophilia has been observed. In chronic myeloid leukaemia also there is often an increase of eosinophils, along with the other types of granular cells, and eosinophil myelocytes may appear in the circulating blood.

Eosinophil leukopenia. Diminution in the eosinophils is a practically constant response to increased secretion of adrenocorticotrophic hormone and of adrenal glucocorticoids; counting the eosinophils has accordingly been employed as a method of estimating the hormonal response to various abnormal conditions, and as a test of adrenocortical function in response to a test dose of ACTH in cases suspected of Addison's disease. The eosinophil count, however, normally shows pronounced variations from person to person and also at different times of day, and adrenocortical function is much more accurately assessed by biochemical methods. A fall in the eosinophil count is often present in cases of acute infections with neutrophil leukocytosis; in lobar pneumonia, for example, eosinophils are practically absent, as a rule, during the period of fever.

The basophil leukocytes

The granules of these cells usually give a purplish metachromatic reaction, and the cells have been known as *"mast-cells"* but this term should no longer be applied because the true mast-cells in the tissues are of a different nature. The roles of the mast-cell in atopic hypersensitivity (p. 101) and also as a secretor of heparin have already been discussed. In chronic myeloid leukaemia basophils sometimes take part in the leukocyte increase and basophil myelocytes may also appear. In various chronic wasting diseases, an increase of basophils in the blood may be present occasionally, but there is no condition known which regularly calls forth a basophil leukocytosis.

Lymphocytes

Recent advances in our understanding of the life cycle and immunological functions of the lymphocyte have been described in Chapter 4. The picture is far from complete, but it is ap-

parent that the lymphocytes in the blood represent at least two functionally different populations, each being concerned, however, with immune responses and reactions; other functions of the lymphocytes, if they exist, are unknown.

Lymphocytosis. Normally the proportion of lymphocytes in the child is higher than in the adult; perhaps in relation to the relative size of the thymus (p. 89), the number is highest shortly after birth and gradually falls in subsequent years; allowance for age must accordingly be made in interpreting lymphocyte counts. As diminution in the number of leukocytes is generally due to a fall in the polymorphonuclears, it is accompanied by a percentage increase of the lymphocytes, and this is termed a *relative* lymphocytosis; it occurs in many virus infections and in the various conditions of leukopenia mentioned above, pernicious anaemia, kala-azar, etc. A true lymphocytosis, that is, an actual increase in the number of lymphocytes per c.mm., also occurs but is less common. Lymphocytosis is a useful diagnostic feature in mild cases of whooping cough. In some cases of this disease, however, the number reaches 100,000 per c.mm. and the blood then presents temporarily a leukaemic appearance. Lymphocytosis also occurs in glandular fever, many of the cells being large and of abnormal appearance (p. 458). It is usually a marked feature in smallpox, especially in moderately severe cases where both the small and large lymphocytes are increased along with the monocytes. An actual increase of lymphocytes is often present in the secondary stage of syphilis, that is, at a time when there are numerous foci of infiltration by these cells, and is common also in myasthenia gravis (p. 810). The outstanding increase of lymphocytes, however, is in lymphatic leukaemia (p. 431), and an increased proportion of lymphocytes may sometimes be observed by a differential count to precede the actual rise in the leukocyte count.

Lymphopenia occurs irregularly in various miscellaneous conditions. In infancy, it is a cardinal feature of some immunological deficiency syndromes (p. 114), in which the near absence of lymphocytes from the blood and lymphoid tissues is associated with a fatal deficiency of the immunological mechanism. Severe lymphopenia results also from X-irradiation and use of cytotoxic drugs for immunosuppressive therapy or treatment of neoplasia.

Monocytes

The monocytes (Fig. 16.8) are circulating cells of the reticulo-endothelial system, and are capable of amoeboid movement and phagocytosis, i.e. they are macrophages (p. 47). There is evidence that the capacity of monocytes and tissue macrophages to destroy ingested bacteria is increased by a factor released by lymphocytes participating in delayed hypersensitivity reactions (p. 106), and they may also be of import-

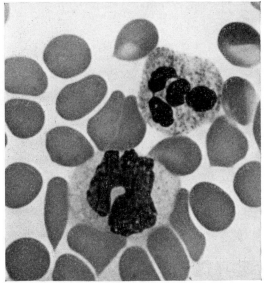

FIG. 16.8.—Monocyte in blood film. The monocyte (lower cell) is larger than a neutrophil polymorph (above), the cytoplasm is more finely granular and the nucleus larger, less condensed, and of irregular shape. × 1400.

ance in the transplant rejection reaction (p. 112).

Like the neutrophil polymorphs, monocytes migrate into inflammatory foci and phagocytose bacteria, damaged tissue elements, dead cells, etc., but they aggregate less rapidly than the polymorphs, and so are seen in increasing numbers in prolonged pyogenic infections, and in chronic inflammations of various types and causes. Monocytosis is commonly present in subacute bacterial endocarditis, and in undulant fever, and sometimes in systemic lupus erythematosus. In tuberculosis, serial studies on individual cases have shown that the numbers of lymphocytes and monocytes in the blood tend to be inversely proportional to one another, and there is some evidence that a high ratio accompanies healing and that a low ratio is associated with extension of the lesions. The monocytes are increased also in typhus and some other rickettsial diseases, and in certain protozoal infections, e.g. malaria, trypanosomiasis, and kala-azar, in which diseases there is no increase of the neutrophils. In chronic malaria, the presence of numerous monocytes is often a striking feature, and some of them may contain small granules of pigment (Fig. 16.21, p. 414).

The abnormal cells which appear in the blood in large numbers in some cases of *infectious mononucleosis* (glandular fever) resemble monocytes, although they are probably altered lymphocytes (p. 458). In *tetrachlorethane poisoning* there is sometimes a progressive increase in the monocytes up to 3–4,000.

The most remarkable example of monocytosis in relation to bacterial infection is attributable to a micro-organism known as *Listeria monocytogenes* recovered from an epizootic amongst rabbits. On experimental inoculation of rabbits these cells numbered, in extreme examples, fully 6000 per c.mm.

Monocytic leukaemia must always be considered in patients with monocytosis (p. 431).

BLOOD PLATELETS

Blood platelets are formed in the bone marrow from megakaryocytes (see Fig. 16.52, p. 445). The platelets are of great importance in blood coagulation (p. 162) by their contribution to thromboplastin formation. They also liberate on disintegration 5-hydroxytryptamine (serotonin), a pressor substance with marked vasoconstrictor properties. Variations in the number of platelets is of common occurrence. Increase is the rule in chronic diseases where there is leukocytosis, especially when associated with anaemia, e.g. malignant disease, chronic suppuration, etc. In acute leukocytosis, however, the number may be normal. Such increase of platelets may conveniently be called *thrombocytosis* and it has merely a symptomatic significance. In most of the anaemias where there is leukopenia the platelet count is reduced and may be markedly so, e.g. in pernicious anaemia, aplastic anaemia, and hypersplenism. In the early stages of chronic myeloid leukaemia the number may be very high; we have seen over 1,000,000 per c.mm. in one case, and similar high figures occur in polycythaemia vera. On the other hand, in the lymphatic and acute types of the disease, scarcity of platelets is the rule.

There are, however, conditions in which there is some fundamental abnormality in platelet formation. A very low count is a feature in one form of purpura—accordingly called thrombocytopenic purpura—which will be described later. There is a very rare disease in which the platelet count is very high, a count of over 3,000,000 per c.mm. having been observed (Fig. 16.9). This condition is associated with a tendency to thrombosis and haemorrhage, and is known as haemorrhagic thrombocythaemia. There is a great increase of megakaryocytes in the bone marrow and the disease is regarded by some as belonging to the myelo-proliferative disorders (p. 429).

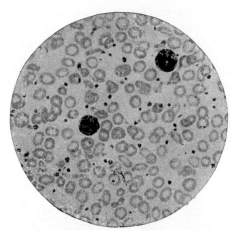

Fig. 16.9.—Blood in thrombocythaemia, showing great increase of platelets, regularly distributed. (The number was over 3,000,000 per c.mm.) × 500.

ANAEMIA

Definition and types of anaemia

Anaemia is defined as a reduction in the concentration of haemoglobin in the blood below the normal level, and is usually but not invariably accompanied by reduction in the number of red cells. Anaemia develops when the rate of regeneration fails to keep pace with destruction of red cells together with any loss from haemorrhage. Accordingly a simple classification of the anaemias can be made as follows:

Anaemia
A. Excessive loss or destruction
- haemorrhage = *post haemorrhagic*
- increased destruction = *haemolytic*

B. Failure of output
- defective haemopoiesis with marrow hyperplasia = *dyshaemopoietic*
- diminished volume of haemopoietic marrow = *hypoplastic* and *aplastic*

The cause of anaemia is often complex, more than one pathogenic mechanism being concerned; for example, in pernicious anaemia, which is due to lack of vitamin B_{12}, there is not only insufficient output of cells but the cells produced wear out too quickly, i.e. excessive destruction is also concerned. Also, hypochromic microcytic anaemia is frequently associated with chronic blood loss, with or without impaired absorption or inadequate intake of iron.

Effects of anaemia

The essential feature of anaemia, however brought about, is a reduction in the level of circulating haemoglobin. If severe, this impairs tissue oxygenation and several compensatory mechanisms operate to prevent this. Thus the haemoglobin releases an unusually high proportion of its oxygen to the tissues, and the plasma volume increases, although seldom enough to prevent a fall in the total blood volume. Of particular importance, however, are the cardiovascular adjustments which accompany anaemia. The stroke volume of the heart, and to a lesser extent the heart rate, increase to augment the cardiac output and the blood circulation time falls, thus increasing the rate of tissue perfusion. Many of the signs and symptoms of anaemia are related to these cardiovascular changes; for example the full bounding pulse, the cardiac systolic (haemic) murmurs, cardiac enlargement, palpitations, dyspnoea on exertion, engorgement of the neck veins and ankle oedema. In severe anaemia, cardiac failure of "high output" type becomes a serious risk; in these circumstances the transfusion of whole blood may, by increasing the load on the heart, precipitate cardiac decompensation, although this danger can be reduced by the slow administration of packed red cells. The maintenance of a hyperdynamic circulation entails increased cardiac demands for oxygen, which, in the presence of impaired tissue oxygenation, occasionally leads to myocardial hypoxia with angina, particularly in patients whose coronary arteries are already diseased. Other effects are more directly related to anaemia, especially tiredness, lassitude, dizziness, headache and paraesthesiae. Pallor of the organs and tissues is evident at operation or *post mortem*. Skin pallor is, however, often misleading, since factors

other than anaemia, and not always pathological, may bring this about; pallor of mucous membranes, especially of the eyelids or mouth, is usually a more reliable sign. Pyrexia and slight splenic enlargement may also be attributable to anaemia *per se*. The most constant morphological manifestation of the tissue hypoxia produced by anaemia is fatty change, often especially marked in the heart and the liver. The mechanism involved in this change is discussed elsewhere (p. 15); it should be mentioned, however, that fatty change in the myocardium, often visible to the naked eye at autopsy ("thrush-breast" heart), is an indication that the metabolism of the heart was in a critical state: this cannot be rapidly reversed by raising the haemoglobin level by pre-operative transfusion. Tissue hypoxia is probably the main stimulus to the release of the erythropoietin which occurs in most forms of anaemia, and to which the compensatory marrow hyperplasia in anaemia is due. Other tissue changes are, of course, often present, but in many instances are related more to the cause of anaemia, e.g. iron deficiency, vitamin B_{12} deficiency, than to anaemia itself, and these are discussed in the appropriate sections.

Post-haemorrhagic Anaemia

The restoration of the fluid part of the blood after haemorrhage has already been dealt with (p. 187); it leads, of course, to dilution of the blood with accompanying fall in the number of erythrocytes per c.mm. The first evidence of regeneration of red cells after a large haemorrhage is a progressive increase in the number of reticulocytes, and the degree of increase is an indication of haemopoietic activity. They show a varying degree of polychromasia in ordinary stained films. Along with them are often a few normoblasts, which, if there are repeated haemorrhages, may become fairly abundant. As regeneration becomes complete the reticulocytes gradually return to their normal level and normoblasts disappear. These changes are the results of proliferation of erythroblasts in the bone marrow, in which they form a larger proportion of the cells than normally (Fig. 16.10). A polymorphonuclear leukocytosis and thrombocytosis, both of moderate degree, appear within a few hours after haemorrhage; they pass off in two or three days, unless the haemorrhage is repeated. Loss of blood,

either acute or chronic, is by far the commonest cause of anaemia and should always be sought.

In certain conditions, e.g. severe epistaxis, repeated bleeding from gastric ulcer, piles, or tumours of various kinds, a *chronic* anaemia of severe iron-deficiency type may result (p. 424). In chronic post-haemorrhagic anaemia the number of red cells may occasionally fall to around one million per c.mm., but levels of $2-4 \times 10^6$ are more common. The red cells vary considerably in size, the smaller forms predominating; there may be a considerable number of poikilocytes, while a few normoblasts may be present. The red cells appear paler than normal, and frequently show ring staining, the MCHC being reduced to 25 per cent or so. The serum iron is lowered (under 70 μg/100 ml.) while the total iron-binding capacity is raised (over 320 μg/100 ml.). In severe and long-continued cases, the number of circulating platelets may rise substantially and there is an increased tendency to thrombosis; the spleen may enlarge slightly and even become palpable.

The process of regeneration after one or two

large hacmorrhages is relatively rapid provided there is the normal reserve of about 1000 mg. iron and half a million corpuscles per c.mm. may be added within a week. Acute loss of a pint of blood (540 ml.) is made good by the withdrawal of 270 mg. of iron from reserve and since the average mixed diet provides only about 4–5 mg. of available iron per day it may take over two months to replace this loss of reserve iron

is more rapid after haemolysis than after haemorrhage, due to the fact that in the former case iron and possibly other substances from the lysed cells are re-utilised. The importance of iron therapy in convalescence after haemorrhage is obvious.

"Secondary anaemia" results from a variety of diseases, usually chronic, in which the fault does not lie primarily in the haemo-

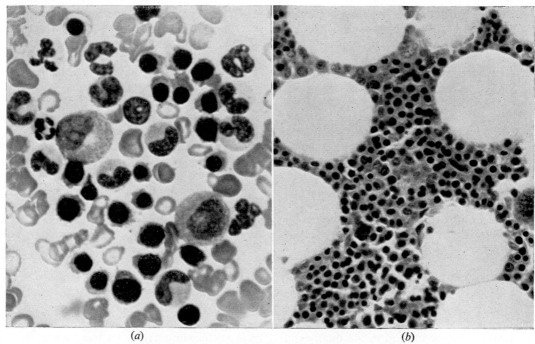

(a)   (b)

FIG. 16.10.—Erythroblastic reaction after haemorrhage.
(a) Smear of sternal marrow, showing numerous normoblasts at various stages of development, also myelocytes. × 1000.
(b) Section of sternal marrow five days after severe haemorrhage; abundant normoblasts encroaching on the fat spaces. × 500.

from the diet alone. When anaemia has existed for some time owing to repeated haemorrhages the marrow undergoes normoblastic hyperplasia, shown by a proportionate increase of the red marrow in the short and flat bones and also by an extension of the red marrow down the shafts of the long bones. Microscopically such marrow contains an increased proportion of early and late normoblasts.

After repeated or continued haemorrhages regeneration becomes slower because of exhaustion of the iron reserves, in spite of the greatly increased capacity for red-cell production in the hyperplastic marrow. Lack of iron thus restricts the output of red cells and such cells as are formed are small and inadequately filled with haemoglobin (see p. 424). Blood regeneration

poietic system. This is so common that the possibility of an anaemia being secondary should never be overlooked in diagnosis. Secondary anaemia is most often encountered in chronic infections, usually but not always suppurative (the "anaemia of infection"), connective tissue disease (especially rheumatoid arthritis), malignant disease, chronic renal and chronic hepatic disease. Anaemia of this type does not respond to haematinic therapy and is likely to improve only when the underlying disease process is cured or ameliorated.

Although the blood picture depends to some extent upon the nature of the underlying disease (see below), the red cells in secondary anaemia are either normochromic and normocytic or show minor degrees of hypochromia. A moderate reduction in the serum iron level is usual but, unlike simple iron deficiency, the total serum iron binding capacity is also reduced and stainable iron is abundant in the reticulo-endothelial cells of the bone marrow and elsewhere, indicating that there is failure of utilisation of iron. The reticulocyte count is usually normal except where haemolysis is a prominent feature, e.g. in the secondary haemolytic anaemia sometimes seen in Hodgkin's disease or other reticuloses. In chronic renal disease a moderate reticulocytosis often associated with the presence of distorted red cells (especially "burr cells", p. 390), is observed in severe cases; target cells (p. 391) and a tendency to macrocytosis may be seen in chronic hepatic disease even in the absence of folate or vitamin B_{12} deficiency and of megaloblastic transformation of the marrow. A neutrophilia and increase in the platelet count may be observed in infection but specific alterations in the white cells and platelets are otherwise uncommon in the absence of complicating factors.

The pathogenesis of secondary anaemia is not entirely clear and is likely to be multifactorial in any case. Blood loss is common and protein synthesis may be reduced by toxic marrow depression. Low grade haemolysis is often present, less commonly blood destruction may be severe. In many cases there is obvious interference with the utilisation of iron and then sideroblasts may sometimes be increased but more commonly the iron accumulates in the reticulo-endothelial cells and not in the red cell precursors. In chronic renal disease it is suspected that the retention of waste products may reduce marrow output while a microangiopathic haemolytic element (see p. 416) may also contribute to the anaemia. Erythropoietin, the hormonal stimulus to red cell formation in the bone marrow (p. 389), is largely formed in the kidney and renal damage may impair its production or release, interfering with the regenerative capacity of the marrow. It is thus evident that secondary anaemia is of complex etiology and that its treatment is clearly that of the causative disease. Drug-induced anaemia is dealt with on p. 426.

Haemolytic Anaemias

The haemolytic anaemias comprise a group in which there is an increased rate of destruction of red cells so that the average red cell survival time is reduced below the normal range of 100–120 days. Variations in the clinical and pathological features depend upon the severity and rapidity of blood destruction, and upon the nature of the causal agent; in all cases, however, there is a compensatory increase in the rate of red cell production, and these two concurrent processes lead to certain changes common to all varieties, irrespective of the cause.

The general features of a haemolytic anaemia may thus with advantage be described before the characteristics which distinguish the individual members of the group are discussed.

The use of radioisotopes ^{51}Cr and ^{59}Fe. Radioisotopes can provide precise data about the fate of the red cells, including both their survival time and the chief sites of destruction. By tagging a small quantity of the patient's red cells with a minute dose of radioactive chromium (^{51}Cr) and returning them to the circulation the fate of the labelled cells can be closely followed. Estimation of the rate of dis-

appearance of the isotope from subsequent blood samples measures the red cell survival time. The "$T\frac{1}{2}$" is the time taken for the initial level of radioactivity to decrease by half and is normally about 25 days. The $T\frac{1}{2}$ value is much shorter than the true mean red cell survival (110 days) due to several factors, including leakage of the ^{51}Cr from the red cells while they are still viable. A reduced $T\frac{1}{2}$ in the absence of blood loss provides conclusive evidence of an increased rate of blood destruction, confirming a diagnosis of haemolytic anaemia. This investigation may be supplemented by surface counting with a scintillation counter over organs such as liver, spleen and bone marrow, to obtain valuable information about the site of blood destruction. A high splenic/liver ratio of radioactivity in the case of a haemolytic anaemia indicates an increased rate of splenic sequestration of red cells and the likelihood that splenectomy may be beneficial. Radioactive ^{59}Fe is much used in studies of iron metabolism and erythropoiesis. The efficiency of intestinal absorption and the incorporation of iron in the haemoglobin molecule can be estimated and, by surface counting, the activity of erythropoiesis in different sites, e.g. medullary and extramedullary, can be assessed.

O

I. The changes resulting from increased destruction of red cells

If destruction outpaces regeneration the consequence is an anaemia in which the fall in haemoglobin is directly proportional to the diminution in number of the red cells; the MCHC therefore remains normal. The mechanism of normal destruction of effete red cells is not fully understood; *in vitro* experiments have shown that when corpuscles are broken up by micro-dissection, the haemoglobin is retained by the cell fragments and does not diffuse into the plasma. It may be that in the normal process of wear and tear the red cells eventually break up into fragments which are then removed from the blood by the phagocytic cells of the reticulo-endothelial system especially in the spleen, bone-marrow and liver. In some pathological forms of increased blood destruction, e.g. black-water fever, incompatible blood transfusion and poisoning with haemolytic chemicals such as arseniuretted hydrogen, lysis of the corpuscles occurs in the circulation and free haemoglobin appears in the plasma, where it is at once bound to the plasma haptoglobins (p. 203). If the haemolysis is of sufficient severity to saturate the plasma haptoglobins some of the released haemoglobin is rapidly converted into methae-malbumin, whilst the remainder appears in the urine—haemoglobinuria. After incompatible transfusion, this may be associated with renal damage and acute renal failure (p. 724). The renal threshold for haemoglobin is thus determined to a considerable extent by the amount of haptoglobin present in the plasma. In other conditions, e.g. hereditary spherocytosis, excessive blood destruction is not associated with release of free haemoglobin into the plasma in detectable amounts, although the reduction in haptoglobin levels clearly indicates that this has occurred; in such conditions, the blood destruction results not from intravascular haemolysis, but mainly from phagocytosis of large numbers of red cells in the spleen and other organs. It is probable that there is a fundamental difference between those forms of increased breakdown in which haemoglobinuria occurs and those in which it is usually absent; in the latter splenectomy is likely to be beneficial, whereas in the former group it is useless.

Whatever the mechanism of increased red cell destruction, any haemoglobin not excreted is broken down by reticulo-endothelial cells into haemosiderin and haemobilirubin (i.e. unconjugated bilirubin). The fate of these two pigments is discussed on pp. 201 *et seq.*, but it may be recalled here that the haemobilirubin passes into the blood stream, rendering the plasma yellow and giving an indirect positive van den Bergh reaction. If, as frequently happens, the rate of formation of haemobilirubin exceeds the ability of the liver to conjugate it with glucuronic acid and to excrete it into the bile the concentration of haemobilirubin in the plasma rises; when it exceeds 3 mg. per 100 ml. jaundice becomes clinically apparent, but the haemobilirubin, being bound to plasma albumin, does not pass into the glomerular filtrate, and the condition is accordingly known as *acholuric jaundice*. Although the liver is unable to keep pace with the excessive bilirubin production, there is nevertheless a great increase in the bilirubin content of the bile, and in chronic haemolytic anaemia pure pigment stones are commonly formed in the gallbladder. The increased amount of bilirubin passing into the intestine is associated with reabsorption of an increased amount of pigment in the form of stercobilinogen which the liver may be unable to excrete, consequently it is excreted by the kidney as urobilinogen. Increased excretion of stercobilinogen and urobilinogen in the faeces and urine provides reliable evidence that increased red cell destruction is taking place, and the quantitative estimation of the daily excretion of these substances is sometimes helpful in determining the nature of an anaemia, when the amount excreted is related to the total red cell mass.

The haemosiderin derived from excessive destruction of red cells is stored in various organs, notably in the spleen where it accumulates in the reticulum cells and macrophages of the pulp, and also occasionally in the endothelial cells of the sinuses; in longstanding cases the reticular and collagenous framework of the organ, including the elastic laminae, may be saturated with iron in a patchy distribution. In the liver, haemosiderin accumulates in both Kupffer cells and hepatic parenchyma, in the marrow in the endothelial and reticulum cells, while in the kidney the cells of the primary convoluted tubules may become impregnated (Fig. 16.30). If the haemolytic process diminishes, then the excess of stored iron is largely re-used in the synthesis of haemoglobin, and in such a remission there may be comparatively little iron in the organs.

Increased red cell destruction, when acute, is usually accompanied by fever and jaundice, with enlargement and tenderness of the spleen and neutrophil leukocytosis.

II. The changes associated with increased red cell production

As already mentioned, it is a characteristic of haemolytic anaemias that there is hyperplasia of the bone marrow, with increased production of red cells. This rapid replacement results in an increased number of young red cells in the blood; in a Leishman-stained film many of the erythrocytes show polychromasia, and there may be both early and late normoblasts. Reticulocytes are always increased, often up to 20 per cent or more (Fig. 16.4). In any untreated case of anaemia such a reticulocytosis is strong presumptive evidence of a haemolytic process provided blood loss can be excluded. The MCHC is not diminished and the anaemia is usually of normocytic and normochromic type, although in severe chronic cases there is a distinct tendency for the blood to become macrocytic, perhaps because the requirements of folic acid exceed the available supply. The red cell precursors commonly show *partial megaloblastic transformation*, also termed *macronormoblastic erythropoiesis* (Fig. 16.11).

The marrow shows an erythroblastic hyperplasia and may extend down the shafts of the long bones while the medullary cavity may eventually become widened with loss of bony trabeculae and thinning of the cortical bone. In extreme cases of long duration, extramedullary haemopoiesis occurs in the spleen, and extra-osseous masses of haemopoietic tissue have been found under the pleura in the costo-vertebral angles.

Types of haemolytic anaemia

Although recent advances in our understanding of the metabolism of glucose by red cells has helped to clarify the modes of red cell destruction, the causation of the different types of haemolytic anaemia is by no means fully understood, and classification is therefore tentative.

Reduced red cell survival time is the essential feature of haemolytic anaemia; it may be either the result of an intrinsic abnormality in the red cells, or of an extrinsic haemolytic mechanism. The distinction is based on red cell survival times in cross transfusion experiments (Fig. 16.12). Such methods are not usually required for routine hospital diagnosis as

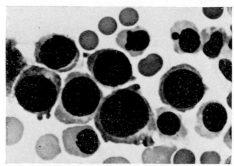

FIG. 16.11.—Marrow smear in hereditary spherocytosis, showing normoblastic hyperplasia. × 900.

A cluster of erythroblasts, ranging from early basophil cells to small pyknotic normoblasts; also spherocytes.

the various different forms of the disease present other distinctive characteristics. However, the availability of radioactive chromium (^{51}Cr) as a means of labelling red cells has brought the red cell survival time into general use as a diagnostic measure. For descriptive purposes, the following subdivisions may be made:

CLASSIFICATION OF HAEMOLYTIC ANAEMIA

I. Intrinsic defects in the red cells

A. *Genetically determined*
(1) Hereditary spherocytosis (familial acholuric jaundice).
(2) Hereditary elliptocytosis.
(3) Hereditary non-spherocytic haemolytic anaemia (a group of conditions including (4) and (5) below).
(4) Glucose-6-phosphate dehydrogenase deficiency.
(5) The haemoglobinopathies.

B. *Acquired*
(1) Paroxysmal nocturnal haemoglobinuria.
(2) Dyshaemopoietic anaemias.

II. Abnormal extra-erythrocytic haemolytic mechanisms

A. *Auto-antibodies to red cells*
(1) Auto-immune haemolytic anaemia of "warm" antibody type.
(2) Auto-immune haemolytic anaemia of "cold" antibody type.

B. Iso-antibodies to red cells

    (1) Erythroblastosis fetalis.

    (2) Transfusion reactions.

C. Parasitic invasion of red cells

    (1) Malaria.

    (2) Oroya fever.

D. Haemolytic toxins and chemicals

    (1) Bacterial toxins, e.g. *Cl. welchii, Strep. pyogenes.*

    (2) Chemicals, e.g. phenacetin, phenylhydrazine, potassium chlorate, arseniuretted hydrogen, lead.

    (3) Vegetable poisons, e.g. favism.

E. Mechanical damage to red cells

    (1) March haemoglobinuria.

    (2) Microangiopathic haemolytic anaemia.

NOTE: The groups and types of haemolytic anaemia listed above are not entirely independent. For example, subjects with glucose-6-phosphate dehydrogenase deficiency are abnormally susceptible to haemolysis by various chemicals.

I.A. Genetically determined red cell defects

(1) Hereditary spherocytosis (familial acholuric jaundice). This is a common type of chronic haemolytic anaemia occurring in most parts of the world. It results from a genetically determined abnormality of the red cells which is transmissible by either parent, generally affects more than one member of the family, and can be traced in more than one generation. The essential abnormality lies in excessive permeability of the red cell membrane to sodium ions (p. 8). Ageing of the red cells is accompanied by reduction in glycolytic activity, and as this provides the energy to pump out excess of sodium, the cells swell because of sodium retention and concomitant uptake of water; they become microspherocytic, and undergo sequestration mainly in the spleen. It may be that the defect is accentuated in the splenic red pulp, where the amount of plasma and therefore of glucose is diminished, and so intrasplenic destruction of the cells results. Such a mechanism would certainly account for the remarkably beneficial effects of splenectomy in this disease. Microspherocytes are also believed to be less resistant to the action of lysolecithin in the spleen than are normal cells. They may be identified in a blood film as small cells which, owing to their increased thickness and full haemoglobin saturation, stain intensely and do not exhibit the central pallor of the normal erythrocyte (Fig. 16.13). This spherocytic shape is

I. Intrinsic red cell defects

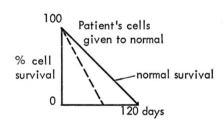

and II. Path. haemolytic mechanisms

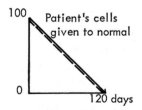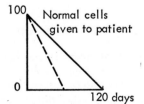

FIG. 16.12.—The survival of red cells in cross-transfusion experiments in haemolytic anaemia. The continuous lines indicate the rate of disappearance of transfused red cells from normal donors to normal recipients. The interrupted lines show the rates of disappearance of transfused red cells in the stated circumstances.

responsible for a diminished resistance to hypotonic solutions, for such cells cannot swell to the same extent without rupturing as can normal biconcave red cells. Spherocytosis is much less apparent in the reticulocyte than in the more mature forms.

The disease is usually detected by a yellowish tinge of skin and conjunctivae in the early years of life, although sometimes not until later. There may be at first little disturbance of health, but later there are exacerbations in which red cell destruction is sufficiently severe to produce a moderate degree of anaemia

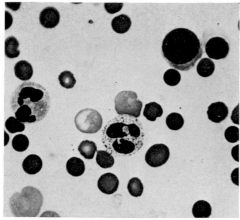

FIG. 16.13.—Blood film in hereditary spherocytosis. Note the small, densely staining spherocytes. × 650.

with acholuric jaundice, while increased red cell production is reflected in an abnormally high proportion of reticulocytes in the blood, perhaps 20 per cent or more; the leukocytes and platelets show little change. The disease usually pursues a fluctuating course; remissions may occur during which jaundice is absent, the red cells are little reduced in number, and reticulocytes only slightly increased: acute exacerbations are, however, common and may be fulminating; such a crisis is marked by fever and leukocytosis, a rapidly increasing jaundice, profound fall in the red cell count, and increase in the size of the spleen which is the chief site of red cell destruction. Hypoplastic crises also occur, in which reticulocytes are virtually absent from the peripheral blood and the marrow contains chiefly early basophil normoblasts. It is uncertain whether this signifies a degree of "maturation arrest" or whether it is due to simultaneous destruction of the more mature nucleated red cells in the marrow. Survival from

such an exacerbation is followed by reticulocytosis, sometimes amounting to 80 per cent or even more of the total red cells with numerous normoblasts both early and late, and thereafter the red cell count gradually rises.

It has been shown that when cases of hereditary spherocytic anaemia are transfused with normal blood, the transfused cells have a normal life span, whereas if blood from such a patient is transfused into an individual not suffering from the disease, the transfused cells are destroyed with abnormal rapidity (Fig. 16.12). Excessive osmotic fragility of the red cells may be found in other, apparently healthy, members of the family, and such individuals may later suffer from fulminating haemolytic attacks, sometimes precipitated by pregnancy, by minor infections, or occurring without known cause. In the absence of a significant family history, the condition may be mistaken for the other relatively common type of chronic haemolytic anaemia, which is due to auto-antibody (p. 411), but a negative Coombs' test helps to differentiate the two disorders.

The changes in the marrow and other organs are those found in any chronic haemolytic condition (see above) and the urine contains excess urobilinogen. Chronic ulceration of the skin of the leg sometimes accompanies the condition, and is resistant to treatment unless splenectomy is performed. The spleen is constantly enlarged, but does not often exceed 1400 g. and adhesions are usually absent. Microscopically, the pulp is distended with red cells, while the venous sinuses are somewhat collapsed (Fig. 16.14); the degree of iron storage depends on the rate of blood destruction at the time.

The essence of the disease is an increased destruction of abnormal red cells in the spleen, and the absence of haemoglobin and methaemalbumin from the plasma, even in a fulminating attack, indicates that intravascular haemolysis is not a feature of the condition although the plasma haptoglobins are much reduced: moreover, splenectomy leads to disappearance of the excessive red cell destruction almost at once: the number of red cells and the percentage of reticulocytes return to normal: these favourable effects are usually permanent, although the spherocytosis and increased fragility persist.

(2) **Hereditary elliptocytosis** presents a much less pronounced sequestration of cells in the spleen pulp

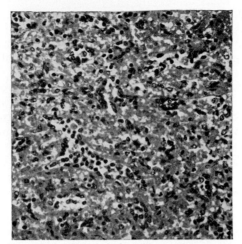

FIG. 16.14.—Spleen in hereditary spherocytosis.

The pulp is intensely congested and the sinuses are small and appear somewhat collapsed. × 230.

and the anaemia is usually mild. This defect exhibits genetic linkage with the Rh blood group genes.

(3) Hereditary non-spherocytic haemolytic anaemia. This is a general term applied to hereditary forms of haemolytic anaemia in which the osmotic fragility of the erythrocytes is normal. Two main etiological groups have been recognised. In one group, deficiency of different types of enzymes concerned in the metabolism of glucose is the fundamental abnormality which shortens the life span of the cells. The other is due to an *abnormal haemoglobin* of "unstable" type, of which again several different forms are known.

In one form of the enzyme deficiency type, an absence of pyruvate kinase is transmitted as a recessive character, the heterozygotes being recognisable by having only half the normal amount of the enzyme. In another type, the enzyme defect is a severe lack of glucose-6-phosphate dehydrogenase. Both these metabolic defects result in a reduced life span of the red cells, but there is no specific sequestration in the spleen and accordingly splenectomy is not usually therapeutically worthwhile.

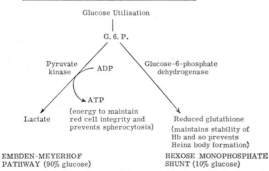

ENZYMIC FACTORS IN RED CELL SURVIVAL

Glucose Utilisation
|
G. 6. P.

Pyruvate kinase — ADP — Glucose-6-phosphate dehydrogenase

→ ATP

Lactate — (energy to maintain red cell integrity and prevents spherocytosis) — Reduced glutathione (maintains stability of Hb and so prevents Heinz body formation)

EMBDEN-MEYERHOF PATHWAY (90% glucose) HEXOSE MONOPHOSPHATE SHUNT (10% glucose)

(4) Glucose-6-phosphate dehydrogenase deficiency and Heinz body anaemia. In most of the common types of G-6 PD deficiency spontaneous haemolysis does not occur but the red cells are susceptible to the haemolytic action of the broad bean and to certain drugs, notably antimalarials, e.g. primaquine, sulphonamides, etc. The deficiency results in a decrease in reduced glutathione, which allows the drugs to oxidise the haemoglobin and so produces within the cells granules of denatured haemoglobin—

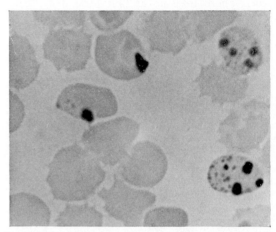

FIG. 16.15.—Blood film in sodium chlorate poisoning, stained with methyl violet to show Heinz bodies. × 1400.

Heinz bodies (Fig. 16.15 and p. 393). The deficiency is genetically determined and is common in the Negro and in the Mediterranean peoples, where the incidence may be as high as 50 per cent of the population (the incidence in Caucasians is less than 1 : 100,000). Sensitivity can be determined *in vitro* by exposing the cells to phenylhydrazine and observing the numbers of Heinz bodies produced, or by a dye test for enzyme activity.

(5) Haemoglobinopathies

Sickle-cell or haemoglobin-S disease. First recognised in America, this condition is found in Negroes, or in those with Negro ancestry, even though this may be remote. In conditions of reduced oxygen tension, e.g. following the addition of a reducing agent *in vitro*, the red cells assume a peculiar crescentic shape (Fig. 16.16). Haemoglobin-S $\alpha_2\beta_2^{\ 6val}$ may be distinguished from normal haemoglobin by electrophoretic and chromatographic methods, and it differs chemically in the substitution of valine for glutamic acid in the sixth position of the amino-acid sequence of the β-chain. When the β-chains move apart on giving up oxygen, the amino-acid substitution results in locking of the adjacent ends of the α-chains with the abnormal β-chains, and the haemoglobin molecules become stacked in rows: this accounts for the characteristic distortion of the red cells in the de-oxygenated state.

In vitro sickling can be demonstrated in approximately 12–18 per cent of persons in certain communities of African Negroes, and family studies show that the trait is inherited as a Mendelian dominant.

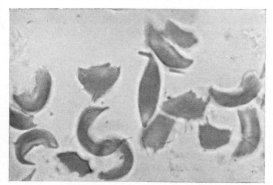

FIG. 16.16.—Sickle cells showing characteristic shapes in low oxygen tension. × 1000.

The majority showing this trait (heterozygotes) are apparently healthy and have a normal red cell survival time, but some, who have both Hb-S and Hb-C, develop a mild form of anaemia, in which target cells are very prominent. There is some evidence that persons with Hb-S have a diminished susceptibility to malaria and that this is an advantage in highly malarious districts. This situation, in which the presence of an otherwise deleterious gene (i.e. the gene for Hb-S) confers a survival advantage, is known as *balanced polymorphism*. In homozygotes, however, sickling occurs *in vivo* and a chronic haemolytic anaemia with the usual characteristics (p. 404) is present; the manifestations tend to diminish in severity in older subjects, perhaps because many homozygotes die in childhood or in early adult life; pregnancy may precipitate a haemolytic crisis. Chronic leg ulceration, like that seen in spherocytic anaemia, is sometimes associated, and the spleen may be much fibrosed and shrunken from repeated infarction.

Thalassaemia major *and* minor. This hereditary anaemia is due primarily to defective globin synthesis but the abnormal cells also have a reduced life span. Thalassaemia *major*, seen in those homozygous for the trait, is a severe anaemia manifest within a few weeks of birth and splenomegaly is prominent. There is a reticulocytosis and many nucleated red cells are present together with a leukocytosis and occasional myelocytes. Target cells (p. 391) are numerous (Fig. 16.17) and the blood shows increased osmotic resistance owing to the flattened shape of the cells (leptocytes). Many such

cases die in infancy or early childhood and are found to show accumulation of haemosiderin in the liver, spleen, pancreas, stomach wall, etc.; in cases of long survival hepatic cirrhosis tends to develop. The marrow is actively hyperplastic and in consequence of the long duration and severity of this the bones show structural changes with thickening of the calvarium and great increase in the diploë so that the child may have a rather mongoloid appearance; myeloid metaplasia is present in the spleen and other organs. The *minor* form (target cell anaemia) occurs in the heterozygote; it is much less serious and presents in adult life merely as a mild anaemia of hypochromic microcytic type highly resistant to treatment with iron. Sometimes, owing to the variable penetrance of the gene, the condition may be symptomless and such cases are described as *trait carriers*.

The defect in haemoglobin synthesis may affect either the α or β polypeptide chains of the globin molecule (see p. 391). In the classical form of the disease the β-chains are affected. In consequence, production of Hb-A ($\alpha_2\beta_2$) is reduced while Hb-A$_2$ ($\alpha_2\delta_2$) and Hb-F ($\alpha_2\gamma_2$) are "compensatorily" increased; no abnormal haemoglobin is formed. In

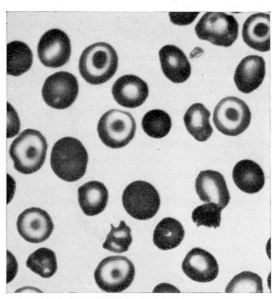

FIG. 16.17.—Target cells in a case of thalassaemia minor. × 1000.

α-chain thalassaemia all three normal haemoglobins are affected since they all contain α chains and so low A, A$_2$ and F values are present but excess β, γ and probably δ units are produced. Although these β, γ and δ chains are normal, their abnormal combination, e.g. as tetramers, results in the appearance of the abnormal haemoglobins Hb-H (β_4) and Hb Bart's (γ_4) (Fig. 16.18).

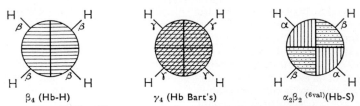

FIG. 16.18.—The structure of some abnormal haemoglobins.

Thus the two biochemical forms of thalassaemia contrast:

α-chain —low A_2 and F. Bart's or H present.
β-chain —High A_2 and usually high F also. No abnormal haemoglobin present (see Fig. 16.19).

The disease most frequently affects inhabitants of the Mediterranean littoral (hence "thalassaemia") but is seen also in parts of the world where other haemoglobinopathies occur. When a mixed heterozygous state is encountered, as in thalassaemia—Hb-C or E disease, a clinical picture similar to thalassaemia *major* results. The disease is rare in Great Britain.

I.B. Acquired red cell defects

(1) Paroxysmal nocturnal haemoglobinuria (PNH) is a rare chronic haemolytic disease of insidious onset, most common in early middle life and characterised by haemoglobinuria, weakness, fever, slight jaundice and moderate splenomegaly. Intra-vascular haemolysis occurs mostly during sleep and is attributable to a remarkable sensitivity of some of the red cells, but not all, to slight lowering of the pH; this is the basis of Ham's test for haemolysis with acidified serum. The urine passed at night or on rising contains haemoglobin whereas the daytime urine contains less or even none. Lysis is now attributed to an abnormal sensitivity of the red cells to complement. There is also a tendency to venous thrombosis, the cause of which is not clear. Transfusion is dangerous owing to the risk of a haemolytic crisis. Repeated haemolytic episodes cause a marked degree of anaemia with reticulocytosis, marrow hyperplasia and siderosis of the organs, especially the kidneys (Fig. 9.11, p. 203); granules of haemosiderin are abundant in the urine both day and night. After a few years death results from thrombosis in the portal or cerebral veins, but milder forms occur and spontaneous permanent remissions have been observed. The essential abnormality in the red cells has not yet been clearly defined but pits in the red cell surface have been detected by electron microscopy and the stromal lipoproteins are abnormal. Occasional patients present with hypoplastic anaemia, the

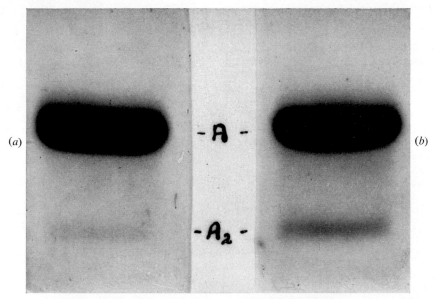

FIG. 16.19.—Starch-gel electrophoresis of haemoglobins.
(a) Normal. (b) Thalassaemia minor, showing increase in Hb-A_2.

marrow being hypocellular, and it may be that PNH arises as an acquired red cell abnormality following an aplastic episode.

(2) Dyshaemopoietic anaemias. In many anaemias due primarily to underproduction of red cells, there is also a haemolytic element, the average life span of the red cells being shortened. This occurs in the macrocytic anaemias, iron-deficiency anaemia, in some cases of aplastic anaemia, and in leukaemia. Apart from the macrocytic anaemias, in which the mechanical injury to abnormally large cells during their passage through capillaries may be a factor (p. 419), the nature of the damage to the red cells in the above conditions is unknown.

II. Abnormal extra-erythrocytic haemolytic mechanisms

There are several conditions in which excessive blood destruction results from the presence of an abnormal antibody, which combines with the red cells, rendering them susceptible either to phagocytosis by cells of the reticulo-endothelial system, or to the lytic action of complement.

II.A. Auto-antibodies to red cells

There are a number of conditions in which auto-antibody develops which is capable of reacting with the individual's own red cells, and which brings about an increased rate of their destruction. The clinical features depend largely on whether red cell destruction takes place mainly by erythrophagocytosis in the reticulo-endothelial tissues (extravascular "haemolysis"), or by lysis of circulating red cells (intravascular haemolysis). In the former, there is acholuric jaundice but little or no detectable haemoglobin-aemia except during haemolytic crises, while in the latter haemoglobin and methaemalbumin are present in the plasma and haemoglobin may pass into the urine. In general, extravascular haemolysis predominates in patients who develop antibody, usually of IgG class, which reacts at normal body temperature ("warm" antibody), and is non-haemolytic, while intravascular haemolysis is observed when the auto-antibody, usually of IgM class, reacts at temperatures below 37° C, and fixes complement, so that haemolytic attacks occur on exposure to cold. This latter type of antibody may also cause intra-vascular haemagglutination and give rise to Raynaud's phenomenon (p. 283).

1. Auto-immune haemolytic anaemia of "warm" antibody type. This is a relatively common form of haemolytic anaemia which occurs in both sexes, and at all ages, being commonest after the age of 40 and in women.

The blood picture is typical of a chronic haemolytic anaemia, often with exacerbation—sometimes fulminating—and remissions. Spherocytosis is usually not marked, except during a severe exacerbation, and the osmotic fragility may not be greatly increased. Most cases are "idiopathic", but the condition occurs also as a complication of systemic lupus erythematosus, rheumatoid arthritis, or lympho-reticular malignancies—Hodgkin's disease, lymphosarcoma and chronic lymphatic leukemia—and occasionally with carcinomatosis. Associations have also been described with tuberculosis and various other infections, and also with the presence of an ovarian dermoid cyst. In both idiopathic and secondary cases, a "false" positive Wassermann reaction is sometimes observed, but more specific serological tests for syphilis are nearly always negative.

The antibody in this condition is of IgG class, and in some cases has been shown to react with a red cell antigen resembling one of the known iso-antigens, e.g. antigen *e* of the Rh system. This may be of some practical importance, for transfused red cells will be destroyed as rapidly as the patient's own (Fig. 16.12) unless a donor can be found whose red cells do not contain the antigen to which the patient has responded: however, it is often very difficult to find such an individual. The antibody is commonly termed "incomplete"; it does not usually cause intravascular agglutination of red cells, fixes little or no complement, and is non-haemolytic. It reacts optimally at 37° C, and erythrophagocytosis in the reticulo-endothelial tissues appears largely responsible for the increased rate of red cell destruction. Free antibody is seldom present in high titre in the patient's serum, and commonly cannot be detected. Its presence on the surface of the red cells is demonstrated most easily by the direct Coombs test, using anti-IgG. In some cases splenectomy is beneficial, but not nearly as regularly as in hereditary spherocytosis, and initial response may be followed by relapse. Splenic enlargement varies up to 1000 g. in idiopathic cases; the cut surface is firm and congested, and microscopy shows engorgement of the splenic cords, and sometimes enlarged germinal centres in the Malpighian bodies. Erythrophagocytosis is often difficult to find, although there is usually abundant haemosiderin in macrophages. In secondary cases, the features of the spleen depend on the nature of, and extent of its involvement in, the disease process which has preceded the haemolytic anaemia.

2. Auto-immune haemolytic anaemia of the "cold" antibody type. In this group of conditions, the auto-antibodies are usually of IgM class and react only at temperatures below 37° C. Accordingly, they produce their effects following exposure of the individual to cold. Because of the low thermal reactivity of the antibodies, they are often present in the serum in high titre, of the order of 1 in 1000. Their presence is associated with two fairly distinct clinical syndromes. Firstly, *paroxysmal cold haemoglobinuria*, which consists of attacks of haemolysis following exposure to cold, due to union of the antibody with the red cells, and subsequent fixation of complement, causing intravascular lysis. Secondly, *cold haemagglutinin disease*, in which the antibody causes also strong haemagglutination, resulting in attacks of cyanosis and Raynaud's phenomenon on exposure to cold, and also chronic haemolytic anaemia in cold weather: this latter is due to complement fixation and also to the increased mechanical fragility of the agglutinated red cells.

Paroxysmal cold haemoglobinuria. The classical type of this condition occurs in association with syphilis, particularly congenital syphilis. The auto-antibody is unusual in being of IgG class, and reacts with antigens of the P system, present in the red cells of nearly all individuals: it is capable of strong complement fixation and causes intravascular haemolysis. The mechanism of haemolysis was elucidated by Donath and Landsteiner, who demonstrated haemolysis *in vitro* by first chilling the blood to allow the cold antibody to react with the red cells, followed by warming to allow complement activity. This was the first demonstration of an auto-immune disease mechanism, and the test is still used, although paroxysmal cold haemoglobinuria must now be extremely rare as a complication of syphilis, at least in this country. Indeed, most cases of paroxysmal cold haemoglobinuria encountered nowadays are not associated with syphilis, although a false-positive Wassermann reaction is not uncommon.

Cold haemagglutinin disease. This tends to affect middle-aged or older individuals, and while it is sometimes idiopathic, more commonly it is secondary to various diseases, especially lympho-reticular malignancies, connective tissue diseases, or following certain infections, especially *primary atypical pneumonia* due to infection with *Mycoplasma pneumoniae*. The antibody is of IgM type and commonly reacts with the antigen I, which is present in the red cells of nearly all individuals. The thermal amplitude of antibodies of this type varies, and the disease occurs only in those subjects with antibody reacting at temperatures up to about 30° C. The Coombs test is usually positive using anti-IgM or antibody to complement (e.g. anti-β_{1C}), but negative with anti-IgG. The haemagglutinin titre of the serum is usually 2,000–64,000 when tested at 2° C. When the condition follows primary atypical pneumonia it is self-limiting, the antibody disappearing within a few months.

II.B. Iso-antibodies to red cells

(1) Haemolytic disease of the newborn. When an Rh-negative mother has one or more Rh-positive pregnancies she may become immunised by the Rh antigen of the fetus and in a subsequent pregnancy the Rh antibodies in her blood may cross the placenta and damage the fetal red cells (Fig. 5.4, p. 103). Three varieties of disease occur of which the most severe is *hydrops fetalis*, a uniformly fatal condition (if untreated) comprising severe anaemia, oedema and ascites; many such fetuses are prematurely stillborn. *Icterus gravis neonatorum* is the most important variety because it often requires urgent treatment. Jaundice comes on within a few hours of birth, the infant is usually anaemic and many normoblasts and primitive erythroblasts are present, together with a high reticulocyte count. The liver and the spleen are enlarged and contain haemosiderin, the liver cells may show widespread necrosis and bile appears in the urine, the stools then becoming pale. The central nervous system may show necrosis and bile-staining, especially the hippocampus, corpus Luysii, lentiform and olivary nuclei—*kernicterus* (p. 605)—and, if the infant survives, choreoathetosis and mental deficiency may result. The third and mildest variety is *congenital haemolytic anaemia*: the infant is only slightly jaundiced, but develops progressive anaemia, often with little sign of regenerative marrow activity; ultimately recovery follows. In the severer forms, extramedullary haemopoiesis is abundant in the liver, spleen, adrenals, kidneys, etc., and numerous erythroblasts appear in the blood, justifying the former name of *erythroblastosis fetalis*. The etiology of all three varieties lies in iso-immunisation of the mother, usually against the Rh factor but occasionally against some other blood group antigen. Two kinds of Rh antibodies may be evoked; agglutinins of IgM class appear first but later "incomplete" antibodies of IgG class, which attach themselves to the Rh-positive cells of the fetus without causing visible agglutination and which are responsible for the damage of the fetus because only they pass readily through the placenta. A high titre of such antibodies in the mother's serum is of grave prognostic significance and is usually followed by the birth of a macerated or stillborn fetus.

Unless the Rh-negative mother has been sensitised by transfusion with Rh-positive blood, it is usual for at least one pregnancy to be successfully completed, but when once the disease has appeared all subsequent Rh+ children are likely to be affected; but if the father is heterozygous Rh+ (e.g. CDe/cde), there is an equal chance of an Rh-negative pregnancy, the fetus then being unaffected. Haemolytic disease due to Rh incompatibility occurs less frequently, but with undiminished severity, in cases of heterospecific pregnancy, i.e. pregnancy in which the fetal red cells contain either A or B group antigens not present in the maternal corpuscles.

It is now known that fetal red cells gain entrance to the maternal circulation mainly during labour, and this explains why maternal iso-immunisation does not usually occur *during* the first Rh+ pregnancy. Trials initiated by Clarke (1963) have demonstrated conclusively that intravenous injection of Rh antibody (anti-D) of IgG class into the mother after delivery greatly reduces the chance of her developing Rh antibodies, and thus lessens the risk of haemolytic disease in subsequent pregnancies.

(2) Transfusion reactions. When incompatible blood is transfused into a recipient in whose circulation the appropriate antibodies are already present, a haemolytic transfusion reaction results and the transfused cells are rapidly destroyed. The results of an incompat-ible transfusion depend to some extent on the speed of destruction of the transfused red cells and this is likely to be greater when abundant iso-antibody is present, e.g. in ABO incompatibility, especially transfusion of Group A blood into a Group O recipient, or of Rh positive blood into an Rh negative *immunised* recipient. These are not the only incompatibilities encountered, but are so much the most common that stringent precautions must be taken to avoid them. The patient is likely to suffer a rigor, pain in the back and pyrexia; shortly thereafter haemoglobinuria appears, followed by jaundice. In a severe reaction death from shock may occur within a few minutes. If the patient survives, a hypofibrino-gaemic state with haemostatic failure may ensue. Later the urinary output may diminish and death may result from acute renal failure (p. 724).

Similar clinical effects may result from the transfusion of blood that is too old, or contaminated by gram-negative organisms, some of which grow freely at refrigerator temperature (cryophilic bacteria).

II.C. Parasitic invasion of red cells

In malaria and oroya fever the parasites invade and destroy large numbers of red cells, thus producing an anaemia.

(1) Malaria. There are three types of malarial fever caused by four different parasites. These are (a) the tertian, with paroxysms of fever every other day, caused by *Plasmodium vivax* and by *Plasmodium ovale*, (b) the quartan, with paroxysms at 72 hr. intervals, caused by the *Plasmodium malariae* and (c) the subtertian or malignant malaria caused by *Plasmodium falciparum*, in which the fever is without a regular cycle. These parasites belong to the *Haemosporidia*, a sub-class of the *Sporozoa*. The first three are closely allied, being of the same genus, and the gametocytes or sexual cells are of spherical form; in the fourth the gametocytes are crescentic. Each parasite passes through two cycles of development—an asexual one or *schizogony* in the human subject, and a sexual one of *sporogony* in the mosquito. In the former cycle, the gametocytes are formed, but undergo no further development in man, whilst in the latter, conjugation of the gametes formed from the gametocytes takes place in the mosquito. Several species of mosquito of the genus *Anopheles* have been found to be capable of carrying infection. The onset of a febrile attack of malaria coincides with the setting free of a new brood of young parasites (merozoites) by the asexual division of the adult forms within the red cells, and the period of the fever depends on the time taken for the full development from the young to the adult form. Multiple infection occurs when

Malarial anaemia. With each attack of pyrexia in malarial infection a large number of red cells are destroyed by the parasites, and the dark brown pigment formed from the haemoglobin is taken up by monocytes and by phagocytic cells in the spleen, liver and other organs. It is accordingly not surprising that when the disease is chronic, anaemia results and may be severe. The occurrence of *blackwater fever*, due to intravascular haemolysis, will of course greatly

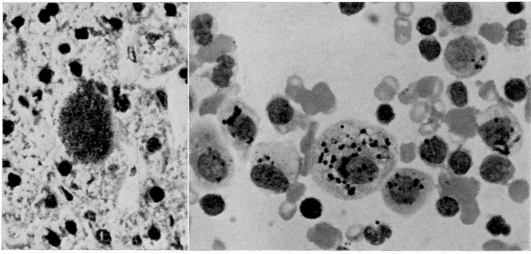

FIG. 16.20.—Development of malaria parasites within a liver cell. × 550. (Preparation kindly lent by Prof. P. C. C. Garnham.)

FIG. 16.21.—Malaria; monocytes containing pigment.

parasites are introduced by mosquitoes on more than one occasion, so that parasites at different stages of development are present. Sometimes also mixed infection occurs, e.g. by the tertian and subtertian parasites.

Cycle of development in man. It has now been conclusively shown that when the human subject is bitten by infected mosquitoes, sporozoites are injected from the infected salivary glands and are carried to the liver, where they undergo a stage of development within the hepatic cells (Fig. 16.20). Schizogony takes place and culminates after 6–9 days in the liberation of merozoites in large numbers into the blood, where they enter the red cells. This pre-erythrocytic development constitutes the incubation period of the disease of about 6–9 days. Within the red cells the parasites go through further cycles of asexual proliferation which cause the paroxysms of fever. It is highly probable that in benign tertian malaria there are persistent exoerythrocytic forms of the *P. vivax*, from which the relapses so characteristic of the disease are derived.

intensify the anaemia. Malarial anaemia is generally of the normochromic or mildly hypochromic type and, at an early stage, the blood destruction leads to a reticulocyte response, but in chronic cases deficient formation of red cells may be present. A few normoblasts may sometimes be found. When severe, malarial anaemia may become macrocytic, especially in malignant falciparum infections. This may, in some cases at least, be due to excessive demands for folic acid. The leukocyte count is usually somewhat reduced, though it varies, and a noteworthy feature is the increase of the monocytes which often exceed 15 per cent. Some of these may contain malarial pigment (Fig. 16.21).

Blackwater fever. This occurs in subjects, usually Europeans, who have, or have previously suffered from malaria. It consists of an acute intravascular haemolysis, with consequent haemoglobinaemia, methaemalbuminaemia and hyperbilirubinaemia, and the urine is dark from the presence of haemoglobin and methaem-oglobin. It is accompanied by fever, vomiting, shock, and sometimes convulsions and coma, and is often fatal. Acute renal failure with anuria is common (p. 724). The haemolytic agent is not known: in some cases quinine may precipitate an attack, but in others it has not been ingested.

The possible relationship between malaria and Burkitt's lymphoma (p. 220) is of considerable interest. The geographical distributions of the two conditions in Africa coincide fairly closely, and it seems likely that either malaria in child-hood, or an infective oncogenic agent trans-mitted by insects, plays a carcinogenic role.

(2) Oroya fever. This is caused by infection with a small gram-negative bacillus—*Bartonella bacilli-formis*—which colonises the red cells and the mac-rophages of the reticulo-endothelial tissues. Infec-tion is transmitted by certain species of sandfly (*Phlebotomus*) and is limited to the slopes of the Andes. The infected red cells show increased mechanical fragility and become sequestered in the liver and spleen, haemolytic anaemia resulting. The organisms can be seen in Romanowsky-stained blood films. Fever, joint and muscle pains, and enlarged lymph nodes are followed by a papular skin eruption.

II.D. Haemolytic toxins and chemicals

(1) Bacterial toxins. The toxins of certain bacteria have haemolytic properties; those of the *Streptococcus pyogenes* and *Cl. welchii* are noteworthy examples.

(2) Chemicals. There are many chemical poisons which have a haemolytic effect, such as phenylhydrazine, lead, arseniuretted hydrogen, saponin, potassium chlorate, and some of these have been extensively investigated. In *chronic lead poisoning* the effect of lead is upon the red cell surface, rendering the cells brittle and in-creasing the mechanical but diminishing the osmotic fragility. Accordingly they are short-lived, and anaemia results. Lead also inter-feres with haemoglobin synthesis and the utilisa-tion of iron. Consequently the red cells tend to be hypochromic although iron is plentiful in the marrow. The iron accumulates in the nucleated red cell precursors which are then called sideroblasts (Fig. 1.12, p. 11). Lead also precipitates the RNA of young polychro-matophilic erythrocytes in the form of punctate

basophilia. The anaemia is rarely severe, and the diagnostic feature is the presence of punctate basophil (stippled) cells which are most easily detected in smears from the lower part of the buffy coat. The detection of punctate basophilia is now seldom used in the diagnosis of lead poisoning, which can be achieved earlier and with more certainty by the more specific method of estimating the concentration of lead in the blood. The disorder in haemoglobin synthesis induced by lead is reflected in the high levels of erythrocyte protoporphyrin, urinary copropor-phyrin and aminolaevulinic acid, the estimation of which can be valuable in diagnosis.

Drug-induced haemolytic anaemia of Heinz body type is common, and many drugs have been incriminated, e.g. phenacetin, sulphonamides, dapsone, primaquine, etc. This has already been mentioned in describing the effects of G-6 PD deficiency. It is important to realise however that simple overdosage with oxidative drugs, of which phenacetin is the commonest in use in Britain, can overwhelm the hexose monophos-phate shunt in the absence of G-6 PD deficiency, with the production of Heinz bodies and methaemoglobin in sufficient concentration to produce distinct cyanosis: the anaemia is usually only moderate, but may be severe. Reticulocytes, being more active metabolically than older red cells, are more resistant to this kind of drug damage. In consequence haemoly-sis tends to lessen in severity as the concentration of reticulocytes rises. Withdrawal of the drug is curative.

Not all drugs inducing haemolysis cause the formation of Heinz bodies. Others, notably methyldopa (Aldomet), can cause haemolysis by inducing auto-antibody formation with red cell specificity and the direct Coombs test is positive. Only a small proportion of those in whom sensitisation occurs actually develop a haemolytic anaemia. Other drugs, e.g. penicil-lin, can on occasion act as haptens and so pro-duce haemolysis.

(3) Vegetable poisons. Historically, the best known condition in this group is *favism*, which results from eating broad beans (*Vicia faba*). As already stated, it occurs mainly in subjects with a glucose-6-phosphate dehydrogenase deficiency (p. 408), and is therefore observed chiefly in those of Mediterranean or Negro ancestry, the inci-dence in Malta, for example, being 3·5 per cent of the population. In Mediterranean peoples, the haemolytic anaemia may be severe and even fatal. Negroes have a different form of G-6 PD deficiency, and the haemolysis is milder. In both populations, the deficiency is sex-linked, being carried in the X chromosome and this accounts for the higher incidence in men. Various pollens, fruits and other vegetables give rise to a similar condition, and the term *alimentary haemolysis* is now used in place of the more restricted term *favism*. The chemical nature of the haemolytic agents is unknown, but they induce oxidative denaturation of haemoglobin with appearance of Heinz bodies in the red cells (p. 393).

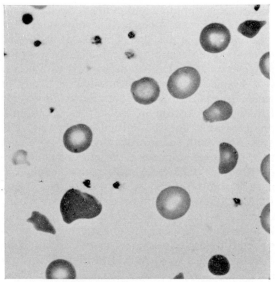

FIG. 16.22.—Fragmentation of red cells in microangiopathic haemolytic anaemia. × 1000.

II.E. Mechanical damage to red cells

(1) March haemoglobinuria. This consists of acute haemoglobinuria, usually mild, resulting from long marches. The haemolysis is now believed to be due to mechanical injury to the red cells sustained in the circulation through the soft tissues of the plantar aspect of the feet and brought on by the prolonged mild trauma of long walks, particularly on hard surfaces and carrying heavy loads.

(2) Microangiopathic haemolytic anaemia. For many years the presence of mis-shapen red cells has been associated with various disease states in which, however, no other common pathological feature seemed evident. These damaged erythrocytes, termed variously "burr, leaf, helmet or irregularly-contracted cells" (Fig. 16.22), are found in malignant hypertension with uraemia, eclampsia, carcinomatosis, thrombotic thrombocytopenic purpura and, curiously, gastro-intestinal bleeding. Very little was known about the precise pathogenesis of this form of red cell damage until Dacie reproduced experimentally the red cell changes by giving animals snake venom to induce intravascular fibrin deposition. He suggested that the red cell damage in man might be caused by the cells impinging on fibrin strands at points of arteriolar damage (hence microangiopathic) associated with thrombosis. Since platelets would tend to be consumed by such a process the hypothesis also explains the known association between thrombocytopenia and the appearance of these irregularly-contracted red cells in the blood.

Dyshaemopoietic Anaemias

Introduction

The essential feature of anaemia of dyshaemopoietic type is failure by the marrow to deliver to the blood adequate numbers of normal red cells. This can come about in different ways. Obviously if the precursor cells in the marrow are deficient in number, as in aplastic and hypoplastic anaemia, the result will be underproduction of erythrocytes. But failure of output can occur even when the marrow is grossly hypercellular either because of delayed maturation of the cells, or because the erythrocytes produced are being destroyed within the

marrow; to this latter process the term *ineffective erythropoiesis* is applied and radioactive isotope studies using ^{51}Cr and ^{59}Fe are required for its detection. Aplastic anaemia is a relatively rare condition and anaemia of dyshaemopoietic type is much more commonly the result of failure of the marrow to obtain substrates which it requires to achieve its normal output. Anaemias of this type are of peculiar importance for, in many cases, the nature of the deficient substance can be deduced from appropriate investigations. Most important is the fact that, in simple deficiency states, complete cure can be obtained by replacement therapy. As will be seen, the classification of the dyshaemopoietic anaemias is based logically on differences in etiology of this kind. However, these anaemias are often more complex than simple failure of output. Commonly the cells produced are themselves defective. They may be lacking in haemoglobin and so be functionally defective or they may have a reduced life span in the circulation.

(a) Macrocytic type

This type of anaemia is fundamentally due to deficiency of vitamin B_{12} or folic acid, as a consequence of which erythropoiesis becomes megaloblastic, and diminished output of abnormally large red cells results in the development of macrocytic anaemia. These deficiencies can be brought about in various ways, e.g. impaired metabolism, failure of absorption, etc., but pernicious anaemia is the outstanding example of this type and the term should be restricted to the anaemia first described by Addison, other conditions with a similar blood picture being entitled megalocytic or macrocytic anaemia with whatever qualification may be appropriate.

Pernicious anaemia (Addison's anaemia)

This is mainly a disease of late adult life and affects men slightly more often than women. There is intense pallor of the skin and mucous membranes, often with a lemon tint; there is little or no emaciation. Until the introduction of treatment with liver, pernicious anaemia was usually a progressive and fatal disease, although remissions were not un-

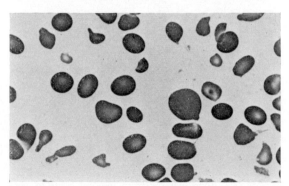

FIG. 16.23.—Red cells in pernicious anaemia, prepared from below buffy coat. Gross anisopoikilocytosis. × 650.

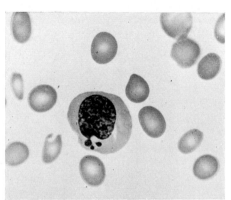

FIG. 16.24.—Blood in pernicious anaemia showing a megaloblast with Howell-Jolly bodies. × 1000.

common and sometimes marked temporary improvement took place. The disease is now highly amenable to treatment (see below). It results from a deficiency of the so-called "intrinsic factor" in the gastric secretion (p. 421), which is necessary for the absorption of cyanocobalamin (vitamin B_{12}).

Blood changes. In the advanced stage the blood is pale and distinctly watery, and coagulation occurs slowly. The number of red cells is greatly reduced, not infrequently being below 1×10^6 per c.mm., and may fall to less than half that figure before death. The individual erythrocytes are well coloured, the MCHC being normal. There is usually, though not always, great variation in their shape, numerous poikilocytes being present. While cell size varies greatly, macrocytes are generally conspicuous (Fig. 16.23), and the average diameter is distinctly above normal (8·5 μ), as is also the MCV, 100–140 cμ. In stained preparations, some of the erythrocytes usually show polychromatophilia (p. 392), and punctate basophilia may be associated with it. The number of reticulocytes varies considerably according to the progress of the disease; in the stage of relapse it is usually about 3 per cent, which taken in conjunction with the low red cell count indicates that the total marrow output is reduced. Nucleated red cells can usually be found, especially by examining the buffy coat after centrifuging, and sometimes they are numerous: they may be of both megaloblastic and normoblastic type, and often show considerable nuclear variation. The presence of macrocytes and megaloblasts along with a raised MCV is thus an important feature of this type of anaemia (Fig. 16.24). Cabot's "ring-bodies" are some-

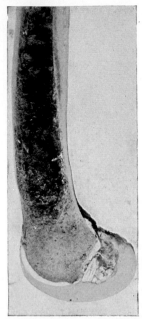

FIG. 16.25.—Section of femur in pernicious anaemia, showing the dark red marrow throughout the shaft. × ½.

times present. Leukopenia of about 2000 per c.mm. is usual, and the decrease is mainly of the polymorphonuclear cells. There is often an increased proportion of the older neutrophils with lobes well separated—"a shift to the right" (Cooke)—and some are of large and hypersegmented type—*macropolycytes*; in addition sometimes a few myelocytes and metamyelocytes are present. The *blood platelets* also are reduced in number. Thus whilst the chief changes are in the erythrocytes, the diminished number of leukocytes and of platelets is evidence of a more generalised disturbance of marrow function.

In pernicious anaemia, the concentration of vitamin B_{12} in the serum is reduced from the normal range of 160–900 pg. per ml. to 100 pg. or less. The plasma bilirubin is increased and gives an indirect van den Bergh reaction. During a severe relapse it may rise to 2 mg. per 100 ml. or even higher, indicating a greatly increased rate of red cell destruction. The urine is often dark from excess of urobilin and urobilinogen.

Morphological changes. In addition to the general pathological changes of severe anaemia (p. 400), the following features are observed in pernicious anaemia.

The bone marrow shows gross hyperplasia.

The yellow fatty marrow of the long bones is replaced, to a varying extent, by dark red cellular marrow (Fig. 16.25). In the long bones, the change starts at the upper end and extends downwards. The whole medullary cavity may ultimately be occupied by red marrow and there is often a considerable absorption of bone trabeculae (Fig. 16.26), so that portions of marrow can readily be cut out; this indicates prolonged hyperplasia and the more chronic and severe the anaemia the greater is the red marrow increase.

Microscopic examination of the red marrow shows *megaloblastic erythropoiesis*. There is a large proportion, 50 per cent or more, of megaloblasts showing variable degrees of haemoglobinisation, together with their more primitive precursors with basophil cytoplasm. The proportion of cells at different stages of maturation varies greatly and many intermediate polychromatic cells are seen; in general the more severe the anaemia and the longer its duration the higher the proportion of primitive basophil cells. The nucleus of the more primitive cells shows the finely reticulate arrangement of the chromatin that is diagnostic (Fig. 16.27, 16.28), but some of the fully haemoglobinised cells show nuclear condensation, pyknosis and fragmentation. The marrow is not, however, entirely megaloblastic, and normoblasts are usually present also in small numbers.

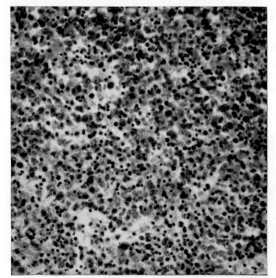

FIG. 16.26.—Bone marrow from femoral shaft in pernicious anaemia, showing an extreme degree of megaloblastic hyperplasia with complete loss of fat and absorption of the bony trabeculae. × 250.

Although the marrow is hyperplastic there is a deficiency in output of red cells; megaloblasts mature too slowly to maintain the erythrocyte count. Moreover, instead of normal-sized erythrocytes, they provide macrocytes and these undergo early destruction in the

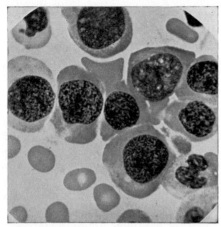

FIG. 16.27.—Film of bone marrow from a case of pernicious anaemia, showing large megaloblasts. × 1000.

circulation, perhaps in consequence of increased mechanical buffeting owing to their large size. Because of the erythropoietic hyperplasia, myelocytes form a *reduced percentage* of the marrow population but their *total numbers* may actually be increased. The earlier myelocytes may also be enlarged and a conspicuous feature is the formation of giant metamyelocytes, with abnormal nuclei and disproportionately underdeveloped cytoplasm; possibly the macropolycytes in the blood are derived from these cells. Accordingly there is defective development and maturation of both granulocytes and red cells in pernicious anaemia. Megakaryocytes are usually scanty, thus accounting for the paucity of platelets in the blood.

Within the marrow there is also evidence of the excessive destruction of red cells by erythrophagocytosis and accumulation of haemosiderin granules in excess in the reticulo-endothelial cells. This, however, varies greatly, depending probably upon the amount of recent red cell destruction.

Alimentary tract. Lesions of the mouth are common, especially glossitis with formation of small vesicles and ulcers, followed by atrophy of the papillae. The tongue is smooth and has often a red and raw appearance. Such lesions are not always present and are not peculiar to the dis-

ease; they occur also in microcytic anaemia and in sprue (p. 525). The essential defect in pernicious anaemia is severe atrophic gastritis, of auto-immune nature (p. 488), affecting the acid-secreting mucosa, with virtually complete loss of parietal and chief cells. This results in gross deficiency or absence of the intrinsic factor, a mucoprotein secreted by the parietal cells. In most cases the serum contains an auto-antibody to a microsomal constituent of the parietal cells, while in over half the cases a second antibody is detectable which reacts with human intrinsic factor. Not only is secretion of intrinsic factor greatly diminished, but antibody to intrinsic factor has been shown to gain entrance to the gastric lumen, where it reacts with what little intrinsic factor is available, interfering with its union with vitamin B_{12}, and thus further impairing B_{12} absorption from the ileum (see p. 421). Histamine-resistant achlorhydria is always present and is usually associated with achylia gastrica—complete absence of the gastric digestive enzymes. Such defects precede the onset of pernicious anaemia and they are not reversed by B_{12} treatment.

Haemosiderosis. During a relapse there is a deposit of iron in various organs, but during remissions, either naturally occurring or induced

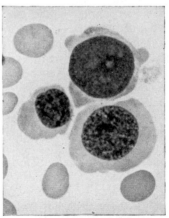

FIG. 16.28.—Bone marrow in pernicious anaemia.
A very primitive cell (haemocytoblast) is shown, together with two typical haemoglobinised megaloblasts. × 1000.

by treatment, most of the iron is re-utilised to make haemoglobin. The *liver*, generally a little enlarged, is browner than usual, and the central parts of the lobules stand out yellowish from fatty change. It gives a marked iron reaction with the usual reagents, the colour being deepest at the periphery of the lobules (Fig. 16.29). Haemosiderin granules are abundant in the liver cells in the outer two-thirds of the lobules around the portal tracts, chiefly in the parts of the cells adjacent to the bile canaliculi; some may be present also in the Kupffer

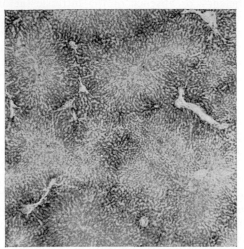

FIG. 16.29.—Liver in pernicious anaemia, showing haemosiderosis in the periportal areas demonstrated by the prussian blue reaction. × 20.

cells. The *spleen* is usually of about normal size but, depending on the increase in red cell destruction, it may become palpable during relapse; it is then dark red and gives an iron reaction. The haemosiderin occurs in coarse granules within cells in the pulp, the Malpighian bodies being free; phagocytosis of red cells may be present, together with splenic haemopoiesis.

The renal tubule cells, particularly of the proximal limb, may contain haemosiderin granules, and in some cases the amount is large (Fig. 16.30). The raised serum bilirubin level in pernicious anaemia is indicative of increased red cell destruction, and the renal tubular siderosis suggests that in some cases there is intravascular haemolysis: this now receives support from the virtual absence of haptoglobins from the plasma (see p. 203). Free haemoglobin is not, however, present in the plasma in sufficient concentration to be readily detectable.

Other changes. Capillary haemorrhages or petechiae are present often in the serous membranes, leptomeninges, and especially in the retinae, rarely in the skin: occasionally haemorrhagic manifestations including haematemesis, are prominent, usually in severely anaemic

patients who show also marked leukopenia and a thrombocytopenia with less than 50,000 platelets per cm. The haemorrhagic state responds well to the administration of vitamin B_{12}. In pernicious anaemia changes are often present in the *spinal cord*, constituting *subacute combined degeneration*, with disturbances of sensation and motion, ataxia, etc. (p. 660). Such lesions were commonly present in pre-liver-therapy days. In addition minor nervous disturbances, chiefly sensory, are common, and have been found to be due to peripheral neuritis. The nerve lesions in pernicious anaemia like the marrow changes are due to lack of vitamin B_{12}. Some patients develop the neural lesion before the appearance of anaemia. Usually in such cases the marrow is not entirely normoblastic, showing transitional changes towards megaloblastic erythropoiesis, but assessment of this may be difficult. The serum B_{12} level is, however, always very low.

Cause of the anaemia. Definite knowledge on this subject dates from 1926, when the efficacy of liver treatment was discovered by Minot and Murphy.

This discovery was promoted by the experimental work of Whipple and others on diets

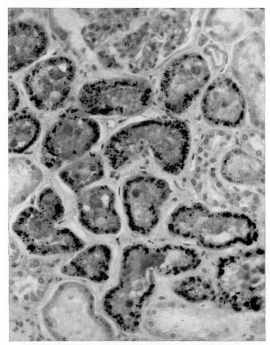

FIG. 16.30.—Kidney in pernicious anaemia showing pronounced iron storage in the convoluted tubules (prussian blue). × 400.

most favourable for blood regeneration after haemorrhage, one result being that liver was specially efficacious. The active substance in liver has been isolated as reddish needle-shaped crystals of a non-protein complex containing cobalt. Now known as cyanocobalamin or vitamin B_{12}, it has been found not only in liver, beef muscle, and abundantly in autolysed yeast, but also in various fermentation liquors. By the addition of radioactive cobalt to such a medium a radioactive vitamin B_{12} has been obtained which has been of great value in tracing the absorption of this essential substance.

Vitamin B_{12} is absorbed mainly in the ileum, and only in the form of a complex with *intrinsic factor*, a mucoprotein secreted into the gastric juice by the parietal cells. As already explained (p. 419) the essential lesion in pernicious anaemia is atrophic gastritis, probably of an auto-immune nature, which destroys the parietal cells and thus abolishes secretion of intrinsic factor. As a result, absorption of B_{12} from the gut falls below the daily requirement of 1 μg., and in time deficiency results. If very large amounts of B_{12} (e.g. 1000 μg.) are administered some absorption occurs even in the absence of intrinsic factor. Cyanocobalamin is now recognised as the extrinsic factor originally postulated by Castle. Addition of gastric mucoprotein (containing intrinsic factor), even to a diet not specially supplemented in B_{12}, brings about a remission in pernicious anaemia, but if foreign (e.g. hog or bovine) gastric mucosa is used, resistance to this form of therapy commonly develops. The part played by the intrinsic factor in promoting the absorption of B_{12} is utilised in the *Schilling test*, in which radioactive B_{12} is given by mouth, first without, and then together with, intrinsic factor. Absorption of B_{12} is estimated on each occasion from the radioactivity in the urine following a "flushing dose" of B_{12} given parenterally. In pernicious anaemia absorption of the radioactive test dose is greatly enhanced when intrinsic factor is given with it. When liver therapy was first discovered its great curative value by mouth was probably due to its content of B_{12} and folic acid (see below). Even in the absence of intrinsic factor, consumption of large amounts of liver probably resulted in the absorption of sufficient B_{12} for physiological needs.

Pernicious anaemia is, therefore, due to failure of absorption of vitamin B_{12} because of lack of intrinsic factor. Theoretically a similar state of deficiency might result from absence of B_{12} from the diet, or from failure of absorption from some cause other than the intrinsic factor deficiency, or from failure to store it in the liver or to utilise it after storage. There is evidence that almost all these possibilities are realised and the conditions in which they occur are considered later. These theoretical possibilities harmonise well with what is known about the frequent association of macrocytic anaemia with various gastric and intestinal lesions, as described below.

The mode of action of B_{12} at the cellular level is still obscure (p. 14), but it has a highly complex metabolic activity. B_{12} plays an important part as a co-enzyme in the synthesis of deoxyribonucleic acid (DNA) and also of ribonucleic acid (RNA). Thus, in the marrow, lack of B_{12} would be expected to influence adversely, through absence of its DNA effect, the cells which normally divide very actively, and morphological confirmation of this adverse effect is visible in the consistent failure of nuclear maturation that characterises the megaloblast series and also the precursors of the granular cells. Lack of B_{12} leads also to disorder of ribonucleic acid synthesis (RNA) and thus to deficiencies in the formation of proteins. In the posterior and lateral columns of the spinal cord it is the long fibre tracts that are especially affected, perhaps on account of their high metabolic turnover for which the diminished protein synthesis consequent upon lack of B_{12} is inadequate, and the integrity of the axons suffers; accordingly breakdown of the long-fibre tracts follows in the form of subacute combined degeneration (p. 660).

Pernicious anaemia affects more than one member of a family (blood relations) more often than would be expected by chance, and, further, the incidence of achlorhydria, of gastric parietal-cell auto-antibody, and of iron-deficiency anaemia, have been found to be higher in such families than in the general population. The auto-immune gastritis which leads to pernicious anaemia may then have genetically-determined predisposing factors, but the causation of chronic gastritis may be multifactorial, and environmental factors could be important or even predominant. It is of interest that families and individuals with chronic gastritis tend to develop also chronic thyroiditis (p. 490).

Effects of treatment. The parenteral administration of even a few micrograms of B_{12} per day leads to a remarkable remission in pernicious anaemia. Within a few days there is great subjective improvement and a feeling of well-being, the number of reticulocytes in the blood rises from a previous 2–3 per cent to 25 per cent or higher, the maximum number appearing usually in 4–6 days. The reticulocytosis after the injection of B_{12} is so constant that its absence should throw doubt on the diagnosis. The lower the initial red cell count the higher the percentage and absolute number of reticulocytes after treatment with B_{12}, since the output depends on the degree of marrow hyperplasia existing at the onset of treatment. This rise soon disappears, but it is accompanied by an increase in the haemoglobin level and in the red and white cell counts, whilst the mean corpuscular diameter falls and the serum bilirubin level drops to normal, indicating return to a normal rate of red cell destruction. These changes reflect a dramatic return of the marrow to normoblastic erythropoiesis, megaloblasts being rapidly transformed into normoblasts with disappearance also of the abnormalities of the myeloid series. With adequate treatment the number of red cells should rise to normal in two to three months, and neurological symptoms should cease to develop and may even improve. The atrophic gastritis is, however, permanent, and treatment must be continued for life, otherwise relapse will occur.

Another substance which has a striking therapeutic effect in all megaloblastic anaemias is folic acid (pteroyl-monoglutamic acid), a member of the vitamin B group present in yeast, crude liver and in spinach and other green vegetables. It is not present in purified liver extracts or in gastric juice and it is converted *in vivo* to the physiologically active form folinic acid (5-formyl-5.6.7.8. tetrahydrofolic acid) by vitamin C. Folic acid administered by any route to cases of macrocytic anaemia in relapse rapidly induces a remission provided that the stores of B_{12} are not completely exhausted, but for maintenance increasing doses are required and relapse follows when total exhaustion of B_{12} has finally occurred. The neurological complications of pernicious anaemia are not relieved, indeed they may develop or be exacerbated under folic acid therapy despite improvement in the blood picture. This suggests that folic acid has the effect of mobilising the last traces of B_{12} in the body and diverting them to the active marrow, to the detriment of the nervous system. Its use is therefore contra-indicated in pernicious anaemia.

Other forms of macrocytic anaemia

Macrocytic anaemia is the consequence of megaloblastic erythropoiesis in the marrow and results from deficiency of B_{12} or folic acid, however brought about, and also from vitamin C deficiency (p. 446). We have no precise knowledge of any other cause of megaloblastic transformation of the marrow, although cases due to unknown cause do occur, and are classified loosely as *refractory megaloblastic anaemias* (p. 428). Since deficiency of B_{12} or folic acid can arise in various ways, macrocytic anaemia is encountered in several different conditions, in all of which the changes in the blood, though not identical, are closely similar and the clinical picture depends on the associated disorder. Subacute combined degeneration of the spinal cord is rarely seen except in true pernicious anaemia.

Gastrectomy (partial or complete) may induce macrocytic anaemia due to failure to absorb vitamin B_{12} owing to lack of intrinsic factor. The onset of anaemia is usually deferred for three years or more, the time required to deplete the liver store of B_{12} which is used up at the rate of about 1 μg. per day.

"Pernicious anaemia" of pregnancy. Some degree of anaemia is common in pregnancy, usually of the iron-deficiency type (p. 424), but anaemia is often more apparent than real owing to the hydraemia and increased blood volume that is present. In megaloblastic anaemia of pregnancy, the red cell count falls rapidly and a *severe* type of anaemia results. Owing to the greatly diminished output of cells from the marrow the megaloblastic picture is not fully reflected in the state of the peripheral blood during the pregnancy, macrocytosis is often inconspicuous and the MCHC may actually be reduced owing to concurrent iron deficiency. The serum bilirubin is also less markedly raised than in true pernicious anaemia. The blood picture is therefore misleading, and the diagnosis can be made in some cases only by biopsy of the marrow when a fully developed megaloblastic state is revealed. Examination of films made from the buffy coat of the peripheral blood will usually reveal the presence of megaloblasts and then the need for marrow puncture will be obviated. Spontaneous recovery usually follows delivery of the child but may be delayed, e.g. in the presence of sepsis; and in such prolonged cases the blood picture eventually may be identical with that of true pernicious anaemia. The nature of the defect in this severe anaemia of pregnancy is uncertain and may be complex; during gestation there is often hypochlorhydria but absence of intrinsic factor has been excluded since radioactive B_{12} is absorbed normally, the serum level is normal, and the anaemia is refractory to parenteral B_{12} administration. It does, however, respond to folic acid, and the increased folic acid requirement in pregnancy is probably an important factor, as the high incidence in twin pregnancies indicates.

Dietary deficiency of either B_{12} or folic acid is a possible cause of megaloblastic anaemia. B_{12} deficiency is probably the cause of the megaloblastic anaemia developing in some strict vegetarians (vegans). Dietary deficiency of folic acid, uncomplicated by other factors, rarely causes megaloblastic anaemia in Britain, although it does so in India, the condition being known as tropical nutritional anaemia; it responds to administration of folic acid, or autolysed yeast (Marmite) rich in folate.

The malabsorption syndrome. In idiopathic steatorrhoea and sprue, anaemia is a prominent and sometimes the presenting feature. At first it is of iron-deficiency type but later the blood picture may become partly macrocytic, i.e. a dimorphic anaemia develops as the effects of folic acid deficiency are superadded and become severe. The marrow then shows typical megaloblastic transformation and the blood picture may become indistinguishable from pernicious anaemia. Laboratory confirmation of folic acid deficiency is less readily achieved than that of vitamin B_{12} deficiency, where serum assay is conclusive, but the *Lactobacillus casei* assay to determine the folate content of the red cells ("tissue" folate assay) has been shown to reflect folic acid deficiency more accurately than serum levels which are merely an indication of the immediate dietary past. In approximately one third of cases of the malabsorption syndrome there is an associated deficiency of vitamin B_{12}, and both assays should be performed.

Folic acid is very effective in relieving not only the macrocytic anaemia but also many of the alimentary symptoms in sprue and in idiopathic steatorrhoea, without, however, notably improving fat absorption.

Vitamin C and anaemia. Vitamin C influences haemopoiesis in two ways; it potentiates the conversion of folic acid to folinic acid, and it is required for the incorporation of iron in the haem molecule. In *scurvy*, anaemia is usually mild and of normocytic normochromic type but may become microcytic if blood loss is pronounced. Occasionally a macrocytic anaemia develops owing to failure of conversion of folic acid, and thrombocytopenia may be severe. Reticulocyte response, reversion of the marrow and restoration of the haemoglobin and platelets follow the administration of vitamin C alone.

Competition for B_{12} in the intestine may reduce the amount available for absorption in cases of diverticulosis of the small intestine and the blind loop syndrome following surgical operation or tuberculous ulceration (pp. 512,526).

In Finland, macrocytic anaemia is found in a small proportion of individuals harbouring the fish tapeworm *Dibothriocephalus latus*. The effects of infestation depend on the site of the worm in the intestine and the amount of B_{12} available, because the worm absorbs considerable amounts of B_{12} and thus deprives the host. Only a small percentage of individuals harbouring the parasite develop the anaemia and the presence of the worm is no more than a precipitating cause in persons on the borderline of B_{12} insufficiency.

Drugs. Anticonvulsants of the phenytoin type and folic acid antagonists used in the treatment of leukaemia, etc., may by competitive inhibition of folic acid induce megaloblastic changes in the marrow.

Megaloblastic change in haemolytic anaemia. Finally, deficiency of folate arises when excessive demand outstrips supply, even when the latter is sufficient to meet normal needs. This explains the megaloblastic transformation of the marrow occasionally seen in cases of chronic haemolytic anaemia. We have observed a case of fatal megaloblastic anaemia in an adolescent girl addicted to ingestion of naphthalene (mothballs). A thick deposit of inspissated mucus on the mucosal surface of the ileum was found *post mortem*, and may have impaired B_{12} absorption.

The essential metabolic abnormality which results in megaloblastic erythropoiesis in the diseases considered above resides in interference with the formation of nucleic acids. Folinic acid is necessary for the formation of purines and pyrimidines, a stage in the production of nucleosides, from which the elaboration of nucleic acids is mediated by B_{12}. Thus deficiency in either folic acid or vitamin B_{12} will reduce the synthesis of nucleic acids that is required for DNA synthesis in the progressive division and maturation of red cell precursors. This deficiency has its clear morphological expression in the characteristic alteration of nuclear structure to the fine reticular pattern that is the earliest microscopic indication of megaloblastic transformation in a primitive nucleated red cell.

In some rare cases which present a macrocytic blood picture, nucleated red cells are practically absent from the blood throughout the disease and there is a great diminution in the number of polymorphonuclear leukocytes and platelets. There is a lack of cellular proliferation in the bone marrow and on marrow examination a state of hypoplasia is found. The marrow of the long bones is yellow or there may be small islets of reddish marrow here and there, while the marrow in the short bones may also be deficient. The appearances suggest a progressive failure of the marrow during which some of the primitive cells revert to megaloblastic type. Such cases usually do not benefit from vitamin B_{12} or folic acid and their real nature is unknown; probably they belong more to the group of aplastic anaemias.

Hypochromic microcytic anaemia

This form of anaemia is due to iron deficiency and is much commoner in women than men because of the increased iron loss from menstruation and reproduction. Chronic blood loss is the most important single etiological factor in the development of iron deficiency in adults but lack of iron in the diet or defective absorption from the gut also play a part in some cases. There is thus no sharp distinction between chronic post-haemorrhagic anaemia (p. 401) and anaemia due to dietary deficiency of iron or impaired absorption or utilisation of iron, the relative importance of these factors varying between individual cases. There is also a nutritional microcytic anaemia of infants, especially in those born prematurely.

Conditions of occurrence. This type of anaemia affects women mainly during the reproductive period of life, and tends to be aggravated by repeated pregnancies and by prolonged or excessive menstrual loss, often exceeding 150 ml. per month. After the menopause it may disappear. In an otherwise healthy person blood loss averaging 8 ml. per day can be made good. Important predisposing factors in patients with iron deficiency include chronic gastritis, a low intake of available iron, and malabsorption syndrome (p. 523). Iron absorption is impaired in subjects with chronic atrophic gastritis (probably from lack of hydrochloric acid secre-

tion) which is of auto-immune nature (p. 419). Occasionally iron deficiency anaemia is observed in men, usually in circumstances of repeated blood loss combined with one or more of the additional factors outlined above, and sometimes after partial gastrectomy.

The blood picture. The anaemia is of the microcytic hypochromic type, the cells being of smaller diameter than normal and of reduced volume (e.g. 50–70 cu.μ); they are inadequately filled with haemoglobin so that the MCHC is low, 30 per cent or less. The fall in the number of red cells is usually not so great; many of the red cells show ring-staining owing to deficiency in haemoglobin, but some are normochromic (Fig. 16.31). Poikilocytes are less common than in megaloblastic anaemia and erythroblasts are rarely found. The leukocyte count is usually normal. The platelet count is also normal, but in long-standing cases it may be increased and venous thrombosis may occur. The concentration of serum bilirubin is below normal and there is no evidence of increased haemolysis, but if blood loss is an important factor, there may be a reticulocytosis. The serum iron is reduced to below 70 μg./100 ml. but the total iron-binding capacity is increased. Accordingly the anaemia is due mainly to faults in the quality of the erythrocytes—they are undersized and deficient in haemoglobin. The bone marrow examined by sternal biopsy shows a degree of normoblastic hyperplasia, an increased number of early forms being accompanied by a high proportion of small, poorly haemoglobinised pyknotic normoblasts (Fig. 16.32): the marrow responds to the stimulus of anoxia by hyperplasia, but is

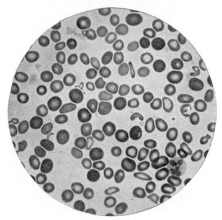

Fig. 16.31.—Film of blood from a case of microcytic anaemia. Some of the erythrocytes show ring-staining owing to deficiency in haemoglobin, others are larger and uniformly stained. × 400.

unable to produce red cells of normal size and haemoglobin content because of lack of enough iron to make the required quantity of haemoglobin. The bone marrow is devoid of stainable iron.

Associated conditions. The spleen as a rule is slightly enlarged but is only rarely palpable. In a high proportion of cases the nutrition of the nails is affected; they are longitudinally striated, hollowed and unduly brittle, the condition being known as *koilonychia*. Achlorhydria or hypochlorhydria is usually present, but the degree of atrophic gastritis is often less severe than in pernicious anaemia; the gastric juice contains the intrinsic factor, and often some pepsin and mucus is usually present in excess. In about 20 per cent of cases antibodies to gastric parietal cells (see p. 490) have been found. Digestive disturbance is usually present, also *glossitis* with redness and soreness of the tongue and *cheilosis* with atrophy and fissuring of the angles of the mouth are fairly common, similar to that in riboflavin and nicotinic acid deficiency. Whether due to lack of these vitamins or to deficiencies in the iron-containing cytochrome enzymes is uncertain; however, all respond to iron therapy. There is some evidence also that in some cases improvement in gastric

secretion results from iron therapy. Sometimes there is dysphagia, which is now usually attributed to contraction of the cricopharyngeus muscle or at least to its non-relaxation during the act of deglutition. The dysphagia depends on structural changes, both hypertrophic and atrophic, in the epithelium of the mouth, pharynx and oesophagus. The association of the three symptoms, anaemia, glossitis and post-cricoid dysphagia, was first recorded by Kelly and Paterson in 1919 but is generally known as the Plummer–Vinson syndrome. Carcinoma supervenes in this part of the oesophagus (p. 485) too often to be merely coincidental, as Paterson first pointed out. The anaemia is amenable to treatment with large doses of iron, but it must be emphasised that an essential part of the management is a careful search for a source of chronic blood loss. As with pernicious anaemia, a familial element has been observed in a proportion of cases, and depends presumably on the tendency of auto-immune gastritis to be familial (p. 490).

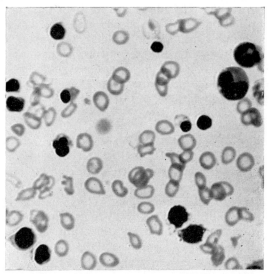

Fig. 16.32.—Sternal marrow in hypochromic microcytic anaemia, showing normoblastic hyperplasia. There had been considerable post-partum haemorrhage, superimposed on long-standing iron-deficiency anaemia. × 1000.

Nutritional anaemia in infancy. This is seen especially in premature infants whose insufficient prenatal stores of iron may be reduced still further by clamping of the umbilical cord as soon as the infant is born. Anaemia or iron deficiency in the mother during pregnancy is rarely an important factor because the fetus receives priority over maternal needs for iron. The maternal supply must suffice until dietary iron begins to be utilised towards the end of the first year. The anaemia is of microcytic type with low MCHC, low MCV, and scanty or no nucleated red cells. A similar type of anaemia is present in infantile scurvy (p. 446). As in the adult with malabsorption syndrome, the anaemia associated with coeliac disease, usually of the microcytic type, sometimes becomes macrocytic later. Macrocytic anaemia has been encountered also with nutritional deficiencies involving lack of folic acid and vitamin C.

The anaemia of ankylostomiasis. In warm climates intestinal infestation with hookworms is an extremely common and important cause of anaemia and in a community in which infestation is prevalent the chronic ill-health produced may be a factor of economic importance. The anaemia is now thought to be the result of chronic blood loss from the bites of the worms in poorly nourished individuals; it can be relieved by the administration of iron without removal of the worms. The blood picture is of the hypochromic microcytic type characteristic of iron deficiency, but an important observation of diagnostic value is the presence of eosinophil leukocytosis (sometimes 3000 per c.mm. or so) due to the parasitic infestation. The diagnosis is made by finding the ova in the faeces.

Drugs and the haemopoietic system

The haemopoietic system is one of the most susceptible tissues to the toxic effects of various chemicals, and blood disorders are among the most frequent and serious manifestations of toxic drug reactions. So varied are the effects that almost any form of blood dyscrasia may on occasion prove to be drug-induced.

Mode of action. Marrow failure is the most serious of the drug-induced blood dyscrasias. A drug may be directly cytotoxic, suppressing haemopoietic activity so that the marrow becomes fatty everywhere and there is peripheral pancytopenia, i.e. anaemia, neutropenia and thrombocytopenia. Resultant effects include agranulocytic angina (p. 396) and purpura (p. 446). While a large number of compounds is capable of producing aplasia, the precise mode of action is known in only a few instances,

e.g. aminopterin and amethopterin, which interfere with the utilisation of folic acid. The mortality varies with various agents; with some, e.g. chloramphenicol, recovery of the marrow is unusual.

Drugs may also act by inducing *sensitisation* (p. 109) sometimes rapidly, sometimes only after prolonged administration. Once sensitisation is established, even a minute dose will produce a profound effect, e.g. agranulocytosis following the administration of amidopyrine (p. 396) and thrombocytopenia following the use of Sedormid (p. 446).

Haemolytic anaemia due to drugs is commonly associated with the production of Heinz bodies. Reference has been made to deficiency of the enzyme G-6 PD in this connection (p. 408) but drug-induced Heinz body anaemia can occur in the absence of this enzyme deficiency if enough of the drug, e.g. phenacetin, is ingested. The induction of auto-immune haemolytic anaemia by methyldopa has already been mentioned on p. 415.

As mentioned on p. 423, megaloblastic anaemia also may result from taking certain drugs, and sidero-achrestic anaemia, giving a picture resembling iron deficiency, may also result from drugs (p. 428).

The true incidence of drug-induced blood dyscrasias is not known and the risk to an individual patient cannot therefore be calculated. Once marrow damage has occurred there is no certain means of reversing it. In most cases the use of marrow-depressing drugs can be avoided as innocuous alternatives exist and these should be employed in preference wherever possible.

Hypoplastic and aplastic anaemia. Anaemia due to diminution in the volume of haemopoietic marrow is termed *aplastic* when little or no cellular marrow exists, and *hypoplastic* when the marrow is merely of reduced cellularity, as is more commonly the case. Two varieties of the condition are described:

(*a*) The *primary* or *idiopathic* form, which may be genetically-determined, as in the Fanconi type, and

(*b*) a *symptomatic* or *secondary* form, due to the toxic action of drugs and chemical poisons or physical agents on a previously healthy marrow.

In aplastic anaemia the characteristic findings in the peripheral blood are a marked deficiency in all the formed elements produced by the marrow—erythrocytes, granular leukocytes and platelets. Reticulocytes are usually diminished or absent, but may be increased in a minority of cases where an element of increased red cell destruction is also present. There is, however, usually no evidence of increased blood destruction, the anaemia being due to failure to replace

or for immunosuppression; X-rays; chloramphenicol; butazolidine; antithyroid drugs; anticonvulsants and gold salts. In some of these toxic varieties the marrow is hypoplastic or even aplastic as in the primary form of the disease, but in others it is surprisingly cellular and actual hyperplasia, but with diminished output, may be found. Such dyspoietic cases

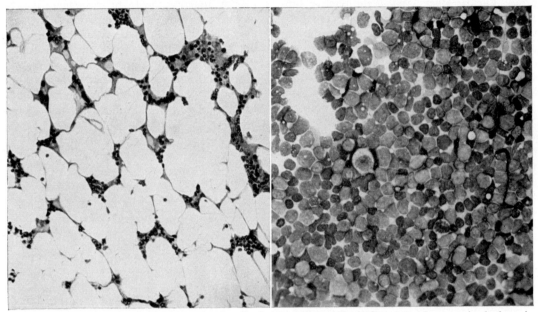

FIG. 16.33.—Sternal marrow biopsy in aplastic anaemia due to chloramphenicol. There is great reduction in the numbers of all the cellular elements. × 250.

FIG. 16.34.—Smear from sternal marrow in aleukaemic lymphatic leukaemia. The clinical picture was that of aplastic anaemia. × 400.

the cells as they wear out. The MCHC and MCV are normal. Associated with the deficiency of platelets a purpuric eruption may be present, and while this is often terminal, it is occasionally the presenting feature: similarly the agranulocytosis may lead to ulcerative lesions about the mouth and throat (p. 396). Spontaneous cases of this kind are rare; they occur most often in early life, and are termed *primary*. In such cases there is little or no red marrow in the body, even the short and flat bones being filled with pale fatty marrow, or sometimes with watery gelatinous tissue devoid of haemopoietic elements, but usually containing plasma cells and an excess of haemosiderin. In adults a similar diminution in all the formed elements of the peripheral blood is seen both without known cause and more commonly secondary to the effects of cytotoxic agents. A great number is known, including nitrogen mustards and other cytotoxic agents used to treat malignancy

have been called "refractory anaemias" because of the failure of the cellular marrow to respond to haematinics (see p. 428), and toxic industrial solvents, such as benzol, have been thought to be concerned in their pathogenesis. A diagnosis of aplastic anaemia cannot be made on the results of examination of the peripheral blood alone, and examination of the marrow by films and sections of the marrow biopsy (Fig. 16.33) is essential to establish the diagnosis during life and to separate cases of true aplasia from those of refractory anaemia with hypercellular marrow. Also in aleukaemic leukaemia, the pancytopenia may suggest marrow aplasia, but sternal puncture will reveal the lymphoblastic replacement of the marrow (Fig. 16.34). Some cases of aplastic anaemia go through a phase of partial megaloblastic change in the hypocellular marrow so that in its morphology the blood resembles that of pernicious anaemia. Such cases were formerly regarded as examples of pernicious anaemia in which the marrow had become exhausted but, since B_{12} and folic acid therapy is without effect, it is probable that they are of a fundamentally different nature.

Those exposed to external irradiation by radium or X-rays may develop marrow aplasia, the leukopoietic tissues usually being first affected. On the other hand, if radioactive substances are ingested, the heavy metals are stored in the bones and continuous internal irradiation of the marrow results in different effects. An outstanding example of this condition was the anaemia observed in America in girls working with luminous paint containing radium and mesothorium. From the practice of pointing with the lips the brushes used in applying the paints, minute amounts of the radioactive metals were ingested; a severe and fatal anaemia resulted, usually of macrocytic type. Necrosis of the bones, especially of the jaws, was also observed and in some cases bone sarcoma developed (see p. 759).

In some cases of paroxysmal nocturnal haemoglobinuria (p. 410) the marrow is hypoplastic at an early stage in the disease.

Pure red cell aplasia. In this rare form of marrow failure erythrocyte production alone is affected. Thrombocytopenia and agranulocytosis, which accompany the usual form of aplastic anaemia, are absent and these patients survive for long periods when supported by blood transfusion. Remissions usually occur and considerable periods of good health may be enjoyed. In some cases the disease has been associated with a thymic tumour, removal of which has resulted in a reticulocytosis and remarkable improvement in the anaemia.

Thrombocytopenic purpura. Rarely, aplasia affects mainly the megakaryocytes, resulting in thrombocytopenic purpura. The true nature of such cases is obscure, but the prognosis is much worse than in idiopathic thrombocytopenia in which there is hyperplasia of the megakaryocytes (p. 444).

Agranulocytosis (p. 396) may also dominate the clinical picture in aplastic anaemia.

Refractory anaemia. Anaemia resistant to treatment is a common association of infections, uraemia, neoplasia, connective tissue diseases and various other conditions, and may also result from drug treatment (see p. 426); but refractory anaemia due to a primary marrow dysfunction is less common. Cases in which the

marrow is hypercellular (p. 427) would seem from cytological examination to be attributable to an arrest of cellular maturation but investigations using radioactive isotopes have demonstrated intramedullary destruction of newly formed red cells. This process has been called *ineffective erythropoiesis* and accounts well for the apparent discrepancy between the hyperplastic marrow and the aregenerative blood picture. In some the neutrophils and/or the platelets may also be reduced in number but whether similar mechanisms account for this is unknown. Erythropoiesis is commonly normoblastic and sometimes iron-containing normoblasts (sideroblasts) are numerous (Figs. 16.35, 1.12, p. 11), the anaemia then being termed

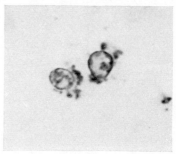

Fig. 16.35.—Sternal marrow smear in sidero-achrestic anaemia in a patient with carcinomatosis. Two normoblasts containing iron-rich granules are shown (Prussian blue reaction). × 1500.

sideroblastic or *sidero-achrestic*. Failure of utilisation of iron is evident from the association between the presence of a hypochromic blood picture and excess iron in the marrow. In one form, *hereditary hypochromic anaemia*, the disease is genetically determined, being sex-linked and carried on the X chromosome, but usually the cause of these sideroblastic anaemias, when drug action has been excluded, is obscure. In a few instances some improvement has followed the administration of pyridoxine but the significance of this is uncertain.

In another form of refractory anaemia, erythropoiesis is megaloblastic and the blood macrocytic, the appearances closely resembling the findings in pernicious anaemia but there is no response to either B_{12} or folic acid. Among the haemoglobinised megaloblasts giant forms with multiple nuclei (polyploidy) are to be found, and the cytoplasm of a variable proportion of the most mature forms may show a positive periodic acid-Schiff reaction. Such cases, first described by Di Guglielmo, are believed to be related to erythraemia (red cell leukaemia) although only in a minority does this disease eventually develop. The prognosis is poor and few survive for many months. Although primary refractory anaemias are rare, their study yields valuable illustrations of pathological mechanisms in dyshaemopoiesis, and it may be that with better understanding of these improved management will become possible.

THE MYELOPROLIFERATIVE DISORDERS

This term embraces a group of diseases which have certain features in common and thus appear to be interrelated. It was first applied to the conditions in which excessive numbers of red and white cells and/or their precursors appeared in the blood in varying proportions. Such conditions include polycythaemia vera, myeloid leukaemia and certain disorders with a leuko-erythroblastic blood picture such as myelofibrosis with hepatosplenomegaly due to myeloid transformation. Later haemorrhagic thrombocythaemia, erythroleukaemia (Di Guglielmo's syndrome) were also included. These diseases of the haemopoietic system are peculiar in that what appear to be transitions between one and another are not rarely encountered but opinion is still divided as to their exact relationships and on whether such appearances indicate genuine transitions or mere superficial resemblances. Recent observations on the myeloid cell series do not wholly support the view that polycythaemia vera, splenomegaly with myeloid metaplasia and chronic myeloid leukaemia are merely variants or phases of one fundamental disorder. The neutrophils in polycythaemia vera are rich in alkaline phosphatase whereas in chronic myeloid leukaemia the enzyme is reduced. The 22 Ph' chromosome of myeloid leukaemic cells (p. 436) is not found in the formative cells of polycythaemia or other leuko-erythroblastic states. The term "myeloproliferative disorder" may be a convenient way of indicating that many hyperplastic conditions of the bone marrow and lympho-reticular organs may share certain features, and that this can be attributed to an origin from the primitive lympho-haemopoietic stem cells which pass into the blood and reach the organs and tissues (p. 125). But it would be a mistake to infer too close a relationship or assume an etiological connection that is as yet unproven and there is a real danger that the term may be used to cover too wide a variety of conditions of fundamentally different nature.

Marrow replacement syndrome. This condition occurs when the formative marrow is replaced by some abnormal tissue, e.g. in fibrous transformation (Fig. 16.36), in osteosclerosis (marble bone disease), in secondary carcinomatosis of bones (Fig. 16.37) and rarely in multiple myelomatosis. The anaemia is characterised by the appearance in the blood of primitive cells of both red and white series rather than by a severe fall in the haemoglobin level, although this commonly occurs later. There may be a considerable number of early and late normoblasts and rarely a few megaloblasts may appear; the number of reticulocytes is usually considerably increased. The leukocyte count is raised (20,000 or more per c.mm.) owing to increase of polymorphonuclears with some myelocytes and intermediate forms,

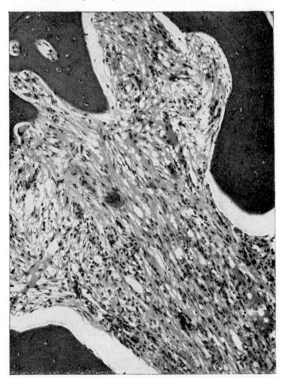

FIG. 16.36.—Myelofibrosis associated with leuko-erythroblastic blood picture.

and sometimes these may be so numerous as to simulate leukaemia, especially when there is pronounced extramedullary haemopoiesis and splenomegaly is conspicuous (p. 453). The anaemia is termed *leuko-erythroblastic* or *osteosclerotic*. In myelofibrosis, sternal puncture results in a "dry tap" and iliac crest biopsy may be required. In some cases there may be actually an increase of red marrow, e.g. around cancer nodules, and the anaemia in these cannot be ascribed to a replacement of haemopoietic tissue by the neoplastic cells. In other cases the sclerotic changes in bones may lead to marrow deficiency but it is

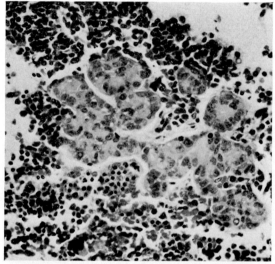

Fig. 16.37.—Section of sternal marrow aspirate showing metastatic breast carcinoma. × 250.

then likely that myeloid tissue will form in the spleen, liver, etc. In such extramedullary haemopoietic foci megakaryocytes are often very numerous.

The leukaemias

In these diseases there is generally a remarkable increase of the leukocytes in the blood, which is of neoplastic nature. There are three main varieties of leukaemia: one in which the cells in excess are of the myeloid series—*myeloid leukaemia*; one in which the cells are of the lymphoid series—*lymphatic leukaemia*, and there is a third less frequent type in which the monocytes are in excess—*monocytic leukaemia*. The leukocyte-forming tissues are hyperplastic in varying degree and leukocytic infiltrations of

various organs are common, especially in the lymphatic form. The disease may be chronic, lasting sometimes three or four years, but in all three types there are cases which run a comparatively rapid course. The term "acute" applied to leukaemia usually implies not only a more rapid clinical course, but also the presence of more primitive cells in the blood stream. Along with the leukocyte increase in the blood there is a varying degree of anaemia, which is more marked and advances more rapidly in the acute cases.

In all forms of leukaemia the changes in the blood are secondary to the neoplastic changes in the leukocyte-forming tissues. In some cases the marrow changes occur without a blood leukocytosis, and the term "aleukaemic leukaemia" is then usually applied. No doubt an aleukaemic (or pre-leukaemic) stage may occur in every case of leukaemia.

The blood

In *chronic myeloid leukaemia* the number of leukocytes may be enormously increased. A count of 300,000 per c.mm. is common, and even higher figures occur; in consequence of this and the anaemia often present, the blood may be paler and rather more opaque-looking than the normal. The main increase is on the part of the finely granular neutrophil cells, including mature polymorphonuclear leukocytes, myelocytes, and metamyelocytes (Fig. 16.38). The proportion of the two types of cells varies much, and the myelocytes may even exceed the polymorphs, especially in the less chronic cases (Fig. 16.39). Occasionally eosinophils and/or basophils are especially numerous, but usually neutrophils predominate. In addition to the ordinary neutrophil myelocytes, there are earlier stages, promyelocytes with basophil granules, and also still younger cells, without granules—*myeloblasts*. These last are especially numerous in the more acute cases (Fig. 16.40), and they sometimes appear in large numbers in the terminal stages in chronic cases—the so-called "acute myeloblastic" termination, when the effects of anaemia, thrombocytopenia and agranulocytosis become prominent, and ulcerative lesions occur in the mouth and throat.

In the more chronic cases of myeloid leukaemia there is only a moderate reduction in the number of the red cells and polycythaemia may be present initially. The blood platelets may be much increased.

There is thus in myeloid leukaemia an overflow of the neoplastic leukocytes of the marrow into the blood, and the circulating cells represent different stages in the formation of the granular

the chronic lymphatic type is often about 100,000 per c.mm., i.e. less than in the myeloid type, and anaemia tends to be only slight when the patient is first seen. Normoblasts are in general scanty and may be absent, in contrast to myeloid leukaemia. Occasionally there is a concomitant auto-immune haemolytic anaemia of either

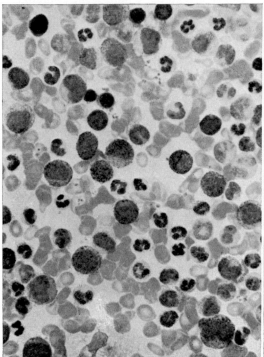

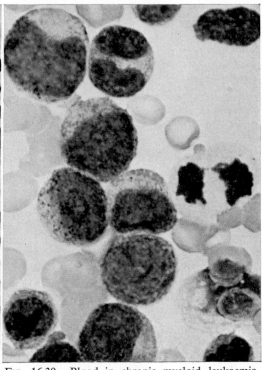

Fig. 16.38.—Blood in chronic myeloid leukaemia, showing myelocytes, polymorphonuclear leukocytes and intermediate forms; two erythroblasts are seen above centre of field. × 500.

Fig. 16.39.—Blood in chronic myeloid leukaemia, showing finely granular myelocytes and polymorphonuclear leukocytes. One cell is in mitosis. × 1000.

leukocytes. Further, the more rapidly progressive a case is, the more do the more primitive cells predominate, and aberrant polyploid types, unlike normal myeloblasts, may be numerous. Sometimes, under treatment, the number of leukocytes may fall greatly and may reach the normal level; but even then myelocytes are usually still present.

In *lymphatic leukaemia* the blood picture is much simpler and presents a marked increase on the part of the lymphocytes, which often number more than 95 per cent of the cells present. In the chronic cases nearly all may be small lymphocytes (Fig. 16.41), or there may be an admixture of larger forms; the myeloid cells and monocytes are not increased and are often actually diminished in number. The leukocyte count in

cold or warm antibody type, as mentioned on pages 411 and 412.

Monocytic leukaemia. This variety is relatively common, is usually acute or subacute, and is associated with necrotic inflammatory conditions of mouth and fauces and sometimes of the rectum. There is irregular pyrexia, advancing anaemia, petechiae and bleeding from the mucous membranes. The leukocyte count is usually not very high but occasionally it is over 250,000 per c.mm. The percentage of monocytes and "blast" cells may be 70 or higher and the more mature cells give the characteristic segregation granules on supravital staining with neutral red. In addition to ordinary monocytes there may also be larger monocyte precursors, the cytoplasm of which often shows a projection of pseudopodia. Unlike the more mature cells, these larger cells are often oxidase-negative. This pure monocytic form is termed the *Schilling type* of leukaemia (Fig. 16.42). An admixture of myeloblasts and myelocytes is present in

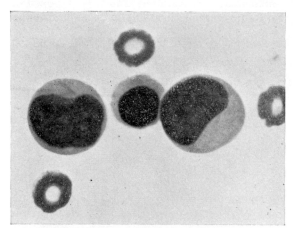

Fig. 16.40.—Blood in acute myeloid leukaemia, showing two large myeloblasts; the one on the left contains an Auer rod. × 1000.

some cases in the blood and these cells predominate in the enlarged, infiltrated lymph nodes, spleen, liver and bone marrow. This myelo-monocytic form of leukaemia is termed the *Naegeli type* (Fig. 16.43). Leukaemic infiltration is often scanty but tumour-like nodules may occur, and leukaemic masses may invade the wall of the rectum and give rise to necrotic and ulcerative infection there.

Acute leukaemia

This is the commonest form of leukaemia in children and adolescents, but it also occurs in adults at all ages.

Clinical features. In *children*, in whom the acute lymphatic form is commonest, the disease appears abruptly with fever, weakness, pallor, bleeding from the gums and often petechial haemorrhages in the skin. Intercurrent infections are very common and the whole course from onset to death may occupy only a few weeks. In *adults* the onset is more often insidious and the symptoms are commonly of tiredness and dyspnoea on exertion owing to concomitant anaemia. The inclusion of such cases in the acute leukaemia group refers mainly to the primitive cell types that dominate the blood and bone

marrow picture which may be fully developed when the disease is first recognised. Markedly swollen spongy and bleeding gums are especially associated with the monocytic form of the disease.

The blood picture. The peripheral blood shows a moderate increase in the total white cell count, 20,000–50,000 per c.mm. being common, but in over one third of the cases the total count may be little raised or even be reduced although 90 per cent of the leukocytes are primitive cells with prominent nucleoli. These patients present clinically like cases of aplastic anaemia with rapidly advancing normocytic anaemia, severe agranulocytic angina and severe thrombocytopenia responsible for the purpuric state.

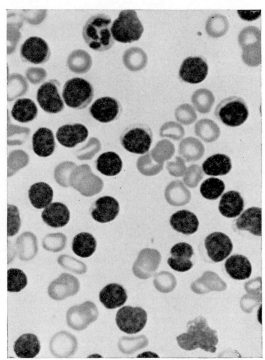

Fig. 16.41.—Blood in chronic lymphatic leukaemia, showing increase of small lymphocytes.

The erythrocytes are scanty and show 'ring-staining' owing to deficiency of haemoglobin. × 750.

The nature of the primitive cells can sometimes be distinguished by the presence of some that have differentiated sufficiently for recognition, e.g. the presence of appreciable numbers of lymphocytes suggests that the blast cells are lymphoblasts (Fig. 16.44). Similarly, the presence of promyelocytes suggests acute myeloid leukaemia. Changes in the organs in acute

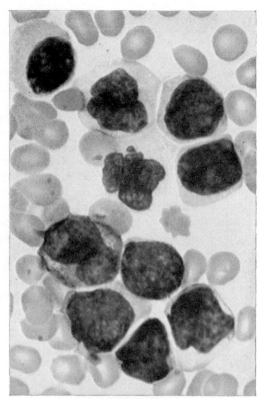

FIG. 16.42.—Acute monocytic leukaemia (Schilling type). × 1000.

leukaemia are usually less pronounced than in chronic forms but are of the same general nature.

Cytochemical tests of value in the diagnosis and classification of leukaemia include: (1) the *leukocyte alkaline phosphatase reaction*. The amount of the enzyme is low in chronic myeloid leukaemic leukocytes and raised in the granulocytes in other myeloproliferative disorders and in reactive leukocytosis. (2) the *periodic acid Schiff (PAS) reaction*, which helps to classify acute leukaemia: lymphoblasts may contain coarse cytoplasmic PAS-positive clumps, whereas myeloblasts and monoblasts are negative or contain finer PAS-positive granules. (3) the *oxidase reaction*, which is positive for promyelocytes, myelocytes and polymorphs, and negative for blast cells and lymphoid cells.

Chloroma. The term is applied to a greenish cellular tumour which is associated with acute leukaemia, usually in childhood. The growth, which is often multiple, starts usually under the periosteum of the bones of the head, occasionally projecting into the orbit or cranial cavity, and afterwards may appear in other parts. The greenish colour disappears on exposure to the air and its nature and significance are unknown. As has been said, a leukaemic condition of the blood is present, and is usually myeloblastic. We have, however, observed multiple chloromata in the breasts in association with acute leukaemia of monocytic type. The leukocyte count may not be much raised. The cells of the growths correspond with those in the blood, and the condition is of interest as suggesting an intermediate stage between acute myeloid leukaemia and ordinary tumour growth.

Changes in the organs

Bone marrow. *In chronic myeloid leukaemia* the fatty marrow is replaced by a pale cellular marrow, and there is considerable absorption of bone trabeculae, so that it is easy to cut out large portions (Fig. 16.45). The colour is usually pinkish-grey with redder streaks and patches, and sometimes it has a slightly greenish tint; autolytic softening may be present *post mortem*, so that the marrow appears almost purulent. On microscopic examination, there is an enormous hyperplasia of the cells of the marrow, including in the early stages the megakaryocytes. The finely granular myelocytes and myeloblasts, however, markedly preponderate, and the latter are the chief cells in acute cases. Erythroblasts are still present, but are relatively reduced in number. It is of particular interest that the Ph' chromosome is present in cases of chronic myeloid leukaemia not only in the myeloid cells but also in the red cell precursors and megakaryocytes (p. 436).

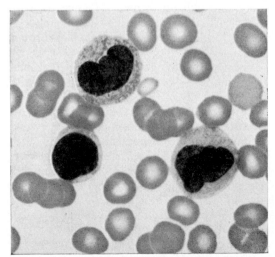

FIG. 16.43.—Monocytic leukaemia (Naegeli type). × 1000.

In the lymphatic type, the cells proper to the marrow may have almost disappeared and been replaced by masses of lymphocytes, between which run blood vessels with thin and badly defined walls, from which there may be much haemorrhage, so that the marrow is dark red. Erythroblasts and megakaryocytes are very

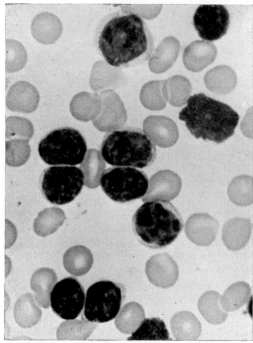

FIG. 16.44.—Blood in acute lymphatic leukaemia, showing increased numbers of immature lymphocytes. × 900.

scanty, and difficult to find. The marrow tissue is thus virtually destroyed by the lymphocytic invasion, and in this way the anaemia is brought about.

The marrow changes described in leukaemia are sometimes associated with a dull pain in the bones, especially in the sternum.

The spleen. Great enlargement of the spleen is a feature in chronic leukaemia. It is greater in the myeloid type, where the weight of the organ may reach 3 kg. or more, but occasionally it may be almost as large in chronic lymphatic leukaemia. In the more acute types, the enlargement is only moderate, or may even be slight. A large spleen in leukaemia is usually moderately firm and, on section, shows a fairly uniform or somewhat mottled pale red surface, in which the Malpighian bodies, as a rule, cannot be distinguished. Pale infarcts are often

present and may be large. In acute cases, the organ is of normal or even soft consistence. The essential histological change in all cases is packing of the pulp with leukocytes of the same types as those in the blood. Thus, in the myeloid type the pulp is occupied chiefly by myeloblasts, myelocytes and granular leukocytes. There is also erythropoiesis in the spleen, and megakaryocytes can be found. The Malpighian bodies usually take no part in the change and are small; they appear scanty owing to their being separated by the enlarged pulp. In the lymphatic type, the pulp is so packed with lymphocytes that the Malpighian bodies are indistinguishable. Sometimes a considerable amount of haemosiderin is present in the spleen pulp.

Lymph nodes. In the myeloid type, the nodes may be of normal size or slightly enlarged. On microscopic examination, in chronic myeloid leukaemia it is common to find accumulation of myeloid cells, including megakaryocytes.

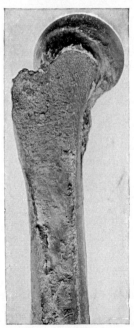

FIG. 16.45.—Section of femur in leukaemia.
The fatty marrow is replaced by a pale cellular tissue and there is also absorption of bone. × ½.

In the lymphatic form there is usually marked enlargement of the lymph nodes. In chronic cases this enlargement may be gross and affect many groups, while in the more acute cases the enlargement is often localised to a particular region, and is less marked or may be slight. The nodes are soft and highly cellular and usually greyish or pinkish-grey, although occasionally haemorrhages are present, especially in the more acute cases. The enlargement is due to an overrunning of the nodes with lymphocytes similar to those in excess in the blood. The

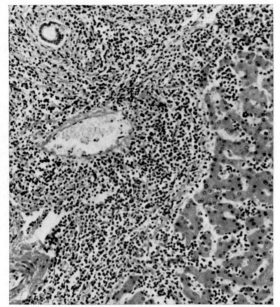

FIG. 16.46.—Section of liver in lymphatic leukaemia, showing infiltration of lymphocytes around the portal tracts. × 60.

normal architecture of the nodes is lost, and they have a uniformly cellular appearance, with loss of the normal differentiation into germinal centres, follicles, deep cortex and medulla. There is little or no tendency to fibrosis even in very chronic cases.

In monocytic leukaemia, also, a moderate enlargement of lymph nodes occurs, the cervical nodes being those most commonly affected.

Changes in other organs. These are chiefly infiltrations of leukaemic cells, and are most prominent in lymphatic leukaemia. Such infiltrations may be general and produce uniform enlargement of organs with pallor, irregular pale areas, or sometimes even to rounded tumour-like masses. A periportal infiltration of lymphocytes in the liver, with encroachment on the parenchyma, is common in lymphatic leukaemia (Fig. 16.46), and a similar condition is occasionally present in the kidneys, which may become greatly enlarged as a result; but the appearances and distribution of such infiltrations vary

P

greatly in different cases, and practically any organ in the body may be affected. In the myeloid type, collections of myelocytes, etc., are occasionally present in the sinusoids, and to a lesser extent in the portal tracts of the liver and around capillaries in various organs.

In leukaemias generally, especially when there is marked anaemia, fatty change and capillary haemorrhages are common in various organs, on serous surfaces, etc. In the brain, haemorrhage of considerable size is occasionally observed, and is apparently the result of blocking of the vessels with leukocyte thrombi. Such haemorrhage is often in multiple foci and irregularly distributed in the brain substance. The local effects of leukaemic infiltrates are largely responsible for the varied symptomatology encountered in cases of leukaemia.

In chronic leukaemia the amount of uric acid in the blood and in the urine is usually increased, and in the spleen there has been found an increase of uric acid and xanthine bases. These substances are derived mainly from nucleic acid, and their increase is no doubt due to the excessive breaking down of leukocytes that occurs in the disease.

The etiology of leukaemia

The cause of leukaemia in man is still unknown but much has been learned recently about factors that are concerned. The mortality in England and Wales attributed to leukaemia increased from 17 per million in 1931 to 54 per million in 1957. Subsequently, this rate of increase has not been maintained and this provides support for the belief that part at least of the increase was due to improved diagnosis. The disease occurs at all ages, but is most common over the age of 60 years. Until early adult life acute leukaemia is by far the commoner, but as age advances chronic myeloid, and then over the age of 60 years chronic lymphatic leukaemia, predominate, although there is a second peak of incidence of acute leukaemia. Males develop leukaemia only slightly more than females except in the chronic lymphatic form where the ratio is about 2 : 1.

Acute leukaemia occasionally undergoes temporary spontaneous remission but there have been recent striking advances in treatment, particularly of the acute lymphatic, and stem cell varieties of uncertain cytogenesis in childhood. In over 90 per cent of cases therapeutic agents, alone or in combination, can induce a remission which can be maintained for months or years, and then remission can be re-induced so that in some, survival may be prolonged for two to five years or even longer. These therapeutic agents fall into three classes: (1) steroids; (2) antimetabolites such as folic acid antagonists and antipurines, both of which interfere with the metabolism of the cells by blocking nucleic acid synthesis; (3) cytotoxic agents, of which a considerable number have been employed. No form of curative treatment has, however, yet emerged.

It has long been customary to regard leukaemia as a form of malignant neoplasia and there are many points of resemblance such as the development in the course of the disease of tumour-like masses composed of leukaemic cells or conversely a lymphosarcoma may after a time be accompanied by lymphatic leukaemia.

The clearly defined etiological factors in human leukaemia are few. There is, however, an undoubted association with ionising radiation, seen in (a) increased liability to chronic myeloid leukaemia in patients given deep X-ray therapy over the spine for ankylosing spondylitis; (b) the 8-fold increase in the incidence of chronic myeloid leukaemia in radiologists as compared with physicians; (c) the increased incidence of myeloid leukaemia amongst survivors of the atomic explosions at Hiroshima and Nagasaki. The incubation period between exposure to irradiation and the appearance of the disease is from 6 to over 20 years, and it has been shown that any considerable exposure to X-radiation produces recognisable chromosome damage which may persist for many years. Less certain are the suggestions that exposure of the fetus *in utero* to diagnostic X-ray examination in the late stages of pregnancy increases the risk of leukaemia in childhood, or that treatment of patients with polycythaemia with radioactive phosphorus increases the incidence of myeloid leukaemia. In all these examples there is a strong indication that the leukaemogenic effect is proportional to the total dose of irradiation.

Certain chromosomal abnormalities are associated with myeloid leukaemia in two possibly related ways. In mongolism, due to trisomy of the chromosome pair 21 in the Denver classification, there is a substantially increased risk of *acute* myeloid leukaemia. In most untreated cases the primitive cells of *chronic* myeloid leukaemia show a chromosomal abnormality consisting of partial loss of the long arm of one of the small acrocentric chromosomes, now classified as pair 22; this is seen both in "spontaneous" cases and in those thought to be induced by radiation. The abnormal 22 chromosome has been named the Philadelphia chromosome (Ph' for short) and its formation is regarded as an integral part of the leukaemic process, rather than as a mere epiphenomenon; it is not yet known whether this is the primary change in the induction of the disease process. A high rate of concordance for leukaemia has also been reported in identical twins, but strong evidence of a genetic factor is lacking.

Leukaemia in lower mammals has been studied especially in inbred strains of mice and guinea-pigs. In mice it is a common disease, especially the lymphatic type, and is often associated with lymphomatous tumours of the thymus, in which the leukaemic process seems to begin. Lymphatic leukaemia becomes more frequent in mice treated with carcinogenic agents. Pure-line strains have been bred with a very high incidence, and the disease can readily be transmitted from one animal to another of the same strain by inoculation of cells or cell-free filtrates. Certain types can be transmitted by inoculating cell-free filtrates into newborn mice (but not to older animals) of a strain which does not develop leukaemia spontaneously (Gross). By such experimental studies it has been established that the pathogenic agents are members of a group of murine leukaemia viruses. The disease is transmitted "vertically" in leukaemia-prone strains, i.e. from the mother to fetus, the tissues of which carry the virus *in utero*, although the pathogenic effects are not manifest until the animal is mature.

Virus particles morphologically identical to the viruses of mouse leukaemia have recently been identified in lymphoid neoplasia, including lymphatic leukaemia, arising spontaneously in cats (Jarrett, 1970). The virus has been passaged in cell cultures of various species including man, and inoculation of kittens has been folfowed by multiplication of the virus and development of a spectrum of lymphoid neoplasia which includes lymphosarcoma, reticulum-cell sarcoma, chronic lymphatic leukaemia and also acute leukaemia. Conditions resembling Hodgkin's disease and chronic myeloid leukaemia have not so far been observed. The interest of this work resides particularly in the ability of the virus to infect several species and to thrive and produce disease in outbred animals under natural conditions.

In fowls, too, leukaemia is comparatively common, different forms occurring, and being transmissible to other fowls by a cell-free filtrate, resembling in this respect the filterable tumours of birds. In leukaemia, as in tumours, the more undifferentiated the cell is, the more rapid is the course of the disease. If all these facts are considered it appears highly probable that leukaemia is an example of neoplasia, and that a number of different etiological factors are concerned in the different types.

Polycythaemia vera or erythraemia

This is a disease of middle and later life in which there is a marked increase in the number of red cells per c.mm., and also a marked increase in the percentage of haemoglobin. The patient has commonly a florid appearance, and there is a tendency to cyanosis, especially on exposure to cold. Peptic ulceration of stomach or duodenum is a commonly associated complaint, also gout.

The blood picture. The blood volume is considerably increased, so that the total increase of red cells is greater than is indicated by the number per c.mm. The red cells tend to be small and the MCHC is usually distinctly lowered; some polychromatophil corpuscles and normoblasts are occasionally to be found in films. The leukocytes may show little change, but a moderate increase of polymorphonuclears is usually observed and a white cell count of 25,000 per c.mm. is fairly common with many young cells and occasional myelocytes. The platelets are increased and multiple thromboses are not uncommon, but nevertheless undue bleeding may follow minor wounds. The spleen is enlarged, often considerably. The left ventricle of the heart undergoes compensatory hypertrophy. The blood pressure may be raised from an early stage and arteriosclerosis may develop.

Morphological changes. There is increase in the haemopoietic marrow which usually extends down the shafts of the long bones and produces an abnormally great number of erythrocytes. This is not compensatory but rather of neoplastic nature, analogous to the increase of leukocytes

in leukaemia. There is indeed much to support the view that polycythaemia vera is a *panmyelosis* with increased formative activity of *all* the cellular elements, and in a proportion of cases the blood picture comes to resemble myeloid leukaemia terminally, but the polymorphs, unlike those in leukaemia, are rich in alkaline phosphatase. In some cases of erythraemia the marrow eventually becomes fibrous and myeloid transformation occurs in the spleen and other sites so that a leuko-erythroblastic blood picture (p. 429) results. Acute myeloid leukaemia may also supervene.

Other neoplastic conditions of the bone marrow

Multiple myeloma (myelomatosis)

This is a neoplastic condition of plasma cells or their precursors, usually confined to the bone marrow, and occurring in elderly subjects, more commonly in men than women. Death results within 2–3 years, mainly from anaemia, infection, renal failure or skeletal lesions. Plasma cells are normally present in the bone marrow and may be increased in chronic infections, connective tissue diseases, etc. The proportion in such reactive states rarely exceeds 10 per cent.

Although not a common disease, multiple myeloma is of considerable interest and investigation of the so-called myeloma proteins, which are produced by the neoplastic cells, has contributed significantly to our understanding of both antibody production and neoplasia.

Morbid anatomy. The neoplastic tissue occurs usually in the form of numerous reddish nodules throughout the bones which normally contain red marrow (Fig. 16.47), but also throughout the long bones. It is therefore called multiple myeloma or myelomatosis. The nodules exert an osteolytic effect so that absorption and rarefaction of the affected bones take place and spontaneous fractures are common, especially in the ribs (Fig. 16.48). The effects of localised rarefaction are characteristically seen in the skull where the myeloma nodules in the diploë erode the tables, producing sharply punched-out defects in the bone. Occasionally a solitary discrete growth, usually in a long bone, may appear first, but only rarely does the disease fail eventually to become generalised throughout the skeleton. Amputation is therefore unlikely to effect cure, though a few successful cases have been recorded. The term *plasma-cell myeloma* is often used and *plasmacytoma* for the solitary form, but it should be remembered that plasmacytoma may occur elsewhere, e.g. the nasopharynx, stomach, etc., and its relation to the true myeloma is uncertain.

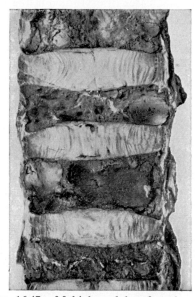

Fig. 16.47.—Multiple nodules of myeloma in vertebral column.
Note the collapse of the vertebrae with shortening.

Myeloma cells may be widely and diffusely distributed through the marrow without the formation of discrete nodules. Generalised osteoporosis may then develop and we have seen the vertebral bodies much collapsed and so softened that the tissue could be scooped out with the finger.

Microscopic appearances. The nodules or diffuse infiltrates of myelomatosis are highly cellular and vascular. The appearance of the cells is variable, but most commonly many of them are recognisable as plasma cells (Figs. 16.49, 16.50), having the typical eccentric cartwheel nucleus, and cytoplasm of various grades of basophilia and pyroninophilia due to their content of RNA. There may also be a pallid crescentic area of cytoplasm adjacent to the nucleus, and bi- and tri-nucleate cells are often seen. More primitive cells—plasmablasts—are also present in varying proportions. As with tumours in general, the cells may not be well differentiated, and in some cases they are

rounded, with a round nucleus, but do not show the characteristic features, outlined above, of plasma cells: cells of intermediate appearance between small lymphocytes and plasma cells may also predominate. There is usually little fibrous stroma.

Myeloma proteins. In most cases the myeloma cells, like normal plasma cells, synthesise and secrete immunoglobulin, but when this has been tested for immunological reactivity, it has not been shown to react strongly and specifically with any one of a large number of antigens, and it cannot therefore be regarded as an antibody; nor is there any other evidence to indicate that myeloma cells have proliferated as a result of an antigenic stimulus. In most cases, the level of serum immunoglobulins is raised, in some instances exceeding 10 g. per 100 ml.

A feature of considerable interest is the remarkable homogeneity of the myeloma protein in each particular case: it is entirely of one or other immunoglobulin class (IgG, IgA, etc.), and its uniformity of electrophoretic migration is shown by a narrow dense band or "peak", contrasting with the broader less well-defined bands of normal serum immunoglobulins. Moreover, evidence from chemical analysis suggests that the individual molecules are identical in the amino-acid sequences of their polypeptide chains. These findings indicate that, in any one case, most or all of the secreting myeloma cells are producing identical molecules of immunoglobulin and this in turn suggests that they have all originated from a single plasma

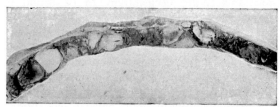

Fig. 16.48.—Multiple nodules of myeloma in a rib; numerous spontaneous fractures were present. $\times \frac{2}{3}$.

cell or plasma-cell precursor—hence the term *monoclonal gammopathy*. Not only is the conclusion that myeloma cells comprise a single clone of importance in relation to the nature of neoplasia, but it provides also strong support for Burnet's clonal selection theory of antibody production (p. 82). In more than 50 per cent of cases of myelomatosis, the cells secrete IgG; secretion of IgA is less common, IgD rare, and only two cases have so far been reported to secrete IgE. Comparison of myeloma immunoglobulins of the same class (e.g. IgG) from a number of cases shows that, in contrast to the homogeneity of the protein in each case, the proteins from different cases all differ from one another in their amino-acid sequences.

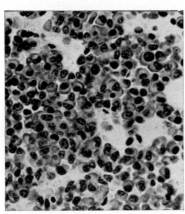

Fig. 16.49.—Section of sternal marrow aspirate in myelomatosis: clumps of plasma cells with eccentric nuclei and basophil cytoplasm, showing a marked perinuclear halo. × 360.

Another feature of myeloma cells is that they may produce immunoglobulin light chains in addition to whole molecules, and in 50 per cent of cases light chains in the form of monomers and dimers, of molecular weights 20,000 and 40,000 respectively, are demonstrable in the urine where they are known after their discoverer as *Bence–Jones proteins*. Adjustment of the pH of the urine to 4–6 and heating results in precipitation of the light chain molecules at about 50° C, and they re-dissolve at about 80° C. This test is positive in some cases where there is relatively little myeloma immunoglobulin in the serum, and so is of diagnostic value: it is rarely positive in macroglobulinaemia (see below) and lymphatic leukaemia.

Associated changes. *Skeleton.* Myelomatosis causes pronounced bone resorption with focal or generalised osteoporosis, a rise in the level of blood calcium, and increased excretion of calcium and phosphorus in the urine; the serum alkaline phosphatase, however, is usually not much raised.

Blood. The increased level of immunoglobulin in the plasma results in a tendency to unusually strong rouleaux formation and a high ESR, while the increase of protein may cause background staining in blood films. Anaemia

results from extensive infiltration of the marrow by myeloma cells, and is usually of normochromic normocytic type, although blood loss from a haemorrhagic tendency may bring about an iron-deficiency anaemia. The tendency to haemorrhage may be due to formation of complexes between myeloma immunoglobulin and several of the clotting factors. The neoplastic plasma cells sometimes appear in the blood in numbers which warrant the term *plasma cell leukaemia*. Infiltration of various organs may also occur.

Renal changes are common, and result from precipitation of Bence–Jones protein in the lumen of the renal tubules to form dense hyaline casts: these cause tubular obstruction and also stimulate a foreign-body giant-cell reaction, and consequent tubular destruction may bring about renal failure. Nephrocalcinosis may also result from the bone resorption.

Immunological deficiency. Patients with myelomatosis show an increased tendency to bacterial infections, produce relatively low titres of antibodies in response to various antigenic stimuli, and commonly have a low serum level of non-myeloma immunoglobulin. These features are attributable in part to the increased rate of catabolism of immunoglobulins which has been observed in myelomatosis, but it is

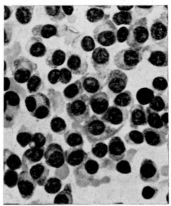

Fig. 16.50.—Smear of sternal marrow aspirate showing almost total replacement of the haemopoietic elements by plasma cells. × 520.

likely that antibody production is also impaired.

Amyloid deposition is a common complication of myelomatosis, and usually presents the pattern of "primary" amyloidosis (p. 195); the underlying condition is usually apparent from skeletal X-rays, but diffuse myelomatosis may remain undetected unless further diagnostic procedures, including marrow biopsy, are undertaken.

Conditions resembling myelomatosis

In some elderly individuals, excessive numbers of plasma cells appear in the bone marrow, accompanied by myeloma-like immunoglobulin in the serum and/or Bence–Jones protein in the urine, and yet the condition does not progress to fully developed myelomatosis.

Heavy-chain disease. This is a very rare condition in which the marrow and lymphoid tissues become infiltrated with lymphocytes, plasma cells, reticulum cells and eosinophil polymorphs. An abnormal protein is present in the plasma and urine and has been shown to be the Fc fragment of immuno-globulin heavy chains (see p. 77).

Macroglobulinaemia. This uncommon condition, originally described by Waldenström, occurs in individuals over 50 years of age, in men more often than women. The primary form of the disease, which is described below, runs a prolonged course; it is basically a monoclonal gammopathy of IgM class, and may be regarded as a low-grade neoplasm of lymphoid cells. In some cases, however, the syndrome is associated with a frankly malignant lymphoid neoplasm, and the outlook is then poor.

The clinical features include weakness and tiredness; spontaneous haemorrhage of the respiratory, urinary or alimentary tracts and in the periphery of the retinae; susceptibility to bacterial infections, and a variable degree of enlargement of the liver, spleen and lymph nodes. The plasma protein level is usually raised to 8 g. per 100 ml. or more, and the increase is due to the presence of immunoglobulin of IgM class with a molecular weight of approximately 10^6, and seen as a narrow myeloma-protein-like band on serum electrophoresis. It is insoluble in water, and precipitates when plasma is diluted with water (Sia test). In some instances, the IgM behaves as an auto-antibody, reacting with the patient's red cells to produce a haemolytic anaemia, while in others it has been shown to react *in vitro* with extracts of human and animal tissues. The macroglobulinaemia renders the blood unduly viscous, with resulting circulatory embarrassment, and in some instances it gels on cooling (*cryoglobulin*), so that exposure of the patient to cold may result in ischaemia, and even gangrene, of the extremities. The cells often show a strong tendency to aggregate *in vitro* which renders cell counting difficult, and the ESR is raised. The haemorrhagic tendency may be due to the IgM coating the platelets and preventing release of platelet Factor III, but the increase in macro-molecular globulin itself interferes with the poly-merisation of fibrin and thus impairs haemostasis.

Structural changes. The marrow is diffusely infiltrated with small lymphocytes, plasma cells, mast cells, and cells with vacuolated cytoplasm which appear intermediate between lymphocytes and plasma cells: there are no focal lesions in the bones, which are either normal on X-ray or show diffuse osteoporosis. The lymph nodes are moderately enlarged and are over-run with cells resembling small lymphocytes, but with more cytoplasm: unlike lymphosarcoma, the reticulin pattern of the lymph nodes is preserved. Similar cells infiltrate the portal tracts of the liver and Malpighian bodies of the spleen, and in some cases infiltrates are present also in the brain (Bing–Neel syndrome).

Solitary plasmacytoma has already been considered on p. 438.

Secondary tumours of bone marrow

Metastatic deposits, both of carcinoma and sarcoma, are fairly common in the bone marrow; and in malignant melanoma and carcinoma of certain organs, especially the breast, bronchus, prostate, and thyroid, the nodules may be very numerous and widespread. They occur especially in the red marrow. When the marrow of the short bones is extensively invaded, there is often a compensatory hyperplasia of red marrow in the long bones. The changes which occur in the blood are described on p. 429. Further, in some cases of carcinoma, especially of the prostate, there may be a remarkable condition of overgrowth and sclerosis of the bone around the nodules, and the bone marrow may be greatly encroached upon by the new bone, with resulting anaemia, often called *osteosclerotic anaemia* (p. 430); the blood picture is commonly of leuko-erythroblastic type.

HAEMORRHAGIC DISEASES

Under this heading we have grouped together a number of conditions of different etiology, which have the common feature of a liability to the occurrence of haemorrhages into the tissues and from mucous membranes. They fall into two broad classes, the *purpuras* and the *coagulation defects*. In purpura, the bleeding is chiefly in the skin and mucous membranes and is spontaneous. In coagulation defects, haemorrhage is usually initiated by trauma and is characterised by its persistence rather than by its severity.

A haemorrhagic tendency may be present also in some of the diseases already described, notably in acute leukaemia and in aplastic anaemia.

Before reading the following account of haemorrhagic disorders, it is essential to have a basic understanding of the physiological mechanisms and the various factors involved in haemostasis and coagulation of the blood. A brief account of this subject has been provided in relation to thrombosis on pp. 162–5.

Deficiency of coagulation factors

The combined deficiency of Factors II, VII, IX and X is common as an acquired abnormality due to the administration of oral anticoagulant drugs or as a result of vitamin-K deficiency, as in obstructive jaundice, malabsorption, or haemorrhagic disease of the newborn. The common genetically-determined coagulation defects are deficiency of Factor VIII or anti-haemophilic globulin (haemophilia), and Factor IX or Christmas factor (Christmas disease). Genetic deficiencies of the other coagulation factors are very rare.

Laboratory investigation of defects in prothrombin conversion. The activity of the tissue (extrinsic) thromboplastin system (p. 163) is studied in the *one-stage prothrombin time* in which calcium and tissue extract are added to citrated plasma and the time taken for a clot to form is measured. An overall screening test for the blood thromboplastin system is the *kaolin–cephalin clotting time* in which the clotting time of citrated plasma is measured after the addition of standard amounts of kaolin to produce maximum contact activation, cephalin to ensure an adequate amount of lipid, and calcium. A third

screening test is the *thrombin clotting time* which measures the time taken for a clot to form in citrated plasma on addition of a standard amount of thrombin: this is a measure of the thrombin–fibrinogen reaction.

These three screening tests permit the rough localisation of a clotting defect. Precise definition of the abnormality then depends on assay of single coagulation factors. Fibrinogen deficiency may also occur and can be detected by chemical estimation of the fibrinogen.

Defects of coagulation

Haemophilia. This disease is characterised by a congenital deficiency in the coagulating property of the blood. From almost any trifling wound there is persistent bleeding, while a larger one, especially that caused by tonsillectomy, may, in severe haemophilia, cause death. Haemorrhage occurs into the joints and into the subcutaneous tissues, and this may happen either "spontaneously" or as the result of slight injuries. Especially dangerous is bleeding into the tissues of the floor of the mouth, as this may cause death by suffocation. Within the joints, absorption of the blood is slow and often imperfect; fibrous adhesions leading to partial ankylosis with secondary erosion of cartilage, etc., are apt to follow, and thus permanent interference with movement may result. Spontaneous haemorrhages occur also from mucous membranes, such as those of the nose, alimentary and urinary tracts, etc., but the skin petechiae of purpura do not occur.

In its typical form, haemophilia is restricted to the male sex and is transmitted through a female carrying the defect. It is clearly genetically determined, half of the sons being affected and half of the daughters being carriers. Haemophilia results from a defect in a gene carried by the X chromosome and controlling the development of Factor VIII, the anti-haemophilic globulin normally present in the plasma. In the female with two X chromosomes the abnormality (X') is represented as XX' and the normal X is sufficient to prevent the bleeding tendency; such a heterozygous female is not haemophilic although some can be shown to have an abnormally low plasma level of Factor VIII, a feature which is explicable on the Lyonisation hypothesis.

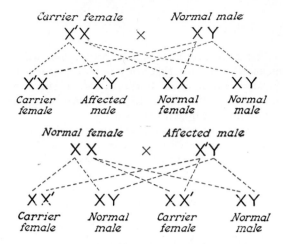

The male sex chromosome Y does not carry the normal gene and accordingly an X′Y male is haemophilic. The union of a haemophilic male with a normal female never results in haemophilia—there is always one X to prevent it—but all daughters would be carriers and would transmit the disease to half of their grandsons. A haemophilic female X′X′ could arise only from the union of a haemophilic male X′Y with a female carrying the gene abnormality XX′. Such a union must be very rare, though it might occur from intermarriage, e.g. of cousins, in a haemophilic stock. The great rarity of such individuals suggests that X′X′ is usually a lethal gene combination. Experimentally the homozygous condition has been produced by selective breeding of haemophilic dogs with carrier bitches.

In haemophilia there is no important change in the cells of the blood. The *coagulation time* of the blood, when estimated between the bleedings, is usually lengthened and may be up to an hour by the capillary tube method; after a haemorrhage, however, it may approach normal. The *bleeding time* is usually normal, since in a wound such as a prick, bleeding from the capillaries is stopped by vasoconstriction and by accumulation of platelets, the number of which in haemophilia is normal.

The platelets in shed haemophilic blood are much more slow to undergo viscous metamorphosis than those of normal blood, and this is due to the absence of Factor VIII. Deficiency of this Factor interferes with the intrinsic system of blood coagulation by causing deficient formation of thromboplastin, and can be corrected by the transfusion of *fresh* blood or *fresh* concentrated plasma. Factor VIII is very labile, and unlike Christmas factor (see below) does not keep well

in stored blood. After repeated transfusions a refractory state sometimes develops and this appears to be due to immunisation of the recipient against Factor VIII, supplied in the transfused blood. There are also quantitative differences in the severity of Factor VIII deficiency from one affected family to another, but the same degree of severity is likely to be shown by all the affected members of any one family, and the severity of the defect remains the same in different generations.

Christmas disease (Haemophilia B) is due to deficiency of Factor IX *plasma thromboplastin component* (PTC, Christmas factor) in the absence of which thromboplastin formation fails and thus a haemorrhagic disorder clinically identical with haemophilia results. It shows a similar sex-linked inheritance, and is named after the patient in whom the defect was first recognised.

When Factors VIII and IX are transfused to persons in whom they are deficient, they may disappear very rapidly from the plasma in patients who have become sensitised to them by repeated transfusions.

Factor V and Factor VII are determined by autosomal genes and occasionally are congenitally defective; acquired deficiency is more common and occurs in various pathological states, in which it contributes to a haemorrhagic tendency. Anticoagulant drugs, e.g. warfarin, administered to prevent thrombosis, act mainly by causing a deficiency of Factor VII.

In rare instances following irradiation or as a complication of pregnancy, and also in systemic lupus erythematosus, defective blood coagulation may be attributable to the presence of abnormal circulating anticoagulants which inhibit the formation of thromboplastin, or act as antithrombins. Other less well defined conditions exist in which there is a tendency to excessive haemorrhage following trauma: these are grouped together as the "pseudohaemophilias", for the coagulability of the blood is apparently normal. One type (von Willebrand's disease) is characterised by a prolonged bleeding time; there is apparently a primary capillary defect but also a partial deficiency of Factor VIII. In another type (thromboasthenia) the platelets are normal in number but morphologically abnormal and functionally inadequate in some way; the bleeding time is prolonged and there is failure of clot retraction.

Combined deficiency of Factors II, VII, IX and X in various combinations is seen most commonly in patients on anticoagulant therapy, but occurs also in the following conditions.

(1) *Haemorrhagic disease of the newborn.* This condition, characterised by spontaneous haemorrhages from the umbilicus and mucous membranes, often causes severe melaena; it occurs in about 0·3 per cent of live births. The condition may be due to inadequate supplies of vitamin K before the intestinal bacterial flora is established and administration of this substance to the infant rapidly restores the coagulation time to normal and bleeding ceases. Lack of vitamin K results in the combined deficiency of Factors II, VII, IX and X. Administration of 5 mg. of vitamin K to the mother in the 24 hours before labour raises the plasma prothrombin of the infant above the danger level. However, if given direct to a premature infant, the dose must be carefully regulated on account of the danger of increasing haemolysis and thus of raising the load of bilirubin which the immature liver cannot conjugate and excrete: the risk of kernicterus is thereby increased.

(2) *Malabsorption.* In prolonged obstructive jaundice, or malabsorption from other causes, impairment of absorption of vitamin K may be sufficiently severe to result in the continued deficiency of clotting factors; tests for impaired coagulation are therefore of importance before surgical procedures in these conditions.

(3) *Liver failure.* The liver is responsible for production of Factor II and other clotting factors. Severe liver insufficiency may thus result in the combined defect, and also in deficiency of fibrinogen (Factor I). Needle biopsy of the liver may, in the circumstances, result in severe and even fatal haemorrhage.

Hyperplasminaemic states and the defibrination syndrome. Excessively rapid activation of plasminogen (p. 164) may result in the appearance of free plasmin in the circulation with digestion of plasma proteins, including fibrinogen and coagulation factors. The breakdown products of digested fibrinogen interfere with haemostasis by inhibiting polymerisation of fibrinogen, and there is also accelerated lysis by plasmin of any fibrin which may form. Hyperplasminaemia may occur as a *primary* event where tissues rich in plasminogen activator have been traumatised, but is also encountered as a *secondary* phenomenon in response to generalised intravascular coagulation. Release of thromboplastic substances producing intravascular coagulation may occur as a complication of surgical operations, certain tumours and obstetric accidents. Treatment of

a low fibrinogen level depends on identification of the cause; where primary fibrinolysis is responsible, a fibrinolytic inhibitor (e.g. ε-aminocaproic acid) may be used, but if the primary problem is intravascular fibrin formation then either conservative measures, or in some circumstances a heparin infusion, may be indicated.

Afibrinogenaemia occurs also as a rare congenital abnormality; the condition is inherited as a recessive character, and the blood is virtually incoagulable. In severe liver failure, production of fibrinogen by the liver may be reduced sufficiently to interfere with coagulation, and afibrinogenaemia may occur also in the cachexia accompanying widespread carcinoma.

Purpura

This term is applied to various conditions in which small haemorrhages occur spontaneously from capillaries throughout the body, resulting in haemorrhagic spots (petechiae) in the skin, mucous membranes and serous surfaces, etc., while more gross bleeding may occur from the mucous membranes of the alimentary, respiratory and genito-urinary tracts. In some cases, the platelets are normal, and the defect resides in the walls of small blood vessels. In others the primary defect is gross diminution in the number of blood platelets, and there is no readily demonstrable vascular defect. Accordingly it is customary to classify purpura into *non-thrombocytopenic* and *thrombocytopenic* types, and further classification depends upon the nature of the condition bringing about the vascular defect or the thrombocytopenia.

Non-thrombocytopenic purpura

Here the vascular defect may be of (*a*) *toxic nature,* illustrated by the development of petechiae in haemorrhagic smallpox, acute septicaemia or severe scarlatina, (*b*) *nutritional* as in scurvy, and (*c*) *allergic* as in *anaphylactoid purpura.* This last condition occurs mostly in children, and frequently the purpuric rash develops explosively 2–3 weeks after a streptococcal respiratory infection, but the high titres of anti-streptolysin O found in rheumatic fever are not present. Common accompaniments are acute polyarthritis similar to that of rheumatic fever, colic, haemorrhage and serosanguineous effusion into the gut, and an acute haemorrhagic glomerulonephritis (p. 711), which sometimes progresses to renal failure. It is unnecessary to sub-divide the condition into purpura rheumatica, Henoch's purpura and Schönlein's purpura. The preceding streptococcal infection and the lesions resembling rheumatic fever and glomerulonephritis all suggest that this type of purpura is the result of hypersensitivity. Common articles of food, e.g. chocolate, may be responsible for sensitisation, and also certain drugs, e.g. carbromal, the purpura being accompanied by an itchy dermatitis.

Dysproteinaemic purpura. Abnormalities in the plasma proteins which are a feature of certain diseases are now known to be a rather uncommon cause of purpura. In most of the conditions there is a high level of immunoglobulin, for example the raised IgG of multiple myeloma or the increase in IgM of the macroglobulinaemias. Various factors are concerned in the production of purpura in these conditions: the excessive globulin may complex with coagulation factors or they may interfere with the circulation through small vessels by causing sludging of the red cells or by gelling on exposure to cold (cryoglobulin). Vascular injury may be brought about by these and other complex phenomena, resulting in purpura.

Hereditary haemorrhagic telangiectasia. This rare disease is transmitted as a simple dominant in both sexes. Symptoms vary greatly in severity and time of onset, but epistaxis is usually a prominent feature. Multiple small telangiectatic spots, which are, in fact, arteriolar-venular anastomoses, occur in the skin and mucous membranes and from them repeated haemorrhages occur so that a severe degree of anaemia may result. In the lungs similar lesions may give rise to profuse haemoptysis.

Thrombocytopenic purpura

This may be secondary to diseases causing disturbance of haemopoiesis, e.g. pernicious and aplastic anaemias, myelomatosis or leukaemia. In these conditions there is a diminished production of platelets.

Idiopathic thrombocytopenic purpura (Werlhof's disease) occurs chiefly in children and young adults; it is often a self-limiting disease which disappears spontaneously within three months of onset and does not recur, but chronic relapsing cases also occur for which splenectomy may be necessary. The acute form begins with a petechial skin rash, haemorrhages into and from the surface of mucous membranes, and there is a danger of haemorrhage into the central nervous system. Occasionally, death may result from haemorrhage in the acute stage but in most cases the condition subsides completely or becomes chronic and less severe, but with a liability to acute exacerbation. During acute attacks, the platelets are usually very much reduced, sometimes below 10,000 per c.mm., and they often show abnormalities in size and in shape; during remissions the platelets increase but frequently remain below the normal range. There is usually little or no increase in the coagulation time of the blood outside the body, but the *bleeding-time*, that is, the time during which bleeding occurs from a prick or small wound, is much prolonged, owing to the insufficient number of platelets which, by apposition on the damaged capillary endothelium, should plug the gap and thus stop the capillary bleeding. The coagulum formed in extravascular clotting has the peculiarity that it does not retract from the wall of the container and owing to this it remains soft and friable. In a wound, clot of this nature must form a less efficient seal and this is probably a factor in the continuation of haemorrhage. Failure of clot retraction is related to the paucity of platelets and it appears that while small numbers of these are sufficient to cause blood to clot in the usual time, large numbers are required to produce a firm clot.

Increased numbers of megakaryocytes are usually present in the marrow (Fig. 16.51), and although the cytoplasm of some is agranular and hyaline, there is no clear evidence of lack of platelet production in idiopathic thrombocytopenic purpura. There is, however, strong evidence of increased destruction of circulating platelets, and it has been shown by American workers that in over 50 per cent of cases the plasma contains a substance which is capable of agglutinating platelets *in vitro* and also of causing temporary thrombocytopenia and purpura when administered to a normal individual. Accordingly it has been suggested that the increased platelet destruction results from development of autoantibody active against the patient's own platelets. This interpretation is still open to some doubt, since the majority of cases of chronic or relapsing thrombocytopenic purpura have been transfused, and they have developed platelet iso-antibodies. It is therefore necessary to demonstrate antibody active against the patient's *own* platelets before assuming an immunological etiology; in some cases, auto-antibody has been demonstrated, but the techniques of its demonstration are difficult and not altogether satisfactory. The favourable effects of glucocorticoids or ACTH

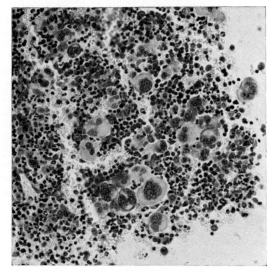

FIG. 16.51.—Marrow biopsy in thrombocytopenic purpura.

The marrow contains an excessive number of megakaryocytes, many of which are immature. × 205.

are also consistent with an immunological pathogenetic mechanism, although the mode of action of these drugs is complex and by no means fully understood.

Some abnormality of the capillary endothelium has been postulated in this type of purpura, and Macfarlane has shown that the capillaries lack contractile power after injury. It is uncertain whether this is related to the deficiency in platelets, but the appearance of purpura and thrombocytopenia in healthy volunteers transfused with plasma from patients with idiopathic thrombocytopenic purpura suggests that this is so.

The injection of an anti-platelet serum pro-

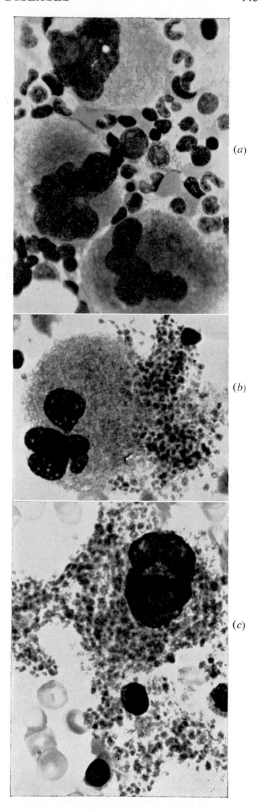

(a)

(b)

(c)

FIG. 16.52.—Megakaryocytes and platelets.

(a) Young megakaryocytes with commencing granulation. × 900.

(b) More advanced cell showing early platelet formation. × 600.

(c) Mature megakaryocyte with fully formed platelets. × 600.

duces purpura in guinea-pigs, as well as a rapid fall in the number of platelets. Bedson, in investigating this phenomenon, found no evidence that the haemorrhages are due to platelet thrombosis, and he came to the conclusion that the serum produces some slight lesion of the vascular endothelium, possibly by reacting with antigenic factors common to both platelets and vascular endothelium. The fact remains that severe thrombocytopenia, however produced, is very likely to be accompanied by purpura, and it may be that platelets are essential to the maintenance of the integrity of capillary walls. It is appropriate to draw an analogy between idiopathic thrombocytopenic purpura and acquired haemolytic anaemia of immune auto-antibody type. In one case auto-antibody reacts with the platelets, in the other with the red cells, and cases of acquired haemolytic anaemia with a positive Coombs' test and simultaneous thrombocytopenic purpura are by no means rare.

Clinical course. Idiopathic thrombocytopenic purpura runs a very variable course. Most patients suffer only one or two attacks and the disease is self-limited. In chronic relapsing purpura with exacerbations, splenectomy is followed by a remarkable improvement, but in acute cases with marked anaemia the administration of suitable corticosteroids may cut short an attack and should be tried preferentially. The operation may be followed not only by disappearance of the purpuric state but by a rapid increase in number of platelets, in some cases up to normal: the bleeding time becomes shortened and the blood coagulum shows normal retraction. There is often also a remarkable reticulocyte response with rise in the number of erythrocytes. The results are most satisfactory in cases in which marrow biopsy reveals abundant megakaryocytes, whereas when these cells are scanty, dramatic improvement is less probable. In some cases relapse following splenectomy has been recorded, but undoubtedly in many instances the favourable effect has lasted for some time and probably is permanent, although the number of platelets may not remain at the high post-operative level. The effects of splenectomy in the disease indicate that the essential abnormality is in the abnormally rapid removal of platelets by the spleen, but whether this is always due to sensitisation of the platelets by an auto-antibody is not yet certain.

Secondary (symptomatic) thrombocytopenic purpura may arise in the course of any condition which severely disturbs haemopoiesis. Thus pernicious anaemia, aplastic anaemia, or replacement of haemopoietic marrow in leukaemia, secondary carcinoma, myelofibrosis, may all exhibit purpura of thrombocytopenic type, attributable to reduced output of platelets by the disturbed marrow.

Purpura due to drugs. Drugs and toxic chemicals may induce thrombocytopenic purpura either by causing depression of haemopoiesis, affecting especially the megakaryocytes, with consequent diminished platelet production, or by combining with the platelets and rendering them auto-antigenic. Sedormid, quinine, and certain other drugs have been shown to have this latter effect in occasional individuals. It has been demonstrated that lysis of platelets depends on the presence of complement, the patient's serum or plasma, and the drug to which sensitisation has developed. The drug, e.g. Sedormid, unites with the platelets, rendering then antigenic, and the antibody which develops promotes their phagocytosis in the spleen or lysis by complement. The sensitised patient develops purpura only when the drug is taken, and transfusion of his plasma to a healthy volunteer will likewise be without effect on the recipient's platelets unless he too takes the drug.

Scurvy

In this disease, the well-marked haemorrhagic tendency is due to lack of vitamin C, present mainly in fresh vegetables and fruit. Cases of mild scurvy are occasionally encountered amongst the poor, especially in old people living alone, whilst infantile scurvy is now rare owing to antenatal care and dietary supervision. The changes in the bones and the other features of the latter condition are described later. The anti-scorbutic property in vegetables, etc., depends upon the presence of vitamin C, L-ascorbic acid, which is heat labile, and together with hyaluronic acid and calcium, is essential for the maintenance of the integrity of the vascular endothelium. Vitamin C converts folic acid to folinic acid (p. 423) and is also concerned in the synthesis of collagen; it appears to promote the polymerisation of mucopolysaccharides in conjunction with the phosphatase of fibroblasts. When vitamin C is deficient, wounds fail to heal firmly, owing to deficient collagen formation. Anaemia of microcytic type is often present and this is as a rule readily amenable to treatment by vitamin C and iron.

Scurvy is characterised by the occurrence of petechiae in the skin, haemorrhages or sanguineous effusions under the skin, in the muscles, under the periosteum, and into the joints of the lower limbs. Another characteristic feature is swelling and sponginess of the gums, especially around carious teeth, and later there may be extensive ulceration with exuberant granulations. In severe cases haemorrhages occur from the mucous membranes, the subcutaneous swellings may become infected and ulcerated, and blood-stained effusions into the serous sacs may occur.

In scurvy there is no abnormality in the coagulation of the blood or in the number of the platelets, the haemorrhages being due to increased vascular fragility. Accordingly the capillary resistance test is strongly positive. Although the platelet count is usually normal, occasionally a true thrombocytopenia occurs in those cases with a macrocytic anaemia and megaloblastic marrow (p. 423). In borderline cases scurvy may be precipitated by administration of ACTH, presumably as a result of depletion of ascorbic acid in the adrenal cortex and tissues.

Scurvy can be readily produced in guinea-pigs by feeding them with a diet composed of cereals and water, to which autoclaved milk may be added; and by this method the distribution and properties of the anti-scorbutic factor have been further defined.

CHAPTER 17

SPLEEN, LYMPH NODES, THYMUS

THE SPLEEN

Functions

The spleen is a composite organ, composed of two types of tissue and with two major functions. The first function consists of *specific immunological responses*, and is related particularly to the focal aggregates of lymphoid tissue in the spleen, known collectively as the *white pulp* and individually as the *Malpighian bodies* or *splenic follicles*. The second is a scavenging function, performed by the vascular reticulo-endothelial tissue which comprises the bulk of the spleen and is termed the *red pulp*: it consists of phagocytosis by macrophages of foreign material, especially particles (bacteria, etc.) in the blood, and also abnormal or effete red cells, leukocytes and platelets. It is thus apparent that the spleen performs functions in relation to the blood stream which are similar to those of the lymph nodes in relation to the lymph stream.

The spleen is not an essential organ, and indeed in adults it may be removed without any obvious impairment of health. In infants, however, there is evidence that splenectomy is followed immediately by increased susceptibility to infections by pyogenic bacteria which is probably attributable largely to the capacity of the spleen to phagocytose micro-organisms in the blood before there has been time for the development of a specific immune response with production of protective antibody. Splenectomised animals, e.g. sheep, are abnormally susceptible to various parasitic infections, and it is known that, in both animals and man, the spleen is an important site of formation of antibodies in response to *intravascular* injection of antigens, and considerably less antibody is produced by splenectomised individuals. The spleen is of less importance than the lymph nodes in the response to antigens injected into the tissues.

The spleen plays an important physiological role in the removal from the blood of effete or injured red cells, which are phagocytosed and digested by macrophages in the cords of the red pulp. The bilirubin formed from the breakdown of haemoglobin is secreted into the blood, to be extracted, conjugated and excreted by the liver cells, while the iron is re-utilised in haemoglobin synthesis in the marrow. The average life of the red cells and the number in the blood are not increased following splenectomy, and it is apparent that reticulo-endothelial cells in the liver, marrow and other tissues also destroy old red cells. However, the macrophages in the red pulp of the spleen have a special function in extracting from the red cells various cytoplasmic inclusions, and also in removing the nuclei of any normoblasts which have gained entrance to the circulation, the cells then being returned to the blood. Loss of this function, which is known as "pitting", is observed following splenectomy, when normoblasts and red cells containing Howell–Jolly bodies may be found in blood films (p. 393).

It is less certain that the spleen is an important site of physiological destruction of leukocytes and platelets, but splenectomy is commonly followed by a polymorphonuclear leukocytosis, sometimes of up to 30,000 per c.mm., a monocytosis, and a thrombocytosis which may reach 1×10^6 per c.mm. The polymorphs reach a peak level during the few days following splenectomy, the platelets 2–3 weeks later. The levels decline thereafter, but monocytes and platelets may remain above the normal ranges for months or even years.

Structure

The vascular arrangements of the spleen are of particular importance in relation to its two major functions. The larger arteries branch within the trabeculae, and give off arterioles of approx. 200 μ diameter which leave the trabecula and become ensheathed in a cuff of lymphoid tissue—the Malpighian bodies—to which they supply capillaries. At the periphery of the lymphoid tissue, each central arteriole divides into several penicillar arterioles, many of which show a fusiform swelling of the wall, termed an ellipsoid. The ellipsoid consists of an inner layer of prominent capillary endothelium surrounded by layers of large pale cells and a basement membrane. The red pulp consists of vascular channels termed *sinuses*, lined by elongated endothelial cells with their long axes parallel to that of the sinus. The sinuses traverse the continuous spongework, termed the *splenic cords*, of the red pulp. The sinus endothelial cells are supported by circular reticulin fibres: cells of the blood and particulate material may enter the sinuses from the splenic cords by passing between the endothelial cells. The vascular arrangements of the red pulp are not fully understood. Blood may pass from the central arterioles through the penicillar arterioles and thence directly along the sinuses to enter the trabecular veins—the so-called *closed circulation*. A second pathway—the *open circulation*—is through the splenic cords, blood entering directly from capillaries in the Malpighian bodies and then passing through the walls into the sinuses. The distribution of the blood through these two pathways may be controlled by the ellipsoids, which are believed to be contractile, or by contraction of the distal ends of the sinuses. The splenic cords consist of stellate cells, many of which are macrophages, supported on a network of reticulin fibres: in fact, the cords form a continuous spongework through which blood can filter between the stellate cells, eventually draining into venules. The "open" circulation through the red pulp clearly provides opportunity for phagocytic removal of abnormal materials or cells from the blood, whereas the sinuses provide a more direct route. In animals, the spleen is a storage organ for blood, and has a muscular capsule which contracts in response to catecholamines. In man this function is not important, and the spleen normally contains only 20–30 ml. of blood although it can become enlarged and engorged with blood in disease.

Shrinkage of the spleen

Atrophy of the spleen occurs in old age, affecting both red and white pulp, and is sometimes a feature of wasting diseases. Hyaline thickening of the walls of the small arteries and arterioles of the spleen is very common and increases in incidence and severity with increasing age; it is by no means confined to subjects with chronic hypertension or generalised arteriosclerosis. The resulting ischaemia brings about splenic atrophy with some increase in reticulin. Splenic ischaemia is also a feature of *sickle-cell disease* (p. 408) and is due to blockage of sinuses by hypoxic sickle cells; infarcts and atrophy result, and eventually the spleen may be converted into a small fibrous remnant, often heavily pigmented by haemosiderin derived from phagocytosed red cells. Severe splenic atrophy is also a feature of some cases of *malabsorption syndrome* (p. 523), the mechanism being obscure.

Splenomegaly

As already stated, the two known major functions of the spleen are the production of specific immune responses and phagocytosis of abnormal materials in the blood. Accordingly, increased functional activity of the spleen, with hyperplasia of the lymphoid or reticulo-endothelial elements, or of both, commonly results from antigenic stimulation or the presence of abnormal materials, for example micro-organisms, toxins, or abnormal cells, in the blood. Splenomegaly is therefore a very common secondary phenomenon in a great many diseases. In general, enlargement of the spleen is attributable to its phagocytic role, and is due to hyperplasia and hypertrophy of the red pulp. Hyperplasia of the Malpighian bodies, with development of large germinal centres, occurs as an immune response in many diseases, and especially in infections. Another feature of the immune response in many diseases, particularly infections, is the development of large numbers of plasma cells, both in relation to the Malpighian bodies and throughout the red pulp, but these latter changes are seldom if ever sufficiently marked to give rise to significant splenic enlargement.

Because of its vascular nature and phagocytic role, the spleen is prone to blood-borne infection: it has, however, strong defences against pyogenic bacteria, and abscess formation is uncommon except for septic infarcts in pyaemia. However, bacteria are commonly arrested in the spleen and may be recovered from it in non-pyogenic generalised infections, as in typhoid and undulant fevers and in generalised tuberculosis. Colonisation of the spleen with great enlargement is brought about also by trypanosomes, and by micro-organisms which are capable of survival and multiplication within macrophages, as in leishmaniasis and histoplasmosis.

Moderate splenomegaly results also from chronic portal venous hypertension, as in cirrhosis of the liver or hepatic schistosomiasis.

In diseases of the blood, splenomegaly may result from accumulation and phagocytosis of abnormal cells or platelets; also the spleen may re-assume its fetal role of haemopoiesis, as in anaemia resulting from replacement of the haemopoietic marrow by fibrous tissue (myelofibrosis) or by neoplastic deposits. There is evidence also that splenic enlargement from various causes is sometimes accompanied by increased phagocytic activity (hypersplenism) leading to anaemia, leukopenia and thrombocytopenia (splenic anaemia). This is dealt with more fully on p. 452.

Like most other organs, the spleen may be the site of deposits of amyloid, and great enlargement may occur also in those metabolic diseases resulting in storage of abnormal amounts of various metabolites in macrophages of the reticulo-endothelial tissues, e.g. Gaucher's disease. Splenic involvement is common in sarcoidosis, and in the various types of lymphoreticular neoplasia—the leukaemias, lymphosarcoma, Hodgkin's disease, etc.

Bacterial infections

Acute pyogenic infections

The earliest change in the spleen is congestion of the cords of the red pulp. As the number of circulating leukocytes increases, they accumulate progressively in the red pulp of the spleen, and in septicaemia, or severe localised pyogenic infections with a high leukocytosis, they may be present in the spleen in huge numbers. At postmortem examination in such a case, the spleen is slightly enlarged (200–300 g.), acutely congested, and the splenic tissue is so softened that it looks and feels almost like a bag of fluid; the cut surface is pinkish or deep red, and the tissue is semi-fluid. These changes, sometimes termed "septic spleen", are due to congestion, accumulation of polymorphs, and marked terminal and post-mortem autolysis by the digestive enzymes released from degenerate polymorphs.

In fatal septicaemia, the bacteria may be recovered from the spleen, as from other organs, and the macrophages in the red pulp may contain bacteria, red cells, degenerate polymorphs and cell debris. However, microscopic examination is seldom satisfactory owing to severe autolytic changes.

As already stated, abscess formation in the spleen is uncommon except when brought about by septic infarction in pyaemia: occasionally such lesions become gangrenous, the pus being foul smelling. Involvement of the capsule produces perisplenitis, which may progress to perisplenic abscess.

Non-pyogenic bacterial infections

Moderate degrees of splenic enlargement commonly accompany generalised non-pyogenic bacterial infections, and are due to hyperplasia of both the lymphoid tissue and red pulp of the organ, together with granulomatous lesions brought about by arrest and proliferation of bacteria in the red pulp. As enlargement is due mainly to local proliferation of reticuloendothelial cells, infiltrating macrocytes, lymphocytes and plasma cells, together with increase in reticulin, the spleen is usually firm, and postmortem autolysis is not nearly so marked as in pyogenic infections. Some examples are given below.

In **typhoid fever** splenic enlargement is an important feature, the weight sometimes reaching 500 g.; it is usually reddish and only moderately soft, or it may be deep red owing to congestion, with extensive erythrophagocytosis. As in other typhoid lesions, polymorphs are virtually absent. Typhoid bacilli usually occur in clumps in the red pulp, unaccompanied by any sign of damage in their neighbourhood, but sometimes there is necrosis around them.

Undulant fever and relapsing fever are diseases in which there occurs considerable splenic enlargement without much softening, and in both of them the causal organisms abound in the red pulp. In the former, the enlargement becomes more marked as the disease goes on; the average weight is about 500 g., but occasionally much more. In relapsing fever the essential factor in the production of the crisis is the development in the blood of antibodies, which promote phagocytosis of the spirochaetes in the splenic pulp so that they disappear from the blood. The importance of the spleen is exemplified by the fact that animals infected experimentally normally suffer merely a single attack, but relapses occur in previously splenectomised animals.

Tuberculosis. In acute miliary tuberculosis the tubercles are specially numerous in the spleen. They generally appear as minute grey points of about the size of Malpighian bodies, from which they may be distinguished by oblique illumination of the cut surface, upon which the tubercles can usually be seen to project. In less acute generalised tuberculosis in children, the spleen is occasionally studded with yellowish tubercles of 3–5 mm. diameter (Fig. 17.1). In chronic phthisis and other forms of tuberculosis, a few tubercles of various sizes, and occasionally larger nodules, may be present in the spleen. Rarely, the spleen is greatly enlarged and contains tubercles and caseous masses associated with pale infarcts, apparently the result of obliteration of arterial branches; in such conditions the cut surface presents a very variegated appearance, and the blood may present a very striking leukaemoid reaction difficult to distinguish from true leukaemia.

Syphilis. Syphilitic lesions in the spleen are uncommon and difficult to recognise. In congenital syphilis the spleen is enlarged and contains numerous spirochaetes; diffuse fibrosis may result, and miliary gummas have been described. In tertiary syphilis in the adult, gummas may occur rarely; they are wedge-shaped and resemble pale infarcts. The amyloid disease of the spleen produced by syphilis, is usually of the *diffuse* type.

Histoplasmosis is a granulomatous infection of the reticulo-endothelial system by a yeast-like fungus, *Histoplasma capsulatum*, which gains entrance through the alimentary tract and produces prominent lesions in the lymphoid tissues, spleen and liver. The regional lymph nodes may be greatly enlarged and show caseous necrosis, but later the infection may be generalised. Histoplasmosis is common in the U.S.A. but rare in Great Britain and is seen chiefly in persons who have travelled abroad. Formerly regarded as universally fatal, it has been shown by skin tests that many have survived a subclinical infection.

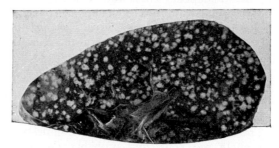

FIG. 17.1.—Subacute tuberculosis of spleen of child, showing numerous and fairly large caseous nodules. × ¾.

Protozoal infections

Massive splenic enlargement is seen in malaria and in kala-azar. In *malaria* swelling of the spleen occurs with each attack of pyrexia from acute congestion due to the accumulation of red cells containing the parasites. After repeated attacks, thickening of the stroma with induration may ultimately occur and in chronic cases the organ becomes firm, brownish-grey owing to accumulation of malarial pigment, and may weigh 1000–1500 g. Many cases of so-called *tropical splenomegaly* are now thought to be due to chronic quartan malaria. Such cases can be recognised on liver biopsy by the presence of pronounced lymphocytic aggregation in the hepatic sinusoids, and have a high titre of antibodies to *Plasmodium malariae*. The other important known cause of tropical splenomegaly is hepatic schistosomiasis with portal hypertension. There may be splenic anaemia (p. 452).

In **kala-azar** there is anaemia, leukopenia and great enlargement of the spleen, 1500 g. or more, and its stroma tends to become much indurated. The meshwork of the pulp is largely occupied by collections of macrophages which contain the parasites known as Leishman–Donovan bodies. These occur also in the bone marrow and in the liver, and diagnosis can be made by sternal puncture, but if this fails, liver biopsy or splenic puncture may be required. The parasites occur in the form of rounded or oval intracellular bodies, sometimes of cockle-shell shape, which measure up to 3.5μ in diameter, though most of them are smaller. Each contains two structures composed of chromatin, the one being larger and somewhat rounded in form, the other more rod-shaped. These two structures represent the macronucleus and the micronucleus of the parasite respectively, as is shown in the further development of the parasite to motile flagellate forms in culture *in vitro*.

Haematological disorders

The normal function of the spleen in destroying effete red cells, and probably also polymorphs and platelets, has been described on p. 448. Numerous abnormalities of the red cells, as for example in various types of haemolytic and macrocytic anaemias, are accompanied by an increased rate of their destruction in the spleen, and as a consequence there is hyperplasia of the reticulum cells, particularly in the red pulp of the spleen. The degree of splenomegaly depends on the severity and duration of the process. Similarly in idiopathic thrombocytopenic purpura there is increased splenic destruction of the antibody-coated platelets, although splenomegaly is usually absent or slight. In contrast to these conditions, in all of which splenic hyperfunction is secondary to an abnormality of the blood cells concerned, splenomegaly from various causes may be accompanied by an increased rate of destruction of normal red cells, leukocytes and platelets. This is termed hypersplenism, or splenic anaemia, and is described below: it is most commonly associated with hepatic cirrhosis.

The haematological disorders accompanied by great splenomegaly, i.e. to about 2 kg., are chronic myeloid leukaemia, the marrow replacement syndrome and sometimes chronic lymphatic leukaemia. Moderate splenomegaly, to about 1 kg., occurs in acute leukaemia, various haemolytic anaemias and polycythaemia vera. The changes in the spleen in these conditions have been described in the previous chapter.

Splenic anaemia and hypersplenism

The concept that certain disorders of the blood might be attributable to overactivity of the spleen was based on the observation that splenectomy is sometimes followed by improvement in the anaemia, leukopenia and thrombocytopenia (either singly or in any combination) commonly associated with splenomegaly. While it is possible that instances of primary hypersplenism occur in which no underlying disorder of the spleen can be established, most cases are secondary to the many well-defined disease states in which there is substantial splenic enlargement. The commonest of these is portal hypertension from hepatic cirrhosis or hepatic schistosomiasis, leading to congestive splenomegaly and sometimes splenic anaemia (the *Banti syndrome*). The anaemia is at first mild and normocytic and is in part attributable to haemodilution, since a rise in plasma volume appears to be a common accompaniment of congestive splenomegaly. After severe or repeated haemorrhage from oesophageal varices the anaemia may become markedly microcytic and hypochromic with a low MCHC. Reticulocytes are scanty and the anaemia responds only slowly to iron. The leukocyte count is generally low, often 2000–3000 per c. mm.; sometimes the fall is chiefly on the part of the polymorphonuclears but more often all the white cells are proportionately affected. The platelets in some cases are about normal in number, in others distinctly decreased. For long it was uncertain whether diminution in the formed elements of the blood was due to marrow inhibition by some splenic hormonal influence or to excessive destruction of cells by an enlarged spleen. The evidence now favours the latter, for excessive sequestration and destruction of red cells by the spleen can be demonstrated by radioactive chromium surface counting methods, while imprints of the cut surface of the spleen sometimes show evidence of phagocytosis of both red and white cells.

In splenic anaemia the marrow exhibits a compensatory hyperplasia and primitive cells tend to predominate. Although this has been attributed to "maturation arrest" it seems more likely to be due to premature release of maturing cells into the blood stream.

The spleen in Banti's syndrome. The weight of the spleen is not often over 1500 g. The capsule is thickened and adhesions are not uncommon. In some cases the organ is congested and blood readily flows out of the excised spleen, leaving the organ somewhat collapsed. In longer-standing cases the spleen is firm, and the Malpighian bodies are usually fibrotic and ill-defined, but may be quite distinct. In many

enlargement. The bone marrow in splenic anaemia shows a marked normoblastic hyperplasia.

The splenic venous pressure is commonly over 300 mm. H_2O, and the view that the condition is essentially due to chronic portal congestion is now widely accepted. However, it

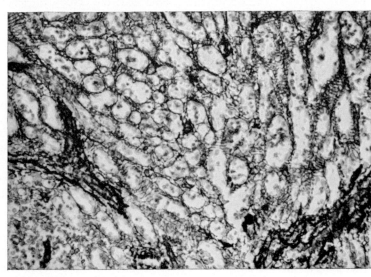

Fig. 17.2.—Spleen in splenic anaemia, showing general increase of reticulum in the red pulp. A Malpighian body in the lower left of the field is unaffected. × 190.

cases siderotic nodules, the so-called Gandy-Gamna bodies, are present. These are organised haemorrhages of the size of pinheads or larger: they often have a yellowish centre surrounded by a brown zone due to deposition of haemosiderin. *Microscopic examination* shows usually a pronounced fibrosis of the spleen. The toughened splenic substance consists mainly of dilated sinusoids with thickened walls and surrounding reticular fibrosis, the intervening cellular tissue of the red pulp being compressed by the distended sinusoids and atrophic. There is, however, an increase in the numbers of reticuloendothelial cells lining the sinusoids (Fig. 17.2). Haemorrhages around the penicillar arteries are common and all transitions may be present between these and the siderotic nodules. McNee regarded them as haemorrhages around ellipsoids as a result of high pressure in the portal system, these structures having a valve-like action and thus being specially exposed to the pressure.

The walls of the dilated splenic and portal veins are often thickened and may show atheroma-like plaques; in some cases thrombosis has been present, which, in the absence of hepatic changes, may be the cause of the splenic

remains unexplained why the Banti syndrome does not invariably occur in chronic portal hypertension.

Splenomegaly with extramedullary haemopoiesis. Great enlargement of the spleen may occur when the bone marrow is extensively destroyed by fibrosis, osteosclerosis, or secondary carcinoma, especially of the prostate. The increase is due to the development of haemopoietic tissue in the red pulp. All the elements of marrow are represented, but in some cases megakaryocytes are present in marked excess. No doubt such extramedullary haemopoiesis is sometimes compensatory for marrow destruction but in cases of myelofibrosis the splenic abnormality is regarded by some authorities essentially as part of a myelo-proliferative disorder. The spleen may reach a huge size—e.g. 2·5 kg. and may contain all the remaining haemopoietic tissue. The organ is of deep red or pinkish red colour but sometimes there are discrete somewhat firm red nodules (10 mm. or more in diameter) in which the haemopoietic tissue is more abundant. The Malpighian bodies are indistinct, infarcts are usually absent and as a rule there are no adhesions. Splenectomy is contra-indicated unless there are unequivocal signs of "hypersplenism", e.g. reduced red cell survival times. The blood commonly contains numerous primitive cells of both the red and white series, suggesting that the extramedullary haemopoietic foci fail to control efficiently the entry of new cells into the circulation. This gives rise to the condition known as leuko-erythroblastosis (p. 430).

Splenic enlargement due to various other causes

Passive hyperaemia. A distinction should be made between this condition as it occurs in general venous congestion and as produced by portal obstruction, since the changes differ considerably in the two cases. The former type, as observed in chronic heart or lung disease, is described on p. 159. In cases of passive congestion resulting from cirrhosis of the liver, the enlargement is much greater, the spleen weighing often considerably more than 500 g. The organ on section has usually the ordinary colour or may be pale and even softened, the red pulp is of increased cellularity and the Malpighian bodies are usually indistinct. In addition to congestive changes, there is often increased cellularity, not only of reticulo-endothelial cells, but also of plasma cells. The changes in the spleen in Banti's syndrome are described on p. 452.

Chronic passive hyperaemia may be produced also by pressure of tumours on the splenic vein, and actual obstruction of the vein, as sometimes happens, leads to intense engorgement of the spleen. The organ then often becomes the site of multiple infarct-like haemorrhages, and its size may be greatly increased.

Amyloid disease. As already stated, this occurs in the spleen in two main forms, the *sago* and the *diffuse* forms, and is, of course, encountered in the conditions which cause general amyloid disease (p. 194 *et seq.*). In the former type the enlargement of the spleen is not great, and the chief change is that the Malpighian bodies stand out against the pulp as somewhat translucent, round homogeneous patches.

In the diffuse form the enlargement is much greater and the weight of the organ may reach 1 kg. or even more. The two types of amyloid disease occur as fairly distinct conditions; it is not known why this should be the case, but we have rarely observed the diffuse form apart from tertiary syphilis.

Sarcoidosis. The spleen is commonly involved in sarcoidosis, although it is not usually enlarged, and frequently the lesions are not visible macroscopically: their histological features are the same as sarcoidosis elsewhere in the body (p. 152), i.e. follicles resembling those of tuberculosis, but showing little or no necrosis, and with multinucleate giant cells which often contain curious stellate and laminated inclusions. In some cases the spleen is extensively affected, and moderately enlarged; the coalescent lesions are then visible macroscopically. Splenic anaemia may complicate the condition.

Disorders involving lipid storage

Storage of lipids in the reticulo-endothelial tissues occurs in human disease in two groups of conditions.

(*a*) One group includes certain diseases associated with high blood levels of β-lipoproteins, and so with hypercholesterolaemia, as in the familial form, diabetes and obstructive jaundice. Marked deposit of lipids of sufficient degree to cause enlargement of the spleen occurs only occasionally. The cells of the red pulp become enlarged owing to the lipid accumulation, and the lipids may be in globules which react variously with fat stains, or in a masked state apparently combined with protein. For example, cholesterol may be present in the spleen in increased amount without doubly refracting esters being detectable in the cells. Although the deposit occurs secondarily to hypercholesterolaemia it is not known what actually determines the extent of deposition.

(*b*) In the second group we have rare diseases of familial and hereditary nature, such as those of the Gaucher and Niemann type, in which the lipid storage becomes excessive in various tissues and the enlargement of the spleen is very great. These conditions result from inborn abnormalities of lipid metabolism (p. 19). The composition of the lipids vary in different types.

Gaucher's disease. This uncommon disease was described first by Gaucher in 1882. In a large proportion it has shown a familial character, two or more members of the family being affected; but the mode of inheritance is uncertain. The disease presents both in adults and in children, but is more severe when in appears in infancy, owing to more widespread changes and involvement of the central nervous system. The enlargement of the spleen may be extreme; in the adult the weight may reach 5 kg., while in a young child is may be a sixth of the body weight. The liver is affected, and also the lymph nodes, especially those in the abdomen and thorax, and the bone marrow, in which the characteristic cells may be detected by sternal puncture (Fig. 17.3). In the last-mentioned situation they may cause

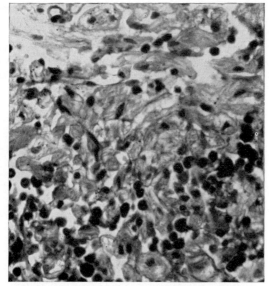

FIG. 17.3.—Section of sternal marrow aspirate in young adult with Gaucher's disease. × 440.

Many of the Gaucher cells show markedly reticulated cytoplasm.

absorption of bone and spontaneous fracture, this sometimes being the first clinical sign. In older cases Gaucher cells may accumulate in the skin and conjunctivae, causing wedge-shaped yellowish-brown patches known in the latter situation as *pingueculae*. The enlargement of these organs is due to collections of large cells with relatively small and sometimes eccentric nuclei which stain deeply; occasionally there are two or more nuclei in one cell. The cytoplasm has a peculiar hyaline or reticulated appearance and sometimes contains small vacuoles (Fig. 17.3). In the spleen the cells occur especially throughout the red pulp, though also within the Malpighian bodies, and they are apparently macrophages, the vascular endothelium being little changed (Fig. 17.4). In the liver they are derived from Kupffer cells especially in the centres of the lobules, and some scarring results.

The essential feature of the disease is an infiltration of cells of the reticulo-endothelial system with lipid material, with subsequent hyperplasia of these cells. The cells give only an imperfect reaction with stains for lipids, and the substances stored in Gaucher's disease are cerebrosides, including an abnormal one, kerasin, in which the sugar present is glucose instead of galactose. There is also a striking increase in the acid phosphatase content of "Gaucher cells",

and a rise in the plasma level. The underlying biochemical abnormality is not known.

Niemann–Pick disease. This condition is an example of abnormal storage, chiefly of the phospholipid sphingomyelin, but also of cholesterol and other lipids. It is a very rare condition presenting in the first two years of life and is soon fatal as a rule. The storage of the lipid is very extensive, occurring in the intestinal mucosa, adrenals, lungs, pancreas, etc., as well as in the liver and spleen, and there is also an accumulation in the histiocytes of the general connective tissues, their cytoplasm being increased and having a foamy appearance. The lipid stains more readily with fat stains than in Gaucher's disease. The nature of the biochemical defect is not known, but it is probably an autosomal recessive trait. Occasionally similar lipid-storage diseases occur in which a different phosphatide accumulates, e.g. a cephalin, and it seems likely they are all founded on defects in the enzyme systems controlling lipid metabolism.

"Histiocytosis X". This term is applied collectively to three uncommon conditions—Letterer–Siwe disease, Hand–Schüller–Christian disease, and eosinophil granuloma of bone—of unknown etiology, and characterised by proliferation of reticulo-endothelial cells which retain some of the histological features of histiocytes.

These conditions are not related to any known abnormality in lipid metabolism, and plasma lipids are not raised. Lipids are, however, present in

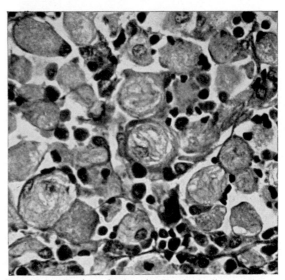

FIG. 17.4.—Section of spleen in Gaucher's disease, showing the characteristic large cells with striated and granular cytoplasm. × 440.

excess in the proliferated histiocytes in longstanding cases, and particularly in Hand–Schüller–Christian disease and eosinophil granuloma.

Letterer–Siwe disease (non-lipid histiocytosis) develops most commonly in infants and usually runs a rapid and fatal course. It is characterised by hepato-splenomegaly, lymph-node enlargement and sometimes nodules in the skin and internal organs. There is usually fever, anaemia, and sometimes leukopenia. The affected organs show massive replacement by proliferated reticulo-endothelial cells; plasma cells, fibroblasts, eosinophil polymorphs and giant cells may be present, but usually in relatively small numbers. There is usually no storage of lipid in the reticulo-endothelial cells, but this is sometimes observed in atypical cases running a more prolonged course.

Eosinophil granuloma of bone (p. 772), the third member of this group, is usually a solitary lesion arising most commonly in adolescents or adults, and composed of a mixture of cells including lipid-laden macrophages, multinucleated giant cells, but predominantly of eosinophils. It is not a cause of splenomegaly, and has a good prognosis, although progression to Hand–Schüller–Christian disease has been described in rare instances.

Although these conditions differ greatly in their behaviour, they are regarded by many as being closely related, and as forming a series of reticuloses in which eosinophil granuloma is the benign counter-

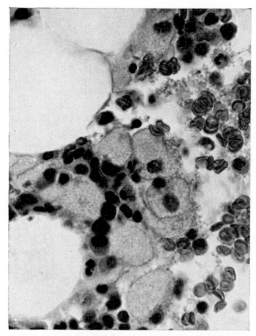

Fig. 17.5.—Familial hypercholesterolaemia. Bone marrow biopsy showing foamy cells. × 540.

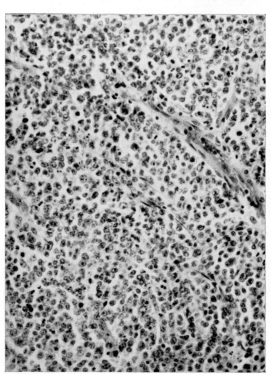

Fig. 17.6.—Reticulosarcoma of spleen.
The lymphoid tissue is replaced by nodules of large round cells of uniform type. × 190.

Hand–Schüller–Christian disease occurs at all ages, but most frequently in children. The proliferated histiocytes accumulate lipids, mainly cholesterol esters, and this is a conspicuous feature in long-standing cases. The lesions are commonly infiltrated with eosinophils, lymphocytes, plasma cells and fibroblasts, and may eventually become extensively scarred: they occur particularly in the bones, but also in the skin, liver, lymph nodes, spleen and lungs. Exophthalmos or diabetes insipidus may result from lesions of the skull adjacent to the orbit or pituitary respectively.

In general, the course is much more prolonged than in Letterer–Siwe's disease, many patients surviving for 10 or more years, but in some instances, particularly when onset is in childhood, it is more acute.

part of the usually rapidly fatal Letterer–Siwe's disease, while Hand–Schüller–Christian disease lies intermediate. The etiology is unknown, but accumulation of lipids appears to follow histiocytic proliferation, and is not the primary change.

Familial haemophagocytic reticulosis. This is a curious familial histiocytic reticulosis, characterised by hepato-splenomegaly with acutely advancing anaemia and pancytopenia. The spleen, lymph nodes, marrow and liver are infiltrated with histiocytes in which active phagocytic destruction of red cells is going on. The condition is usually fatal in infancy. Diagnosis may be made during life by the degree of haemophagocytosis observed in imprints of a needle biopsy of the spleen. Transmission appears to be by a recessive gene.

Essential familial hypercholesterolaemia is a disorder of lipid metabolism, apparently inherited as an autosomal dominant of moderate penetrance, and associated with elevation of the plasma cholesterol and phospholipid levels; the precise biochemical defect is unknown. The condition is associated with deposition of cholesterol esters in reticulo-endothelial cells (Fig. 17.5), in the intima of arteries (precocious atheroma) and as multiple yellowish nodules (xanthomas) in the skin, tendons and eyelids.

Tumours

As in the lymph nodes, the commonest forms of primary neoplasia in the spleen are the various malignant reticuloses (p. 462)—lymphosarcoma, lymphatic leukaemia, reticulosarcoma, Hodgkin's disease, and giant follicular lymphoblastoma. In most instances, widespread dissemination precludes the determination of the sites of origin in these conditions; however, occasional cases of lymphosarcoma and reticulosarcoma (Fig. 17.6) appear to originate in the spleen, and the former may cause general enlargement of the Malpighian bodies.

Benign tumours of the spleen, including fibroma, myoma, haemangioma, and lymphangioma have been described, but all are rarities. *Cysts* of the spleen are occasionally seen. They are usually small and multiple, though one may reach a large size and form a fluctuant swelling on the surface. They contain a clear serous fluid, but there may be an admixture of altered blood. They are regarded as usually of lymphangiomatous origin.

Splenic metastases occur more frequently in sarcoma than in carcinoma, but even in the former they are not common. Secondary carcinoma is rare (p. 239). Metastatic melanoma is observed occasionally. The spleen contrasts with the bone marrow and lymph nodes in the low frequency of secondary splenic tumours.

LYMPH NODES

A brief description of the structure of the lymph nodes has been given in Chapter 4. They consist essentially of two parts, viz. the lymphoid tissue proper with its follicles and deep cortex (paracortex), and the lymph sinuses and paths. The former is concerned in the production of antibodies and delayed hypersensitivity responses, already described in some detail (pp. 85–97); while the lymph sinuses are specially concerned in the destruction of organisms or damaged cells carried from the tissues, as the relatively slow lymph flow gives favourable opportunity for phagocytic action. In fact, the sinus system has much the same relation to the lymph stream as the splenic pulp has to the blood stream. The reticulum cells in both react similarly. In addition to being active phagocytes for particulate material, they exhibit in high degree the capacity for uptake and storage of substances present in solution. The germinal centres are largest and most active in the early years of life; later they are less in evidence, whilst in old age there is marked atrophy of the whole tissue of the nodes.

Acute lymphadenitis

Experimental studies have shown that in normal circumstances lymph nodes are not very efficient in removing particulate elements from the lymph passing through them: for example, bacteria and similar-sized particles have been shown to pass rapidly from the peripheral lymphatics, through the regional nodes, and to reach the blood stream. However, within less than an hour of the establishment of an acute infection, the sinuses of the draining lymph nodes dilate, and neutrophil polymorphs migrate into them from the adjacent small blood vessels and aggregate particularly in the medullary sinuses close to the hilum: these provide a filter by actively phagocytosing bacteria in the sinus lymph, and the efficiency of the nodes in preventing spread of infection to the blood stream is greatly increased. Unless the infection is rapidly overcome, the reticular cells lining the sinuses undergo proliferation (*sinus catarrh*) and they also participate in the phagocytosis of bacteria, degenerate polymorphs, cell fragments, etc., in the lymph.

In addition to the early migration of polymorphs into the sinuses, the lymph nodes draining a focus of acute infection show the other features of acute inflammation, including dilatation of the small blood vessels and inflammatory oedema: these changes are due to the local effects of bacteria or their toxins carried in the increased flow of lymph from the focus of infection. Polymorphs are also carried in the lymph, and supplement those which have accumulated in the nodes by local migration. These inflammatory changes result in swollen, tender and sometimes painful lymph nodes, a common example being in the axillary nodes in acutely infected wounds of the hand.

Other changes in the lymph nodes in acute infections include those associated with immune responses, i.e. the formation of cortical germinal centres and "blast" cell transformation and proliferation of lymphocytes in the deep cortex (p. 93).

Organisms that have invaded a lymph node are often destroyed by the leukocytes and the inflammation then resolves. They may, however, continue to multiply, the leukocytic emigration continues, the tissue of the node gradually softens, and suppuration results, which may spread to surrounding tissues. Such changes may occur in the drainage area of infected wounds of various kinds, particularly when caused by streptococci, and sometimes by staphylococci.

In *lymphogranuloma venereum* suppuration in the inguinal lymph nodes is a conspicuous feature (p. 154) and a closely similar lesion occurs in *cat-scratch disease* or *lymphogranuloma benigna*. Both are produced in the regional nodes by infection with organisms of the genus *Miyagawanella* ("Bedsonia") (p. 358), which gain entrance through trivial superficial scratches on the skin.

In *plague* there is a severe inflammation with infiltration of polymorphonuclears, brought about by the bacilli which are present in enormous numbers; there is much haemorrhage and oedema in the nodes and in the tissue between them, and often considerable necrosis. The so-called bubo is simply an inflammatory mass consisting both of lymph nodes and the tissue around them. In *anthrax* the lesion is mainly an inflammatory oedema with a varying amount of haemorrhage.

In *typhoid fever* there occurs a remarkable proliferation of the endothelial cells along the lymph sinuses and paths, which become distended with such cells, many of which contain cellular remains (Fig. 17.7 and p. 515). The cells of the reticulum react in a similar way and there is also an emigration of monocytes from the blood. Necrosis and autolytic softening may follow (Fig. 18.54), but there is practically no reaction

on the part of the polymorphonuclear leukocytes. If the necrosis is extensive, the dead tissue becomes inspissated and encapsulated.

Infectious mononucleosis (glandular fever). This disease, which is apparently a specific virus infection, occurs sporadically and in small epidemics and affects chiefly children and young adults. It is characterised by swelling and tenderness of cervical lymph nodes, fever lasting a week or two and increase of non-granular cells in the blood. The posterior

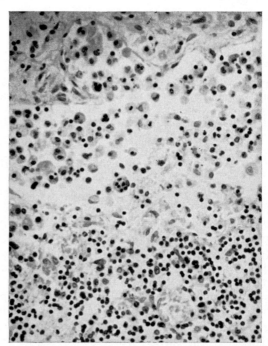

Fig. 17.7.—Section of lymph node in typhoid fever, showing lymph sinus packed with macrophages, some of which contain ingested remains of cells; lymphoid tissue to lower right of field. × 350.

cervical nodes are usually those first affected, but other groups may be involved; some degree of splenic enlargement is not uncommon and rupture may follow a trivial injury. The disease is rarely fatal. In some cases sore throat is a prominent clinical feature and there may be actual ulceration of the mucosa; this is known as the anginose type (monocytic angina). In others there is severe headache and a skin rash. At first there may be a neutrophil leukocytosis, but soon the characteristic blood picture appears, namely a moderate rise in the leukocyte count (up to 20,000 or more per c.mm.) with a high proportion (usually over 50 per cent) of non-granular cells. These cells have been described as lymphocytes, abnormal mononuclears or simply as mononuclears, but most authorities now regard them as abnormal lymphocytes. The lymph nodes show a general hyperplasia with increased mitosis of lymphoblasts, swelling of endothelial cells and atypical lymphocytes in the sinuses. In many cases there is considerable upset of liver function by the usual tests, indicating a degree of hepatitis, and in some cases jaundice develops.

The changes described point to the condition of the blood being the result of increased production of cells in the lymphoid tissues. During or after infection the blood develops heterophil agglutinins for sheep red cells (Paul–Bunnell test) and this may be of value in diagnosis.

A recent chance observation of considerable interest was the development of antibody to the Epstein–Barr virus (EBV, p. 220) in a laboratory technician during an attack of infectious mononucleosis. Subsequent investigations carried out upon students of Yale University, (Niederman *et al.*, 1968) demonstrated that antibodies develop regularly in confirmed infectious mononucleosis, and also in some patients with a similar illness but without the development of heterophil antibodies. Moreover, leukocytes obtained during the illness can be cultured *in vitro* over a long period and can be shown, like those of the Burkitt lymphoma, to contain EBV antigen. Similar observations have since been made by other workers, and there appears a strong possibility that the EB virus is the causal agent of infectious mononucleosis. However, EBV antibody has been demonstrated in a high proportion of healthy individuals, and its incidence increases during childhood. This may possibly be related to sub-clinical attacks of infectious mononucleosis.

There is evidence of a second type of infectious mononucleosis, without sore throat or lymph node enlargement, but sometimes with hepatitis, associated with infection with cytomegalovirus; the Paul–Bunnell test is negative in such cases.

Chronic enlargement of lymph nodes

This occurs in a very large number of conditions and is, of course, a most important clinical sign. The causes may be classified as follows:

(a) Reactive hyperplasia, accumulation of lipid and pigments, etc.

(b) Chronic infections and sarcoidosis

(c) Neoplastic conditions of the lympho-reticular tissues.

Many enlargements of lymph nodes are of known cause and readily classified. Others are of unknown etiology, and some have features which render difficult their classification as either neoplastic or reactive: the term *reticulosis* was usefully applied to this latter group, but has been used indiscriminately for any systematised cellular proliferation of the lympho-reticular tissue. *Malignant reticulosis* is, however, widely used as a group term for malignant lympho-reticular neoplastic conditions.

(a) Reactive hyperplasia, lipid and pigment accumulations

By *catarrh of the sinuses* is meant a reactive proliferation of the reticulo-endothelial cells in the peripheral and especially in the medullary lymph pathways, brought about by the continued action of a mild irritant. It is often seen in the axillary nodes in chronic diseases of the breast, and must not be mistaken for secondary cancer. Lymph nodes draining a focus of chronic infection commonly show also the morphological changes of the immune response (p. 93). These changes, together with catarrh of the sinuses, constitute *reactive hyperplasia* of the lymph nodes. Chronic irritation of long duration leads to a thickening of the stroma; sinuses become obliterated, and ultimately there may be marked fibrosis with atrophy of the lymphoid tissue.

Pigmentary infiltrations. Pigments of various kinds, carried to the nodes, are taken up by macrophages of the sinuses, and afterwards by the cells of the reticulum, in which they may persist for an indefinite period of time, as is seen in tattooing. The lymphocytes take no part in this process. The lymph nodes draining the affected areas in certain skin diseases show marked enlargement with accumulation and phagocytosis of melanin and of fat—so-called *lipomelanic reticulosis*. In cases of *anthracosis* carbon particles are dealt with in a similar way and they come to form black masses which replace the lymphoid tissue with comparatively little stromal thickening. In *silicosis*, on the contrary, marked fibrosis results from the irritation caused by stone particles, and the nodes become enlarged and indurated. Where there has been local haemorrhage an accumulation of blood pigment, especially of haemosiderin, may be seen in the related lymph nodes; and a remarkable accumulation of haemosiderin occurs in certain of the abdominal nodes in *haemochromatosis* and in transfusional siderosis (p. 204). Sometimes the amount is so great that the structure is quite obscured by the masses of pigment, and we have shown that the iron may constitute more than 10 per cent of the dry weight of the nodes. Enlargement of the lymph nodes in lipid storage diseases and "histiocytosis X" is mentioned on p. 455.

(b) Chronic infections and sarcoidosis

Tuberculosis. Tuberculous disease of lymph nodes is a very much less common lesion than formerly. It appears first in the group of nodes draining the site of entry of the bacilli; thus the cervical, bronchial and mesenteric groups are the commonest to be involved, and the disease may spread to others. Infection of the bronchial nodes is nearly always due to lesions in the lungs; much less frequently due to spread downwards from the cervical nodes following tonsillar infection.

As elsewhere, tubercles in the lymph nodes may coalesce and then undergo extensive caseation. The process spreads till ultimately the whole node is destroyed and such nodes form large irregular masses matted together. We have already referred to the regular occurrence of caseating tuberculosis in the tracheo-bronchial nodes in relation to the pulmonary lesions in children and its absence in the chronic phthisis of the adult (p. 145). Caseous lesions, known as *scrofula*, were formerly common in the cervical nodes, but have now become rare in Great Britain since the practice of pasteurising milk has greatly reduced bovine tuberculosis. Such lesions, if untreated, may become adherent to the skin, ulcerate and discharge the softened caseous material, and secondary pyogenic infection may occur. Small sinuses thus formed may discharge intermittently for a long time; and the irregular cicatrices resulting may give rise to considerable disfigurement. Such results are now, however, usually avoided by operation and/or specific chemotherapy. Commonly the disease becomes quiescent; the caseous material undergoes calcification, while great thickening of the surrounding capsule occurs. In children, tuberculosis of the mesenteric nodes, the result of infection from the bowel, may give rise to great swelling and diffuse caseation, the condition being known as *tabes mesenterica*. It is not uncommon to find at necropsies on adults the lower mesenteric nodes transformed into hard calcified masses, which represent a healed tuberculosis of intestinal origin.

Sarcoidosis. This is a granulomatous condition of unknown etiology (p. 152). There is enlargement of lymph nodes and a variable amount of surrounding fibrosis. The pulmonary hilar nodes are usually affected, although other deep and superficial nodes are commonly involved, and also the spleen, lungs and various other organs. The affected nodes may be greatly enlarged, greyish or pinkish, and the condition may readily be mistaken clinically for Hodgkin's disease. On microscopic examination the lesion is seen to consist of aggregates of endothelioid cells closely resembling those seen in tuberculous lesions. The endothelioid cells may form tubercle-like follicles without caseation (Fig. 17.8), although there may be some central fibrinoid necrosis.

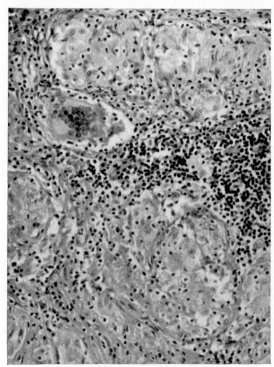

Fig. 17.8.—Lymph node in sarcoidosis.
Note the follicles without caseation. × 75.

Multinucleate giant cells may be present, and sometimes they contain curious stellate or conchoid bodies, which may be calcified. The tuberculin test is usually negative in cases of sarcoidosis, and there is evidence that this is due to defective reactivity of the lymphocytes: delayed hypersensitivity to other antigens, e.g. mumps virus, is also depressed, although the serum contains the usual blood-group and other antibodies, and

general dissemination of the spirochaetes in the skin lesions and is often accompanied by fever. In the tertiary stage, gummas are comparatively rare in the lymph nodes.

Toxoplasmosis. Infection of man by the protozoon parasite *Toxoplasma gondii* is of worldwide distribution and is probably acquired from the mouse. In adult life chronic lymph node enlargement is the commonest clinical feature and

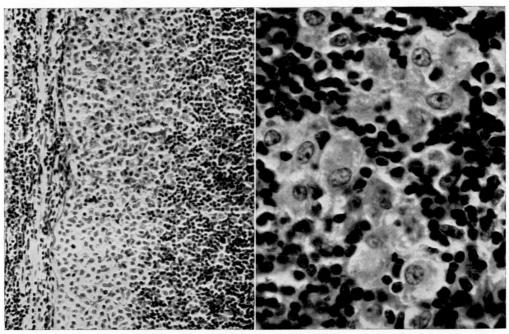

FIG. 17.9.—Toxoplasmosis. The lymph sinus is filled with small macrophages. × 165.

FIG. 17.10.—Toxoplasmosis, showing the characteristic large pale reticulum cells. × 450.

in some cases there is a raised level of serum IgG. In some cases, delayed hypersensitivity to tuberculin has been observed to diminish or disappear following the onset of sarcoidosis, and to re-appear following remission. The Kveim test, a granulomatous sarcoid reaction at the site of intradermal injection of a sterilised extract of sarcoidosis lesions, is useful in diagnosis.

Syphilis. Enlargement with induration of the regional nodes in relation to the primary sore has already been described (p. 148), and also the importance of spread of the spirochaetes by lymphatics and the blood. The lymphadenopathy gradually subsides, but some induration may persist for a considerable time. In the secondary state, there is moderate or slight general enlargement of lymph nodes, though the epitrochlear nodes and those of the posterior triangle are specially prone to be affected. It is related to the

on lymph node biopsy the differential diagnosis from early lymphoid neoplasia may be difficult. The lymph nodes of the neck and axillae are most often involved; they may be as much as 3 cm. in diameter, are usually moderately firm and may be slightly tender. There is no characteristic change in the white cells in the blood. Microscopically there is a pronounced hyperplasia of lymphoid cells with enlarged cortical nodules containing active germinal centres. Two characteristic histological features are (1) the presence of clusters of large palely-staining reticulum cells throughout the cortical nodules and even in the germinal centres, and (2) the intense cellular proliferation and stuffing of the lymphatic pathways with rather small macrophages which fill the sinuses and obscure the architecture, producing a remarkable constant and recognisable picture (Figs. 17.9 and 17.10).

There are also many plasma cells throughout the node and the capsule is thickened. The diagnosis may be confirmed by complement-fixation tests or by the specific dye tests in which the organisms of experimental toxoplasmosis in the mouse are so modified by contact with the antibodies in the serum of an infected person that they fail to take up methylene blue. Congenital toxoplasma infection is dealt with on p. 645.

(c) Neoplastic conditions of lymphoid tissues

Hodgkin's disease

This is the commonest of these neoplasms. The name is unsatisfactory, but neither *lymphadenoma* nor any of the other alternatives suggested has replaced it. The disease is best considered as a neoplastic proliferation of reticulum cells of the lymphoid tissues, but there is commonly an

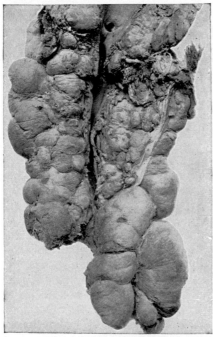

FIG. 17.11.—Mass of retro-peritoneal nodes from a case of Hodgkin's disease.

The aorta is opened from behind and is surrounded by masses of enlarged nodes. × ½.

admixture of neutrophil and eosinophil polymorphs, lymphocytes, plasma cells and fibroblasts, and the true nature of the condition is still obscure. It is characterised most often by a

progressive and usually painless enlargement of lymph nodes and other lymphoid tissues; there may be also nodular and more diffuse formation of Hodgkin's tissue in various organs. It may occur at all ages from early childhood onwards, but affects particularly the

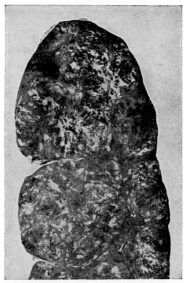

FIG. 17.12.—Section of spleen in Hodgkin's disease, showing the characteristic pale irregular lesions involving the Malpighian bodies and extending into the red pulp. × ⅔.

20–40 age groups. It is usually a chronic disease lasting two or more years, often with anaemia and pyrexia; in some cases it runs a relatively acute, fatal course of a few months, in others the disease may be prolonged over many years. Treatment of localised disease by excision or radiotherapy sometimes results in cure.

Hodgkin's disease usually becomes apparent first in the cervical nodes and spreads to other superficial groups, particularly the axillary, but in some cases there is early involvement of abdominal or thoracic nodes (Fig. 17.11). It may begin in the thorax, first involving the thymus, but in our experience such an occurrence is unusual.

Structural changes. The enlarged nodes are at first moderately soft and uniformly greyish or pale pink, but as the enlargement progresses, they become firmer and may form large masses which produce important results by pressure, e.g. on the trachea, veins, etc. Ultimately they may be densely fibrosed, and may show yellowish areas of necrosis, but there is no suppuration. At an early stage, the lymph nodes

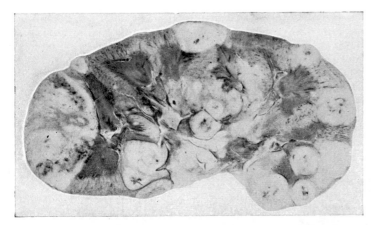

FIG. 17.13.—Nodules of Hodgkin's disease in kidney.

The growth was unusually extensive and the histological features were those of Hodgkin's sarcoma. × ⅔.

are usually not bound together by fibrosis, as occurs in the various granulomatous diseases.

While the lesions are at first mainly in lymphoid tissue, they are found later in various organs. In the *spleen* Hodgkin's disease involves the Malpighian bodies. These become enlarged into irregularly-shaped masses of whitish or yellowish tissue scattered throughout the red pulp; thus a characteristic appearance is produced, resembling the cut surface of a German sausage (Fig. 17.12). The lesions in the Malpighian bodies may occur only in patches, and some of the nodules may reach a considerable size. There is also a general hyperplasia of the red pulp, so that the weight of the organ may be increased to over 1 kg. Rarely there is merely a general enlargement without the characteristic lesion in the Malpighian bodies, and occasionally the organ may be little altered. Nodules of Hodgkin's tissue may occur in other organs, especially in the kidneys (Fig. 17.13), and in the liver there may be diffuse growth along the portal tracts. There may also be focal or more diffuse lesions in the lungs, especially when the bronchial nodes are affected. Lesions in the form of firm plaques, which may ulcerate, are rarely seen in the intestines, and in the stomach. There is generally some extension of the red marrow in the long bones, with both a leukoblastic and an erythroblastic reaction. Nodules of the characteristic tissue are commonly present in the bone marrow. Lesions of the vertebrae or the spinal dura may result in pressure on the spinal cord and paraplegia.

Microscopic examination at an early stage shows that there is proliferation of reticulum cells, with accumulation of various other types

(Fig. 17.14), to produce a cellular tissue of characteristic appearance. The reticulum cells vary considerably in form, are rounded, oval or tailed, and contain a rather pale vesicular nucleus with definite nuclear membrane and prominent nucleoli. Some of these cells increase in size usually up to about 40 μ in diameter, but sometimes to many times this size, and come to contain several nuclei or a large convoluted or ring-shaped nucleus (Fig. 17.15): these enlarged,

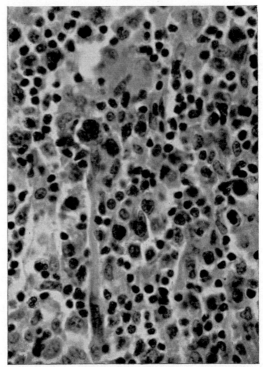

FIG. 17.14.—Lymph node in Hodgkin's disease, early stage; eosinophils and giant cells derived from the reticulum cells. × 450.

often multinucleate forms arc known as Reed–Sternberg cells, although they were described as early as 1878 by Greenfield of Edinburgh. Scattered amongst them are lymphocytes, plasma cells and neutrophil polymorphs in varying proportion, and not infrequently numerous eosinophil leukocytes. Sometimes, however, there are practically no eosinophils in the Hodgkin's tissue.

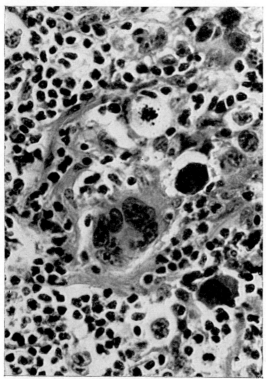

FIG. 17.15.—Hodgkin's disease; showing typical giant-cell and reticulum-cell hyperplasia. × 450.

The Hodgkin's tissue at first occurs in patches, but soon extends through the node, replacing the lymphoid tissue and destroying the architecture. Fibroblasts also appear in the lesions, and at first fine fibres of reticulin are present between the cells, but soon collagen fibres appear, and fibrosis then follows. Ultimately the node may be largely replaced by dense hyaline fibrous tissue in which there are surviving Reed–Sternberg cells and lymphocytes, and necrosis may occur in parts.

The lesions in other organs are similar. In the Malpighian bodies of the spleen, for example, reticulum cells proliferate and encroach upon the pulp at the periphery, where haemosiderin derived from red cells may be present. The cellular proliferation is followed by thickening of the stroma, which usually begins at the margin, and ultimately there is much fibrosis.

Variants and prognosis of Hodgkin's disease

As mentioned above, Hodgkin's disease may cause death within a few months, or may extend over many years: a small proportion of patients have been observed to remain well, without evidence of recurrence, for over 20 years following diagnosis and treatment. These variations in behaviour have prompted attempts to classify the condition into a number of sub-types. The following classification into four types is of proved value, although it does not allow accurate prediction of the prognosis in all cases.

(1) *Hodgkin's granuloma.* This is the classical form of the disease, as described above, and in over two-thirds of cases, death results within 5 years. Approximately 60 per cent of cases are of this type.

(2) *Hodgkin's sarcoma.* This is a highly malignant form. The age-incidence is somewhat higher than thc average for the disease, and the Hodgkin's tissue is composed mainly of aberrant neoplastic reticulum cells, including Reed–Sternberg cells. The lesions extend rapidly and death is invariable, usually within a few months. There is a tendency for the tumour tissue to form large masses, resembling in this respect malignant tumours of non-lymphoid origin. Rapidly progressive haemolytic anaemia is commoner than in the other types of Hodgkin's disease.

(3) *Hodgkin's paragranuloma.* In this variant, the lesions are often, but not invariably, confined to the lymph nodes. The affected nodes do not usually exceed 5 cm. diam., and on section are of uniformly succulent appearance. Microscopy shows replacement of the architecture of the node by a uniformly heavy infiltrate of small lymphocytes, as in lymphosarcoma or chronic lymphatic leukaemia. The distinctive feature is the presence of small numbers of Reed–Sternberg cells scattered singly among the lymphocytes: infiltration with plasma cells, polymorphs, eosinophils and fibroblasts is not a feature (Fig. 17.16). In this form of the disease, the prognosis is much better than average; in

some cases the lesions are localised to one node or group, and over half the patients are then alive and well after 15 years. When more than one group of nodes is involved the outlook is not so good, and classical Hodgkin's disease (granuloma), or even Hodgkin's sarcoma, is more likely to supervene.

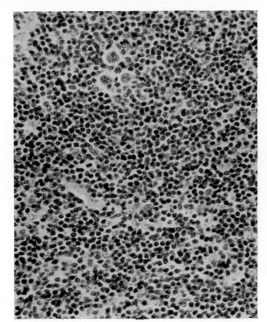

FIG. 17.16.—Lymph node showing Hodgkin's para-granuloma. The cells are nearly all lymphocytes but with occasional Reed-Sternberg cells (upper centre). × 200.

(4) *Nodular sclerosing Hodgkin's granuloma.* This is a more recent and less generally accepted subdivision, with a prognosis intermediate between that of granuloma and paragranuloma. It includes about 15% of all cases of Hodgkin's disease. The lesions present the usual pleomorphic histological picture, but the cellular tissue is divided up into microscopic nodules by dense encircling fibrosis (Fig. 17.17).

While there is undoubtedly considerable prognostic value in classification of this type, individual cases often defy classification, and pathologists often differ widely in their interpretations. The frequency with which new classifications continue to appear is a symptom of this difficulty. (Hanson *et al.*, 1964; Lukes *et al.*, 1966; Harrison, 1960, 1966). On the whole, however, Hodgkin's disease remains a fairly well defined entity.

The extent of the lesions of Hodgkin's disease,

and the clinical features, are also of considerable prognostic importance. When the disease is confined clinically to a single node or group of nodes, the outlook is relatively good. Involvement of lymph nodes in more than one anatomical region, or of the spleen, liver, bone marrow or other non-lymphoid tissues, carries a poor outlook, and pyrexia is also an unfavourable sign. Prognostication based on the extent of the disease is not unrelated to histological assessment, for relatively benign histological types are more likely to be encountered in localised form than the granuloma and sarcoma.

The blood picture. Anaemia of normochromic type is usually present and may reach a marked degree; sometimes an acute auto-immune haemolytic anaemia supervenes, and the red cells give a positive direct Coombs' test. In most cases in the adult, there is fairly well-marked polymorphonuclear leukocytosis but leukaemic changes are invariably absent. An increase of the lymphocytes is sometimes present in children with the disease, but it is rare in adults, and there may be a lymphopenia; increase of eosinophils

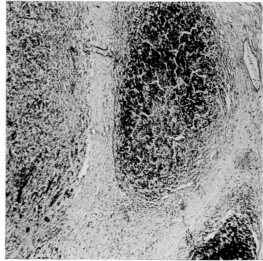

FIG. 17.17.—Lymph node showing nodular sclerosing Hodgkin's disease. Parts of three "nodules" of Hodgkin's tissue are shown, separated by dense connective tissue. × 25.

in the blood is unusual, but may be striking. Amyloid disease has occasionally been observed in association with Hodgkin's disease.

Irregular pyrexia is common, but in some cases it assumes a definitely periodic character known as the Pel–Ebstein type. In this there are bouts of pyrexia of a week or more, separated by remissions of two or three weeks. The pyrexia has no relation to the extent of the lesions and its cause is unknown.

Patients with Hodgkin's disease show a *depression of delayed hypersensitivity reactions*, positive tuberculin and mumps-virus reactions being less common than in the control population: by contrast, they do not exhibit any deficiency

germinal centres but are larger (Fig. 17.18), and usually lack the phagocytes containing ingested nuclear fragments which are usually present in normal germinal centres (Fig. 17.21). The architecture of the affected nodes, including lymphoid sinuses, is lost, and the lymphoid tissue between the "follicles" is replaced by a mixture of lymphocytes and abnormal, although

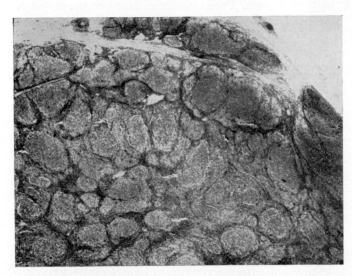

FIG. 17.18.—Lymph node in lymphoid follicular reticulosis.

The architecture is destroyed, the lymph node being replaced by follicles of pale-staining cells around which there are rings of condensed lymphocytes. × 15.

of antibody production, and serum immunoglobulin levels are not reduced. Impairment of delayed hypersensitivity may explain the well-known association of tuberculosis with Hodgkin's disease.

Lymphoid follicular reticulosis (Brill–Symmers' disease)

This is a systematised disease of the lymphoid tissues clinically resembling Hodgkin's disease. It runs a remittent course, appearing usually in adult life, and is characterised by enlargement of successive groups of lymph nodes, splenomegaly and anaemia or even pancytopenia. The Malpighian bodies are much enlarged and follicles of the characteristic tissue occur in the bone marrow and may be recognisable in sections of a sternal marrow biopsy (Figs. 17.19, 17.20). On occasion, the disease appears to begin in the spleen or bone marrow.

The affected nodes are highly cellular, of yellowish-white colour, and the cut surface shows a finely nodular character due to the presence of numerous "follicles" which resemble normal

well-differentiated reticulum cells, the giant "follicles" consisting of dense aggregates of the reticulum cells with scanty lymphocytes. Although highly radio-sensitive for a time, the condition eventually proves fatal. Sometimes lymphosarcoma or leukaemia supervene, and the leukaemic cells may be obviously lymphocytic, or larger and of uncertain type.

Leukaemia

This is dealt with in the previous chapter (p. 430). It will be remembered that lymph node enlargement is usually slight in chronic myeloid leukaemia, variable in acute and monocytic leukaemia and practically always prominent in chronic lymphatic leukaemia. In chronic lymphatic leukaemia there may be a pre-leukaemic, or aleukaemic stage, with lymph node enlargement but a normal white cell count, and diagnosis is then dependent on the histological changes in the lymph nodes, marrow, etc. Usually, however, frank leukaemia supervenes in such cases.

Lymphosarcoma

This is a tumour of lymphocytes or lymphocyte precursors. Lymph nodes are chiefly involved: there may be widespread involvement of numerous nodes, but there is a much greater tendency than in Hodgkin's disease to form localised

The tumour occurs predominantly in old people. It is usually highly sensitive to radiotherapy, but recurrence is the rule and survival usually short. In the early stages there may be confusion between chronic lymphatic leukaemia in the aleukaemic phase and lymphocytic lymphosarcoma, and intermediate forms occur;

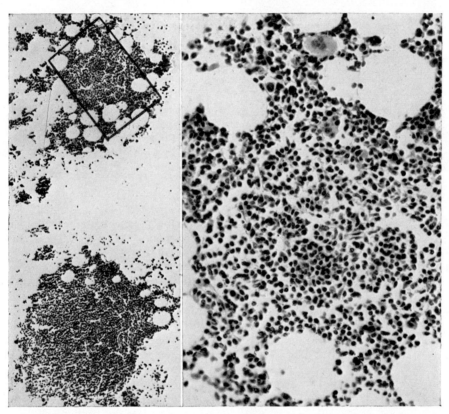

FIG. 17.19.—Marrow biopsy in lymphoid follicular reticulosis. Two marrow fragments contain typical follicles.

FIG. 17.20.—Marrow fragment outlined in Fig. 17.19 is seen to display the characteristic architecture of lymphoid follicular reticulosis.

masses by infiltration of surrounding tissues, with all the destructive characters of a typical malignant tumour. Histologically, there is diffuse replacement of the whole lymph node structure by a strikingly uniform mass of tumour cells: the cells may be small and closely resemble normal lymphocytes (*lymphocytic lymphosarcoma*) or larger with more cytoplasm and less regular nuclei (*lymphoblastic lymphosarcoma*). Little or no reticulin is formed, and no other cell types are present. The tumour cells commonly infiltrate the capsule of the lymph node and invade the surrounding tissue.

but the great majority of cases finally develop clearly into one category or the other.

Lymphosarcoma of the stomach and intestine is histologically very similar, but often remains localised and about a third of cases may be cured by excision: the same applies to other lymphoid neoplasms which also occur, although less often, at the same sites.

Burkitt's tumour (p. 220) is generally described as a lymphosarcoma, but it is entirely different in behaviour and distribution from the much commoner lymphosarcomas described here.

Q

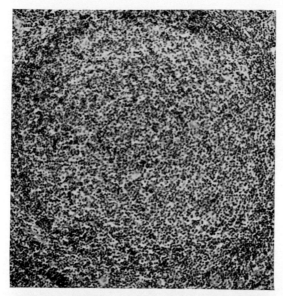

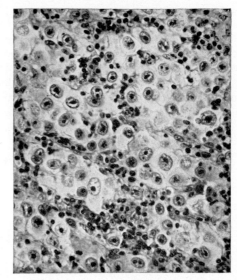

Fig. 17.22.—Reticulosarcoma of lymph node, showing large rounded cells with lymphocytes between. (J. S. F. N.) × 300.

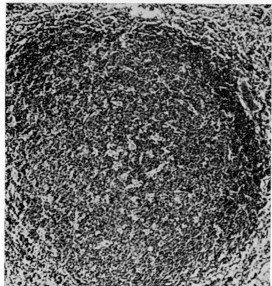

Fig. 17.21.—Lymphoid follicular reticulosis. The follicle above, from a lymph node, is typical of the disease in that there are no phagocytes in its centre. The follicle below, from an apparently unaffected peripheral part of the same node, contains central phagocytes, and is more likely to be reactive. × 100.

Reticulosarcoma

These tumours are similar to lymphosarcoma in their sites of origin, behaviour and naked-eye appearance, though rather less common; they presumably arise from reticulum cells of lymphoid tissues. Most characteristically, they consist of uniform masses of relatively large pale cells, elongated or irregular in shape, with vesicular nuclei (Fig. 17.22), embedded in a network of reticulin fibres which can be demonstrated only by appropriate stains. In less well differentiated forms reticulin may be scanty or absent, and the cell types vary greatly. Diagnosis may then be very difficult, especially when the tumour arises from tissues other than lymph nodes, and distinction from pleomorphic sarcoma or from metastases of poorly differentiated carcinoma may be particularly troublesome.

Other tumours

The lymph nodes may be involved in myelomatosis (p. 437), and also in "histiocytosis X" which is of unknown nature.

Secondary tumours. With the exception of rodent ulcer, lymph node involvement is common in all varieties of carcinoma, and also in malignant melanoma. It may be well to recall and emphasise the wide spread by the lymphatics which may take place, and the involvement of distant nodes—for example, the supra-clavicular group in cases of gastric carcinoma, and of the abdominal group of bronchial carcinoma.

THE THYMUS

The development of the thymus and the advances in our understanding of its major role in the immune response are described briefly in Chapter 4, while the immunological deficiencies resulting from defective thymic development are considered in Chapter 5. (pp. 114–16). The changes in the thymus in myasthenia gravis, and their possible significance, are dealt with on p. 811, and the pathogenic role of thymus-derived lymphocytes in the organ-specific auto-immune diseases on p. 111. It remains to consider the condition known as *status thymico-lymphaticus*, and to provide a brief account of thymic tumours, all of which are rare.

Status thymico-lymphaticus

This term has been applied to cases of sudden death from some cause which is insufficient to account for the death of a normal individual, and in which necropsy has revealed neither adequate cause of death nor any constant abnormality apart from enlargement of the thymus and other lymphoid tissues. In such cases, death has resulted quite unexpectedly from a trivial injury, fright, general anaesthesia, immersion in cold water, etc. The distribution of lymphoid hyperplasia has varied from case to case, and has included the tonsils, follicles at the root of the tongue, groups of lymph nodes, and lymphoid tissue of the alimentary tract. Lymphoid follicles have also been described in abnormal situations, including the liver, kidneys and bone marrow. Hypoplasia has been reported in some cases in other tissues, notably the adrenal medulla and chromaffin system, the aorta and its major branches, and gonadal hypoplasia with alterations in the secondary sexual characters.

Normal weight of the thymus. In considering the size of the thymus, it must be appreciated that the organ reaches a maximal size in relation to body weight at about the time of birth; it continues to enlarge until around puberty, although its weight relative to whole body weight diminishes, and after puberty it undergoes involution, at first rapidly and then more slowly, its absolute weight declining. This involutionary process appears to be dependent on the steroid sex hormones produced by the gonads, and can be inhibited experimentally by castration of young male animals.

A second important consideration in assessing the significance of an enlarged thymus is the accumulation of adipose tissue which occurs in the organ during involution: this proceeds during adult life, until the adipose tissue far exceeds the thymic tissue proper, and crude thymic weights, without an assessment of the proportion of fatty tissue present, are liable to be midleading.

Finally, the thymus, like other lymphoid tissues, is sensitive to the action of glucocorticoid hormones, administration of ACTH, cortisol or cortisone, etc., causing shrinkage of the lymphoid tissues, including the thymus. The reduction in size of the lymphoid organs which occurs during severe illnesses is probable largely attributable to increase in secretion of endogenous corticosteroids as a result of stress. Accordingly, the thymus is larger at necropsy in cases of sudden death than in patients dying after a period of illness.

The total weight of the thymus, and the weight corrected to allow for the proportion of adipose tissue, were determined by Hammar (1926): the mean weights for individuals of various ages, dying suddenly without preceding illness, are given below.

| | *Thymic Weight (grams)* | |
Age (years)	Total	Corrected for Fat
Neonatal	13·26	12·33
1–5	22·98	19·26
6–10	26·10	22·08
11–15	37·52	25·18
16–20	25·58	12·71
21–25	24·73	4·95
26–35	19·87	3·87
36–45	16·27	2·89
46–55	12·85	1·48

Thymic enlargement and sudden death. Considering the factors discussed above, it is not surprising that the thymus and other lymphoid tissues should appear unduly prominent in cases of sudden death, particularly in children, and the term status thymicolymphaticus was introduced on the basis that the enlarged lymphoid tissues predisposed in some way to sudden death from some minor injury or shock. Analysis of data collected by the Committee of the Pathological Society and Medical Research Council has been published by Young and Turnbull (1931) who concluded that an unduly large thymus is not, by itself, associated with a predisposition to sudden death, and that there is little, if any, association between the weight of the thymus and the amounts of lymphoid tissue elsewhere in the body. These views have been supported by other workers, and an analysis of Hammar's observations shows that, in those cases where the weight of the thymus exceeded the mean weight for the age group by more than two standard deviations, death was due not to some trivial incident, but to major trauma, drowning, carbon-monoxide poisoning, etc.

In spite of the evidence against the significance of an enlarged thymus, lymph nodes etc., in sudden death, most pathologists with a large necropsy experience have encountered occasional cases of sudden death from inadequate cause, and have noted thymic and other lymphoid enlargements. One possible explanation is an unsuspected state of adrenocortical hypofunction, which would account for the lymphoid hyperplasia and also for sudden death from minor causes. However, we know of no evidence to support this possibility, nor are we aware of a predisposition to sudden death in patients with known adrenocortical hypofunction, such as untreated Addison's disease or hypopituitarism, although in such conditions the lymphoid tissues may be enlarged.

Tumours of the thymus

Primary thymomas are of several types, all of which are rare.

Epithelial and lymphocytic tumours. Tumours containing both epithelial cells and lymphocytes are least uncommon. They usually consist of nodules, and may be predominantly epithelial, predominantly lymphocytic, or may show widely differing ratios of the two cell types in different parts of the tumour and sometimes within single nodules. The epithelial cells may be plump and ovoid, spindle-shaped or rounded, or they may show acinar formation and resemble tumours of the endocrine glands, and two or more types of epithelium may be present in the same tumour. They are frequently encapsulated, and intersected by dense fibrous stroma, or may extend locally to involve the adjacent tissues, including the major blood vessels, pleura, lung and pericardium. Most tumours are symptomless, and are detected incidentally by X-ray, or cause pressure symptoms, but not uncommonly a thymoma is accompanied by myasthenia gravis, or more rarely by systemic lupus erythematosus, hypogammaglobulinaemia, or pure red-cell aplasia. The significance of these associations is not known, but it is noteworthy that the last two may respond to removal of the tumour, while the response of myasthenia gravis is more variable (p. 812).

The term *lympho-epithelioma* has been applied to thymic tumours of mixed lymphocytic and epithelial type, but should be avoided: they must not be confused with the malignant lympho-epitheliomas of the tonsil and nasopharynx.

Very rarely, tumours of mixed epithelial-lymphocytic type, or purely epithelial tumours, are anaplastic and more highly malignant, and squamous carcinoma has been observed.

Teratoma also occurs in the thymus, and may be wholly well-differentiated or have poorly-differentiated areas.

Seminoma of the thymus resembles closely the commoner testicular tumour, and is highly radiosensitive.

Granulomatous thymoma. This is a thymic lesion which resembles closely Hodgkin's disease, usually of the nodular sclerosing type (p. 465), in its macroscopic and microscopic appearances. Attempts to distinguish between the two conditions on histological grounds are not convincing, and it is uncertain whether the thymic lesion is a separate entity. In some cases, the changes have remained localised over a period of years, but in others involvement of lymph nodes and other tissues has occurred.

Other lymphoid neoplasms, such as lymphosarcoma and reticulum-cell sarcoma, may originate in the thymus, and the organ may also become involved in malignant reticuloses starting in the other lymphoid tissues.

CHAPTER 18

ALIMENTARY TRACT

THE ORAL CAVITY AND PHARYNX

The lips, mouth and tongue

Inflammatory changes

The lips share with the tongue lesions resulting from severe iron-deficiency anaemia and from certain vitamin B deficiencies. In chronic microcytic anaemia with achlorhydria and koilonychia, there are characteristic changes in the labial mucosa resulting in cracks and fissures at the angles of the mouth—*angular stomatitis*—with desquamation, thinning of the epithelium and inflammatory cellular infiltrate in the lips—*cheilosis* and *perlèche*. The tongue is smooth and glazed with loss of the papillae—*atrophic glossitis*. Despite the anaemia it often looks rather fiery red and may be very painful. In pernicious anaemia, atrophic glossitis is also a constant feature.

Similar changes occur in riboflavin deficiency and it is probable that the lesions in both cases are the result of defective intracellular respiration in epithelial cells that have normally a high turnover rate, in the first case from deficiency of the iron-containing cytochrome oxidase and in the second from lack of respiratory flavoprotein.

Herpes simplex. A common inflammatory lesion of the oral mucosa is that due to the virus of herpes simplex. Infection occurs in infancy or childhood and the virus is thereafter carried throughout life, giving rise to the characteristic labial sores from time to time and in circumstances that vary from person to person. Thus labial herpes is almost invariably present in patients suffering from lobar pneumonia, but occurs also in minor infections such as coryza, and it can also be provoked by exposure to cold or excessive ultra-violet light.

The primary lesions consist of groups of vesicles of 1–2 mm. diameter on the mucosa; these rupture and form small shallow ulcers with a red margin and necrotic centre. In subsequent attacks lesions are located chiefly at the muco-cutaneous junction; rupture of the vesicles leads to a painful crusted sore.

Measles. Koplik's spots are small, inflammatory vesicles which appear on the buccal mucosa shortly before the morbilliform rash in the skin. The lesions consist of a central whitish area of thickened epithelium which undergoes necrosis and breaks down to form small shallow ulcers (Fig. 18.1). The measles virus gives rise to multinucleated giant cells of characteristic appearance in lymphoid tissues—Warthin–Finkeldey cells.

Thrush is a superficial infection of the oral mucosa by the monilial fungus *Candida albicans*. It occurs chiefly in children and may be seen in epidemic form in nurseries. It consists of multiple whitish patches from which the fungus is easily recovered. These are irregularly distributed on the oral mucosa, and the surface bleeds on removal. In adults, candida infections of the oral mucosa occur in acute and chronic forms in such conditions as angular stomatitis, denture sore mouth and in a type of leukoplakia. They are however more liable to present in patients who are debilitated or undergoing prolonged treatment with broad spectrum antibiotics, steroids, or cytotoxic drugs. In these circumstances they may occur in severe form and extend to the oesophagus and other sites.

Syphilis. A primary chancre may be contracted by kissing someone with the highly infective secondary syphilitic lesions in the mouth. The primary labial sore is often more exuberant than a typical genital chancre and the lesion

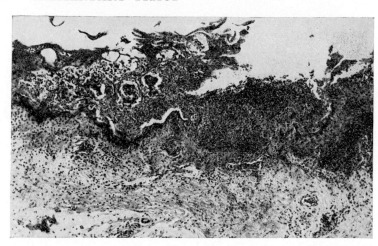

FIG. 18.1.—Buccal mucosa in measles, showing a Koplik's spot, a small central area of ulceration with acute inflammatory reaction. At the margin epithelium is growing over the denuded surface. × 65.

commonly does not present an intensely indurated base, so that its true nature may be unrecognised. In the secondary stage the lips and oral mucosa may show the typical mucous patches and snail-track ulcers, and these are highly infective. In the tertiary stage, the tongue may be the seat of a gumma, usually located centrally in the posterior third of the organ and presenting a deep punched-out ulcer with a yellowish grey wash-leather base. Gummatous ulceration of the hard palate leads to perforation into the nose.

Tuberculosis. Small shallow ulcers with undermined edges occur about the tip of the tongue in cases of chronic pulmonary tuberculosis.

Leukoplakia

Stratified squamous mucosa subjected to chronic irritation of various kinds, e.g. mechanical, thermal, chemical or infective, especially syphilitic, undergoes thickening and hyperkeratosis with the formation of white patches designated *leukoplakia*. The epithelium is thickened, the rete pegs are prolonged and the papillae contain a chronic inflammatory infiltrate. In some cases the epithelium becomes atypical with loss of polarity of the cells and transitions to squamous carcinoma are not uncommon. Leukoplakia on the lip and tongue is a precancerous lesion.

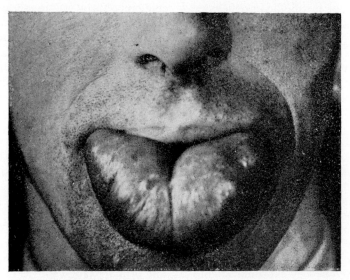

FIG. 18.2.—Haemangioma causing great enlargement of the lower lip.

Pigmentation

Melanotic pigmentation of the lips and buccal mucosa occurs in Addison's disease (q.v.) as brown patches of irregular distribution and of varying severity. In the absence of Addison's disease, marked patchy brown pigmentation of the lips involving both skin and mucosa especi-

young persons it is sometimes viral in origin. There is in general less keratinisation than in the corresponding skin tumour. It rarely becomes malignant. A lesion which may simulate the papilloma macroscopically is the fibroepithelial polyp occurring in the floor of the mouth. This consists of a small nodule of hyperplastic fibrous tissue covered by thinned or acanthotic epithe-

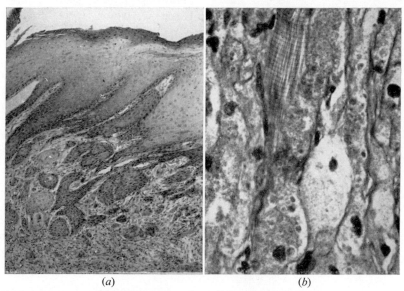

(a) (b)

Fig. 18.3.—Granular cell "myoblastoma".

(a) The characteristic irregular hyperplasia of the overlying squamous epithelium. × 60.
(b) The coarsely granular cytoplasm and small condensed nuclei of the elongated cells amongst the muscle fibres of the tongue. × 450.

ally in an adolescent raises the possibility of the Peutz–Jeghers syndrome (p. 531). In both conditions the pigment is seen in the basal cell layer.

Ingestion of various heavy metals gives rise to a pigmented line in the gums; blue in the case of lead, greyish-black with bismuth and purplish-grey with mercury. The metallic intoxication has to be of long duration to produce these lesions.

Benign tumours

Both haemangioma and lymphangioma may give rise to great enlargement of the lips and tongue and call for plastic surgery (Fig. 18.2). Parabuccal mixed tumours may arise in the lips, palate and fauces as well as in the more usual site in the parotid (see below).

Squamous papilloma is a common tumour of the oral tissues and may occur at all ages although it is most often seen in the elderly. In

lium. It is due to chronic irritation and is not neoplastic.

Granular-cell myoblastoma. In spite of its name, this tumour is probably of neural origin and derived from Schwann cells: it occurs most commonly in the tongue but also in the skin, larynx, breast, etc. It is composed of elongated cells, with nuclei at intervals as in muscle fibres; the cytoplasm is acidophilic and is broken up into innumerable rounded granular masses, and striation is completely absent. The lesion is a true neoplasm and, though not well circumscribed, usually behaves as a benign tumour. We have, however, seen multiple recurrences and undoubted local malignancy; metastases have also been recorded. A remarkable feature is the tendency of the overlying squamous epithelium to be markedly and irregularly hyperplastic (Fig. 18.3), so that an erroneous diagnosis of squamous carcinoma may be made, especially in such situations as the tongue or larynx.

Epulis is the term applied to tumours arising from the gingival margin. Some so designated clinically are inflammatory granulomatous masses, but true tumours also occur.

Congenital epulis is seen in two forms. The better-known arises usually from the maxillary gum margin and forms a soft polypoid mass consisting of cells closely resembling those of the

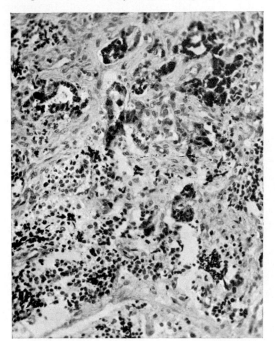

FIG. 18.4.—Congenital melanotic epulis, showing heavily pigmented tubules and masses of small darkly-staining cells. × 180.

so-called granular myoblastoma. It is of interest that similar large granular cells occasionally occur in tumours of the enamel organ (see Fig. 18.15). The other form is the rare, controversial melanotic tumour that occurs chiefly in the maxilla in the newborn or in early infancy and consists of masses of small darkly staining cells resembling neuroblasts and larger paler cells resembling glia. Between these are tubules lined by cubical cells heavily pigmented with melanin granules which may have the rod-like morphology characteristic of retinal pigment (Fig. 18.4). Despite the malignant-looking histology these tumours are clinically simple and do not recur after thorough removal.

The fibrous and bony epulis arises chiefly in connection with the maxilla. It consists of young fibrous tissue amongst which are irregular bony trabeculae and as there is always some inflammatory reaction it is difficult to distinguish the simple variety from reactive lesions. The neo-

plastic nature of such an epulis may be displayed by destructive invasion of the maxilla and antrum and we have seen an example that looked histologically benign undergo repeated recurrence and finally metastasise to the lungs.

The giant-cell epulis or *giant-cell reparative granuloma* arises usually in the mandible in connection with the tooth sockets of the primary dentition. It consists of a loose spindle-celled tissue in which there are numerous multinucleated giant cells which closely resemble those of giant-cell tumour of bone (Fig. 18.5). The surface is often ulcerated and inflammatory cellular reaction may be abundant in the superficial part. It rarely recurs after removal and although it is regarded by many as reactive rather than neoplastic, its true nature is still unknown.

Malignant tumours

Squamous carcinoma can arise anywhere in the mouth, but most often in the following situations. In the *lip* the disease occurs almost exclusively in the lower lip and in males. The lesion may begin as a whitish patch of thickening—

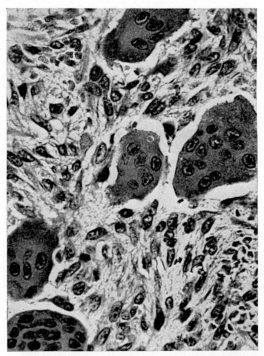

FIG. 18.5.—Giant-cell epulis, showing multinucleated giant cells embedded in spindle-cell tissue. × 400.

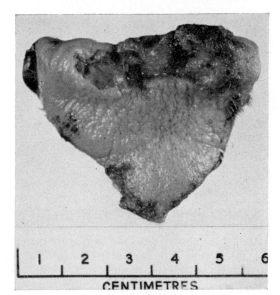

FIG. 18.6.—Squamous carcinoma of lip, showing ulceration and thickened rolled margin. × 1·2.

leukoplakia—or as a warty excrescence which breaks down to form an indurated ulcer with rolled-over edges (Fig. 18.6). Spread to the submental glands is relatively late. Microscopically the growth is usually of well-differentiated keratinising type.

Squamous carcinoma of the tongue arises most often on the lateral margin of the anterior two thirds, beginning as a thickened patch of leukoplakia and going on to a deeply excavated ulcer. Spread to the submental and submandibular lymph nodes is usually early and extends quickly to involve the deep cervical nodes. Squamous carcinoma occurs in the *floor of the mouth* and on the *tonsil* and *pillars of the fauces*. Microscopically the growth is usually fairly well differentiated (Figs. 11.9 and 11.10, p. 243) but despite this it is radiosensitive. The rarer growths on the posterior third of the tongue resemble those on the tonsil and may be more anaplastic or of lympho-epitheliomatous type.

Lympho-epithelioma is a distinctive variety of anaplastic carcinoma. It arises from the modified epithelium overlying the lymphoid tissue of the pharynx. It commonly arises in the region of the Eustachian cushion so that obstruction of the Eustachian tube with deafness may be an early sign. The growth on the surface is often only a small, patch of little thickening, but beneath this there may be widespread invasion and bulky metastases occur in the cervical nodes, often before the primary

tumour is discovered. Invasion of the base of the skull is also relatively common, resulting in cranial nerve palsies. The tumour is composed of poorly differentiated rounded or polyhedral cells, in places recognisable as epithelial. Typically there are many lymphocytes in the tumour (Fig. 18.7). Metastases in internal organs are not uncommon, especially in the cervical spine. In the metastases the large number of lymphocytes is again noteworthy. This type of carcinoma is observed in the earlier years of life as well as later, and for reasons as yet obscure, it is one of the most common types of malignant disease in Chinese. It is markedly sensitive to radiation, but is rarely cured.

Nasopharyngeal carcinoma, including lympho-epithelioma has been shown to be associated with high titres of antibody to the Epstein–Barr virus (see pp. 220, 459).

Sarcoma. While the various types of sarcoma may arise in the oropharynx, two examples are of particular importance.

In the *tonsil* and *adjacent lymphoid tissue*, various highly cellular lymphoid tumours occur, mostly lymphosarcoma and reticulum-cell sarcoma. They can be hard to distinguish from

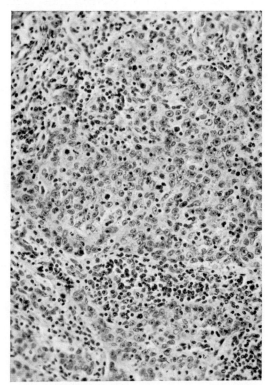

FIG. 18.7.—Lympho-epithelioma, showing tumour cells in trabecular arrangement, interspersed with many lymphocytes. × 220.

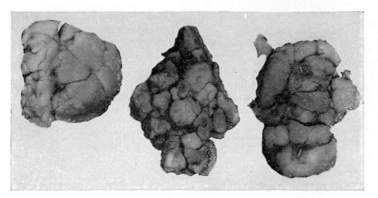

FIG. 18.8.—Rhabdomyosarcoma of the soft palate in a child. The primary tumour on the left with two recurrences. All show the typical blunt clubbed polypoid processes. Natural size.

the lympho-epithelioma; like them they are highly radiosensitive, at least for a time.

In the *soft palate* a distinctive type of rhabdomyosarcoma (p. 249) occurs in children. It is of polypoid form and consists of a number of blunt clubbed processes suspended from a narrow stalk (Fig. 18.8). After simple operative removal, repeated local recurrence in a similar form occurs, sometimes over a number of years, but ultimately spread takes place to the cervical lymph nodes and internal organs. Adequate local excision is therefore an urgent matter.

The salivary glands

Inflammation of the parotid and other salivary glands is most often due to the virus of *mumps*, which gives rise to an early viraemic phase. The chief lesion in mumps is an acute inflammatory swelling, mainly of the parotids, with oedema and interstitial mononuclear cell infiltration. Usually this subsides without permanent damage to the glands. It may be accompanied by orchitis and by pancreatitis, both of which are more prone to result in some degree of atrophy. Mumps virus is also a relatively common cause of meningitis (p. 645).

Suppurative parotitis occurs as a complication of prolonged febrile illnesses, infection usually reaching the gland by way of Stensen's duct. Infection is prone to occur if the duct is partially obstructed by a calculus.

Salivary calculi occur most often in the submaxillary gland. The calculus is round or elongated and may project from the orifice of the duct which it partially occludes. Salivary calculi

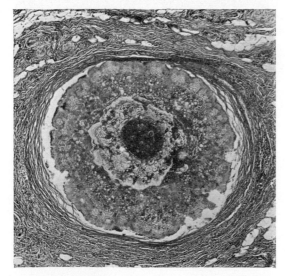

FIG. 18.9(*a*).—Calculus obstructing duct of submaxillary gland. × 55.

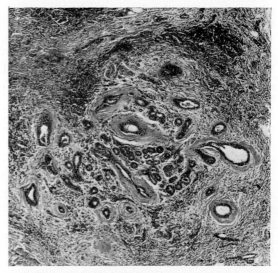

FIG. 18.9(*b*).—Atrophy and fibrosis of submaxillary gland with chronic inflammatory infiltration, resulting from duct obstruction. × 55.

are composed chiefly of calcium carbonate and phosphate. The obstruction thus caused is apt to lead to atrophy and fibrosis of the gland (Figs. 18.9*a* and 18.9*b*).

Sjögren's syndrome. This condition is almost confined to women of middle age and it consists

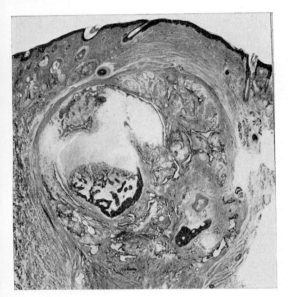

FIG. 18.10.—Parabuccal mixed tumour of lower lip. × 7.

of intermittent swelling of the lachrymal and salivary glands accompanied by attacks of *kerato-conjunctivitis sicca*. Many cases also suffer from chronic polyarthritis of rheumatoid type. The lachrymal, conjunctival and salivary glands are the seat of extensive lymphocytic and plasma cell infiltration and the secretory tissue is much atrophied. Various autoantibodies may appear in the serum, including antinuclear antibodies, precipitins to cellular constituents and rheumatoid factor. The syndrome is sometimes associated with chronic thyroiditis and its immunological accompaniments. The condition long known as Mikulicz's disease is now recognized to be simply a variant of this syndrome with prominent lachrymal gland enlargement.

Uveo-parotid fever. This is one of the important lesions of sarcoidosis (p. 152) in which iridocyclitis and parotid swelling occur, sometimes involving the facial nerve and causing paralysis. The glands may be considerably enlarged due to the presence of chronic inflammatory infiltrates in which sarcoid follicles are found.

Salivary gland tumours

Parabuccal mixed tumour. This type of tumour is commonest in the parotid gland, but tumours of corresponding structure occur in other parts of the mouth, lips and palate. The common "mixed parotid tumour" may reach a large size and produce effects mainly by pressure. As a rule, it is well encapsulated and does not infiltrate the surrounding tissue (Fig. 18.10), but occasionally malignant growth of carcinomatous type supervenes. Histologically, the tumour is found to consist both of epithelial elements and connective tissues, but the former are the essential elements. The epithelial cells are, in places, of a low columnar type and have an acinar arrangement, often with two layers of cells, but occasionally there is transition to squamous epithelium. Cells extend from the acini in solid strands which merge into the stroma, suggesting a transition between stroma and epithelial cells (Fig. 18.12). The epithelial cells appear to secrete mucinous material into

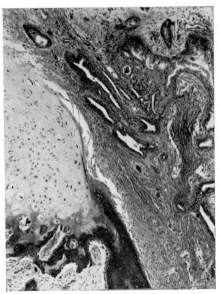

FIG. 18.11.—Parabuccal mixed tumour of lower lip, showing bone, and cartilage undergoing ossification. × 50.

the stroma around them. The stroma may remain gelatinous, or may become condensed and hyaline with isolated cells embedded in it so that it is indistinguishable morphologically and tinctorially from cartilage. Whether the cartilage cells are epithelial elements or altered stromal cells is uncertain but when cartilage has formed in this way true bone may then appear also (Fig. 18.11). Such tumours are fairly common and may be regarded as adenomas in which both the epithelial cells and the associated stroma have a special tendency to undergo metaplasia.

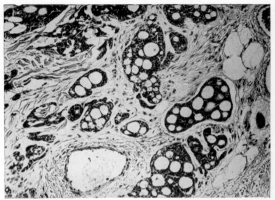

FIG. 18.13.—Cribriform cylindroma, showing the characteristic architecture. × 90.

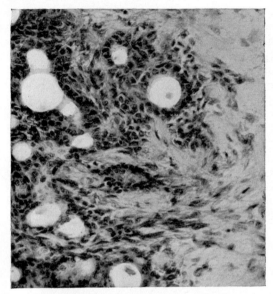

FIG. 18.12.—Parabuccal mixed tumour, showing acinus-like structures above, the cells of which are giving off strands which merge into the connective tissue. × 200.

The range of structural variation among parabuccal tumours is extremely wide, and no histological classification is wholly satisfactory. It is worth distinguishing an acinar tumour with cells resembling those of the serous salivary glands and also a muco-epidermoid type in which large mucin-secreting cells mingle with cells of squamous appearance. The most important variant is the *cribriform cylindroma* (Fig. 18.13). This consists of solid masses of small darkly-staining cells amongst which lie tiny spaces containing clear fluid, either spherical, giving a sieve-like effect on section, or drawn out into little duct-like channels. The prognosis of this tumour type is substantially worse than that of other parabuccal tumours. Despite initial slow growth, local recurrence after excision is the rule. Metastases to local lymph nodes are common in the later stages and blood spread is by no means rare. This type of tumour is relatively commoner outside the parotid than in it. This type of tumour occurs also in the

nose, external auditory meatus and skin (one form of hidradenoma). At all these sites except the last, where the necessary wide excision is usually possible, it has the same slow growth but poor ultimate prognosis.

Adenolymphoma. This is a type of adenoma which occurs in the parotid glands. It is seen especially in males in late adult life and is usually benign. The epithelium is of tall columnar type which is arranged as small glandular acini or as cysts with numerous small papillomatous ingrowths (Fig. 18.14). The stroma is lymphoid tissue with numerous germinal centres. There is apparently a co-ordinated neoplastic growth of both tissues and a developmental abnormality is probably the basis of the tumour.

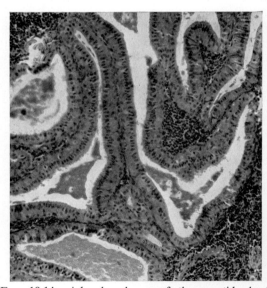

FIG. 18.14.—Adenolymphoma of the parotid gland, showing the papillary architecture, with lymphoid stroma. × 130.

Tumours of dental origin

Adamantinoma (ameloblastoma). This epithelial growth is composed of masses and anastomosing strands of cells (Fig. 18.15). Those at the periphery are usually columnar in type and are believed to represent ameloblasts. The cells within are of more stellate or irregular form and occasionally are distended with granular material. The cell masses may be solid, but not infrequently the central portions undergo softening so that cysts are formed, which are often multiple. Such a tumour was

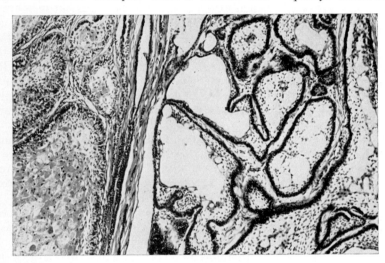

FIG. 18.15.—Adamantinoma, Showing spaces lined by epithelium, some of which contain a loose network of cells resembling the stellate reticulum of the enamel organ. On the left, the alveoli are filled with granular cells. × 56.

formerly called *epithelial odontoma*, but the terms *adamantinoma* and *ameloblastoma* are now used. They originate from the enamel organ, or from small masses of epithelial cells—"paradental remains"—which occur normally in the fetus in the vicinity of the developing teeth. While their behaviour may be benign, they are prone to repeated local recurrences and the more solid types sometimes invade and destroy the surrounding tissues.

Odontoma. The term is applied in a general way to any tumour-like mass developing in connection with the tissues which form the teeth. Such a growth may arise at various stages of development, and may consist of one or several tissues; accordingly odontomata present considerable varieties of structure. We can mention only a few in illustration. Sometimes the tooth follicle forms a *dentigerous cyst*, containing one or more teeth or a large number of imperfectly developed teeth or denticles. In the cyst wall there may be calcium deposition and even formation of bone. In other cases an odontoma consists of various structures containing enamel and cement irregularly admixed and sometimes forming a hard irregular mass; the term *composite odontoma* is applied to such a structure.

Pharynx

Tonsillitis. Acute tonsillitis is a common cause of sore throat. Haemolytic streptococci are the commonest infecting agents and give rise to acute inflammatory swelling with purulent exudate in the tonsillar crypts—*follicular tonsillitis*. The infection occasionally extends more deeply and involves the whole tonsil and adjacent tissues with frank suppuration; this is known as *quinsy*. From such a lesion streptococcal cellulitis may spread widely into the neck—*Ludwig's angina*—or even into the mediastinum or may give rise to a retropharyngeal abscess.

Acute streptococcal tonsillitis occurring alone or in scarlet fever is the usual antecedent infection in rheumatic fever and post-streptococcal glomerulonephritis. Chronic enlargement of the tonsils and adjacent lymphoid tissue commonly results from colonisation by one or other of the many adenoviruses.

Vincent's angina is a painful necrotic ulcerating lesion on the fauces characterised by a patch of yellowish-white false membrane (see p. 134), which later sloughs off, surrounded by an area of acute inflammation. It is due to the symbiotic action of fusiform bacilli and the spirochaete *Borrelia vincenti*. Vincent's infection in its most severe form is probably responsible for the lesions on the cheek known as *noma* or *cancrum oris*, and it also gives rise to a severe ulcerative and necrotic gingivitis. A similar lesion is found in established scurvy, due to vitamin C deficiency. Great swelling, haemorrhage and ulceration of the gingivae are frequently seen in the acute leukaemias, particularly in the monocytic form, and necrotic ulceration occurs on the fauces, pharynx and larynx in various conditions characterised by extreme reduction in the number of circulating polymorphonuclear leukocytes, *i.e.* in *agranulocytosis* (p. 396).

Diphtheria is an acute inflammation which affects most frequently the fauces, soft palate and tonsils, but may also attack the nose, or the larynx and trachea; it occurs chiefly in young children, but may also affect adults. The causal organism, *Corynebacterium diphtheriae*, exists in three main forms, *mitis*, *intermedius* and *gravis*, and infections with the last type tend to be more severely toxic and also to show greater local inflammatory reaction. The organisms remain strictly localised at the site of infection and the systemic effects are due to the formation and absorption of a powerful exotoxin which may cause myocardial damage and toxic fatty changes in the organs; the mechanism of cellular injury is outlined on p. 2. The local lesions are characterised by the formation on the affected surfaces of a false membrane composed of fibrin and leukocytes. In the fauces, palate and tonsils the stratified squamous epithelium becomes permeated by exudate which forms a fibrinous coagulum in which the epithelium is incorporated; it then undergoes extensive necrosis under the influence of the diphtheria toxin. The whole false membrane is dull greyish-yellow and it can be detached only with difficulty owing to the attachment of the dead epithelium to the underlying tissues. When it is removed a bleeding connective tissue surface is laid bare. In *gravis* infections, membrane formation may be less obvious but inflammatory congestion and swelling are more marked and the cervical lymph nodes may be much swollen.

In the larynx and trachea on the other hand the false membrane is formed mainly on a surface of which the covering epithelium is columnar; this becomes detached, so that the coagulated exudate rests on the basement membrane from which it separates easily and is coughed up. Over the vocal cords, however, where the epithelium is of the stratified squamous variety, the membrane is firmly adherent and thus when the membrane is coughed up from the trachea it may fail to become detached from the vocal cords and may then become impacted in the larynx and cause death from suffocation.

In nasal diphtheria the infection is often unilateral and the patient may appear to have a "cold in the head" with discharge from one nostril. This type is often overlooked until toxic manifestations, such as palatal paralysis or myocardial damage appear. Sometimes the diagnosis is made only when secondary cases occur.

Immunisation programmes are largely responsible for the present low incidence of diphtheria in many parts of the world.

OESOPHAGUS

General considerations. The oesophagus is a muscular tube, lined by squamous epithelium and adapted to bear without injury the rapid passing of food over its surface. It has marked powers of resistance and is a rare site of primary bacterial invasion, but damage to the mucosa of the lower end from regurgitated gastric juice is fairly common. Of especial importance are those conditions which interfere with the function of the oesophagus by causing stenosis or obstruction of the lumen, and of these malignant disease is the most important.

Circulatory disturbances

Oesophageal varices. The submucosal veins in the lower oesophagus and cardia of the stomach communicate with both the portal and systemic venous systems. In cases of portal hypertension, most frequently due to *hepatic cirrhosis*, these veins become distinctly varicose and form projections usually called oesophageal varices; these may ulcerate, causing severe and often fatal haemorrhage.

Other causes of oesophageal haemorrhage. Sometimes an *aortic aneurysm* may rupture into the oesophagus, although this is relatively rare on account of the mobility of the tube. A *foreign body*, for example a fish bone or safety pin, may become impacted transversely in the oesophagus, ulcerate through the wall, causing suppurative mediastinitis or empyema and subsequently lead to perforation of the aorta. A *carcinoma* of the oesophagus, especially of the soft and necrotic variety, may ulcerate into the aorta or other large vessel.

Inflammatory conditions

As already mentioned, primary infections of the oesophagus are rare in otherwise healthy individuals. Occasionally the lesion of diphtheria extends into, or arises primarily in, the oesophagus. Tuberculous lesions, resulting from swallowing infected sputum, or arising by extension from an adjacent caseous lymph node, used to be seen. Syphilitic lesions are uncommon, although gumma has been described, and secondary syphilitic lesions of the pharynx may extend to the oesophagus. In the rare but distinctive form of disseminated herpes simplex infection encountered in early infancy, the virus sometimes gains entry through the oesophagus. The characteristic lesion associated with South American trypanosomiasis (Chagas's disease) is described below.

Oesophageal infections may, however, complicate states of immunological deficiency or immaturity, for example in infancy, various chronic diseases, malnutrition or the administration of antibiotics, cytotoxic or immunosuppressive agents. Such "opportunistic" infections are often caused by organisms normally of low virulence. *Thrush*, caused by the yeast-like fungus *Candida albicans*, is the most common infection of this type and is characterised by the formation of irregularly raised opaque whitish patches consisting of swollen and sodden epithelium infiltrated by the septate mycelial threads and spores of the fungus (Fig. 18.16). The infection may have spread from the mouth or throat and can extend more distally in the gastrointestinal tract or even invade the blood stream to produce generalised lesions.

Oesophagitis can, of course, arise from non-infective causes. The most common example of this is peptic oesophagitis caused by regurgitation of gastric juice from the stomach and this is discussed more fully below. Occasionally the self-administration, accidental or otherwise, of irritating fluids is encountered and can give rise to serious and sometimes fatal lesions. Concentrated caustic soda, for example, produces extensive necrosis and sloughing of the oesophageal wall. More dilute solutions lead to superficial destruction followed by inflammatory

changes. The natural consequence of such ulceration and sloughing of necrotic tissue (should the patient survive) is healing by fibrosis, which may later produce fibrous stricture. Rarely the whole of the superficial layers of the oesophagus may become separated as a cast, without obvious cause; clinically this episode is accompanied by great pain and discomfort until the cast is completely separated (oesophagitis dissecans superficialis).

Peptic or reflux oesophagitis. Inflammatory changes and even frank ulceration may be produced at the lower end of the oesophagus by the reflux of acid gastric juice from the stomach. This may take place in severe toxic and infective conditions, particularly after operations, and be accompanied clinically by haematemesis and even oesophageal perforation from acute peptic ulceration. Less severe forms of peptic oesophagitis are seen in about one-third of patients

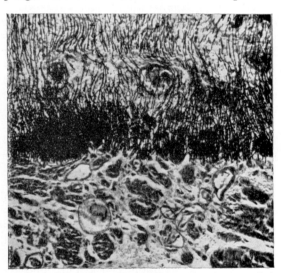

Fig. 18.16.—Thrush of oesophagus, showing mycelial threads penetrating the wall. × 115.

confined to bed for some time before death and give rise to fiery-red oedematous mucosa with superficial ulcers just above the cardiac orifice. It must be appreciated, however, that considerable digestion of the lower oesophagus may take place after death, the wall then being discoloured, softened and shreddy, and often perforated. Recognition of true, antemortem oesophagitis depends upon the histological demonstration of inflammation or haemorrhage.

Hiatus hernia. The most important cause of peptic oesophagitis from the clinical viewpoint is, however, incompetence of the anti-reflux mechanism at the cardia associated with hiatus hernia, i.e. the herniation of part of the stomach through the oesophageal hiatus into the thoracic cavity. The mechanism preventing reflux of gastric juice depends upon three main components: (1) the intrinsic sphincter now thought to exist at the lower end of the oesophagus, (2) the attachment of the cardio-oesophageal junction to the diaphragmatic hiatus, and (3) the maintenance of the cardio-oesophageal angle, probably by a muscular "sling" extending over the body of the stomach. Not all types of hiatus hernia lead to incompetence of this mechanism; for example, in the "rolling" variety, in which part of the fundus of the stomach passes into the thorax alongside the cardia, reflux does not usually take place, although haematemesis and melaena are not uncommonly observed in this condition. It is in the "sliding" type of hernia, which leads to obliteration of the cardio-oesophageal angle with upward displacement of the cardia, that reflux oesophagitis and its complications are most frequently observed. A similar situation pertains in individuals with a congenitally short oesophagus, although this condition is generally considered to be rare, and some doubt its existence.

The primary cause of hiatus hernia is not completely understood. It is certainly a common condition in the middle-aged and elderly although only symptomatic in a proportion of cases, and is usually attributed to increased intra-abdominal pressure coupled with laxity of the diaphragmatic hiatus. Obesity and pregnancy are thus common predisposing conditions and probably account for the higher incidence of hiatus hernia in women.

The principal symptoms, heartburn and regurgitation, are due to diffuse, superficial inflammation, congestion and ulceration caused by reflux of acid gastric juice into the lower oesophagus. Frank haematemesis and melaena are relatively uncommon complications, but chronic blood loss may lead to iron-deficiency anaemia. Perforation of the oesophagus is rare since the ulcers seldom penetrate the oesophageal muscularis. More often healing of the ulcerative lesions leads to the development of a fibrous stricture and dysphagia.

True chronic peptic ulceration of the oesophagus is uncommon. It occurs in the gastric-type mucosa which lines the lower part of the tube in sliding hiatus hernia (Fig. 18.17) or congenitally short oesophagus, and is sometimes known as Barrett's ulcer. Haematemesis, perforation and stenosis are the principal complications.

Spontaneous rupture of the oesophagus

This condition occasionally occurs in previously healthy men, when a heavy meal has been followed by violent vomiting. The lesion takes

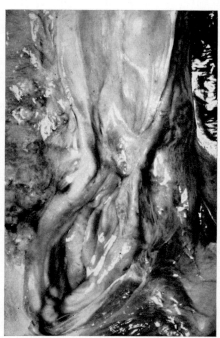

FIG. 18.17.—Hiatus hernia with chronic peptic ulceration in the thoracic portion of the stomach. × ½.

the form of a longitudinal slit, most often in the left posterior position, just above the diaphragm. The acid gastric contents are discharged into the pleural cavity directly or after first distending the posterior mediastinum. The appearance of the lesion indicates that it is essentially a longitudinal burst, brought about by sudden over-distension of the lower oesophagus in the act of vomiting, but the strongly acid gastric juice may also be a factor. In a number of the recorded cases peptic ulceration of stomach or duodenum has also been present.

Severe vomiting, usually associated with heavy alcohol intake, may also lead to brisk haematemesis as a result of laceration of the mucosa in the vicinity of the cardia. The damage, however, usually affects the gastric rather than the oeso-phageal mucosa (Mallory–Weiss syndrome).

Oesophageal obstruction

Obstruction of the oesophagus usually has an *organic* basis. In some instances, however, a primary organic lesion cannot be recognised and obstruction is described as being *functional* in nature.

Organic obstruction

This may arise in a number of different ways. (1) The lumen of the oesophagus may actually be occluded, usually by tumour, either benign or malignant, although occasionally by a foreign body. (2) Disease within the wall of the oeso-phagus may lead to stenosis of the lumen; again malignant tumours are most often implicated. Fibrous stricture may, however, arise as a com-plication of hiatus hernia, the swallowing of irritating fluids, trauma or syphilis, or as a congenital defect. (3) The oesophagus may be compressed from outside, e.g. by a mediastinal tumour or cyst, aortic aneurysm, enlargement of the left atrium following mitral stenosis, con-genital malformation of the great vessels, or pharyngeal diverticulum. (4) Diseases affecting the neuro-muscular co-ordination of the oeso-phagus may interfere with normal deglutition. Progressive systemic sclerosis and Chagas's disease are suitably included in this group, and also disorders of the central nervous system which interfere with deglutition. Most of these diseases are discussed in the appropriate sections.

Progressive systemic sclerosis. This is re-garded as a form of connective tissue disease (p. 814) which may produce widespread systemic lesions, the skin of the hands and face (acro-sclerosis) and the kidneys being especially affected. Dysphagia is a not uncommon feature, and is due to replacement of the oesophageal musculature by fibrous tissue which, if diffuse, leads to pronounced interference with peristaltic activity. Shortening of the oesophagus causing reflux oesophagitis may be an additional com-plication.

Chagas's disease (South American trypano-somiasis). The protozoon parasite, (*Trypano-soma cruzi*) which causes this interesting disease appears to be capable of exerting a toxic effect on the autonomic ganglia of various viscera, especially the heart, oesophagus and colon. In the oesophagus, there may be widespread destruction of the ganglia of the myenteric plexus, leading to disturbance of peristalsis and the development of a clinical picture very similar to that of achalasia (see below).

Functional obstruction

The most important condition falling into this category is achalasia of the oesophagus, although other forms of functional disturbance have been described, e.g. diffuse spasm, sometimes asso-ciated with organic lesions of the gastro-intestinal tract, especially peptic ulcer, gall-bladder disease and hiatus hernia. Dysphagia may also result from functional constriction at the upper end of the oesophagus in anaemic women (Kelly–Paterson or Plummer–Vinson syndrome, p. 425): here it is generally thought to be due to spasm of the crico-pharyngeus portion of the inferior constrictor of the pharynx, associated with an atrophic pharyngo-oesophagitis.

Achalasia of the oesophagus. In this condition, there is pronounced narrowing of the terminal part of the oesophagus with dilatation proxi-mally. It usually develops in early adult life and leads to dysphagia and regurgitation of food; later there may be more serious obstruction. Oesophageal narrowing is usually at the dia-phragmatic level and marked dilatation of the oesophagus results (Fig. 18.18), with compensa-tory muscular hypertrophy of the wall. The narrowing was formerly regarded as due to muscular spasm, hence the term "cardiospasm" commonly applied to the disease; the present view, however, is that there is a primary disturb-ance of motility with defective transmission of peristaltic waves to the cardia and subsequent failure of relaxation of the cardiac sphincter. The cause of this disturbance remains uncertain. Degenerative changes have been described in the myenteric ganglia, and it is probable that the primary lesion in achalasia is an acquired abnormality of autonomic innervation; the close similarity of the disease to Chagas's disease provides indirect support for this hypothesis. Incision of the oesophageal wall through to the mucosa at the level of obstruction (Heller's operation) appears to be the most satisfactory form of surgical treatment in severe cases.

Diverticula

Two varieties of local dilatation are observed in the oesophagus, namely the *pulsion diverticulum* and the *traction diverticulum*. The former is caused by forcible distension during the act of swallowing. It is usually not noticeable till early

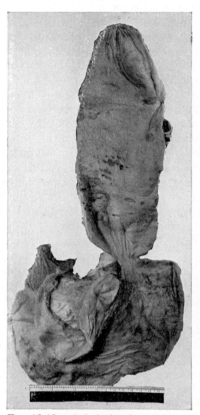

FIG. 18.18.—Achalasia of oesophagus.
Note the great dilatation with numerous superficial ulcers. × ¼.

adult life but the origin of the condition may depend on a congenital weakness or deficiency in the muscle of the inferior constrictor of the pharynx; it is therefore really *pharyngeal* although usually spoken of as oesophageal. Once a diverticulum has formed, as may result from stretching of the deficiency in the wall by a bolus of food, it tends to become distended with food during deglutition and gradually enlarges in a downward direction behind the wall of the oesophagus, tilting the tube forwards so that the

mouth of the sac comes to lie in line with the upper pharynx. The sac ultimately becomes permanently distended by food and may become so large as to prevent the onward passage of food to the stomach. Extreme emaciation may ensue. Such a diverticulum is lined by mucous membrane supported by connective tissue, but its wall usually contains no muscle; occasionally ulceration may take place in it. A diverticulum may also occur anteriorly and bulge between the trachea and the oesophagus; but much more frequently the site is in the posterior wall at the junction of the pharynx and oesophagus.

The *traction diverticulum* of the oesophagus is produced by the contraction of connective tissue pulling the wall outwards, usually by the adhesion to the wall of the tube of a mass of calcified tuberculous lymph nodes or occasionally a mass of silicotic nodes. A pouch with sharp apex is the result, and this is stretched and increased both by the contraction of the connective tissue and by the movements of the oesophagus. Ulceration of the diverticulum may occur and may lead to perforation, resulting in gangrenous mediastinitis which may extend to the pleura and other parts.

In rare cases a local diverticulum opposite the bifurcation of the trachea is due to a congenital abnormality, arising in the same way as a communication between the oesophagus and trachea (p. 485). The congenital diverticula are sometimes lined by columnar epithelium.

Tumours

Benign tumours. These are all rare. Lipoma, fibroma and leiomyoma may all occur, the last mentioned probably being the most common and occasionally reaching a large size. Benign tumours tend to project into the lumen as polyps.

Malignant tumours

Carcinoma of the oesophagus. Carcinoma is by far the commonest malignant tumour in the oesophagus and is comparatively frequent. It occurs usually after the age of forty-five, and is much commoner in men than in women. The commonest site is at the level of the bifurcation of the trachea, the lower and upper ends being next in order of frequency. There is, however, a distinct difference in the sites of incidence in the two sexes. About three-quarters of cases of cancer in the hypopharynx and upper end of the oesophagus occur in women, whereas in oesophageal cancer elsewhere over 80 per cent occur in men.

Oesophageal carcinoma shows remarkable geographical variation in incidence. Although not uncommon in this country its incidence is much greater in certain parts of the U.S.S.R., and in Africa where it is suspected that the consumption of adulterated alcoholic beverages is a contributory factor. Fungal contamination of maize grown upon poor soil has also been incriminated. There is a remarkably high incidence in Curaçao, probably attributable to eating food that is too hot. In this country little is known about the causation of oesophageal cancer apart from a possible association with heavy alcohol intake. There is also the relationship between iron-deficiency anaemia with dysphagia (Kelly–Paterson syndrome) and post-cricoid carcinoma in women.

Naked-eye appearances. There are two chief types. The *hard sclerosing type* is usually comparatively localised, and by its growth round the tube and the resulting contraction a considerable degree of stenosis is produced. The *soft* or encephaloid type involves a greater extent of the oesophagus, forms irregular projections into the lumen, and thus tends to cause occlusion (Fig. 18.19). At the same time, the destruction of the muscular tissue by infiltration interferes with contraction. The tumour not infrequently spreads upwards and downwards in the submucous tissue, and forms secondary growths which raise up the mucosa, giving an appearance of multifocal origin.

In addition to causing obstruction, the tumour may spread to adjacent parts, especially the trachea or a bronchus, and ulcerate through the wall. Infected fluids then are likely to pass down the bronchi and give rise to aspiration pneumonia. In other cases, though less frequently, ulceration into the aorta may result in fatal haemorrhage. Metastases also occur in the lymph nodes, and occasionally also in the internal organs, especially the liver; but death is usually caused by the local lesions.

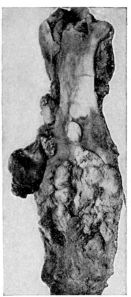

FIG. 18.19.—Extensive ulcerating carcinoma in middle part of oesophagus. × ⅓.

Microscopic appearances. In nearly all cases the tumour is a poorly keratinised squamous carcinoma; rarely it resembles oat-cell bronchial carcinoma. Adenocarcinoma also has been described, but many examples are due to extension of a gastric carcinoma.

Sarcoma. This is rare. It resembles the softer varieties of cancer, but its growth may be more massive. In a few instances rhabdomyosarcoma of the oesophagus has been observed.

Congenital abnormalities

In addition to stenosis or dilatation, already mentioned, there may be various degrees of atresia of the oesophagus. The commonest of these is a condition in which the upper part forms a blind sac which is separated from the lower part, while the latter is patent and communicates with the trachea a short distance above its bifurcation. Sometimes a minor degree of abnormality is observed, the oesophagus being patent throughout, but there is a small communication with the trachea at the site mentioned. In such a condition material from the oesophagus may pass into the trachea and cause a suppurative or gangrenous pneumonia. Occasionally the former site of such an opening is represented by a small pouch or depression.

STOMACH

General considerations. The two most important pathological conditions in the stomach are peptic ulcer and carcinoma. Bacterial infection as a cause of serious disease in the stomach is comparatively rare. Gastric juice rapidly destroys most vegetative bacteria entering with food, and when digestion has been completed, and the stomach contents pass on to the intestine, the stomach soon returns to a state of virtual sterility. Nevertheless ingested tubercle, typhoid, brucella and dysentery bacilli can all successfully evade the chemical barrier of the gastric secretion and no doubt more easily if there is defective acid secretion or stasis. Inflammatory changes in the stomach are, however, attributable to factors other than bacterial infection, such as improper diet or ingested irritants. It is probable, however, that the stomach can be affected by some of the enteroviruses and perhaps other viruses also.

Circulatory disturbances

Acute congestion occurs as part of the acute inflammatory changes produced by various kinds of ingested irritant, but its presence is often obscured by post-mortem autolysis.

Chronic congestion is seen as a result of cardiac and pulmonary disease and is especially marked in obstruction to the portal circulation in cirrhosis of the liver. The mucous membrane becomes swollen, purple or livid and towards the pylorus may be slate-grey, or minute brown points resulting from capillary haemorrhages may be present. Chronic inflammatory changes are often superadded. In long-continued portal obstruction there may be marked varicosity of the veins around the cardiac orifice as well as at the lower end of the oesophagus, and serious haemorrhage may occur from them. Fig. 18.20 shows large varices produced in this way, which caused fatal haemorrhage.

Haemorrhages into the mucosa occur in a variety of conditions such as chronic congestion, purpura, severe anaemia and infective fevers. Sometimes numerous haemorrhagic points 1–3 mm. in diameter are scattered over the mucosa, especially in the fundus and they are often more marked along the summits of the folds. They are usually dark brown; occasionally the overlying mucous membrane becomes eroded with the formation of minute ulcers.

The term *haemorrhagic erosion* is applied to small ulcers of this type (Fig. 18.21). In some of the erosions the pigment may have been removed by ulceration; occasionally, they become confluent and larger and merit the term "acute ulcer". A most important cause is ingestion of

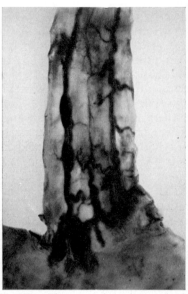

Fig. 18.20.—Oesophagus and cardiac end of stomach, showing large dilated varicose veins from a case of cirrhosis of the liver.

Fatal haemorrhage occurred from the large varicosity at the cardia. × ½.

aspirin. Haemorrhagic erosions occur also in febrile conditions and are thus common in children. In septicaemias small haemorrhages are sometimes due to plugging of small vessels with bacteria, but mostly they appear to be the result of toxic action.

Haemorrhage into the lumen of the stomach—haematemesis. Actual bleeding into the stomach may be the result not only of disease processes in the stomach itself but also in adjacent parts of the gastro-intestinal tract.

The commonest causes of serious haemorrhage are peptic ulcer, either in the stomach or duodenum, and oesophageal varices (Fig. 18.20) due to portal hypertension, usually following hepatic cirrhosis. Carcinoma of the stomach frequently causes haemorrhage, but this is rarely severe. Haemorrhagic erosions, most commonly following ingestion of aspirin, are now recognised as an important cause of gastric haemorrhage. Diffuse haemorrhage may occur from the mucous membrane without any discoverable break of continuity, or from apparently trivial local lesions. This is seen in haemorrhagic diatheses, in severe septic conditions, in yellow fever where

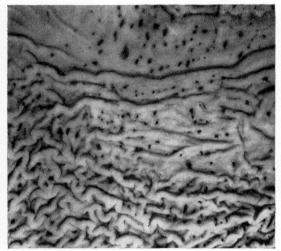

Fig. 18.21.—Multiple minute haemorrhages and erosions in stomach. × ¾.

it gives rise to "black vomit", in acute liver failure, and occasionally without discoverable cause as an agonal event.

Blood effused into the stomach becomes mixed with its contents and acquires a brownish or almost black colour, or there may be fragments of brownish coagulum mixed with the fluid. In cases of rapidly fatal haemorrhage, however, the stomach may be filled by a large coagulum which forms a cast of the interior and the colour of the blood may be little altered. Such a condition may result when blood has passed down from the oesophagus, for example, in rupture of oesophageal varices. When there has been much haemorrhage into the stomach, altered blood is generally found in the small and large intestine.

Inflammatory conditions

Acute gastritis

Acute catarrhal inflammation of a non-specific nature may be produced by the swallowing of irritants, hot fluids, strong alcohol or unsuitable foods. Acute fevers in children, viral infections such as "gastric influenza", and bacterial food poisoning may also be responsible, the latter usually taking the form of acute gastro-enteritis. The pathological changes produced depend on the nature of the irritant and vary in severity but the appearances are often obscured by postmortem change, particularly in the mildest variety, namely *acute catarrhal gastritis* which is, as a result, a poorly defined entity. The condition referred to as *acute erosive gastritis* found particularly in acute fevers in childhood is better defined and has been studied in detail in stomachs fixed shortly after death. The lesion may be localised to the pyloric antrum or may be more diffuse. The mucosa is red and oedematous, covered by patches of adherent mucus and beset with innumerable small (1–2 mm.) erosions on the summits of the rugae. Microscopically there is much infiltration of the mucosa by polymorphonuclears, lymphocytes and plasma cells with some eosinophils and the epithelium of many of the glands shows necrosis and desquamation with polymorphs in the lumen and on the surface (Fig. 18.22). The surface epithelium is altered from tall, clear columnar cells with basal nuclei to a more cubical type with basophilic cytoplasm and shows small foci of superficial ulceration.

Membranous gastritis, characterised by superficial necrosis of the epithelium with fibrinous exudation, is rare apart from the action of chemical irritants. It is sometimes observed in septicaemic conditions and fevers, e.g. typhoid.

Phlegmonous gastritis is a very rare, but distinctive, condition. Three examples observed personally have all been associated with the presence of sharp foreign bodies in the stomach; probably this is related to its alleged prevalence in alcoholics. The lesion is caused by the entrance of organisms, usually streptococci, through some small acute lesion in the mucosa. The organisms subsequently spread widely in the submucosa and produce intense inflammation with a fibrinous or semi-purulent exudate. The changes may be localised or extensive and the affected parts are thickened and stiffened: the mucous membrane on section is raised by the underlying yellow phlegmonous infiltration.

Chronic gastritis

Chronic inflammatory changes in the mucosa of the stomach, with various degrees of loss of the specialised glandular tissue, are extremely common, although often clinically silent. The condition is, however, important, for it is probably a common cause of chronic dyspepsia and, when

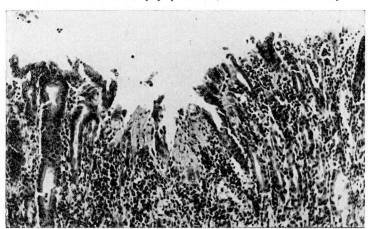

The acid-secreting mucosa

Pathological changes. Macroscopic examination of the gastric mucosa *in vivo* is of little value in diagnosing lesser degrees of chronic gastritis, although in severe degrees the mucosa is extremely thinned. Microscopically, the condition may be divided into *superficial chronic*

FIG. 18.22.—Acute erosive gastritis.

There is superficial loss of the surface epithelium with fibrinoid necrosis and polymorph infiltration. × 205.

it affects the acid-secreting fundal mucosa diffusely and severely, results in achlorhydria which predisposes to iron deficiency; moreover, secretion of intrinsic factor may be lost and this results in pernicious anaemia. There is also an association between chronic gastritis and gastric ulcer, and an increased incidence of gastric carcinoma.

The natural history of chronic gastritis is not well understood, largely because the mucosa undergoes rapid terminal and post-mortem autolysis and so is usually unsuitable for detailed histology. Gastric mucosal biopsies, particularly when obtained perorally, are helpful, but give little indication of the distribution of mucosal changes, and are only justifiable when their examination is likely to influence treatment of the patient.

In considering chronic gastritis in more detail, distinction should be made between the fundal, acid-secreting mucosa and that lining the antrum. Chronic inflammation of the fundal mucosa is, at least in many cases, a specific entity of autoimmune nature, and comparable in its general features to chronic thyroiditis and other organ-specific auto-immune diseases. The antral mucosa is also a common site of chronic inflammation, although little is known about its etiology.

gastritis, atrophic gastritis of various degrees, and *gastric atrophy*.

In *chronic superficial gastritis*, the necks of the gastric glands are increased in length, and the superficial lamina propria is infiltrated with lymphocytes and plasma cells, together with a few neutrophil and eosinophil polymorphs (Fig. 18.23b): the mucosa is of approximately normal thickness and the inflammatory changes are confined to its superficial part. These changes are typically focal.

In *atrophic gastritis*, the inflammatory changes are similar to those of superficial chronic gastritis, but extend more deeply into the mucosa and are accompanied by various degrees of loss of the specialised (i.e. parietal and chief) cells of the mucosal glands. In its extreme degree, the changes affect the fundal mucosa diffusely and there is virtually complete loss of the specialised glandular cells (Fig. 18.23d). The number of glands appears to be diminished, and they are lined by a simple mucus-secreting epithelium similar to the surface mucosa, or show intestinal metaplasia (see below). There is increase in the lamina propria, seen as widened areas of loose vascular connective tissue, heavily infiltrated with lymphocytes and plasma cells, between the glands. The mucosa is appreciably thinned and the rugae are not prominent. In less severe atrophic gastritis the changes are focal, affecting patches of mucosa in a part or the whole of its thickness, while the intervening areas of mucosa may show superficial gastritis, or may be normal.

In *gastric atrophy* the fundal mucosa is diffusely atrophic, with virtually complete replacement of parietal and chief cells by mucus-secreting glandular epithelium, and increase of loose vascular connective tissue in the lamina propria. The appearances resemble closely those of severe atrophic gastritis except for the much smaller numbers of lymphocytes and plasma cells in gastric atrophy.

A very common feature in both atrophic gastritis and gastric atrophy is *metaplasia* of the mucosal glands to resemble closely those of the intestine (Fig. 18.23c), with goblet cells, tall columnar cells bearing a brush border, and Paneth cells. The altered glands may show irregular cystic change, and there may also be abundant lymphoid nodules with germinal centres in the basal part of the mucosa and sub-mucosa: the term "follicular gastritis" has been applied when the lymphoid nodules are promi-

nent, but they occur in variable numbers in the normal stomach.

Etiology. The three types of chronic gastritis described above are merely different degrees of the same process. The destructive inflammatory changes begin superficially, and progress towards the base of the mucosa. At the stage of super-ficial chronic gastritis, the necks of the glands appear lengthened because there has been de-struction of the specialised cells in the superficial part of the glands, and replacement by mucus-secreting cells of the type which normally line the surface and necks of the glands. As the change extends more deeply into the mucosa, the various grades of atrophic gastritis are produced, and finally, when all or virtually all of the specialised cells have been destroyed, the inflammation subsides, leaving the appearances of gastric atrophy. This unitarian view is supported by the frequent finding of superficial chronic gastritis together with various degrees of atrophic gastritis in other areas of the same stomach, and of all grades of inflammation between severe atrophic gastritis and gastric atrophy.

In the past, many causal factors have been

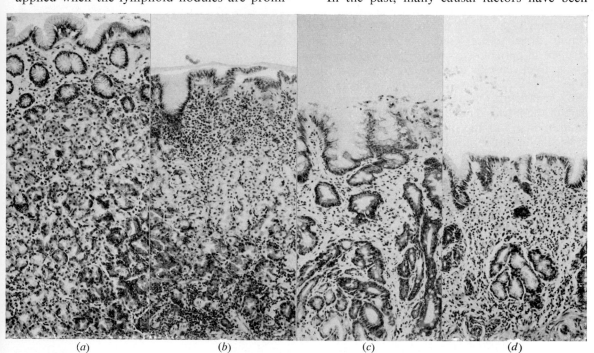

(a)	(b)	(c)	(d)

Fig. 18.23.—Chronic gastritis of acid-secreting mucosa. All × 100.
(a) Normal mucosa.
(b) Superficial gastritis and atrophic gastritis affecting the deep part of the mucosa.
(c) Complete loss of parietal and chief cells with intestinal metaplasia.
(d) Complete atrophic gastritis. The remaining glands are of simple mucus-secreting type.
In (b), (c) and (d), the full thickness of the mucosa is shown.

proposed for chronic gastritis, including dietary indiscretion, stress, oral sepsis, various infections, chronic alcoholism, CVC in heart disease or hepatic cirrhosis, and recurrent acute gastritis. It has, however, become increasingly clear that chronic gastritis of the fundal mucosa is one of the group of organ-specific auto-immune diseases, in which the changes are probably the result of a delayed hypersensitivity reaction against the specialised cells of the target organ. A general description of this group of diseases is provided on pp. 110–12. In the case of chronic gastritis, the evidence may be summarised as follows:

(1) *Auto-antibodies* are commonly present in the serum of patients with chronic gastritis, and their incidence increases with the extent of the gastric mucosal changes. Auto-antibody which reacts with the lipoprotein of the membrane of the endoplasmic reticulum is detectable by immunofluorescence (Fig. 18.24) and by complement-fixation techniques: it is seldom present without chronic gastritis and reaches its highest incidence in patients with severe atrophic gastritis or gastric atrophy. The antibody is present in the serum of over 80 per cent of patients in whom these severe grades of gastritis have resulted in pernicious anaemia. Two auto-antibodies to intrinsic factor, a product of the gastric parietal cells, are also associated with severe chronic gastritis. One of these combines with the part of the intrinsic factor molecule which binds vitamin B_{12}, and the other with a site on the molecule distant from the B_{12}-binding site: they interfere respectively with function of the intrinsic factor-B_{12} complex, and with absorption of the complex from the ileum (p. 421). These antibodies are observed only occasionally apart from pernicious anaemia, in which their combined incidence is rather more than 50 per cent.

(2) *Associated conditions.* The organ-specific auto-immune diseases tend to occur in association with one another (p. 111), and the common association of various grades of chronic thyroiditis and thyrotoxicosis with chronic gastritis supports the auto-immune nature of the latter. Moreover, the rarer members of the group—primary adrenocortical atrophy, and primary hypoparathyroidism—are frequently accompanied by chronic gastritis.

(3) *Familial tendency.* Like the other auto-immune diseases, chronic gastritis shows a familial tendency, and chronic thyroiditis commonly occurs in members of the same families.

(4) *Age and sex.* Like chronic thyroiditis, chronic gastritis occurs mostly in the middle-aged and elderly, and in women more often than men; the female sex preponderance is not, however, nearly so marked as in chronic thyroiditis or thyrotoxicosis.

(5) *Experimental chronic gastritis.* Attempts to induce chronic gastritis in animals by administering immunising injections of gastric mucosal

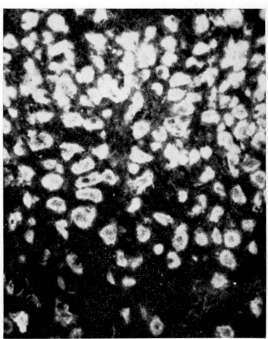

Fig. 18.24.—Indirect immunofluorescence test for parietal-cell antibody. The parietal cells fluoresce brightly, indicating the presence of the antibody in the serum being tested.

preparations together with Freund's adjuvant have given equivocal results. Recently, however, its induction has been reported in monkeys, together with the development of delayed hypersensitivity and antibodies reactive specifically with gastric parietal cells.

The mechanism of the production of the changes in chronic gastritis has not been fully established. In general, auto-antibodies do not appear to play a major pathogenic role in the organ-specific auto-immune diseases, and even severe chronic gastritis is not invariably associated with the presence of circulating auto-antibodies. It is more likely that a delayed hypersensitivity reaction against the specialised gastric glandular cells is largely responsible for the destructive changes, although the auto-antibodies might have a supplementary effect. Auto-antibodies to intrinsic factor may also contribute towards the failure of absorption of B_{12} in pernicious anaemia. These antibodies have been demonstrated in the gastric juice of patients with this condition, and it is likely that their presence there prevents absorption of any intrinsic factor produced by the atrophic mucosa.

Physiological disturbances. The degree to which the specialised gastric glands are lost or replaced in chronic gastritis correlates relatively well with the functional results observed clinically. Thus in superficial gastritis there is little functional upset; with progressing glandular atrophy varying degrees of hypochlorhydria develop, culminating eventually in complete achlorhydria as seen in severe atrophic gastritis. Even at this latter stage, some intrinsic factor is still secreted since megaloblastic anaemia is rarely observed. In the simple gastric atrophy of pernicious anaemia, there is, however, complete achylia with failure to secrete hydrochloric acid, pepsin and intrinsic factor.

The gastric antral mucosa

Chronic inflammation of the antral mucosa is a common condition, but apart from its occurrence locally around a gastric ulcer, the causal factors are unknown. There is no evidence that it is of auto-immune nature, nor is it known whether it tends to occur in association with chronic gastritis of the fundal mucosa. As in the latter condition, the changes may be superficial or extend throughout the thickness of the mucosa, and they consist of atrophic changes in the glands and chronic inflammatory infiltration of the lamina propria.

Although the incidence of *gastric carcinoma* is increased in chronic gastritis of the fundal mucosa, the increase is a small one, and most gastric cancers probably originate in the antral mucosa. It is not known with certainty whether chronic gastritis of the antrum predisposes to carcinoma.

Finally, the condition known as *linitis plastica* may be mentioned. In this disorder there is more or less generalised fibrosis, with thickening and stiffening of the stomach wall resulting in what has been called "leather-bottle stomach". In our experience, this is invariably due to a diffuse scirrhous gastric carcinoma (p. 500).

Action of corrosive poisons

The more powerful corrosives produce much necrosis of tissue, three types of change resulting from their action.

(A) Mineral acids cause extensive destruction of the stomach wall often with much haemorrhage and sometimes actual perforation. Sulphuric acid is specially destructive; some of the parts may be almost black or charred, whilst in less affected parts extravasated blood, variously altered, is present. Perforation is common and the effects of diffusion of the acid into neighbouring parts are then evident. The action of hydrochloric acid is less intense; haemorrhage may be marked and widespread, or necrotic areas of paler colour may be present. Nitric acid usually causes a brownish-yellow or greenish discolouration owing to the formation of xanthoprotein.

(B) The second type of action is extensive necrosis with softening of the tissues, and is seen in the case of the caustic alkalis. Portions of the stomach wall may be changed into soft necrotic gelatinous material; here also perforation may occur.

(C) The third type of action is coagulation of the tissue proteins, by which the lining of the stomach becomes fixed, and the cellular structure may be preserved. This is well seen in carbolic acid poisoning, where the greyish mucosa has a stiff corrugated appearance, and it is a well-marked feature in poisoning by corrosive sublimate or by a strong solution of zinc chloride.

A large number of poisons of less intense action produce chiefly inflammatory changes accompanied by a varying amount of haemorrhage, superficial necrosis or membranous exudate. To this group belong weaker acids, such as oxalic acid or acetic acid, also various metallic salts. Arsenic (arsenious acid) causes an intense inflammation with white patches of tenacious mucus or exudate in which grains of the poison may still be present. Antimony causes a general acute inflammation, while in phosphorus poisoning there are usually haemorrhages and fatty degeneration in the mucosa. For details, however, special works on toxicology must be consulted.

Specific infections

These are comparatively rare in the stomach as compared with the bowel, largely because most spore-free organisms are killed by the action of the gastric juice. Small *typhoid* ulcers arising in the lymphoid tissue have occasionally been observed, but they are very rare. Primary *anthrax* lesions produced by swallowing the spores have occasionally been observed.

Tuberculous ulcers are relatively uncommon; they are seen especially in children with pulmonary cavities. The ulcers are usually superficial and small, and their mode of formation and general features correspond with those of tuberculous ulcers of the intestines. They are apparently the result of swallowing bacilli, but some writers suppose that they may be of haematogenous origin. *Syphilitic lesions*, though rare, occur both in the congenital and acquired forms of the disease. In the latter, the lesion starts in the submucosa in the form of a diffuse infiltration or gummatous mass, and secondary ulceration may follow. The lesion may sometimes reach a considerable size and may simulate carcinoma; sometimes haematemesis with achlorhydria may be produced. Treponemata have been found in such lesions, so that there is no doubt as to their nature. The histological changes correspond with those of syphilitic lesions elsewhere.

Peptic ulcer

Stomach

By far the most important type of ulceration found in the stomach is peptic ulceration, in which the action of gastric juice is primarily concerned. It is often referred to simply as *gastric ulcer*. Peptic ulceration is encountered, however, not only in the stomach but also in other parts of the alimentary tract exposed to gastric juice: it is especially common in the first part of the duodenum and is occasionally found in the lower part of the oesophagus. It is also seen in relation to heterotopic gastric mucosa, e.g. in a Meckel's diverticulum (p. 537) or at the umbilicus. Furthermore, in cases where gastro-jejunostomy has been performed, peptic ulceration may take place in the part of the jejunal walls exposed to the action of gastric juice, especially when this is of high acidity. Apart from these circumstances, however, peptic ulceration distal to the duodenal bulb is rare.

Incidence. The incidence of the different types of peptic ulcer has changed considerably since the beginning of the century. Before that time the prevalent type was the acute perforating ulcer (Fig. 18.31) which was usually found in the anterior wall of the pylorus or duodenum and predominantly affected young women; it was frequently associated with a disease called "chlorosis", a form of anaemia which has long since disappeared. After World War I gastric ulcer became much commoner in men and to a lesser extent in older women. At the present time, gastric ulcer is more common in men than in women at all ages up to 65, but thereafter the sex difference becomes less marked: on the other hand duodenal ulceration, which became more frequent at about the same time, is much commoner in men in all age groups and is between 4 and 10 times as common as gastric ulcer in the general population. Gastric ulcer was formerly considered to be a disease of the lower income groups, but it is doubtful if this is now the case, and duodenal ulcer had never shown any social differentiation. Both types of ulceration show a familial incidence.

Naked-eye appearances. Three main types of peptic ulcer are recognised, namely acute, subacute and chronic. Any such classification, however, is to some extent artificial since intermediate varieties occur.

(*a*) *Acute peptic ulcer.* This type involves only the mucosa and submucosa in the ulcerative process (Fig. 18.25); it is usually small, but may

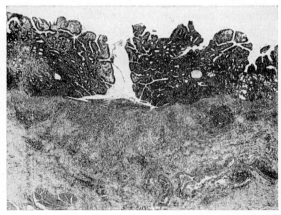

Fig. 18.25.—Acute peptic ulcer.

A small acute peptic ulcer is seen to penetrate through the mucosa to the submucous layer. × 12.

occasionally reach 1–2 cm. diameter. The ulcers may be single, or may occour in large numbers and, unlike chronic ulcers, have a wide distribution. They rarely produce symptoms other than haemorrhage, which on occasion may be severe when a mucosal artery in the base of an acute ulcer is eroded (Fig. 18.32). This type of ulcer usually heals without a visible scar.

(*b*) *Subacute peptic ulcers* are usually fewer in number than the acute type, and not infrequently single. They extend down to the muscular coat the superficial part of which may be involved; like chronic ulcers, they tend to be found on the lesser curvature of the stomach and they may represent a transition from the acute to the chronic type.

(*c*) *Chronic peptic ulcer*. Complete penetration of the muscular coat is regarded as the most important criterion of chronicity in a peptic ulcer. (Figs 18.28, 18.29). This type of ulcer is usually solitary; two opposed peptic ulcers are found in a small proportion of cases and there are practically never more than two in the stomach although there may be a duodenal ulcer as well. The commonest site in the stomach is the lesser curvature between 5 and 10 cm. from the pylorus; the pyloric canal is the next most frequent site. Their occurrence in other sites is rare, and should make one look for some unusual cause.

Chronic ulcers reach a greater size than any of the preceding types; the largest tend to be ovoid (Fig. 18.26), and may measure 5 cm. or more in diameter. The base of the ulcer may be formed by the outer part of the stomach wall, the floor being usually smooth and fibrous with induration of the surrounding tissues. More frequently, however, fibrous adhesions have de-

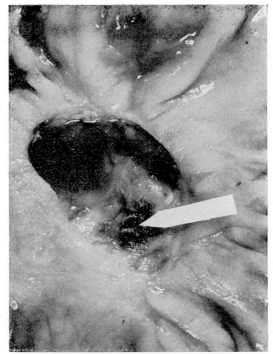

Fig. 18.26.—A large chronic gastric ulcer, showing an eroded artery (arrow) from which fatal haemorrhage occurred. × 1·25.

veloped over the ulcer and the base is firmly fixed; large ulcers may have completely penetrated the wall and extended into adjacent structures, usually the pancreas or liver. When this extreme stage has been reached, the

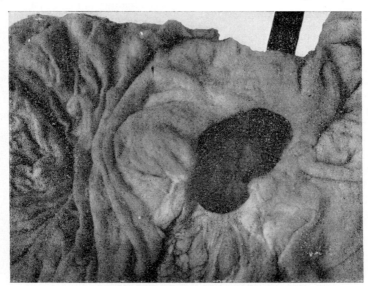

FIG. 18.27.—Large chronic ulcer of duodenum just beyond the pylorus. × ⅘.
The ulcer had perforated at the margin, as indicated by the pointer.

ulcer margin is smooth with overhanging edges, the crater is deep and the floor is firm and nodular, being formed by a fibrosed layer of the adherent viscus. Occasionally an ulcer may burrow into the large bowel, a gastro-colic fistula resulting. Perforation in the chronic type is prevented by fibrous thickening and adhesions but, in about a third of cases, occurs obliquely through one margin of the ulcer beneath the overhanging edge and beyond the adhesions (Fig. 18.27). Occasionally, the actual rupture has been produced mechanically, for example by stretching the body when the stomach is distended with food. Erosion of a large artery in the floor of a chronic ulcer is not uncommon and may lead to a fatal haemorrhage.

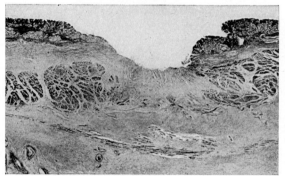

FIG. 18.28.—Early chronic gastric ulcer, showing fibrotic replacement of muscular coat. (J. S. F. N.) × 7.

Duodenum

Peptic ulcers in the duodenum are similar to those in the stomach. The area affected by peptic ulceration is, however, remarkably restricted; over 99 per cent of chronic ulcers arise within the first centimetre of the duodenum.

Acute ulcers may be single or multiple. They tend to be encountered in what might be regarded as "stressful" situations. They are seen, for example, in patients with extensive burns, especially infants, and as a complication of lesions of the central nervous system or chronic debilitating disease both in adults and children.

Chronic ulcers may be as large as those in the stomach (Fig. 18.27), and those arising in the posterior wall of the duodenum tend to be larger than those in the anterior aspect. As a rule there is a single ulcer on the anterior or posterior wall, but in about 15 per cent of cases two ulcers are present, and they may oppose one

another at a corresponding level ("kissing ulcers"). Severe haemorrhage usually occurs from ulcers on the posterior wall, which tend to erode the gastro-duodenal artery.

Microscopic appearances. Active peptic ulcers show relatively little exudate, little more than some necrotic material on the floor and at the margins, as the digestive action of the gastric juice quickly destroys any exudate present. In the severed ends of the muscular coats, leukocytic infiltration with eosinophils is seen but the ulcer generally has a clean-cut appearance.

In the chronic stage, the ulcer crater is lined by a thin zone of fibrinoid necrosis, beneath which is a layer of granulation tissue showing some leukocytic infiltration. The muscular coat is completely severed and replaced by fibrous tissue which at the margin spreads around to form adhesions to adjacent structures. The muscle coat thus ends high up in the lateral walls of the crater (Fig. 18.29). In the floor, obliterative changes are frequently seen in the arteries (Fig. 13.2, p. 263). At the margin of the ulcer, the mucosal epithelium may show active regenerative changes; fragments of mucosa may also be "buried" in fibrous tissue during the ulcerative process, and give a false impression of malignant change (see p. 496).

Results and complications

(1) **Healing and cicatrisation.** The acute peptic ulcers usually undergo healing and leave no visible scar. Healing is the rule also in the subacute type and it is common too in the chronic type, even if the ulcer is of considerable size, as is shown by the presence of scars and contractions. If the ulcer has been superficial, the scar

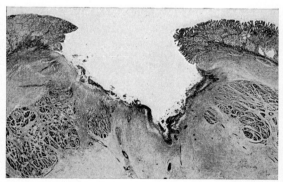

FIG. 18.29.—Chronic gastric ulcer at later stage, showing breach of muscular coat. × 7.

may be merely a small depression with a smooth whitish surface; if, however, it has penetrated more deeply, there is often a radiating indrawing of the surrounding mucous membrane, so that a stellate appearance results (Fig. 18.30). The healing of an ulcer at the pylorus often leads to *stenosis* of the opening owing to the cicatricial contraction, and considerable dilatation of the stomach may follow. The muscle of the pylorus is apt to be thickened and oedematous, and the appearance may suggest scirrhous carcinoma; only microscopic examination can determine

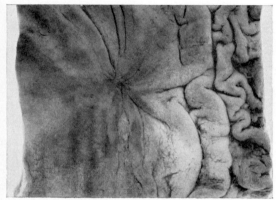

FIG. 18.30.—Healed gastric ulcer with stellate cicatrix. × 1.

the true nature of such a condition. Pyloric stenosis can result from chronic peptic ulceration of either the pyloric antrum or duodenal bulb. This is more likely to happen with ulcers on the posterior wall which tend to be larger. Duodenal stenosis may occasionally occur at a lower level in a similar way.

The healing of an ulcer in the lesser curvature may be accompanied by much fibrous overgrowth both on the anterior and posterior walls, and contraction of the tissue may on rare occasions produce a narrowing of the stomach about its middle—the so-called *hour-glass* deformity. The similar deformity seen most commonly in radiographs is usually attributable to muscle spasm and not scarring.

(2) Perforation. Perforation may occur, and, if rapid, it allows the stomach contents to escape into the general peritoneal cavity or, posteriorly, into the lesser sac. The pain, abdominal rigidity, and symptoms of collapse which follow are caused by the acid gastric contents; these are virtually sterile at first, but organisms soon flourish and acute peritonitis results. The entry

of gas from the stomach causes the liver to separate from the diaphragm, causing loss of liver dullness clinically. After successful surgical treatment of the perforation, there is a risk that infected material lodged between the liver and diaphragm may become sealed off by fibrinous exudate and that consequently a collection of pus—sub-phrenic abscess—may form and may later infect the pleura. In other cases infection of the peritoneum may occur without actual perforation, and thus the peritoneal surface may be glued to adjacent parts by fibrinous exudate. This is more likely to happen posteriorly and in the region of the lesser curvature, where the movements of the stomach are less than in other parts. The inflammation may produce localised fibrous adhesions or rarely localised suppuration may result. Rarely, bacterial invasion of a portal tributary may occur and secondary abscesses be produced in the liver (p. 573). The so-called *acute perforating ulcer*, formerly common but not often seen now, is usually single and situated in the anterior wall of the pylorus or duodenum. They are of 1·5 cm. diameter or

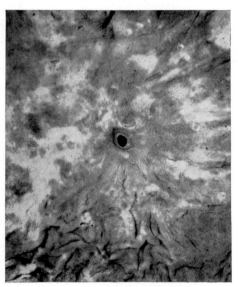

FIG. 18.31.—Acute perforating ulcer. × 1.

less, round or ovoid with a punched-out appearance and a terraced margin (Fig. 18.31), the mucosa being ulcerated over a greater area than the muscle layer. These ulcers are probably subacute, but rapid extension through the deep layers of the gut wall, results in perforation.

(3) Haemorrhage. This is common and varies greatly in degree. Often there is oozing of blood either from an acute or a chronic ulcer. The blood may be scanty and detectable in the stools only by chemical examination, or it may be abundant. The blood may be in considerable quantity and give rise to "coffee-grounds" vomit, or to "tarry" stools. Sometimes an artery of considerable size may be eroded and a large, even fatal, haemorrhage take place. This may

chronic peptic ulcer which has undergone malignant change and a carcinoma which has ulcerated. In the former case, it is necessary to demonstrate clear evidence of pre-existing chronic peptic ulceration, i.e. complete interruption of the muscular coat (Fig. 18.33).

The cancer begins at one margin of the ulcer crater (Figs. 18.33, 18.34) and tends to encircle it, spreading outwards into the submucosa and muscular coat, but not invading the fibrous ulcer

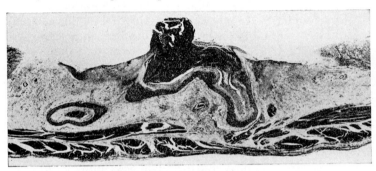

Fig. 18.32.—Superficial acute ulcer of stomach which has eroded an artery and caused fatal haemorrhage. × 10.

occur from a recent acute ulcer (Fig. 18.32) but is seen chiefly in large chronic ulcers which involve an artery lying outside the wall of the stomach, e.g. the gastro-duodenal artery. The artery becomes incorporated in the floor of the ulcer, and is in most cases obliterated by endarteritis (Fig. 13.2, p. 263), but sometimes this does not happen, and the wall of the vessel, weakened by the digestive process, ruptures. Occasionally a small aneurysm forms first. Usually, however, the artery is eroded rather than severed and its wall is so firmly incorporated in the scar tissue that contraction and retraction of the vessel cannot take place to control the bleeding, which ceases only when the blood pressure has fallen and thrombus has formed at the site of erosion. For these reasons, resuscitation by transfusion should be attempted with due care not to raise the blood pressure too rapidly lest further bleeding be encouraged. Severe haemorrhage from duodenal ulcer is commonest when the ulcer is in the posterior wall. In a case of fatal haemorrhage one can usually find the eroded artery in the floor of the ulcer, its mouth partially occluded by thrombus.

(4) Development of carcinoma: ulcer-cancer. Although it cannot be doubted that carcinoma may arise in a chronic gastric ulcer, the frequency of this event has probably been overestimated in the past. One reason for this lies in the difficulty in distinguishing between a

floor to any extent. On the other hand, a primary carcinoma often invades the muscular coat but practically never destroys it entirely and even in advanced cases remains of muscle are to be found between cancer cells. Another important point is that irregular growth and displacement of epithelium at the margin of a peptic ulcer may give a false impression of malignant change.

Taking these factors into consideration, it is unlikely that cancer develops in more than one per cent of chronic gastric ulcers, although it is probable that there is an increased tendency for carcinoma to develop in a stomach bearing a chronic peptic ulcer. Carcinomatous change does not arise in chronic duodenal ulcers.

Etiology

Although it is convenient to discuss the causes of peptic ulceration in general, in many respects such as age and sex distribution, occupational incidence and familial tendency, chronic gastric and duodenal ulcers tend to behave as different diseases and the causes may differ. It may also be necessary to distinguish between acute and chronic ulcers in this respect. In any case, no single factor is clearly responsible and a multiplicity of causes is implicated.

The possible importance of genetic factors in

the pathogenesis is reflected in the familial incidence of the disease referred to on p. 492, and in the relationship between duodenal ulcer and individuals who do not secrete blood-group substances into the gastric juice and belong to blood group O. Environmental factors, however, must be of comparable, if not greater, significance to account for the varying incidence of peptic ulcer during this century and for "epidemics" of the disease which may be localised or affect certain age groups in the community.

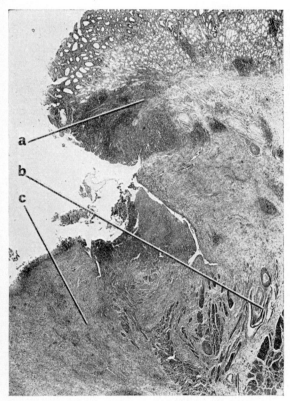

FIG. 18.33.—Ulcer-cancer of stomach. A chronic peptic ulcer showing the characteristic complete breach of the muscle coat. A focus of early carcinoma is seen in the overhanging margin of the near crater.

(*a*) = carcinoma, (*b*) = muscle coat and (*c*) = fibrous base.

Geographical variations in incidence also emphasise the importance of environment. Peptic ulcer is essentially a disease of developed, industrialised communities, although it must be admitted that the reason for this is obscure. Factors such as dietary habits, the ingestion of drugs (especially aspirin) and the "stress" associated with sedentary occupations or social status might, however, be of importance in this context. Cigarette smoking is also a contributory factor, especially in gastric ulcer, and may account for the association between peptic ulcer and chronic bronchitis.

The only entirely consistent finding associated with peptic ulceration is the presence of gastric acid, which is undoubtedly responsible for the special features of this disease. Peptic ulcer does not develop in patients with histamine-fast achlorhydria. The nature of the initial lesion and the cause of its progressive tendency are, however, not understood. The existence of a local lesion in itself is insufficient to explain this process, since wounds heal rapidly in the normal stomach. Local vascular disturbances have been postulated in the genesis of the initial lesion, but there is no evidence that embolism or thrombosis of the gastric vessels are responsible. The anatomy of the blood supply to the gastric mucosa is, however, consistent with the possibility that arterial spasm, or irregular contraction of the gastric musculature interfering with the local blood supply, may be concerned.

It is difficult to accept that the chronic peptic ulcer, which is usually solitary, is always the sole survivor of the multiple acute ulcers sometimes seen in infective or septic conditions. Nevertheless, it is clear that peptic ulceration is caused by interference with the capacity of the gastrointestinal mucosa to resist digestion by gastric acid, due either to impaired mucosal resistance or to hypersecretion of gastric juice, or possibly both. The nature of the mucosal defence mechanism is complex and depends among other things upon the secretion of mucus, the maintenance of normal epithelial cell turnover rates and the presence of inhibitors of gastric secretion. Interference with these factors appears to be of particular importance in the pathogenesis of gastric ulcer. In this disease, gastric secretion may be normal but is often reduced due to the presence of chronic gastritis. Indeed there is some evidence to suggest that gastric ulcers tend to develop during certain phases in the evolution of chronic gastritis, which impairs the defensive capacity of the mucosa. The ingestion of drugs, such as aspirin, which interfere with epithelial cell turnover, might also be of importance in the causation of gastric ulcer.

By contrast, gastric hypersecretion appears to be of major significance in the pathogenesis of duodenal ulcer, and there is a tendency for affected individuals to have an increased parietal-cell mass. The cause of this hypersecretion, which is often nocturnal, is not entirely clear. It is probably mediated by vagal stimulation, and it is of interest in this context that emotional disturbances and "stress" have been invoked as causes of exacerbation of peptic ulcer symptoms, and a "psychological type" of individual has been described in relation to peptic ulceration. Furthermore, acute peptic ulcer not infrequently accompanies lesions of the central nervous system.

Dilatation of the stomach

This occurs in two forms, namely dilatation due to obstruction and dilatation without obstruction. The first results from either scarring due to gastric or duodenal ulcer, carcinoma of the scirrhous type at the pylorus or occasionally from fibrous adhesions outside the stomach at the pyloric region. A degree of congenital stenosis of the pylorus (p. 503) may produce a

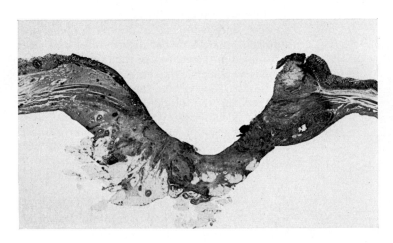

Fig. 18.34.—Ulcer-cancer of stomach. Carcinoma has arisen in the margin of the ulcer on the right, which now has become raised up above the level of the mucosa. × 2.

Although the extent to which humoral stimulants of gastric secretion contribute to the pathogenesis of peptic ulcer in general is uncertain, there is no doubt that the circulation of such substances in excessive quantities is capable of invoking a fulminating ulcer diathesis. Such a situation is observed in the Zollinger–Ellison syndrome (p. 601) the central feature of which is the development of single or multiple pancreatic islet cell tumours which secrete gastrin, a polypeptide and potent stimulant of gastric secretion. These pancreatic tumours may be associated with tumours of other endocrine glands such as the parathyroids, pituitary, adrenals etc. (the multiple endocrine adenoma syndrome) and it has been suggested that this represents a widespread disturbance of polypeptide hormone synthesis. In these syndromes, peptic ulceration takes place not only in the common sites but also in unusual areas e.g. the greater curvature of the stomach and distal duodenum. There is evidence that a raised level of blood calcium promotes an increase in gastric secretion, and this may account for the high incidence of peptic ulceration in patients with hyperparathyroidism.

similar result. In these conditions, dilatation is associated with hypertrophy of the gastric musculature which, owing to the dilatation, often appears less than it actually is.

In the second form a number of factors may be concerned, such as inflammatory change, atony of the muscle and fermentative changes. Any one of these may lead to the others; thus deficiency of gastric juice due to gastritis may lead to abnormal retention of food in the stomach allowing fermentation to take place, and atony of the muscle will have a similar result. Atonic dilatation, which may be a chronic condition, occurs after acute fevers and may also be associated with neurasthenia or hysteria. Under such circumstances the stomach may reach an enormous size and become displaced downwards in the abdominal cavity—*gastroptosis*. The duodenum may become kinked and share in this atonic, dilated state.

A well-recognised form—*acute dilatation of the stomach*—occasionally occurs after abdominal operations; in the absence of sepsis, excessive handling or trauma is probably the cause (cf. paralytic ileus, p. 528). It may also be a feature of diabetic coma and may be relieved by intubation.

In chronic dilatation, the contents of the stomach may show an abundant growth of yeasts, sarcinae, hyphomycetes, etc., leading to fermentation, with the formation of lactic and butyric acids and considerable evolution of gas. There is little growth of bacteria unless there is marked reduction or absence of hydrochloric acid such as is common in cases of carcinoma.

Tumours

Benign tumours

These are rare, the commonest being the *simple polyploid adenoma* or *papilloma* which is most frequently found in the pyloric region. These tumours, composed mainly of mucus-secreting glands with a variable amount of stroma, may have a smooth surface or be covered by papilliform processes. They may be either sessile or pedunculated and are multiple in about one-third of cases. Malignant change frequently supervenes, especially in the larger tumours.

Of the *non-epithelial* tumours, leiomyoma is the most frequent. Although usually small, a leiomyoma may show a characteristic type of clean punched-out ulceration and can produce very brisk bleeding; sometimes it becomes large, and may undergo sarcomatous change with metastasis. Lipoma, fibroma and neuro-fibroma associated with generalised neuro-fibromatosis, and a glomus tumour (p. 251) may also occur.

Gastric carcinoma

Carcinoma is by far the most important tumour in the stomach, both numerically and clinically, and is also one of the commonest malignant tumours in man. There is considerable geographical variation in the incidence of gastric carcinoma, which has shown a slight tendency to become less frequent in this country in recent years. It still, however, remains the commonest malignant tumour in many countries, with a particularly high incidence in Iceland, Finland and Japan. Men are affected more often than women in the ratio of 2 : 1, and the disease is commoner in the poorer economic groups.

R

Men and women exhibit the same gradient of susceptibility in all classes; the maximum incidence is between 50 and 70 years of age.

Etiology. No specific cause for the development of carcinoma has been identified but certain predisposing factors are recognised. Certain families have an unusually high incidence of gastric cancer and *hereditary* influences may be involved in a proportion of cases, perhaps indirectly, as in the association with pernicious anaemia. It has been claimed that in Great Britain people of blood group A show a significantly higher incidence of gastric cancer than those of other blood groups, in contrast to the reputed high incidence of peptic ulcer in those of group O. The virtual absence of gastric cancer in lower animals suggests that some peculiarly human *environmental* factors are of importance, e.g. the cooking of food. There is as yet no well-defined clue as to the possible causal agents but the repeated heating of fats to temperatures used in cooking may lead to the formation of potent carcinogenic or co-carcinogenic agents. The constituents of the soil and the extent of background radiation have been investigated to explain geographical variations in incidence but nothing substantial has emerged; the presence of chromium in soil has been suggested as of possible importance in this respect.

Precancerous lesions. Of *local gastric factors*, the importance of *gastric ulcer* has already been discussed (p. 496). Reference has also been made to the development of carcinoma in *simple adenomatous polyps*, but only a small percentage of malignant tumours appear to arise in these ways (see above). There remains the possible relationship of *chronic gastritis* to carcinoma. Certainly the two lesions co-exist in a high percentage of cases and there is a notable degradation of cell type and replacement of the superficial mucosa by cells of intestinal type, especially in the pyloric antrum. The etiological relationship remains unsettled. The incidence of gastric carcinoma in patients with pernicious anaemia adequately maintained on vitamin B_{12} is about three times that in the general population in a comparable age group.

Macroscopic appearances. The pylorus and the pyloric antrum are the most common sites of carcinoma (85 per cent) which thus differs in distribution from gastric ulcer. Further, carcinoma may occur in any part of the stomach while 94 per cent of gastric ulcers are restricted to the vicinity of the lesser curvature.

Five main types of gastric carcinoma are recognised.

Fungating carcinoma not infrequently arises in the fundus of the stomach and growth is directed mainly towards the lumen to form large friable masses which readily undergo necrosis and ulceration. The gastric wall, is, however, eventually penetrated and spread to adjacent structures takes place.

Scirrhous carcinoma is commonest in the pyloric region, and is characterised by deep infiltration of the gastric wall with marked induration but without obvious protrusion into the lumen. Ulceration is frequent (Fig. 18.35) and despite extensive invasion by cancer cells the muscularis is not wholly destroyed in the base in contrast to the findings in a chronic peptic ulcer. Confusion between the two may, however, occasionally arise. The surrounding muscle is often thickened and hypertrophied and the growth frequently encircles the pylorus, causing stenosis. Extension into the duodenal mucosa is very rare.

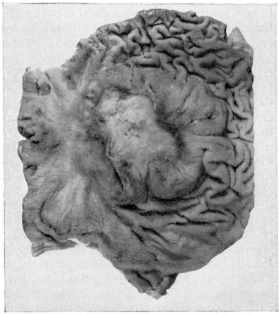

FIG. 18.35.—Carcinoma of stomach, with thick cellular margin and ulcerated base.

Mucoid cancer, like the scirrhous type, usually arises in the pyloric region and is characterised by a diffuse mode of spread and by involvement of the peritoneum. The first leads to marked thickening of the gastric wall (Fig. 18.36) which

has thus a translucent appearance, and the second to enormous growths in the peritoneal cavity in which the organs are embedded in masses of translucent, gelatinous material.

A less common fourth type is recognised,

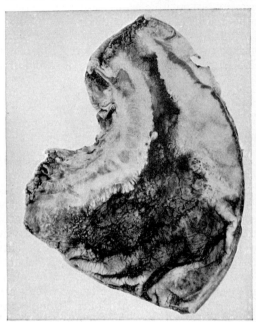

FIG. 18.36.—Mucoid carcinoma at pylorus, showing great infiltration and thickening of the wall (viewed from behind). × ½.

namely *diffuse scirrhous carcinoma* (Fig. 18.37). Growth appears to arise deep in the mucosa and diffuse infiltration of the gastric wall takes place, often without apparent involvement of the mucosal surface. The wall of the stomach is commonly grossly thickened and stiffened (leather-bottle stomach), and extension into the oesophagus proximally is not unusual; more rarely some spread into the duodenum distally may occur.

Superficial spreading carcinoma, which involves only the mucosa and submucosa, is recognised by American authors, particularly in relation to peptic ulcer, but is not well documented in this country.

Spread of gastric carcinoma. Local spread is usually prominent. The muscularis is infiltrated to a varying degree, being most marked in the scirrhous and diffuse types and involvement of the oesophageal and duodenal muscle is not unusual. The duodenal mucosa is rarely invaded, whereas the oesophageal mucosa is often involved in fundal or cardiac growths. The gastric serosa is penetrated at an early stage with direct extension of the growth to surrounding structures such as the greater omentum, lesser omentum, liver, pancreas, spleen, diaphragm and abdominal wall. Invasion of the peritoneum may lead to *transcoelomic spread*. Numerous minute nodules may be scattered throughout the peritoneal cavity and the greater omentum conspicuously infiltrated and drawn up. The ovaries

Spread by the portal venous blood also takes place, giving multiple secondaries in the liver in the first instance and ultimately in the lungs. Less frequently other structures such as the brain and the skeleton may be involved.

Microscopic appearances. In the majority of cases the growth is an *adenocarcinoma* with more or less differentiation towards an acinar structure. Some, however, are composed of

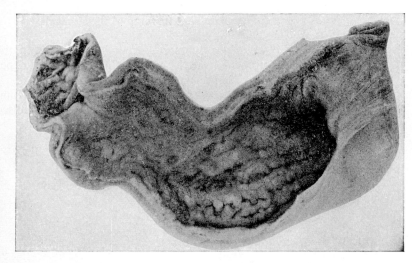

FIG. 18.37.—Diffuse carcinoma of stomach.

Note the general thickening of the wall without the presence of nodular growth and with little ulceration. × ⅔.

are not infrequently involved in this type of spread. If the tumour is of the "signet-ring" cell type with prominent connective tissue reaction, bilateral ovarian metastases are referred to as "Krukenberg tumours" (p. 846).

Lymphatic spread is early and frequent. From the primary focus in the mucosa, the growth spreads to the wide network of submucosal lymphatics (Fig. 18.38) and through the muscularis to the serosal lymphatics and thence to the para-gastric lymph nodes which are usually the first to be involved. Extension may take place into the mucosa from the submucosal lymphatics to form numerous nodules, giving the impression of multiple foci of origin in the stomach. There may be widespread injection of the lymphatic system, involvement of the lymph nodes in the lesser omentum is common, and extension to nodes is occasionally the first sign of disease. Gastric cancer of the diffuse scirrhous (leather-bottle) type may give rise to extensive lymphatic spread in the omentum, mesentery and bowel wall without producing recognisable nodular growth; secondary involvement of the liver is, however, exceedingly rare in this type in contrast to its great frequency in other varieties.

solid masses of anaplastic cells. Mixed patterns are, however, observed in both scirrhous and fungating tumours. In the mucoid type, the cells are bathed in extracellular mucin. In the diffuse leather-bottle type the cells often occur singly or in small groups throughout the thickness of the gastric wall. When there is a marked connective tissue reaction the cancer cells are small and difficult to recognise. At least some of the cells are however "signet-ring" cells (Fig. 18.39) in which the droplets of mucin confirm their identification as cancer cells. The possibility that a diffuse non-neoplastic fibrosis of the gastric wall may occur cannot be excluded but this must be excessively rare.

Associated conditions. Achlorhydria or varying degrees of hypochlorhydria are present in most cases of gastric carcinoma. The hydrochloric acid may be absent when the growth is very small, this being attributed to chronic gastritis which is invariably associated with carcinoma. When carcinoma has developed secondarily to chronic gastric ulcer, hydrochloric acid is likely to be present but may be in reduced amount.

The absence of hydrochloric acid, aided by

stasis due to pyloric stenosis and infection of necrotic tumour tissue, leads to the growth of micro-organisms of various kinds—torulae, sarcinae, lactobacilli, and a large Gram-positive bacillus, the Boas–Oppler bacillus. Bacteria are rarely present unless there is complete achlorhydria. The presence of lactic acid pro-

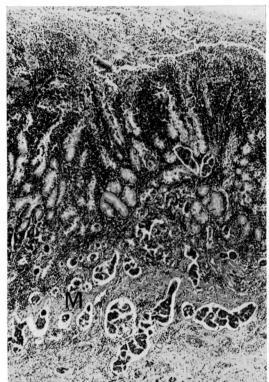

FIG. 18.38.—Stomach wall, showing infiltration of lymphatics by carcinoma cells, which, in places, are growing upwards through the muscularis mucosae (*M*) into the mucosa. Note the severe chronic gastritis. × 30.

duced by micro-organisms in the stomach is suggestive, although not pathognomonic, of gastric cancer.

Secondary bacterial infection of the ulcerating tumour may account, in part, for the *cachexia* and *anaemia* observed clinically in gastric cancer. Anaemia may be either microcytic or normocytic; in the former, blood loss is partly responsible. Macrocytic anaemia is rare, and due to atrophic gastritis, i.e. pernicious anaemia.

Cancer of the stomach is sometimes accompanied by, or even preceded by, the appearance in the skin of multiple warty hyperkeratotic patches, especially about the folds or flexures. This has been named *acanthosis nigricans*. It is

unlikely that this association is purely fortuitous, but the reason for it is obscure.

Finally, mention must be made of the use of exfoliative cytology in the diagnosis of gastric cancer. Although malignant cells are shed into the lumen of the stomach from gastric tumours, the diagnostic value of this phenomenon has proved rather disappointing.

Other malignant tumours of the stomach

Various types of sarcoma may arise in the stomach, but these constitute only about 5 per cent of malignant neoplasms of the stomach.

Leiomyosarcoma (p. 249) is perhaps the commonest of these. It tends to be more localised

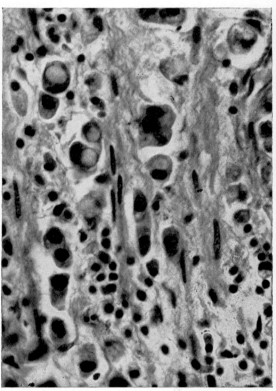

FIG. 18.39.—Diffuse type of carcinoma in muscular coat of stomach. × 600.

Note that the cells are irregularly scattered, some containing mucous globules and others showing atrophic change.

than carcinoma and usually takes the form of a fungating, projecting mass of considerable size. Ulceration and necrosis are common.

Lymphosarcoma may give rise to a localised mass or to a more diffuse infiltrative growth, causing enormous thickening of the whole gastric wall. Lymphosarcoma, when localised to the stomach, may have a relatively good prognosis, if adequate surgical resection is carried out.

Congenital abnormalities

The most important of these is stenosis of the pylorus. It is not uncommon, symptoms appearing usually about two to three weeks after birth, and by obstruction and persistent vomiting may lead to death. The condition is often satisfactorily treated by operation. The obstruction is due to thickening of the wall at the pylorus, and this may extend back over a considerable distance, gradually fading off; or it may be more localised and in the form of a definite band (Fig. 18.40). The thickening is essentially due to hypertrophy of the muscle, the circular fibres especially being increased, whilst the lumen is narrowed to a varying, sometimes marked, degree. It is usually regarded as a hypertrophy produced by spasmodic contraction at the pylorus; but the nature of the exciting agent or neuro-muscular abnormality is not known. Family studies show that this abnormality is of hereditary nature and is due to the action of a pair of recessive genes. In large families the ratio of affected to non-affected is less than the expected Mendelian ratio of 1 in 4 and Cockayne and Penrose have shown that this modification of the effect of the recessive genes depends on sex and on primogeniture. Congenital pyloric stenosis is six times more frequent in male than in female children and, after the first-born, a child is very much less likely to be affected.

Occasionally some degree of congenital pyloric stenosis may persist into adult life, and if symtoms are produced the condition is liable to be confused with carcinoma.

Diverticula occur in connection with the stomach, either in the pyloric portion or in the region of the fundus, but they are rare. Occasionally the stomach is somewhat narrowed

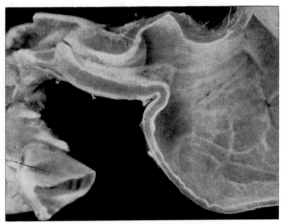

Fig. 18.40.—Congenital stenosis of pylorus. (J. W. S. B.) $\times \frac{5}{4}$.

The anterior wall at the pylorus has been cut away and the greatly hypertrophied muscle at the pyloric antrum is shown.

about the middle, a certain degree of so-called "hour-glass" contraction being produced. Such a condition, however, occurs more frequently as the result of cicatrisation from an old gastric ulcer (p. 495). Persistent vomiting and failure of a neonate to thrive may also be due to congenital deficiency in the enzymes necessary for the metabolism of the sugars, galactose, lactose and sucrose, and these rare conditions may be mistaken for congenital pyloric stenosis.

THE INTESTINES

Introduction

The common and important lesions of the intestines differ from those of the stomach notably in the higher incidence of inflammatory processes, many of which are attributable to the specific effects of known micro-organisms. Although the epidemic and endemic bacterial infections such as typhoid fever, dysentery and cholera have, in this country at any rate, been largely controlled, certain diseases of more ob-

scure etiology, such as ulcerative colitis and the "primary malabsorptive disorders", have assumed greater significance without necessarily becoming more prevalent. Further, the more widespread use of certain operative techniques, drugs and radiotherapy, have introduced a group of factitious or "iatrogenic" intestinal disorders into the community. In the small intestine tumours of clinical significance are surprisingly uncommon; on the other hand, carcinoma of the large bowel is one of the most common malignant neoplasms encountered in Europe and America, both in males and females.

Inflammatory conditions. The pH of the intestinal contents and their high nutritional value provide conditions favourable to the growth of many kinds of bacteria. Not surprisingly, therefore, bacterial infection is the commonest cause of inflammation in the intestinal tract; although viral infection is probably more common than is generally realised, and bacterial toxins e.g. staphylococcal enterotoxin, chemical agents e.g. arsenic, and physical agents e.g. ionising radiation, may also be responsible for inflammatory changes. Damage to the intestine of whatever cause is likely to be exploited by the resident micro-organismal flora, and this must be taken into account in the histological interpretation of inflammatory lesions: thus conditions which are not primarily of an inflammatory origin, e.g. ischaemic lesions, may be confused both grossly and histologically with inflammatory disorders.

As in other organs, inflammatory states in the intestinal tract may be acute or chronic, and vary greatly in severity from a simple "catarrh" at one end of the spectrum to severe necrotising and ulcerative disturbances at the other. In some cases of intestinal inflammation, a single type of micro-organism is the cause of a characteristic lesion. Such conditions are referred to as *specific infections*. In many instances, however, inflammation is *non-specific* in that it can be produced by a number of different micro-organisms or has as yet no identifiable infective cause.

Non-specific Types of Inflammation

Mild forms of acute enteritis, characterised mainly by vomiting and diarrhoea, and probably of viral or toxic origin, are commonly encountered in clinical practice: some of the transient attacks of diarrhoea which frequently complicate visits to foreign localities or countries are probably caused by strains of *Esch. coli* not encountered in one's home environment. The pathological basis for these self-limiting disorders is, however, far from clear, and it is only in more severe and potentially fatal forms of acute enteritis that the pathology (if not the etiology) is known.

Acute gastro-enteritis of infancy. This is an infection that may assume epidemic form in nurseries. In infants under 2 years it carries a high mortality attributable mainly to fluid and electrolyte depletion resulting from diarrhoea and vomiting. Despite this, the pathological changes are seldom impressive—often amounting to no more than areas of mucosal congestion and catarrh in the small bowel—and ulceration is not usually conspicuous. The exact pathogenesis is uncertain, but some serological types of *Escherichia coli*, e.g. types 0111, 055 and 019 are commonly blamed. In fatal cases, the liver usually shows gross fatty change (p. 16).

Membranous forms of enterocolitis. This is a severe condition characterised by the formation of a membrane composed of a fibrinous exudate which incorporates a necrosed layer of the superficial part of the mucosa. The membrane appears first and is most pronounced on the summits of the mucosal folds, and ulceration not infrequently follows. Such an appearance is a common feature of bacillary dysentery due to *S. shigellae* (p. 519) and may rarely occur in cholera (p. 517). It may also be caused by mercuric chloride poisoning. In this country, however, this lesion is encountered more often as a post-operative complication (see below); in association with uraemia and malignant hypertension; in infective states e.g. pneumonia and as a complication of large bowel obstruction ("stercoral" ulceration). The causation is obscure, but it has been suggested that the diffusion of toxic substances or poisons through the mucosa may be of importance in the pathogenesis of the membranous change.

Acute necrotising enterocolitis. This name has been applied to certain severe and often fatal forms of enteritis of uncertain etiology. The small intestine is usually more severely affected, but the colon may be involved, sometimes exclusively. Histologically there is widespread mucosal congestion with patchy necrosis and ulceration associated with haemorrhage and thrombosis of the mucosal and submucosal blood vessels; the mucosal folds may show much irregular deposition of fibrin.

Many cases of necrotising, and in some instances membranous, enterocolitis have followed operative procedures such as partial gastrectomy, although some have complicated medical disorders like myocardial infarction. In the surgical cases the clinical picture is that of severe circulatory collapse, usually with colic and diarrhoea, taking place 5–10 days after operation. In some cases, pre-operative antibiotic therapy is a causal factor by promoting superinfection of the gut with resistant strains of *Staphylococcus aureus; Clostridium welchii* may also be responsible in some cases. Cases also occur in which it is likely that hypoxia of the bowel, possibly related to a hypotensive episode, is responsible. Mesenteric vascular insufficiency may also contribute to this disturbance, since most of the victims are elderly and likely to have degenerative vascular disease.

Certain other necrotising forms of enterocolitis are due to *Clostridium welchii* infection, as in the epidemic disease "darmbrand" described by German workers, and a condition observed in primitive tribes in New Guinea ("pig-bel") due to the ingestion of infected porcine offal. The fatal disease *necrotising jejunitis* found in East African children may also be due to *Cl. welchii* infection.

Phlegmonous enteritis. This rare condition is similar to that described in the stomach (p. 487). It is usually due to the entrance of pathogenic streptococci into the submucosa especially of the caecum and ascending colon. The organisms probably gain access to the submucosa through a superficial lesion and spread widely, causing extensive suppuration and necrosis. The resultant thickening of the bowel may lead to obstructive features. The precipitating causes of this disease are obscure.

Non-specific ulcers of the intestine. Solitary ulcers of a non-specific nature are occasionally encountered both in the small bowel and colon. In most instances the causation is unknown. Recently, however, it has been suggested that administration of enteric-coated tablets of potassium chloride in association with the diuretic chlorothiazide is responsible in some instances.

Regional enteritis (Crohn's disease)

Although this is a relatively uncommon condition it is becoming increasingly recognised as a cause of both small bowel and colonic lesions. Most commonly, however, the terminal part of the ileum is primarily involved.

Clinical features. Young adults of both sexes are most commonly affected, and there is some evidence of familial incidence, although this is not striking. The symptoms are ill-defined at first, mild diarrhoea and vague abdominal pain being the usual complaints. Later signs of subacute or chronic intestinal obstruction develop and necessitate operative intervention. The disease runs a prolonged course, with long remissions, and recurrence after operation occurs in about 50 per cent of cases. Serious consequences can result from repeated and extensive involvement of the small intestine.

Naked-eye appearances. The changes are most often observed in the distal ileum, which is usually involved for a distance of 12 to 20 cm. from the ileo-caecal valve. "Skip lesions" separated from the main lesion by apparently healthy bowel are sometimes found, and distal extension into the caecum and ascending colon is common. The colon may also be involved primarily, especially in the older age groups, and it is probable that many cases of segmental or right-sided forms of colitis, previously classified as cases of ulcerative colitis (p. 507), are examples of Crohn's disease. The lesion is characterised by intensive oedematous thickening of the bowel wall, the submucosa being especially involved, and there is marked narrowing of the lumen (Fig. 18.41). Ulceration of the oedematous mucosa is invariable and often assumes a linear form to produce the typical "cobble-stone" appearance. Fistulae penetrating the entire thickness of the bowel wall, and sometimes involving adjacent organs, are characteristic. The mesentery is usually thickened and oedematous and the regional lymph nodes conspicuously enlarged.

Microscopic appearances. Oedema of all the layers of the bowel wall, but especially of the mucosa, is an early, and always a conspicuous, feature (Fig. 18.42). It is characteristically associated with obstruction and dilatation of lymphatic channels, and it is likely that lymphatic obstruction is of primary importance in the pathogenesis of the disease. Focal lymphocytic infiltration, sometimes with germinal centre formation, is always prominent in the submucosa, but affects all layers and giant-cell systems resembling non-caseating tubercles may develop in these lymphoid aggregates. More often, however, the latter lesions are found in or around lymphatic channels (Fig. 18.43) and may be the initial cause of the lymphatic occlusion. Similar lesions may be found in the mesentery or regional lymph nodes. The mucosal changes, such as ulceration or metaplastic change, and the formation of fistulae, are due principally to secondary infection of the lesions. The affected segments of bowel wall eventually become fibrosed.

tion to the surgical wound and of recurrence of the disease are considerable. Peri-anal fistulae are not uncommon, and are sometimes an early feature of the disease, especially the colonic form, and it is of diagnostic importance that giant-cell systems may be found in these lesions. Hypochromic anaemia due to blood loss is common, and occasionally a macrocytic anaemia

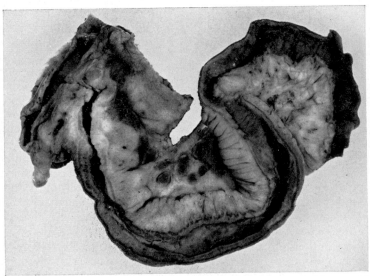

FIG. 18.41.—Regional enteritis, showing diffuse thickening of wall of lower part of ileum with narrowing of its lumen.

Etiology. The cause is unknown. Although the lesions closely resemble ileo-caecal forms of tuberculosis, the two diseases are quite distinct. Even so, it is always necessary to exclude the possibility of tuberculosis by a diligent search for acid-fast bacilli and bacteriological culture of the lesions in any granulomatous disease of the intestinal tract. A relationship to sarcoidosis is suggested by recent reports of positive Kveim tests (p. 153) in patients with regional enteritis, and an inverse relationship in the incidence of tuberculosis (as has been described in sarcoidosis). Sarcoidosis, however, very rarely affects the intestines. Other factors such as the ingestion of irritant substances e.g. silicates, immunological disturbances, and infection by a specific micro-organism, have all been investigated, but their importance remains unproven.

Complications. Intestinal obstruction, initially due to oedema and later to fibrosis of the bowel wall, may ultimately necessitate operative treatment, but the risks of fistula formation in rela-

caused by interference with vitamin B_{12} absorption, which takes place exclusively in the ileum, is encountered. Other features of malabsorption syndrome may develop, especially in diffuse jejuno-ileal forms of the disease (p. 526). As in ulcerative colitis, systemic complications may occur. These include arthritis, uveitis and skin lesions.

Ulcerative colitis

Although no specific cause is known for this common condition it behaves as a distinct clinical and pathological entity, the incidence of which appears to be rising.

Clinical features. The disease mainly affects young adults of both sexes and is characterised by episodes of diarrhoea with the passage of blood per rectum. Constitutional disturbance in varying degrees accompanies these symptoms. Most cases follow a chronic relapsing course with exacerbations and remissions. Some are mild and possibly self-limiting, but a few run a more severe, continuous course and fulminating rapidly fatal forms are by no means rare.

Naked-eye appearances. Ulcerative colitis typically involves the sigmoid colon and rectum (proctitis) either alone or in continuity with the

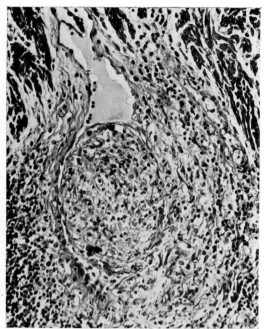

FIG. 18.43.—Regional enteritis, showing a granulomatous lesion occluding a lymphatic in the muscle coat of the ileum. × 200.

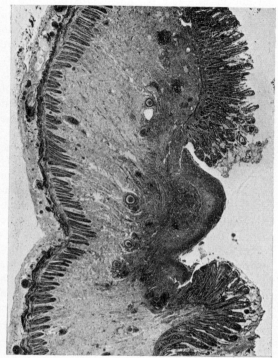

FIG. 18.42.—Regional enteritis showing oedematous thickening of submucosa with focal inflammatory infiltration and ulceration. × 12.

remainder of the colon. The entire colon is affected in about half of the cases, and in such instances the terminal ileum may be involved as a "reflux" phenomenon. Although classically a disease of the distal half of the colon, the proximal colon, with or without the terminal ileum, may be principally affected. It is now recognised, however, that many such "segmental" or "right-sided" forms of colitis are examples of Crohn's disease (p. 505) and others may have an ischaemic origin.

In its early phases, as seen for example through the sigmoidoscope, the colonic mucosa is deeply congested, velvety in appearance and bleeds easily (Fig. 18.44). Punctate erosions herald the onset of ulceration, which usually begins in the rectum or sigmoid and is found initially at the tips of the mucosal folds overlying the longitudinal muscle bands. Later the ulcers coalesce,

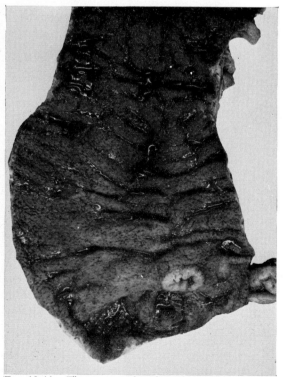

FIG. 18.44.—The caecum in ulcerative colitis. Intense congestion, haemorrhage, and multiple pin-point ulcers of mucosa. The appendicular orifice is shown, and in this case is not affected. × ⅔.

giving rise to large irregular areas of mucosal denudation associated with extensive muco-purulent discharge and haemorrhage. Between the ulcers, especially in chronic cases, the surviving mucosa becomes swollen and hyperplastic (Fig. 18.45) and in some instances numerous polypoid excrescences are seen, a condition known as *pseudo-polyposis*. Attempts at healing take place during remissions, but fibrous thickening and stenosis of the lumen are relatively uncommon. During relapses, the colon is spastic and the early loss of the normal sacculation produces a characteristic radiological appearance.

Microscopic appearances. Unlike Crohn's disease, it is the mucosa which is primarily

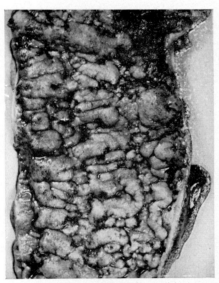

FIG. 18.45.—Ulcerative colitis.

The mucosa is extensively ulcerated and the surviving portions are swollen and hyperplastic with many undermined bridges of mucosa. $\times \frac{4}{5}$.

involved in ulcerative colitis. During active phases it is congested and densely infiltrated with leukocytes, especially plasma cells. The formation of crypt abscesses (Fig. 18.46a), characterised by the accumulation of neutrophils, eosinophils, red cells and mucus within crypt lumina, is a conspicuous feature, although by no means specific for ulcerative colitis. The epithelial lining of the crypts is attenuated and frequently degenerated, and ultimately breaks down, releasing infected material into the lamina propria mucosae. This lesion is a prelude to the appearance of frank ulceration (Fig. 18.46b), which is produced by the coalescence of ruptured

crypt abscesses in the deeper parts of the mucosa. Ulceration seldom extends more deeply than the submucosa and the base is formed by vascular granulation tissue (Fig. 18.46c) containing large numbers of plasma cells and lymphocytes, the latter becoming increasingly conspicuous in chronic cases. The pseudo-polyps observed in chronic cases consist of islands of surviving hyperplastic mucosa and tags of granulation tissue; true polypoid adenomas (p. 533) are rare. Re-epithelialisation of ulcerated areas may take place (Fig. 18.46d) but regeneration is seldom complete. An increase in the number of Paneth cells in the crypts of Lieberkühn is noted especially in the proximal parts of the colon; the significance of this is uncertain.

Complications. Of the local complications, the most urgent is perforation of the colon usually seen in fulminating forms (see above). An association between steroid therapy and perforation has been claimed, but remains unproved. Peri-anal fistulae may be troublesome in some cases. Although simple fibrous strictures are uncommon, it is now recognised that the development of carcinoma of the colon is a considerable risk. It occurs most commonly in cases in which the entire colon is involved, the onset is early in life, and the disease has been present for 10 years or more; the risk is such as to provide an indication for total colectomy in some instances.

Systemic complications are also encountered. In severe cases there is constitutional disturbance with fever and leukocytosis; and debilitating diarrhoea with haemorrhage and exudation leads to protein depletion and anaemia. Arthritis, iridocyclitis and skin lesions, such as erythema nodosum and pyoderma gangrenosum, are seen in a proportion of cases. There appears to be an association between joint disease, especially ankylosing spondylitis, and chronic inflammatory disease of the intestine. Liver disease, of which chronic pericholangitis is the most characteristic and frank cirrhosis the most severe, is not infrequent in ulcerative colitis.

Etiology. The cause of ulcerative colitis remains an unsolved problem. No specific microorganism has been isolated, although it is notable that certain types of colonic infection, especially amoebiasis (p. 520) may closely resemble ulcerative colitis pathologically. A search for *Entamoeba histolytica* and other known pathogens should always be undertaken in suspected cases. The possibility that ulcerative colitis has an immunological basis is gaining increasing acceptance. The finding of antibodies to human colonic epithelium in the serum of patients has not, however, been universally confirmed; and the auto-immune hypothesis of causation must be regarded as speculative at the present time.

Acute appendicitis

This lesion is of the highest importance on account of its frequency and the serious results which often follow. Individuals of either sex and of virtually any age may be affected but the

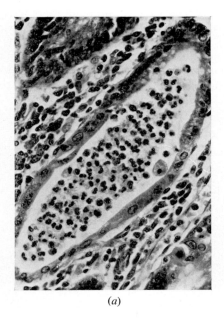

(a)

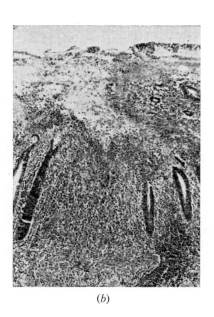

(b)

FIG. 18.46.—Ulcerative colitis.

(a) Crypt abscess. × 350.
(b) Early mucosal ulceration with purulent exudate. × 55.
(c) Chronic stage: complete loss of mucosa on the left, with undermining of surviving mucosa on the right. × 13.
(d) Healing stage showing granulation tissue covered by a simple mucosa. × 115.

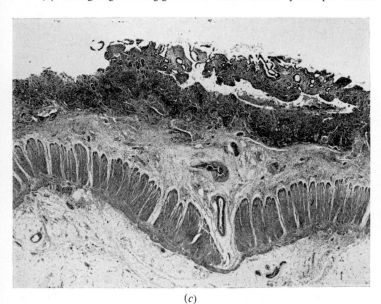

(c)

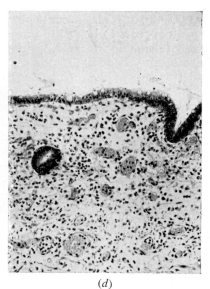

(d)

disease is commonest in children and young adults.

Naked-eye appearances. The condition occurs in three forms: simple acute appendicitis, suppurative or phlegmonous, and gangrenous appendicitis. The first two of these types may be regarded as different degrees of severity of the same condition; the third has special features of its own. Perforation may occur in both suppurative and gangrenous types.

In all cases, the whole thickness of the wall is involved. In the earlier stages of *acute appendicitis*, the appendix is swollen, tense and markedly congested, and there may be a little fibrin on the surface. When the appendix is cut into, the mucosa bulges owing to the swelling, and purulent-looking material may exude from the lumen.

In other cases the changes are of greater severity. The primary inflammatory lesion may increase in intensity and lead to a small abscess in the wall, and this may perforate. There may occur also more general suppuration and necrosis with multiple abscesses and perforations. This mode of perforation by intramural suppuration may take place quite apart from the presence of a concretion. When a concretion is present it may in some cases simply escape through such a perforation. The swollen wall will, however, become stretched over a large concretion and the circulation in the wall will be impaired, so that a perforation is liable to take place at that point.

Gangrenous appendicitis. In the course of acute appendicitis, gangrene may affect the distal portion, sometimes in relation to a concretion (Fig. 18.48), or it may occur in patches. In some cases it appears to be due to thrombosis of the veins in the meso-appendix, which, aided by the inflammatory condition, leads to haemorrhage and stoppage of the circulation. But in other cases the gangrenous change develops early and rapidly and affects the whole appendix apart from any vascular lesion. The two factors determining gangrene are obstruction at the outlet of the appendix and distension with faecal material. Experimentally a closed portion of small intestine filled with faecal material becomes gangrenous within a short time, and general gangrene of the appendix may be produced in a similar way. The term "acute appendicular obstruction" is now applied to such a condition and many cases of so-called fulminating appendicitis are of this nature. In any case of gangrenous appendicitis with or without perforation there is apt to occur

an early general infection of the peritoneum; the organisms are of great variety, including anaerobes.

Microscopic examination. The lesion begins as a focus of inflammation at the foot of one of the indentations of the mucosa, where bacterial infection leads to ulceration (Fig. 18.47). The infection is focal at first, although there may be several foci. Around such a small lesion extension of inflammation into the other coats is found, and a little later the whole thickness of the wall may be involved and infiltrated with polymorphonuclear leukocytes. At the same time

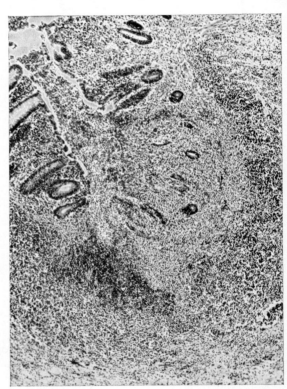

Fig. 18.47.—Acute appendicitis, showing a local ulcerative lesion in mucosa with commencing abscess formation beneath. × 60.

inflammatory exudation from the blood vessels increases the swelling, and a thin fibrinous layer is often formed on the peritoneal surface. The condition is thus an acute interstitial inflammation secondary to one or more focal lesions in the mucosa. We consider that this mode of infection is of prime importance in the various types of appendicitis.

Clinical features. Acute appendicitis presents typically as colicky abdominal pain in the umbilical region, due to spasmodic contractions of the inflamed appendix. This is followed by a continuous "burning" pain, tenderness, and rigidity of the abdominal muscles, in the vicinity of the appendix. These latter features are due to irritation of the parietal peritoneum by the inflamed appendiceal serosa, and they may be inconspicuous or absent when the appendix is retrocaecal. Vomiting, pyrexia, increased pulse rate and leukocytosis are inconstant, and not of great diagnostic value.

The diagnosis of acute appendicitis is often difficult and gangrenous appendicitis may be accompanied by remarkably slight clinical upset. The results of delay in removing an acutely inflamed appendix (see below) are so serious that exploratory laparotomy is often necessary in cases where the diagnosis is anything but certain.

Results. Acute appendicitis gives rise to important complications. In some cases there is merely a slight amount of fibrinous exudate on the surface, which does not spread and may afterwards give rise to local adhesions. In others, a localised collection of pus may form around the appendix—*appendix abscess*—which in many cases shows perforation of the wall. Sometimes an escaped concretion is present in the pus. The suppuration may spread upwards alongside the caecum and ascending colon and between the surface of the liver and the diaphragm. Alternatively, an abscess may develop in, or extend into, the pelvic cavity. Cases of this kind may run a prolonged course. In other cases, a fatal generalised peritonitis may result. This is specially apt to occur at an early stage in gangrenous appendicitis. Other complications of appendicitis are due to infection of the veins. There may be a local septic phlebitis, and from this emboli may be carried to the liver, where they set up secondary abscesses. Rarely, a spreading thrombosis with secondary suppuration may extend up the portal vein—*pylephlebitis suppurativa* (p. 573).

Etiology. Although appendicitis is essentially a bacterial infection, the particular conditions which lead to its occurrence are still largely unknown. There is even doubt about which organisms primarily invade the tissues, although there is no doubt that the important effects are produced by coliform bacilli, streptococci and occasionally various anaerobes; some of the most virulent infections are due to streptococci. Foreign bodies, such as cherry or date stones,

bristles or pins, have no relation to the etiology of appendicitis in general, and the same is true of the presence of the common intestinal threadworm *Oxyuris vermicularis*, often found in operative specimens. It is difficult to say exactly what part concretions play in appendicitis. These bodies, which vary in size and consistence, are essentially composed of faecal remains and inspissated mucus, in which there is often deposition of calcium salts (Fig. 18.48). In some cases without inflammatory change an appendix contains fluid faeces, in others a cylinder of inspissated faeces, and all intermediate stages to ordinary concretions may be observed. Concretions or faecal collections, containing, as they do, abundant bacteria, will not always be harmless. They favour infection of the mucosa,

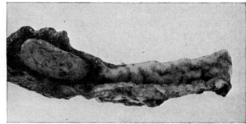

FIG. 18.48.—Acute appendicitis. A concretion is lying in the distal extremity and the wall of the appendix around it is gangrenous. × ¾.

and they also play an important part in gangrenous appendicitis, as already described. It must be admitted, however, that the factors determining the onset of acute appendicitis are imperfectly understood.

Chronic appendicitis and mucocele of the appendix

Fibrous thickening of the wall of the appendix, especially in young people, may be a consequence of acute inflammation. Occasionally, fibrosis may be the result of persistent chronic infection—the so-called *chronic appendicitis*—and there may be no history of an acute attack. It is conceivable that mild attacks of abdominal pain in the region of the appendix are due to this ("appendicular dyspepsia"). It should be emphasised, however, that in older individuals asymptomatic appendicular fibrosis is extremely common and can almost be regarded as a normal ageing process.

A common result of a localised lesion of the appendix is obliteration of the lumen at that point, whilst elsewhere the mucosa may be comparatively well preserved. Such a condition may be readily explained by the commonly focal nature of acute appendicitis. When localised obliteration is present dilatation of the distal portion of the tube may follow (Fig. 18.49). This may be slight, or there may be a cyst-like enlarge-

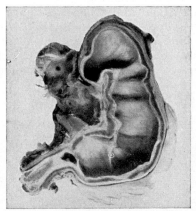

FIG. 18.49.—Chronic appendicitis with obliteration at proximal end and mucocele of the distal portion.

ment or *mucocele*. Another not uncommon result, owing to the distension acting on a localised lesion in the muscle, is the production of a diverticulum, which may project on the surface of the appendix. Occasionally rupture of a mucocele takes place and a communication is established between the lumen and the peritoneal cavity into which the contents, which are generally of mucoid nature, continue to escape. Reactive phenomena follow and the thick mucus is invaded by young connective tissue cells and by new blood vessels; this is known as *pseudomyxoma peritonei*. It is a serious complication when the mucus is abundant, and adhesions form with collections of mucus between. The microscopic appearances may simulate those of a mucoid carcinoma.

Diverticular disease

A diverticulum when fully formed consists of protrusion of the mucous and submucous coats through the muscle of the wall, and since the sac has no muscle coat, it is properly called a "false diverticulum", in contrast to a true diverticulum,

e.g. Meckel's (p. 537), which has a complete layer of muscle like the bowel.

(a) Small intestine. Diverticula are uncommon in the small bowel. The duodenum is most often involved, followed by the jejunum and ileum in that order. The diverticula may be single or multiple and are invariably found along the mesenteric border of the bowel in close relationship to the entry-sites of the blood vessels. They may measure 3 cm. or more in diameter (Fig. 18.50).

Pathological effects. Small-bowel diverticula are seldom encountered before adult life; they probably cause abdominal symptoms more often than is generally realised. Frank inflammatory change, haemorrhage and obstruction are, however, rare complications; more often a malabsorptive disturbance related to the "blind-loop syndrome" (p. 526) is the principal feature. The latter is mainly caused by abnormal and excessive bacterial proliferation in the diverticula. Bacterial uptake of vitamin B_{12} before it can reach its main absorptive site in the distal ileum leads to vitamin B_{12} deficiency and megaloblastic anaemia, and it is probable that bacteria are also responsible for the steatorrhoea which is sometimes observed. Oral broad-spectrum antibiotics lead to improvement in both vitamin B_{12} and fat absorption.

(b) Colon. Diverticula are comparatively frequent in the large bowel in later adult life: in

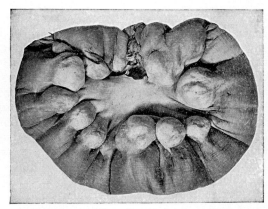

FIG. 18.50.—Multiple diverticula of small intestine situated in mesenteric attachment. $\times \frac{1}{3}$.

this country about one person in ten is affected, although in only 20 per cent of cases does the condition produce symptoms. The sigmoid colon is most often involved, although diverticula may occur at a higher level, including the caecum,

They may be present in large numbers, characteristically lying in two rows between the mesenteric and the anti-mesenteric taeniae and are related to the entry of blood vessels into the colonic wall. They commonly extend into the appendices epiploicae. Small depressions at first, they enlarge and become spherical or flask-shaped, but are rarely more than 1 cm. in diameter. Diverticula frequently contain inspissated faeces and it is notable that muscle hypertrophy and thickening of the peri-colic fat are commonly observed in affected parts of the bowel.

Pathological effects. Inflammatory change in the diverticula (*diverticulitis*) is the common cause of clinical symptoms, which are usually encountered in the older age groups. Acute inflammation leads to a syndrome resembling appendicitis with localisation of pain to the left side of the abdomen. This condition may progress to peri-colic abscess formation and even to free perforation into the peritoneal cavity and acute peritonitis. The development of fistulae between the colon and adjacent organs, especially the bladder, is not uncommon. More chronic diverticulitis leads to fibrous thickening of the colonic wall with some degree of intestinal obstruction, and the lesion may be mistaken macroscopically for carcinoma. There is no evidence that diverticular disease is a pre-cancerous condition. Rarely severe rectal haemorrhage occurs, probably due to erosion of blood vessels in the diverticular wall.

Etiology. It is generally accepted that diverticula are caused by high pressure within the bowel lumen leading to protrusion of the mucosa through points of weakness in the bowel wall. The latter are usually related to the entry of blood vessels from the mesentery. Recent studies suggest that, at least in the colon, diverticula are associated with the generation of localised areas of unusually high intraluminal pressure by abnormal segmental contraction of the bowel musculature, and that the muscle hypertrophy related to diverticula is a morphological expression of this effect. The cause of this disordered muscle activity has however, yet to be elucidated.

Specific infections

Many inflammatory conditions of the intestines, both acute and chronic, are produced by bacilli of the typhoid-coli group. These organisms affect chiefly the small intestine with special localisation in the lymphoid tissue. The food-poisoning bacilli (*Salmonella typhimurium* and others) cause acute diffuse catarrhal enteritis, especially of the small intestine, and the para-typhoid organisms sometimes have a similar effect; the dysentery bacilli affect chiefly the large intestine and cause both acute and chronic lesions. In all these cases, and also in cholera, infection is acquired by ingesting the specific micro-organisms in food or water contaminated by the excreta of cases of the disease or of carriers of the infection. Contamination by handling of food, or by the activities of flies, gives rise to sporadic cases or small outbreaks, but major epidemics are virtually always due to seepage of sewage into water supplies. In the case of food-poisoning organisms an additional source of infection is the soiling of food by the faeces of infected mice or rats. Other organisms which produce important effects are the anthrax bacillus, actinomyces, and the tubercle bacillus, and it is known that many viruses that produce no local lesion have their habitat in the intestinal contents, and gain entrance to the tissues chiefly from this source, e.g. poliomyelitis virus, Coxsackie virus.

The enteric fevers

This term is used to describe the illnesses caused by acute infections with *S. typhi* (typhoid fever) or *S. paratyphi* (paratyphoid fever).

Typhoid fever

This disease is caused by the Gram-negative bacillus *Salmonella typhi*. Corresponding with the definite course of this fever there are inflammatory changes in the lymphoid tissue of the bowel, leading to destructive effects which may be followed by healing.

Course. After an incubation period of about two weeks, the ingested organisms, which have invaded the lymphoid tissues of the small intestine, enter the blood stream. There is then progressive fever of insidious onset, sometimes with a "staircase" rise; after a further week the characteristic rose spots appear in the skin. In the first week of the fever the organisms are invariably present in the blood, from which they may be recovered in culture to confirm the diagnosis. Thereafter they persist in the liver and biliary passages and re-enter the small intestine in large numbers from the bile so that they are then readily detected in the faeces. About the end of ten days, immunity begins to develop and the organisms disappear from the blood stream, but during the bacteraemic phase they may settle in various sites and later produce localised lesions. It is significant that the gallbladder bile is invariably infected during the early phase, and the wall of the viscus may become inflamed, producing a typhoid cholecystitis with serious secondary effects. These phases in the distribution of the organisms are of decisive importance in the bacteriological diagnosis of the disease. The course may be modified considerably by previous immunisation, and diagnosis may then be difficult clinically and on occasion bacteriologically.

Naked-eye appearances. Re-infection of the lymphoid tissue of the gut by organisms in the bile leads to the development of lesions in the Peyer's patches and solitary follicles in the lower ileum. The lesions may be restricted to several centimetres above the ileo-caecal valve or may occur also more proximally, in diminishing severity; the higher ones may not pass beyond the stage of inflammatory swelling. The solitary follicles in the proximal large intestine are usually affected, and sometimes also the lymphoid tissue of the appendix. The typhoid lesion progresses through the following stages: (*a*) acute inflammatory swelling of the lymphoid tissue followed by (*b*) necrosis, (*c*) the separation of the dead tissue, with the formation of ulcers, and lastly (*d*) the process of healing. As a general rule, necrosis becomes conspicuous about the tenth day of the disease. The process of healing, after the separation of the sloughs, begins about the end of the third week and may be completed in the fifth week in uncomplicated cases. The necrosis, however, does not affect all the inflamed lymphoid tissue; in parts resolution occurs.

In the early stage the lymphoid tissue becomes swollen and prominent. The Peyer's patches come to have a somewhat convoluted appearance, as parts are fixed by connective tissue bands, whilst the intervening portions swell. Necrosis then occurs irregularly in the inflamed patch and the swelling becomes more marked; the epithelium gives way and ulceration starts. The dead tissue then imbibes the bile pigments and becomes yellowish-brown and ultimately almost black, though alterations in the effused blood also play a part in producing this appearance. Sometimes a whole Peyer's patch may be affected in this way, sometimes only a part (Fig. 18.51). Ulceration commences at the margin as the dead tissue is gradually digested and separated. If the whole patch has sloughed, the ulcer corresponds to it in shape and extent; its margins

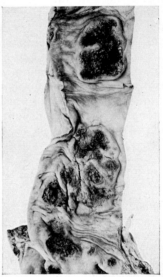

FIG. 18.51.—Lower end of small intestine in typhoid fever, showing the necrotic change in the Peyer's patches and solitary follicles. × ½.

are somewhat soft, shreddy, and undermined. If sloughing is incomplete necrotic material may be seen on the floor, but later the floor is comparatively smooth, and shows the transverse markings of the internal muscular coat.

The process of healing begins when the necrotic debris has been separated; epithelium grows over the surface and underneath it a layer of fibrous tissue forms. The lymphoid tissue and the mucosal glands are not usually fully restored so that a completely healed typhoid ulcer has a smooth silky appearance often studded with minute pigmented points. There is never any tendency to cicatricial narrowing of the bowel. The comparatively rapid spread of necrosis, not uncommonly causes *perforation* and fatal general peritonitis. Perforation of a typhoid ulcer is not usually attended by the dramatic onset of acute abdominal symptoms seen in gastro-duodenal perforations and the onset may be clinically silent; the mild alkaline reaction of the intestinal contents may be responsible for this difference. Severe *haemorrhage* may also occur.

In the proximal *large intestine*, the lymphoid follicles similarly undergo marked swelling, become necrotic in the centre, and small rounded ulcers with swollen margins result (Fig. 18.52). When the *appendix* is involved, there may be considerable necrosis and sloughing, and occasionally perforation follows.

Microscopic appearances. These are characteristic. The enlargement of the Peyer's patches (Fig. 18.53) is due to congestion, oedema, and a great increase of non-granular cells including lymphocytes, and phagocytes derived from histiocytes and monocytes (Fig. 17.7, p. 458). Similar cells may be seen extending along the lymphatics of the mucous and submucous coats for a considerable distance around, and also deep down in the muscular coats and in the subserosa. Haemorrhages occur and increase the swelling; there may also be some fibrinous exudate. Polymorphonuclear leukocytes are virtually absent from the affected area, except at the margin, when the dead tissue is in process of separation. Patchy necrosis appears and gradually extends; the patches appear amorphous from loss of cellular structure; there is often much karyorrhexis in the adjacent cells, whilst many of the phagocytes digest remains of cells and nuclei as well as red cells. Necrosis in the affected tissue may be due to a delayed hypersensitivity reaction, and to bacterial toxins.

The *mesenteric nodes* undergo pronounced inflammatory swelling. At an early stage they are pinkish and rather soft, but later become greyish or even yellowish owing to the occurrence of necrosis (Fig. 18.54). Suppuration does not occur unless there is infection with other organisms. Typhoid bacilli are present in large numbers in the nodes, which occasionally soften and rupture, giving rise to peritonitis.

Associated lesions. The comparative absence of emigration on the part of the polymorphonuclear leukocytes and the absence of the neutrophil reaction in the blood (p. 124) and bone

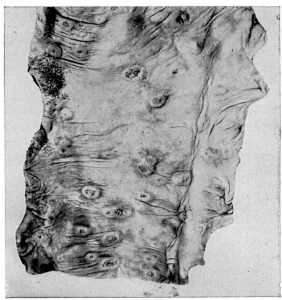

Fig. 18.52.—Large intestine in typhoid fever, showing multiple small ulcers. $\times \frac{1}{2}$.

marrow are noteworthy features. In the enlarged spleen also there is an absence of the accumulation of polymorphonuclear leukocytes which usually accompanies severe acute bacterial infections (p. 450).

Typhoid fever is associated with a great variety of lesions throughout the body, arising during the disease or later. These are referred to more

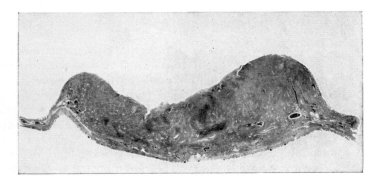

Fig. 18.53.—Peyer's patch in early stage of typhoid fever, showing the marked inflammatory swelling and commencing necrosis. $\times$ 5.

fully in connection with the different systems. In the production of lesions in other parts, two main factors are concerned, viz. *toxaemia*, from the liberation of the powerful endotoxin, and *bacteraemia*, i.e., the actual presence of *S. typhi* in the blood. **Toxic action** is shown by the occurrence of fever and degenerative changes in the heart and other organs, which may lead to myocardial weakness, and in severe cases death from heart failure. Patchy necrosis of the abdominal muscles in typhoid, the so-called Zenker's degeneration, degenerative changes in the renal tubules and inflammatory foci in the liver (p.549), are further evidence of toxic action, although, in the production of the latter, the typhoid bacilli may actually be present. The toxaemia of typhoid also appears to lower the resistance to invasion by other bacteria. Thus laryngitis, bronchitis (sometimes an early

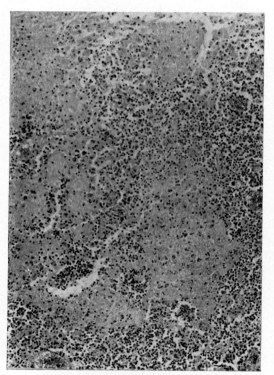

FIG. 18.54.—Mesenteric lymph node in typhoid fever, showing extensive necrosis. × 115.

symptom) and pneumonia are common and typhoid bacilli may be present along with pneumococci and other organisms.

Bacteraemia brings about the acute enlargement of the spleen (p. 450), and may lead to infection of various parts, e.g., the bacilli have been found in the rose-coloured spots in the skin. The gall bladder and the urinary tract often become infected with or without distinct inflammatory changes, and the bacilli may persist there for various periods, accounting for "faecal" and "urinary" carriers respectively. Such carriers are the common source of outbreaks of enteric fever. Later, calculi may form in the gall-bladder. Endocarditis, meningitis or arthritis may occasionally develop in the course of the blood infection. The periosteum of bones, and occasionally the perichondrium of the costal and laryngeal cartilages, may become inflamed and the ribs have a special liability to suppurative periostitis caused by typhoid bacilli several months after the initial attack; occasionally it may recur in another part after operative treatment.

Paratyphoid infections

Infections caused by the paratyphoid organism are not uncommon, paratyphoid B being the most frequent of the enteric fevers in Great Britain. In some cases the disease has the general characters of typhoid, though usually less severe. There is a similar involvement of the lymphoid tissue, especially the Peyer's patches and solitary glands of the small intestine, with swelling of mesenteric nodes and spleen; but the necrotic and ulcerative processes are less marked and usually limited to a small part of the intestine. In other cases, however, a general acute catarrhal condition of the intestine is the characteristic feature and there is little implication of the lymphoid tissue; sometimes enteritis is associated with marked gastritis. The "carrier" condition may result also from paratyphoid infections, as has been described above in typhoid fever.

Food poisoning

This term is widely applied in a restricted sense to include acute gastro-enteritis due either to infection with *Salmonellae* other than those which cause enteric fever, or to ingestion of bacterial toxins. The *Salmonellae* most commonly responsible are *S. enteritidis* and *S. typhimurium*, harboured by rats and mice respectively, but a very large number of other *Salmonellae* cause local outbreaks in all parts of the world. Characteristically, acute gastro-enteritis, with fever, vomiting and diarrhoea, develops 12–24 hours after eating contaminated food. The inflammation is of catarrhal type and affects the ileum most severely; in most cases, recovery is complete within 3–4 days, but death can result from water and electrolyte depletion. Blood culture is usually negative although in fatal cases the organisms may be recovered from the spleen.

The commonest cause of toxic food poisoning is *staphylococcal enterotoxin* in foods contaminated by *Staph. aureus*: this toxin is highly resistant to heat and produces acute gastro-enteritis within 1–6 hours. It is rarely fatal.

Botulism. Small outbreaks of botulism occur in North America and other countries where home bottling or canning is popular. The organism, *Clostridium botulinum*, grows in inadequately cooked fruit or vegetables, or in sausages, and produces the most powerful toxin known. Within 12–36 hours of its ingestion, muscular weakness and paralysis develops, particularly in the muscles of the eye, pharynx and neck. Death commonly results from respiratory paralysis and aspiration pneumonia. Alimentary symptoms are slight, and constipation is more usual than diarrhoea.

Cholera

This disease is caused by the *Vibrio cholerae* or its subtypes and is a classical example of a waterborne infection capable of causing explosive epidemics. Profuse watery diarrhoea is the outstanding clinical feature and the stools are often described as having a colourless "rice-water" appearance. Diarrhoea leads to the loss of about 30 litres of fluid during an illness lasting 3–6 days, and the depletion of water and electrolytes, especially sodium and potassium, from the extracellular fluid compartment may be so marked as to cause peripheral circulatory failure (p. 179).

Until recently it was considered that the pathological basis for the severe diarrhoea was an acute inflammation of the small intestine, especially its distal part, and occasionally of the large bowel in addition. Intense mucosal congestion associated with desquamation of the superficial epithelium, and sometimes with membrane formation and frank ulceration, have

been described histologically. Intestinal biopsies have failed, however, to demonstrate loss of the integrity of the surface epithelium, and it is now thought that *Vibrio cholerae*, which is present in large numbers in the intestinal lumen, causes diarrhoea by producing an exotoxin which increases the net flow of fluid and electrolytes from the plasma into the lumen of the gut, particularly in the jejunum. The mechanism differs from that of inflammatory exudation, and the fluid has a low protein content: there appears to be an increase in permeability of the mucosal epithelium for water and sodium ions. Oral administration of glucose and electrolyte solutions has been shown to be of great therapeutic value. Although the organisms are largely confined to the intestinal tract, there can now be no doubt that they can become established in the gall-bladder and lead to a carrier state which, although usually of short duration, may last as long as four years. It has also become apparent that the number of cases of cholera is far exceeded by the number of individuals who become infected and excrete the vibrio without developing the disease.

The El Tor vibrio, first isolated in Sinai, is closely related to *V. cholerae* and has been responsible for recent outbreaks of a cholera-like illness in various parts of the world.

Tuberculosis

In the past the intestinal tract was a common site of tuberculous lesions. This is no longer the case in this country, partly as a result of measures taken to prevent infection with bovine tubercle bacilli, and partly as a consequence of the falling incidence of pulmonary tuberculosis. Three main forms of intestinal tuberculosis are recognised.

(a) Primary infection. The small bowel was formerly a common site for the primary tuberculous complex, especially in children who had ingested cow's milk containing bovine tubercle bacilli. As elsewhere, the site of entrance of the organisms is inconspicuous, although this probably means that the lesion has been minute and has not spread, rather than that the bacilli have been absorbed without producing any lesion. The prominent change is produced by spread to the mesenteric lymph nodes, which become greatly enlarged and caseous (tabes mesenterica). In favourable circumstances, the condition remains localised, and the calcified mesenteric nodes still quite often observed in adults represent the result of intestinal infection in early life. Occasionally, however, the disease spreads from the nodes to the peritoneal cavity leading to tuberculous peritonitis. (p. 540).

(b) Secondary infection. Intestinal lesions used to be a common complication of open pulmonary tuberculosis, especially in children. This secondary form of intestinal tuberculosis, caused by swallowing sputum containing tubercle bacilli, presents different pathological features from the primary form in that the changes are more conspicuous in the bowel wall itself than in the related lymph nodes.

The small intestine is the common site of the lesions, which usually occur in the Peyer's patches or solitary lymphoid follicles. Initially, caseating tubercles develop in the mucosa and the submucosa, and subsequent mucosal breakdown leads to the formation of small ulcers, which become progressively enlarged by direct spread of the organisms to adjacent parts of the mucosa. Ultimately large ulcers are produced and these tend to extend by spread of infection along the lymphatics, transversely to the longitudinal axis of the bowel; sometimes indeed they encircle the gut (Fig. 18.55). The larger ulcers have an irregular outline, undermined edges and raised nodular margins (Fig. 18.56). The floor is uneven or granular and may be coated by caseous material, but tubercles are rarely visible. The serous coat overlying the ulcer is often thickened and opaque and the presence of visible tubercles along the lines of serosal lymphatics may be of diagnostic value. Histologically, the tuberculous lesions are similar to those observed elsewhere: the ulceration is seen to extend through the mucosa into the submucous layer and there may be varying degrees of fibrous replacement of the muscular coat. Tubercles are

usually found throughout the entire thickness of the bowel and in the related mesenteric lymph nodes. These, however are seldom as grossly affected as in the primary form.

Tuberculosis ulceration rarely causes gross haemorrhage, and perforation into the peritoneal cavity is uncommon. The formation of fistulae between adjacent loops of bowel, initiated by the development of adhesions,

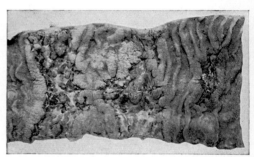

FIG. 18.55.—Tuberculous ulceration of small intestine. × ¾.

Note the irregular ulceration with transverse spread.

may, however, lead to short-circuiting of bowel contents and malabsorption. In these respects there is a contrast with typhoid ulceration. The peritoneum may show frank tuberculous lesions (p. 540) or simply multiple fibrous adhesions which may cause mechanical obstruction of the bowel.

(c) "Hyperplastic caecal tuberculosis". The large bowel is a less common site of tuberculous ulceration apart from a curious lesion localised to the vicinity of the caecum and characterised by ulceration and marked thickening of the bowel wall (Fig. 18.57). This condition is associated with pronounced narrowing of the bowel lumen and leads to intestinal obstruction. It bears a close macroscopic and histological resemblance to regional enteritis (p. 505) with which it may have been confused in the past.

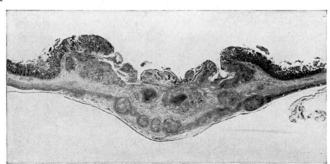

FIG. 18.56.—Small tuberculous ulcer of small intestine with thickened and irregular margins and floor. Note tubercles in serous coat. × 6.

Indeed regional enteritis must now be regarded as the commonest cause of ileo-caecal granulomas; nevertheless, it is always important to exclude tuberculosis as a cause of caecal disorders of this type both by histological and by cultural methods (p. 506). Hyperplastic caecal tuberculosis is usually secondary to pulmonary disease, but in some instances it appears to be a variant of the primary form.

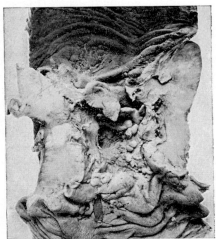

FIG. 18.57.—Chronic tuberculosis of ascending colon. × ½.

The lesion has produced great thickening of the wall with resulting obstruction.

The *appendix* is occasionally affected in cases of intestinal tuberculosis. The changes are of the usual kind, and in a proportion of cases a faecal fistula has developed post-operatively. More often this sequence is attributable to Crohn's disease.

The dysenteries

The term dysentery was originally used clinically to denote conditions of severe inflammation and ulceration of the colon, attended by diarrhoea, tenesmus and the passage of blood and mucus in the stools. Two main types of dysentery are distinguished, namely, *bacillary* and *amoebic*.

Bacillary dysentery

Bacillary dysentery is produced by bacilli of the *Shigella* group, of which there are several varieties, distinguishable by their serological and fermentative reactions. The mildest type is usually caused by *Shigella sonnei*, and in children is often called ileo-colitis; more severe infections are caused by the *Sh. flexneri* type, and the most severe tropical form by the *Sh. dysenteriae* (*Sh. shigae*) type, which produces a powerful exotoxin. The lesion is essentially inflammation of variable intensity in the colon, though the lower end of the ileum is sometimes affected. In milder cases it is mainly an intense catarrhal inflammation accompanied by much formation of mucus, oedema of the mucosa and haemorrhage into it; but even in these there tends to be formation of fibrinous exudate on the summits of the folds of the mucous membrane. In the severer infections of Shiga type this change is more marked, and there is extensive formation of false membrane in small patches along the ridges of the mucosa. Patches then become confluent and necrosis of the underlying mucosa follows. The dead tissue then separates, with formation of ulcers which begin over the ridges and then extend in an irregular manner, having a shreddy margin. In this way, large areas may become denuded of mucous membrane and the submucous layer becomes involved.

Microscopically there is intense inflammation with infiltration of polymorphonuclear leukocytes, escape of red cells, etc. Leukocytes also pass in large numbers on to the surface and are present in the faeces mixed with blood and mucus; they can readily be found on microscopic examination of the stools, and this fact is of great service in rapid tentative diagnosis.

When the acute stage passes off, the process of healing may commence, but the disease may pass into a subacute or chronic stage, where attempts at healing and repeated ulceration occur side by side. When healing is effected, the ulcerated areas become covered over by epithelium and assume a comparatively smooth and even appearance as occurs also in ulcerative colitis (Fig. 18.46d). They thus present a contrast to the surviving mucosa, which is relatively raised, and in addition may show thickenings and even small polypoid growths. In chronic cases considerable fibrous contraction with stenosis of the bowel may result. The disease is often prolonged and relapses are fairly frequent. Bacillary dysentery may occasionally lead to pyogenic infection of the portal blood and foci of suppuration in the liver.

Amoebic dysentery

This form is produced by the *Entamoeba histolytica*. The disease is only rarely acquired in Great Britain, but is common in tropical and subtropical countries, a fact not easily explained since cysts of the entamoeba are found in the faeces of a small proportion of people who have not been abroad.

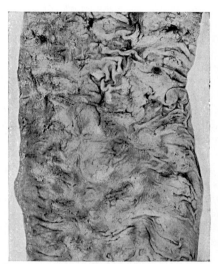

FIG. 18.58.—Portion of large intestine in amoebic dysentery at early stage before ulceration, showing the irregular swelling of the mucosa. × ⅔.

Naked-eye appearance. The organisms, swallowed in the cystic stage in food or water, are freed in the gut by digestion of the cyst wall, and enter the wall of the large intestine through the mucosa and settle in the submucous tissue where they liberate a proteolytic enzyme causing tissue necrosis. Accordingly, the first lesion visible to the naked eye is the formation of swollen congested patches in the mucosa, the central parts of which become soft and somewhat yellowish as necrosis occurs (Fig. 18.58). The mucosa then gives way and an ulcer is formed with shreddy and undermined margins. Such ulcers, as they spread, become confluent first in their deeper parts, so that a probe may be passed under the mucosa from one to the other; the bridges then give way and the ulcerated areas are greatly increased. Accordingly a considerable part of the bowel may have lost its mucosa, while in the intervening parts fragments of mucosa in process of disintegration and separation are present (Fig. 18.59). Gangrene of the mucosal patches may be superadded.

Microscopically the most prominent feature is an intense inflammatory oedema, which is accompanied by remarkably little leucocytic infiltration. Subsequent necrosis takes place in the tissues around the entamoebae which multiply and spread in the submucous tissue and thus necrosis extends. The amoebae are to be found at the margins of the ulcers, often in considerable numbers, chiefly in the submucous coat, but also extending more deeply (Fig. 18.60). Occasionally they penetrate the small intestinal veins and sometimes in sections they may be seen within the blood vessels (Fig. 18.61).

Results and complications. When the acute stage of amoebic dysentery has passed off, attempts at healing may occur. The necrotic tissue is thrown off and the epithelium grows over the denuded areas. But the process is often interrupted, and just as in bacillary dysentery, the disease may become protracted and passes into a chronic condition. Overgrowth of fibrous tissue is apt to occur in the

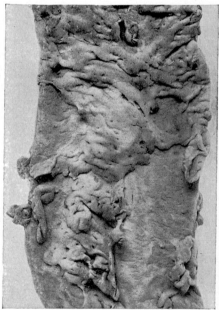

FIG. 18.59.—Large intestine in chronic amoebic dysentery, showing irregular smooth areas where the mucosa has been destroyed. × ¾.

deeper coats with resulting narrowing of the bowel at places. Enterostomy or faecal fistula in the presence of active amoebic infection may be followed by spread of amoebae into the skin, where they produce a severe necrotising ulceration. The passage of entamoebae to the liver in the portal blood gives rise to amoebic hepatitis and in some cases a tropical abscess is produced (p. 576).

Diagnosis. In the acute phase the stools contain blood and mucus but, in contrast with bacillary dysentery, pus is absent. The mucus is thus clear and in it vegetative amoebae showing

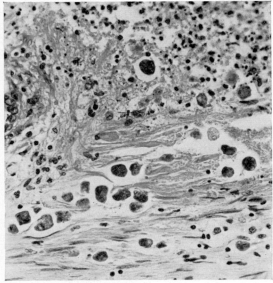

Fig. 18.60.—Section through the base of an amoebic ulcer of the colon. The amoebae are seen lying in spaces with no surrounding inflammatory reaction. × 200.

active movements are readily found on microscopic examination of a fresh preparation, examined without delay on a warm stage; the ingestion of red cells by the amoebae is diagnostic. In the chronic phase, vegetative forms are absent, and the diagnosis depends on the detection of cysts in the faeces or from the base of ulcers seen on sigmoidoscopy.

Actinomycosis

As a path of entry for the streptothrix *Actinomyces bovis*, the intestine comes next to the mouth in order of frequency. The lesions are found in the wall of the large intestine, and sometimes ulcers with suppuration of the submucous coat have been present usually with extension beyond the wall of the gut, especially in the region of the caecum and in the tissues around the rectum. More commonly, the organism seems to gain entrance to the appendix, from which it spreads to give rise to an inflammatory

mass containing multiple abscesses. In the peritoneum it may cause loculated collections of pus between the coils of intestine, which may discharge into the bowel. Diagnosis can usually be made by finding colonies of *Actinomyces* on microscopic examination. Secondary actinomycotic abscesses (p. 573) may occur in the liver, and suppurative pylephlebitis due to secondary invasion by other pyogenic organisms has been recorded.

Intestinal schistosomiasis (bilharziasis)

This disease, which is common in various tropical and sub-tropical parts of Africa and other countries, is produced by the dioecious trematode, *Schistosoma mansoni*. The adult parasites lodge in the tributaries of the portal vein (Fig. 18.62), especially those in the colonic wall, and the females there lay ova which escape into the surrounding tissues. The ova give rise to much irritation and lead to lesions in the large intestine, especially in the rectum (Fig. 18.63), similar to those caused in the bladder by the *Schistosoma haematobium* (p. 743). The eggs are oval, measuring about 140 μ in the long diameter, and have a small lateral spine near one extremity. The lesions are of chronic inflammatory nature and produce general thickening of the mucous and submucous coats and

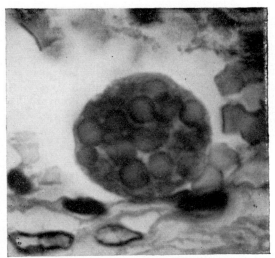

Fig. 18.61.—Amoebic dysentery: an entamoeba containing red cells is seen in a venule in the base of an ulcer of the colon. × 1000.

usually there are also nodular thickenings which enlarge and give rise to polypoid projections (Fig. 18.64). Ulceration with haemorrhage occurs, and sometimes there is gross fibrous thickening of the wall.

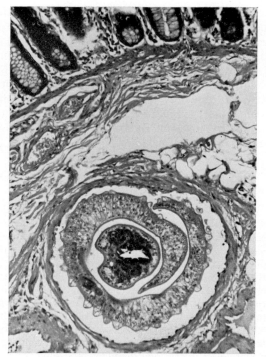

FIG. 18.62.—Schistosomiasis. Wall of colon, showing *S. mansoni* adults in cross section. The female lies in the gynaecophoric canal of the male. × 200.

Histologically the disease is characterised by a focal granulomatous lesion centred upon the ova, which are surrounded by concentric rings of fibrous tissue and are occasionally calcified. Inflammatory cells, especially eosinophils and histiocytes (sometimes containing haematin pigment), are noted round the periphery of the lesion. Similar lesions may be observed in other tissues, particularly the liver and lungs. In the liver, they develop in relation to the portal tracts and lead to a condition sometimes referred to as "pipe-stem cirrhosis" (Fig. 19.35, p. 578); portal hypertension with splenomegaly arises from obstruction of the portal radicles (p. 577). Unlike

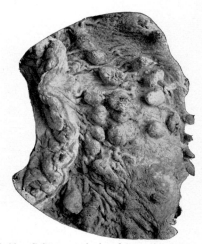

FIG. 18.64.—Schistosomiasis of large intestine, showing multiple polypoid nodules projecting from mucosal surface. × ½.

the vesical type, intestinal schistosomiasis does not appear to predispose to the development of carcinoma; even so, it is an all too frequent cause of chronic ill-health in the tropics.

The life-cycle of the parasite is similar to that of *S. haematobium* (p. 743).

Functional disorders of the colon

In clinical practice it is by no means uncommon to encounter patients who have symptoms associated with constipation and excessive mucus secretion, although organic lesions cannot be demonstrated.

"Mucous colitis", in which membranous structures composed of inspissated mucus are passed by the bowel, is probably a variant of this syndrome.

Although a variety of names has been attached to such states, the term "irritable colon syndrome" is most commonly employed, and finds

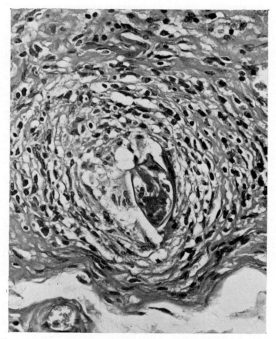

FIG. 18.63.—Ovum of *S. mansoni* with surrounding granulomatous reaction in the wall of the colon. × 300.

justification in the fact that the colon may be found to exhibit unusual irritability or hyper-motility. The causation is obscure—indeed this syndrome may possibly include more than one disease entity—although previous organic disease, for example dysentery, psychological disturbance and dietary indiscretion might be of etiological significance.

Inflammatory stricture of the rectum

In the tertiary stage of *syphilis*, lesions are sometimes present in the large intestine, the rectum being by far the commonest site, but it is probable that many of the lesions formerly so classified are really due to *lymphopathia venereum* (p. 154) which, in women, tends to spread by the lymphatics from the genitalia to the rectum and peri-rectal tissues. It is significant that gumma of the rectum is said to be commoner in prosti-tutes, who might well harbour both infections. Whatever the true nature of the lesion, there is first formed a raised patch of inflammatory in-filtration in the mucosa and submucosa, which tends to spread transversely to the length of the bowel and undergoes ulceration. Ultimately the whole circumference of the bowel may be in-volved and extreme stenosis may result from scarring, the condition sometimes simulating a malignant tumour. In the rectum, perforation of the ulcer is not uncommon, and suppura-tion may occur in the surrounding tissues. Pus occasionally makes its way into the bladder or tracks to the perineum, thus leading to the forma-tion of fistulae.

In congenital syphilis, multiple lesions are not infrequent, especially in the ileum. The in-flammatory patches may undergo ulceration and resemble tuberculous lesions. Sometimes the infiltration is more diffuse, or miliary gummas may occur.

The malabsorption syndrome

The products of digestion of food are absorbed almost exclusively from the small intestine, and accordingly most pathological processes in the small intestine, if at all extensive, interfere with this important function to some degree. The absorption of some nutrients may be restricted to certain relatively well-defined parts of the small bowel; iron, for example, is absorbed mainly from the duodenum and vitamin B_{12} from the distal ileum. Depending thus upon the extent, site or nature of the disease process, the absorp-tion of some constituents of the diet may be affected more than others. In severe cases, all nutrients including protein, fat, carbo-hydrates, vitamins, minerals and even water may fail to be adequately absorbed. Failure to absorb fat is the most prominent feature in most cases and on it depend some of the other de-ficiencies.

Clinical features. The clinical manifestations of malabsorption vary accordingly. The most common symptom is chronic diarrhoea; the stools are pale, bulky and foul-smelling and contain an excess of fat (steatorrhoea) and of nitrogenous material. In severe cases, loss of weight, muscle wasting, dehydration and hypo-tension are prominent features. Hypoglycaemia, with a low glucose tolerance curve (p. 899) indicates failure of carbohydrate uptake. Hypo-proteinaemia, associated with oedema, may be the result not only of impaired amino-acid ab-sorption, but also of protein leakage into the bowel lumen (protein-losing enteropathy)—a feature of primary malabsorptive disorders (see below). Vitamin deficiencies are common, and symptoms of beri-beri, pellagra, scurvy and rickets in children, may be presenting features of the syndrome. Anaemia frequently dominates the clinical picture, usually microcytic and attri-buted to iron deficiency but macrocytic anaemia following failure to absorb vitamin B_{12} or folic acid is by no means unusual. It is rare for all of those features to be noted together, and any one deficiency may predominate; biochemical tests, however, usually reveal more extensive malab-sorption than is clinically evident.

Classification of the causes of malabsorption is to some extent unsatisfactory, since in any one case several factors may operate. Two main groups, however, are recognised: (*a*) primary malabsorptive conditions, without known cause, and (*b*) secondary malabsorption, which may follow a variety of recognised disease entities.

Peroral intestinal biopsy. This technique has only been in widespread use over the last decade and has proved of considerable value in the diagnosis and investigation of malabsorptive disturbances. Biopsy makes it possible to assess not only the morphological state of the mucosa but also the enzyme content of the absorptive epithelium and the bacterial content of the intestinal lumen.

Under the dissecting microscope, the normal jejunal mucosa has tall, slender finger-shaped

in the digestion of many nutrients takes place in the vicinity of the innumerable microvilli which form the epithelial surface. Malabsorptive disturbance may be caused by deficiency of intestinal enzymes, especially the disaccharidases.

Villous atrophy (Fig. 18.65) is the commonest pathological change in villous pattern. In the *partial* form (PVA) the villi show extensive

(a)

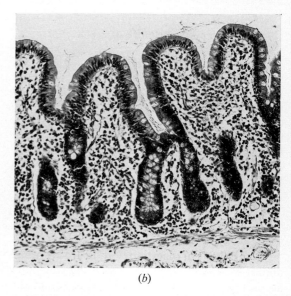

(b)

FIG. 18.65.—Villous atrophy of jejunum: *a*, normal jejunal mucosa: *b*, partial villous atrophy; *c*, complete villous atrophy. × 150. (Material obtained by peroral biopsy.)

villi interspersed with occasional broader leaf-shaped villi, which are more conspicuous in the duodenum. The villi measure about 400μ in height and usually account for about 70 per cent of the total mucosal height. In tropical residents, however, the villi are more often leaf-shaped and may even fuse to form short ridges. Histologically, moreover, they appear shorter and broader than their temperate counterparts. The cause of this geographical variation in jejunal morphology is not known.

The absorptive epithelial cells clothing the villi are formed in the crypts of Lieberkühn and gradually ascend the villi before becoming extruded into the lumen after a life-span of about 5 days. It is now known that these cells are the principal source of the digestive enzymes of the succus entericus, and that the final stage

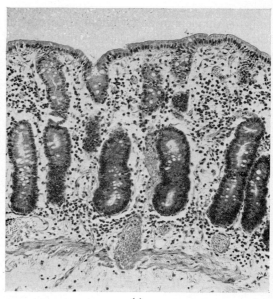

(c)

fusion with the formation of long ridges or convolutions; histologically they appear shorter and broader than normal, although the crypts are enlarged and hyperplastic. The villous epithelium often shows degenerative change, and there is little doubt that the fundamental disturbance is a shortening of the life-span of these cells with compensatory hyperplasia of the generative crypt cells. There is often increased cellular infiltration in the lamina propria mucosae, plasma cells being most conspicuous. In the more severe *subtotal* form (SVA) villous fusion is more advanced and the mucosa appears completely flat both histologically and under the dissecting microscope. Epithelial degenerative changes are also more prominent.

Villous atrophy is not a specific change; it is, however, most often seen in the primary malabsorptive diseases. Less commonly it is seen in a number of other disease processes such as malignant lymphoma, hypogammaglobulinaemia (p. 114), kwashiorkor, skin diseases, especially dermatitis herpetiformis, ulcerative colitis, hepatic disease, helminthic infestations, following drug therapy especially with neomycin, and in some patients with carcinomatous cachexia.

Primary malabsorptive disorders

This group includes gluten-enteropathy (coeliac disease and idiopathic steatorrhoea) and tropical sprue.

(a) Gluten-enteropathy. This term includes *coeliac disease* of childhood and *idiopathic steatorrhoea*, which is considered to be its adult counterpart. In both conditions the exclusion of the wheat protein gluten from the diet leads to remission in the malabsorptive disturbance; and, although the exact nature of the defect is not known, mucosal damage is produced by a toxic peptide released by the breakdown of gluten. Possibly there is deficiency of an enzyme required during a critical phase in gluten digestion. The mucosal damage takes the form of villous atrophy, which is most marked, and usually subtotal, in the proximal small bowel and becomes progressively less severe or partial distally. Institution of a gluten-free diet leads to reversal of the changes, initially in the distal small bowel and only latterly in the upper jejunum, which may never revert entirely to

normal. Recovery appears to be more often attainable in coeliac disease than in the adult form.

In coeliac disease, the most common cause of malabsorption in childhood, impairment of growth and development become superadded to symptoms of generalised malabsorption. The changes of late rickets may thus be a feature. Idiopathic steatorrhoea, or non-tropical sprue, is an important cause of malabsorption in adults in temperate climates. In some cases there is a history of coeliac disease in childhood, and it is probable that in these instances the mucosal defect has been present from an early stage in life.

(b) Tropical sprue is a disease encountered in certain areas in the tropics and sub-tropics, Africa being an exception. There is malabsorption resulting in severe emaciation and chronic diarrhoea, and anaemia which is often macrocytic may arise from deficiency of B_{12}, folate or both. Villous atrophy, usually partial and less often subtotal, is the characteristic change found at jejunal biopsy. This lesion, and the malabsorptive disturbance, are relieved by removal of the patient from the tropical environment and by oral broad-spectrum antibiotics, but a gluten-free diet has little or no beneficial effect. Folic acid may also cause some improvement. The cause of the disease remains uncertain, but it is likely that abnormal bacterial colonisation of the upper small bowel is implicated.

(c) Whipple's disease. This rare and interesting disease, which is suitably included in the primary malabsorptive states, predominantly affects adult males in middle age. Malabsorption is usually the presenting feature, although other signs and symptoms such as generalised lymphadenopathy, arthropathy, skin pigmentation and chronic cough may be encountered. Jejunal biopsy is diagnostic: the mucosal lamina propria is stuffed with large granular macrophages containing material staining strongly with the periodic acid-Schiff technique for mucopolysaccharides (Fig. 18.66). The regional lymph nodes, and occasionally other tissues, e.g. brain and heart valves, contain similar cells. Neutral fat accumulates in lymphatic channels. Electron microscopy has demonstrated that the abnormal macrophages contain unidentified bacteria and bacterial debris. Moreover, the disease responds to oral antibiotics. It would, however, be premature to assert that Whipple's disease is a form of specific infection, especially in view of the unusual age and sex incidence of the condition.

Secondary malabsorption

Numerous disease processes are capable of interfering with absorption. Most of these are discussed elsewhere, and only a brief account will be given here. Classification is most rationally based upon the mechanism thought to be mainly involved in causing malabsorption, although it should be appreciated that more than one mechanism may be operating in any individual disease.

(a) Chronic intestinal disease may cause malabsorption if extensive areas of the mucosa are affected. Examples of this include regional enteritis, tuberculosis, tumours, especially malignant lymphoma, connective tissue disorders such as systemic sclerosis, radiation damage and amyloidosis.

(b) Abnormal bacterial proliferation in the small bowel interferes not only with the absorption of vitamin B_{12} but also to some extent with fat absorption. It results from stasis in the intestinal lumen, especially that produced by short-circuit operations which leave stagnant loops of bowel (the blind-loop syndrome). Stasis is also seen in jejunal diverticulosis (p. 512) and chronic intestinal obstruction and may contribute to the development of malabsorption following partial gastrectomy if there is stasis in the afferent loop.

(c) Other mechanisms which may cause malabsorption include *biochemical defects* such as disaccharidase deficiency, agammaglobulinaemia and abetalipoproteinaemia; *endocrine disturbances*, including the carcinoid syndrome (p. 532) and the Zollinger–Ellison syndrome (p. 601); *lymphatic obstruction*, congenital or acquired, e.g. as a result of tuberculosis or tumour; *circulatory disturbance*, especially mesenteric vascular insufficiency; and *drug therapy*, e.g. phenindione, neomycin.

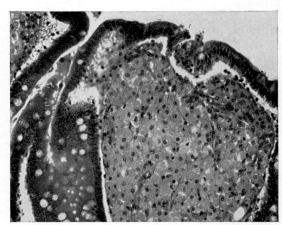

Fig. 18.66.—Whipple's disease of small intestine, showing infiltration of the mucosa with granular macrophages. × 230.

(d) Inadequate digestion must always be considered as a cause of malabsorption and may be due to disease of the liver and biliary tract or to pancreatic deficiency (p. 598). Malabsorption following gastro-jejunostomy, alone or with partial gastrectomy, is largely a consequence of disordered digestion. There is inadequate mixing of food with pancreatic enzymes or bile as a result of interference with the normal anatomical relationships.

Intestinal obstruction (ileus)

Interference with the passage of the intestinal contents may be complete or incomplete, slowly or suddenly produced; it may occur in the small or in the large intestine and it may be brought about in a variety of ways, *mechanical*, *nervous* or *vascular*.

The following are the chief mechanical causes of intestinal obstruction:

(*a*) *Constriction from outside*—for example, by a hernial sac, by special conditions such as volvulus or intussusception, or by fibrous peritoneal adhesions. This is the commonest cause of acute mechanical obstruction.

(*b*) *Stenosis caused by thickening and contrac-* *tion of the wall* usually takes place in the large intestine and is produced by such conditions as scirrhous carcinoma or a cicatrising ulcer, e.g. rectal stricture following lymphopathia or in chronic dysentery. The obstruction from this cause is ordinarily incomplete and chronic, but an acute state may be added by the impaction of inspissated faecal masses in the narrowed portion of bowel. In the small intestine, obstruction may result from an ingrowth of secondary cancer from the peritoneal aspect.

(*c*) *Actual obstruction of the lumen.* This may result from impaction of a large gall stone or other foreign body or by the growth of a tumour into the lumen, usually malignant but sometimes a simple polyp.

(*d*) *Pressure from outside*, for example by a large tumour in the pelvis; obstruction is not often complete from such a cause.

The *nervous type* of intestinal obstruction is called *paralytic* or *adynamic ileus* and may occur after handling of the intestines at operation, or it may result from peritonitis. The principal *vascular* lesions producing intestinal obstruction are occlusion of the mesenteric vessels by embolism or thrombosis. In the type of mechanical obstruction seen in group (*a*) above, vascular obstruction is commonly superadded and the subsequent course is then modified. When the blood supply is intact the obstruction is said to be *simple*, when it is impaired the term *strangulation* is applied.

The results of intestinal obstruction

The site of the obstruction plays an important part in determining both the effects and the prognosis. High intestinal obstruction is in general more acute in onset, more rapid in its progress and more likely to be complete than low intestinal obstruction which is usually of slow onset, is often incomplete and is less rapidly fatal.

Acute obstruction. When a portion of the small intestine is suddenly obstructed, e.g. by passing under a fibrous band, the part above contracts actively for a time and then passes into a condition of paralytic distension. There are probably both increased secretion from the wall and diminished absorption, and thus the bowel becomes distended with fluid contents in which there is abundant growth of bacteria. The fluid is passed back to the stomach by antiperistalsis and is vomited. Its exact composition depends on the site of the obstruction, but since nearly 8 litres of fluid are secreted into the gut daily, of which all but 100 ml. are normally reabsorbed, the volume of fluid available for loss by vomiting or by pooling in the gut is obviously considerable.

If the obstruction is at the *pylorus* or *duodenum* the fluid lost is predominantly acid in reaction with a high Cl^- content. This results in a depletion of plasma chloride, and the urinary excretion of chlorides is then diminished or absent. Since sodium, the ion which normally balances the Cl^- ion, is not lost, carbonic acid is retained to take the place of the lost chloride and the plasma bicarbonate content therefore rises. This state of *alkalosis* is shown clinically by drowsiness and slow shallow respiration and can be demonstrated on analysis by a rise in the CO_2 combining power. A further complication is the development of *tetany* due to a fall in the ionised serum calcium, as a result of the alkalosis. Intracellular potassium deficiency may be superadded—*hypokalaemic alkalosis*. If the fluid loss is great enough, oliguria and extrarenal uraemia may follow, the blood urea being markedly raised terminally.

Obstruction in the *jejunum* results in the loss by vomiting of a fluid which contains saliva, gastric juice, bile, pancreatic juice and succus entericus. This leads to depletion of Na^+, K^+, and Cl^-. The CO_2 combining power remains normal, without marked disturbance of the acid-base balance. Although in high obstruction there is a tendency towards acidosis, it is the loss of fluid and electrolytes that leads rapidly to a fall in blood volume, dehydration, haemoconcentration and finally death. Fluid and electrolyte replacement is therefore essential to prolong life until surgical intervention can be undertaken.

Chronic obstruction. In low intestinal obstruction there is a large surface area of gut proximal to the obstruction which allows of reabsorption of much of the regurgitated fluid. Loss by vomiting is less severe, but ultimately the vomit becomes brown and foul-smelling, the so-called faecal or stercoral vomit, and there is dehydration by loss of water and electrolytes into the lumen of the bowel, which becomes increasingly distended. The contents of the bowel above the obstruction are fluid faecal material and gas, much of which consists of swallowed air. Distension is a vitally important factor. The effect of prolonged, increased intraluminal pressure is to impair the viability of the bowel wall, and under these conditions toxic bacterial products diffuse into the peritoneal cavity where they are absorbed and produce toxaemia and death. It is unlikely that the intestinal contents in an obstructed gut are more toxic than those normally present, and it has been shown experimentally that the intestinal contents from normal and obstructed dogs are equally toxic when given parenterally. Death in low obstruction is thus ultimately due to the distension and if this can be relieved by intubation, the life of the patient may be prolonged long enough to allow surgical intervention.

The fluid lost—through intubation and ileal drainage—is predominantly alkaline, and this leads to acidosis with a low CO_2 combining power. In addition to sodium and chloride the patient should receive lactate or bicarbonate parenterally. Depletion of potassium may also result from loss in the intestinal secretions, and lead to weakness and even muscular paralysis, thus aggravating the state of ileus. Since potassium is chiefly an intracellular cation, the amount present *in the plasma* at any moment may not accurately reflect the state of the cells and caution must be exercised in interpreting the results of biochemical analysis of plasma as the basis for potassium replacement.

Partial chronic obstruction of the large intestine. Here the wall above, in addition to becoming distended with faeces, undergoes hypertrophy in a varying degree. The pressure of the faecal accumulation on the distended wall interferes with the blood supply and impairs the nutrition, and hence bacterial invasion may occur and an exudate may form on the mucous surface. In other cases the stretched mucosa gives way and so-called "stercoral ulcers" form. Perforation of such an ulcer may occur, and in a case of chronic stricture may be at some distance above the obstruction. Thus perforation of the caecum may occur in cases of carcinoma of the sigmoid colon. The large intestine tolerates obstruction much better than the small intestine, and chronic stricture may lead to complete obstruction for some days with comparatively slight symptoms.

In obstruction with strangulation the viability of the bowel wall is impaired early and its permeability is therefore increased. If unrelieved, death results rapidly from toxic absorption and peritonitis. A strangulating intestinal obstruction is therefore always an acute surgical emergency.

Vascular causes. Apart from strangulation these are chiefly embolism or thrombosis of the superior mesenteric artery, but thrombosis of the mesenteric veins will produce the same result. This is sometimes seen when a thrombus occluding the portal vein extends backwards to obstruct the mouths of the splenic and superior mesenteric veins. Haemorrhagic infarction with gangrene of a segment of bowel quickly supervenes, and death follows from toxic absorption and peritonitis.

Obstruction due to nervous causes: paralytic or adynamic ileus. In this condition the motor activity of the bowel is impaired without the presence of a physical obstruction. Sometimes it is due to over-activity of the sympathetic nervous system, and may then be relieved by antagonistic drugs, but in other cases toxic damage to the bowel muscle causes the paralysis. Lowering of the potassium level of the plasma greatly aggravates the condition. It is seen most often in association with peritonitis or it may follow operations on the abdomen, frequently of a minor nature. It may result also from intestinal infections or severe toxaemia. The whole intestine may be implicated and there may be a great distension of the bowel. The condition is serious and if untreated will result in death in much the same way as in acute mechanical obstruction. The advent of intestinal intubation has improved the outlook—once the distended bowel is decompressed its contractility may return, and intubation enables restoration of the electrolyte balance to be achieved more quickly.

Hernia

The term really means a rupture, but it is applied to any protrusion of a portion of viscus outside its natural cavity. Protrusion of the bowel usually occurs in a pouch of the peritoneum, which projects on the surface of the body, forming an *external hernia*. The term *internal hernia* is applied when the swelling does not present to an external surface. In the occurrence of hernia two prime factors are concerned, *local weakness* and *increased pressure*, the latter being usually brought about by muscular exertion, coughing or straining at stool. The local weakness is usually congenital, notably at the umbilicus or the inguinal canal; occasionally it results from the stretching of the scar of an operation wound—*incisional hernia*.

Of the *external* types of hernia, the commonest are the *inguinal, femoral* and *umbilical*. Others, less common, are the *ventral*—through any portion of the abdominal wall other than the sites mentioned—*obturator*, etc. The inguinal herniae are of two varieties, the indirect, where the hernia follows the inguinal canal lateral to the inferior epigastric artery, and the direct, which passes medial to the latter vessel and comes through the external abdominal ring. The femoral hernia passes under Poupart's ligament medial to the femoral vessels. Examples of *internal* hernia are seen when the protrusion occurs through an aperture in the diaphragm, through the foramen of Winslow, or into a pouch in the jejuno-duodenal fossa, the pouch then passing behind the peritoneum. In the ordinary external herniae, the contents are usually a portion of small intestine, though in the larger ones omentum or other structures may be present. So long as it is possible to return the contents into the abdominal cavity, the hernia is termed "reducible". When this is impossible owing either to the bulk of the contents or to adhesions which have formed, the hernia is said to be incarcerated.

The most serious result of hernia is strangulation, seen when the circulation in the protruded bowel is interrupted. This may occur by the addition of a fresh loop of bowel to the sac or by accumulation of faeces and gas. Strangulation may develop when the hernia is first formed, a portion of bowel being forced into a tight aperture; this is not uncommon in a femoral hernia. The changes following strangulation have already been described (p. 528).

Intussusception

This is a condition in which one portion of the bowel is pushed down or invaginated into the portion below. This often happens in the small intestine in children at the time of death, and several intussusceptions may be present owing to irregular contraction of the bowel; the term *agonal intussusception* is applied, but it is of no clinical importance.

Intussusception may, however, occur in health and lead to very serious results; here again it is observed chiefly in infants and young children. Irregular contraction and spasm of the intestinal wall are thought to be the chief factors concerned. Recently the mesenteric lymph nodes and intestinal contents of infants with intussusception have been found commonly to harbour ECHO, adeno- or other viruses. These may play a part in causing the lesion by producing such swelling of the Peyer's patches that they act like polyps over which the intestine contracts and which it then endeavours to pass along like a foreign body. The intestinal wall is thus drawn in and intussusception results. A Meckel's diverticulum or a true polyp of any type also acts in this way.

Naked-eye appearances. In intussusception of the ordinary type three layers of bowel are seen on section, two layers formed by the doubling of the bowel invaginated, and one layer consisting of the wall of the bowel into which the intussusception has occurred. Thus it consists of four parts, (1) the apex, (2) an entering tube, (3) a returning tube, and (4) an ensheathing tube. The commonest site is at the ileo-caecal valve, and usually the valve forms the apex of the intussusception and is passed along the large intestine (Fig. 18.67). The apex

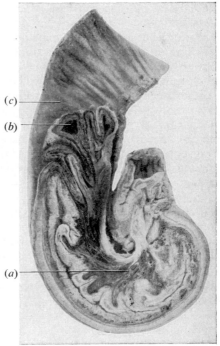

Fig. 18.67.—Longitudinal section of ileo-caecal intussusception.

(*a*) Mesentery drawn in and haemorrhagic, (*b*) apex of intussusception, and (*c*) colon. (J. W. S. B.) × ⅔.

may ultimately reach the rectum, and the bowel affected forms a fairly firm sausage-shaped mass, which is palpable during life. This type of intussusception is called *ileo-caecal*. More rarely the small intestine is passed through the orifice into the colon—*ileo-colic* type—and there may also be combinations of these two types with more complicated invaginations. For example, the ileo-caecal valve may be passed along for only a short distance, so that the tip of the appendix may be still visible, and then coils of the small intestine may be passed down through the valve and firmly impacted. Intussusception occurs in other situations, for example, in the small intestine or the transverse colon, but it is comparatively rare. Intussusception of the appendix has been recorded, but it is very rare; it occurs chiefly in children.

Results. The important effects of intussusception are interference with the blood supply and mechanical obstruction of the bowel. The vessels of the invaginated part are pulled upon and also constricted; intense venous engorgement is the result, and this is followed by diffuse haemorrhage into the tissues of the bowel. Accordingly the passage *per anum* of a mixture of blood and mucus is a common sign of intussusception, but pure blood may be passed. Following upon the haemorrhagic infarction of the bowel, necrosis takes place and the part undergoes gangrenous softening. It will be noted that, at the upper part of the intussusception, the serous surface of the invaginated part is in contact with that of the bowel receiving the invagination. At this point adhesions may form and prevent extension of organisms to the peritoneum. The dead tissue of the invaginated bowel may gradually slough away and a process of natural cure follow. In most cases, however, death occurs from obstruction or from organisms gaining access to the peritoneum and causing a diffuse peritonitis. When a favourable result follows without operation, portions of sloughs from the dead bowel may be passed for a considerable time after the intussusception has occurred.

Volvulus

This is a condition in which a loop of bowel is twisted or rotated through two right angles or more, so that obstruction and a varying degree of strangulation result (Fig. 18.68). It is most apt to occur when a loop has a long attachment and the ends are comparatively close together; rotation is then facilitated. Most cases involve the sigmoid colon, and the occurrence of the volvulus is aided by a long mesocolon and by a loaded sigmoid due to constipation. Usually the upper part of the sigmoid passes forwards and downwards to lie in front of the upper part of the rectum. Once the twist has occurred, passage of faeces is prevented. The bowel becomes more and more distended, the venous return is interfered with, and the wall becomes

congested and haemorrhagic; ultimately it may become almost black. In some cases a portion of bowel is found to be enormously distended, filling a large part of the abdominal cavity. Volvulus of the small intestine may occur also, but it is less common; the favouring conditions are the same, and sometimes the approximation of the ends of the loop is due to local adhesions around calcified mesenteric lymph nodes. In children, however, volvulus of the small bowel is much commoner than

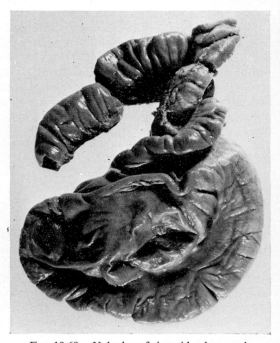

Fig. 18.68.—Volvulus of sigmoid colon. × ⅓.

in adults. More rarely two loops of intestine become intertwined and then the symptoms are very severe.

Intestinal obstruction due to foreign body

The most common cause of this type of obstruction is a large composite gallstone, which has entered the duodenum through a fistulous track developing between gallbladder and bowel; commonly there is little or no history of symptoms to indicate cholelithiasis. The calculus passes along the intestine but may become impacted at some point, this being aided by spastic contraction of the bowel, as even the largest stones is smaller than the diameter of the fully relaxed bowel. In our experience the point of impaction is usually about a metre proximal to the ileocaecal valve, corresponding roughly to the site of the omphalo-mesenteric duct. Unmasticated food may act similarly, for example obstruction of the ileum by a mass of dried fruit. Gastro-enterostomy predisposes to the passage of large masses of undigested food into the intestine, with resulting obstruction.

Hirschsprung's disease

This is a rare condition seen in the earlier years of life and apparently of congenital origin; it is distinguished from other forms of megacolon in infancy on clinical and radiological grounds. It is characterised by an enormous distension and enlargement of the colon which then forms a large portion of the abdominal contents and gives rise to great swelling from accumulation of faeces, which may be voided only at considerable intervals. Repeated attacks of obstruction are common. The distension may extend as far as the caecum, but at first affects mainly the lower colon. In true Hirschsprung's disease the rectum is not involved in the distension and the grossly hypertrophied and dilated colon tapers rather abruptly into a narrow segment joining sigmoid to anus. There is congenital absence of the para-sympathetic ganglion cells of both Auerbach's and Meissner's plexuses for a distance of 5–20 cm. below the dilated sigmoid, i.e. corresponding to the narrow segment of rectum. In consequence there is overaction of the sympathetic, which normally inhibits the propulsive contraction of the intestinal wall and stimulates contraction of the internal anal sphincter. The disease is thus one of neuromuscular inco-ordination. While lumbar sympathectomy has proved helpful in some cases, the results have not always been permanent and excision of the defective narrow segment and anastomosis of the sigmoid to the anus has proved more effective.

Tumours of the intestines

Benign tumours. Leiomyoma and lipoma are the least rare in both small and large bowels. Leiomyoma may present on the mucosal surface and ulcerate, resembling in appearance a fungating carcinoma. Multiple tumours sometimes occur. Both haemangioma and lymphangioma (Fig. 12.23, p. 254) also occur, and may be multiple. These simple connective tissue growths may be subserous or submucous in position, and like the much commoner adenomatous growths of the colon to be described, they may become polypoid and may give rise to an intussusception (p. 529).

Small Intestine

Epithelial neoplasms of the small bowel are rare, forming less than 2 per cent of all intestinal tumours. Three distinct types are, however, worthy of mention.

(a) The Peutz-Jeghers syndrome. This interesting hereditary disorder is transmitted as a Mendelian dominant of high penetrance. Multiple polypi of highly differentiated structure are found in the small intestine, especially the jejunum, and are associated with pronounced melanotic pigmentation of the lips and oral mucosa which is the key to diagnosis. The polyps cause recurring attacks of intussusception and sometimes iron deficiency anaemia due to blood loss, but rarely if ever undergo malignant transformation; indeed they are perhaps better regarded as hamartomatous (p. 250) rather than truly neoplastic in nature.

Carcinoma. This is surprisingly uncommon in the small bowel, being scarcely more frequently encountered than lymphoid tumours. Length for length, the proximal parts of the small bowel are more often affected than the distal, and we have seen several examples in the duodenum. In appearance and behaviour carcinomas of the small intestine are very similar to those of the colon (p. 535). Intestinal obstruction and the effects of haemorrhage are the most common modes of presentation; curative surgical treatment is often not possible, however, since the tumour growth is commonly in an advanced stage when diagnosed. The causal factors are unknown, although occasionally carcinoma arises as a complication of a primary malabsorptive disorder.

Carcinoid tumour: argentaffinoma

This interesting tumour arises from the argentaffin cells of Kulschitsky in the base of

S

the crypts of Lieberkühn. They were named *carcinoids* because in their commonest site in the appendix they are clinically benign in spite of the appearance of infiltration. They occur occasionally in the stomach, frequently in the ileum

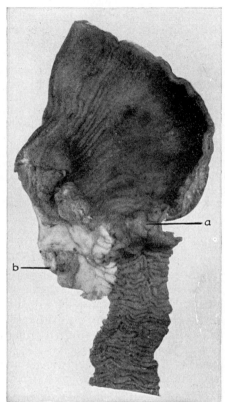

FIG. 18.69.—Argentaffinoma of ileum causing obstruction. × ½.

Note dilatation and hypertrophy of bowel above the tumour (*a*) and secondary deposit in the mesenteric lymph node (*b*).

and rarely in the rectum. In the routine examination of appendices removed surgically it is not uncommon to find at the tip a yellowish-brown nodule of carcinoid a few millimetres in diameter, or even filling the distal lumen. In the small intestine, especially in the lower ileum, carcinoids are commonly multiple. They form small button-like swellings in the mucosa one or more of which shows deep penetration of the muscular wall which may be locally hypertrophied (Fig. 18.70). Lymphatic invasion is often widespread in the affected segment. Ileal carcinoids are not benign like those in the appendix, and as a consequence both intestinal obstruction (Fig. 18.69) and metastases to the mesenteric lymph nodes and

liver occur; characteristically these secondary deposits grow exceedingly slowly.

Microscopically. Carcinoid tumours consist of small clear cells, closely packed in alveolar formation (Fig. 18.71), throughout the whole thickness of the appendicular or ileal wall. The yellowish colour is due to the presence of lipids, some of which are doubly refracting. The tumour cells contain granules which reduce silver salts—hence called argentaffin cells. In the appendix, carcinoid tumours are commonly related to old inflammatory lesions and the cells are often associated with proliferated nerve fibres.

The carcinoid syndrome. Massive hepatic secondary growths of carcinoid tumours are sometimes, but not invariably, accompanied by a remarkable clinical syndrome characterised by flushing, diarrhoea, asthmatic symptoms and cardiac disease, especially pulmonary stenosis. These effects are largely, but not exclusively, due to the secretion of large amounts of

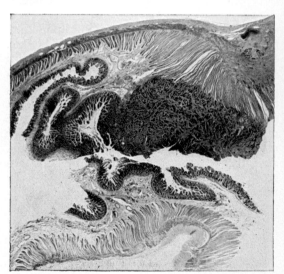

FIG. 18.70.—Carcinoid tumour of ileum, showing stenosis of lumen and great hypertrophy of circular muscle coat. There were hepatic metastases and the carcinoid syndrome developed. × 2·5.

5-hydroxytryptamine (5HT) by metastatic tumour cells in the liver. 5HT is inactivated by amine oxidase in the liver cells, and so long as the tumour is confined to the drainage area of the portal circulation systemic effects are not produced. Massive hepatic metastases, however, set free 5HT into the systemic circulation. 5HT is a potent vasodilator, and smooth-muscle stimulant; it may also stimulate fibroblastic proliferation, which is possibly the cause of the subendocardial fibrosis in the right atrium and ventricle. This leads ultimately to pulmonary stenosis, observed in the later phases of the syndrome. The left side of the heart is less often involved, since 5HT is inactivated also in the lungs. Excessive diversion of tryptophane to the

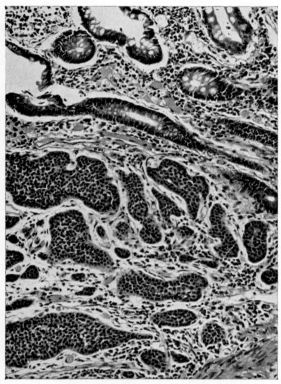

FIG. 18.71.—Carcinoid tumour of ileum, showing clumps of small polygonal epithelial cells in alveolar spaces infiltrating the mucosa. × 125.

metabolism of massive secondary deposits may induce symptoms of pellagra. 5HT is converted by the enzyme amine-oxidase to 5-hydroxy-indole-acetic acid (5HIAA), which is excreted in the urine where its quantitative estimation affords a valuable clinical test for the presence of massive argentaffin tumours. It should be noted, however, that the flushing attacks, often precipitated by alcohol or sympathetic stimulation, may be due to other secretory products of the argentaffin cell, especially kallikrein, a proteolytic enzyme which releases the vasoactive polypeptide bradykinin from its circulating inactive precursor.

Carcinoid tumours arising from endodermal tissues outwith the small intestine may be atypical both morphologically and with regard to secretory activity. Many, for example, do not exhibit the true argentaffin reaction, and only take up the silver stain when an external reducing agent is applied (argyrophilia). Other carcinoid tumours, e.g. those arising from the bronchi (p. 379), secrete 5-hydroxy-tryptophane, possibly because they lack the enzyme decarboxylase required to convert this substance to 5HT. Carcinoids of the stomach may also secrete histamine in addition to 5HT and kallikrein. Rectal carcinoid tumours rarely give rise to the syndrome.

Lymphoid neoplasms

Although generalised forms of lymphoma may metastasise to the intestinal tract, it is important to realise that lymphomas may arise primarily in the small intestine, where they are at least as common as carcinomas. These primary intestinal lymphomas, which may be multiple, frequently cause perforation, less often intestinal obstruction; most are found to be reticulosarcomas or lymphosarcomas, although plasma-cell tumours may also be encountered. Malabsorption is sometimes a feature, and it has been suggested that gluten enteropathy (p. 525) predisposes to the development of lymphoid neoplasia, and occasionally carcinoma.

Tumours of the large intestine

This is a very common site of simple epithelial tumours of which two principal types are recognised.

(a) Villous papilloma occurs chiefly in the rectum; it forms a sessile usually solitary tumour with a frond-like structure (Fig. 18.72). The base may occupy a considerable area of the colonic mucosa and the growth may secrete a large amount of watery mucoid fluid which is sometimes so rich in potassium that muscular weakness and paresis result from hypokalaemia.

(b) Polypoid adenoma is the commonest simple tumour of the large bowel. In the adult, its age incidence and distribution in the large intestine are similar to those of carcinoma. Thus the recto-sigmoid region is the most common site, followed by the caecum and ascending colon. They usually have a lobulated or globular shape with a narrow pedicle (Fig. 11.6, p. 231). Histologically the epithelial cells show pronounced

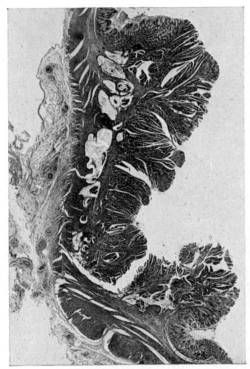

FIG. 18.72.—Villous papilloma of rectum. There is early malignant infiltration of the wall by mucoid carcinoma. × 3.

de-differentiation and hyperchromatism, expecially towards the tip of the polyp. Provided such changes (which might otherwise be regarded as malignant do not involve the pedicle of the polyp, simple excision by transection of the base is an effective form of treatment. Even so there is considerable circumstantial evidence that the presence of these tumours, which are often multiple, predisposes to the development of carcinoma, with which they are often associated. This relationship is particularly strong in the hereditary condition polyposis coli.

Polyposis coli. This hereditary disorder is usually transmitted by either sex as a Mendelian dominant but in some families either with very poor penetrance or as a recessive character. It is characterised by the development of hundreds of adenomatous polyps in the large intestine (Fig. 18.73). The condition is not usually manifested until late childhood or early adult life. Since

each of the many polyps appears to share the predisposition to become malignant, the onset of carcinoma of the colon is almost inevitable, usually about 15 years after the development of symptoms of polyposis.

Other polypoid lesions are encountered in the large bowel, and are not to be confused with the true tumours already described. The *metaplastic polyp* is a small, raised, pale, sessile lesion not infrequently encountered in middle or later adult life. Histologically there is localised papilliform hyperplasia of the epithelium lining the surface and upper parts of the crypts. This lesion lacks the hyperchromatism of the polypoid adenoma and does not appear to be pre-malignant. In childhood globular polypoid lesions, sometimes

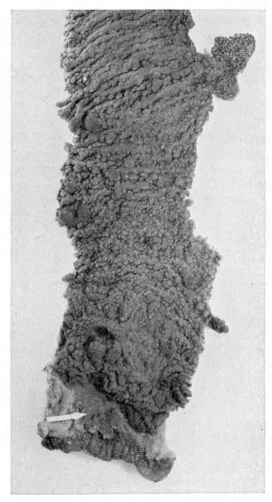

FIG. 18.73.—Polyposis coli. Innumerable small polyps and several larger ones are present. Two small cancers have developed just above the anal margin. × ⅔.

quite large, are encountered in the rectum: histologically they consist of intensely inflamed mucosa in which the crypts are markedly dilated and cystic, and are frequently ulcerated. Usually referred to as *juvenile polyps*, they do not show epithelial de-differentiation and are probably inflammatory in nature. Apart from polyposis coli, true adenomatous polyps are seldom observed in children. Finally, mention must be made of the condition known as *benign lymphoid polyposis of the rectum*, in which multiple polypi, consisting of masses of lymphoid tissue, showing numerous germinal centres and covered by normal rectal epithelium, develop in the rectum especially in young women. The condition is of unknown causation but, as the name implies, does not have malignant potential.

Carcinoma of the large intestine

This is one of the commoner malignant tumours. It occurs mainly amongst older people. The rectum is the commonest site, especially in males; next follows the sigmoid colon, the caecum and ileo-caecal valve and the flexures. The overall incidence is about the same for males and females.

Etiology. For the most part this is unknown, although carcinoma of the large bowel is principally a disease of urban communities. Three conditions already discussed are regarded as precancerous states, namely simple polypoid adenoma (especially polyposis coli), villous papilloma and ulcerative colitis. In ulcerative colitis, and in polyposis coli, carcinoma tends to develop 10–15 years after the onset and thus may affect relatively young individuals.

Naked-eye appearances. When carcinoma begins in an adenomatous polyp, infiltration of the stalk and base occurs so that the growth appears like a button fixed to the bowel wall; subsequently the centre breaks down leaving a necrotic ulcer with raised everted ("rolled") edges. The base is then fixed to the muscular coat, which is ultimately breached by progressive ulceration. Spread in the submucous and subserous lymphatics also occurs (Fig. 18.74) so that the growth gradually encircles the bowel wall. The majority of cancers of the colon are of the scirrhous type, resulting in some degree of contraction and stricture; some, however, are soft and fungating, and others are mucoid and gelatinous. The

more slowly growing types have a great tendency to encircle the bowel, forming a ring-shaped growth and thus producing narrowing or complete obstruction. The bowel above the obstruction undergoes great, sometimes enormous

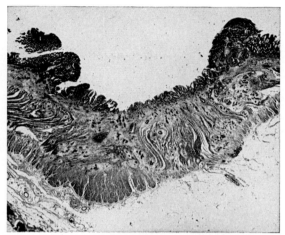

FIG. 18.74.—Ulcerating adenocarcinoma of colon, showing the rolled-over edge and the widespread permeation of the lymphatics in the wall. × 4·5.

dilatation, while its wall becomes hypertrophied (Fig. 18.75). The pressure of the contained faeces interferes with the nourishment of the mucosa and a pseudo-membranous inflammation may be superadded. In other cases, the wall becomes thinned and a so-called stercoral ulceration may follow, and may undergo perforation with resulting peritonitis. The softer type of cancer forms an irregular mass which in its turn may bring about obstruction by projecting into the lumen (Fig. 18.76). The mucoid type may, as in the stomach, lead to widespread infiltration and thickening of the wall, and may give rise to secondary growths in the peritoneum. It is of interest to note that this type of cancer is sometimes seen in the earlier years of adult life.

Microscopic appearances. Practically all intestinal cancers are adenocarcinomas, some being highly differentiated, while others are anaplastic and the arrangement of the cells is irregular (Fig. 11.12, p. 235). This is the usual variety that complicates ulcerative colitis.

In cases of cancer of colon and rectum, invasion of the lymphatics takes place at an early period, while secondary growths in the liver usually occur relatively late. This is of importance in surgical treatment. The tumour occasionally spreads to the peritoneum, and results similar to those described in the case of the stomach are produced. Squamous carcinoma may occur in the mucosa of the anal canal, and tumours containing both squamous and adeno-

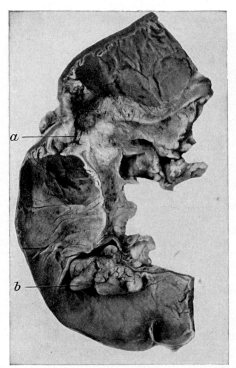

FIG. 18.75.—Carcinomatous stricture (*a*) of colon. × ⅔.
Note the hypertrophy of the wall above; below there is a simple polypoid adenoma (*b*).

carcinomatous elements are occasionally seen. True carcinoma may originate in the appendix, but this is very rare.

Sarcoma

Sarcoma of the intestine is comparatively rare, the commonest form being *lymphosarcoma* (Fig. 18.77). We have observed several examples taking origin in the ileo-caecal region, in young people, where it forms a bulky mass causing rapidly progressive obstruction. Sometimes the growth is diffuse, converting a considerable length of bowel into a rigid tube. There is diffuse infiltration of the mucosa and submucosa with soft whitish tumour. The coats being much thickened, and ulceration follows. Another type is that in which multiple

foci of apparently independent growth occur; these become ulcerated and deeply excavated (Fig. 18.78) so that localised perforation occurs. This lesion may be difficult to recognise as neoplastic and is commonly mistaken for an inflammatory lesion; repeated perforations may occur, requiring multiple resections. Ultimately widespread dissemination occurs, the mesenteric lymph nodes are extensively involved and become enormously enlarged, the whole condition being described as *intestinal lymphosarcomatosis*. Sarcoma of spindle-celled type is also encountered. Some appear to arise in leiomyomas, others in neurofibromas; both tend to become pedunculated, and may bleed severely.

Secondary tumours

Secondary growths in the intestine, apart from invasion by way of the peritoneum or lymphatic spread, are extremely uncommon though metastatic melanoma is seen occasionally, and also

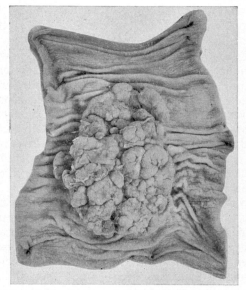

FIG. 18.76.—Large polypoid adenocarcinoma of descending colon. × ⅔.

the lymphoid neoplasm *struma reticulosa* of the thyroid (p. 897) has a notable tendency to metastasise to the gut. The peritoneum is a common site for secondary carcinoma (p. 541) and the bowel may become invaded from the serous surface and its lumen considerably contracted.

Congenital abnormalities

The commonest of these is the Meckel's diverticulum, which represents the proximal end of the omphalomesenteric duct. The diverticulum usually measures about 2–3 cm. in length, and is somewhat narrower than the small intestine. Occasionally it is adherent at the umbilicus and in some cases a fistula is present; or again, there may be obstruction at the proximal end, sometimes merely by a fold, and accumulation of mucus occurs so that an *enterocyst* results. A Meckel's diverticulum rarely leads to any serious results, but when it is adherent it may cause volvulus of the small intestine or, even more serious, strangulation. Acute inflammation of a Meckel's diverticulum presents features similar to those of acute appendicitis, and requires similar surgical treatment. Sometimes heterotopic acid-secreting gastric mucosa is present and may lead to peptic ulceration of the diverticulum with perforation or haemorrhage. In the adult the diverticulum occurs usually about a metre above the ileo-caecal valve, and at about half that distance in young children. Carcinoma has very rarely been observed to develop in the apex of a Meckel's diverticulum.

Stenosis or actual *atresia* may occasionally occur in the intestines. In the small intestine, the commonest site is at the orifice of the common bile duct or at the ileo-caecal valve. Occasionally a part of the intestine is completely absent, a condition which is usually associated with other malformations. The commonest site of atresia, however, is at the lower end of the rectum. Sometimes a dimple in the skin, representing the anus, is separated from the lower end of the rectum by a thin layer of tissue—the condition being known as *imperforate anus*. In other

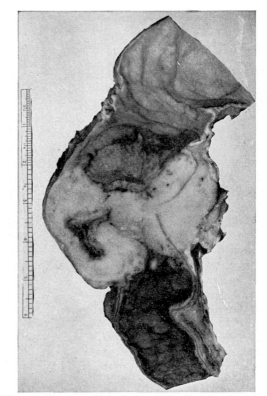

FIG. 18.77.—Lymphosarcoma of the ileo-caecal region. × ⅔.

cases, however, the lower end of the rectum may be absent for some distance—*atresia recti*. In association with the latter condition, there may also be a fistulous opening between the lower end of the bowel and the bladder or urethra in the male; in the female the communication is with the vagina.

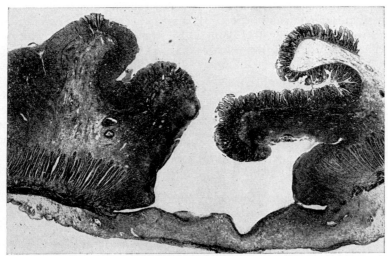

FIG. 18.78.—Lymphosarcoma of small intestine, showing deep but sharply localised ulcerative penetration of the wall. × 6·5.

THE PERITONEUM

Acute peritonitis

Infection of the peritoneum by organisms takes place in a great variety of ways and the effects are of all degrees of severity. The resulting lesion may be a relatively slight inflammation in a restricted area, the exudate afterwards becoming absorbed or undergoing organisation to form fibrous adhesions. This is especially liable to happen if at operation the peritoneal surfaces are contaminated by surgical talc (Fig. 2.18, p. 49), the siliceous particles exercising a powerfully irritating effect in some cases, and preventing resolution and absorption of fibrinous exudate between loops of bowel and so tending to provoke intestinal obstruction (p. 526), with all its dangerous complications. In other cases, however, virulent organisms rapidly invade the peritoneal sac widely, and lead to death, even when inflammatory changes are at an early stage. At a necropsy in such a case, the intestines are usually in a state of paralytic distension and contain much fluid material and gas. The bacterial toxins apparently act on the muscle directly and lead to the dilatation, whilst absorption by the bowel is interfered with. At the same time there is probably increased secretion leading to accumulation of fluid. The surface of the bowel is intensely congested, small haemorrhages are present, the serosa is dull, and the coils are stuck together by flakes and strands of fibrin. Fluid exudate may also be present, especially posteriorly and in the pelvic cavity, but the amount and type of exudate vary greatly. Sometimes there is merely a blood-stained turbid fluid, in which there are swarms of bacteria; such a condition may occur in streptococcal and in mixed infections. The profound toxaemia and rapidly fatal collapse can be readily understood, because not only is the area of bacterial multiplication extensive but also absorption takes place rapidly from the peritoneal cavity both by blood vessels and by the lymphatics of the diaphragm. In some cases the organisms give rise to septicaemia. While the general effects in peritonitis are chiefly the result of toxic absorption, symptoms are also due to the paralytic ileus which occurs in varying degree.

In acute peritonitis there is evidence of marked toxic cellular injury in the various organs throughout the body and in the liver this not infrequently amounts to zonal necrosis (Fig. 19.5, p. 550).

Varieties. The varieties of peritonitis, described according to the characters of the exudate as *serous, fibrinous, haemorrhagic, fibrinopurulent* and *suppurative*, correspond with those seen in other serous sacs, and accordingly do not need to be described in detail. There is, however, a special form of peritonitis, resulting from perforation, in which gastric, intestinal or biliary contents escape into the cavity. In such cases a varying amount of the escaped material is found mixed with a serous or haemorrhagic exudate with numerous bacteria. Gastroduodenal perforation is usually accompanied by symptoms of shock, but perforation of a typhoid ulcer may be almost silent clinically.

One point of importance in connection with the peritoneum as compared with other sacs is that, owing to the complicated arrangement of the serous membrane, the inflammatory process may either remain localised or it may become generalised. The resulting effects are very different in the two cases. The peritoneum, by virtue of the cells which pass into it, has great powers of resisting bacterial invasion, but once bacteria have gained a foothold there they may spread and infect a large surface. The spread is often prevented by fibrinous adhesions, aided by immobility of the abdominal wall and a varying degree of local paralysis of the intestine.

Predisposing conditions. Some of these have already been noted in connection with lesions of the stomach and bowel, and others will be referred to later, especially in relation to diseases of the female genital tract. The causes are very numerous but the sources of infection may be conveniently arranged in three main groups: (*a*) lesions of the alimentary tract, (*b*) lesions of the pelvic organs, and (*c*) lesions of the solid viscera, retro-peritoneal tissue, etc.

(*a*) In the majority of cases of acute peritonitis, the bacteria reach the peritoneum from a lesion of a hollow viscus, usually the stomach or the bowel, but occasionally the gallbladder. This occurs in such conditions as peptic ulcer, typhoid, dysentery, ulcerated tumours, stercoral ulcers (p. 528), whilst acute appendicitis is the commonest cause of all. Accordingly, in investigating any case of peritonitis at necropsy, all these parts must be carefully examined. There is also the whole group of cases where there is some mechanical interference with the bowel, e.g. strangulated hernia and intussusception, as has already been described. Peritonitis may also occur secondarily in infarction of the small intestine due to occlusion of the superior mesenteric artery. If these lesions are considered as a whole, it is to be noted that in some cases there is actual *perforation*, whilst in others the bacteria reached the peritoneum by spread through the wall at the site of the lesion. Acute peritonitis in connection with an inflamed gallbladder, for example, occurs in both these ways. Lymphatic extension with localised peritonitis is the more common, but occasionally rupture of a necrotic portion of the wall takes place and the contents escape; a fatal general peritonitis then usually results. A similar statement applies to the urinary bladder affected by septic cystitis.

(*b*) Peritonitis extending from the pelvic organs takes origin most frequently in infections of the female genital tract. Here there are two chief modes of spread, namely, (1) by direct extension from the serous covering of a viscus, and (2) by way of the Fallopian tubes. Although in most cases the mode of extension of the inflammatory process can be traced, this may sometimes not be possible. Peritonitis may occur secondarily to gonorrhoeal salpingitis; it is usually a local acute condition which often leads to adhesions, but occasionally localised suppuration may follow. Various other inflammatory conditions of the uterus and tubes may lead to peritonitis, the most important occuring during the puerperium. These are often caused by streptococci and in the absence of specific treatment are sometimes rapidly fatal. Peritonitis due to pneumococcus is not infrequently observed in children. It is more common in the female sex, the infection taking place by way of the genital tract. In most cases the pneumococci belong to types I and II. Again, peritonitis, either localised or general, may arise in connection with septic cystitis, this occurrence being commoner in the male sex.

(*c*) Peritonitis due to infection from solid viscera is less common, but there are a considerable number of lesions which may give rise to it. For example, suppuration in the liver, haemorrhagic pancreatitis, septic infarction of the spleen, a ruptured mesenteric lymph node in typhoid fever and extra-peritoneal suppuration. As a rule, in such cases the origin of the infection can be readily traced.

Haematogenous infection of the peritoneum also occurs, but is much rarer than in the other serous sacs. It is seen occasionally in septicaemia and infective fevers, but the possibility of spread of the organisms from a local source must always be considered.

Many types of bacteria may cause peritonitis, including the pyogens, *S. typhi*, *Proteus sp.*, and various anaerobes from the gut. However, when infection originates from the alimentary tract without perforation, bacilli of the coli group and streptococci are most frequently concerned; and many of the most acute cases are due to the latter, though the virulence varies greatly. The effects of *Esch. coli* are usually less severe, and a diffuse suppurative peritonitis due to this organism may exist for some time before causing death.

Chronic peritonitis

This is usually localised in distribution; it may occur secondarily to an acute attack, a common variety being the development of a subphrenic abscess after perforation of a hollow viscus, usually due to peptic ulceration: air from the perforated viscus lies between the liver and the diaphragm, as is shown clinically by the loss of liver dullness. Gastric contents containing bacteria then become lodged in the subphrenic space thus created. Later the air is absorbed, the surfaces again come in contact and are first glued together by fibrin, thus walling off the inflamed site. Suppuration then occurs around the infected material and the resulting collection of pus constitutes a subphrenic abscess. A similar condition occurs more rarely as a sequel to an appendix abscess (p. 511). Peritonitis may be chronic from the beginning, as a result of extension of infection of a chronic nature from a viscus—for example, chronic cholecystitis. It is common also as a result of peritoneal invasion by carcinoma and is a well-marked feature in tuberculosis of the peritoneum, as described below.

Chronic hyperplastic peritonitis. This is a comparatively rare condition in which, along with adhesions between the viscera, there occurs great hyaline thickening of the visceral peritoneum. The distribution of the lesion varies considerably, but the liver is often specially affected and may be covered by smooth, shiny laminated connective tissue of whitish appearance, which at places may reach half an inch in thickness or even more. The term "sugar-iced liver" (Zuckergussleber) has been applied. The thickening may be attended by a certain amount of subcapsular fibrosis and occasionally there is more extensive hepatic fibrosis. A similar change may occur on the surface of the spleen and there is often fibrous thickening with retraction of the omentum and mesentery. The chief effect is an intractable ascites requiring repeated tappings. Such a condition is often associated with similar changes in the pericardium, pleurae and mediastinal tissues, and great thickening of the serous membranes, especially of the lower parts of the pleurae, may be present—polyserositis. (Other names have been applied, e.g. *Concato's disease* when all the serous sacs are involved, *Pick's disease* when the pericardium and peritoneum over the liver are implicated; but these seem to be merely varieties of the same condition.) Microscopic examination of the thickened area shows merely laminated hyaline connective tissue in a relatively avascular state. With regard to the etiology, it is not possible to say anything definite but in *Pick's disease* tuberculosis is thought to be responsible in some cases. Rheumatism or chronic renal disease have been associated with some cases.

In the *carcinoid syndrome* (p. 532) there may be a very striking diffuse fibrous thickening of the peritoneum especially that covering the posterior abdominal wall, but extending also to other parts. This has been attributed to the action of 5-hydroxytryptamine in liberating histamine from the tissue mast cells, the resultant increase of capillary permeability and consequent increased protein in the tissue fluid exerting a stimulating influence on the fibrocytes.

Tuberculous peritonitis is much less common than formerly: it may be general or localised. The origin of the generalised type may be a caseous lymph node in tabes mesenterica, or the bacilli may reach the peritoneum from a tuberculous Fallopian tube, either directly through its covering or by way of its abdominal opening. In other cases where no gross lesion can be found, the infection is probably by the blood-stream, a small focus forming from which dissemination afterwards occurs. The appearances vary widely in different cases. There may be an eruption of minute grey tubercles all over the peritoneum, with or without a sero-fibrinous effusion. The omentum is often extensively involved and forms a large mass across the upper part of the abdomen. In other cases, there may be caseation, either in scattered foci or diffusely. Lastly, cases are encountered in which the tubercles are comparatively scanty and where the chief result is formation of adhesions, sometimes with serous effusion between them. When chronic tuberculous peritonitis is associated with ulcers of the intestine, ulceration between adjacent loops of the bowel may lead to the formation of multiple fistulae, and may result in the malabsorption syndrome.

Ascites

Serous effusion into the peritoneum occurs in cases of general oedema of both the cardiac and renal types, and is sometimes abundant; some fluid may accumulate also in severe anaemias and wasting diseases. The most severe ascites, however, results from portal obstruction, and the accumulation of fluid often leads to enormous distension of the abdomen: the commonest cause is cirrhosis of the liver, and in cases which develop primary liver cancer thrombosis of the portal vein often occurs, the ascitic fluid then accumulating very rapidly and becoming bloodstained. Ascites *may* sometimes result from conditions outside the liver which lead to pressure on the portal vein, such as tumour growth, chronic inflammation with contraction, etc., but it does not necessarily follow them, and in portal vein thrombosis with cavernous transformation there may be little or no ascites. Ascites is always most severe and intractable when the site of obstruction is intra-hepatic, as in portal cirrhosis. Thus endophlebitis of the hepatic veins (Chiari's syndrome) is accompanied by pronounced ascites. In the above conditions the fluid is a transudate and there is no formation of fibrin in the peritoneum, but in cases of portal cirrhosis it is not uncommon for a mild infection to become superadded, and occasionally this is tuberculous. Ascites may also result from some lesion of the peritoneum—for example, disseminated carcinoma or tuberculosis; in such cases there is usually an inflammatory reaction and the fluid is at least partly an inflammatory exudate, though the protein content is relatively small,

Polymorphonuclear leukocytes are then found, and not infrequently there is blood in the fluid.

Tumours

Primary tumours of the peritoneum are rare, and in most cases they take origin not from the serous layer but from some adjacent structure. For example, *lipoma* may arise from the *appendices epiploicae*; *fibroma* takes origin from the connective tissue and sometimes from the sheaths of the nerves in *neurofibromatosis*; and *lymphangioma* occasionally arises from the lymphatics of the mesentery. *Mesothelioma* of the peritoneum presents features like those of the mesothelioma of the pleura but is less frequent, and the same caution in the interpretation of the appearances is required. In both situations, asbestos has been implicated in some cases (p. 385).

Secondary tumours of the peritoneum are comparatively frequent, especially from gastric and ovarian carcinoma. They may be extremely numerous and very minute, often producing a haemorrhagic and inflammatory reaction; or there may be larger nodules and diffuse infiltration. The omentum is very frequently involved and becomes contracted into a hard irregular mass. In some cases of cancer the chief lesion is a very diffuse infiltration with thickening of the serous layers, but with little nodular formation; by such a process the mesentery may become greatly thickened and shrunken. This often results from *linitis plastica* of the stomach, and is accompanied by marked ascites. In mucoid carcinoma the peritoneum is sometimes overgrown by enormous soft translucent tumour masses (Fig. 18.79). Metastases of melanoma are not infrequent and the peritoneum may be studded with enormous numbers of small black nodules; these tend to be specially numerous in the omentum and mesentery.

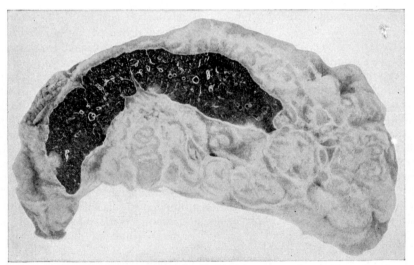

FIG. 18.79.—Section of spleen embedded in large mass of mucoid carcinoma.

CHAPTER 19

LIVER, BILIARY TRACT AND PANCREAS

THE LIVER

General Considerations

The liver is unique in the large number of its important functions, notably in the metabolism of proteins, carbohydrates and fats, in the detoxication of endogenous waste products and drugs, and in the formation and secretion of bile. Accordingly, the liver cell is liable to injury from many causes, discussion of which forms a large part of this chapter.

While the anatomical changes in the liver in disease have long been extensively studied *post mortem*, histological changes are best studied in biopsy material, for in no organ does autolytic change occur with greater rapidity than in the liver. This must always be borne in mind in interpreting structural changes in post-mortem material, for the appearances of damage may thus be greatly exaggerated.

Injury from metabolic disturbances. In experimental animals, specific dietary deficiencies can cause fatty change, progressing to loss of liver cells, compensatory hyperplasia, and fibrosis, i.e. to hepatic cirrhosis. Acute, extensive necrosis of liver cells can also be brought about experimentally by dietary deficiency. In man, the factors concerned in the causation of similar lesions are not fully understood, although geographical surveys suggest that dietary factors may be of great importance.

Injury from toxins and poisons. The liver cell is especially liable to injury because of its function of taking up and dealing with many metabolites, toxic substances, drugs and poisons. The vast number of chemicals used industrially and pharmacologically provide an ever-increasing hazard to the liver, particularly as it has been shown that certain chemicals are harmless to most individuals, but can cause extensive liver damage in individuals with a special susceptibility as, yet unpredictable. The liver also receives blood draining the gastro-intestinal tract, and is exposed to poisons and toxins absorbed from the gut.

A succinct account of hepatotoxic chemicals has been provided by Weinbren (1966). Their effects include liver cell injury and necrosis, inflammatory changes and cholestasis, and various clinical pictures are thus produced. In this chapter these are described along with the diseases they mimic. Meanwhile it is important to appreciate that a careful history of any administration of drugs or exposure to chemicals is an essential part of the investigation of patients with liver disease.

Lesions of the biliary tract affect the liver in two ways. Biliary tract obstruction if sufficiently prolonged results in obstructive biliary cirrhosis, and secondly the bile ducts are also the most common route of bacterial infection of the liver.

Certain virus infections damage the liver severely, causing acute hepatitis with extensive necrosis of liver cells. The most important of these, because of their ubiquity, are the viruses of infective hepatitis and homologous serum jaundice (serum hepatitis).

Hypoxia. Owing to their active and complex metabolism, liver cells are readily injured by hypoxia, as in CVC or anaemia. Swelling of the liver cells in acute liver damage may, by compressing the sinusoids, account for the centrilobular necrosis which is a common feature of chemical poisoning, and interference with the hepatic circulation by the scar tissue present in the cirrhotic liver may contribute to the progressive liver damage commonly associated with cirrhosis.

Tumours. The liver is a common site of metastatic carcinoma, particularly from primary tumours of the gastro-intestinal tract. Primary carcinoma of the liver is much less common in Great Britain though of great frequency in Africa and the Far East: it arises commonly in association with the long continued liver-cell destruction and regeneration of cirrhosis.

Pathological disturbances of liver function

Just as hepatic functions are numerous and complicated, so the disturbances of function resulting from lesions of the liver and biliary tract are varied and complex in their effects. Disturbances of function may be considered under three major headings; hepato-cellular failure (p. 571), portal hypertension (p. 572) and biliary obstruction (p. 591). These are described more fully later in this chapter, as indicated, but brief summaries of their main features are helpful at this point.

Hepato-cellular failure arises when total liver cell function falls below the minimum required to maintain a physiological state. It results from loss of a large number of liver cells from various causes, and from impaired function of liver cells, usually attributable to chronic interference with hepatic blood flow. The more important effects include (1) a rise in the blood level of toxic nitrogenous compounds produced by bacteria in the gut and normally metabolised by the liver cells; these compounds affect especially the central nervous system, causing locomotor disturbances, confusion and delirium, and finally "hepatic" coma; (2) hormonal disturbances attributable to failure of the liver to metabolise various steroid and probably other hormones; (3) failure to remove bilirubin from the blood, to conjugate it and excrete it in the bile; (4) failure to produce the normal amounts of various plasma proteins, particularly albumin and eventually fibrinogen; also prothrombin and various other clotting factors; (5) increased rate of blood flow throughout the body, of obscure nature.

Portal hypertension. This is caused by obstruction of the hepatic veins, sinusoids, or portal veins. As a result, veins which provide an anastomosis between the portal and systemic systems enlarge, and much of the portal blood passes directly into the systemic circulation instead of through the liver. The enlarged anastomotic channels in the wall of the oesophagus may rupture and bleed, and also the bypassing of the liver increases the blood level of toxic nitrogenous compounds absorbed from the gut, thus aggravating the effects of hepatocellular failure on the central nervous system.

Biliary obstruction. This results from obstruction of the major hepatic or bile ducts (extrahepatic cholestasis), or from stagnation of bile in the biliary canaliculi without major duct obstruction (intrahepatic cholestasis). The effects include (1) re-absorption of conjugated bilirubin into the blood, causing *obstructive* or *regurgitative jaundice*; some of the bilirubin escapes into the urine, which is dark; (2) re-absorption of other constituents of bile, such as bile salts and cholesterol; (3) malabsorption of fats and fat-soluble vitamins resulting from lack of bile in the intestines; the faeces are pale and fatty (steatorrhoea), and there may be effects arising from deficiency of vitamins A, D and K; (4) prolonged cholestasis resulting in liver cell injury and eventually in cirrhosis. Bacterial infection of the biliary tract (cholangitis) and gallbladder (cholecystitis) is an important complication of major duct obstruction, particularly when due to gallstones.

CIRCULATORY DISTURBANCES

Approximately three-quarters of the blood supplied to the liver comes via the portal vein, and one quarter via the hepatic artery. In spite of these proportions, the arterial blood is the more important to liver-cell survival, and ligation of the hepatic artery usually results in fatal liver necrosis, whereas portal venous obstruction has only a temporary effect upon the structure and function of the liver.

The internal vascular arrangements of the liver are such that the centrilobular liver cells have the poorest supply of oxygenated blood, and are therefore most severely affected in hypoxia, as in CVC or anaemia.

Chronic venous congestion

Chronic venous congestion of the liver is most commonly seen in congestive heart failure. The pathological changes have already been described (p. 158). In longstanding cases, especially when the condition has started in early life and there have been repeated attacks of cardiac decompensation with intervals of recovery, the surviving peripheral tissue undergoes compensatory hyperplasia, and, as this is of irregular distribution, the pattern becomes still more irregular, as is well seen in Fig. 8.4 (p. 159). Rarely, fibrosis may develop in the congested centrilobular zones; this seldom, if ever, progresses to true cirrhosis, although it has been termed "cardiac cirrhosis".

Although the functions of the liver are not seriously impaired by CVC, there may be mild jaundice, the serum transaminase levels may be raised, and the rate of hepatic inactivation of various drugs may be reduced.

Hepatic venous obstruction. Obstruction of the *major hepatic veins*, by endophlebitis with superadded thrombosis, known as the *Budd–Chiari syndrome*, is rare. Obstruction may result either at the junction of the hepatic veins and inferior vena cava, or in the intrahepatic tributaries. Intense engorgement of the liver results, resembling severe CVC, and leads to centrilobular liver cell loss. The liver is enlarged, there is often abdominal pain, ascites is usually severe, and death results from hepato-cellular failure. Invasion and pressure by malignant tumours, e.g. primary liver-cell carcinoma, which is particularly prone to grow extensively in the portal and hepatic veins within the liver (p. 579), may occasionally have similar effects.

Obstruction to the flow of blood through the liver is an important feature of advanced cirrhosis, and is in part due to constriction of hepatic venules by fibrous tissue, although the sinusoids and portal veins are also affected.

Veno-occlusive disease of the liver occurs in Jamaica and certain other tropical countries probably as a result of drinking "bush tea", an infusion of various plants. The active agents are alkaloids of the pyrrolizidine group present in plants of the genera *Senecio* (ragwort), *Crotalaria* and *Heliotropium*. Sub-intimal fibrosis of the centrilobular hepatic veins develops, and may progress to complete occlusion. The effect on the liver resembles severe CVC, with centri-

lobular liver-cell necrosis and intense sinusoidal congestion. Death may result from liver failure, particularly in young children, and some of the survivors develop cirrhosis; the centrilobular areas become fibrosed and unite, while the surviving cells in the periphery of the lobules undergo compensatory hyperplasia to form small nodules. Liver damage occurs also in animals that eat these plants and it has been induced experimentally by this means. A similar condition may result from irradiation of the liver (see Harrison, 1960).

Portal venous obstruction

Impairment of the portal venous blood flow can arise from obstruction of the hepatic veins, hepatic sinusoids, portal branches within the liver, or the portal vein itself. The commonest, and most important cause, is cirrhosis of the liver, already referred to above in relation to hepatic venous obstruction. Obstruction of the branches of the portal vein within the liver is an important consequence of schistosomiasis of the intestine (p. 521), and results from scarring around ova deposited in the liver (p. 577). As already mentioned, portal and hepatic veins within the liver may be obstructed by metastatic tumour deposits or primary liver-cell carcinoma. Obstruction of the portal vein itself is uncommon. It can result from pressure of enlarged lymph nodes in the porta hepatis or invasion by tumour; also from conditions predisposing to thrombosis, e.g. polycythaemia vera, chronic myeloid leukaemia, carcinoma of the pancreas. Splenectomy in an individual with a normal platelet count both raises the platelet count and slows the portal blood flow, and thus predisposes to thrombosis; there is also an increased frequency of portal vein thrombosis in patients with portal hypertension, e.g. due to cirrhosis.

The most important effect of portal venous obstruction, whatever the site or cause, is portal hypertension, which is discussed on p. 543. As already stated, the supply of portal blood is not essential to the functioning of the otherwise normal liver, although there may be some temporary impairment of liver function in acute portal obstruction.

The effects of complete portal vein obstruction, as by thrombosis, depend on the site. If it is in the portal vein *alone* nothing dramatic

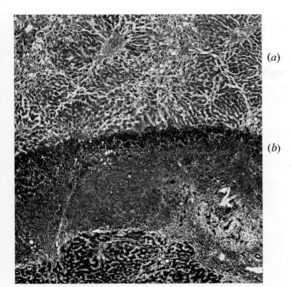

(a)

(b)

Fig. 19.1.—Infarction of liver in polyarteritis. The dead liver lobules (a) are separated from the liver by a zone of inflammatory cells (b). × 38.

happens, but when it extends backwards and occludes the ostium of the splenic vein, then the blood cannot be drained away via the splenic and gastro-oesophageal anastomoses and haemorrhagic infarction of the bowel follows. In cases of longstanding portal thrombosis, there may be an abundant formation of new vascular channels in the portal fissure, so that a cavernous type of tissue is formed. Closure of a branch of the portal vein may sometimes be followed by "red infarction", especially when there is also systemic venous congestion. Such lesions are, however, not complete infarcts, but are due to an engorgement by blood from the adjacent vessels, with ischaemic atrophy of liver cells, the blood vessels and supporting tissue surviving (p. 175).

Hepatic arterial obstruction

The hepatic artery is rarely severely obstructed by disease. Occasionally it is accidentally ligated at operation, and we have seen fatal liver necrosis following ligation of the main trunk or its branch to the right lobe. Obstruction of a smaller intrahepatic branch is usually without effect, owing to collateral anastomoses, but sometimes small areas of ischaemic atrophy may form from blocking of the smallest terminal twigs. We have, however, observed both local infarction (Fig. 19.1) and extensive necrosis of the central zones of the liver lobules in polyarteritis nodosa, apparently from hypoxia due to multiple obstructions of small branches of the hepatic artery. All such infarcts are apt to be colonised by anaerobic bacteria from the gut.

Traumatic infarction. In laceration of the liver, death is likely from haemorrhage into the peritoneum and from shock, especially if fragments of the liver are sequestrated and become free in the peritoneal cavity, where they exercise a profoundly toxic effect.

The liver in eclampsia. The liver is not usually injured in eclampsia (toxaemia of pregnancy), but in fatal cases there are often foci of haemorrhage, necrosis and deposition of fibrin in the parenchyma lying adjacent to portal tracts (Fig. 19.2), and sometimes much larger areas of necrosis. These lesions are probably ischaemic, and due to hepatic involvement in disseminated intravascular coagulation with fibrinoid change and endothelial swelling in the small blood vessels.

Acute ischaemia. In severe shock, and particularly in patients with recent myocardial infarction, acute ischaemic liver injury may be severe, with extensive centrilobular necrosis of liver cells, and features of liver failure may complicate the picture.

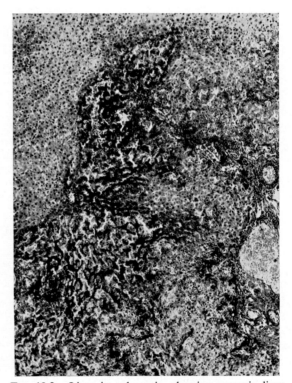

Fig. 19.2.—Liver in eclampsia, showing necrotic liver cells (darkly stained), fibrin and haemorrhage. × 75.

ATROPHY AND HYPERTROPHY

Atrophy. The chief cause of general atrophy of the liver is starvation, in which it becomes shrunken and brown. This is seen in lesser degree in senility. The cells, especially in the central parts of lobules, are shrunken, and often contain granules of the brownish-yellow pigment, lipofuscin (p. 205).

The so-called *cough furrows* occur in chronic bronchitis, and consist of antero-posterior grooves on the upper surface of the liver. They have been attributed to atrophy due to the pressure, during coughing, of hypertrophied bands of diaphragmatic muscle, and are of little importance.

Atrophy from pressure also occurs around tumours and hydatid cysts of the liver, and also in amyloidosis. Focal atrophy of the liver is widespread in cirrhosis (p. 561).

The condition formerly known as *acute yellow atrophy* is not in fact atrophy, but a massive acute necrosis of liver cells.

Hyperplasia and hypertrophy occur commonly as a compensatory process, the cells both multiplying and enlarging, and often becoming multinucleate, e.g. when part of the liver is removed experimentally, and in many lesions causing death of a large number of liver cells. These processes are prominent in the stage of recovery from infective hepatitis (Fig. 19.3), in multiple nodular hyperplasia, in cirrhosis, and sometimes in chronic venous congestion where there has been much loss of liver tissue (p. 159). The changes are often focal, and the surrounding liver cells may be stretched and even atrophied (Fig. 19.20a, p. 562). Experimentally, when as much as two-thirds of the liver is removed, the weight of the organ may be restored within a few weeks. In fact, restoration occurs so rapidly that attempts to study diminished hepatic function by this method have usually failed. The restoration of liver tissue occurs by means of hypertrophy and hyperplasia of the cells of the surviving lobules, but no new lobules are formed (p. 70).

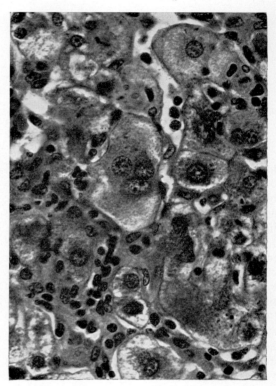

Fig. 19.3.—Multinucleated liver cells, in the stage of recovery after acute hepatitis. × 450.

DEGENERATIONS

As already explained, the liver cells are very susceptible to injury, not only by certain viruses, bacterial toxins and hypoxia, but also by known chemical substances, which may be introduced into the body by the alimentary tract, e.g. various drugs: by inhalation, e.g. halothane; by the normal skin, e.g. trinitrotoluol, or through damaged skin in the now abandoned tannic acid treatment of burns. The liver occupies a special position in being the organ first exposed to enteroviruses, bacterial toxins and poisons passing into the portal blood. It acts as a detoxicating organ and often suffers in consequence. Accordingly, degenerative changes are common and frequently result in permanent liver damage. Fatty change and necrosis of liver cells present special features which were not included in the general account of these changes in Chapter 1, and these are considered below.

Fatty change and malnutrition

Because of their central role in fat meta-bolism, the liver cells are particularly prone to undergo fatty change, i.e. to accumulate in their cytoplasm droplets consisting mainly of neutral fat. In addition to the causes of general fatty change—hypoxia, various chemicals, bacterial toxins and starvation (p. 15)—fatty change in the liver can result from chronic malnutrition, and this must now be considered. The subject is important because of the prevalence of malnutrition in many parts of the world.

In his treatise on the effects of malnutrition on the liver, Himsworth (1953) made a systematic attempt to explain liver disease in malnourished peoples in terms of experimental observations. The investigations of Himsworth and Glynn, Gyorgy, Goldblatt, Best and others had estab-lished that two distinct liver lesions could be produced in rats by dietary deficiencies. Firstly, massive hepatocellular necrosis, which is de-scribed on p. 551. Secondly, gross fatty change which developed in rats maintained on a diet deficient in lipotropic factors, notably choline and its precursor methionine: after some weeks, the fatty change gradually diminished and cirrhosis of the liver supervened. Both the fatty change and cirrhosis were prevented by admin-istration of choline or high-grade protein (which supplies methionine). There is evidence that lipotropic factors are of importance in the hepatic synthesis of phospholipids, which are essential for lipoprotein synthesis in the liver (p. 15). The development of fatty change of the liver in lipotrope-deficient animals is thus attributable to accumulation of neutral fat which would normally have been incorporated into lipoprotein and secreted into the plasma. These experimental findings provided a possible explanation for the fatty liver of childhood, and the supposedly high incidence of cirrhosis, in parts of the world where the diet is low in high-grade protein, and particularly in the amino-acid methionine. In severe form, malnutrition gives rise to a syndrome termed *kwashiorkor*, which affects infants and young children in many parts of southern and central Africa, in tropical America, and extensively in the Far East. The syndrome is a complex one, attributable to a diet severely deficient in high-grade protein, less deficient in total calories, and with additional features due to vitamin deficiencies. Growth is

impaired, the liver is grossly fatty (Fig. 19.4), the pancreas is atrophic, the plasma albumin is low and there is nutritional oedema. Other features include depigmentation of the skin and hair, and dermatoses. Childhood fatty liver is much commoner than the fully developed picture of kwashiorkor, and probably represents less severe malnutrition. While of considerable interest at the time, Himsworth's suggestion that the liver lesion might be due to dietary lack of lipotropic factors has not been established by subsequent observations. In fact, administration of choline has little effect on the fatty liver of kwashiorkor,

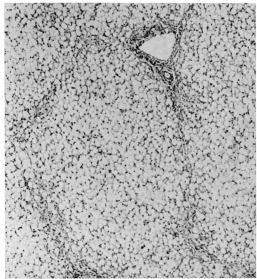

Fig. 19.4.—Fatty liver in kwashiorkor. In addition to vacuolation of each liver cell by a large globule of fat, there is an increase in connective tissue in the form of fine strands running through the parenchyma. × 40. (Preparation kindly lent by Dr. R. S. Patrick.)

whereas it is reversed by administration of a diet of adequate calories and rich in skimmed milk or other high-grade protein, and when supple-mented by vitamins, such a diet is curative unless the syndrome is too advanced or com-plicated by severe infection. In gross protein deficiency, the liver may lose over 40 per cent of its protein, and it is likely that the fatty liver of kwashiorkor results from failure of the liver cells to synthesise sufficient protein for the incorporation of neutral fat into lipoprotein. Another factor may well be starvation, for the child with kwashiorkor eventually loses his appetite and this, together with impaired pan-creatic exocrine secretion, leads to a fall in carbohydrate intake: the blood sugar is often abnormally low, and, as explained below, failure of carbohydrate metabolism leads to deposition of fat in the liver cells. The age incidence of kwashiorkor is attributable to the high protein requirements of growing infants and young children. The protein requirements and the incidence of protein deficiency in adults are difficult to determine, for there is no measurable protein store comparable to the fat deposits, and while protein deficiency in childhood can be measured in terms of impairment of growth, deficiency in adults results in atrophy of the cells of the various organs and of the skeletal muscles, and is not readily measurable *in vivo*.

The possible relationship between the fatty liver of malnutrition and cirrhosis is discussed on p. 570, and fatty change in alcoholism on p. 553.

The liver in obesity. In pathological obesity (p. 18), fat is deposited mainly in adipose tissue, and does not accumulate in other types of cell. The liver, however, is exceptional in this respect. The accumulation of fat usually begins and is greatest in the liver cells round the portal tracts (Fig. 1.17, p. 17); thence it extends inwards, and in severe cases involves all the liver cells. The fat appears first as a few small globules which run together, and ultimately the cell becomes distended with a single large globule of fat, while the nucleus is flattened and pushed to one side. In extreme cases almost every liver cell is distended with a fat globule, the microscopic appearance coming almost to resemble adipose tissue. When there is great accumulation of fat the liver becomes much enlarged, greasy and yellow.

The gross fatty change in the liver in pathological obesity results from the special role of the liver cells in normal fat metabolism. Not only do they take up a high proportion of dietary fat absorbed from the intestine and fatty acids released from the depots, but they are active in the synthesis of fat from glucose and amino-acids. The relative importance of these processes will depend on the amounts of carbohydrate, fat and protein in the diet, but the essential cause is a caloric intake which exceeds the body's requirements.

Pigmentary changes

As these have been described in other chapters, only a summary need be given. The following are the chief varieties of pigment observed in the liver:

Lipofuscin is deposited in the cells towards the centres of the lobules as yellow-brown granules in conditions of liver cell atrophy, and in old age.

Bile pigment. This accumulates in cholestasis (p. 592) and particularly in major bile duct obstruction. It is seen within the liver cells as greenish-brown granules, especially in the central parts of the lobules, and also within the bile canaliculi as irregular hyaline olive-green casts from which branches are seen passing between the liver cells (Fig. 19.25, p. 567). These are composed of inspissated bile, probably in combination with protein, and are called *biliary thrombi.*

Haemosiderin. This pigment, which gives the iron (prussian blue) reaction, is found mainly in conditions of excessive blood destruction or absorption from haemorrhages. It usually appears first in the Kupffer cells and is found also as brownish-yellow granules within the liver cells, especially at the periphery of the lobules: at an early stage the cells may give only a diffuse iron reaction. This pigment is prominent in pernicious anaemia in relapse, but it may occur in leukaemia, subtertian malaria and various haemolytic anaemias. The greatest deposits of haemosiderin occur, however, in haemochromatosis (p. 204). The pigment is present in large quantities in the liver cells, bile duct epithelium, the walls of capillaries and in macrophages. Normal liver tissue contains about 0·08 per cent of iron (dry weight); in untreated pernicious anaemia the amount is about 0·3 per cent, while in haemochromatosis it may reach 5 per cent or more. In infancy the liver normally gives an iron reaction and this becomes more marked in wasting conditions.

Malarial pigment. This occurs especially in chronic malaria and may be sufficient to give the liver a dusky greyish-brown appearance. It consists of minute dark brown granules which do not give the iron reaction, present chiefly in histiocytes in the connective tissue of the portal tracts and in the Kupffer cells.

Amyloid disease

In this condition the liver becomes larger, firmer and elastic and is often palpable during life. The structural changes and causation have already been dealt with (p. 196). Amyloid disease does not produce jaundice, nor, as a rule, ascites; but the latter may occur as part of the general oedema in the nephrotic syndrome due to accompanying amyloid disease of the kidneys and the hypoproteinaemia is possibly aggravated by the liver damage.

LIVER CELL NECROSIS

Necrosis of liver cells, of greater or lesser extent, occurs in many diseases of the liver, and also in many other conditions, such as severe infections, wasting diseases, and congestive heart failure, in which liver cell injury is neither the most important nor the most characteristic feature. In most of the conditions, liver cells degenerate or atrophy and die one by one—*necrobiosis*—when they can be recognised as smaller, deeply eosinophilic, rather granular cells with shrunken nuclei. The present account is limited to conditions in which death of large numbers of liver cells occurs simultaneously or within a short period. Necrosis due to sudden deprivation of arterial blood supply (e.g. ligation of the hepatic artery, laceration of the liver, polyarteritis nodosa) takes the form of infarction (Fig. 19.1) and needs no further description here.

There remains a group of conditions in which necrosis of liver cells occurs rapidly, while the supporting tissue, including the blood vessels and bile ducts, survives; this group is considered below.

Causal agents

Necrosis of hepatic parenchymal cells occurs in *certain virus diseases* which affect especially the liver, e.g. infective hepatitis, yellow fever, in *acute bacterial infections* associated with severe toxaemia, and as a result of *poisoning* with various, mostly organic, chemicals. The same chemical compounds which cause fatty change in the liver can, in larger dosage or in unusually susceptible individuals, cause liver cell necrosis.

Liver cell necrosis can also be produced in animals by diets deficient in vitamin E and selenium, and the possible role of dietary deficiencies in predisposing to extensive necrosis in man is discussed below (p. 551).

Classification

Liver cell necrosis is usually classified according to the distribution of the lesions. Thus microscopic foci of necrosis not related to any particular part of the liver lobules is termed *focal* necrosis; necrosis occurring mainly in a particular part of the lobules is termed *zonal* necrosis,

and is further subdivided according to whether the lesions are situated centrally, peripherally, or in the mid-zones of the lobules. Necrosis also occurs in *massive* form in which large areas of liver cells, comprising many lobules, and sometimes involving almost the whole organ, are affected.

Focal liver cell necrosis

This is common in severe toxaemias, particularly those resulting from infections within the drainage area of the portal vein, e.g. typhoid fever, peritonitis, severe bacillary dysentery. The lesions consist of minute pale yellowish foci, irregularly distributed and most easily detected by microscopy, when they are seen to consist of groups of necrotic liver cells, some of which may have disappeared as a result of autolysis, leaving a patch of congestion and inflammatory cell infiltration. Focal necrosis of single liver cells and small groups of cells occurs in the important virus infections, infective hepatitis and serum hepatitis (pp. 555–8). On recovery, restoration to normal occurs by proliferation of the adjacent surviving liver cells.

Zonal liver cell necrosis

Centrilobular necrosis is caused by certain chemicals, e.g. the chlorinated hydrocarbons, chloroform and carbon tetrachloride, and is sometimes seen in streptococcal and pneumococcal infections (Fig. 19.5).

Peripheral zonal necrosis is uncommon. It is seen in phosphorus poisoning, in which the outstanding lesion is the intense fatty change described on p. 17. Necrosis of cells is seen especially in patients dying after about a week; it appears at the periphery of the lobules, and as the dead cells undergo absorption, there occurs an ingrowth of bile duct epithelium from the free ends of the minute ducts. Thus numerous new bile ducts may be seen at the margin of the lobules, and their growth is accompanied by condensation of the connective tissue and by lymphocytic and monocytic infiltration. As this process goes on, the liver shrinks and the resulting condition is known as the "atrophic phosphorus liver".

Mid-zonal lobular necrosis is also uncommon. It occurs consistently in fatal cases of yellow fever (p. 558) and is seen occasionally in fatal acute peritonitis (Fig. 19.6).

Results of zonal necrosis. The necrotic liver

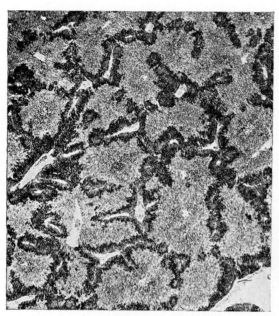

FIG. 19.5.—Centrilobular necrosis and peripheral fatty change. A case of streptococcal peritonitis. × 15.

cells are rapidly autolysed and disappear, provided that the circulation of the blood through the affected tissue is maintained, while the adjacent surviving liver cells multiply and repair the columns. Thus the central necrosis produced in dogs by chloroform inhalation may be followed by replacement of cells and a return to normal within ten days, and no doubt the same result would follow mid-zonal necrosis. Where the damage is more severe, involving whole lobules, and especially where the periphery of the lobules is involved, collapse of the lobular supporting tissue and fibrosis follow, accompanied by bile duct proliferation. When repeatedly damaged by carbon tetrachloride, the liver has remarkable powers of recovery by regeneration of the central necrotic zones within 10–14 days; if the doses of poison are closely spaced, complete regeneration does not occur and a permanent fine fibrosis, periportal as well as central in distribution, results (Fig. 19.19b).

Massive liver cell necrosis (formerly **acute yellow atrophy**)

This consists of necrosis of all or nearly all the parenchymal cells in large areas of liver tissue, often more severe in the left lobe. When almost the whole of the parenchyma is destroyed, death results from acute liver failure within three weeks. If sufficient parenchyma remains to allow survival, within a few months of the acute incident the areas of liver deprived of parenchymal cells become fibrosed and contracted, while the surviving cells enlarge and proliferate to form hyperplastic nodules. Eventually—within months or years—death results from chronic liver failure, portal hypertension, or both: there is also a liability to further attacks of acute necrosis.

Etiology. The disease occurs in "idiopathic" form, without either a preceding illness or exposure to known hepatotoxic agents. This is commoner in females and occurs especially in

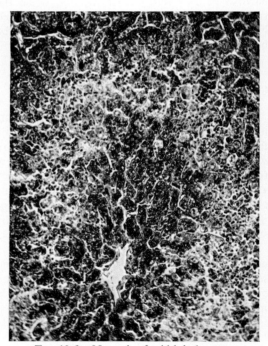

FIG. 19.6.—Necrosis of mid-lobular type.

The necrotic part, which appears pale, occupies the intermediate zone, though closer to the portal tracts. × 105.

pregnancy or early in the puerperium. Epidemiological studies have shown that some cases are due to infective or serum hepatitis, and while the incidence in the former disease is low, recent outbreaks of serum hepatitis among the staff of dialysis units in this country have included fatal cases of massive necrosis which, as shown by the demonstration of "Australia antigen" (p. 558) are without doubt of viral nature. It is quite apparent that, in these outbreaks, the hepatitis is particularly severe, but the explanation is at present obscure. Certain chemicals used therapeutically and in industry produce massive liver

Hadfield and Garrod (1947), was of major importance in providing a possible explanation of the disease in man: it suggested that dietary deficiencies were a predisposing cause, and that superadded liver injury, due to virus hepatitis, chemicals, etc., although producing only relatively mild injury in the well-nourished, might cause massive necrosis in malnourished indivi-

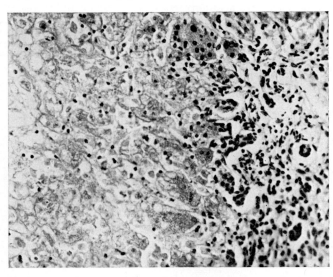

FIG. 19.7.—Massive necrosis of liver. Margin of necrotic area showing remains of dead liver cells and junction with small bile ducts. × 200.

necrosis in a small proportion of the individuals at risk; the therapeutic substances include cinchophen, plasmoquin and dinitrophenol, the industrial agents trinitrotoluol, tetrachlorethane, chlorinated naphthalenes and certain nitrobenzol compounds. Massive necrosis is only an exceptional complication of infective hepatitis, and its incidence in chemical poisoning is not related to dosage alone, but also to some form of idiosyncrasy of unknown nature. Ingestion of the poisonous mushroom *Amanita phalloides* is fatal chiefly owing to massive hepatic necrosis.

Experimental dietary necrosis. In experimental studies, Himsworth and Glynn and other workers showed that rats, kept on a diet lacking in high grade protein and deficient in vitamin E for some weeks, developed acute massive hepato-cellular necrosis resembling the human disease. This was preventable by adding to the diet either vitamin E or sulphydryl-containing amino-acids: the latter could be cystine or methionine or high grade protein, e.g. casein. It was thus concluded that deficiency in two dietary factors (vitamin E and SH-amino-acids) resulted in massive necrosis.

This work, which was well reviewed by

duals. There is some evidence to support this; for example, infective hepatitis has been observed to run a more severe course, with a higher mortality from massive necrosis, in malnourished people. In general, however, malnutrition could not be implicated in cases of massive necrosis in this country, and there has been little progress in elucidating the factors which determine the occurrence of the human disease.

More recently, it has been shown that deficiency of a selenium compound is of importance in the experimental massive necrosis produced by dietary deficiency. Initially it was believed that this was a third factor, and it is still known as Factor III, but the protective effects of sulphydryl-containing amino-acids or high grade protein have been shown clearly to depend on contamination with trace-amounts of selenium. Addition of SH-amino-acids free of Factor III to the diet delays the onset of massive necrosis but does not prevent it. Accordingly, the two important factors are vitamin E and Factor III. The combined deficiency of these two factors produces massive hepato-cellular necrosis in rats, but has different effects on other species, for example, muscular dystrophy in the mink and an exudative diathesis in the chick. The effects of deficiency of either vitamin E or Factor III alone are quite distinct from each other and from the combined deficiency.

The amount of Factor III-selenium which must be present in casein to prevent massive necrosis in rats is only 1 atom per 350,000 molecules of casein; certain other selenium compounds are effective in larger amounts, and the hepatotoxic dose of selenium in animals is rela-

may occur from a recurrence of massive necrosis (Fig. 19.10), from chronic hepato-cellular failure or portal hypertension.

The acute necrosis is usually accompanied by renal tubular injury, particularly when chemicals are responsible, and acute renal failure may result. Owing to the liver injury the blood urea level does not rise rapidly, and occasionally crystals of leucine and tyrosine may be present in the urine (p. 572).

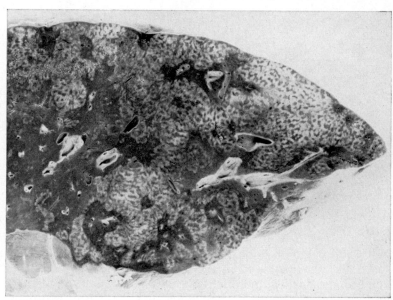

FIG. 19.8.—Massive necrosis of liver, three weeks after the onset of jaundice.

Note the irregular dark areas from which the dead liver cells have been absorbed, and the portions showing persisting liver structure which were deeply jaundiced. These latter areas had undergone necrosis shortly before death.

tively huge. These experimental advances have so far contributed little to the elucidation of massive necrosis in man, and it is not known whether vitamin E and selenium deficiencies are contributory factors.

Pathological changes. When death occurs within a few days, before autolysis of the dead liver cells, the liver is approximately normal in size, diffusely yellow owing to bile-staining, and necrotic (Fig. 19.7). After 2–3 weeks, the dead cells have disappeared, and the affected areas of the liver are shrunken, soft and red (Figs. 19.8, 19.9). If the patient survives for weeks or months, proliferation of the surviving parenchyma produces pale nodules varying in size to over a centimetre, and scarring occurs in the areas of liver cell loss. These changes result in a shrunken nodular liver (*multiple nodular hyperplasia* or *post-necrotic scarring*) (Fig. 19.11). The variation in size of nodules, and the breadth of sheets of fibrous tissue, are much greater than in cirrhosis. The outlook is poor, and death

Alcohol and the liver

The commonest abnormality in the liver in the chronic alcoholic is *fatty change*, which may be severe and diffuse. Other changes include the so-called *alcoholic hepatitis*, which may follow a particularly heavy bout of drinking. *Cirrhosis* of the liver develops in approximately 10 per cent of severe chronic alcoholics. Elucidation of the mechanism of these abnormalities is rendered difficult by their inconstant occurrence in the alcoholic, by the complex and variable dietary imbalances which frequently are associated with alcoholism, and by the inability or unwillingness of the alcoholic to provide accurate information on the amount of alcohol consumed, diet, etc. It is therefore not surprising that investigators attempting to solve the mechanisms of alcoholic liver disease have turned largely to studies on experimental animals. Valuable advances have resulted from experimental studies under carefully controlled conditions, but some of the major problems remain unsolved, and in particular an experimental model of alcoholic cirrhosis has not been produced.

Fatty change. As in fatty change from other causes, most of the fat in the alcoholic fatty liver

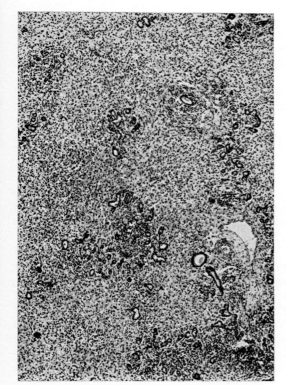

FIG. 19.9.—Massive necrosis of liver; portion of red area from which the liver cells have completely disappeared and the lobules consist of dilated capillaries. Early formation of new bile ducts is seen around the portal tracts. × 60.

is neutral triglyceride, and its accumulation must therefore be considered against the background of the normal metabolism of neutral fat and the disturbances which can lead to its accumulation in the liver cells (p. 14). Most of the alcohol reaching the liver is oxidised by alcohol dehydrogenase to acetaldehyde and then to acetyl co-enzyme A: this is broken down to acetate which is largely released and oxidised by the other tissues of the body. However, some of the alcohol is utilised in the synthesis of fatty acids, and the possibility arises that the fatty liver results merely from the high caloric intake of the alcoholic. This can be ruled out as the sole cause of the fatty liver by experimental studies in which it has been shown that alcohol in the diet results in appreciably more fatty change than

occurs with isocaloric diets containing carbohydrates or fat in place of alcohol. Another possibility is that the fatty liver results from dietary deficiency of lipotropic factors (e.g. choline or methionine) or of protein. There is some evidence to support this possibility in man, and fatty liver can be produced in rats by moderate alcohol intake associated with such dietary deficiencies. However, fat accumulates in the livers of rats given larger amounts of alcohol, equivalent to that consumed by the chronic alcoholic, even when the diet is adequate, and is not fully or constantly prevented by large amounts of lipotropes. Here again, alcohol is more lipogenic than equivalent amounts of carbohydrate or fat. These and similar experiments do not rule out the importance of dietary

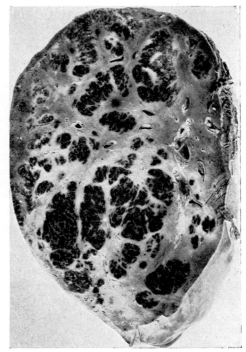

FIG. 19.10.—Massive necrosis of liver with fatal recurrence. The pale areas consist of fibrous tissue, the liver cells having undergone necrosis in the initial attack and subsequent autolysis. The dark areas consist of tissue in which the liver cells survived the initial attack, but were destroyed in a rapidly-fatal recurrence. × 0·9.

deficiency in the alcoholic, but they demonstrate that alcohol also has a specific effect, other than as a source of calories, in inducing fatty liver, and that if enough alcohol is administered, this effect is not prevented by other dietary constituents,

Recent experimental studies have demonstrated that most of the fat accumulating in the liver cells in alcoholism is of dietary origin, and not from the depots, and that fatty change is aggravated by a high fat diet. When fatty liver is evoked by alcohol in animals on a fat-free diet,

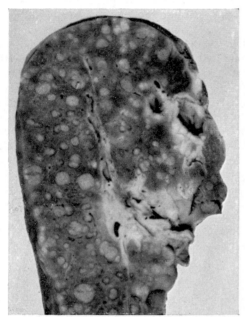

FIG. 19.11.—Multiple nodular hyperplasia of liver.

Note the pale round nodules composed of hypertrophied parenchyma, lying in a background of scar tissue from which the liver cells have disappeared. × ¾.

most of the fat is probably synthesised in the liver, and again little of it is provided by release of fatty acids from the depots. In both man and experimental animals, the available evidence suggests that synthesis and secretion of lipoproteins by the liver cells is not impaired, and in this respect the condition differs from fatty liver from various other causes (p. 15). There is also evidence that oxidation of alcohol in the liver may be associated with an unusually high rate of reduction of nicotinamide adenine dinucleotide

(NAD) to NADH, but the significance of this, and of various other possible metabolic effects of alcohol on the liver, are uncertain.

The accumulation of fatty droplets in the liver cell cytoplasm precedes all other changes observed by light and electron microscopy in experimental alcoholism. In acute experiments the fat accumulates in small droplets in the more peripheral parts of the lobules, but in chronic experiments the droplets enlarge and the centrilobular cells are most severely affected. In man, the droplets are large and appear first in the peripheral cells. Other changes, observed in man and experimentally, are enlargement, distortion and clumping of the mitochondria, formation of phagosomes, and changes in the endoplasmic reticulum. Mallory bodies (p. 564) are rarely seen in man apart from alcoholic cirrhosis, and have recently been produced in animals by administration of alcohol. The onset of fatty change precedes all those other structural changes.

Alcoholic hepatitis. Following a particularly heavy bout of drinking, the chronic alcoholic may develop an acute illness with upper abdominal pain, nausea and vomiting, enlargement of the liver, fever and sometimes jaundice. The liver shows extensive fatty change, enlargement and clumping of mitochondria, an acute inflammatory reaction with leukocytic infiltration, and in some instances cholestasis. The liver cell injury may progress to focal or massive necrosis, and the condition is sometimes fatal.

Cirrhosis. The nature of the association between chronic alcoholism and cirrhosis is discussed on p. 570. It is worth emphasising that cirrhosis develops in only a small proportion of alcoholics and usually after more than ten years of heavy drinking: this long latent period may explain why alcoholic cirrhosis has not been produced in experimental animals. The parts played by fatty change and alcoholic hepatitis in the development of cirrhosis remain obscure.

VIRUS HEPATITIS

Minor degrees of injury to the liver cells occur in virtually every acute generalised viral or other infection; there are, however, three virus infections which affect especially the liver: they are *infective hepatitis*, *serum hepatitis*, and *yellow*

fever. In most parts of the world, infective hepatitis is endemic and thus it is the commonest acute disease of the liver, and is of great importance. Yellow fever is endemic in certain tropical latitudes, and is a severe, often fatal disease, which can become epidemic in a susceptible population but can be prevented by prophylactic immunisation; it is spread by insect vectors.

Since infective hepatitis and serum hepatitis are similar, only infective hepatitis will be described in detail, the account of serum hepatitis being limited to its special features.

Infective hepatitis

Definition. An acute virus infection, characterised by an acute hepatitis with liver cell necrosis. Diagnosis is presumptive, and is made on clinical and epidemiological considerations.

Pathological changes. Infective hepatitis is typically a non-fatal disease, from which the patient recovers completely, and so the pathological changes have been studied mainly by percutaneous needle biopsy of the liver. In the early stages, the liver cells are seen to be detached from one another, giving an appearance of trabecular disruption: by contrast, appropriately stained sections show the reticulin framework to

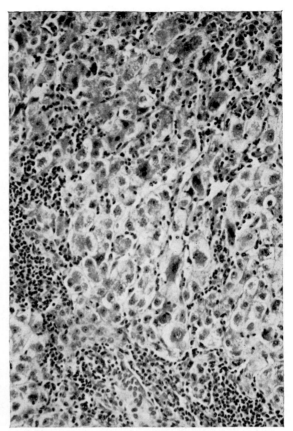

FIG. 19.13.—Liver in infective hepatitis. Scattered liver cells are shrunken, hyaline and pyknotic; others are ballooned. Cellular infiltrate, predominantly lymphocytic, is heavy in the portal areas (lower and left margins) and lighter within the parenchyma. × 185. (Dr. R. S. Patrick.)

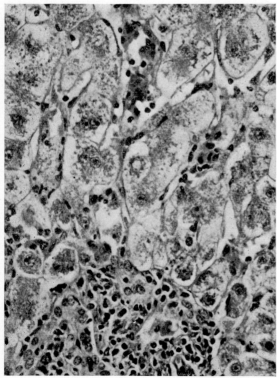

FIG. 19.12.—Liver in infective hepatitis, showing ballooning of liver cells, and the remains of a group of shrunken, hyaline cells (upper centre). × 465. (Dr. R. S. Patrick.)

be intact. Although the liver is diffusely affected, there is great variation in the degree of injury of individual liver cells: many appear normal, but single scattered cells are enlarged and rounded (ballooned) and the cytoplasm is condensed into feathery strands between vacuoles (feathery degeneration) (Fig. 19.12). Other liver cells are shrunken, the cytoplasm is eosinophilic and homogeneous, and often bile-stained: this hyaline change may affect part of the cytoplasm, which is similar to the Councilman body (p. 558), or may involve the whole cell, while the nucleus appears pyknotic (Fig. 19.13).

Many of these more severely damaged cells die, but autolysis is so rapid that it is unusual to see more than an occasional dead cell. Electron microscopy shows irregular swelling of the endoplasmic reticulum to form vesicles and detachment of the membrane-associated ribosomes.

Enlarged lysosomes containing altered mitochondria and organelle debris (phagosomes) are seen, but none of these electron microscopic changes is specific, and virus particles have not been identified. These changes in the liver cells are accompanied by proliferation and enlargement of the Kupffer cells, which accumulate lipofuscin pigment. There is a widespread infiltration with lymphocytes and smaller numbers of monocytes, plasma cells and eosinophil polymorphs, with few neutrophil polymorphs: these cells aggregate most densely in the portal tracts, but are present also among the liver cells (Fig. 19.13). Biliary stasis is not severe, but here and there canaliculi are distended with bile.

The acute liver cell injury is brief, and before the attack has subsided clinically, hypertrophy and hyperplasia are seen among the surviving liver cells (Fig. 19.3, p. 546) and the trabeculae are thus restored. The inflammatory cellular infiltrate may, however, persist for weeks or even months. In unusually severe cases, there may be more extensive loss of liver cells, sometimes affecting especially the centres of the lobules (Fig. 19.14), sometimes groups of liver cells anywhere in the lobule. There is also epidemiological evidence that massive liver cell necrosis

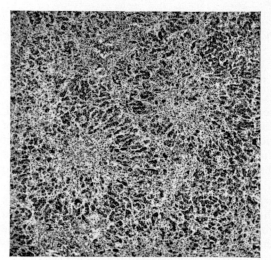

Fig. 19.14.—Liver in infective hepatitis, showing centrilobular loss of liver cells. × 45.

Accidental death on 7th day of illness.

(p. 550) can result from infective hepatitis (Fig. 19.15), and alcoholic drinks appear to predispose to this.

Clinical and biochemical features. The early features of infective hepatitis are severe nausea, anorexia, often retching and vomiting, and sometimes fever. The inflamed liver is often enlarged, tender and uncomfortable. The urine is dark with bilirubin, the faeces pale, and jaundice appears within a day or two. The serum bilirubin level is usually between 5 and 15 mg. per 100 ml., and is mainly conjugated, giving a

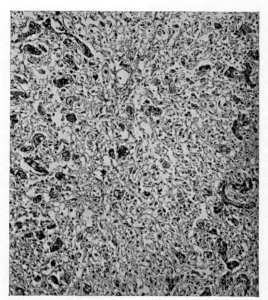

Fig. 19.15.—Liver in infective hepatitis, showing complete destruction of the liver lobule and prominence of bile-duct structures. × 100.

From a case dying in relapse in the fourth week.

direct van den Bergh reaction, and indicating that the jaundice is mainly of regurgitative type, attributable presumably to swelling of the liver cells and cholestasis. Serum alkaline phosphatase levels rarely exceed 30 K-A units per 100 ml. As would be expected, serum transaminase levels are high at an early stage, reflecting liver cell injury. The major symptoms usually subside after a few days. In some cases, vague upper abdominal symptoms persist, with nausea and poor appetite, and may continue for months (post-hepatitic syndrome); liver biopsy in many cases has shown no evidence of continuing hepatitis and eventual recovery is complete.

Relapses occur in a small percentage of cases, and drinking alcohol appears to increase the risk of this.

In outbreaks of hepatitis, mild anicteric cases are common, and may outnumber overt cases: liver biopsy has shown the usual changes, although in milder degree.

Blood picture. An initial leukopenia is sometimes succeeded by lymphocytosis, with many large abnormal cells recalling the picture in infectious mononucleosis, thus indicating a widespread involvement of the lymphatic and reticulo-endothelial systems. As infectious mononucleosis is sometimes complicated by hepatitis, its distinction from infective hepatitis may rest upon the finding of a positive Paul-Bunnell test.

Etiology and epidemiology. Study of the epidemiology of virus hepatitis has hitherto been handicapped by failure to transmit the disease to animals, or to grow the virus in tissue cultures. Indeed, confirmation of the presence of the hepatitis virus has until recently been demonstrated only by its infectivity for susceptible human volunteers. Immunological studies, so often helpful in epidemiological investigations, have also proved difficult, for although the serum γ-globulin of recovered patients protects susceptible volunteers, there is no generally available *in vitro* test capable of demonstrating immunity in this disease.

Growth and serial passage of the viruses of both infective hepatitis and serum hepatitis in cultures of human cells have been reported, but other attempts have been unsuccessful, and no standard procedure has yet emerged. Very recently, reports have appeared of a precipitin test which may be capable of detecting the virus in the serum of early cases; the observations concern mainly serum hepatitis, and are described on p. 558.

During an attack the virus is present in the blood and faeces, and the disease is spread by faecal contamination of food. The incubation period is 15–40 days, and the duration of infectivity following recovery is probably short.

Idiosyncracy to various drugs and chemicals, including hydrazines (e.g. Iproniazid), TNT and cinchophen, can produce liver injury resembling infective hepatitis.

Atypical "infective hepatitis"

In some cases, jaundice is deeper and persists for weeks or even months. Distinction from drug cholestasis or duct obstruction may be difficult clinically, but needle biopsy shows the usual inflammatory changes of infective hepatitis, with more pronounced cholestasis: eventually recovery is complete. A form of hepatitis termed *cholangiolitic hepatitis* has previously been regarded as a variant of infective hepatitis. It is characterised by injury to the smaller bile ducts, and is possibly primary biliary cirrhosis (p. 567).

Rarely infective hepatitis may continue for a year or more, with continued liver tenderness and mild symptoms: liver biopsy shows continued injury of individual liver cells and inflammatory infiltration, but without significant fibrosis. Complete recovery ensues.

In unusually severe cases, death may occur in the acute stage from hepato-cellular failure and the changes are those of massive liver cell necrosis: in other cases, particularly in middle-aged women, the hepatitis is progressive and is fatal in 1–3 months. Some cases of *active chronic hepatitis* (p. 559) start with an acute hepatitis indistinguishable from infective hepatitis, and progress to post-hepatitic cirrhosis.

The evidence that the virus of infective hepatitis is responsible for these various illnesses is insecure, and is based on the observations that, in some cases, the illness has started during an epidemic of infective hepatitis, or that there has been contact with a typical case of infective hepatitis. As infective hepatitis is widely endemic, the situation must remain obscure until the difficulties of virological study of the disease have been overcome.

The possibility that a typical attack of infective hepatitis predisposes to cirrhosis is unlikely (p. 571).

Serum hepatitis
(Homologous serum jaundice)

Definition and epidemiology. This is a virus infection with clinical and pathological features similar to infective hepatitis but differing in having a longer incubation period (50–140 days) and in being more often severe or fatal; it is transmitted by parenteral injection of blood or plasma from an individual carrying the virus. There is no cross-immunity against the virus of infective hepatitis.

As with infective hepatitis, repeated attempts to infect animals, or to grow the virus in tissue cultures have failed. At the time of writing, reports are appearing which describe the detection of an antigen in the serum of patients with, or following, serum hepatitis; the antigen is demonstrated in an agar-diffusion test, by means of antibody present in the serum of very occasional patients who have received numerous transfusions, e.g. haemophiliacs. There is strong presumptive evidence that the antigen is of viral nature, and it has been detected also in the serum of a small proportion of early cases of infective hepatitis, in a proportion of cases of active chronic hepatitis and in some cases of Down's syndrome in institutions. Curiously, the *antibody* has not usually been found in the serum of recovered cases of virus hepatitis, nor in active chronic hepatitis. Neither antigen nor antibody has been observed in post-hepatitic cirrhosis or other liver diseases. Originally detected in the serum of an Australian aborigine, the antigen was first thought to be an allotypic lipoprotein factor, and was termed by Blumberg and his co-workers the Australia ("Au") antigen; subsequently it has been referred to as "SH" (serum hepatitis) and "hepatitis-associated" antigen. Reviews and references relating to this work, which is likely to be of great importance in the elucidation of virus hepatitis, are readily available (Lancet, 1969, 1970).

Infection may be transmitted by as little as 2×10^{-6} ml. of the blood, serum or plasma of carriers, and also by preparations of fibrinogen and thrombin, but γ-globulin prepared by certain techniques appears to be non-infective. The virus is present in the blood for the greater part of the long incubation period, and sometimes for long periods thereafter. It is not present in the faeces during the illness. The risk of transmitting the virus is not confined to the intravenous transfusion or injection of blood, plasma or serum, but occurs also when needles or syringes used to inject drugs, vaccines, etc., are not adequately sterilised between each injection, and even needles used for vaccinia vaccination or for obtaining finger-prick samples of blood may transmit the infection from one individual to another. Outbreaks have occurred recently among the staffs and patients in haemodialysis centres where a lot of donated blood is used, and apparatus contaminated with blood is handled. The viruses of both infective and serum hepatitis may be involved.

Prevention. The incidence of the carrier state and of the disease itself is not known, and as there is no fully reliable method of detecting the virus in blood or of sterilising blood or plasma, the risk of transmitting infection is a valid reason for not giving unnecessary transfusions of blood, and especially of large-pool plasma. Of even greater importance is the efficient sterilisation, after use on each individual, of needles, syringes and other apparatus employed to give injections, to withdraw blood or to scratch or puncture the skin. The danger of transmitting the virus of homologous serum jaundice is one of the more important reasons for the institution of central supply and sterilisation services and for the use of disposable syringes and needles. There are indications that the scrupulous practice of hygienic measures and the use of disposable dialysis membranes are effective in reducing the risk of outbreaks in haemodialysis centres.

Yellow fever

This is an acute disease, caused by a Group B arborvirus, which occurs sporadically and in epidemics in certain parts of Africa and tropical America. Monkeys, and perhaps other animals, develop the disease, which is transmitted among them and to man by the bites of *Aedes aegypti* and certain other mosquitoes. In epidemic form the disease has a high mortality rate, but serological evidence suggests that between epidemics a high incidence of infection occurs but that most cases are mild.

Pathological changes. In severe cases, there are acute degenerative changes and haemorrhage into the various internal organs and tissues. Vomiting of altered blood is usual. The liver lesion consists of mid-lobular zonal necrosis, haemorrhages, and fatty change in the surviving liver cells. The first change is the appearance of hyaline eosinophilic areas in the cytoplasm of the liver cells, ultimately embracing the entire cell (the "Councilman lesion") and by coalescence of adjacent degenerate foci the zonal necrosis is built up. Tubular degeneration, sometimes progressing to necrosis, occurs in the kidneys.

Confirmation of the disease is provided by the development of encephalitis in mice injected intracerebrally with serum from a suspected early case, or later by demonstrating a rise in the titre of antibody protective to mice.

Cytomegalovirus hepatitis is a feature of the generalised form of infection with this virus which occurs in neonates from intra-uterine transmission. In older children and adults the virus causes hepatitis either alone, or as part of an illness resembling infectious mononucleosis (p. 458).

Active chronic hepatitis (Lupoid hepatitis)

In many cases of cirrhosis the presenting features are those of hepato-cellular failure or portal hypertension, but in others there is evidence of liver disease for some years before cirrhosis finally develops. Two such pre-cirrhotic conditions are primary biliary cirrhosis (p. 567) and active chronic hepatitis.

Although active chronic hepatitis is not a well-defined entity, its occurrence predominantly in adolescent females and young women, its usual relentless progress to cirrhosis within a few years of onset, and the common occurrence of certain associated extra-hepatic features, suggest that it may be a specific disease.

Clinical features. While more than half the patients are females between 10 and 30 years of age, it occurs also in males and older women. The onset may be indistinguishable from an attack of infective hepatitis or may be more insidious. The hepatitis persists, but tends to fluctuate, so that there are periods of fever, jaundice and malaise, with raised serum transaminase levels, alternating with periods of comparative well-being and subsidence of the above abnormalities. In the later stages, appropriate tests show impairment of liver functions, and in most cases death results from cirrhosis.

In addition to the features of chronic hepatitis, arthralgia, various skin rashes, pleural effusions, thrombocytopenia, leukopenia and proteinuria attributable to glomerular lesions, are encountered in various degrees and combinations. These miscellaneous associations are similar to the features of systemic lupus erythematosus (SLE), and there is moreover a high incidence of antinuclear and other auto-antibodies in the serum, as in SLE. For this reason, the condition is sometimes called *lupoid* or *auto-immune hepatitis*. There is evidence also of an increased incidence of ulcerative colitis and of chronic thyroiditis in patients with active chronic hepatitis.

Glucocorticoid therapy induces a fall in the serum bilirubin and transaminase levels, and may prevent or delay cirrhosis, and prolong life.

Pathological changes. The liver may be of normal size or enlarged. For a long time the surface is smooth but eventually it becomes nodular. There is a heavy infiltrate of lymphocytes and plasma cells in the portal areas, and irregular infiltration of the parenchyma with these cells. Individual liver cells and groups of liver cells, sometimes lying in or adjacent to the

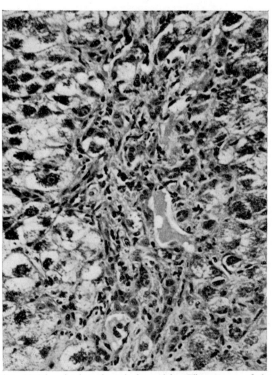

FIG. 19.16.—Active chronic hepatitis. The centre of the field is occupied by an enlarged portal area with irregular margins, and the adjacent liver cells show feathery degeneration. There is an infiltrate of lymphocytes in the portal area and among the liver cells. × 350.

lymphoid cell infiltrates, show feathery degeneration: they are swollen, show irregular vacuolation of their cytoplasm, and nuclear enlargement or pyknosis. These changes progress to piecemeal loss of liver cells and the limiting plates (the margins between the liver cells and portal areas) become irregular and ill-defined (Fig. 19.16). In foci of liver cell destruction, the sinusoids and reticular framework collapse, new reticulin fibres form, and fibrous tissue gradually develops and extends out irregularly from the portal areas into the adjacent parenchyma (Fig.

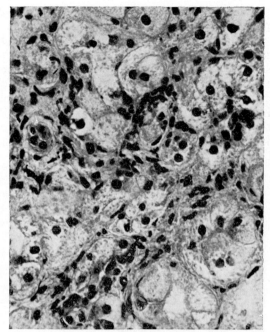

FIG. 19.17.—Active chronic hepatitis. Connective tissue has extended irregularly through the parenchyma. Note the lymphocytic infiltration and feathery degeneration of the liver cells. × 560.

19.17). Eventually the parenchyma becomes broken up into irregular-sized nodules, and the picture is that of macronodular cirrhosis (p. 564). Although the lymphoid cellular infiltration may decrease at this stage, the cirrhosis is progressive and usually fatal.

The spleen is enlarged and often palpable from an early stage: this is due to hyperplasia of the red pulp, and occurs before cirrhosis leads to portal hypertension.

Etiology. In a minority of cases, the onset of active chronic hepatitis is indistinguishable from infective hepatitis, but until specific diagnostic tests for infective hepatitis are available the part it plays in initiating or perpetuating active chronic hepatitis must remain undecided.

The various extra-hepatic features suggest a relationship with SLE and rheumatoid arthritis, and various auto-antibodies are commonly present in the serum: these include antinuclear factors, occasionally a positive LE cell test, rheumatoid factor, antibody to smooth muscle fibres and antibody to mitochondrial membrane. None of these antibodies is invariably present, and none is specific for active chronic hepatitis. Antibody detectable by immunofluorescence (p. 80) and reacting with the canalicular margins of the liver cells has been demonstrated in some cases, but it is not yet known whether it is specific for active chronic hepatitis, nor whether the antibody responsible reacts solely with liver cells.

While the above features indicate auto-immunity to various cell constituents, their etiological significance is unknown. The postulated relationship between active chronic hepatitis and SLE is ill-defined. Most of the features suggestive of SLE are relatively mild, and differentiation between the two conditions is usually not difficult. It has been suggested that the condition may occur in individuals who contract infective hepatitis and who have latent SLE or a predisposition to SLE, but when infective hepatitis develops in a patient with overt SLE, it usually runs the typical self-limiting course with complete recovery.

In our experience, active chronic hepatitis is not common, and this agrees with the small number of deaths from cirrhosis which we have encountered in young women. In its typical form, active chronic hepatitis does not appear to be the explanation of most cases of post-hepatitic cirrhosis. In most, there is either little evidence of pre-cirrhotic illness, or a rather vague history of ill-health without the various additional features of active chronic hepatitis: when biopsy has been performed in such instances it has shown chronic hepatitis, but there is little justification at present for considering chronic hepatitis as a single disease, and active chronic hepatitis is not a well-defined entity.

CIRRHOSIS OF THE LIVER

Definition. Cirrhosis is a condition in which long-continued loss of liver cells, accompanied by fibrosis and compensatory hyperplasia, has resulted in conversion of the hepatic parenchyma into a large number of nodules separated from one another by irregular branching and anastomosing sheets of fibrous tissue. The progressive loss and regeneration of liver cells is focal and leads to disruption of the normal lobular architecture, so that the portal tracts and hepatic veins are spaced irregularly in the nodules of surviving parenchyma, as well as being embedded in the fibrous septa. The condition is irreversible and the fibrosis and distortion of lobular architecture interfere with the flow of blood through the liver, with the result that, in most cases, loss of liver cells continues, and death usually results eventually from hepato-cellular failure, portal hypertension, or a combination of both.

lipochrome, and the nodules are thus often paler than normal liver parenchyma.

Microscopy of the nodules shows loss of lobular architecture, the portal tracts and central veins having lost their regular spacing. This is associated with foci of liver cell atrophy and loss, and foci of hypertrophy and hyperplasia, so that in some parts of a nodule the cells are small, and in others they are enlarged and include binucleate forms (Fig. 19.20*a*).

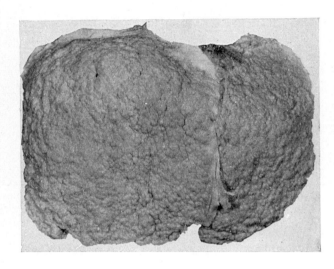

FIG. 19.18.—Cirrhosis of liver showing diffuse nodularity of the surface. $\times \frac{2}{5}$.

It is important to emphasise that the changes of cirrhosis affect the whole liver. Localised scarring caused, for example, by syphilitic gummas, is not included within the term cirrhosis: nor are mild degrees of more generalised hepatic fibrosis unaccompanied by loss of lobular architecture.

Pathological features of cirrhosis

The liver may be enlarged, usually due to fatty change of the liver cells, or of normal size, but it tends to shrink as the disease progresses, due to loss of liver cells exceeding regeneration, and terminally may weigh less than 1 kg. The surface is diffusely nodular (Fig. 19.18) and on section the parenchyma is seen to be divided up everywhere into rounded nodules, separated by bands of fibrous tissue (Fig. 19.19). The colour varies considerably, depending on whether or not there is severe fatty change, on the presence or absence of jaundice, and on the degree of congestion. Recently-divided liver cells are deficient in

The fibrous tissue runs in septa between parenchymal nodules: it may contain fine or dense collagen fibres, and varies in its vascularity depending on the duration of the cirrhotic process. It tends to involve the portal tracts, but also envelops central veins. Some nodules are seen to be partially divided by incomplete septa extending into them. The fibrous tissue appears to develop in relation to damaged liver cells, which presumably stimulate proliferation of fibroblasts, although these cells are not conspicuous in the early stages of experimentally-induced cirrhosis. Commonly, single and small groups of liver cells are entrapped within the fibrous septa (Fig. 19.20*b*). Increased numbers of small bile ducts are also present in the fibrous tissue (Fig. 19.21). Cholestasis is not usually marked (except in biliary cirrhosis, p. 565) but is seen focally in some cases.

Lymphocytes, and less commonly plasma cells, infiltrate the connective tissue and less frequently the parenchymal nodules. The infiltrates tend to be focal, and vary considerably in degree from case to case.

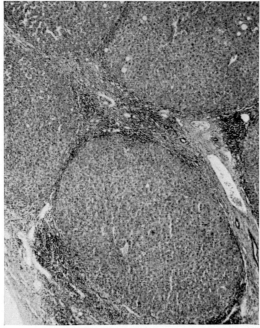

(a) Section showing connective tissue strands (in this case heavily infiltrated with lymphocytes) enclosing areas of hepatic parenchyma. × 56.

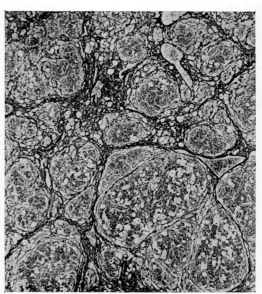

(b) Cirrhosis produced in a rat by repeated inhalation of carbon tetrachloride (see p. 550). Reticulin fibres stained black. × 40.

FIG. 19.19.—Cirrhosis of the liver.

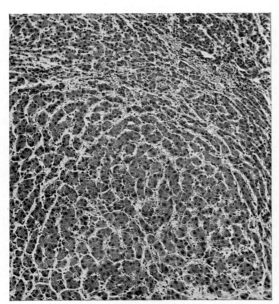

FIG. 19.20a.—Early cirrhosis of liver, showing hypertrophy of the liver cells in part of a nodule, and stretching and atrophy of the adjacent cells in upper part of field. × 90.

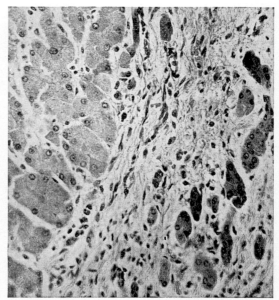

FIG. 19.20b.—Advanced cirrhosis of liver. Left, hypertrophied liver cells; right, atrophic liver cells, resembling bile-duct epithelium, lying in the fibrous tissue.

Although cirrhosis is the result of necrosis of liver cells, it is a slow process, the cells dying one by one, and necrotic cells are not usually seen in biopsy material unless there has been recent circulatory collapse, e.g. as a result of haemorrhage. In necropsy material, there is often extensive recent liver cell necrosis, attributable to terminal failure of the circulation.

Feathery degeneration of liver cells (p. 555) may be observed especially at the margins of the nodules, and this, particularly if associated with heavy lymphocytic infiltration, is an indication that the cirrhotic process is actively progressing.

Effects of cirrhosis

Cirrhosis has two major effects, *hepatocellular failure* and *portal hypertension*. It is the major cause of these conditions, particularly when they occur together.

Hepato-cellular failure is due in part to loss of liver cells, which gradually outstrips regeneration as cirrhosis progresses, and partly due to interference with the blood supply of the surviving liver cells. This latter effect is caused by the constricting effect of the fibrous tissue and also by the focal hypertrophy and hyperplasia of liver cells, which disorganises and compresses

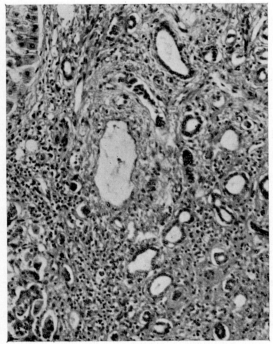

FIG. 19.21.—Cirrhosis of the liver. Proliferation of bile ducts in the connective tissue. × 250.

T

the sinusoids. Also, in areas of liver-cell loss, portal and hepatic arterial blood may pass into hepatic veins without first perfusing liver cells. This has been termed *internal Eck fistula*, and can impair the effectiveness of the blood supply to the liver.

Portal hypertension also is due to the impairment of blood flow through the liver, and wedged hepatic venous pressure measurements indicate that a major site of constriction is in the hepatic venules, although it undoubtedly affects also the portal venules and sinusoids.

The manifestations of hepato-cellular failure (pp. 571–3) and of portal hypertension (pp. 543, 572) are described elsewhere. Their association in cirrhosis gives rise to the additional feature of *ascites*, and the oesophageal and gastric varices resulting from portal hypertension can rupture and bleed, thus aggravating the features of hepato-cellular failure, as explained on p. 572.

Apart from biliary cirrhosis, which is associated with cholestasis, jaundice is usually no more than latent or mild in cirrhosis, but it may increase as a result of acute hepatic necrosis, either of unknown cause or resulting from the circulatory collapse following haemorrhage.

Haematological changes. Cirrhosis is often accompanied by a mild or moderate anaemia. Occasionally this is of macrocytic type, but more commonly it is microcytic and attributable to repeated haemorrhage from oesophageal varices or to the generalised haemorrhagic tendency of hypoprothrombinaemia in liver failure.

In the syndrome known as Banti's disease (p. 452) the splenic enlargement and cirrhosis of the liver are associated with normocytic anaemia, with leukopenia and thrombocytopenia, but the inter-relationships of the liver and spleen in this syndrome are not yet clarified. Not all cases of cirrhosis with portal hypertension develop the features of Banti's disease.

Liver cell carcinoma arises in approximately 10 per cent of cirrhotic patients in Great Britain, the incidence varying in different types of cirrhosis. It is an example of the tendency of long-continued hyperplasia to progress to neoplasia.

Types of cirrhosis

The differentiation of cirrhosis into various types is not entirely without clinical significance, and elucidation of the causes of cirrhosis, and thus eventually its prevention, are dependent on distinguishing between various types and etiologies. Cirrhosis may be classified on an etiological basis or by the appearances of the liver. Neither method is very satisfactory. The etiological factors are complex and poorly understood, and in many cases completely unknown (*cryptogenic cirrhosis*). Pathological classification is based on various features, including lymphocytic infiltration and fatty change. The main division is, however, into *macronodular* and *micronodular* types. These features are of most value in the early stages of the disease. In the later stages, the distinctive hepatic features of most etiological types of cirrhosis tend to disappear, and in particular the nodules of micronodular cirrhosis tend to enlarge. In our experience, the correlation between etiological factors and post-mortem hepatic changes is poor, However, it is becoming increasingly apparent that examination of liver biopsy material reveals features which correlate with etiological factors, and it now seems appropriate to give an etiological classification and describe the pathological features most commonly found in each type.

Type of Cirrhosis	Synonyms
Alcoholic	Portal, atrophic, nutritional, multilobular, Laennec's, fine.
Post-hepatitic	Post-necrotic, juvenile, coarse.
Cryptogenic	Multinodular, portal, etc.
Biliary:	
(a) Primary	Hanot's, non-obstructive biliary.
(b) Secondary	Obstructive biliary.
Miscellaneous	

Alcoholic cirrhosis

This is commoner in men than in women, and develops mainly between 40 and 70 years of age. Cirrhosis is often, but not always, preceded by gross fatty change in the liver cells (p. 570), and although this tends to diminish as the disease progresses, focal fatty change may persist into the final stages. Reduction in size of the liver, if present, is usually slight, the weight being 1200 g. or more. The size of the nodules in biopsy material is of the order of 1 mm. diameter and they tend to be uniform, but they become more

irregular in size as cirrhosis progresses, and at death they may average 3–4 mm., some exceeding 5 mm. Since the total liver weight tends to diminish, this change is attributable to loss of some nodules and enlargement of others. The increasing size and variation in size of the nodules as alcoholic cirrhosis progresses is one reason for the common difficulty in classifying a cirrhotic liver, at necropsy, as macro- or micronodular.

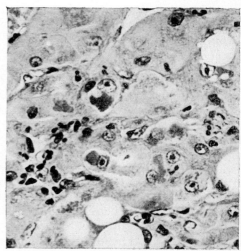

Fig. 19.22.—The liver in chronic alcoholism. "Mallory bodies" ("alcoholic hyaline"), are seen as irregular dark cytoplasmic inclusions. × 745. (Dr. R. S. Patrick.)

Variation in liver cell size is not as marked as in post-hepatitic cirrhosis; in some cases the cells contain cytoplasmic hyaline material of unknown nature but possibly derived from mitochondria (*Mallory bodies—alcoholic hyaline*, Fig. 19.22) which is seldom seen in other types of cirrhosis apart from Wilson's disease and the childhood cirrhosis common in India. The margins between nodules and fibrous septa are in most places sharply defined, the septa are narrow and composed of mature connective tissue, bile duct proliferation is slight, and lymphocytic infiltration is usually not heavy and may be almost absent.

Jaundice and fever are relatively common in alcoholic cirrhosis, probably due to alcoholic hepatitis (p. 554). The spleen is usually not palpable, and hepatic encephalopathy is less common than in post-hepatitic cirrhosis. Additional common features are muscle wasting, anaemia, vitamin B and C deficiencies, alcoholic gastritis and peptic ulceration, chronic pancreatitis, and the mental changes of chronic alcoholism.

The clinical importance in recognising this type of cirrhosis lies in its slower progress than most other types, and the possibility of effecting improvement by eliminating alcohol and instituting a balanced diet.

Post-hepatitic cirrhosis

This seems the least objectionable term for cirrhosis resulting from chronic or recurrent hepatitis (p. 571). The term "post-necrotic cirrhosis", although widely used, should be avoided, for all types of cirrhosis result from necrosis of liver cells, and moreover the term tends to be confused with multiple nodular hyperplasia which results from massive necrosis and is not a true cirrhosis (p. 569).

The liver is usually smaller than in alcoholic cirrhosis, and fatty change is slight or absent. It may be reduced to about 1 kg. The surface is more coarsely nodular, and section shows the nodules to vary more in size, often up to 10 mm. or more in diameter, and to average more than 5 mm. The lobular architecture is not completely lost, and can be detected in parts of some of the nodules. The liver cells vary considerably in size, multiple and large nuclei being common, and in places the margin between nodules and fibrous septa is irregular. The septa are thicker than in alcoholic cirrhosis, are often composed of younger, more cellular connective tissue, and are often, but not always, heavily infiltrated with lymphocytes. Bile duct proliferation is usually marked.

Post-hepatitic cirrhosis is commoner in women than in men, and occurs usually at a younger age than alcoholic cirrhosis, although the range is wide. In those cases which result from active chronic hepatitis (p. 559), many of the additional features of this condition may persist. For example, the spleen is often palpable at an early stage, there may be skin rashes, arthropathy, leukopenia, etc., the serum IgG may be high and there may be various auto-antibodies. The disease has a poor prognosis, progressive portal hypertension and hepato-cellular failure usually being more rapid than in alcoholic cirrhosis. There is also a higher incidence (about 15 per cent) of liver cell carcinoma.

Cryptogenic cirrhosis

About half the patients developing cirrhosis in this country must be placed in this category, in which the causal factors remain unknown. The group is a heterogeneous one. It includes patients with cirrhosis resembling that of the alcoholic, but without a history of alcoholism: in other patients the liver changes are macronodular, resembling post-hepatitic cirrhosis, but without any history to suggest a preceding chronic hepatitis. In some cases, the liver presents mixed features of macro- and micronodular cirrhosis.

Biliary cirrhosis

Long-continued cholestasis, whether extra- or intra-hepatic, can lead to cirrhosis. Two varieties are recognised. (a) Obstructive or secondary biliary cirrhosis, resulting from prolonged mechanical obstruction of the larger biliary passages, and (b) primary biliary cirrhosis, so-called because obstruction of the larger biliary passages is absent: this variety was described in 1876 by Hanot, and is sometimes called Hanot's cirrhosis. Its etiology is unknown.

General features. In both types, the liver is enlarged and finely nodular (Fig. 19.23), and there is jaundice with biochemical changes indicative of biliary obstruction. The serum cholesterol is high and multiple xanthomas may appear in the skin. Lack of bile in the intestine causes malabsorption syndrome (p. 592). The spleen is enlarged, at first by reticulum cell hyperplasia and sometimes accumulation of cholesterol: later, hepato-cellular failure, or less commonly portal hypertension supervenes, but the course is slow and often extends over several years.

Obstructive (secondary) biliary cirrhosis

Unrelieved obstruction to the outflow of bile from the liver from any cause results, in time, in biliary cirrhosis. The rate of development of cirrhosis is extremely variable, and depends partly on the degree of obstruction. In some cases, particularly those with calculous obstruction, bacterial cholangitis is superadded and, if severe, leads to necrosis and abscess formation, while in neoplastic obstruction the period of survival is limited, and death often results before cirrhosis has developed.

Structural changes. The early changes following biliary obstruction consist of cholestasis, the

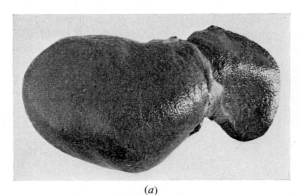

(a)

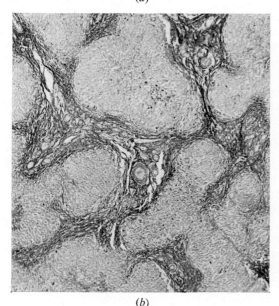

(b)

Fig. 19.23.—Secondary biliary cirrhosis. The liver of a child with congenital atresia of the biliary tract. (Dr. A. M. MacDonald.)

(*a*) Uniform fine nodularity of the surface. × ⅔.
(*b*) Fine cirrhosis with cholestasis. × 25.

bile canaliculi, particularly in the centrilobular zones, and the small bile ducts, becoming distended with bile. The larger bile ducts are dilated (Fig. 19.51, p. 588) and filled with dark inspissated bile or with white bile, depending on the site, completeness and duration of obstruction (p. 582). After weeks or months, a progressive inflammatory reaction develops in the portal tracts, which become infiltrated with lympho-

cytes, plasma cells and polymorphs, while fibroblasts proliferate and new connective tissue develops and extends irregularly between and into lobules, linking up with adjacent portal tracts (Fig. 19.24). These changes are accompanied by bile duct proliferation to form many small ducts and groups of cells within the newly-formed connective tissue. Individual liver cells, particularly in relation to dilated bile canaliculi, become atrophic, sometimes pigmented, and undergo necrosis. Bile-stained foci of necrosis ("bile lakes") are seen at the periphery of lobules, and probably result from the necrotising effect of bile escaping from ruptured canals of Hering. Biliary granulomas are also a feature. Eventually loss of liver cells and fibrosis result in disturbance of lobular architecture.

Naked-eye appearance. The liver is enlarged and firm from the increase in fibrous tissue; it is deeply jaundiced, and the surface is granular or

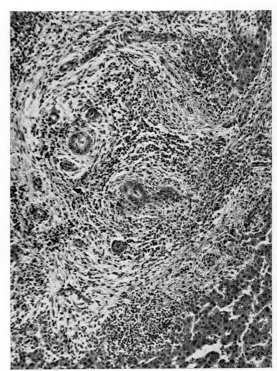

Fig. 19.24.—Obstructive jaundice and cholangitis. From a case of early biliary cirrhosis. × 100.

finely nodular. The cut surface is olive-green and the parenchyma is divided by fine strands of connective tissue into irregular-sized areas, the pattern being usually microdular. The larger intra-hepatic ducts are often much dilated. Regenerative nodules are not conspicuous until a late stage when the loss of liver cells is severe, and the appearances may then differ from micronodular cirrhosis only in the greater degree of cholestasis and jaundice (Fig. 19.25). Portal hypertension may eventually supervene, but death results more often from liver failure or intercurrent infection. Biliary

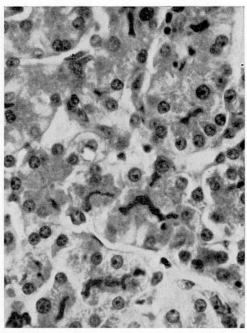

Fig. 19.25.—Cholestasis with biliary thrombi. × 390.

cirrhosis appears to be due to the irritant effect of inspissated stagnant bile upon the liver parenchyma; in some cases this is aggravated by the occurrence of a mild bacterial cholangitis, but in others infection is absent. Experimental occlusion of the main duct in animals results in cirrhosis only in some species, e.g. in the rabbit, in which multiple "bile lakes" soon appear around the portal tracts and overgrowth of connective tissue into the damaged areas follows. In man the best example of pure obstructive biliary cirrhosis without infection is seen in *congenital obliteration of the bile ducts* which causes marked jaundice and, unless relieved, leads to death within a year or so of birth. Patchy atresia in smaller, intrahepatic bile ducts may have a better prognosis. Infants surviving for several months develop a cirrhosis with features similar to those described above, but of finer, more truly monolobular pattern (Fig. 19.23).

Primary biliary cirrhosis

This uncommon condition, of unknown etiology, is characterised by the features of chronic obstructive jaundice in the absence of mechanical obstruction of the major bile ducts. After a duration varying from months to many years, it causes death from liver failure or occasionally from portal hypertension. It occurs at all ages and in both sexes, but especially in middle-aged women. Clinically, the onset is insidious, sometimes with a period of vague ill-health before jaundice appears. The degree of jaundice and of illness may fluctuate and bouts of fever are uncommon. The clinical and biochemical features of obstructive jaundice are present with a reduced amount of bile pigment in the faeces. The serum level of conjugated bilirubin may be disproportionately low when compared with the rise in alkaline phosphatase and cholesterol. Serum transaminase levels (p. 594) are usually only slightly raised. In longstanding cases, osteomalacia, osteoporosis, hypercholesterolaemia, anaemia and hypoprothrombinaemia may develop and death is preceded by overt liver failure, usually with increase in the degree of jaundice and with haemorrhages.

Pathological changes. The major bile ducts, both intrahepatic and extrahepatic, are usually normal but collapsed. The most conspicuous changes are the marked reduction in the smaller (50 μ or less) intrahepatic ducts and the abundant infiltration with lymphocytes and plasma cells around the medium-sized bile ducts and within their epithelium, which may be degenerate in places (Fig. 19.26) and heaped up in others. Early proliferation of the minute bile ducts, which are so prominent in secondary biliary cirrhosis, is uncommon. Miliary granulomas resembling sarcoid follicles are found in about one third of the cases (Fig. 19.27). At an early stage, before the development of cirrhosis, the liver is smooth and enlarged, destruction of liver cells is not apparent in biopsy material, and there may be little or no dilatation of the bile canaliculi. Later, individual liver cells may be seen undergoing degeneration and necrosis, and cholestasis is apparent. Fibrosis accompanies the inflammatory and destructive changes and eventually nodular regeneration of liver cells completes the picture of cirrhosis. The late appearances of the liver are those of micronodular cirrhosis, but jaundice is more intense and microscopy reveals cholestasis and a scarcity of smaller intrahepatic bile ducts.

Etiology. In this condition cirrhosis is attributable to prolonged cholestasis and this in turn is due to destruction of the smaller bile

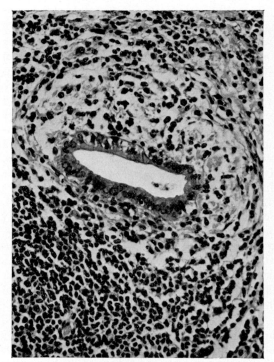

FIG. 19.26.—Primary biliary cirrhosis. Showing an intrahepatic bile duct with surrounding inflammatory reaction. The duct epithelium is unduly basophilic with vacuolation of the cells along the upper margin. × 350.

ducts. The nature of the latter is quite obscure, and it is clear that the condition has been confused with other forms of biliary cirrhosis. In the great majority of cases the serum contains in high titre an antibody against a non-organ specific mitochondrial antigen and this immunological feature is a valuable confirmatory test. The lymphocytic and plasma-cell infiltration of the portal tracts and walls of the medium-sized bile ducts raises the possibility that this is an auto-immune disease, but this is highly speculative and the anti-mitochondrial antibody may be merely a secondary phenomenon. Recent reports have described detection of SH antigen–antibody aggregates in the serum of a minority of patients with primary biliary cirrhosis.

Cirrhosis in infancy and childhood

This can arise from various causes, including genetically-determined metabolic defects such as galactosaemia, Fanconi's disease and a rare form

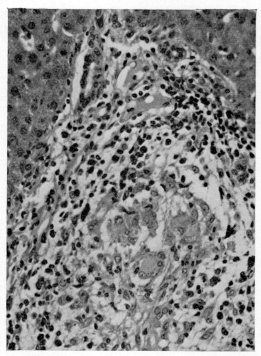

FIG. 19.27.—Primary biliary cirrhosis, showing a miliary granuloma with formation of giant cells, lying in a portal area which is heavily infiltrated with lymphoid cells. × 350.

of glycogen storage disease: mucoviscidosis (p. 599) is a rare cause of childhood cirrhosis of biliary type.

A form of hepatitis termed *neonatal giant-cell hepatitis* develops in fetal life and may progress to micronodular cirrhosis: it may be due to various virus infections. Cirrhosis is common in children of 1–3 years in India, and is of unknown etiology, and in the tropics veno-occlusive disease (p. 544) may lead to childhood cirrhosis. Of the types of cirrhosis described in other sections, hepato-lenticular degeneration and some cases of post-hepatitic cirrhosis following active chronic hepatitis occur in childhood. Finally, congenital atresia of parts of the biliary tract can cause chronic cholestasis and thus lead to biliary cirrhosis in childhood.

Diseases which include cirrhosis

Cirrhosis of the liver occurs together with other characteristic features in two rare diseases, haemochromatosis and hepato-lenticular degeneration (Wilson's disease).

Haemochromatosis

The term "pigment-cirrhosis" is applied to some cases of cirrhosis in which there is a pronounced accumulation of iron in the liver together with some iron-free brown pigment. This condition is much commoner in males. The liver may be the only organ affected or there may be siderosis and fibrosis of the pancreas and other viscera amounting to the complete picture of haemochromatosis (p. 204). The liver is usually somewhat enlarged and typically shows a cirrhosis of micronodular, less commonly of macronodular, pattern. The incidence of primary liver cell carcinoma is higher than in micronodular cirrhosis unassociated with haemochromatosis. The degree of cirrhosis and the intensity of iron storage are not closely correlated and there is no evidence that the cirrhosis results from the accumulation of haemosiderin. In cases of aplastic anaemia repeatedly transfused with blood we have found that intense haemosiderosis of the liver, spleen, pancreas, bone marrow, etc., has no harmful effect and, in contrast to haemochromatosis, fibrosis in the liver and pancreas does not usually develop.

Hepato-lenticular degeneration (Wilson's disease)

This is a familial disease affecting young people, in which cirrhosis of the liver is associated with bilateral degeneration of the lenticular nuclei. It is an inherited disorder of copper metabolism determined by a pair of autosomal recessive genes and characterised in some cases by an abnormally low level of the copper-binding serum α-globulin (caeruloplasmin). Consequently copper is absorbed from the gut in excess and is carried in the plasma in loose combination with serum albumin from which it is too easily deposited in the tissues, especially the liver and brain, and in the kidneys where it leads to amino-aciduria by defective tubular absorption. It is unlikely, however, that loss of amino-acids plays any part in the development of the hepatic lesions. The liver proteins have a high affinity for copper and this leads to the deposit of copper in the liver in greatly increased amounts. Treatment with penicillamine is of value in chronic cases. The cirrhosis is of macronodular type, but, like micronodular cirrhosis, is often accompanied by quite marked fatty change. Mallory's "alcoholic hyaline" (p. 564) is seen in some cases. Distension of the liver-cell nuclei with glycogen is said to be more prominent than is usual in cirrhosis. The changes in the nervous system are described on p. 572.

Other diseases which give rise to cirrhosis in infancy and childhood are mentioned on p. 568.

Conditions confused with cirrhosis

The rare condition *multiple nodular hyperplasia* (p. 552) is sometimes misnamed postnecrotic cirrhosis. Like cirrhosis, it leads to death from hepato-cellular failure and portal hypertension. In typical form, it is clearly distinguishable macroscopically, and the lobular pattern is maintained in the surviving areas of parenchyma. It must be admitted that the dividing line between this condition and macronodular cirrhosis is not sharp, some cases presenting intermediate features.

"Pericellular cirrhosis" is wrongly used to describe the pericellular granulomatous reaction in the liver in congenital syphilis, also now a rare condition in this country.

"Cardiac cirrhosis". As already stated (p. 159), congestive cardiac failure can result in focal hyperplasia and fibrosis of the liver but true cirrhosis seldom, if ever, ensues.

Etiology of cirrhosis

Cirrhosis results from long-continued loss of liver cells, accompanied by fibrosis and compensatory liver cell hyperplasia with formation of "regenerative nodules". It is, in fact, the outcome of prolonged hepato-cellular injury, and its prevention depends on the elucidation and elimination of the various agents responsible for such injury.

Setting aside specific metabolic abnormalities which are associated with cirrhosis, e.g. galactosaemia and the disturbances of iron and copper metabolism in haemochromatosis and hepatolenticular degeneration respectively, and the causal role of prolonged cholestasis in biliary cirrhosis, we are still left without an explanation for the great majority of cases of cirrhosis. The three factors most likely to be concerned are *alcohol, malnutrition* and *virus hepatitis*.

Alcohol. Chronic alcoholism is an important cause of cirrhosis: the incidence is much higher than in the general population, and about half the patients with micronodular cirrhosis in this country are known severe chronic alcoholics. Also, there is some correlation between the duration and amount of alcohol consumed and the incidence of cirrhosis. Nevertheless, only about 10 per cent of severe chronic alcoholics develop cirrhosis, and it is apparent that other factors are involved. The commonest hepatic abnormality in the chronic alcoholic is gross fatty change, and this frequently precedes cirrhosis, the transition involving a gradual diminution of the fat and concurrent liver cell loss, hyperplasia and fibrosis. The same train of events was produced experimentally (Himsworth and Glynn, 1944) in rats maintained on a diet poor in lipotropic factors (e.g. choline and methionine) and in first-class protein, and was preventable by adding choline to the diet. These experiments focussed attention on dietary deficiencies as a cause of cirrhosis, and certainly the alcoholic often lives on a poor diet: he is often impoverished, has a high intake of calories from alcohol, and also a poor appetite from alcoholic gastritis. However, it has not been shown that the 10 per cent of alcoholics developing cirrhosis are more severely malnourished than the others, and the role of dietary deficiencies is uncertain. It must be added that cirrhosis can apparently develop in the alcoholic without gross fatty change of the liver. Much experimental work has failed to demonstrate that alcohol can produce liver injury unless its administration is associated with dietary deficiencies, but there is recent evidence that it is indeed cytotoxic (p. 553), and this may explain alcoholic hepatitis in man (p. 554), which develops in the chronic alcoholic after a particularly heavy bout of drinking. It is not yet known whether either of these features of chronic alcoholism—fatty change and alcoholic hepatitis—is important in the pathogenesis of cirrhosis, or whether other factors are mainly concerned, The effects of alcohol on the liver are considered more fully on p. 552.

Malnutrition. The possibility that malnutrition may be of importance in alcoholic cirrhosis has been discussed above. As already stated, micronodular cirrhosis resembling that in the alcoholic, and sometimes associated with fatty change, is encountered also in non-alcoholics, and must be classed as cryptogenic. In this country, there is no evidence that the patients concerned are deficient in any major dietary constituent, and if malnutrition is an important factor it is likely to be of a more subtle nature.

In populations living on a diet poor in high grade protein, gross fatty change in the liver is common in young children, and is attributable to the protein deficiency (p. 547). In extreme cases, it is accompanied by depigmentation of the skin, a patchy skin rash, pancreatic damage and nutritional oedema—*malignant malnutrition* or *kwashiorkor*. The induction of gross fatty change experimentally, and its progression to micronodular cirrhosis (p. 547) suggested that the supposedly high incidence of cirrhosis in protein-deficient populations might be a consequence of prolonged severe fatty change in the liver. However, there are serious objections to this view. Firstly, there is a lack of convincing statistical evidence on the incidence of cirrhosis in those African, Asian and Central American countries where severe protein deficiency exists. A high incidence of cirrhosis is based on the impression of clinicians and pathologists, but what figures are available suggest that the death rate from cirrhosis is appreciably lower than in some European countries and some cities in the U.S.A. Moreover, with the exception of cirrhosis accompanying haemosiderosis in parts of Africa (p. 205), cirrhosis in Africa, India and South East Asia is mainly of a macronodular pattern, resembling post-hepatitic cirrhosis more closely than the micronodular cirrhosis which may follow fatty change in adults in this country. Secondly, kwashiorkor is seen mostly in children 1–3 years old, whereas cirrhosis occurs mainly in adults. Follow-up of treated cases of kwashiorkor has failed to demonstrate progression to clinically-apparent cirrhosis: if cirrhosis does ensue, it must take 20 years or more to develop, and this is unlike the experimental findings referred to above. Nor is there evidence that malnourished children with a grossly fatty liver but without the other features of kwashiorkor develop cirrhosis.

It may be concluded that (i) fatty liver is a common feature of chronic protein deficiency in children, (ii) it has not been shown to progress to cirrhosis, and (iii) the type of cirrhosis commonest in malnourished peoples is more likely to have resulted from chronic hepatitis than from fatty change.

Chronic hepatitis. There is no doubt that many cases of cirrhosis of macronodular pattern result from the liver injury of chronic hepatitis. These cases are classified here as *post-hepatitic cirrhosis*, and the main problem concerns the etiology of the hepatitis. In some cases, it is accompanied by additional features which justify the diagnosis of *active chronic hepatitis* (p. 559), but in others these features are lacking, and it is not known whether we are dealing with one or more entities.

A problem of great importance is the possible role of the viruses of infective hepatitis and serum hepatitis in the production of post-hepatitic cirrhosis. As already pointed out (p. 560) in relation to chronic hepatitis, the answer to this question awaits the development and application of laboratory methods for detecting these viruses and antibodies to them. At present, all that can be said is that many cases of chronic or recurrent hepatitis, whether or not accompanied by the additional features of active chronic hepatitis, often start off with an illness which on clinical and histological grounds is an acute hepatitis and could well be a virus infection, and in some instances the onset has occurred during an outbreak of infective hepatitis.

It is necessary to take into account also the fact that cryptogenic cirrhosis, developing in patients without a history of alcoholism or chronic hepatitis, is often of macronodular pattern, resembling post-hepatitic cirrhosis. In such cases, there is the possibility of a smoulder-ing sub-clinical chronic hepatitis leading to cirrhosis, and there is evidence, based on serial liver biopsies, that this does happen.

The problem of the relationship of infective hepatitis to cirrhosis has also been investigated by studying the long-term outcome of epidemic cases of infective hepatitis. No evidence has been provided of the development of cirrhosis in British and American soldiers who had infective hepatitis during the 1939–45 World War, and of an estimated 95,000 cases among British servicemen there were, by 1956, only four individuals who suffered from a single typical attack of infective hepatitis and who had subsequently been awarded a disability pension for cirrhosis. Investigations on American soldiers contracting infective hepatitis during the Korean war have likewise failed to demonstrate an increased incidence of cirrhosis. It might be argued that the individuals in these surveys were well nourished, healthy young adults at the time of contracting infective hepatitis, but an epidemic of infective hepatitis occurred among the general population of Delhi in 1955, and five years later, investigation of 304 cases, including liver biopsy on selected cases, showed no evidence of continuing liver damage or cirrhosis. Clearly, cirrhosis is not a significant sequel of at least some outbreaks of infective hepatitis. By contrast, an increased incidence of cirrhosis has been reported in women following an outbreak of infective hepatitis in Denmark. The possibility that cirrhosis is more likely to develop from infective hepatitis in malnourished individuals cannot be discounted, but does not receive strong geographical support, for although most cases of cirrhosis in malnourished peoples in Africa and India resemble post-hepatitic cirrhosis, the overall incidence of cirrhosis has not been shown to be high (see p. 570).

HEPATO-CELLULAR FAILURE
(LIVER FAILURE)

Although the liver has a large functional reserve and a high regenerative capacity when injured, liver insufficiency, manifested by failure of the liver cells to perform adequately their various functions, occurs both in patients with severe acute liver injury and in advanced cases of chronic progressive liver disease. Acute failure occurs in severe virus hepatitis, in poisoning by certain hepato-toxic chemicals and drugs, and in massive liver cell necrosis of unknown cause. By far the commonest cause of chronic liver failure is cirrhosis.

The degree of failure of the liver depends mainly upon (*a*) the amount of surviving liver tissue, and (*b*) the blood supply to the liver cells. In severe acute liver disease, e.g. massive necrosis, the extent of damage is the most important factor. In chronic liver disease, e.g. cirrhosis, liver failure may occur even in cases with a relatively large amount of surviving liver tissue, and is attributable in part to the interference with hepatic blood flow which results from the deranged architecture and fibrosis of the liver (see p. 563): this further impairs liver function and also brings about portal hypertension.

Portal hypertension, which is common in cirrhosis, results in enlargement of venous anastomoses between the portal and systemic systems, and much of the blood from the intestines by-passes the liver and enters the systemic veins. Consequently toxic substances, which would normally be intercepted and metabolised by the liver, enter the general circulation and some of the features of liver failure are thereby aggravated, or even develop in spite of relatively good liver function.

Because of the multiple functions of the liver, hepatic insufficiency gives rise to a complex syndrome, which includes disturbances of nitrogen metabolism and of formation of bile, upsets of blood coagulation, and defective functioning of the nervous, circulatory and endocrine systems. In individual cases, the features depend largely upon the nature of the liver injury, whether it is acute or chronic, and whether it is accompanied by obstruction of the biliary tract or portal flow, and by injury to other organs, e.g. the kidneys. In addition to general ill-health, with anorexia, vomiting and fever, the main functional disturbances of hepato-cellular failure are as follows:

Nervous disturbances often dominate the clinical picture, and include emotional upsets— apathy, disorientation or excitement, a coarse "flapping" tremor of the extended arms, muscular rigidity, mental confusion and finally coma. These symptoms are accompanied by abnormalities in the electroencephalogram. All these features are reversible, and are not accompanied by any obvious structural changes in the neurones, whereas the nuclei of astrocytes are enlarged, sometimes to 25 μ in diameter: the chromatin is condensed around the nuclear membrane, and the nucleolus is conspicuous.

In occasional cases, however, progressive brain damage may occur (p. 605).

All these changes are attributed to failure of the liver to detoxicate nitrogenous bacterial metabolites absorbed from the gut. In acute liver disease, they parallel the degree of injury. In chronic failure, they are dependent also upon the degree of porto-systemic shunt, and may be precipitated by performing porto-caval anastomosis to relieve portal hypertension, by a nitrogen-rich diet, or by haemorrhage into the gastro-intestinal tract from ruptured oesophageal varices, which provides a rich source of protein, and thus increases the amounts of toxic bacterial metabolites coming from the gut.

In most cases, there is an increased level of ammonia in the blood, and nervous disturbances can be induced in patients with advanced cirrhosis by oral administration of ammonium salts. It has been suggested that the nervous tissue is especially susceptible to ammonia intoxication, possibly because of interference in the metabolism of glutamic acid. However, the blood ammonia levels do not correlate closely with the clinical state, and other nitrogenous compounds formed in the intestines by bacterial action may be concerned. The liver has a very great capacity for converting ammonia to urea, and abnormally low levels of blood urea are unusual, occurring only in very severe acute liver injury. Excessive amounts of amino-acids appear in the urine, especially in acute liver failure, due to failure of deamination by the liver.

Jaundice is usual in acute hepato-cellular failure, but in very severe cases death may result before jaundice has become conspicuous. In chronic failure, the degree and type of jaundice depend upon the nature of the liver disease. In cirrhosis, it is usually absent, latent or mild until the late stages. Biliary cirrhosis, however, develops in individuals with chronic cholestasis, and jaundice of regurgitative type precedes and accompanies it. The types of jaundice associated with various liver diseases are described on pp. 590–3.

Ascites does not result from hepato-cellular failure unless there is also portal hypertension, as in cirrhosis. In chronic liver insufficiency, there is diminished production of plasma albumin, the level of which falls progressively. This contributes to the production of ascites by lowering the plasma osmotic pressure, while cirrhosis contributes by raising the intravascular hydrostatic pressure in the liver. Other factors, including increased production of aldosterone by the adrenal cortex, may also play a part.

Circulatory and vascular changes. In liver failure, there is diminished capacity to produce prothrombin and a clotting defect results which, unlike that of biliary obstruction, cannot be corrected by injection of vitamin K. Other clotting factors may also be deficient. These features are of particular significance if operation or needle biopsy of the liver is contemplated, or if haemorrhage occurs from a ruptured oesophageal vein.

In some cases, particularly those of acute liver injury, the circulation rate and cardiac output, and sometimes the blood volume, are increased; the pulse is bounding, and there is vasodilation, notably in the skin, skeletal muscles and lungs. These circulatory changes are attributable either to release of vasodilator substances by the injured liver cells, or to failure of the cells to metabolise vasodilators produced elsewhere. A well known feature of the circulatory changes is exaggerated mottling, due to patchy congestion, of the skin of the palms—the so-called "liver-palms". Another very common feature is the "spider naevus". Both these features may occur in pregnancy in the absence of liver disease, and they probably have a hormonal basis. Spider naevi consist of small leashes of dilated vessels in the superficial dermis, radiating out from a central arteriole. They are visible on the skin surface, nearly always in the drainage area of the superior vena cava; they fade temporarily on pressure and permanently after death.

Endocrine disturbances. In chronic liver failure there is in both sexes a tendency to depression of libido, sterility and loss of body hair. In men, the testes are frequently atrophic, and occasionally one or both breasts are enlarged (gynaecomastia), probably due to failure of the liver to inactivate oestrogens, which have a stimulating effect upon the breast and may also suppress the production of pituitary gonadotrophin, thus explaining the testicular atrophy. In women, the menstrual cycle becomes irregular and often the breasts atrophy, but the underlying hormonal changes are obscure.

Other features. In hepato-cellular failure, and also in portal hypertension without failure, the breath has a sweetish smell, termed *foetor hepaticus*, which is probably due to bacterial products absorbed from the gut and normally extracted from the blood and metabolised by the liver.

Fever is common in hepato-cellular failure, and occurs apart from obvious infection. *Bacteraemia*, particularly with coliform organisms, is also a complication.

BACTERIAL INFECTIONS OF THE LIVER

Pyogenic infections

Suppuration in the liver is rare except as an extension of suppurating infection in the bile ducts above an obstruction: infection is particularly common when the obstruction is due to gallstones. The condition is described on p. 588.

Rarely, multiple abscess formation in the liver results from suppurative phlebitis affecting the veins around a septic focus in the abdomen, e.g. acute appendicitis or diverticulitis of the colon; the infection may reach the liver by septic emboli or by septic thrombosis extending along the portal vein and its branches in the liver—*pylephlebitis suppurativa* (Fig. 19.28). Umbilical sepsis in the neonate sometimes reaches the portal vein and liver by the umbilical vein.

Abscesses may also develop in the liver in generalised infections, septicaemia or pyaemia, but they are less frequent and less important than in various other organs.

Actinomycosis

In actinomycosis in and around the appendix, the liver may be infected by the portal venous system, with multiple abscesses separated by granulation and fibrous tissue, and having a honeycomb appearance (Fig. 19.29). The abscesses contain thick greenish-yellow pus in which may be found the small granular colonies ("sulphur granules") of *Actinomyces israelii* which are yellowish or greyish and are sometimes visible to the naked-eye, particularly in early cases (p. 151). They may be detected by spreading some of the pus on a glass slide and looking at it by transmitted light. If a colony is crushed and stained by Gram's method, the branching filaments of the organism are readily recognised.

Weil's disease

The spirochaete *Leptospira icterohaemorrhagiae* causes a chronic renal infection endemic among rats, and can survive for some time after excretion in rat urine. It can penetrate the intact human skin, and after an incubation period of 10–15 days causes a febrile illness with albuminuria, rise in blood urea level, a haemorrhagic tendency and jaundice. The disease occurs chiefly in fish handlers and sewage

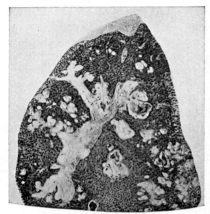

FIG. 19.28.—Section of liver, showing pylephlebitis suppurativa and numerous small abscesses. × ½.

workers and has caused epidemics in certain insanitary conditions, e.g. trench warfare. Liver biopsy may show liver cell degeneration, sometimes necrosis, cholestasis and haemorrhages. In some cases, however, the changes are slight. After death, the liver cells are often rounded and separated from one another: this may be a post-mortem change, but it is seen when necropsy has been performed within a few hours of death. Another feature is mitotic activity of the liver cells, which is sometimes striking. Death may occur in the first week, when haemorrhagic consolidation of the lungs may be the most conspicuous lesion, or after three weeks from renal tubular necrosis and renal failure. There may be haemorrhages into the skin and mucous membranes, and vacuolation, necrosis and haemorrhages in the skeletal muscles and heart. A mild lymphocytic meningitis is also common. Infection with *Leptospira canicola* from dogs causes a similar disease, with fever, mild meningitis, albuminuria and uraemia, and commonly purpura. The liver lesion is not usually severe and jaundice may be absent.

Relapsing fever

This is a spirochaetal disease, caused by various species of *Borrelia*. Large epidemics have occurred in the past and sporadic outbreaks are encountered in various parts of the world. The species of parasite and its vectors differ in different places. In Europe, *Borrelia recurrentis* or *B. obermeieri* are transmitted by lice or ticks, the spirochaete gaining entrance through scratches. In parts of Africa *B. duttoni* is transmitted by tick bites and the reservoir is in rodents and other animals. After an incubation period of 1–2 weeks a febrile illness develops and lasts for about a week, during which *Borrelia* are present in the blood, cerebrospinal fluid and urine. The attack of fever may recur once or more. The liver is congested with centrilobular necrosis, the kidneys show tubular degeneration with fatty change, the spleen is enlarged with foci of necrosis and there may be petechial haemorrhages in the skin and internal organs. Severe cases are deeply jaundiced and may die of liver failure.

Syphilis

The liver is frequently affected in syphilis, in both the congenital and acquired forms. In

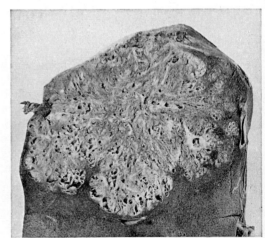

FIG. 19.29.—Actinomycotic abscesses in liver, showing the characteristic loculated arrangement. × ⅔.

congenital syphilis, the commonest lesion is the so-called pericellular cirrhosis, which is an extensive proliferation of fibroblasts, not only along the portal tracts but also throughout the lobules, between the capillary endothelium and the liver cells, both of which are compressed; thus the liver cells are atrophied and separated from one another by cellular connective tissue in which monocytes and lymphocytes are interspersed (Fig. 19.30). Occasionally compensatory hypertrophy may be present at places, the liver cells being enlarged and multinucleated. *Miliary gummas* are not uncommon. These are minute foci of necrosis in which the hyaline remains of

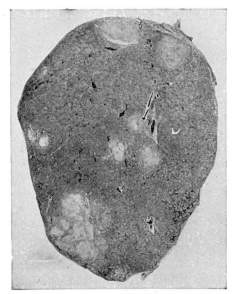

FIG. 19.31.—Multiple gummas of liver, showing the characteristic necrotic centre with fibrous capsule. × ⅔.

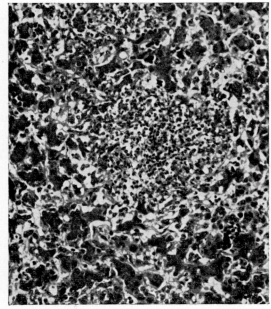

FIG. 19.30.—Congenital syphilis of liver with miliary gumma. × 130.

necrotic liver cells are surrounded by inflammatory cells (Fig. 19.30). The liver is enlarged and firm with a smooth capsule; commonly it is slightly jaundiced. On the pale or mottled cut surface the lobules are indistinct or unrecognisable. Miliary gummas, when present, are seen as minute paler points, but the smallest ones can be found only on microscopic examination. Rarely, large gummas occur in congenital syphilis. In cases dying in the neonatal period spirochaetes are usually abundant throughout the liver even when reactive changes are less pronounced than those shown in Fig. 19.30.

In *acquired syphilis*, gummas are comparatively common in untreated cases and may be very large, especially when several coalesce. In the early stage they are usually rounded and reddish grey, with central necrosis; later, they are dull yellowish and are encapsulated by

translucent fibrous tissue (Fig. 19.31). Gummas have a special tendency to undergo healing, and fibrous scars result. As elsewhere in syphilis, fibrosis may occur without necrosis, usually in irregularly distributed bands, which, together with the gummatous cicatrices, lead to indrawing of the surface at places, and thus to great deformity of the organ. This type of lesion—known as the *hepar lobatum*—is peculiar to syphilis (Fig. 19.32), and is often accompanied by chronic perihepatitis with adhesions. Compensatory changes occur, and the liver tissue forms rounded

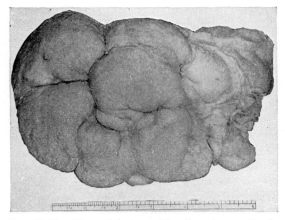

FIG. 19.32.—Hepar lobatum. The liver is greatly deformed as a result of deep scarring from tertiary syphilis. × ⅓.

projections between fibrous bands. Amyloid disease, sometimes irregular in distribution, may also be present.

Tuberculosis

Tuberculous lesions are less common than in most other organs. In generalised tuberculosis, *miliary tubercles* occur chiefly in the periportal tissue and the capsule: they may be scarcely visible, or larger and with a caseous, bile-stained centre. Rarely, a few large caseous lesions result from blood spread, and these can be distinguished from gummas only by the finding of tubercle bacilli. Another rare finding is *bile duct tuberculosis*, which probably results from ulceration of a tuberculous nodule of the liver into a bile duct. Clusters of comparatively large tuberculous nodules, with softened bile-stained centres, may involve much of the liver, and by discharging into bile ducts may lead to cavitation.

Tubercle-like follicles in the liver

Lesions resembling tubercle follicles occur in the liver in several non-tuberculous conditions. They consist of minute collections of epithelioid cells, often with one or more multinucleated giant cells which may contain various cytoplasmic inclusions, and show little or no central necrosis. Such lesions occur in most cases of *brucellosis*, in many cases of *sarcoidosis* (p. 152), and sometimes in *chronic berylliosis*. Their presence is not usually accompanied by clinical evidence of liver disease, but is sometimes helpful in diagnosis by liver biopsy when simpler methods have failed. Tubercle-like granulomatous follicles occur also as a feature of *primary biliary cirrhosis* (p. 567), but are found on biopsy in less than half the cases. Occasionally, tubercle-like follicles are found incidentally in the liver in individuals not obviously suffering from any of the above conditions, nor from tuberculosis: their significance is unknown.

PROTOZOAN PARASITES

Hepatic amoebiasis

This is a complication of amoebic dysentery (p. 520), brought about by amoebae entering colonic venules and passing by the portal vein to the liver, which they then colonise. Liver lesions may be the presenting clinical feature, or may occur only many years after the colonic lesions have apparently subsided.

The early stage of hepatic involvement is called *amoebic hepatitis*. Amoebae become arrested and multiply in the sinusoids, and cause a sufficient degree of vascular obstruction, either by their size and number or by promoting thrombosis, to produce small areas of infarction. This stage may be clinically silent. The amoebae may die off, and the necrotic areas be replaced by insignificant scars, or the condition may progress to *"tropical abscess"* formation.

Usually there is a single "abscess" of up to 15 cm. diam.; the commonest site is the upper part of the right lobe where it forms a dome-shaped swelling. It may ulcerate through the diaphragm into the lung and discharge via the bronchi. Sometimes there are several "abscesses", but they are rarely numerous. Although

the term "abscess" is used, the lesion is a necrosis of liver tissue followed by softening, and not suppuration. The cavity may have a distinct fibrous capsule, and contains thick glairy fluid, often chocolate-coloured or showing admixture

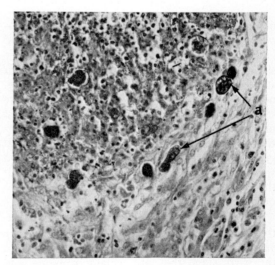

Fig. 19.33.—Amoebic abscess of liver showing numerous amoebae (*a*)—in the necrotic margin of a small recent lesion. × 200.

of blood. On microscopic examination the contents include necrotic liver cells, granular debris and a varying number of red cells; only a few leukocytes are present. Secondary bacterial infection with suppuration may occur. *Entamoeba histolytica* has a necrotising action on the liver cells similar to that seen in the colonic submucosa (p. 520). At the early stage amoebae may be present in the necrotic wall (Fig. 19.33), but when the abscess is encapsulated they are present only in the inner layer of the granulating wall. Accordingly, when a liver abscess is aspirated, amoebae are rarely present in the fluid.

Malaria

The pre-erythrocytic stage of the malarial parasites develops within the liver parenchyma cells (Fig. 16.20, p. 414), but does not appear to bring about permanent damage. Cirrhosis is sometimes attributed to chronic malaria, but this is improbable, and certainly there may be great accumulation of malarial pigment in the liver without any distinct increase of connective tissue.

Kala-azar (visceral Leishmaniasis)

In this condition, the liver is usually enlarged, and the Kupffer cells are distended by large numbers of Leishman–Donovan bodies. There may be some intralobular fibrosis, but cirrhosis does not result.

METAZOAN PARASITES

Schistosomiasis

Infestation with *Schistosoma mansoni*, in which the adult worms colonise the veins of the colon, is prevalent in Egypt and various other parts of Africa, in the West Indies, and parts of South America. *S. japonica* infestation occurs in Japan, China and the Phillipines, and the worms live in the veins of the small intestine. Both

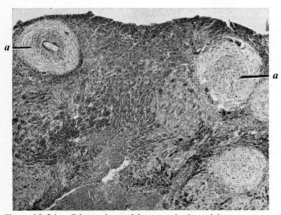

FIG. 19.34.—Liver in schistosomiasis with numerous granulomas (*a*), two of which are seen to contain schistosome eggs. × 45.

species lay large numbers of ova, some of which escape into the mesenteric veins instead of passing into the gut; these misplaced ova pass along the portal vein and impact in the liver where they give rise to reactive foci of endothelioid cells resembling tubercles, around which dense

fibrosis develops (Fig. 19.34). This inflammatory reaction is probably of an immunological nature, in which both antibody and delayed hypersensitivity are involved. Adult worms may also colonise portal veins within the liver and large numbers of eggs are deposited around the veins. The result is dense periportal fibrosis commonly termed "pipe-stem cirrhosis" (Fig. 19.35). Liver function is well maintained, but portal hypertension may develop with marked enlargement of the spleen and there may be haemorrhage from oesophageal varices. The life-cycles of the parasites are similar to those of *S. haematobium* (p. 743).

Hydatid disease

Hydatid or echinococcus is the cystic stage of *Taenia echinococcus*, and occurs most commonly in sheep, but also in cattle, pigs and man. Infection results from swallowing the ova shed in the faeces of dogs, which harbour the strobila or adult worm stage in the small intestine. The liver is the commonest site of hydatid disease in the human subject, but hydatids occur also in the lungs, brain and various other organs and tissues. Dogs become infected by eating the offal of infected sheep, thus enabling the life cycle to be completed. The disease in man results from a combination of poor hygiene and close contact with infected dogs, it occurs in many sheep-farming communities, and infection probably

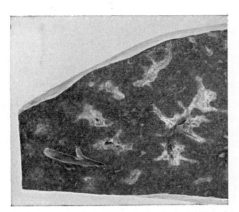

FIG. 19.35.—Liver in schistosomiasis, showing the pale areas of fibrous tissue around the portal veins.

occurs mostly in childhood. The parasite is widely distributed throughout the world; in the United Kingdom it is uncommon except in parts of Wales. The commonest type of hydatid is a cyst of up to 20 cm. diameter, containing secondary or daughter cysts, and sometimes within these again grand-daughter cysts. The cyst wall consists of a laminated ectocyst of chitinous substance, and cellular or parenchymatous endocyst, and becomes surrounded by a layer of host granulation tissue. In the endocyst, smaller cysts or brood capsules are formed, and within them numerous scolices with double rows of hooklets develop. The cyst is filled with a clear, almost colourless fluid, containing some protein (very little of which, however, is coagulable by heat). Aspirated cyst fluid usually contains some scolices or separated hooklets, and thus a diagnosis may be made from it (Fig. 19.36). When the parasite dies, the fluid becomes absorbed and the cyst wall collapses and disintegrates, and later may calcify. In a dead hydatid the hooklets persist and are recognisable for a long time. Sometimes there is secondary infection by pyogenic organisms and suppuration occurs.

Variations include a single unilocular cyst, containing brood capsules but no daughter cysts, or a mass of small cysts, most of which are not more than 6 mm. in diameter, separated by the connective tissue of the host: it is somewhat gelatinous with a nodular surface, and has been mistaken for a mucoid cancer.

The adult worm, *Taenia echinococcus*, which usually occurs in the intestine of the dog, is only 3–6 mm. in length. The small head has a rostellum with two rows of hooklets and four suckers. There are only three or four segments, and the terminal one, which is much the largest, contains the genital organs. The eggs, which are about 35 μ in diameter, have a distinct covering or embryophore with radial striation. When swallowed by man or by some animal, the covering of the ovum is dissolved and the minute embryo or oncosphere, which possesses three pairs of small spines, bores its way into the blood vessels of the alimentary canal and passes to the liver or other organs. The oncosphere there enlarges and a space containing fluid forms in its centre, while the peripheral part becomes differentiated into ectocyst and endocyst, and then the formation of brood capsules follows.

Diagnostic immunology. Absorption of antigenic proteins from a hydatid evidently takes place, for antibodies appear in the blood of infested individuals. These antibodies act as precipitins and also fix complement (p. 81). The individual also exhibits hypersensitivity to the hydatid antigen and may suffer severely from anaphylaxis when a hydatid cyst ruptures. This hypersensitivity is used in the diagnostic *Casoni reaction*, in which a minute amount of hydatid antigen is injected intradermally. Positive reactions are complex, and may include an immediate (atopic, type I) reaction (p. 99), an Arthus (type III) reaction (p. 104) and a delayed hypersensitivity (type IV) reaction (p. 106). This last is regarded as most likely to be indicative of infection, but both the skin test and the complement-fixation test may give false positive reactions in the presence of infestation by other tapeworms.

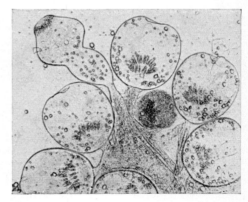

FIG. 19.36.—Scolices of *Taenia echinococcus* in fluid removed from hydatid cyst. The scolices show the point of attachment to the brood capsules, and all but one are in the invaginated condition.

Note the characteristic rings of hooklets. × 125.

TUMOURS

Benign tumours of the liver are rare. Only adenoma and cavernous angioma need be considered.

Adenoma (benign hepatoma). This occurs in childhood and is probably always congenital. It may be single or multiple, is round or oval on section and usually well circumscribed. It is generally paler than the surrounding liver tissue, although red vascular areas may be present. In most instances the tumour is composed of trabeculae of liver cells, but the arrangement is somewhat irregular and usually no bile ducts are present. Sometimes the tumour cells abstract bile-pigment from the blood, but in the absence of bile ducts are unable to discharge it, and the growth has then a greenish tint. It is usually small, but may exceed 10 cm. in diameter, and we have seen much of the liver occupied by irregular adenomatous formation, distinctly bile-stained. Adenomas may become malignant, even in childhood. Adenomas composed of bile-duct epithelium have been described, but are very rare.

Cavernous angioma. This lesion (p. 251) is dark purple owing to the contained blood, and is sharply demarcated from the surrounding tissue. Although probably starting from a congenital abnormality, the angioma apparently grows gradually. It is usually an incidental finding.

Malignant tumours

Liver cell carcinoma. (Malignant hepatoma.) This is the commonest primary malignant tumour of the liver. Occasionally a congenital adenoma becomes malignant, but in most cases liver cell cancer is preceded by cirrhosis. It is common in Africa and the Far East. Occasionally the tumour forms a single large mass which may appear to be encapsulated with central necrosis, haemorrhage and irregular bile-staining (Fig. 19.37). In other cases several nodules are present, and there is moreover a type in which an extensive nodular infiltration involves a considerable part of the liver. The tumour often grows extensively into the branches of the veins of the liver; occasionally metastases occur in the lungs, lymph nodes and elsewhere.

There has been considerable discussion about the relation of cirrhosis to cancer. We believe that cancer develops secondarily to the liver-cell hyperplasia of cirrhosis, the compensatory proliferation, for some reason, becoming neoplastic. The cells of the tumour are undoubtedly derived from liver cells, and their arrangement is more or less trabecular (Fig. 19.38); ultimately, irregularities in arrangement and aberrant cells appear (Fig. 19.39). Malignant transformation may also occur in several independent foci.

Liver cell carcinoma is a commoner complication of macronodular than of micronodular cirrhosis, the incidences in this country being approximately 15 and 1 per cent respectively. In the South African Bantu, and in some parts of the Far East, liver cell carcinoma is extremely common; this may be due in part to high incidences of macronodular cirrhosis, but there is no doubt that carcinoma develops in a much higher percentage of cirrhotic patients in these areas than in most other parts of the world.

A high incidence of liver tumours has been demonstrated in ducks, rats and trout fed on mouldy peanuts, and this has been attributed to *aflatoxins*, which are products of the mould *Aspergillus flavus*: the significance of this to the high incidence of liver cancer in parts of Africa and the Far East is unknown, but it obviously deserves the most careful attention.

Experimental production. Cancer of the liver can be produced experimentally in animals by various carcinogens, notably by *o*-amino-azotoluol and *p*-dimethyl-amino-azo-benzene (butter-yellow). These agents produce severe initial liver damage by combining with the liver cell

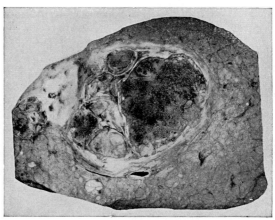

FIG. 19.37.—Primary carcinoma in a cirrhotic liver.
The tumour is chiefly in one large mass which is partly necrotic.

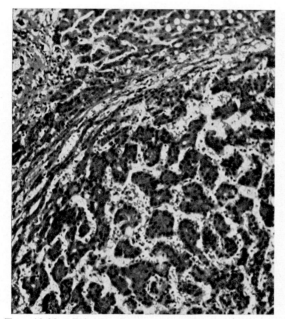

FIG. 19.38.—Primary liver cell carcinoma, secondary to cirrhosis, showing well differentiated trabeculae. × 130.

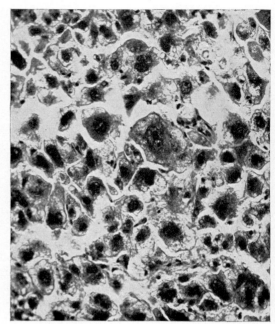

FIG. 19.39.—Primary carcinoma of liver in cirrhosis. The large aberrant cells bear some resemblance to liver cells. × 200.

proteins, followed by regeneration and compensatory hyperplasia, which in a high proportion of animals goes on to carcinoma. The tumours induced by "butter-yellow" include liver cell carcinoma, cholangiocarcinoma and cystadenoma. It is of particular interest, in relation to the high incidence of liver cell carcinoma in parts of Africa, etc., that these effects occur only in animals on a deficient diet, poor in protein and insufficient in riboflavin, cystine and choline, adequate supplements of which inhibit or at least greatly delay the onset of neoplasia.

Cholangiocarcinoma. Primary cancer derived from the smaller bile ducts—cholangiocarcinoma—has the structure of adenocarcinoma (Fig. 19.40); like liver cell carcinoma, it is seen occasionally as a complication of cirrhosis, but is the less common type of cancer. In the Far East, where it is not uncommon, about 65 per cent of cases are associated with infestation by the liver flukes *Clonorchis sinensis* or *Opisthorchis Viverrini*.

Secondary tumours

The liver is a common site of secondary tumours of all kinds. In carcinoma of the

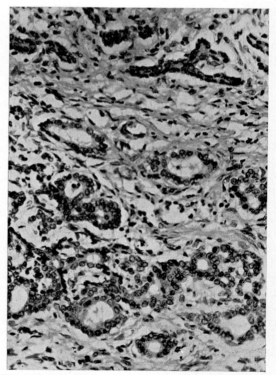

FIG. 19.40.—Cholangiocarcinoma. An adenocarcinomatous architecture with some small bile duct-like structures. × 230.

stomach, hepatic metastases are the rule. Secondary carcinoma may be in one or two main masses, but often the whole organ is permeated by tumour nodules (Fig. 19.41). The liver becomes enlarged and its surface is beset with nodular elevations, some of which may show umbilication owing to central necrosis. In encephaloid carcinoma, the liver may be enormous, 4 kg., or more; the individual masses are sometimes huge with extensive central necrosis. Jaundice may result from involvement of numerous or large bile ducts, or there may be complete obstruction of the main bile duct by pressure of tumour in the portal fissure. Sometimes, however, there are very extensive metastases without jaundice. In cases of malignant melanoma, secondary nodules may occur in enormous numbers; some nodules are almost jet-black, but others contain less pigment and are only greyish. The liver becomes greatly enlarged by leukaemic infiltration and is commonly involved in Hodgkin's disease. Secondary sarcomas are not uncommon and the liver may become greatly enlarged.

Congenital malformations

Cystic liver. Congenital cysts are rare in the liver, and are usually associated with cystic disease of the kidneys; the latter condition, however, occurs much more commonly alone. The cysts vary greatly in size and number; there may be only a few, or the liver may be studded with them. They usually contain a clear fluid, have a cubical epithelial lining, and probably originate from the bile ducts. Other congenital abnormalities such as hydrocephalus, spina bifida, etc., may also be present.

Congenital hepatic fibrosis is being increasingly recognised, many cases in the past having been misdiagnosed as cirrhosis. It is present at birth and consists of bands of fibrous tissue with a peri-lobular distribution. The condition does not progress to cirrhosis, nor to hepato-cellular failure; it may, however, give rise to portal hypertension, and when this is relieved surgically the prognosis is excellent. For this reason, it is important to distinguish the condition from cirrhosis. The hepatic lesion may be familial and is sometimes accompanied by cystic disease of the kidneys.

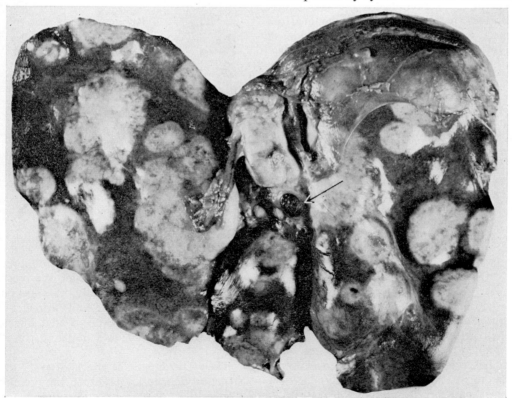

FIG. 19.41.—Under surface of liver showing multiple nodules of secondary cancer with marked umbilication. Note the thrombosed portal vein (arrow). × ½.

THE GALLBLADDER AND BILE DUCTS

Function of the gallbladder

The relatively watery bile from the liver is normally reduced to one-tenth of its volume or less in the gallbladder by the absorption of water, sodium chloride and cholesterol, the last being concentrated only about six-fold because of partial absorption. Accordingly, with the addition of mucin from the lining, gallbladder bile becomes thick and mucoid. The normal structure of the mucosa is well suited to this absorptive function (Fig. 19.42). Concentration of the bile is of importance in the formation of gallstones. It has also been established by clinical and experimental methods that the gallbladder practically never empties itself completely. When the acid chyme enters the duodenum the gallbladder discharges a certain proportion of its contents, and thereafter only small quantities are passed at intervals, but there is always a relatively large amount of bile retained in the gallbladder. Between these periods of discharge the bile from the hepatic ducts probably enters the bladder in a fairly steady flow, there to be concentrated. When the gallbladder is removed some dilatation of the common bile duct and hepatic ducts is usually observed, and this indicates an action of the sphincter of Oddi at the lower end of the common bile duct. It seems doubtful whether the normal intermittent flow of bile into the duodenum is effectively restored in this way, but there is usually no obvious disturbance of digestive function. This dilated state of the common bile duct may predispose to an ascending infection, but this is not a frequent complication.

Obstruction of biliary passages

Obstruction of the major biliary passages is common, resulting most often from impacted gallstones or tumour. The **common bile duct** is most frequently obstructed, and if the gallbladder has retained its ability to concentrate, the bile above the obstruction becomes very thick, dark and tarry, especially when obstruction is intermittent or incomplete. If the gallbladder has been removed, or has lost its concentrating power as a result of cholecystitis, or if the obstruction is in the common hepatic duct, i.e. proximal to the junction with the cystic duct, the pressure of the bile rises rapidly above the secretion pressure of about 25 cm. water. Secretion of bile quickly ceases and the unconcentrated hepatic bile is absorbed and replaced by a thin colourless mucoid secretion derived from the biliary tract epithelium and mucous

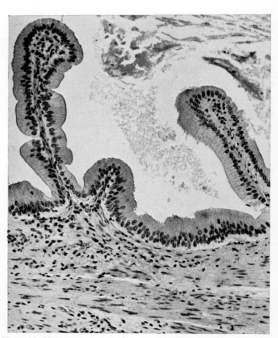

Fig. 19.42.—Normal human gallbladder, showing delicate villous folds of mucosa covered by tall columnar epithelium. × 180.

glands of the ducts—the so-called "white bile". In complete obstruction of the common duct, even with a healthy gallbladder, the pressure of the retained bile eventually rises beyond the secretion pressure of bile and ultimately secretion of bile stops; the inspissated bile is then gradually absorbed and replaced by "white bile".

The cystic duct. The effects of cystic duct obstruction depend largely upon the presence and degree of associated infection. Following ligation of the cystic duct in a healthy animal, the gallbladder becomes rather shrunken and contains highly concentrated gelatinous mucus. Following cystic duct obstruction in man, the gallbladder may become distended by a clear mucoid fluid—*mucocele* of the gallbladder. The biliary constituents become absorbed and a mucin-containing fluid is formed by the gallbladder lining. In such cases there is usually evidence of previous inflammatory change in the wall, and this probably explains the difference from the result of experimental obstruction. If the gallbladder is actively inflamed and infected, cystic duct obstruction may result in an exacerbation of the cholecystitis with the possibility of serious complications (see p. 587).

The features of the jaundice resulting from obstruction of the common bile or hepatic ducts are described on p. 591. Prolonged obstruction by stone is likely to be complicated by fatal suppurative cholangitis (p. 588), but if this does not supervene, biliary cirrhosis may eventually develop (p. 565).

Cholecystitis

Causal factors. Inflammation of the gallbladder is produced by bacteria, chiefly non-haemolytic streptococci and bacilli of the coli-typhoid group. In many cases organisms may be cultivated from the gallbladder wall or from the cystic lymph node when the bile is sterile. The organisms usually reach the gallbladder by the blood. It is possible that infection may come by the bile from the liver when the organisms are present there, as in typhoid fever. An ascending infection from the duodenum can hardly occur apart from obstruction and cholangitis. It is often impossible to state the path of infection in an individual case, but cholecystitis has been produced experimentally by tying the cystic duct and then injecting bacteria intravenously. In man, bacteria may presumably be carried in the blood to the gallbladder wall from infected foci elsewhere in the body. The presence of metabolic (cholesterol or pigment) stones in the gallbladder is an important predisposing factor in the development of cholecystitis by haematogenous bacteria. Conversely, the presence of chronic cholecystitis predisposes to the formation of mixed stones (see below).

Infection by *typhoid or paratyphoid bacilli* occurs frequently by the blood stream, and the organisms may persist for a long time with little or no inflammatory change resulting. The formation of gallstones may follow, especially when there is catarrhal inflammation, which is often associated with the additional presence of *Esch. coli.*

Acute cholecystitis. This may be merely a mild, catarrhal inflammation, or more severe—fibrinous, pseudo-membranous, haemorrhagic, or suppurative. These more severe types occur especially when the cystic duct is obstructed by impaction of a stone or by inflammatory oedema and exudate, and the lumen may become filled with pus (empyema of the gallbladder). Ulceration of the mucous lining is a frequent result and may pass into a chronic stage leading to great fibrous thickening. Abscesses may also form in the wall, or there may even be necrosis or gangrene of the wall with rupture into the peritoneal cavity. Apart from the latter occurrence, local inflammation of the serous surface is not uncommon, and adhesions around the gallbladder are thus often produced.

Chronic cholecystitis is usually an insidious infection accompanied by dyspepsia; sometimes it may be traced to a previous acute attack. More often acute attacks occur as exacerbations in a chronically inflamed gallbladder. The appearances vary according to the presence or absence of gallstones and of obstruction, but the all-important change is thickening of the wall. When there is obstruction the bladder may be dilated and its wall thinned and smooth; more commonly it shows distinct and sometimes great fibrous thickening and contraction (Fig. 19.43). The lining is often irregular and there may be distinct pouches, especially when numerous gallstones are present. The contents may be clear, turbid or frankly purulent. In many cases of chronic cholecystitis the bile is sterile, but organisms can often be cultured from the wall of the gallbladder. A common result of chronic cholecystitis is the formation of multiple gallstones, and some of the most serious complications result from their presence.

In some cases of chronic cholecystitis, the lining epithelium extends as downgrowths between the muscle bundles giving rise to deeply situated gland-like structures, known as Rokitansky-Aschoff sinuses (Fig. 19.44). Sometimes the epithelial growth is considerable and numerous gland-like spaces lined by epithelial cells are

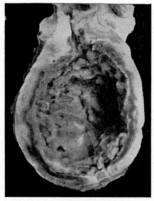

FIG. 19.43.—Chronic cholecystitis, showing great thickening of wall. The gallbladder was packed with small rounded stones. × 1.

present not only in the inner part of the thickened and fibrous wall, but throughout its entire thickness and even beneath the serous coat. The term "cholecystitis glandularis proliferans" has been applied to such a condition. In this way an appearance suggestive of malignant infiltration may be produced, although no tumour is present.

Tuberculosis of the gallbladder with ulceration has been described, but it is very rare.

Gallstones

These are concretions formed from constituents of the bile—chiefly cholesterol, bile

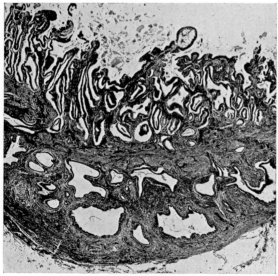

FIG. 19.44.—Chronic cholecystitis showing extensive penetration of fundus of gallbladder by epithelial-lined spaces lying between muscle and serosa. (Rokitansky-Aschoff sinuses.) × 20.

pigments and calcium salts—in various proportions in different cases, along with organic material. They form usually in the gallbladder, but sometimes a dilated hepatic duct or its branches become filled with crumbling, friable deposits composed mainly of bile pigment (Fig. 19.45). Occasionally also small and more compact dark stones composed chiefly of bile pigment are found in dilated ducts.

The following are the chief types of gallstones:

The cholesterol stone. This is usually solitary, oval, and may reach a few centimetres in length.

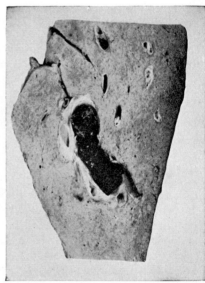

FIG. 19.45.—Intrahepatic gallstone, lying in dilated duct in liver. × ¾.

It is pale yellow or almost white, soapy to the touch and of low specific gravity, often floating in water. Some are almost transparent with a frankly crystalline surface (Fig. 19.46a). When broken across, the stone shows a crystalline structure composed of sheaves of cholesterol crystals which radiate outwards from the centre. The latter is sometimes dark owing to the incorporation of bile pigment between the crystals, but there is no break in the continuity of their formation, and no trace of lamination. Some specimens of solitary cholesterol stones, however, have a laminated cortex (i.e. concentric deposits) composed of bile pigment and calcium salts, the pigment causing the darker markings (Fig. 19.46b). This is due to a secondary deposit, which occurs when the gallbladder wall becomes inflamed by superadded

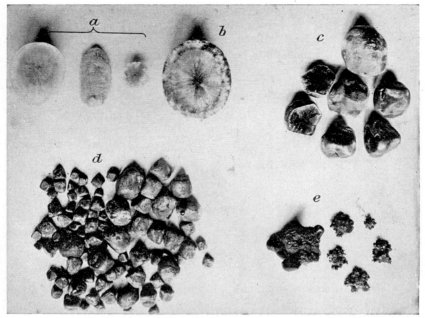

FIG. 19.46.—Types of gallstones.

(*a*) Three cholesterol stones; (*b*) cholesterol stone with mixed deposit on surface—combination stone; (*c*) and (*d*) multiple faceted mixed gallstones; (*e*) bile-pigment stones. × ⅔.

bacterial infection. Stones of this class may be called *combination* or *compound cholesterol stones*. They constitute the largest gallstones.

Cholesterosis of gallbladder. Normally absorption of some cholesterol takes place from the gallbladder. In certain states cholesterol, in combination as doubly-refracting esters, becomes deposited within the histiocytes in the mucosa (Fig. 19.48), a condition of *cholesterosis* resulting. The lipid is seen also in the deepest parts of the epithelial cells. Deposition occurs in patches, giving rise to distinct yellowish spots visible to the naked eye and a speckled appearance of the mucosa (Figs. 19.47, 19.48), The lipid deposits may increase in size, forming small polypoidal nodules. These may occasionally become free and form centres around which cholesterol crystallises. Deposition of cholesterol in the mucosa seems to depend chiefly on metabolic changes leading to excess of cholesterol in the blood and thus in the bile. It occurs in otherwise normal gallbladders, quite apart from inflammatory changes, though these are believed by some to intensify the process. The mucosa flecked with yellow has been described as *strawberry gallbladder*, but usually there is no congestion and the description is appropriate only to an unripe fruit.

About 30 per cent of cases of cholesterosis are associated with the formation of cholesterol stones, solitary or mulberry. The latter may be few in number and over 1 cm. in diameter or they may be numerous and smaller, mostly under

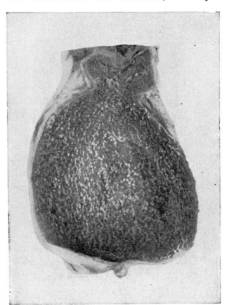

FIG. 19.47.—"Strawberry gallbladder", showing characteristic pattern due to deposition of cholesterol esters. Nat. size.

1 cm. in diameter. The surface of the larger ones is nodular and on section they show a radiate crystalline structure, there being sometimes a considerable amount of bile pigment incorporated in the central parts.

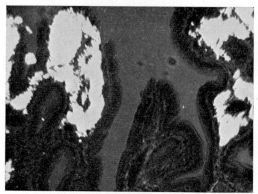

FIG. 19.48.—Section of wall of "strawberry gallbladder", showing deposits of cholesterol esters in papillae, viewed by polarised light. (Professor W. A. Mackey.) × 90.

Mixed or laminated gallstones. These, the commonest type, are always multiple and often very numerous (Fig. 19.46*c,d*). They are sometimes associated with and secondary to a solitary cholesterol stone. They vary greatly in size—from 1 cm. or more in diameter to the size of sand grains, are irregular in form and often faceted. On section they have a distinctly laminated structure, dark brown and paler layers alternating. These layers consist chiefly of cholesterol and bile pigment respectively, both containing also an admixture of calcium salts and organic material. The layers are thicker at the angles. The facetting is due to formation of the stones in contact with one another. Their colour varies greatly from white, grey, brownish-yellow, pinkish, brown or almost black according to the nature of the covering layer and the stage of oxidation of the bile pigment. Mixed gallstones occur in very variable numbers; occasionally there may be hundreds of small stones. They may lie free in the bile, which may be mixed with inflammatory exudate or pus, or they may be tightly packed together within a contracted gallbladder with thickened wall (Fig. 19.49). Occasionally a contracted bladder contains two or three barrel-shaped combination cholesterol stones placed end to end.

Bile-pigment stones. Such stones are comparatively rare; they are usually multiple, black,

irregular in form or occasionally somewhat stellate (Fig. 19.46*e*). They are composed chiefly of bile pigment, and may be friable or hard. They are often present in chronic haemolytic anaemias and are due to excess of bile pigment in the bile, but are encountered also occasionally in the absence of increased red cell destruction and in apparently normal gallbladders.

Calcium carbonate stones. These also are rare. They are multiple, small, pale yellowish and fairly hard.

Predisposing factors

Gallstones are very common, and while they may give rise to serious effects, very often they are unsuspected during life. Especially is this so with the solitary cholesterol stone. They are commonest in late adult life, especially in obese individuals, and are much commoner in women than in men; further, they are said to occur more

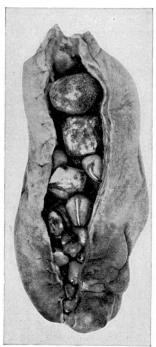

FIG.19.49.—Gallbladder filled with numerous gallstones of mixed type. × ⅔.

frequently in women who have borne children than in nulliparae. The three chief factors concerned in their production are (*a*) *stasis or stagnation of the bile*, (*b*) the *composition of the bile* and (*c*) *bacterial infection*. Biliary stasis is produced by atony of the gallbladder, which occurs in association with constipation, common in stout women, and is favoured by conditions causing pressure on the gallbladder. Some degree of atony probably also occurs in pregnancy, as part of the general diminution in the tone of smooth muscle during gestation (cf. atony of the ureters).

The importance of the composition of the bile and of infection have been established by more recent work. Cholesterol is formed in various parts of the body, is secreted into the blood, and is excreted by the liver cells, being held in solution in the bile by the action of the bile salts. The cholesterol content of the blood is increased chiefly in pregnancy, obesity, the nephrotic syndrome, diabetes, myxoedema and in typhoid fever, and a corresponding increase occurs in the bile. The solitary cholesterol stone forms in a sterile gallbladder with a normal wall or with cholesterosis, and is due to crystallisation of cholesterol from bile containing it in excess. This occurrence is favoured by stagnation of the bile and over-absorption of water. Deficiency of bile salts is a factor. Bacterial infection results in exudation, and impairment of the selective power of the gallbladder mucosa to retain bile salts within the lumen while removing water. The ratio of bile salts to cholesterol, normally 20 to 1, may fall to 6 to 1, and this favours precipitation of cholesterol, mixed with bile pigment and calcium salts.

Solid constituents of the inflammatory exudate —fibrin and cellular material—may also provide nuclei on which such precipitation occurs. Accordingly, infection predisposes to the formation of multiple mixed stones. The presence of a cholesterol stone predisposes to infection, the result being deposition of mixed constituents upon the surface of the stone, converting it to a combination or compound cholesterol stone, while multiple mixed stones may also develop (Fig. 19.50).

Bacteria can often be demonstrated within mixed stones, and Aschoff suitably applied the term "inflammatory stones" to them, and the term "metabolic stones" to the solitary cholesterol and bile pigment stones.

Effects of gallstones

Gallstones, single or multiple, may lead to no noticeable symptoms, but effects of varying severity may follow. These are partly mechanical and partly inflammatory; the latter, due mainly to the associated presence of bacteria, have been described above under cholecystitis. A stone may become impacted in Hartmann's pouch, and great distension of the gallbladder result; the bile pigments become absorbed and the contents may be a clear mucoid fluid. In other cases, and especially when multiple stones are present, the blocking is associated with more severe inflammatory change, and the contents of the gallbladder are turbid or purulent. If inflammation of the wall progresses to necrosis, the contents may escape into the peritoneal

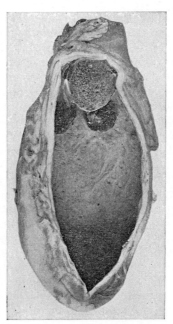

Fig. 19.50.—Enlarged gallbladder with impacted solitary cholesterol stone.

Two mixed gallstones are seen behind. Chronic cholecystitis was present. × ⅔.

cavity, resulting in localised or general peritonitis. A gallstone may pass into the common bile duct and give rise to biliary colic and jaundice. It may then pass into the duodenum or may be arrested in the ampulla for a varying length of time. If, as often happens, the stone remains loose in the duct, the jaundice is often partial or intermittent. If the stone is impacted, jaundice becomes deep, and there is complete absence of bile from the faeces. The stone may gradually dilate the sphincter, or it may be of such size that its passage is effected only by ulceration. Occasionally, when the stone is arrested at the ampulla, bile may pass along the pancreatic duct and haemorrhagic pancreatitis may develop (see p. 597). Biliary colic may also occur apart from the passage of a stone, apparently due to spasm of the gallbladder when the outlet is obstructed by inflammatory products.

The presence of a stone often leads to bacterial infection and cholangitis, which may be suppurative, especially when the stone is impacted: this may extend backwards to the liver and give rise to biliary abscesses. As has been mentioned, only in a small proportion of cases does the obstruction of the duct lead to biliary cirrhosis (p. 555). The bile ducts above an arrested gallstone or other obstruction sometimes become dilated (Fig. 19.51) and then effects follow according to the site of the obstruction and the condition of the gallbladder (p. 582). When the obstruction is below the entrance of the cystic duct there may be precipitation of bile pigment from the concentrated bile, and the formation of secondary biliary concretions which are usually elongated and comparatively soft.

In chronic cholecystitis the wall becomes thickened and may be contracted over a mass of closely packed stones: there are often adhesions around the gallbladder and a stone or stones may ulcerate in one of several directions. A large stone of the compound cholesterol type may, for example, ulcerate through into the duodenum or less frequently into the colon. It may pass along the bowel, or may become arrested at some part of the small intestine, chiefly by contraction of the muscular coat, and may produce acute intestinal obstruction, which is then termed *gallstone ileus*. Ulceration into the portal vein with the setting up of portal pyaemia has been recorded.

Lastly, the irritation produced by gallstones may lead to carcinoma of the gallbladder, or, more rarely, of the large ducts

Congenital abnormalities

Minor abnormalities of the gallbladder which concern its size, shape, mode of attachment to the liver, etc., are not uncommon, but of more importance is congenital obliteration of the bile duct. There may be merely a local obliteration or narrowing above the ampulla or at a higher level, or a length of the duct may be absent, and it may be impossible to find any trace even on microscopic examination. The condition of the gallbladder varies

considerably; sometimes it is dilated, sometimes small. It may be absent entirely. There is, of course, absence of bile from the bowel, intense jaundice coming on soon after birth, and death usually follows within a year or so. According to some observers, including Muir, the condition represents a developmental abnormality, while others regard it as the result of inflammatory change. Occasionally secondary obliteration may follow obstruction of the main ducts by inspissated bile in icterus gravis neonatorum. The condition may possibly therefore arise in two ways which may be difficult to distinguish when death occurs after several months. In a large proportion of cases, biliary cirrhosis develops.

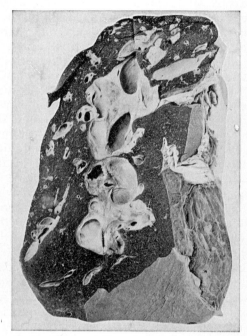

Fig. 19.51.—Section of liver, showing greatly dilated bile ducts, the result of obstruction due to carcinoma involving the main bile duct. $\times \frac{2}{3}$.

Tumours of the biliary tract

Benign tumours, such as fibroma, lipoma and papilloma, are all very rare. Rarely, a large papilloma may obstruct the outflow with much distension of the gallbladder.

Carcinoma is uncommon, and gallstones are an important factor in its causation, being present in fully 80 per cent of cases of cancer. The commonest site is the fundus and next is the neck of the gallbladder. It is usually of the slowly-growing, infiltrating type, but sometimes it is a soft growth with a tendency to necrosis. Occasionally the gallbladder may be practically destroyed and its cavity represented by a small irregular space in which gallstones may be present. It may invade the liver, and may also give rise to numerous metastases. In most cases the growth is an adenocarcinoma, sometimes a cancer of spheroidal cell or the mucoid type. Squamous carcinoma, arising secondarily to metaplasia of the lining epithelium, also occurs.

Carcinoma occurs also in the *large bile ducts* and is usually a small and slowly growing tumour. The two commonest sites are the lower end of the common bile duct (Fig. 19.52) and the junction of the cystic and hepatic ducts, the latter being more frequent; this site is also commonly involved by secondary lymphatic spread from carcinoma of the gallbladder.

Of the very many individuals who develop gallstones, less than two per cent develop carcinoma: the incidence of bile-duct carcinoma is also low, although it is often not possible to determine whether a tumour around the ampulla has originated from bile duct or pancreas.

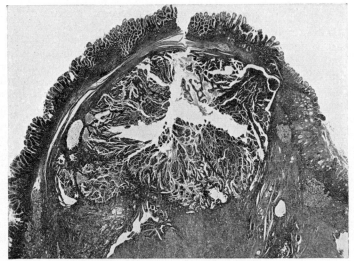

Fig. 19.52.—Primary carcinoma of the ampulla of Vater causing obstructive jaundice. × 6.

JAUNDICE

Staining of the tissues with bilirubin or bilirubin complexes is known as *jaundice* or *icterus*. When the serum level of these pigments rises above 2 mg. per 100 ml., generalised jaundice develops. According to the severity and duration of the condition the skin presents various degrees of yellow staining up to deep orange colour and in very chronic cases it becomes olive-green owing to formation of biliverdin. The internal organs also are pigmented except the brain and spinal cord, which are not usually affected. In *icterus gravis neonatorum*, however (p. 412), there may be bile staining of areas in the central nervous system, usually localised to the grey matter of the basal nuclei—the so-called *kernicterus* —but sometimes affecting the cortex (p. 605). The presence of the pigment in the blood in a case of marked jaundice is readily shown by the colour of the serum. Bile pigment may also be excreted in the urine and in the sweat; the tears, however, are not coloured, nor are the saliva, gastric juice or secretion of the bile-duct epithelium (p. 582). When the cause of the jaundice has been removed the skin may remain stained for some time after the serum bilirubin level has returned to normal, owing to the strong affinity of the elastic tissue for bilirubin. A rise of serum bilirubin from the normal level of 0·2–0·8 mg. up to 2 mg. per 100 ml. is not usually accompanied by visible jaundice, but is sometimes called "latent jaundice". The term "localised jaundice" is seldom used but it is seen around a bruise, the escaped haemoglobin being broken down to bilirubin.

Before considering further the features and types of jaundice, it is necessary to give an outline of the normal bile pigment metabolism.

Bile pigment metabolism

Most of the bile pigment is derived from the breakdown of effete red cells. Normally, about 6 g. of haemoglobin are broken down daily, with formation of approx. 300 mg. of bilirubin. This takes place in the cells of the reticulo-endothelial system—in man chiefly in the spleen, bone-marrow and liver, and the steps have already been described (p. 201). *Unconjugated* or *haemobilirubin* is water-insoluble, but it circulates as a bilirubin–albumin complex: it is taken up by the hepatic parenchymal cells and conjugated with glucuronic acid, yielding bilirubin mono- and di-glucuronides. These pigments are both water-soluble, and are referred to as *cholebilirubin* or *conjugated bilirubin*; they are secreted directly into the bile canaliculi and hence pass into the bile. Conjugated bilirubin is converted in the intestine into stercobilinogen, the normal faecal brown pigment. A small fraction of the stercobilinogen is reabsorbed from the gut and most of this passes back to the liver, where it is re-excreted, possibly after reconversion to bilirubin, into the bile (the entero-hepatic circulation of bile pigment). A minute amount (1–3 mg. daily) of the reabsorbed stercobilinogen passes into the urine, where it is termed *urobilinogen*.

The above brief account refers to the main metabolic pathway of bile pigment. It is now recognised that a small proportion of the total bilirubin is produced not from the breakdown of effete red cells, but from other haem pigments and during synthesis of haemoglobin. Moreover, conjugation of a small proportion of the bilirubin to the monoglucuronide may take place in the kidneys. Although the liver conjugates bilirubin mainly with glucuronic acid, some is converted to water-soluble bilirubin sulphate.

To understand the clinical, biochemical and morbid anatomical features of the different types of jaundice, it is necessary to appreciate that unconjugated bilirubin is water-insoluble and remains in solution in the plasma only as a rather firm complex with albumin. Consequently, it does not readily pass through capillary walls, and its increase in the plasma is not accompanied by bilirubinuria. Nevertheless, unconjugated bilirubin is capable of staining the tissues, although the form in which it escapes from the plasma remains unknown. Another feature of unconjugated bilirubin is its solubility in lipids, which may explain the bilirubin-staining of the brain in neonates with high plasma levels of unconjugated bilirubin. The brain damage which may result is due to the toxic effects of bilirubin on nerve cells. By contrast, conjugated bilirubin is water-soluble, and increased levels in the plasma are always accompanied by its appearance in the urine: it is relatively insoluble in lipids and causes neither staining of, nor damage to, the central nervous system.

The van den Bergh reaction. When Ehrlich's diazo reagent—a mixture of sulphanilic acid and sodium nitrite—is added to a solution of bilirubin, the pigment becomes diazotised to give a blue-violet compound. Water-soluble, i.e. conjugated, bilirubin gives an *immediate* colour (direct reaction) whereas unconjugated bilirubin gives a *delayed* reaction unless it is first separated from plasma protein by alcohol—the indirect reaction. A mixture of the two pigments gives an immediate colour which gradually deepens (biphasic reaction).

Classification of jaundice

Most cases of jaundice are found to belong to one or other of the following categories:

1. *Haemolytic* or *acholuric jaundice*—from increased red cell destruction.
2. *Regurgitative*, *obstructive* or *cholestatic jaundice*—from obstruction of the biliary tract.
3. *Hepato-cellular jaundice*—from damage to the hepatic parenchyma.

While it is of diagnostic and therapeutic importance to determine which of the above three factors is responsible for the development of jaundice, in practice it is found that more than one factor is often concerned. For example, the anaemia resulting from increased red cell destruction may cause liver cell injury, as also does prolonged obstruction of the biliary tract, whether or not accompanied by infection. Thus jaundice is frequently attributable to more than one factor, and diagnosis of the underlying condition is sometimes very difficult.

Haemolytic (acholuric) jaundice

Increased red cell destruction, either acute or chronic (see p. 404), results in the production in the reticulo-endothelial system of increased amounts of bilirubin, up to 1·5 g. daily. Normally, the liver is capable of extracting, conjugating and excreting such large amounts of bilirubin, and jaundice is often latent or mild. The agent causing the haemolysis may, however, also damage the liver, or the anaemia resulting from haemolysis may depress liver function, and in these circumstances jaundice is more pronounced. In infants, the rate of red cell destruction is relatively high, and the liver is deficient in the enzymes necessary for conjugation of bilirubin, particularly when birth is premature. Accordingly, *icterus neonatorum* is a common condition, and is likely to be especially severe in infants with haemolytic anaemia due to maternal iso-antibodies (p. 412). Exchange blood transfusions may be necessary to keep the plasma bilirubin below 20 mg. per 100 ml., the level at which there is a real danger of brain damage from kernicterus.

In haemolytic jaundice, most of the bilirubin in the plasma is unconjugated, and thus bile pigment is absent from the urine (acholuric jaundice). The amount of urobilinogen in the urine is, however, usually much increased and its estimation is used in the investigation of haemolytic states. The faeces are dark from the excessive amounts of bile pigment excreted. Urinary urobilinogen is also raised in various conditions in which liver function is impaired.

Familial non-haemolytic acholuric jaundice

(a) *Gilbert's disease.* Although rare, this is the commonest form of familial non-haemolytic acholuric jaundice. It is apparently due to a "dominant" defect of a single autosomal gene which impairs either transport of bilirubin to the liver, or uptake of bilirubin by the liver. Mild intermittent acholuric jaundice results. The condition is, however, rather poorly defined.

(b) *Defective bilirubin conjugation.* In this very rare but severe condition, described by Crigler and Najjar, the capacity of the liver to form glucuronides and thus to conjugate bilirubin is impaired and consequently there is severe acholuric jaundice. Kernicterus within the first two years of life is the usual cause of death.

Both these conditions cause jaundice in infancy; they can be distinguished from haemolytic jaundice by the absence of anaemia and of reticulocytosis.

Obstructive jaundice (regurgitation or retention jaundice)

Causes. This results from obstruction of either the major, usually extrahepatic, bile passages, or from cholestasis in multiple small intrahepatic biliary ducts without major duct obstruction. The distinction is important, as in the former case the obstruction can often be relieved surgically.

Major duct obstruction is caused chiefly by gallstones lodging in the common bile duct, and by carcinoma of the head of the pancreas or of the lower end of the common bile duct. Less commonly, it arises from scarring of bile ducts due to previous inflammation and ulceration by gallstones, and from accidental injury or ligation of the common bile duct during operations in this area. Other causes include congenital malformations of the major duct system, and involvement of the ducts in carcinomas, Hodgkin's disease, or tuberculosis affecting the lymph nodes and surrounding tissues in the portal fissure.

When due to gallstones, the obstruction may be sudden and complete, or intermittent if the stone or stones move along the common bile duct; it is often accompanied by biliary colic. In carcinomatous involvement or scarring of the ducts, obstruction, and hence jaundice, are usually of more gradual onset, progressive and often painless.

Apart from jaundice and its effects, major duct obstruction, particularly if caused by gallstones, is likely to be complicated by superadded suppurative cholangitis (p. 588), and in unrelieved obstruction the patient does not usually survive long enough to develop secondary biliary cirrhosis (p. 565).

Cholestasis without major duct obstruction. This occurs as a chronic "idiopathic" fatal disease, known as primary biliary cirrhosis (p. 567), and also as a complication of therapy with certain drugs.

Drug-induced cholestasis occurs as an idiosyncrasy in a small proportion of patients taking phenothiazine derivatives, notably chlorpromazine, and appears unrelated to dosage. It is reversible, at least in most cases, on discontinuing the drug. Cholestasis results also from administration of methyl testosterone and certain other C17-alkyl-substituted testosterones, and does not depend upon idiosyncrasy, being produced regularly by a sufficient dosage of such compounds. Cholestasis is also a prominent feature in some cases of infective (virus) hepatitis, and develops sometimes in infants with haemolytic disease of the newborn.

Apart from biliary cirrhosis, cholestasis is not usually a prominent feature of cirrhosis, in which jaundice, if present, is likely to be attributable to liver cell necrosis and hepato-cellular failure.

Pathological features. When obstruction of ducts occurs, the liver cells go on forming and secreting bile, and this leads to distension of the bile canaliculi between the liver cells. In long-standing cases these may be filled with hyaline greenish plugs of inspissated bile, which often show branching processes passing between the liver cells (Fig. 19.25, p. 567). In major duct obstruction, the large intrahepatic ducts also become dilated and the appearances of their contents vary according to the position of the obstruction (p. 582). The accumulated bile in the liver contains only a part of the pigment formed, the rest being absorbed and carried into the circulation. There has been dispute as to the path of absorption. Some experiments point to its being via the lymphatics; others no less clearly seem to prove that the pigment passes directly into the blood. Probably both paths are concerned in the absorption. Conjugated bilirubin diffuses readily through the capillary walls into the tissues, and it is very likely that similar diffusion occurs from the surcharged liver cells into the related capillaries. There is often microscopic evidence of phagocytosis of plugs of inspissated bile by Kupffer cells.

The distinction between major duct obstruction and cholestasis without major duct obstruction is difficult to make from liver biopsy material. In the former, the biliary ducts are usually more prominent in the portal tracts, and polymorphs are often fairly numerous in their vicinity; in some cases, rupture of canals of Hering at the margins of lobules leads to foci of bile-staining and necrosis of liver cells—the so-called *bile lakes* (p. 566).

In obstructive jaundice, not only is there a great accumulation of conjugated bilirubin in the blood, with consequent excretion in the urine, but there is also regurgitation into the blood of bile salts and cholesterol (cholaemia). The bile salts are usually abundant in the urine, though after a time they may disappear; apparently they

may cease to be formed by the liver. The cholesterol content of the blood is usually considerably increased, and cholesterol esters may be deposited in macrophages in the skin as yellow patches or nodules—*xanthomas* (p. 19), or in the spleen, causing splenomegaly. The serum level of alkaline phosphatase is also much raised owing to its re-absorption, and estimations of blood cholesterol and alkaline phosphatase levels are helpful in distinguishing obstructive from other types of jaundice. The serum van den Bergh reaction is direct, but this is a less helpful finding in differential diagnosis. It should be noted that biochemical tests fail to distinguish between major duct obstruction and intrahepatic cholestasis.

The absorption of the constituents of the bile leads in itself to comparatively little toxic effect. There is usually bradycardia, mental depression, and itchiness of the skin often occurs.

In addition to the above features resulting from regurgitation of bile constituents, prolonged obstructive jaundice is associated with malabsorption owing to exclusion of bile from the intestine. Fats and fat-soluble vitamins are poorly absorbed, and this may lead to vitamin K deficiency and consequently to a clotting defect due to hypoprothrombinaemia, a complication of importance in surgical intervention. This is remediable by injection of vitamin K unless biliary cirrhosis and liver failure have supervened, when the liver may fail to produce sufficient prothrombin even when vitamin K is provided. Calcium deficiency, osteomalacia and osteoporosis may also result from malabsorption.

Dubin-Johnson syndrome. In this rare condition, there is a partial failure of the liver cells to secrete conjugated bilirubin into the bile canaliculi, and as a consequence conjugated bilirubin is regurgitated into the blood and intermittent jaundice results. The other constituents of the bile are secreted normally, and the serum alkaline phosphatase level is not raised. A curious feature is accumulation of granules of brown pigment, apparently lipofuscin, in the liver cells. Little or no disability results from this syndrome, which is believed to be due to a single gene defect with "dominant" transmission. A second, and genetically related condition, is the *Rotor syndrome* in which there is failure to secrete conjugated bilirubin but no accumulation of lipofuscin in the liver cells.

Hepato-cellular jaundice (toxic jaundice)

This type of jaundice results from damage to liver cells, for example by viruses, bacterial toxins or hepatotoxic chemicals. It is a feature of infective hepatitis, yellow fever and leptospiral jaundice (Weil's disease), where the organisms are actually present in the liver, and it occurs occasionally in typhus, pneumonia, septicaemia, relapsing fever, smallpox, etc. It is seen also in some forms of snake-bite and in poisoning with trinitrotoluol, phosphorus, amanitine and amanita toxin from poisonous fungi, etc.

Two factors are concerned in the production of hepato-cellular jaundice.

(*a*) Damage to the liver cells may interfere with the passage of bile along the bile canaliculi; in other words a degree of intra-hepatic cholestasis arises. Focal necrosis or swelling of the liver cells, and disorganisation of the columns of liver cells and fibrosis (as in cirrhosis), may thus cause focal cholestasis. (*b*) Removal of unconjugated bilirubin from the blood, its conjugation and discharge into the bile canaliculi, may all be impaired as a result of liver-cell injury. The relative importance of these two factors varies in different cases, and may also change, as liver-cell injury progresses, in the individual case.

In infective hepatitis, the commonest cause of hepato-cellular jaundice, most of the serum bilirubin is conjugated; the urine is bile-stained and the faeces pale, indicating that regurgitation, and not failure to take up or conjugate bilirubin, is the major factor. Accordingly, the van den Bergh reaction is usually direct, and is of little or no value in differentiating the condition from obstructive jaundice. In some cases of hepato-cellular jaundice, bile salts are absent from the urine, the term "dissociated jaundice" being then applied. By contrast with obstructive jaundice, patients with hepato-cellular jaundice have more severe symptoms—nausea, vomiting, anorexia and malaise—owing to the parenchymal damage which has caused jaundice. Some of the chemical poisons cause haemolysis also, and the increased formation of bilirubin accentuates the jaundice.

Liver function tests

When we consider the many different functions of the liver, and the various methods available for their assessment, it is hardly surprising that a great number of tests have been proposed. Such tests are often misapplied, and some are unsatisfactory, but the consensus of opinion is that helpful information is obtainable from the procedures enumerated below, especially if repeated tests can be carried out.

According to the aspect of liver function they are designed to assess, liver function tests may be conveniently grouped as follows:

(*a*) *Estimation of the blood level of substances excreted by the liver.* Either products of normal metabolism, such as bilirubin, alkaline phosphatase and cholesterol, or foreign substances introduced intravenously, may be used. Of the latter "bromsulphthalein", a constant proportion of which is normally removed by the liver per unit of time, is frequently employed.

(*b*) *Plasma protein estimations.* The liver is the source of a number of plasma proteins, and their production tends to diminish in prolonged hepato-cellular insufficiency. For example, the serum albumin level is low in decompensated cirrhosis, while a fall in plasma prothrombin level (in the presence of adequate vitamin K) is also an indication of liver failure, and is of particular importance where operation or liver biopsy is being considered. Other proteins made in the liver include fibrinogen, transferrin and caeruloplasmin, but assay of these is of less value.

The immunoglobulins are produced mainly by plasma cells in the lymphoid tissues, and their serum levels are not directly related to liver disease. However, increased levels are encountered in various types of prolonged hepatitis and cirrhosis (as well as in many chronic non-liver diseases).

The levels of serum α_2- and β-globulins, which include lipoproteins, are usually raised in obstructive jaundice, along with a general rise in cholesterol and other lipids.

A rapid and useful method of investigating the serum proteins is provided by electrophoresis on paper or cellulose acetate strips. This shows the relative concentrations of the various protein fractions, and if necessary can be supplemented by quantitative techniques, including the increasingly popular radial immuno-precipitation method of Mancini. A number of empirical tests depend upon precipitation of various substances in colloidal solution on addition of the patient's serum: they include the cephalin–cholesterol flocculation test, colloidal gold and zinc sulphate reactions, and the thymol turbidity and thymol flocculation reactions. The mechanisms of precipitation are complex, depending on the levels of immunoglobulins, albumin and probably other plasma proteins: they are being replaced gradually by serum protein determinations, transaminase estimations, etc.

(c) *Estimation of the amount of urobilinogen excreted in the urine.*

(d) *Estimation of the blood level of transaminases.* The cells of many tissues, including the liver, myocardium, skeletal muscle and lung are rich in enzymes termed transaminases. There are many such enzymes, and their function is to convert amino-acids to keto-acids; the two which have received most attention are glutamic-oxalacetic (GOT) and glutamic-pyruvic (GPT) transaminases, which convert glutamic acid to oxalacetic and pyruvic acids respectively. Injury of transaminase-rich cells results in their release into the blood, and accordingly assay of the serum levels (SGOT and SGPT) is used to detect and determine the extent of destructive changes in liver, skeletal muscles, myocardium, etc. Because of the size of the liver and its richness in these enzymes, acute liver injury is accompanied by very high serum transaminase levels, while smaller increases occur in chronic liver injury, e.g. cirrhosis.

For details of these tests, manuals on laboratory procedures should be consulted. Only a brief general summary of their significance can be given here. The chief problems clinically are (1) *diagnostic*, i.e. the detection of liver cell injury in the absence of jaundice, as in mild virus hepatitis; the differentiation of obstructive from other types of jaundice, and the differentiation of alcoholic cirrhosis, primary biliary cirrhosis, active chronic hepatitis and post-hepatitic cirrhosis. (2) *prognostic*, in cases of diffuse liver damage. Some assistance is obtained by comparing the results of a number of the above tests. In addition to quantitative estimation of serum bilirubin, urinary urobilinogen and plasma proteins, three tests which should always be performed, it is usual to carry out at least one additional test in each category in order to procure information over a range of hepatic functions. The most consistently useful tests appear to be the following: in *group* (a) the alkaline phosphatase, which gives consistently higher figures in obstructive jaundice than in toxic-infective states. There is, however, a considerable zone of equivocal results. Also the clearance from the blood of bromsulphthalein after intravenous injection is especially useful in assessing impairment of function in the absence of jaundice. A severe fall in the albumin level, e.g. to less than 3 g. per 100 ml., has a very unfavourable prognostic significance. The levels of the immunoglobulins are of some help in distinguishing between various types of chronic hepatitis and of cirrhosis, although changes in their levels are neither consistent nor characteristic of any particular type of disease, nor indicative of hepatic abnormality. The IgG level is usually high in persistent infective hepatitis, active chronic hepatitis and post-hepatitic cirrhosis; a marked rise of IgM is usual in primary biliary cirrhosis and common in alcoholic cirrhosis; IgA levels are raised in some cases of cirrhosis of various types.

Serum transaminase levels are of value in distinguishing between obstructive and hepatocellular jaundice. They are also raised in liver damage which has not resulted in jaundice. Raised levels are helpful in the early diagnosis of acute liver injury, e.g. in infective hepatitis, and continued high levels indicate disease activity; but subsequent to the initial rise, the levels may fall in spite of extensive liver cell necrosis, and falling levels alone are of little prognostic value.

The various tests of liver functions are in general likely to yield positive evidence of impairment in conditions of diffuse generalised damage to the organ, and they are often of value in following the progress of a case. When there are extensive secondary malignant deposits or other infiltrations in the liver the results of liver function tests are commonly within normal limits owing to the substantial functional reserve. In post-necrotic scarring and in cirrhosis and other fibrotic conditions following diffuse damage to liver cells, certain abnormalities are likely to be revealed by a judicious selection of the above tests so that it is often, though not invariably, possible to distinguish diffuse involvement of the liver cells from other causes of hepatic enlargement. Decisive information may sometimes be obtained by percutaneous needle-biopsy of the liver. The method is, however, not without some risk, and the information gained may be misleading if an unrepresentative sample of liver tissue is obtained. Biopsy by laparotomy is often more satisfactory and if exploratory laparotomy is performed the opportunity should be taken to secure a representative portion of liver for microscopic examination.

DISEASES OF THE EXOCRINE PANCREAS

The pancreas is composed of two kinds of tissue with distinct functions—the acinous or exocrine glandular tissue, which produces the digestive secretion of the gland, and the islets of Langerhans, which secrete several hormones of importance in carbohydrate metabolism, including insulin and glucagon and also probably gastrin (Chapter 24, also p. 600).

Pancreatic function can be assessed with a fair degree of accuracy by measuring the volume and enzyme content of pancreatic juice obtained by duodenal aspiration. The response of the organ to a secretory stimulus can be assessed by administration of secretin or pancreozymin. Radiographic techniques such as arteriography, air insufflation, pancreatography and duodenography, assist in the diagnosis of structural abnormalities.

Degenerative changes. Cloudy swelling and even focal necrosis occur in infections, fatty change in various poisonings, and sometimes amyloid change from the usual causes. Lipomatosis occurs in obesity, and is often a marked feature when the glandular tissue becomes atrophied, e.g. after obstruction of the duct. Atrophy of the gland accompanies fibrotic lesions and obstructions of the duct, described below; it occurs also in wasting diseases, and to a lesser degree as a senile change. Abnormal smallness of the pancreas without any other change occurs in some cases of diabetes in young subjects, but its nature and significance are doubtful. Pigmentation from deposition of granular haemosiderin, sometimes considerable, is common in haemochromatosis (p. 204) and may be accompanied by diabetes. When the pancreatic tissue is injured in various ways, it is attacked by its own enzymes, and necrosis results. Thus small circumscribed areas of dull yellowish necrotic tissue are a common necropsy finding. They are seen especially after operations on the pancreas, in acute and chronic pancreatitis, and in obstruction of the ducts; they are often accompanied by patches of necrosis in the fat around the pancreas (Fig. 19.53*b*). Fine fibrosis and dilatation of the pancreatic ducts and acini may occur in uraemia ("uraemic pancreatitis").

Experimentally the administration of ethionine to rats has resulted in pancreatic degeneration and necrosis, apparently by antagonising methionine and interfering with protein synthesis.

U

Acute haemorrhagic necrosis of the pancreas (acute pancreatitis)

In most cases this condition is essentially an acute necrosis with haemorrhage in greater or lesser degree; in the later stages secondary infection leading to *suppuration* and even to *gangrene* may occur. These changes characterise stages in the condition rather than distinct varieties. In cases dying very rapidly after the onset of symptoms there may be patchy necrosis of the pancreas with only a light haemorrhagic speckling, indicating that necrosis precedes thrombosis and haemorrhage, but in others of longer duration the whole organ may be deep purple-black owing to diffuse interstitial haemorrhage.

Clinical features. Haemorrhagic necrosis is somewhat rare. It occurs most frequently after the age of forty, has a distinct association with obesity, alcoholism, diabetes, cholecystitis and gallstones, and is commoner in women than in men. The disease comes on suddenly with abdominal pain, vomiting and collapse, and it may simulate gastro-duodenal perforation. The cause of the rapid and fatal collapse is not clear; it has been ascribed to the pressure by the blood on the sympathetic ganglia and coeliac plexus, or to the absorption from the damaged pancreas of products of tryptic digestion of protein. The latter is probably the correct explanation as the symptoms may occur when there is little haemorrhage. The peritoneal cavity generally contains bloodstained serous fluid, and numerous patches of *fat necrosis* result from the liberation of pancreatic lipase from the damaged parenchyma; the fat is split, the glycerol being absorbed, while the firm yellowish-white patches represent fatty acids. These patches are specially numerous in the region of the pancreas and in the greater omentum, (p. Fig. 19.53*b*), but occur elsewhere. Amylase is also set free and is absorbed into the blood, which then shows enhanced amylolytic power; it is also excreted in the urine, and estimation of the serum and urinary amylase may be of diagnostic help. The haemorrhage into the pancreas and tissues around may be so extensive that a dark mass is seen through the peritoneum of the lesser peritoneal sac. The cut surface of the pancreas varies; in some cases it is almost uniformly haemorrhagic, in others there is a mixture of dull yellowish areas of necrosis with haemorrhage between and around (Fig. 19.53), and sometimes necrosis predominates.

On **microscopic examination**, necrosis, haemorrhage and inflammation are associated in varying proportions. Haemorrhage may be the outstanding feature, the whole tissue of the gland being infiltrated with blood, while diffuse

necrosis of the acini is seen at places. Many of the small veins and capillaries contain packed red cells owing to extreme loss of plasma; later their walls become necrotic and this may play a part in causing haemorrhage. In other cases there are areas of well-defined necrosis, affecting all the tissues, both glandular and interstitial, and accompanied by heavy neutrophil polymorph infiltration (Fig. 19.54). The inflammatory reaction seems to occur later, and is most marked in the less acute cases. All the appearances may be interpreted as the result of some

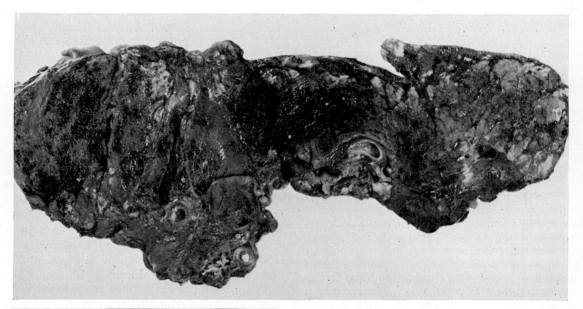

FIG. 19.53*a*.—Acute haemorrhagic pancreatitis. × 0·6.

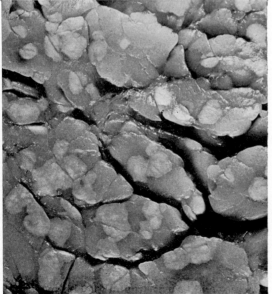

FIG. 19.53*b*.—Part of the greater omentum from the same case, showing pale patches of fat necrosis. × 1·7.

toxic agent, which kills the parenchyma and also acts on the vessels, leading to thrombosis and haemorrhage. Clumps of bacteria, chiefly bacilli, may be seen at places, but these are to be regarded as secondary invaders, as it is common to find large areas in which none can be seen.

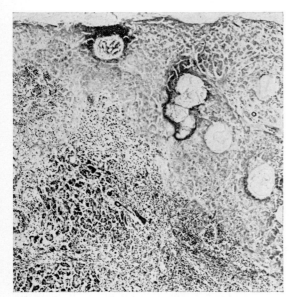

FIG. 19.54.—Acute haemorrhagic necrosis of pancreas.
The pale-staining necrotic area with fat necrosis is seen top right, with surviving pancreas below. × 38.

Gangrenous pancreatitis is generally regarded as merely a late stage of the condition. The haemorrhagic and necrotic tissue becomes secondarily invaded by putrefactive organisms which lead to softening and disintegration of the tissue, and may spread to the peritoneal cavity and cause a local or general peritonitis.

The etiology of haemorrhagic pancreatitis is, in most instances, obscure. It is thought to be due essentially to liberation of activated trypsinogen either as a result of damage to the parenchyma or perhaps from rupture of distended ducts, the free enzymes leading at first to an acute inflammatory oedema, and later to necrosis of the vessel walls, sludging of red cells, haemorrhage and thrombosis. There is recent evidence that low molecular-weight dextran administered intravenously may arrest the experimentally-induced condition at the stage of inflammatory oedema, and preliminary reports on the clinical use of dextran are encouraging.

Pancreatic enzymes may be activated by several agents, including bile, dilute hydro-

chloric acid and bacteria. Cases have been reported in which obstruction of the ampulla of Vater, usually by a gallstone, has resulted in bile passing along the pancreatic duct, and it has been shown that spasm of the sphincter of Oddi, which can be induced by dilute hydrochloric acid, can have a similar effect. However, in most cases of acute pancreatitis the bile and pancreatic ducts have been found to open separately into the duodenum, and this mechanism cannot operate. The reflux of duodenal contents along the pancreatic duct has recently received much attention, and some workers believe that increased intra-abdominal pressure may play an initial role in acute pancreatitis.

Partial obstruction of pancreatic ducts by squamous metaplasia has been suggested as a predisposing cause. Such changes are not, in

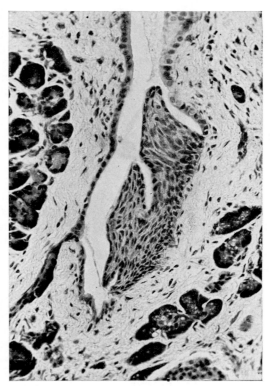

FIG. 19.55.—Squamous metaplasia of lining of pancreatic duct, an incidental finding in an otherwise normal organ. × 210.

our experience, very frequent, and their significance is uncertain, but we have seen partial blockage of the ducts by squamous metaplasia (Fig. 19.55) in cases of acute pancreatitis.

In addition to cholelithiasis, diabetes mellitus, obesity, alcoholism and pregnancy, which are the commoner associations of acute pancreatitis, less common but nonetheless significant associations have been reported for a large number of conditions. These include mumps, acute renal failure, the connective tissue diseases, abdominal trauma and conditions causing a raised level of plasma calcium. It has also been reported in patients being treated with thiazides, cortisone or anticoagulants, and in families transmitting certain genetically-determined diseases, including familial hyperlipidaemia, muco-viscidosis, and renal tubular defects.

Suppurative pancreatitis may occur apart from secondary infection of an established pancreatic necrosis. It is then usually caused by passage of organisms along the ducts, but sometimes results by extension from the surrounding tissues or by blood spread; the lesions lack the characteristic enzymatic tissue destruction of haemorrhagic necrosis. We have seen one case where there was ulceration of a diverticulum in the duodenum, and from this the organisms had spread to the pancreas. The suppuration may occur in one or several foci, and may produce considerable destruction of the gland. Fat necrosis may be present in the tissues around, but it is usually less marked than in the more acute haemorrhagic lesions.

Chronic pancreatitis

It is important to distinguish between recurrent attacks of acute pancreatitis, which do not necessarily lead to pancreatic deficiency, and chronic pancreatitis, which is usually progressive.

Chronic pancreatitis is fairly common, and its etiology is often obscure. Frequently, however, it appears to follow an ascending infection of the ducts. Thus it may be associated with cholelithiasis, and it occurs also when the pancreatic duct is obstructed, as will be described below. It may occur in chronic alcoholics, and it is certainly fairly often associated with cirrhosis of the liver. Chronic pancreatitis with calcification is reported to be common in Uganda, the Congo and Nigeria. Alcoholism and a high-carbohydrate, low-protein diet have been suggested as causal factors. The combination of chronic pancreatitis and cirrhosis of the liver with accumulation of haemosiderin is seen also in

haemochromatosis ("bronzed diabetes"). The evidence is against the view that deposition of haemosiderin is the cause of the overgrowth of the connective tissue. Muir and Dunn recorded several cases in which the chronic pancreatitis had begun, while there was practically no deposit of pigment, although the liver was cirrhotic and extensively pigmented. Areas of fibrosis in the pancreas may be produced, as in other organs, by arteriosclerosis and this may account for some cases of healed mild pancreatitis. Lastly, there is a form of diffuse interstitial pancreatitis in congenital syphilis.

In chronic pancreatitis the gland becomes firmer. Sometimes it is enlarged, but more frequently shrunken and atrophic. The histological changes comprise fibrosis and atrophy of the glandular elements. The fibrosis may be chiefly between the lobules—*interlobular*—or there may be a more diffuse fibrosis between the acini—*intralobular*. In the connective tissue, the small ducts may be unduly prominent, and some of these may be newly formed in the same way as the small bile ducts in cirrhosis of the liver. The islets of Langerhans suffer less than the glandular acini, but they also may be implicated in the fibrosis when it is intralobular in distribution, and thus diabetes may result.

Chronic pancreatitis is associated with varying degrees of malabsorption, and the stools contain an excess of *unsplit* fat and of undigested muscle fibres. Other features of the *malabsorption syndrome* (p. 523) may be present. In some cases, the serum amylase and lipase levels are raised, and a radiograph of the abdomen may show calcification.

Obstruction of pancreatic ducts

Obstruction of the main duct may be caused by a pancreatic calculus, occasionally by a gallstone filling the ampulla of Vater, by cicatricial contraction, or by pressure of a tumour, most frequently cancer of the head of the pancreas. When obstruction is produced in any of these ways, there is some irregular dilatation of the large ducts. The smaller ducts may be similarly affected and may occasionally show cyst-like distension. The result, as in other organs, no doubt depends on whether the obstruction is constant or intermittent, but two changes are prominent, atrophy of the exocrine cells and overgrowth of the connective tissue. In long-standing cases only shrunken remains of the parenchyma are found in the connective tissue. Sometimes the atrophy is accompanied by extensive replacement of the gland by adipose tissue (lipomatosis) (Fig. 24.18, p. 900). The islets of Langerhans are not affected by the atrophic process, but, on the contrary, they are more prominent and appear more numerous than usual, owing to the shrinking of the other tissues (Fig. 19.56). Even when the exocrine tissue has

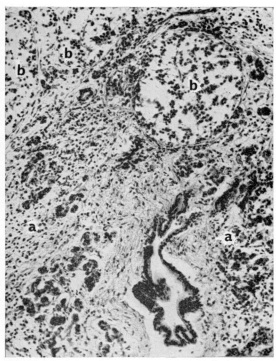

FIG. 19.56.—Fibrosis of pancreas secondary to obstruction of the duct. Note marked atrophy of the parenchyma (*a*), while the islets of Langerhans (*b*) are relatively normal × 140.

almost gone, groups of virtually unchanged islets remain. Similar results have been obtained by experimental ligation of the pancreatic duct in animals; here also the persistence of the islets is outstanding. This explains why diabetes does not as a rule follow ligation of the main duct.

In view of the effects of pancreatic duct obstruction, it is curious that pancreatic tissue of normal microscopic appearance is sometimes seen in teratomas of the thymus: it seems most unlikely that such tissue could have a patent duct system.

Pancreatic calculi

These are small concretions composed of calcium carbonate and a little phosphate, which form in the pancreatic ducts, though their occurrence is rare. They seldom exceed 5 mm., and they may be numerous and minute. They are irregularly rounded or elongated, whitish and usually hard. In addition to causing obstruction in varying degree, they may lead to secondary bacterial infection, with acute or chronic inflammatory change as the result.

Cysts

The most important variety is the single "pancreatic cyst" which forms a large rounded swelling, sometimes of over 10 cm. diameter. The cyst usually contains a colourless fluid, clear or slightly turbid, though sometimes there may be an admixture of altered blood. The pancreatic enzymes are present in the fluid for a time, and may be detected by the usual tests; later, however, they disappear. The formation of such a cyst has been observed after injury, and this is regarded as the usual origin. The layer of peritoneum over the pancreas is torn and there then occurs an escape of blood and pancreatic secretion into the lesser peritoneal sac, the fluid becoming localised by adhesions. The condition is thus really a *pseudo-cyst* which is situated outside the pancreas. A similar condition has been ascribed to an attack of pancreatitis with escape of secretion, but the cause is often obscure. A cystic form of adenoma sometimes occurs in the pancreas. In *Lindau's disease*, multiple cysts may occur in the pancreas—along with vascular growths in the cerebellum. Hydatid cysts also occur in and around the pancreas.

Fibrocystic disease of the pancreas

Fibrocystic disease of the pancreas in the newborn (**mucoviscidosis**) is associated with intestinal obstruction and sometimes perforation due to inspissated meconium—so-called *meconium ileus*. In surviving infants this is followed by respiratory disease, notably pneumonia and bronchiectasis. In older children respiratory symptoms remain prominent, and malabsorption, with symptoms like those of coeliac disease, is also an important feature. The pancreas is small, firm and gritty, the cysts rarely being visible to the naked eye. On section the acini and ducts are dilated and filled with tough yellowish eosinophilic secretion which contains abundant mucin (Fig. 19.57). Subsequent fibrosis, both inter- and intra-lobular, may lead to loss of the normal lobulation. Rarely hepatic cholestasis

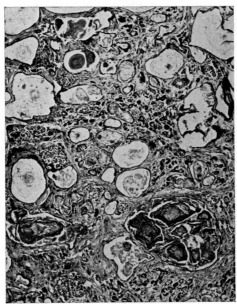

FIG. 19.57.—Fibrocystic disease of the pancreas. The ducts are filled with eosinophilic laminated secretion; the acini are either markedly atrophied or much dilated. × 50. (Prof. G. L. Montgomery.)

and biliary cirrhosis may develop. The nature of the disease is obscure but Farber suggests that it is a fundamental disorder of secretion affecting both pancreas and respiratory tract, in which an abnormal mucopolysaccharide is secreted, or possibly insufficient mucolytic enzymes. An increased sodium chloride concentration in sweat was observed by di Sant 'Agnese, with consequent loss of salt by the skin, and use is made of this in the diagnostic fingerprint tests. Roberts showed that excessive secretion and the consequent pathological changes are common to all the glands with cholinergic secreto-motor innervation and he postulates that many of the morbid histological changes are the result of exhaustion of the glands from prolonged overstimulation, the fibrosis and cystic changes being secondary to obstruction by the altered viscid secretion. Accordingly this disease might be due to excessive acetylcholine activity such as

would result from insufficient production of cholinesterase, and the disease would then be the physiological antithesis of myasthenia gravis. Roberts' familial studies gave data which cannot be reconciled with the hypothesis of recessive inheritance by a single gene pair, although this view is widely held by other workers. It is not uncommon, occurring once per 2,000 live births in Europeans.

Tumours

Apart from carcinoma, tumours are rare in the pancreas. Fibroma, lipoma, lymphangioma, adenoma and cystadenoma have been described; the last mentioned may reach a considerable size.

Carcinoma of the pancreas. In the great majority of cases carcinoma occurs in the head, less frequently in the body, whilst cancer in the tail is rare. The growth is usually of the scirrhous variety, though occasionally of more encephaloid type; as a rule it is an adeno-carcinoma, which may mimic the pancreatic structure, but sometimes the cells are quite irregularly arranged. The growth in the head practically always leads to obstruction of the main ducts, with exclusion of the pancreatic secretion from the intestine, and usually the common bile duct also is obstructed. Thus jaundice, clay-coloured stools, interference with digestion, etc., are brought about.

Carcinoma of the pancreas is one of the most commonly obscure forms of malignant disease clinically, and is one in which bizarre symptoms such as unexplained venous thrombosis, peripheral neuropathy and myopathy may be the presenting ones. It is sometimes accompanied by anomalies of carbohydrate metabolism, and is twice as common in diabetics as in the general population. The possibility of pancreatic cancer should therefore be considered in late-onset unstable diabetes, or development of instability in a previously stable diabetic.

Tumours of the islets of Langerhans. These tumours are of particular interest and importance because of their hormonal effects. Adenoma, sometimes called *nesidiocytoma*, commonly contains a predominance of β-cells and secretes insulin; a minority of tumours are mainly composed of non-β cells and secrete gastrin.

Insulin-secreting tumours. These are associated with attacks of hypoglycaemia during which the blood sugar is reduced to 20–50 mg. per 100 ml., and symptoms of hypoglycaemia then appear. Somnolence, dizziness, loss of consciousness and other nervous symptoms occur from time to time and can be abolished by taking sugar, but long intervals of freedom from symptoms occur spontaneously. When the condition has not been recognised, prolonged hypoglycaemia may lead to coma from which the patient cannot be roused even by intravenous glucose, and death follows. The tumour is usually a solitary adenoma in which the structure of the islets is reproduced (Fig. 19.58). Occasionally multiple tumours are present or even a widespread adenomatosis of the islet tissue, the latter sometimes being associated with multiple adenomatous tumours in the other endocrine glands. In *pluriglandular adenomatosis*, tumours arise in various combinations in the pituitary, parathyroids, thyroid, adrenals and pancreas.

In islet-cell tumours, the cells, which are arranged in trabeculae or irregularly, are of both the α- and β-types, with the latter usually preponderating, and these have been found to have a high content of insulin. Areas of hyaline fibrosis may be present in the tumour tissue and even calcification may occur. Malignancy with metastatic growth has been observed but is a rarity. Removal of the tumour is curative, but some adenomas are minute and unrecognisable at operation; in such cases it is justifiable to resect the tail of the pancreas in the hope that it contains the tumour. It is clear that we have here an example of a tumour of an endocrine tissue producing the specific hormone, and in this respect there is a similarity to other endocrine tumours for example of the anterior pituitary lobe or adrenal cortex.

Gastrin-secreting tumours. These contain a preponderance of α-cells or a mixture of α- and δ-cells. By secreting excess of gastrin, they stimulate the gastric mucosa to secrete very large amounts of hydrochloric acid, more than the pancreatic secretions can neutralise; accordingly not only is there severe peptic ulceration of the stomach and duodenum, and even extending into the jejunum, with persistent and severe diarrhoea, but also steatorrhoea from inhibition of lipase. This leads to excessive depletion of the

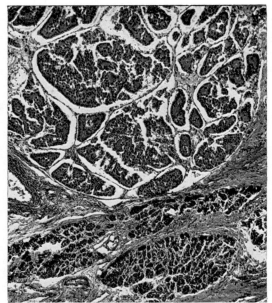

Fig. 19.58.—Islet-cell adenoma of pancreas. The tumour consists of highly differentiated cells, arranged in groups and forming occasional duct-like structures. Death was due to hypoglycaemia. × 75.

serum sodium and potassium levels and results in uncontrollable dehydration. Most of the cases reported have been in women (Zollinger and Ellison), but the disorder is not confined to women as was at first suggested. In a few cases, also usually women, watery diarrhoea is the only symptom (Vernier–Morrison syndrome).

More than 50 per cent of islet tumours in patients with Zollinger–Ellison syndrome have proved to be malignant.

Congenital abnormalities. Variations in the configuration of the pancreas and in the arrangement of its ducts are not uncommon. Occasionally the tissue of the head surrounds the adjacent part of the duodenum as a circular band, and stenosis may be produced. This is known as "annular pancreas". Foci of ectopic pancreatic tissue also occurs, and may be single or multiple. The commonest site is the submucous tissue of the jejunum, though occasionally they occur in the duodenum and even in the stomach. Ectopic pancreas is sometimes found in the apex of a Meckel's diverticulum and also in an ordinary "false diverticulum" of the small intestine. In the latter situation it has been supposed that its presence may cause the diverticulum.

CHAPTER 20

THE NERVOUS SYSTEM

I. THE BRAIN

Introduction

The nervous system is composed of two types of tissue both of which are involved in varying degree in disease processes. The first consists of the highly specialised nerve cells and their processes together with the neuroglial cells, all of which are of neuro-ectodermal origin: the second comprises the meninges, the blood vessels and their supporting connective tissue, and phagocytic cells, all derived from mesoderm and similar in many respects to corresponding tissue found in other systems of the body. Many of the morbid changes of the nervous system correspond in their nature with those observed in other organs —for example, those produced by infections, diseases of the blood vessels and tumours. Others are primary diseases of the neurone involving the cell body, its axon or its myelin sheath and in this group the etiology is often obscure although virus infections, metabolic disturbances and nutritional deficiencies, particularly of the vitamin B group, are known to cause direct damage to nerve cells. Even in those diseases where the primary damage is to the neurone, the most conspicuous pathological changes are often secondary to reactive changes in the neuroglia, the microglia or the blood vessels. On the other hand, the histological lesions produced in the nervous system by known bacterial toxins, e.g. tetanus toxin, are insignificant in comparison with their profound clinical effects, and there is no doubt that severe derangement of the function of a nerve cell can occur in the absence of any identifiable abnormalities in the cell as seen by the light microscope using current techniques. It seems likely that further progress in these fields will depend on the development of more highly specialised histochemical and neurochemical techniques and perhaps on information yielded by studies with the electron microscope.

Applied anatomy

In connection with the pathological changes in the brain, some anatomical facts are of particular importance. In the first place the arrangement of the meninges and the distribution of the cerebrospinal fluid (CSF) are intimately concerned with the spread of pathological processes. The dura mater is to be regarded as a structure quite separate from the pia-arachnoid. It acts as a periosteum to the cranial bones but it can be separated from the skull by collections of blood or pus in the potential *extradural space*, the former secondary to tearing of a meningeal blood vessel by a fracture and the latter from spread of an inflammatory process in the adjacent bone. The dura and the outer surface of the arachnoid are normally in contact but the *subdural space* can also be distended by blood or exudate in some pathological processes. The pia and arachnoid may be considered as virtually parts of one membrane. The arachnoid forms a continuous membrane in contact with the dura, while the pia follows the windings of the convolutions of the brain. The space between them, known as the *subarachnoid space*, is broken up by trabeculae of connective tissue into a series of intercommunicating spaces filled with cerebrospinal fluid. The subarachnoid space includes the cisterna magna and the cisterns at the base of the brain; apart from these it is broadest in the sulci, and within it lie the main vessels, the veins superficially, the arteries at a deeper level. The arterial branches ultimately break up in the pia into minute twigs from which the small *nutrient* vessels pass into the grey matter. The nutrient arteries to the basal ganglia and other deep structures enter the base of the brain at the *perforated spots*.

As an artery penetrates the brain substance, it carries with it a thin layer of the connective tissue of the pia: the resulting potential perivascular space (often known as the Virchow–Robin space) between the vessel wall and the invaginated pia is continuous with the subarachnoid space but it is present around only the larger vessels (Fig. 20.1). As the vessels become smaller the two layers fuse to form a reticular perivascular sheath which can be followed as far as precapillary vessels but not to the capillaries themselves.

The existence of a second space, the space of His, between the prolongation of the pia around the vessels and the adjacent brain tissue is not now generally accepted, and studies by the electron microscope have shown that the foot processes of astrocytes form a cuff in apposition to and completely surrounding the Virchow–Robin space and the capillaries of the brain.

These arrangements are of importance in connection with the spread of pathological processes. Thus organisms and their toxins readily diffuse throughout the subarachnoid space, which may become filled with inflammatory exudate. The inflammatory process may then spread into the brain around the nutrient blood vessels which are often seen to be surrounded by collections of leukocytes. The perivascular space also forms a path by which products of degeneration may be removed from the brain.

The ventricular system communicates with the subarachnoid space by means of the foramina in the roof (Magendie) and lateral recesses (Luschka) of the fourth ventricle. Cerebrospinal fluid passes freely through these foramina and, in certain disease processes, so also do blood, pus, micro-organisms or, more rarely, tumour cells. The circulation of the cerebrospinal fluid is dealt with in greater detail in relation to hydrocephalus (p. 611).

Examination of the cerebrospinal fluid often provides valuable information in diseases of the nervous system. Specimens are ordinarily obtained by lumbar puncture but cisternal or ventricular puncture may sometimes be indicated. The pressure of the CSF should always be measured, as either an increase or a decrease may be of diagnostic value. Microbiological, serological, cytological and biochemical investigations on the CSF are routine procedures. As the changes may be many and varied, only the most important can be given in the accounts which follow.

Normal cerebrospinal fluid is clear and colourless, does not coagulate and has a specific gravity

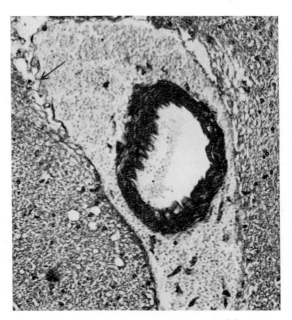

Fig. 20.1.—Haemorrhage into Virchow–Robin space.
The blood shows the relation of the small artery to the brain tissue. Note the pia (arrow). (A. C. L.) × 100.

of 1·006. It contains about 15–40 mg. protein per 100 ml., about 50–100 mg. glucose per 100 ml. and approximately 750 mg. sodium chloride per 100 ml. A few mononuclear cells may be found in normal fluid but rarely more than 4 per c.mm. (see Table, p. 652).

THE REACTIONS OF THE NERVOUS SYSTEM TO DISEASE

1. Neurones

Neurones are extremely complex cells and, as they exhibit great metabolic activity, they are highly sensitive to alterations in their environment. As mitotic division of neurones ceases within a few weeks after birth, dead cells cannot be replaced, and the alterations observed within nerve cells are generally of a retrogressive or degenerative nature.

Primary degenerations

Under the term primary degeneration we include the structural changes produced directly by toxic action or impairment of oxygen supply. The latter may result either from vascular disease or from hypoxaemia, as in carbon monoxide poisoning, but might be considered also to include the serious damage to the nervous system which is brought about by interference with the intracellular oxidation-reduction enzyme systems. When there is deficiency in the intake or in the absorption of the vitamin B group, various disturbances of neural function result from interference with the utilisation of carbohydrates by the nervous tissue owing to faulty intracellular respiration.

Before discussing the various primary degenerations of the nervous system it is important to consider the part played in the metabolism of nervous tissue by the vitamin B complex. Vitamin B_1 (aneurin or thiamine) is essential for intracellular respiration as it constitutes, in conjunction with pyrophosphoric acid, the enzyme co-carboxylase which is concerned in the final degradation of carbohydrate on which the nervous tissue is chiefly dependent for its energy. Vitamin B_2 consists of several components, including riboflavin, nicotinic acid and pyridoxin, which also participate in intracellular respiration. Riboflavin phosphate complexed with protein takes part in oxidative processes, and if this enzyme is deficient, avascular tissues which are dependent upon it for oxidation may become vascularised as a reaction to tissue hypoxia, e.g. vascularisation of the cornea in B_2 deficiency. Nicotinic acid (niacin) is a constituent of co-enzymes I and II and thus participates by reversible oxidation and reduction in intermediary metabolism; deficiency in niacin is the principal but not the only disturbance in pellagra.

Deprivation of cyanocobalamin (vitamin B_{12}) leads to degeneration of the long spinal tracts of the cord in the form of subacute combined degeneration (p. 660). Its mode of action is complex, but in addition to its part in protein synthesis, vitamin B_{12} participates in sulphydryl and glutathione metabolism, in carbohydrate metabolism and in the synthesis of phospholipids.

It is not yet possible to say how far these metabolic disturbances may form the foundation of various obscure nervous disorders and little is known about the factors determining their localisation, but it is clear that deranged metabolism underlies the pathogenesis of disorders apparently so diverse as peripheral neuropathy, Korsakoff's psychosis, Wernicke's encephalopathy, pellagra and beri-beri, and subacute combined degeneration of the cord.

Degenerative changes in neurones result from the action of a great many poisons, but they are in no way specific to the particular agent. As has been indicated, a clear distinction cannot as yet be made between the morbid changes in cells affected by toxic action and those damaged by faulty metabolic processes. Accordingly it is convenient to refer to such changes in a general way as "toxic". They may be of acute or of chronic nature.

Acute toxic action is manifested chiefly by a swelling of the cell and diminution or disappearance of the Nissl granules (chromophil substance), and by enlargement and pallor of the nucleus, which assumes an eccentric position. Such changes correspond in a general way with the central chromatolysis seen in secondary degeneration (p. 606). Actual *necrosis* of nerve cells with disappearance of nuclei and homogeneous staining followed by disintegration occurs chiefly in infarcts and in acute viral encephalitis. Necrosis of neurones occurs also when the supply of blood or oxygen to the brain as a whole is impaired as in cardiac arrest, severe hypotensive episodes or carbon monoxide poisoning. Certain neurones are particularly vulnerable to *hypoxia*, e.g. the Purkinje cells of the cerebellum and the neurones in the hippocampus and in the third and fifth layers in the cerebral cortex, while the less susceptible supporting tissues of the nervous system survive. Very similar selective necrosis of neurones can be brought about by *hypoglycaemia* as glucose is essential for their metabolism. In this latter instance the absence of the essential fuel produces the same effects as the lack of oxygen.

The effects of *chronic toxic action* are shown by shrinkage of the cells, often with loss of finer structure and apparent density of Nissl granules, loss of normal outline and processes, vacuolation, etc., and these changes may be followed ultimately by death and disappearance of the cells. Accumulation of brownish pigment of lipid nature, the so-called "fuscous degeneration", is sometimes a prominent feature in senile atrophy of the cells but is not in itself of much significance. The actions of various poisons may be indicated by change first of all in the extremities of the axons; these degenerate and the degeneration gradually ascends towards the cell body or perikaryon—the so-called "dying back" process. Degenerative changes in the nerve cells may therefore be partly the direct result of the toxic action on them and partly secondary to damage to their axons.

In addition to these non-specific reactions of the neurone to disease, more specific abnormalities are observed in some other diseases. Examples are ballooning of the cells by lipid in certain metabolic disturbances such as Tay–Sach's disease (p. 652), degeneration and coarsening of neurofibrils in Alzheimer's presenile dementia (p. 653) and inclusion bodies in some virus diseases (p. 639).

Wernicke's encephalopathy. This is a symmetrical disorder of the brain involving the mamillary bodies, the structures in the walls of the third ventricle, and the tissue around the aqueduct and in the floor of the fourth ventricle. The affected parts show marked congestion and numerous petechial haemorrhages, which mark them off from the normal tissue. The microscopic changes are chiefly vascular—marked irregular dilatation and proliferation of capillaries and small haemorrhages. The parenchyma is oedematous, but there is relatively little damage to nerve cells. There is microglial reaction with accumulation of lipids in macrophages to form compound granular corpuscles and later there is an increase in astrocytes.

Clinically the disease presents as an acute or subacute disorder characterised by disturbances of consciousness, ophthalmoplegia and ataxia with, if untreated, terminal coma. Peripheral neuropathy is present and there is a raised pyruvate level in the blood. The condition was thought at one time to be mainly due to chronic alcoholism but it can occur also as a complication of other diseases in which the stomach is involved, e.g. gastric carcinoma,

and in other conditions of persistent vomiting such as hyperemesis gravidarum. The disorder was rather common among prisoners of war in the Far East and was attributed to dietary deficiencies. It is now generally accepted that insufficient intake of thiamine and nicotinic acid and perhaps other members of the B complex is responsible, and dramatic improvement often follows their administration. Its relation to alcohol is like that of peripheral neuropathy.

Hepatolenticular degeneration. This affection, first described by Kinnier Wilson, is a rare condition, in which the changes are of very striking character. It occurs mainly in adolescents and young adults, shows a familial tendency, and is probably due to an autosomal recessive character which determines an inborn error of copper metabolism (see p. 569). The principal abnormalities are in the putamen and caudate nucleus, which become soft, shrunken, and ultimately cystic. The neuronal loss is accompanied by a fibrillary gliosis and the occurrence of large astrocytes with strikingly vesicular swollen nuclei. These are Alzheimer astrocytes and in hepatolenticular degeneration they may be widely distributed throughout the grey matter. The lesions in the nervous system are due to metabolic disturbances dependent partly on deposition of copper. The greenish-brown discoloration of the cornea near the limbus, known as Kayser–Fleischer rings is due to deposition of copper. The resulting symptoms are mainly muscular tremors and spasticity. The condition is associated with cirrhosis of the liver, and both the hepatic and nervous lesions are attributable to the defect in copper metabolism described on p. 569.

An acquired type of *hepatocerebral degeneration* is also recognised. The acute forms are associated with massive liver-cell necrosis when the principal abnormality in the brain is the occurrence of Alzheimer astrocytes. A chronic form is seen in individuals with a large porto-systemic venous shunt as occurs in cirrhosis (p. 572). Alzheimer astrocytes again appear in the brain but there may also be microcystic degeneration in the caudate nucleus, the putamen, and the deeper layers of the cortex.

Nuclear jaundice. In icterus gravis neonatorum about 40 per cent of cases dying between the second and fifth days of life show signs of damage to the nervous system. This is more likely to occur when there is a considerable reduction of the fetal haemoglobin at birth and when there has been difficulty in establishing respiration; hypoxia may therefore be a significant factor in precipitating the cellular damage. The nervous lesions can be prevented by adequate exchange transfusion within a few hours of birth. Grossly, there is yellow (bilirubin) staining of the hippocampus, subthalamic, olivary and dentate nuclei, globus pallidus and sometimes the cerebral cortex; this is known as *kernicterus* or *nuclear* *jaundice*. The affected areas are often remarkably symmetrical and in them the neurones are shrunken and encrusted with unconjugated bilirubin.

Pathogenesis. The damage occurs soon after birth rather than *in utero*, because the fetal bilirubin is excreted through the placenta into the maternal circulation and a marked rise in the infant's plasma bilirubin level occurs only after birth. It is generally agreed that the danger of kernicterus is greatly increased if the unconjugated bilirubin level reaches 15–20 mg. per 100 ml. The cause of the specific localisation of the nerve cell damage is obscure but its occurrence in full-term infants is practically confined to cases of maternal iso-immunisation by Rh incompatibility and it is usually associated with severe liver damage in the infant. In premature babies the danger is increased because the immature liver is deficient in the ability to conjugate bilirubin. The administration of vitamin K in excess to premature infants to counteract haemorrhagic disease of the newborn, lowers the level of reduced glutathione in the red cells and thus increases lysis and raises still further the level of unconjugated bilirubin. Kernicterus also occurs occasionally in feeble premature infants without any associated blood group incompatibility. Infants surviving kernicterus later show choreo-athetosis, spasticity and often mental deficiency, and in such cases the destroyed nervous tissue is absorbed and replaced by a neuroglial scar.

Secondary degenerations

Secondary degeneration can be defined as changes occurring in one part of a neurone as a result of damage to another part. The first of these is *Wallerian degeneration* which occurs in its most typical form when axons in a peripheral nerve are transected. The axon distal to the point of transection shrinks, becomes varicose and granular, and then breaks up into fragments which are later absorbed. The myelin sheath reacts at the same time and the complex lipids are broken down into simpler lipids and, ultimately, neutral fat. Products of myelin degeneration may be seen three or four days after damage to the axon and thereafter the fatty globules are gradually absorbed, mainly by phagocytes from the endoneurium. The Schwann cells proliferate to form cords of cells within endoneural tubes. Degeneration of the central part of the axon usually extends for only a short distance proximal to the level of transection. The sequence of changes in the nerve cell is described below. An essentially similar degeneration occurs in axons within the central nervous system when they are transected for any reason but, possibly because of the absence of Schwann cells, the entire length of the axon degenerates. The lipids produced by the degeneration of myelin are absorbed by microglia and when large tracts are affected, these cells persist for a considerable time; ultimately, however, they disappear.

In peripheral nerves axonal sprouts from the proximal stump proliferate rapidly and, unless the cut ends of the nerve lie in close apposition, form a *traumatic neuroma* (p. 67). If they are in apposition, however, the axons grow along the degenerated part of the nerve where they may ultimately affect contact with motor endplates and terminal sensory organelles. Regeneration of axons with restoration of function does not occur in the central nervous system.

Wallerian degeneration of the long tracts in the spinal cord will be dealt with in more detail later (p. 654) but it should be observed here that two principal staining techniques are used to demonstrate loss of myelin. The first of these— the Marchi technique—is used as a positive technique to demonstrate recent or active breakdown of myelin as the unsaturated fatty acids formed during this process are stained black, while normal myelin remains unstained. In the later stages, when most of the breakdown products have been removed, the demyelinated areas remain pale with conventional stains—the Weigert–Pal method and its modifications— which stain normal myelin black. These techniques are used also to demonstrate loss of myelin in conditions other than Wallerian degeneration, e.g. multiple sclerosis (see p. 649).

The other form of secondary degeneration is that which occurs in the body of the nerve cell when its axon has been destroyed or injured— *retrograde degeneration*. When a motor nerve, for example the hypoglossal, is cut across, changes begin to appear in the related nerve cell bodies two or three days afterwards, and reach their maximum about two weeks later. The Nissl granules gradually lose their configuration and break down into small dust-like particles, some of which disappear. The process, which is called *central chromatolysis*, appears first round the nucleus and then extends to the periphery. The whole cell becomes pale-staining and at the same time somewhat swollen; its nucleus becomes eccentric in position, and may even form a slight bulging on the surface of the cell.

These changes may be followed by a period of restitution which may not be completed till the end of three months, the appearance of the cell then returning to normal. In some cases, however, this does not occur and the nucleus may break down or be extruded from the cell which then distintegrates and disappears. Similar changes occur in sensory neurones but take place more rapidly than in the motor neurones. To what extent these two results—repair or ultimate loss of the cell—occur, is not fully determined. It is well established, however, that destruction of fibres within the central nervous system is followed by gradual disappearance of the corresponding nerve cell bodies. This has been found to be the case, for example, in the motor neurones in the cortex when the pyramidal fibres have been interrupted, and also in the thoracic nucleus when the posterior spino-cerebellar tract has been interrupted. Among the lower motor neurones, restitution after the occurrence of chromatolysis appears to be the rule; it is evident, of course, that if the nerve cell bodies are destroyed the process of regeneration in the peripheral axons cannot take place.

Another form of secondary degeneration is transneuronal or trans-synaptic atrophy. This occurs in neurones whose principal afferent connections have been destroyed: examples are atrophy of the neurones in the external geniculate body after lesions in the retina or optic nerves, or in the nucleus gracilis and nucleus cuneatus when the posterior columns of the spinal cord have degenerated. Trans-synaptic degeneration is sometimes "retrograde", i.e. it can occur in cells which make synaptic connections with cells which have been destroyed.

Atrophy

Diffuse atrophy of the brain is usually due to a progressive loss of neurones. The cerebral cortex is most frequently affected and, when the process is advanced, the convolutions become more rounded and firmer than normal and the sulci widened, so that there is an excess of fluid in the subarachnoid space. The pia-arachnoid, especially over the vertex, is thickened and opalescent in appearance, and, owing to the excess of fluid in the subarachnoid space, the sulci appear to be filled with semi-gelatinous material.

The full extent of the atrophy is often not apparent until the meninges have been stripped from the surface of the brain. As the neuronal loss is accompanied by the disappearance of their axons and myelin sheaths, the white matter also becomes reduced in amount and this is accompanied by enlargement of the ventricles. The histological changes underlying atrophy vary with the many different causes, e.g. senile and pre-senile dementia, ischaemia, subacute encephalitis and, to a more limited degree, as part of the changes in old age, but the two constant abnormalities are loss of neurones and neuroglial overgrowth. Less commonly there may be atrophy of the basal nuclei: this may be primary as in hepatolenticular degeneration or secondary to destruction of axons as in prefrontal leucotomy.

2. Neuroglia

The neuroglia includes astrocytes, oligodendrocytes and ependymal cells, and constitutes one of the "connective tissues of the brain", the other being the true connective tissue of the meninges and the blood vessels (*vide infra*). With the neuroglial cells, which are derived from spongioblasts, it is convenient to describe the microglia, the histiocytes of the brain.

Astrocytes. The astrocytes, which form the astroglia, and constitute the principal supporting tissue of the central nervous system, are stellate cells with numerous fine branching processes, which lie in a mucopolysaccharide ground substance. Protoplasmic astrocytes and fibrillary astrocytes may be distinguished; the latter have fibres in their cytoplasm, which join cell to cell, and their processes are longer and straighter. In normal conditions the protoplasmic astrocytes are found mainly in the grey matter, the fibrillary astrocytes in the white matter and subpial glial layer. Both forms are attached to the walls of capillaries and other small vessels by one or more processes with swellings at their ends, the so-called "sucker feet". Under the pia similar expansions unite with the fibres of this membrane. These swellings or sucker feet thus represent the union of ectodermal and mesodermal tissues.

In general, the reactions of astrocytes resemble those of fibroblasts. They are less susceptible to noxious processes than neurones but where the process is severe, as in an infarct or an acute inflammatory lesion, they undergo necrosis and disintegration. In less severe injury or when adjacent to an area of tissue necrosis, astrocytes enlarge, proliferate and produce glial fibrils in increased amount. This process is known as *gliosis* and it occurs in almost all conditions where damage is inflicted on any part of the central nervous system. Where gliosis is recent and active, many enlarged cell bodies are seen, but in the late stages the cell bodies disappear and all that can be seen is a dense network of glial fibrils. The brain tissue is then firmer than normal and may have a grey translucent appearance.

Oligodendrocytes. The oligodendrocytes, which form the oligodendroglia, are small cells so named because of their few short protoplasmic processes. They are extremely numerous and occur as perineuronal satellites in the grey matter, and as rows of closely apposed nuclei in relation to myelinated nerve fibres where they constitute the interfascicular oligodendroglia. This close juxtaposition to myelin sheaths has always led to the assumption that they play an important part in the nutrition of myelin. Further evidence of this is derived from recent electron microscope studies which suggest that developing axons invaginate into oligodendrocytes which then form the characteristic laminated myelin sheath.

Further, in some of the leukodystrophies (p. 651), loss of the interfascicular oligodendrocytes appears to precede obvious degeneration of myelin. Very little is known about the causes or significance of reactive changes in the oligodendrocytes apart from the *acute swelling* which occurs in many acute toxic processes and the proliferation of perineuronal satellites around degenerating neurones. The latter process is known as *satellitosis* and it is important to distinguish it from neuronophagia (*vide infra*).

Ependyma. The ependyma is a single layer of columnar cells lining the ventricular system and the central canal of the spinal cord. Cilia are attached to their free, i.e. ventricular surface immediately deep to which there is a line of small oval bodies known as blepharoplasts. Processes from the deep surface of the cells merge with the underlying neural tissue.

Ependymal cells show few reactive changes. Thus when the ventricles distend as in hydrocephalus, the ependyma is stretched and then broken, but the ependymal cells do not proliferate to fill the defects. One common but non-specific reaction of the ependyma to chronic inflammation is the appearance of numerous small excrescences on the surface, the condition being known as a *granular ependymitis*. However, this is consequent on focal proliferation of groups of subependymal astrocytes and not to reactive changes in the ependymal cells themselves (Fig. 20.32).

Microglia. The microglial cell is small, with an elongated hyperchromatic nucleus, scanty cytoplasm, and delicate cytoplasmic processes. They may be regarded as the homologues of the histiocytes of ordinary connective tissue (p. 48), i.e. they are part of the peripheral reticulo-endothelial system.

With regard to the development of the microglia, these cells do not appear in the central nervous system until the vessels are formed, and they are few in number till shortly before birth, when they invade the neural tissue from the pia especially at spots where the pia is close to the white matter. The columns of invading cells are referred to as "fountains" and they travel in the white matter and afterwards become diffused through the grey matter. They also are often closely related to nerve cells and to blood vessels.

The microglia play an important part in disease; these cells, ordinarily inconspicuous, become enlarged and spherical. After they have taken up the products of degeneration they may pass into the perivascular sheaths of the small vessels where they may be found in large numbers. In other conditions, e.g. subacute encephalitis, the microglial cells increase in length but do not become ovoid: they are then referred to as *rod cells*. Another important function of the microglia is the phagocytosis of neurones which have undergone necrosis as in hypoxic brain damage or active virus infection. The effete nerve cell becomes obscured by a group of enlarged elongated microglial cells, and often also by polymorphonuclear leukocytes, this process being known as *neuronophagia* or neuronophagy (Fig. 20.35, p. 640). It must be distinguished from satellitosis by oligodendroglia (*vide supra*).

3. The meninges and blood vessels

These constitute the true connective tissue of the brain. Whereas gliosis readily occurs when there is any damage to the brain, proliferation of ordinary connective tissue is seen only in grosser lesions where the blood vessels and their sheaths are involved. For instance, when suppuration occurs within the brain, proliferation of this connective tissue along with new formation of blood vessels leads to the production of a distinct capsule around an abscess cavity. Gliosis occurs also and this combined glial and fibroblastic reaction is often known as a *gliomesodermal scar*. Proliferation of capillary blood vessels is often seen also in association with severe ischaemic or anoxic lesions and in relation to rapidly growing cerebral tumours. The reactions of the meninges to disease will be considered in the section on meningitis (p. 625).

Leukocytes are extremely scanty in the substance of the brain and spinal cord under normal conditions, but may occur in large numbers when pathological changes are present.

THE PATHOLOGY OF AN INTRACRANIAL EXPANDING LESION

Diverse pathological processes, such as tumour, haematoma, or a massive recent cerebral infarct, have in common the feature of increasing the bulk of the brain. As the brain is enclosed within the rigid cranium, there is very little free space to accommodate these various *expanding lesions* with the result that they ultimately produce an increase of intracranial pressure. An essentially similar state is produced by an extracerebral intracranial expanding lesion such as an extradural or subdural haematoma or a meningioma, but there is a stage of spatial compensation during which the intracranial pressure remains within normal limits. This compensation is brought about principally by a reduction in the volume of cerebrospinal fluid both within the ventricles and within the subarachnoid space, possibly by a reduction in the volume of blood within the cranium, and less commonly by actual loss of brain tissue. When all the available space has been utilised there is a critical point at which a further slight increase in the volume of the intracranial contents causes an abrupt increase of intracranial pressure with subsequent and often rapid deterioration in the patient's condition. Near this critical point, arteriolar vasodilatation consequent on a short period of increased arterial $p\mathrm{CO_2}$ may be sufficient to produce this effect. Clearly the compensatory mechanisms will fail more rapidly when the lesion is expanding rapidly, e.g. an intracerebral haematoma, than one of similar size that has developed slowly, e.g. a meningioma. Indeed in the latter instance there is often also local pressure atrophy and loss of brain tissue. Expanding lesions also cause distortion of the brain and it cannot be emphasised too strongly that distortion and displacement of the brain and any associated increase in intracranial pressure are often of much greater significance with regard to the immediate survival of the patient than the nature of the lesion or the amount of cerebral tissue destroyed by it.

The sequence of changes in the brain caused by an intracerebral expanding lesion follows a fairly standard pattern. As the lesion expands so also does the hemisphere. The cerebrospinal fluid in the subarachnoid space is displaced and the convolutions become flattened against the dura, the sulci are progressively narrowed and the surface of the brain, when exposed *post mortem*, is dryer than normal. Cerebrospinal fluid is also displaced from the ventricular system with the result that the lateral ventricle on the same side as the lesion becomes smaller while the contralateral ventricle may become larger. Further expansion of the affected hemisphere leads to distortion of the brain and a shift to the opposite side of the midline structures, viz. the interventricular septum, the anterior cerebral arteries and the third ventricle (Fig. 20.2). Such displacement is readily seen radiologically by air encephalography or carotid arteriography. Then, depending to some extent on the site of the expanding lesion, internal herniae develop. Thus the cingulate gyrus frequently herniates under the free margin of the falx cerebri above the corpus callosum—the so-called *supracallosal hernia* (Fig. 20.2). However, the most important hernia associated with a supratentorial expanding lesion is a *tentorial hernia*, viz. protrusion of the medial part of the ipsilateral temporal lobe through the tentorial opening (Fig. 20.3). The herniated hippocampal gyrus compresses and displaces the midbrain which is pushed against the contralateral rigid edge of the tentorium. The pressure may be sufficient to produce a dis-

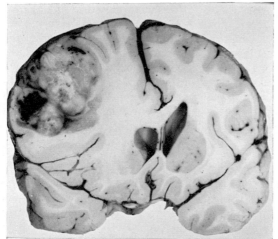

FIG. 20.2.—Increased intracranial pressure due to
parietal lobe tumour. × ½.

Note displacement of lateral ventricles, mid-line shift and
supracallosal hernia.

tinct groove (Kernohan's notch) on the surface
of the midbrain at this point. Compression of the
aqueduct may then block the free flow of cerebrospinal fluid from the lateral ventricles and
this further increases the intracranial pressure.

Other features frequently associated with a
tentorial hernia are caudal displacement of the
brain stem, compression of the third and sixth

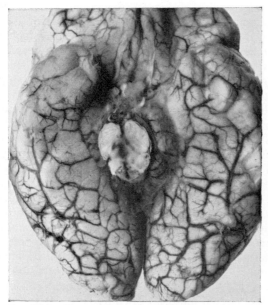

FIG. 20.3.—Increased intracranial pressure due to a
supratentorial tumour. × ½.

Note displacement of brain stem and medial and downward
displacement of the hippocampal gyrus—a tentorial hernia.
The deep groove indicates the position of the edge of the
tentorium.

cranial nerves with resultant disturbances of
eye movement and pupillary reflexes and, less
commonly, infarction of the ipsilateral medial
occipital cortex due to kinking of the posterior
cerebral artery over the tentorium. A common
terminal event in raised intracranial pressure is
haemorrhage into the midbrain and pons (Fig.
20.4), usually involving the tegmentum adjacent
to the midline. The precise pathogenesis of this
lesion is obscure but it is presumably a combination of caudal displacement of the brain stem,
obstruction to venous drainage and to stretching
and spasm of arteries.

Similar abnormalities may be brought about

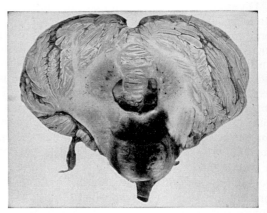

FIG. 20.4.—Increased intracranial pressure.
Secondary haemorrhage into pons. × ⅔.

by extracerebral intracranial expanding lesions,
although flattening of the convolutions is often
not so pronounced. If the increase in volume of
the brain is more diffuse, as in generalised cerebral oedema, both lateral ventricles and the
third ventricle are reduced in size. There may
also be bilateral tentorial herniae. A frequent
clinical sign of raised intracranial pressure is
papilloedema due to compression of the central
vein where it traverses the subarachnoid space in
the optic nerve sheath.

A supratentorial expanding lesion may also
cause a *tonsillar hernia* (*cerebellar cone*), viz.
impaction of the cerebellar tonsils in the foramen
magnum (Fig. 20.5) but this type of hernia is
more constant when the lesion lies below the
tentorium cerebelli. The tonsils compress the
medulla oblongata and interfere with the function
of the vital centres adjacent to the floor of the
fourth ventricle. The cone, by obstructing the
flow of cerebrospinal fluid through the fourth
ventricle and the exit foramina, may in turn

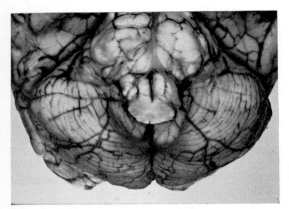

FIG. 20.5.—Increased intracranial pressure.
Cerebellar cone resulting from a diffuse glioma of the pons.
× ⅔.

Prolonged increase of intracranial pressure may result in erosion of certain parts of the skull and these changes can often be seen on radiological examination. The most common examples are erosion of the posterior clinoid processes and, in children, thinning of the inner table of the skull over the convolutions, the so-called convolutional markings or beaten-brass appearance (Fig. 20.6).

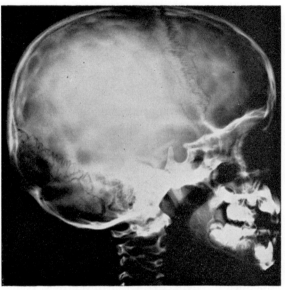

FIG. 20.6.—Prolonged increase of intracranial pressure.
Note thinning of the inner table of the skull.

further increase the intracranial pressure so that a vicious circle is set up.

In a patient with an intracranial expanding lesion, either a cerebellar cone or a tentorial hernia can be precipitated by removing CSF from the spinal subarachnoid space at lumbar puncture. Even if only a small quantity of CSF is removed, there is commonly a leakage of CSF into the spinal extradural space through the puncture in the meninges after the needle has been withdrawn. Lumbar puncture is therefore strongly contra-indicated in all cases where an intracranial expanding lesion is suspected; the procedure is very often followed by a sudden deterioration in the patient's general condition.

HYDROCEPHALUS

Definition. Hydrocephalus denotes an increase in the amount of cerebrospinal fluid. This may arise when production of CSF exceeds absorption, and consequently the volume increases at the expense of the other intracranial contents (*primary hydrocephalus*). *Secondary hydrocephalus* is an increase in CSF which is compensatory to loss of neural tissue, e.g. from infarction, and is a relatively unimportant phenomenon. Hydrocephalus may be further classified into *internal hydrocephalus* in which the ventricles are distended with fluid, and *external hydrocephalus* in which there is an increased amount of cerebrospinal fluid in the subarachnoid space. The term hydrocephalus, when used without qualification, usually connotes internal hydrocephalus and this can be either *communicating* or *noncommunicating* in type. In the former, cere-brospinal fluid is still able to pass from the lateral ventricles to the subarachnoid space while, in the latter, it is unable to do so owing to the site of the obstruction. The two types may be distinguished during life by cerebral pneumography by injecting air either into the lumbar subarachnoid space or directly into the ventricles. The air extends wherever there is free communication, and can be seen as dark areas on the X-ray plate. By varying the position of the patient's head the air can be made to pass from the ventricles to the subarachnoid space in cases of communicating hydrocephalus, or in the reverse direction if air has been introduced by the lumbar route. This technique can also be used to locate the site of obstruction in the ventricular system, or in the subarachnoid space. A more accurate technique is to introduce a radio-opaque fluid into the lateral ventricles after withdrawing an equivalent volume of CSF.

The source and circulation of cerebrospinal fluid

The main source of CSF is the choroid plexuses of the ventricles but some may be formed on the surface of the brain and spinal cord, for it is known that ionic exchange between blood and cerebrospinal fluid can occur widely and is not restricted to the choroid plexuses. Dandy was the first to show convincingly that the CSF is derived from the choroid plexuses by demonstrating experimentally, (*a*) that obstruction of one foramen of Monro in the dog caused enlargement of the corresponding lateral ventricle and, (*b*) that if, in addition to obstruction, the choroid plexus was removed, the ventricle became smaller than that on the normal side. It is thought that the total volume of the CSF is about 120–150 ml. and that it is renewed several times per day. When, however, it is able to escape freely, as in a fracture of the base of the skull, the amount formed may be enormous. The mechanism of production is by secretion, and the fluid formed in the lateral ventricles passes by the foramina of Monro to the third ventricle and then by the aqueduct of Sylvius to the fourth ventricle, being added to by the choroid plexuses on its way. It then passes through the foramina of Magendie and Luschka in the roof and lateral recesses respectively of the fourth ventricle to reach the subarachnoid space of the cisterna magna and basal cisterns. Thereafter it spreads through the subarachnoid space over the surface of the brain and spinal cord and is absorbed into the blood through the arachnoid granulations (arachnoid villi) which project into the dural venous sinuses (Fig. 20.64, p. 667), the amount absorbed by the spinal arachnoid being relatively small.

Primary hydrocephalus

By far the most important cause of primary hydrocephalus is obstruction to the free flow of cerebrospinal fluid. Obstruction is most likely to occur where the structures permitting the flow are smallest, as in the aqueduct or at the exit foramina in the fourth ventricle, but the obstruction may also be in the subarachnoid space itself.

Dandy demonstrated this by placing a strip of gauze soaked in iodine around the brain stem; the resulting inflammation produced thickening of the meninges and obliteration of the subarachnoid space with the subsequent development of hydrocephalus.

Obstruction to the flow of CSF results in expansion of that part of the ventricular system which lies proximal to the obstruction. Thus, if the obstruction is in the third ventricle, both lateral ventricles enlarge symmetrically; if at the exit foramina in the roof of the fourth ventricle, the entire ventricular system enlarges; if in the subarachnoid space around the brain stem, the entire ventricular system again enlarges but the hydrocephalus in this instance, in contrast to the two preceding examples, is of communicating type, as cerebrospinal fluid can flow from the lateral ventricles to the subarachnoid space.

It is convenient to divide obstructive hydrocephalus into congenital and acquired types but the separation of the two varieties is not always clear-cut.

Other possible causes of primary hydrocephalus are increased production of cerebrospinal fluid or impaired absorption. Increased production of fluid is rare but may be the cause of the hydrocephalus associated with a secreting papillary tumour of the choroid plexus (Fig. 20.79, p. 673). Decreased absorption of fluid is theoretically and experimentally possible, but its existence in man has been questioned.

Congenital hydrocephalus

This condition may be marked at the time of birth and be of such a degree as to interfere with parturition, but more frequently it is only slight at birth and afterwards increases. The head may become enormously enlarged and tends to become quadrangular, the vertex becomes flattened, and the frontal bone projects over the orbits. The sutures are greatly widened and the fontanelles much enlarged, their closure being long delayed. There is a corresponding enlargement of the brain, the convolutions being broadened and flattened and the sulci shallow. The accumulation of fluid in the lateral ventricles may be so great that the brain substance around them may be less than a centimetre wide (Fig. 20.7). If the third ventricle is involved its floor can become greatly ballooned and extremely thin. It is remarkable how the brain substance can adapt itself to its altered configuration and although considerable interference with mental function is usual, in a very few cases the child may be surprisingly intelligent.

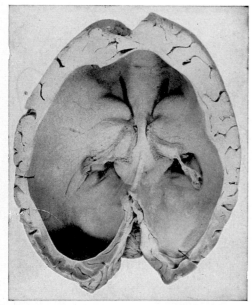

FIG. 20.7.—Section of brain in congenital hydrocephalus, showing enormous dilatation of the lateral ventricles. $\times \frac{2}{3}$.

Congenital hydrocephalus is frequently associated with the Arnold–Chiari malformation (Fig. 20.8): this consists of a tongue-like prolongation of the inferior cerebellar vermis through the foramen magnum and lying dorsal to the greatly elongated medulla. The lower part of the fourth ventricle thus lies in the upper part of the vertebral canal and the foramen magnum is blocked by the misplaced tissue from the posterior fossa. Cerebrospinal fluid can flow out of the main exit foramina in the fourth ventricle—the hydrocephalus is, therefore, by definition, of communicating type—but as it is unable to re-enter the cranial cavity, it cannot reach the main sites of reabsorption. The entire ventricular system thus becomes grossly enlarged. A meningomyelocele (see p. 666) is an almost invariable accompaniment of the Arnold–Chiari malformation.

Other relatively common congenital abnormalities which give rise to hydrocephalus are faulty development of the aqueduct of Sylvius and atresia of the foramina of Luschka and

Magendie: in the former, hydrocephalus is confined to the third and lateral ventricles; in the latter there is in addition enlargement of the aqueduct and of the fourth ventricle. The ballooning of the roof of the fourth ventricle in these cases is usually so severe as to cause distortion of the inferior surface of the cerebellum.

Congenital hydrocephalus occurs also in the absence of any apparent developmental malformation. One cause of this is intra-uterine

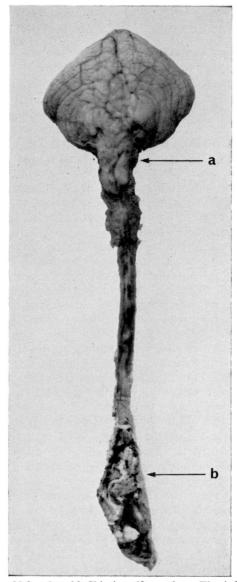

FIG. 20.8.—Arnold–Chiari malformation. The inferior part of the cerebellum protrudes as a tongue-like mass (*a*) into the foramen magnum. Note the characteristic meningo-myelocele (*b*). $\times \frac{7}{12}$.

meningitis or ventriculitis, of which toxoplasmosis is an example, when the inflammation has resulted in obliterative change in the subarachnoid space or in the ventricular system, particularly in the aqueduct. It seems likely, too, that some cases of hydrocephalus which are apparently congenital in type are in fact a consequence of neonatal meningitis or subarachnoid haemorrhage from cerebral birth injury, either of which may evoke a fibroblastic reaction leading to obliteration of the subarachnoid space and obstruction to the flow of CSF.

Acquired hydrocephalus

Any expanding lesion within the skull can obstruct the flow of CSF but the nature of the lesion, e.g. a tumour, an abscess, a haematoma or a granuloma is much less important than its location. Even a small lesion, if it lies in a vital site, e.g. adjacent to a foramen of Monro or close to the aqueduct (Fig. 20.85, p. 676), will cause hydrocephalus, whereas lesions elsewhere within a cerebral hemisphere require to be large in order to interfere with the circulation of the cerebrospinal fluid. In general, expanding lesions in the posterior fossa are particularly prone to cause hydrocephalus because they readily compress the aqueduct and the fourth ventricle. Common examples are a tumour of the acoustic nerve, a meningioma or a tumour within the fourth ventricle. Acquired obstruction of the exit foramina or the subarachnoid space is almost always due to inflammation; this may be acute, as in an acute purulent meningitis, or subacute, as in tuberculous meningitis, since, in both, the subarachnoid space is at least partly occluded by exudate. If the inflammation does not resolve, fibroblastic proliferation proceeds to obliteration of the subarachnoid space particularly in the basal cisterns (Fig. 20.9) and around the midbrain which is closely embraced by the rigid tentorium cerebelli. Such an occurrence is common in the later stages of tuberculous meningitis and sometimes is a late result of acute purulent meningitis particularly if there has been some delay in instituting effective treatment. Quite frequently, in cases of hydrocephalus which on histological examination are obviously of post-inflammatory type, a clear history of previous meningitis cannot be obtained: in Dorothy Russell's series this was so in

19 of 23 cases and there is good reason for supposing that the hydrocephalus was the result of an unrecognised neonatal meningitis or birth injury. In post-inflammatory hydrocephalus, a granular ependymitis is frequently prominent (see p. 608).

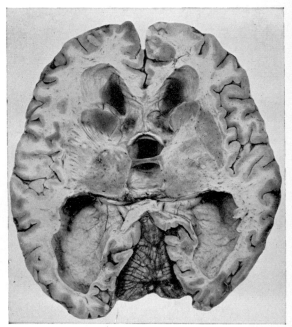

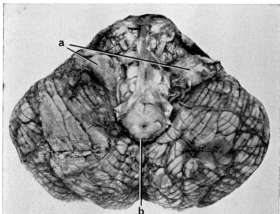

Fig. 20.9.—Hydrocephalus due to occlusion of the foramina of Luschka (*a*) and Magendie (*b*) by fibrous adhesions. $\times \frac{7}{9}$.

Note the enlargement of the third ventricle and stretching of the massa intermedia.

A relatively uncommon cause of hydrocephalus occurring after early childhood is progressive gliosis around the aqueduct. The etiology of this is obscure but it is probably a hamartomatous proliferation of astrocytes,

Secondary hydrocephalus

Enlargement of the ventricles may be a secondary phenomenon. If there is a generalised reduction in the amount of brain tissue, as in senile dementia or general paralysis of the insane, the ventricles enlarge symmetrically. If there is local loss of cerebral tissue, the adjacent ventricle enlarges; a frequent example of this is enlargement of one lateral ventricle when there is an old infarct in the territory supplied by the ipsilateral middle cerebral artery. External hydrocephalus is almost invariably secondary to a general or local reduction of brain tissue.

HEAD INJURIES

The clinical and pathological aspects of head injuries have become increasingly important because of their great frequency as a result of road traffic accidents. All degrees of injury may occur but the important basic concepts are that when the head is struck the calvaria is momentarily deformed, and may fracture, and the brain, because of the sudden change of velocity, moves within the skull. Similarly, when the skull is suddenly arrested in a deceleration injury, the brain again moves within the skull. Rotational movements appear to be the most prone to cause injury and the consequent shearing strains on neuronal pathways within the brain can produce a marked decrease in cerebral electrical activity as demonstrated by the electro-encephalogram. The importance of the sudden alteration in the velocity of the skull and brain is clearly demonstrated by the fact that when the head is fixed, as in a crush injury, consciousness is often not lost unless the blow has been sufficiently severe to smash the skull.

Fractures of the skull

The significance of a fracture of the skull has been exaggerated in the past. However, it does indicate that the blow has been of considerable force and that there is a greater likelihood of concomitant injuries to the brain. Aird states that a fracture can be detected in only 30 per cent of all head injuries yet it is present in 90 per cent of fatal cases.

There are some specific features related to fractures which are important. The fracture may be depressed thus causing pressure on the brain; furthermore many depressed fractures are compound and therefore liable to be followed by intracranial sepsis, or the inner table of the skull may fragment, the spicules of bone then impinging on the brain or penetrating its substance to produce laceration of the underlying cortex. Fractures at the base also provide a potential route of entry for micro-organisms from the outside air or from the nasal passages, the para-nasal air sinuses or the middle ear to the sub-arachnoid space with the subsequent development of meningitis. The presence of a fracture of the base of the skull is often indicated by bleeding from the nose or ear, or by rhinorrhoea or otorrhoea of cerebrospinal fluid. A serious although rare consequence of a fracture of the base of the skull is injury to the carotid artery within the cavernous sinus giving rise to an arteriovenous fistula.

Extradural haematoma

An especially important aspect of a fracture of the squamous part of the temporal bone is that it can cause laceration of the middle meningeal artery, but other vascular channels may be torn when the fracture is at another site. The blood from the torn vessel separates the dura from the bone and ultimately a large saucer-shaped extradural haematoma (Fig. 20.10) develops which, as it may attain a thickness of more than 2 cm., can produce severe compression and distortion of the brain and a rapid rise in intracranial pressure. In such cases the patient may, after regaining consciousness, subsequently relapse into coma and die from the effects of raised intracranial pressure. Diagnosis of this condition is of the utmost importance as it is amenable to surgical treatment. Occasionally, an extradural haematoma occurs in the absence of a fracture, particularly in children.

Subdural haematoma

A subdural haematoma is a collection of blood in the subdural space caused by laceration of small "bridging" veins or of venous channels running to the main venous sinuses.

Acute subdural haematoma covering one or both cerebral hemispheres is a common necropsy finding if death has occurred soon after a head injury. The haematoma is often thin and may not have significantly contributed to the patient's death. In some cases, however, it attains a considerable thickness and, unless

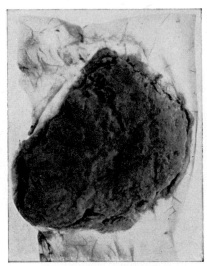

FIG. 20.10.—Large saucer-shaped extradural haematoma due to rupture of middle meningeal artery. × ¾.

surgically evacuated, can cause a serious rise in intracranial pressure, resulting in coma and death.

Chronic subdural haematoma is the name applied when the haematoma is of insidious onset and of considerable duration. In some cases symptoms do not develop until some weeks or even months after a head injury, which may have been of a rather trivial nature. In fact such lesions may occur in the absence of a history of injury, e.g. in various chronic dementias, particularly in general paralysis of the insane, and in chronic alcoholics, but it seems probable that a previous minor head injury has remained unnoticed.

Chronic subdural haematomas are commonest over the convexities of the cerebral hemispheres, are not uncommonly bilateral and can attain a thickness of up to 3 cm. The haematoma becomes organised very slowly from the dura; new blood vessels, connective tissue cells and phagocytes penetrate the layer of clot and gradually organise it, whilst the red blood cells dis-

integrate and form the various breakdown pigments; a layer of endothelium also grows over its inner surface from the lining of the dura. In this way a brownish membrane of varying thickness is formed. The new vessels are usually wide and thin-walled and consequently haemorrhages may occur again into its substance and the haematoma may come to have a somewhat laminated appearance. The membrane is usually not adherent to the surface of the arachnoid, but sometimes adhesions form. Because these haematomas enlarge so slowly, presumably as a result of further small haemorrhages, symptoms of distortion and compression of the brain usually do not appear until weeks or months after the injury.

Subdural haematomas occur also in patients with haemorrhagic diatheses, and, in recent years, there have been several reports of their occurrence in people on prolonged anticoagulant therapy. Again the haemorrhage may have been the result of a minor head injury.

Trauma to the brain

The most characteristic feature of a recent head injury is the presence of contusions or lacerations on the crests of gyri. They are often found at the site of injury, particularly if there is a fracture, but the most characteristic sites are

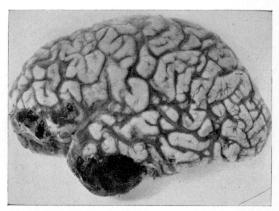

FIG. 20.11.—Acute head injury: contusions at frontal and temporal poles. × ½.

the frontal poles, the orbital surfaces of the frontal lobes, the temporal poles (Fig. 20.11), the under aspects of the anterior parts of the temporal lobes, and less commonly the under aspects of the cerebellar hemispheres. This distribution is due to the fact that it is in these regions that movement of the brain within the skull brings the surface of the brain into contact with bony protuberances in the base of the skull. Rotational movements may also cause tearing of small meningeal vessels in these regions. The concept of *contre-coup* lacerations which are said to occur at the pole of the brain opposite the site of injury should not be taken too literally: what does matter is that the most severe contusions are often seen at sites other than the site of injury.

In the acute stage the crests of the affected gyri are haemorrhagic and, if the pia is torn, blood enters the subarachnoid space. It may be extremely dangerous to perform lumbar puncture on a patient with a severe acute head injury (see p. 611), but if this is done, the cerebrospinal fluid is almost invariably bloodstained. If the patient survives, the lacerated tissue is removed by phagocytes, although a considerable amount of haemosiderin invariably remains, and the original sites of contusion are represented by well-demarcated depressions involving one or more convolutions, covered by thickened golden-yellow leptomeninges.

Sections of the brain after a fatal acute head injury confirm that cortical damage is usually restricted to the crests of gyri but may show numerous other haematomas in the white matter as well as in the basal ganglia. In some cases, well-defined infarcts, single or multiple, may be observed and these are presumably caused by tearing or spasm of arteries. In severe head injuries a haemorrhagic tear in the corpus callosum or tearing of one or both superior cerebellar peduncles is not uncommon. Oedema of the brain is another important factor in acute head injuries: this is most marked adjacent to lacerations and infarcts but it can be more diffuse and cause a considerable rise in intracranial pressure.

Microscopic examination of the brain in acute head injuries is often rather unrewarding apart from confirming the presence of destruction of tissue at the sites of laceration, infarcts and haemorrhage, although evidence of damage to nerve cells in the cortex and brain stem has been observed in the absence of gross changes. Important observations on the nature of the brain damage due to head injury have however been made by Sabina Strich who has demonstrated widespread tearing of nerve fibres with subsequent Wallerian degeneration of their myelin sheaths in the white matter of the cerebral hemispheres and in the brain stem in patients permanently incapacitated and more or less demented after a head injury.

Although the wide variety of macroscopic abnormalities which can be caused by a head injury have been described, it is not uncommon to observe only apparently minor damage in fatal cases. The current tendency is to attach increasingly greater significance to the rotational movements which occur at the time of injury and to the various shearing forces which are produced. As Strich has shown that these strains and stresses can disrupt nerve fibres, it seems probable that less severe injuries may stretch nerve fibres which, in consequence, lose their power of conduction for varying periods. Thus many neuronal pathways in the brain are temporarily or permanently blocked.

Intracranial haemorrhage may also occur during a difficult labour due to excessive moulding of the fetal head; most often it results from tearing of the edge of the tentorium or falx cerebri. There may be widespread haemorrhage and, if the infant survives, permanent neurological defects are usual.

Functional effects. The symptomatology of head injuries is a complex subject. A sufficiently severe blow is followed by *concussion*, there being sudden loss of consciousness, general flaccidity of muscles, etc. There may be rapid recovery as in the "knock-out" blow of boxers, or it may be prolonged and followed by the symptoms of shock which in severe cases may be complicated by the symptoms of raised intracranial pressure. The mechanism of concussion is still a matter of dispute but molecular disturbance and stretching of the nerve cells and fibres are probably the most important factors. When a patient regains consciousness after concussion there sometimes follows a period of cerebral irritation which has been ascribed to oedema of the brain. There is usually amnesia for the events immediately preceding the injury (post-traumatic amnesia).

When death follows within a day or two after severe injury, it is often due to raised intracranial pressure and distortion of the brain, brought about partly by effused blood and partly by oedema of the injured brain substance. The combined effect of these two leads to interference with the cerebral circulation, to deficient supply of blood to important centres, and thus to coma. The principal cause of death may also be a specific expanding lesion, such as an extradural haematoma.

When the patient recovers from the earlier effects of the injury, healing occurs in the lacerated areas, resulting in gliosis, and this may later give rise to post-traumatic epilepsy. This is readily understood in the case of the grosser lesions, but it is important to realise that there are also in head injuries multiple minor effects on the brain substance, discoverable only on microscopic examination as Strich has shown, and that healing of these may lead to later functional disturbances. It is, however, remarkable that in cases of fracture of the skull with evidence of severe brain injury there may be complete return to normal function after a time, particularly in children.

Trauma to the spinal cord

Injuries of the *spinal cord*, like those of the brain, are of all degrees of severity. In cases of fracture-dislocation, bullet wounds, etc., the cord may be directly lacerated, or even torn across. Apart from such extreme cases, the cord may be damaged from severe concussion, blows on the back, falls on the feet, etc., and haemorrhage may occur either outside or inside the dura. Lesions may be encountered within the cord itself, either infarction or haemorrhage or a combination of both. Haemorrhage occurs especially immediately dorsal to the grey commissure, and tends to extend upwards and downwards through several segments. In cases of haemorrhage into the cord, or haematomyelia, the blood is broken down and ultimately an elongated pigmented encapsulated cavity may result, which may simulate syringomyelia (p. 660). Apart from these grosser effects it is not uncommon to find partial degeneration of fibres in the cord, sometimes extending through several segments. This is apparently the result of sudden bending or stretching of the cord at the time of injury. Functional disturbance may be produced in this way.

CIRCULATORY DISTURBANCES

Of these, by far the most important are *intracranial haemorrhage* and *occlusive vascular disease*. Before discussing these, some general points will be considered. The amount of blood present in the intracranial veins and sinuses *post mortem* varies greatly, and assessment of this requires that the cranial cavity be opened first. When the thorax is opened and the heart removed, a considerably amount of blood drains off. Pallor of the brain is seen in severe anaemia, deaths due to external haemorrhage and sudden heart failure, from aortic disease, and in association with oedema in nephritis.

Intense congestion of small vessels occurs in chronic cardiac and pulmonary disease, and the degree of venous engorgement probably depends mainly on the oxygen and carbon dioxide content of the blood at the time of death as both hypoxia and hypercapnia cause marked arteriolar dilatation. Thus intense congestion may also be a marked feature in cases of prolonged coma. The same basic mechanism may also account for the extreme congestion of grey and white matter which we have observed in fatal strychnine poisoning. *Acute congestion* of the meninges may represent the earliest stage of an acute meningitis whereas acute congestion of the brain itself, most noticeable in the grey matter, may be seen adjacent to recent haemorrhagic infarcts, in fevers and other infective conditions, and especially locally in the region of inflammatory changes, e.g. in encephalitis. The significance of acute congestion must be judged in connection with the other conditions present.

General cerebral oedema can occur especially in acute head injuries and is seen in cases of nephritis, particularly where there is generalised "renal" oedema. The accumulation of fluid occurs especially in the white matter, and when the brain is cut with a dry knife the cut surface becomes wetter afterwards, owing to the gradual escape of the fluid from the tissue on to the surface. Oedema probably plays a part in producing convulsions in cases of hypertensive encephalopathy, arteriolar spasm leading to ischaemic damage in the walls of capillaries, increased capillary permeability and oedema. In some cases the oedema may be so great as to cause internal herniae (see p. 610). Local oedema is often seen in the neighbourhood of gross lesions, such as a tumour or an abscess and may contribute very significantly to the volume of the expanding lesion. When the oedema has lasted for some time the nerve fibres suffer, their myelin is broken up into globules, a certain amount of demyelination resulting. The brain substance is paler, moister and rather less firm, and, when the circulatory disturbance is more marked, merges into frank infarction. A true *inflammatory oedema* may occur around a cerebral abscess.

Intracranial haemorrhage

There are five possible sites for intracranial haemorrhage—extradural, subdural, subarachnoid, intracerebral and intraventricular. The first two of these are usually due to trauma and have already been described (p. 615). *Subarachnoid haemorrhage* may also be due to a head injury but other common causes are rupture of an aneurysm on one of the major cerebral arteries in the subarachnoid space at the base of the brain or bursting of an intracerebral haematoma on to the surface of the brain and into the subarachnoid space: rarer causes are a vascular malformation on the surface of the brain or haemorrhagic diseases. *Intracerebral haemorrhage* is most often due to hypertension but it is also commonly a sequel to a head injury: rarer causes are rupture of an aneurysm on one of the major cerebral arteries at the base of the brain, haemorrhage into an intracerebral tumour, an intracerebral vascular malformation or haemorrhagic diatheses. *Intraventricular haemorrhage,* although not uncommon, is rarely a primary event as it is almost always due to rupture of an intracerebral haematoma into the ventricular system or rarely to a vascular malformation in the choroid plexus.

The two commonest types of intracerebral haemorrhage other than those caused by head injury will now be discussed in more detail.

Intracerebral haemorrhage

Haemorrhage into the brain is due to the rupture of a nutrient perforating artery. The resulting haematoma usually increases rapidly, producing destruction of brain tissue, distortion of the brain, and often a rapid increase in intracranial pressure. The term *apoplexy* is frequently applied and the mortality rate is high. By far the commonest cause is hypertension associated with arteriosclerosis and hypertrophy of the myocardium of the left ventricle, but it may also occur in old age as a result of degenerative changes in small arteries. Almost a century ago Charcot came to the conclusion that the haemorrhage occurred from miliary aneurysms on the perforating cerebral arteries, but his hypothesis gained little support. It has however been clearly demonstrated recently by Yates and his colleagues in Manchester, as a result of postmortem microangiographic studies and by histological examination, that microaneurysms do in fact develop on perforating cerebral arteries. These microaneurysms, which are usually multiple, tend to occur on arteries less than 25 microns in diameter and may attain a size of 2 mm. They occur mainly in hypertensive individuals over the age of 50. In con-

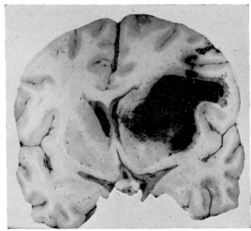

Fig. 20.12.—Large haematoma in basal ganglia, resulting from chronic hypertension. × ½.

trast, microaneurysms are rare in normotensive subjects although a few can be demonstrated in some people over the age of 65. Yates believes that hypertension is the principal cause of these microaneurysms and that their subsequent rupture is the commonest cause of intracerebral haemorrhage (Cole and Yates, 1967).

By far the commonest site of this type of cerebral haemorrhage is the region of the basal ganglia (Fig. 20.12); the pons and cerebellum come next in order of frequency, whilst haemorrhage into the superficial parts of the brain or into the crura and medulla are rare. A deeply placed haematoma may rupture into the ventricles. Haemorrhage into the basal ganglia usually occurs from the lenticulo-striate artery, which arises from the middle cerebral artery. It enters at the anterior perforated spot, passes upwards in the external capsule and then curves inwards through the lentiform nucleus and internal capsule. Charcot applied the term "artery of cerebral haemorrhage" to the lenticulo-striate artery, though there are several arteries to which the former term is applicable. Haemorrhage is not uncommon from the lenticulo-optic and other branches in the thalamus and adjacent territories.

When haemorrhage occurs, the effused blood forms a large oval blood clot, which may measure up to 10 cm. in its long axis. It tears up and destroys the adjacent structures, and at the margin there are often small secondary haemorrhages. When a haematoma bursts into the lateral ventricles they become distended with blood, the ventricle on the same side as the haemorrhage usually to a greater extent, and the blood passes down the aqueduct of Sylvius and through the foramina in the roof of the fourth ventricle. The blood then reaches the subarachnoid space and may there spread widely over the structures at the base of the brain and pass downwards over the spinal cord. An intracerebral haematoma may also break through directly to the surface of the brain.

At post-mortem examination in a case with a large cerebral haematoma, the convolutions are seen to be flattened and dry in appearance because of expansion of the brain and this is often more marked over the affected hemisphere. Primary haemorrhage into the pons may be sufficient to cause obvious enlargement. Rupture into the fourth ventricle frequently follows (Fig. 20.13).

In a recent cerebral haemorrhage, the blood forms an ordinary dark-coloured clot and retains this appearance for several days. At the end of about a week it comes to have a brownish colour at the periphery, and this change in colour extends and becomes more marked as time goes on. The clot becomes softened at the margin and is thus surrounded with a brown fluid, whilst neuroglial proliferation leads to the formation of a capsule. Ultimately the clot disappears and fluid remains, which gradually becomes paler. The ultimate result is the so-called *apoplectic cyst* (Fig. 20.14), which has a pigmented wall owing to the presence of bilirubin

and haemosiderin in the tissue; the contents may ultimately be yellow. If the haemorrhage is relatively small, it may be entirely replaced by proliferated neuroglia, which contracts and forms an orange or brown glial scar, in which bilirubin crystals may persist for very long periods (Fig. 9.7, p. 201).

In a case of cerebral haemorrhage, it is not uncommon to find in the unaffected basal ganglia evidence of previous haemorrhages in the form of small spaces containing brownish fluid. Small infarcts, due to occlusive arterial disease, may also be present.

The effects of cerebral haemorrhage may be both focal and general in character. The former

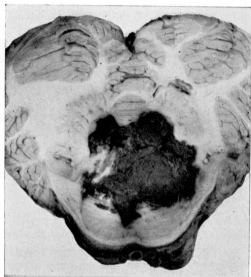

FIG. 20.13.—Hypertensive haemorrhage into pons. × 1.
Note typical rupture into fourth ventricle.

effects are produced by the destruction of cells and fibres which results in paralysis and permanent loss of function. However, a large intracerebral haematoma may cause a rapid and often fatal rise in intracranial pressure and frequently there is a tentorial hernia and terminal secondary haemorrhage in the brain stem (see p. 609).

Haemorrhage from an aneurysm in the subarachnoid space

When the haemorrhage is from the circle of Willis or one of its primary branches, a ruptured aneurysm can usually be found. The features and conditions of occurrence of aneurysms in this situation have already been discussed (p. 287); it is sufficient to recall that these, though commonest in middle life, may occur in younger people quite apart from any general arterial disease; they are generally known as *congenital* or *berry aneurysms* though only the defect in the muscle coat is congenital, and the resulting aneurysm develops gradually as age advances. Rarer causes of aneurysms on the cerebral vessels are infected emboli (mycotic aneurysms) and atheroma, while dissecting aneurysms have also been described.

Berry aneurysms arise at points of bifurcation of the cerebral arteries and while they can occur

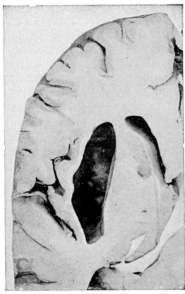

FIG. 20.14.—Old apoplectic cyst on left side of brain.
The cyst involves chiefly the external capsule and the outer part of the lentiform nucleus. × ⅔.

in any position, the commonest sites are on the middle cerebral artery in the Sylvian fissure, at the junction of the anterior communicating artery with an anterior cerebral artery, and on the terminal portion of the internal carotid artery. Aneurysms of this type occur also on the basilar artery and its branches. In most cases of rupture of an aneurysm, there is diffuse and extensive subarachnoid haemorrhage, most abundant adjacent to the ruptured aneurysm, particularly when in the Sylvian fissure or between the frontal lobes. This haematoma may be large enough to act as a significant expanding lesion

leading to a rise in intracranial pressure. Leakage of blood from a cerebral aneurysm is not invariably fatal, and the lesion may become fibrosed and healed by organisation of the clot. In many cases, however, a further haemorrhage takes place which proves fatal, and post-mortem examination reveals evidence of previous leakage by the presence of altered blood pigment in the adjacent thickened and pigmented leptomeninges.

The aneurysm sac may be embedded in the adjacent brain tissue, and subsequent rupture is attended by haemorrhage directly into the brain. The resulting intracerebral haematoma may track into the ventricles, or intraventricular haemorrhage may be direct as when an aneurysm on the anterior communicating artery ruptures through the rostrum of the corpus callosum. A rupture of a cerebral aneurysm may thus simulate an ordinary apoplectic haemorrhage and the presence of an aneurysm should always be suspected when investigating an intracerebral haematoma in an unusual site. Another important complication of a ruptured aneurysm is cerebral infarction in the tissue supplied by the artery on which the aneurysm is situated. This is apparently due to arterial spasm, and the swelling which always occurs in an early infarct (*vide infra*) causes further displacement and distortion of the brain.

When the haemorrhage is from a vascular malformation in the brain, the pathological findings are very similar to those of a ruptured congenital aneurysm.

It should be emphasised that ruptured cerebral aneurysm and subarachnoid haemorrhage are not synonymous terms: the latter may be the result of an acute head injury, or haemorrhage from a vascular malformation, or it may be subsequent to a primary intracerebral haemorrhage tracking into the ventricles or through the surface of the brain; whilst a ruptured aneurysm may cause an intracerebral haematoma or a cerebral infarct without any significant subarachnoid haemorrhage.

Multiple small haemorrhages are encountered chiefly in certain blood diseases and in severe infective conditions; examples of the first are pernicious anaemia, purpura, scurvy, leukaemia, and of the second septicaemia, typhus, smallpox, etc. They also occur in caisson disease (p. 661) and in fat embolism (p. 171), in traumatic asphyxia, and in various disorders, e.g. Wernicke's encephalopathy (p. 605), haemorrhagic leuko-encephalitis (p. 648) and polyarteritis. They are usually in the form of petechiae, though sometimes they are larger, and occur especially in the leptomeninges. In leukaemia, haemorrhages of considerable size, single or multiple, occasionally occur in the brain substance and have been attributed to the formation of leukocyte thrombi in the vessels, but this is uncertain. In most cases of infection the haemorrhages are the result of toxic action on the capillary walls, but sometimes organisms are present. In some cases of very acute staphylococcal infection, for example, capillaries plugged with cocci may be found in the haemorrhagic spots in the brain substance. Haemorrhage may also be a concomitant of meningitis, and diffuse haemorrhage in the subarachnoid space is a prominent feature of meningitis caused by the anthrax bacillus. Multiple small areas of haemorrhage in the brain are a constant finding when a major venous sinus and its tributaries are occluded by thrombus.

Cerebral infarction

The brain receives its blood supply from the internal carotid and vertebral arteries, frequently referred to as the *extracranial* cerebral arteries, from which the major *intracranial* cerebral arteries arise. A *cerebral infarct* occurs when the blood flow to any part of the brain falls below the critical level necessary to maintain the viability of brain tissue: it is essentially *focal* in nature, in contrast to the *diffuse* selective neuronal loss that may occur in hypoxic states with preservation of the cerebral blood flow, and may be restricted to a small discrete lesion in the grey or white matter or may affect a large part of the brain. The reduction in blood flow may be of such a degree as to result only in the death of the most susceptible cells, *viz.* the neurones, but usually it is more severe, producing necrosis also of the neuroglial cells and, slightly less commonly, of microglia and blood vessels also. Occlusion of a cerebral artery is not a prerequisite for a cerebral infarct: indeed an episode of severe hypotension or transient cardiac arrest may cause cerebral infarction in the complete absence of any occlusive arterial disease, but more usually there is stenosis and/or occlusion of a major extracranial or intracranial cerebral artery. The critical reduction in the blood flow to a particular region of the brain needs to extend over a period of only

several minutes to produce an infarct. If this reduction is transient the blood flow may even return to normal through the infarct. When the cerebral circulation is already compromised by pre-existing arterial stenosis, infarction is particularly liable to occur in any state of generalised circulatory insufficiency, such as hypotension due to a myocardial infarct or massive haemorrhage, even although there is no actual arterial occlusion.

The principal local causes of a deficient cerebral blood flow are intrinsic structural abnormalities in the arteries, embolism, or spasm. By far the commonest abnormality is atheroma: this may result only in stenosis, but actual occlusion of a cerebral artery is usually produced by the formation of thrombus on an atheromatous plaque. Other vascular diseases leading to a reduced arterial lumen with or without thrombosis are arteritis (polyarteritis nodosa, giant cell and temporal arteritis), tuberculosis and syphilitic endarteritis. A cerebral embolus usually comes from vegetations on the mitral or aortic valve cusps in cases of subacute bacterial endocarditis or from mural thrombus in patients with auricular fibrillation or a myocardial infarct. Transient neurological symptoms, the so-called "transient ischaemic attacks" are often attributed to small cholesterol emboli from atheromatous plaques in the carotid or vertebral arteries. Spasm of intracranial cerebral arteries is probably only of significance in association with a ruptured aneurysm of a major cerebral artery or in acute head injuries.

Sites. An infarct may occur in almost any part of the brain although the middle cerebral arterial territory is most frequently involved. The size of the infarct depends to a considerable extent on the degree of occlusive arterial disease and the available collateral circulation. Collateral channels exist between the major cerebral arteries on the surface of the brain and by way of the circle of Willis, but similar channels do not exist within the substance of the brain. An infarct may therefore affect an entire arterial territory or only part of it, while if the blood flow through two adjacent arterial territories is affected, infarction may be restricted to the boundary zone between them.

Arterial obstruction

Occlusive arterial disease leading to a cerebral infarct may lie within the skull or in the neck. In a recent study Yates and Hutchinson could find no evidence of occlusion or significant stenosis of the intracranial cerebral arteries in 16 out of 35 cases of cerebral infarction. However, in a post-mortem study of 100 cases which were selected because the clinical picture had suggested that cerebral ischaemia was either the cause of death or else contributory to it, they found serious stenosis or occlusion of the internal carotid and vertebral arteries in 33 cases, of the internal carotid arteries alone in 18 and of the vertebral arteries alone in 7. The commonest site of occlusion of the extracranial cerebral arteries is in the carotid sinus and, if the collateral circulation is or becomes inadequate, the usual site of infarction is in the distribution of the middle cerebral artery on the same side. In a few cases the infarct is caused by thrombosis extending from the carotid sinus along the internal carotid artery into the middle and anterior cerebral arteries. When the vertebral arteries are the more severely involved, ischaemic changes occur characteristically in the brain stem, cerebellum and the part of the cerebral hemispheres supplied by the posterior cerebral arteries, i.e. the occipital lobes. Yates and Hutchinson concluded that cerebral infarction is usually the result of a combination of systemic circulatory insufficiency and stenosis of the extracranial or intracranial cerebral arteries, or both, and that in cerebral infarction, stenosis of the extracranial cerebral arteries is more often a major factor than stenosis of the intracranial arteries. Although occlusion of the internal carotid artery in the neck is usually secondary to atheroma, attention has recently been drawn to its occurrence after closed injuries to the neck.

Structural changes in a cerebral infarct

A cerebral infarct may be pale or haemorrhagic (Fig. 20.15:) this depends (*a*) on whether or not some blood flow has been restored through the infarct and (*b*) on whether or not necrosis of vessel walls has occurred, thus allowing the extravasation of blood into the necrotic tissue. An intensely haemorrhagic infarct may superficially resemble a haematoma but the distinctive feature of an infarct is the preservation of intrinsic architecture. A pale infarct less than 24 hours old may defy recognition macroscopically. Thereafter the dead tissue becomes slightly soft and swollen and there is a loss of the normal sharp definition between grey

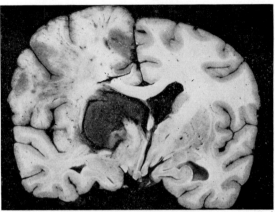

FIG. 20.15.—Recent infarct in left cerebral hemisphere. The basal ganglia show the features of haemorrhagic infarction; the posterior part of the frontal lobe above the Sylvian fissure shows those of pale infarction. Note that the affected hemisphere is swollen and that there is displacement of the mid-line structures to the right.

and white matter. At this stage histological examination will show ischaemic necrosis of neurones, pallor of myelin staining and sometimes polymorphonuclear leukocytes in relation to necrotic vessel walls. If the infarct is large, it may swell to the extent of producing all the typical features of an acutely expanding lesion and raised intracranial pressure (see p. 609). Within a few days the infarct becomes distinctly soft and the dead tissue disintegrates: hence a cerebral infarct is often referred to loosely as a "softening" (Fig. 20.16). Microscopic examination at this stage will show phagocytes (p. 608), filled with globules of lipid produced by the breakdown of myelin (Fig. 20.17), enlarged astrocytes, and early capillary proliferation. Eventually the dead tissue is removed, lipid phagocytes become scanty, a fibrillary gliosis occurs and the lesion ultimately becomes shrunken and cystic. The cysts are often traversed by small vessels and glial fibrils (Fig. 20.18). If the infarct has been of the haemorrhagic type, a proportion of the phagocytes will contain haemosiderin. Shrinkage of the affected region is usually accompanied by enlargement of the adjacent lateral ventricle, this being an example of secondary hydrocephalus

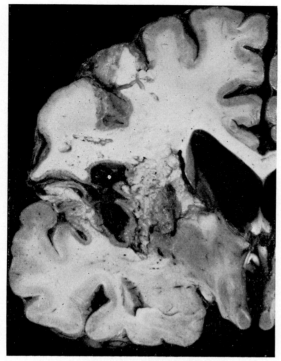

FIG. 20.16.—Infarct of a week's duration in the left cerebral hemisphere. The dead tissue is disintegrating and there is already some shrinkage of the affected cortex.

cortex is usually cystic and traversed by strands of thick astrocytic fibres. An important result of infarction is Wallerian degeneration in the nerve fibres that have been destroyed. Thus if the infarct involves the internal capsule, there is progressive degeneration and shrinkage of the corresponding pyramidal tract in the brain stem and in the spinal cord.

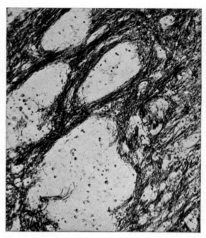

FIG. 20.18.—Margin of cerebral softening at a later stage, stained to show thickened neuroglia and spaces containing fluid. × 80. (A. C. L.)

(Fig. 20.19). In the case of an old cortical infarct, the overlying meninges are somewhat thickened and opaque and underneath there is usually an adherent layer of brownish-yellow cortical tissue composed of enlarged astrocytes and occasional lipid phagocytes. Beneath this the

Other aspects of ischaemic brain damage

A diminished blood supply to the brain may lead to loss of nerve cells without frank infarction. The neuroglia in such circumstances retains its vitality with the result that focal neuronal loss is accompanied by a fibrillary gliosis. This process is analogous to the ischaemic atrophy with fibrosis which follows as the result of arterial narrowing in the kidneys and other organs. Areas of sclerosis produced in this way are a prominent feature in dementia of arteriopathic type, and they are common also in general arterial disease, especially in old people.

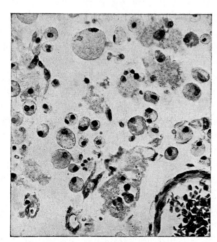

FIG. 20.17.—Margin of cerebral softening showing characters of "compound granular corpuscles"—enlarged microglial cells. × 250. A.C.L.

Venous obstruction

The most important form of this occurs as a result of thrombosis in one of the sinuses. Two types of thrombosis are usually distinguished, the *marantic* and the *infective*: in the latter there is often suppuration within the sinus. *Marantic thrombosis* is most frequent in poorly nourished children during the course of acute infections, e.g. gastro-enteritis; but it may occur in adults in conditions of cachexia, e.g. from malignant disease, or as a complication of infective fevers. Impaired circulation and possibly bacterial infection of mild virulence may be causal factors. The commonest site is the superior longitudinal sinus, and, when obstruction is complete, intense engorgement of the superficial veins occurs. There may also be irregular zones of intensely haemorrhagic infarction in the para-saggital parts of the cerebral hemispheres. In cases of thrombosis of the straight sinus, similar haemorrhagic areas are present in the walls of the third ventricle. *Infective thrombosis* is the result of direct spread of organisms from an inflammatory or suppurative condition in the neighbourhood. This is described on p. 629.

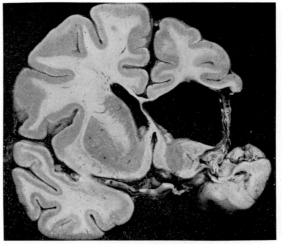

FIG. 20. 19.—Infarct of several years' duration in the right cerebral hemisphere. The dead tissue has been completely removed. The lateral ventricle is separated from the surface of the brain by a narrow web of tissue composed of leptomeninges, ependyma and a few glial fibrils.

INFLAMMATORY CHANGES

Meningitis

Inflammation of the meninges, viz. *meningitis*, and inflammation of the substance of the brain, viz. *encephalitis*, are considered separately for, although both are commonly involved in any severe inflammatory process, one is almost always much more severely affected than the other. Meningitis may involve the dura—pachymeningitis, or the pia and arachnoid—leptomeningitis, but the term meningitis is frequently used as implying only leptomeningitis.

Pachymeningitis

Acute inflammation of the dura is practically always due to an extension of septic inflammation from the bones of the skull. It formerly occurred most frequently as a result of chronic middle ear or mastoid disease, and also as a complication of disease of the nasal sinuses. These conditions, however, are now largely controlled by chemotherapy and consequently a larger proportion of cases of pachymeningitis now appear as a sequel to compound fracture of the skull, which permits access of pyogenic organisms. When pyogenic organisms spread from the bone, suppuration occurs between bone and dura and an *extradural abscess* may form. The dura becomes swollen, softened and infiltrated with pus, and if the infection spreads to its inner aspect, pus will accumulate in the subdural space: the infection can then spread widely over the hemisphere to form a *subdural abscess*. The organisms may also spread to the arachnoid, setting up either localised or general leptomeningitis. Further effects of spread, such as the production of cerebral abscess, are described below. Considerable thickening of the dura may occur in relation to chronic inflammation in the bone. The dura is occasionally the site of gummatous lesions in syphilis (p. 634), but it is rarely affected by tuberculosis except in the case of direct spread, for example, from the petrous bone or from the vertebral column.

Leptomeningitis

This condition is due essentially to the spread of micro-organisms in the meshwork of the sub-arachnoid space. When the organisms reach this situation they set up an inflammatory reaction, and thus exudate is added to the cerebrospinal fluid, producing a medium in which organisms can multiply freely. Owing to the wide inter-communicating system beneath the arachnoid, they readily spread, and in this they are no doubt aided by the normal movements of the cerebrospinal fluid. The exudate is most abundant where the subarachnoid space is widest, and thus tends to accumulate in the cisterns at the base of the brain. In most cases the exudate is confined to the subarachnoid space but in severe purulent cases, particularly in children, there may be extension to the subdural space. Pus in the subdural space can be easily scraped off the surface of the brain whereas this is not possible when the exudate is confined to the subarachnoid space.

Causes and modes of infection. Acute bacterial meningitis is most commonly caused by the meningococcus, giving rise to cerebrospinal meningitis (sometimes in epidemic form), the pneumococcus, and the haemophilus group. Some viral diseases of the nervous system and also the presence of blood in the subarachnoid space are accompanied by many of the clinical signs of acute meningitis. Infection of the meninges by tubercle bacilli was formerly very common and the ensuing reaction was not infrequently acute with exudation of fibrin and polymorphs, but tended to pass into a subacute state. Less frequent causal agents are the ordinary pyo-cocci, the bacilli of the coli-typhoid group, the anthrax bacillus, *Treponema pallidum*, leptospirae, and various fungi.

(*a*) *Infection by the blood stream.* In cerebrospinal fever (meningococcal meningitis) infection is spread by droplet infection from carriers who harbour the micro-organism in the nasopharynx. Spread is favoured by poor hygienic conditions, especially overcrowding, and thus the disease tends to occur in epidemic form amongst recruits in overcrowded barracks, refugees in camps, etc. In susceptible persons the meningococci pass from the nasopharynx to the meninges by the blood stream and during epidemics cases of fatal meningococcal septicaemia can occur without meningitis, death sometimes occurring within a few hours of infection. In cases of primary pneumococcal meningitis in the adult, without other discoverable lesion, the infection is evidently blood-borne. Spread by the blood stream is seen also in cases of suppurative inflammation elsewhere in the body, in septicaemia, bacterial endocarditis, pneumonia, etc. In acute staphy-

lococcal pyaemia, due for example to suppurative osteomyelitis, the infection of the meninges commonly occurs from a small abscess in the cerebral cortex.

(*b*) *Infection by spread from an adjacent lesion.* Examples are seen of extension of infection from septic inflammation of the bones and dura, resulting from compound fractures or from middle ear disease, suppurative infection of the nasal bones or of the frontal sinuses, etc. The spread may take place in such instances directly through the dura to the meninges, or along an emergent vein, with or without the formation of an abscess in the brain. In young children, pneumococci may spread by the Eustachian tube to the middle ear, giving rise to acute otitis media, and thence to the brain; this is the usual sequence of events in cases of pneumococcal meningitis in early life. Pneumococci of Group IV are the ordinary causal agents. It should be emphasised that acute leptomeningitis is a not infrequent complication of a fracture of the base of the skull as a result of direct spread of organisms from air sinuses or the roof of the nasopharynx.

(*c*) *Iatrogenic infection* happens occasionally, by the introduction of micro-organisms at operation or by lumbar puncture with non-sterile instruments. This is a rare occurrence but as the infecting agents are introduced into the subarachnoid space, a generalised meningitis rapidly ensues.

Structural changes. The exudate occurs in the subarachnoid space and tends to be most marked where the spaces are largest (Fig. 20.20). Thus it is most abundant along the sulci, where it obscures the blood vessels to a varying degree, and at the base of the brain, where it accumulates around the optic chiasma and in adjacent cisterns. It varies markedly in character, even in the same type of infection. There may merely be excess of fluid of turbid appearance along the sulci, or the exudate may be abundant, yellowish and fibrinous, or it may be distinctly purulent.

The inflammation frequently extends to the ventricles: they contain turbid fluid and a varying amount of fibrinous exudate is seen on their walls and on the choroid plexuses. Some degree of internal hydrocephalus is a common result.

In anthrax infection of the meninges, the exudate is serous and contains a considerable admixture of blood—in fact the effused blood may be so abundant as to simulate diffuse subarachnoid haemorrhage. In meningitis due to the yeast *Torula histolytica*, the exudate is notably gelatinous in character, and in it the infecting organisms can be recognised as refractile bodies about the size of red cells, surrounded by a wide capsule giving a clear zone around the organisms.

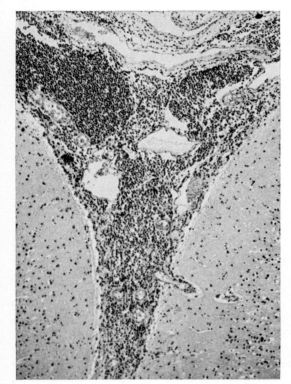

FIG. 20.20.—Acute pneumococcal meningitis: section of cerebral cortex from a case of acute meningitis, showing distension of the subarachnoid space with polymorphonuclear leukocytes. × 55.

In all varieties of meningitis the *spinal meninges* are involved to a variable degree, owing to the direct continuity of the cerebral and spinal subarachnoid spaces. The latter, despite its size, becomes distended in cases of meningitis, and when lumbar puncture is undertaken to establish the diagnosis, the cerebrospinal fluid is often found to be under considerable pressure, 300 mm. H₂O or more. The cerebrospinal fluid presents varying degrees of turbidity and may even be distinctly purulent. Microscopic examination shows it to contain numerous polymorphonuclear leukocytes. The protein content is raised and the sugar reduced or absent (Table, p. 652). The causal organisms are often apparent, although in some cases they can be obtained only by culture. At necropsy, the

X

appearances of the spinal cord correspond in their general features with those described above: fibrinous or purulent exudate when present is usually most abundant over its dorsal aspect, and may obscure the vessels to a considerable extent.

In acute meningococcal meningitis—*cerebrospinal fever*—there is often a haemorrhagic rash from which the old name "spotted fever" is derived (Fig. 20.21). The degree of inflammation observed over the brain and cord and in the ventricles varies greatly. The exudate may be abundant, and then it has a yellowish purulent appearance, or if death has occurred early in the disease it may be only a turbid serous fluid. Both brain and spinal cord are affected. As a rule, meningococci can be readily found in the cerebrospinal fluid, most being contained within

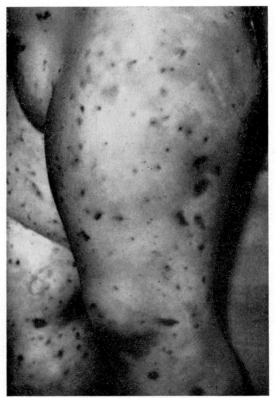

FIG. 20.21.—Acute meningococcal meningitis, showing the haemorrhagic rash.

polymorphonuclear leukocytes; in some cases, however, especially those of less severe degree, they are very scanty and may not be found on microscopic examination. In this type of meningitis, extensive phagocytosis of the polymorphonuclear leukocytes by macrophages is often a striking feature in the exudate.

If treatment has been inadequate or has been commenced too late for resolution of the inflammatory exudate to occur, the disease may pass into a subacute or chronic phase. Formerly this was not uncommon in young children and the disease was then referred to as *posterior basal meningitis.* The leptomeninges become thickened and oedematous and the exudate undergoes organisation leading to obliteration of the foramina in the roof of the fourth ventricle and/or some degree of obstruction in the subarachnoid space. Either process leads to the occurrence of progressive internal hydrocephalus which is often the cause of death. Various cranial nerves may be involved with resulting paralyses. Similar chronic changes can occur in the spinal meninges with widespread involvement of nerve roots. Organisms are usually scanty in such chronic cases, but the meningococcus was most commonly the infecting agent. Closely similar structural changes may be brought about by the tubercle bacillus (see p. 630) and by *Haemophilus influenzae.*

Bacterial encephalitis

Some degree of acute generalised encephalitis is an almost invariable accompaniment of acute bacterial infection of the meninges, both pyogenic and tuberculous, but apart from this, bacteria are not an important cause of encephalitis. Viruses, however, are very frequently concerned; these are considered separately.

Bacterial encephalitis may be suppurative (i.e. a *brain abscess*). *Non suppurative* encephalitis usually results from extension of inflammation from an acute meningitis. The degree to which this occurs varies greatly. In some cases it is striking how little leukocytic infiltration may be present along the blood vessels; in others the perivascular spaces are crowded with leukocytes which may extend a considerable distance into the brain substance, whilst exudate, haemorrhage and foci of cortical infarction may be present. In tuberculous meningitis there is usually marked involvement of the cortex due to obliterative arteritis and thrombosis in many of the arteries in the subarachnoid space. Similarly the spinal cord is almost invariably implicated to some extent in meningitis.

Brain abscess

The causative organisms vary greatly, anaerobic strains of streptococci, diphtheroids and coliforms, etc., being encountered in addition to the common pyogenic cocci. The organisms reach the brain, as in meningitis, by direct spread or by means of the blood stream.

Direct spread of organisms. This is usually a consequence of pyogenic infection in the bones or sinuses of the skull or of a compound fracture. In our experience the commonest and most important cause is spread of an infection in the middle ear or the mastoid air cells. The carious process reaches the dura and may produce a local pachymeningitis, an *extradural abscess,* or a *subdural abscess* (p. 625). The inflammation extends to the leptomeninges and a generalised meningitis may ensue but more frequently the inflammation is limited by local adhesions. The organisms may then cause superficial destruction of the cortex before extending more deeply into the brain, but frequently the subsequent abscess is separated from the surface of the brain by an intact layer of cortex; in fact, in some cases of middle ear disease, the caries may not even have reached the surface of the bone. The precise route of infection in these cases is open to doubt but it is probably via small blood vessels or their perivascular spaces. It is to be noted that the emergent veins from the bone drain into a venous sinus, into which the veins of the brain also discharge, and in this way a path of infection is provided. It is of course evident that the existence of septic thrombus in the particular sinus will aid the spread of infection, but an isolated cerebral abscess often occurs without sinus thrombosis. Similarly, an abscess may follow disease of any of the other air sinuses, or a compound fracture of the skull.

If middle ear infection spreads upwards through the tegmen tympani, it comes into relation with the under surface of the temporal lobe, and thus the abscess occurs in this lobe (Fig. 20.22). If the disease has spread from the mastoid antrum, or from the middle ear to the posterior aspect of the petrous bone, the abscess occurs in the cerebellum; in such cases the sigmoid sinus often becomes implicated and may be thrombosed. In some cases with chronic middle ear disease, abscesses may be found both in the temporal lobe and in the cerebellum.

As elsewhere, an abscess in the brain becomes limited by a pyogenic membrane which, unless the septic process extends very rapidly to involve the meninges or ventricles, soon becomes a well-defined capsule composed of young connective tissue, new capillaries, proliferated astrocytes and lipid phagocytes: i.e. there is a gliomesodermal reaction. In the adjacent cerebral tissue there are varying degrees of oedema,

membrane is perforated allowing access of a very mixed bacterial flora. The bone becomes eroded and infection may reach the dura, giving rise to one or more of the lesions mentioned—local pachymeningitis, acute leptomeningitis, cerebral abscess, sinus thrombosis, etc. A similar sequence of events may follow acute suppuration in the frontal sinus, the resulting abscess being in the frontal lobe, but this is more rare.

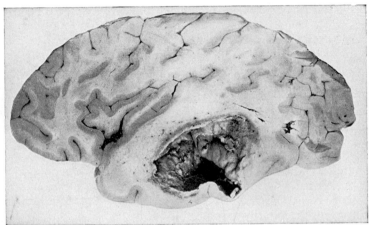

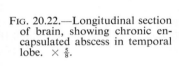

FIG. 20.22.—Longitudinal section of brain, showing chronic encapsulated abscess in temporal lobe. × ⅝.

reactive gliosis and infiltration by inflammatory cells, the latter being particularly prominent in the perivascular spaces. Plasma cells often predominate. These changes are commonly silent clinically and, by the time the patient presents with symptoms, the abscess is likely to contain thick greenish-yellow pus commonly with a foul odour because of the mixed bacterial flora. The abscess can exist for a considerable time in a virtually latent state but localised extension to form a multilocular abscess is not uncommon. Without effective treatment, spread to the ventricles or the subarachnoid space often occurs as a terminal event.

Otitis media and mastoiditis. Disease of the middle ear, mastoid antrum and air cells is the result of infection spreading and ascending by the Eustachian tube from the pharynx, especially in children, but also in adults. Not infrequently it starts as a complication of scarlet fever or other streptococcal tonsillitis; in infants pneumococci of Group IV are often concerned but many other organisms are soon superadded. Acute suppurative inflammation of the lining of the tympanic cavity develops and, if this progresses, the mucous membrane is destroyed and replaced by a layer of granulation tissue; commonly the tympanic

Sinus thrombosis. This is the result of an extension of septic inflammation to the wall of a sinus, and occurs most frequently in the sigmoid sinus in cases of mastoid or middle ear disease. The first effect is the production of acute phlebitis with secondary formation of thrombus on the damaged intima. At the very earliest period the thrombus may be free from organisms, but it soon becomes invaded by them and then suppurative softening of its substance occurs. Once thrombosis has started it tends to spread, and it may pass into the internal jugular vein. The oldest part of the thrombus thus comes to be occupied by purulent material, while the process of ordinary thrombosis continues to spread at the end, and thus may prevent the detachment of infected portions. Accordingly, while septic emboli may become detached, and cause secondary abscesses in the lungs, this occurs only in a relatively small proportion of cases of septic sinus thrombosis.

Haematogenous abscesses. These occur most frequently in the parietal lobes but they may be found in any part of the brain and they are not infrequently multiple. When solitary they may attain a large size and develop a thick gliomesodermal capsule before being diagnosed. The source of the septic embolus may be anywhere in the body but the primary site is often in the lung as a result of septic involvement of small pulmonary veins. There is a particularly close association between suppurative bronchiectasis and brain abscess, but fortunately most cases of bronchiectasis can now be adequately controlled by antibiotics. Individuals with congenital cyanotic heart disease are particularly prone to develop a brain abscess. Multiple small acute abscesses occur in pyaemia, while in a patient dying with subacute bacterial endocarditis numerous small perivascular inflammatory foci are almost invariably found in the brain. Such lesions may sometimes be seen as minute haemorrhagic foci but frequently they are identifiable only on microscopic examination.

Occasionally the yeast *Torula histolytica* may set up a chronic granulomatous "abscess", the source of infection, as in torula meningitis, being probably the lung. Abscesses in the brain, single or multiple, and sometimes of considerable size, may occasionally be produced by the actinomyces and other streptothrix organisms; they usually occur secondarily to similar lesions in the lungs.

Tuberculosis

Involvement of the nervous system is a not uncommon feature of tuberculosis. It may take the form of tuberculous meningitis or, less commonly, one or more large caseating lesions—tuberculomata—embedded in the brain. These latter may present clinically as expanding lesions.

Tuberculous meningitis

This is always preceded by an active tuberculous infection in some other organ in the body, usually the lung. In the meninges inflammation with exudation is associated with the presence of tubercles. The bacilli may reach the meninges from the blood stream in generalised miliary tuberculosis, or, less commonly, by direct spread from tuberculous disease in any of the bones related to the central nervous system (e.g. vertebrae).

Another mode of infection is from small haematogenous caseous lesions in the cortex which are secondary to active tuberculous disease elsewhere in the body. Such cortical foci

often contain abundant tubercle bacilli, and it has been suggested that such small foci are a commoner cause of tuberculous meningitis than direct haematogenous infection of the meninges. Another possible source of infection is miliary tubercles in the choroid plexus.

Tuberculous meningitis is most likely to occur in association with the primary complex and was, therefore, most frequently encountered formerly in young children in whom miliary spread had occurred. This preponderance is now rather less as the primary complex is no longer so restricted to this age group. The disease can also arise as a complication of adult fibrocaseous tuberculosis but miliary tuberculosis in the adult does not invariably lead to tuberculous meningitis.

Structural changes. When the bacilli reach the meninges they spread in the perivascular connective tissue of the arteries which become ensheathed in a cellular reaction in which tubercles develop as small grey nodules along the lines of the vessels. These tubercles are rounded aggregations of cells with central caseation (Fig. 20.23)

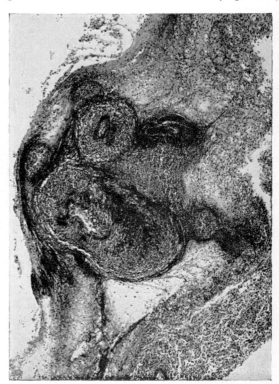

FIG. 20.23.—Tuberculous meningitis showing serofibrinous exudate in the subarachnoid space and cellular exudate, most abundant around vessels; caseation is beginning. × 48.

rather than typical follicles; endothelioid cells are poorly developed and giant cells are usually scanty or absent, except in subacute cases. There is a generalised inflammatory reaction in the pia-arachnoid, often with a fibrinous exudate (Fig. 20.24), containing at first many polymorphonuclear leukocytes, which are soon replaced by lymphocytes, monocytes and desquamated arachnoidal cells. Leukocyte emigration is abundant not only in the meninges but also around the nutrient twigs as they extend into the brain substance (Fig. 20.24). Necrosis and caseation affect also the unaggregated cells in the exudate, so that in certain areas both fibrin and cells are blended into a homogeneously eosinophilic mass. The presence of necrotic and caseous exudate on the wall of an artery causes a reactive endarteritis, which leads to great thickening of the intima and not infrequently actual occlusion; caseous necrosis of the wall may follow. A considerable amount of softening of the superficial grey matter is often present; this is the result in part of toxic action and in part of focal infarction from occlusion of the vessels. Obliterative endarteritis

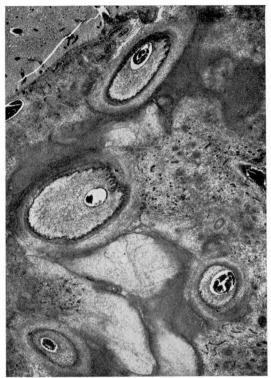

FIG. 20.25.—Cerebral arteries in chronic tuberculous meningitis, showing severe obliterative endarteritis. × 15.

is more marked in chronic cases and is very pronounced in cases in which antibiotics have prolonged life but failed to effect a cure (Fig. 20.25).

The exudate is usually greatest at the base of the brain. Occasionally, the meningitis is chiefly over the vertex, and may be asymmetrical; for example, there may be a local eruption of tubercles over one hemisphere (Fig. 20.26) perhaps representing spread from a local cortical focus.

Post-mortem appearances. The dura is usually tense, and the convolutions are markedly flattened and somewhat dry in appearance, as the result of raised intracranial pressure and hydrocephalus. The abundant exudate at the base of the brain obscures the optic chiasma, anterior surface of the pons, etc. The exudate may be soft and yellowish, with much fibrin, or the chief change may be more an inflammatory oedema with greyish opacity and thickening of the meninges. The ventricles are greatly distended with fluid which is often cloudy. Tubercles may often be found in the choroid plexuses and also in the lining of the ventricles.

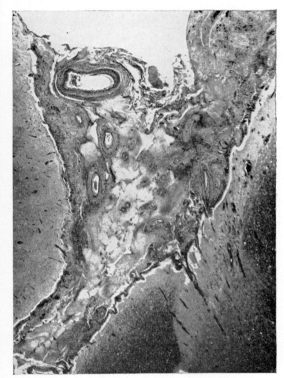

FIG. 20.24.—Tuberculous meningitis. Chiasmal cistern, showing soft fibrinous exudate filling the subarachnoid space, with cellular exudate in the walls of vessels. × 8.

Tubercles are most readily seen in the congested areas just beyond the exudate, especially between the frontal lobes and extending from the Sylvian fissure (Fig. 20.27). A hand lens greatly assists the search for them. In adults, the disease may run a relatively chronic course, the meninges

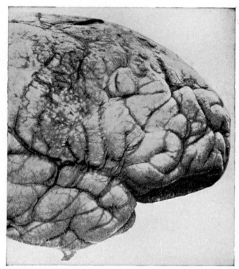

Fig. 20.26.—Tuberculous meningitis: localised eruption of tubercles on surface of hemisphere in region of Sylvian fissure. $\times \frac{2}{3}$.

being greyish, opaque and rather firm from fibroblastic proliferation, often with implication of the roof of the fourth ventricle. Tubercles may be found only with difficulty; in fact, occasionally the true nature of the case can be determined only by microscopic examination.

The spinal meninges are always affected, and the tubercles have the same characters as, and produce results similar to, those in the brain. Sometimes involvement is most marked in the cervical region, indicating a downward spread. But sometimes, as has been said, the cord is more affected than the brain, and the appearance of the lesions suggests that the spinal meninges have been primarily involved.

The cerebrospinal fluid. On lumbar puncture, in most cases of tuberculous meningitis, the cerebrospinal fluid is found to escape under increased pressure.

The cerebrospinal fluid in tuberculous meningitis as obtained by lumbar puncture is never turbid; often it is clear but it may have an opalescent appearance. A fine fibrin web may appear on standing. The number of cells is raised, often being 200 per c.mm. or even higher; the majority are lymphocytes as a rule,

with a small proportion of macrophages, but polymorphonuclears may be quite numerous and may occasionally exceed the lymphocytes, especially in the earliest stages. The polymorphonuclears often show signs of degeneration. The protein is increased but in variable amount, and the glucose and chlorides are diminished, the latter due to the persistent vomiting which reduces the general body chlorides. Tubercle bacilli can usually be found on microscopic examination of the centrifuged deposit or of the fibrin web which forms in the fluid. They may be scanty and difficult to find and, as they grow only slowly in culture, it is essential to treat immediately with the appropriate antibiotics all suspected cases in which the general picture is strongly suggestive of

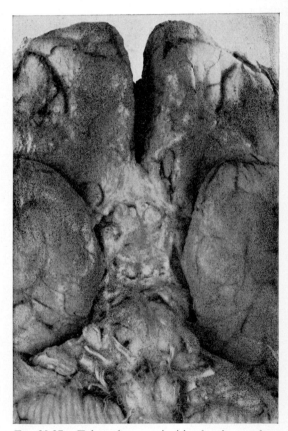

Fig. 20.27.—Tuberculous meningitis, showing exudate which obscures structures at base of brain.
A few tubercles can be seen on the frontal lobes. $\times 1$.

the diagnosis. Delay in instituting treatment may allow the pathological changes to progress to a point from which complete resolution and restoration to normal are impossible.

Metastatic *tuberculosis of the dura mater* is very rare. In tuberculous leptomeningitis, as a rule, the dura mater is quite unaffected. Secondary infection of the dura mater of the spinal cord from tuberculosis of the vertebrae is of common occurrence; in some cases the spinal cord is affected in a mechanical way by the angular curvature which takes place, but in others the dura may be infiltrated by tubercles which extend inwards, involving the leptomeninges and leading to tuberculous lesions of the cord.

Clinical features. The symptomatology of tuberculous meningitis varies greatly; the onset is usually gradual; occasionally it may be acute with neck retraction and rigidity, from liberation into the subarachnoid space of numerous bacilli. The inflammation at the base of the brain leads to implication of various cranial nerves, the oculomotor often being involved; thus ptosis and various forms of squint and other

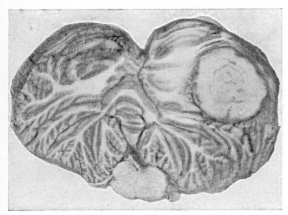

Fig. 20.28.—Tuberculoma in cerebellum.

paralyses are common early signs. The growth of tubercles in the cortex leads to irritation, and focal fits may result, whilst infarction of the cortex due to obliterative changes in vessels may lead to paralytic symptoms. Lastly, the accumulation of fluid in the ventricles produces the symptoms of raised intracranial pressure and ultimately coma.

Tuberculomas

The occurrence in the brain of masses known as tuberculomas is nowadays uncommon in Europe. They are, however, frequently seen in East Africa, India and South America where they can account for as many as 20 per cent of all intracranial expanding lesions. They are

often multiple, are encountered especially in young subjects, and their commonest sites are the cerebellum (Fig. 20.28), medulla, pons and mid-brain. Unlike gummas, they occur within the brain and are often 5–20 mm. in diameter, though they may exceed 5 cm. Their consistence is usually firm and they present a dull yellowish centre which is surrounded by a pinkish-grey capsule, though sometimes there may be a considerable degree of vascularity at the periphery. Calcification in such a mass is rare. Such nodules produce their effects partly by pressure and partly by destruction of nerve nuclei and tracts. In the region of the fourth ventricle or in the pons, they may cause interference with the flow of the cerebrospinal fluid, and thus give rise to hydrocephalus. Occasionally tuberculous meningitis follows. When the capsular tissue is very abundant, the tuberculous mass may resemble a glioma with some central necrosis.

Syphilis

Syphilitic lesions of the central nervous system were formerly both frequent and serious. They fall conveniently into two groups. The first includes lesions found in the late secondary and in the tertiary stages, which involve the ordinary connective tissues and the blood vessels; these comprise meningitis, gummas and endarteritis, and various combinations of these. In the second group are tabes dorsalis and general paralysis; these occur much later than the tertiary stage, and in them the nervous tissue is involved from the outset.

Syphilitic meningitis

At a relatively early period syphilitic meningitis may involve either the dura or the leptomeninges, or both. Syphilitic *leptomeningitis* is commonest at the base of the brain, where it causes a diffuse thickening of the meninges with, as a rule, superficial involvement of the brain substance. The affected meninges are swollen and gelatinous, with patches of necrosis, the condition being then known as *gummatous meningitis*. Various cranial nerves, especially the optic and oculomotor nerves, become implicated, and thus symptoms of irritation or paralysis result. The process may obstruct the foramina of the fourth ventricle and give rise to hydrocephalus.

Microscopic examination reveals proliferation of connective tissue cells accompanied by abundant infiltration of lymphocytes and plasma cells (Fig. 20.29); reactive endarteritis is a common accompaniment (Fig. 20.30). Cellular infiltration occurs round the small penetrating vessels and there is gliosis in the outer layers of the cortex. Syphilitic *pachymeningitis* occurs especially over the hemispheres and all stages of transition to gumma may be observed.

Corresponding lesions occur in the spinal cord and may affect a considerable part of the cord accompanied by some superficial gliosis. Arterial

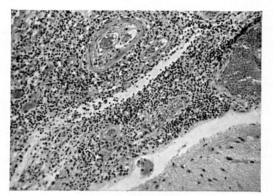

Fig. 20.29.—Syphilitic leptomeningitis. There is a lymphocytic infiltrate and endarteritis of the small vessels. × 100.

changes are prominent and infarction may follow from lack of blood supply (p. 654). The rare condition of *hypertrophic cervical pachymeningitis* is produced mainly by syphilis. In this condition the dura becomes markedly thickened, and generally adherent to the arachnoid. The leptomeninges also become thickened, a varying amount of gliosis occurs in the spinal cord, and the nerve roots may be compressed or invaded by the dense connective tissue and undergo atrophy.

Gummas occur in the meninges and are to be regarded as an extension and intensification of meningitis. Not infrequently they are multiple. When originating in the leptomeninges, they extend inwards and have a somewhat rounded or irregular shape; the central parts may be diffusely necrotic or multiple foci of necrosis may be present. Gummas originating in the dura are usually flattened and may cover a large part of a

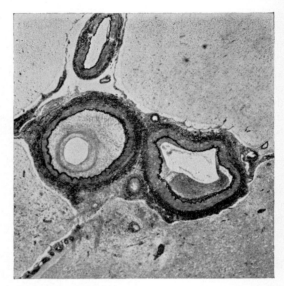

Fig. 20.30.—Syphilitic endarteritis of the anterior cerebral arteries. There is also a well-marked syphilitic meningitis. Multiple small softenings (infarcts) were present in both hemispheres. × 20.

hemisphere (Fig. 20.31). The meninges become adherent, and there may be superficial infarction of the brain, probably from endarteritis. A gumma growing from the outer aspect of the dura affects chiefly the bone, leading to erosion; or it may grow inwards and press on the brain.

The arterial changes are mainly an obliterative endarteritis usually accompanied by cellular infiltration in the perivascular tissue (Fig. 20.30). Great thickening of the intima occurs and sometimes actual obliteration, while thrombosis is a common result. These lesions are pronounced in the areas of syphilitic meningitis and in relation to gummas, but they may affect vessels in otherwise healthy areas. Small gummas

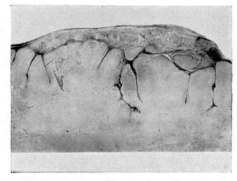

Fig. 20.31.—Section of hemisphere showing a large gummatous mass arising in the dura. × ½.

may occur along the lines of the small vessels and involve their walls—the so-called *gummatous arteritis*, the narrowing or thrombotic occlusion of the affected vessels then leading to infarction.

General paralysis of the insane (GPI)

This disease is a chronic encephalitis with very widespread lesions in the nervous system; the resulting symptoms are motor and sensory as well as psychiatric. Like locomotor ataxia it is a late or quaternary syphilitic condition, occurring some years after the period at which tertiary manifestations are encountered; it is much commoner in the male and it comprises about 10 per cent of all cases of neuro-syphilis (Biggart). Occasionally, as a sequel to congenital syphilis, it may appear about the age of ten or somewhat later. *Treponema pallidum* has been found in the brain even apart from the lesions, and is irregularly distributed, being present in some areas in large numbers, whereas in others it cannot be demonstrated. The Wassermann reaction is usually positive in both blood and CSF. The chief changes are degeneration of nerve cells and fibres, especially in the grey matter, reactive proliferation of the astroglia and leptomeninges and perivascular lymphocytic and plasma cell infiltration.

Structural changes. In an advanced stage of the disease the dura mater is usually abnormally adherent and somewhat thickened. There are often unilateral or bilateral chronic subdural haematomas. The arachnoid over the hemisphere shows thickening and opacity, while the sulci are widened and contain an excess of fluid; the subarachnoid space has a somewhat gelatinous character, but collapses as the fluid runs out. Sometimes the pia-arachnoid cannot be stripped from the surface of the convolutions in the normal way, and small portions of the grey matter are removed along with it, leaving a worm-eaten appearance on the surface of the convolutions particularly over the frontal lobes. The cerebral cortex is often narrow. The ventricles are enlarged and contain an excess of fluid, this being the result of cerebral atrophy. Not infrequently minute excrescences or granulations, composed of local proliferations of neuroglia, are present beneath the ependyma (Fig. 20.32). The floor of the fourth ventricle is a common site of these, the condition being termed

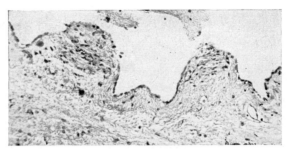

Fig. 20.32.—Granular ependymitis in the floor of the fourth ventricle. × 112.

granular ependymitis, but it is not peculiar to cerebral syphilis (see p. 608).

On *microscopic examination*, the cortical grey matter is much more cellular than the normal, owing chiefly to increase of neuroglial cells. The small nutrient vessels stand out more prominently, surrounded by lymphocytes and plasma cells. There is a general increase of glial fibres, whilst the astrocytes are much enlarged and branched, constituting the well-known "spider-cells". These cells are specially abundant in the superficial parts where, with the increased fibres, they constitute the sub-pial felting (Fig. 20.33). They are abundant also round the small vessels. The microglial cells also are enlarged and increased in number, and many

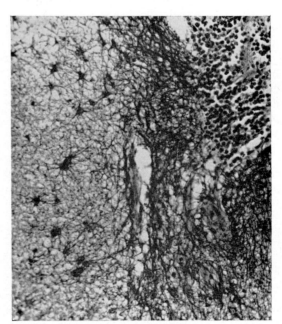

Fig. 20.33.—Cerebral cortex in general paralysis of the insane, showing giant astrocytes and subpial felting.
Note the syphilitic meningitis also present. × 230.

contain granules of iron pigment. The normal arrangement of nerve cells is disturbed, and many disappear; of those surviving, many show signs of damage. Gliosis may also be present in the subjacent white matter and in other parts of the brain. There may be degeneration in the spinal cord, a degree of lateral sclerosis being not uncommon, and occasionally the typical lesions of tabes dorsalis are superadded (see below), the combined disorder being known as *taboparesis*.

Clinical features. The resulting *symptoms* are very varied. Amongst the earliest are disturbances of mental function, alteration in disposition and in moral qualities, loss of memory and, especially, grandiose ideas. Ultimately there is dementia. These symptoms are related to the progressive changes in the neurones, there being interruption of the association fibres, degeneration and ultimately disappearance of the cells. Corresponding changes in the motor neurones lead to disturbances of finer movements; tremor of the lips and tongue, interference with articulation, inequality of the pupils, etc., are examples. General weakness of progressive nature develops, and minor convulsive seizures with loss of consciousness are common.

In more acute cases, degeneration and loss of nerve cells is less marked and neuroglial proliferation is noteworthy only under the pia. Perivascular infiltration with lymphocytes and plasma cells are the most conspicuous features.

In cases in which the disease has been arrested by treatment, e.g. by malarial pyrexia or by chemotherapy, the signs of active inflammation disappear and gliosis, both general and subpial, together with loss of nerve cells, indicate the previous damage.

In GPI there is usually an increase in the cell content of the CSF, the number of cells being 50 per c.mm. or more. They are chiefly lymphocytes, but small proportions of macrophages and plasma cells also are present. There is a considerable increase of the protein, the level of IgG is usually raised, and the fluid almost invariably gives a positive Wassermann reaction. The Lange colloidal gold test usually gives a paretic reaction (p. 652).

In *trypanosomiasis* or *sleeping sickness* changes somewhat similar to those of GPI, though of minor degree, are present in the nervous system. These are of proliferative type with lymphocytic infiltration in the meninges and superficial parts of the brain, in fact a mild meningo-encephalitis is present. In this disease the trypanosomes are found in the cerebrospinal fluid.

Tabes dorsalis or locomotor ataxia

This disease of the lower sensory neurones is characterised by degeneration of the posterior root fibres and their upward prolongations in the spinal cord, though there are changes in other parts of the nervous system also. *Tabes dorsalis*, like GPI, is a late result of syphilis. The Wassermann test is positive in both blood and cerebrospinal fluid in most cases, and when the symptoms of tabes appear, a previously negative Wassermann reaction may become positive, indicative of renewed activity of the syphilitic process. *Treponema pallidum* has been found in the cord in only a few instances. Occasionally tabes and GPI occur together, though one is usually more marked than the other.

Tabes is much commoner in men than in women (in a proportion of about 9 : 1), and usually a period of about ten years intervenes between the primary syphilitic infection and the appearance of symptoms, though both shorter and longer intervals are observed. Rarely, it has developed as a result of congenital syphilis, the symptoms then commencing in childhood—juvenile tabes. The disease usually starts in and affects the lower portion of the cord—the lumbar enlargement—and gradually fades off in an upward direction, so that the upper thoracic roots may be practically healthy. In a small proportion of cases, however, tabes affects chiefly the region of the cervical enlargement, where the posterior roots show the characteristic changes; such cases constitute the *cervical type* of tabes.

Structural changes. In the common type of tabes, the posterior columns in the lumbo-sacral region of the cord are somewhat shrunken and greyish; the pia-arachnoid over them is thickened. The posterior roots appear wasted and many have a distinctly grey tint contrasting with the white colour of the anterior roots, these changes gradually diminishing in the upper segments of the cord.

Microscopically, in sections of the lumbar enlargement of a severe case stained by the Weigert–Pal method, the posterior roots proximal to the ganglia exhibit considerable degeneration and loss of fibres, as indicated by the pale staining, and this degeneration becomes still more marked in the root fibres inside the cord. The posterior horns also lose myelinated fibres to a severe degree and thus appear pale (Fig. 20.34). The posterior columns show marked degeneration and gliosis, though there are usually a considerable number of non-degenerated fibres just behind the commissure; these represent endogenous or commissural fibres which are not affected. At higher levels it is found that the root fibres gradually become less affected, until ultimately they appear healthy. At this level the degenerated fibres of the posterior columns have become separated from the posterior horns by a layer of healthy fibres, which represent the root fibres which have entered the cord above the level of the actual disease. Thus, in the cervical region the changes

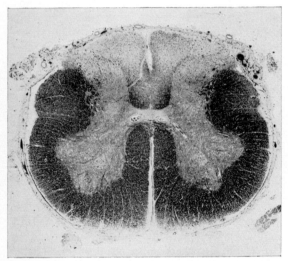

FIG. 20.34.—Tabes dorsalis: section through lumbar enlargement of cord, showing the degeneration in the posterior roots and dorsal columns. × 8.
(Weigert–Pal method.)

represent merely an ascending degeneration as the result of the disease at a lower level. In the *cervical form* of tabes the posterior roots show degeneration similar to that described, and the outer parts of the posterior columns are then chiefly involved. The degeneration in tabes does not extend higher than the nucleus gracilis and the nucleus cuneatus, that is, the upper terminations of the long fibres of the posterior columns.

The affected parts of the cord show the usual changes secondary to degeneration of nerve fibres. The neuroglia becomes thickened, as do also the walls of the small vessels, and corpora amylacea are often present in the sclerosed tissue. In the posterior root ganglia degenerative changes may be found in neurones. The thickened pia-arachnoid over the affected part of the cord is merely a secondary change.

Changes occur also in the sensory neurones in the higher parts of the central nervous system. Atrophy of the optic discs and optic nerves is common, as is also the Argyll–Robertson phenomenon, in which there is a loss of the light reflex while contraction of the pupils in accommodation is retained. Degenerative changes may be present also in the sensory cranial nerves and in their nuclei—the trigeminal, auditory, glossopharyngeal and vagus. Similar changes in the sympathetic system may explain the severe attacks of pain and sickness—the "gastric crises"—which are sometimes a marked feature of the disease, though the lesions of the vagi also may be concerned in their production.

Clinical features. These widespread lesions are necessarily attended by marked disturbances of sensory function. The afferent fibres first affected are chiefly those from the deeper structures, muscle sense being impaired early, loss of co-ordination and ataxia resulting. The sensation of pain, especially in the deeper structures, is affected before tactile sensation, though the latter also becomes impaired and paraesthesia is common. Severe shooting pains in the limbs—"lightning pains"—also occur, and there is often a "girdle sensation", or feeling of constriction, round the trunk at a level corresponding to the upper limit of the disease. The lesions in the posterior root fibres necessarily interrupt the reflex arc and accordingly the tendon reflexes disappear; absence of the knee-jerk is thus a well-recognised clinical sign.

The CSF shows fairly constant changes. The cells are increased, often to 50 per c.mm. or more; they are chiefly lymphocytes but large macrophages may be found. The protein is normal or slightly raised and there is usually an increase of globulin. The Lange colloidal gold test as a rule gives a luetic reaction, and the Wassermann reaction is usually positive (See Table, p. 652).

Other effects. In addition to interference with the sensory functions and irritation of the sensory nerves, various trophic disturbances are common. Thus in the skin, zoster and pemphigoid eruptions are encountered, and a fairly common lesion is a perforating ulcer which starts in the sole of the foot, passing deeply into the tissue, and is of a very intractable nature. Important lesions occur in the joints and bones constituting what is known as "Charcot's disease". The hip-joint and the knee-joint are those most commonly affected, though the ankle-joint and more rarely the joints of the upper extremities may be affected. Charcot's disease occasionally occurs in association with other diseases of the spinal cord and the pathological changes are described on p. 798.

The precise pathogenesis of the lesions of tabes is uncertain. Tabes occurs in only a small proportion of cases of long-standing syphilis, and we do not know what factors, in addition to the presence of syphilis, are important in determining the site of the lesions.

VIRUS INFECTIONS OF THE NERVOUS SYSTEM

It has already been explained that superficial encephalitis is an invariable accompaniment of acute bacterial meningitis and that bacteria can also cause suppurative encephalitis. In most cases of acute encephalitis, however, the causal agent is a *virus*. Many viruses can attack the nervous system: some are neurotropic, i.e. they show a marked tendency to invade the nervous system and to parasitise and destroy nerve cells, causing a true encephalitis or myelitis, e.g. the viruses of herpes simplex and anterior poliomyelitis. Others, often associated with a less severe clinical picture, cause a generalised meningitis and are accompanied by little more encephalitis than in acute bacterial meningitis: examples of the latter are the enteroviruses (polioviruses, echoviruses and Coxsackie viruses) and mumps virus.

The mode of access of viruses to the nervous system is not always clear. The virus enters the body either by ingestion, e.g. polioviruses and other enteroviruses; by inhalation, e.g. mumps; or by insect vectors from an animal reservoir, e.g. the viruses of St. Louis encephalitis and Russian spring–summer encephalomyelitis. Most viruses reach the nervous system by the blood stream but some neurotropic viruses, e.g. rabies, can also travel along nerve tracts, both those within the central nervous system and along peripheral and autonomic nerves. For example, the virus of equine encephalomyelitis, after experimental intra-ocular injection, constantly travels along the optic pathways to the contralateral visual cortex. Greenfield suggested that the more purely neurotropic viruses such as rabies may spread only along nerves whereas those with a more general tissue affinity may be conveyed either by the nerves or by the blood-stream. Within the central nervous system a neurotropic virus may quickly become general-ised, even in the absence of lesions, but this is clearly not by way of the cerebrospinal fluid, which rarely contains virus. Payling Wright has speculated that virus or toxin may be carried by the tissue fluid of the interneuronal spaces which show a certain alignment with the well-defined fibre tracts, the motive force for this fluid transport being provided by changes of pressure resulting from respiratory and other movements, from the propagation of the arterial pulse in the highly vascular neural tissue and perhaps from the pumping action engendered by rhythmic contractions of oligodendroglial cells.

There are at present a large number of infections of the nervous system from which specific viruses have been isolated. Some occur sporadically, others in epidemic form. In addition there are other forms of encephalitis with specific clinical and pathological features which are almost certainly viral in origin but the virus has not been isolated, e.g. encephalitis lethargica.

There is a certain similarity in the structural changes brought about in nervous tissue by viruses but fortunately the variation in distribution and intensity of the changes allows several types to be distinguished when the nervous system is examined *post mortem*.

General features of virus encephalitis

There may be no macroscopic abnormalities in the nervous system in a fatal case of acute virus encephalitis but in some varieties there may be congestion, swelling, softening, or focal haemorrhage in the more severely affected regions. If the patient lives for some time after the acute illness, the areas that have borne the brunt of the damage may be shrunken and cystic. In the acute stage the most prominent and widespread abnormality on microscopic examination is the presence of lymphocytes, large mononuclear cells and plasma cells in the meninges and around small vessels (often referred to as *perivascular cuffing*), in all parts of the brain and spinal cord. The next most characteristic feature is necrosis of nerve cells and neuronophagia, when the dead neurones become engulfed by hypertrophied microglia and other macrophages, and less commonly by polymorphonuclear leukocytes. In the more florid types of encephalitis, necrosis may not remain restricted to nerve cells but may spread to involve grey and white matter, e.g. in herpes simplex encephalitis. In certain forms of encephalitis, e.g. herpes simplex encephalitis and subacute sclerosing panencephalitis, intranuclear inclusion bodies may be found in neurones or astrocytes. Another feature of encephalitis is focal or diffuse hypertrophy and hyperplasia of microglial cells.

Examination of cerebrospinal fluid obtained by lumbar puncture often demonstrates some increase in pressure: in virus encephalitis there is characteristically an increase of leukocytes (50–200, usually lymphocytes, plasma cells and large mononuclear cells) and of protein (70–200 mg./100 ml.) whereas the sugar content is normal.

Acute demyelinating encephalomyelitis is an uncommon sequel to various acute virus infections (p. 647).

Acute anterior poliomyelitis

This is an acute inflammatory condition affecting chiefly, though not exclusively, the anterior horns of the spinal cord, and leading to destruction of the motor neurones, with corresponding paralysis and atrophy of the related muscles.

Epidemiology and virology. Before the introduction of poliovaccine, this was probably the commonest acute encephalomyelitis caused by a neurotropic virus. It may occur sporadically but also in both major and minor epidemics. Three strains of polio virus have been distinguished. Most cases of paralytic poliomyelitis are caused by type I virus: immunity to one type does not protect against the others. A similar paralytic illness may be caused by other enteroviruses.

Until comparatively recently poliomyelitis was a disease affecting, in urban communities, young children almost exclusively, whereas in sparsely populated rural areas there were proportionately more cases in older subjects. Recent observations have indicated that infection with the virus of poliomyelitis is much more prevalent than was formerly suspected. Most infections, however, are symptomless or cause a mild febrile illness. Only a few develop severe neurological lesions which may appear after a brief temporary remission of fever. There is good evidence that this recrudescence of infection may be determined by factors such as muscular fatigue during the initial stage of the illness or by local tissue damage, e.g. by intramuscular injections, such as those used in the immunisation of children by combined prophylactics, especially those containing alum. In developing countries with poor hygiene and living standards there is a high proportion of young children amongst the cases, since the majority of adults are immune as a result of previous non-paralytic and subclinical infections acquired during childhood. The rise in the proportion of adult cases in recent years is a reflection of improved hygiene, which has resulted in a greater number of people escaping infection in childhood and thus constituting an increased element at risk among the higher age groups. Adults are also more likely than children to develop paralysis when infected with poliovirus. This change in incidence has not been shared by more primitive communities.

In man the natural route of infection is by the mouth and the virus multiplies in the alimentary tract. It is often present in the nasopharyngeal secretions of a person suffering from the disease but is most readily isolated from the faeces, where it may persist for long after the disease has been overcome. There is an early viraemia and the infection reaches the central nervous system by crossing the blood–brain barrier. There is no longer any doubt that the principal natural mode of spread is by the faecal–oral route. Once infection has been established, the virus enters the blood from initial sites of multiplication in the lymphoid tissue of the gut.

Structural changes. The virus displays a remarkable predilection for the neurones in the ventral horns of the spinal cord (Fig. 20.35), especially in the lumbar and cervical enlargements, and these in an asymmetrical manner. On macroscopic examination in an acute case, there is little to be observed beyond congestion of the meninges over the affected part of the cord, and of the ventral horns with, in severe cases, some softening and haemorrhage.

Microscopic examination reveals an extensive inflammatory infiltration of the leptomeninges, with lymphocytes, plasma cells, and some poly-

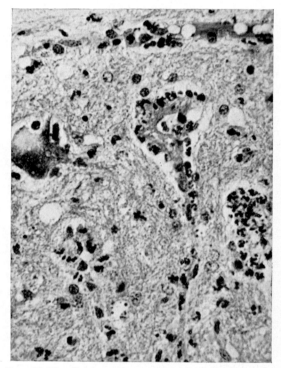

FIG. 20.35.—Section of ventral horn in acute experimental poliomyelitis in the monkey. Destruction of nerve cells, infiltration by neutrophil polymorphs and intense neuronophagia are seen. × 400.

(From a preparation kindly lent by Dr. Weston Hurst.)

morphonuclear leukocytes, but no fibrin. The infiltrate extends along the nutrient vessels, especially the anterior spinal arteries and their branches (Fig. 20.36).

In the anterior horns, where inflammation is usually most marked in the medially placed cell groups, there is much congestion and oedema along with the cellular infiltration; some of the minute vessels may be thrombosed and small capillary haemorrhages are not uncommon. The nerve cells are affected in varying degree. Some undergo acute necrosis, and disappear by the action of phagocytes—neuronophagia (Fig. 20.37). If the nerve cell dies, disintegration of its axon and myelin sheath follows. Other nerve cells show varying degrees of chromatolysis,

though it is remarkable how little altered some of them are, even when surrounded by inflammatory change. There may be little change in the adjacent white matter beyond perivascular leukocytic infiltration. Cell damage extends upwards and downwards in the grey matter, so that this may be seriously involved through several segments above and below the site of maximum injury. In very intense cases, necrosis rather than leukocytic infiltration may be the main feature.

The lesions are usually much more widespread in the nervous system than might be thought on the basis of clinical signs, and the neurones of the reticular formation of the medulla are probably always involved; this may in part account for the spasm of many non-paralysed muscles. Sometimes the virus affects severely the motor

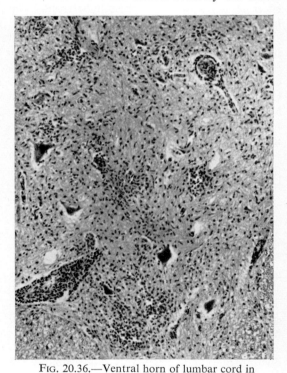

FIG. 20.36.—Ventral horn of lumbar cord in poliomyelitis fatal on the 5th day.

Note the perivascular cuffing, the general inflammatory infiltration and neuronophagia of dead nerve cells.

nuclei in the medulla, causing acute bulbar paralysis. There are also lesions in the cerebral cortex, characteristically localised to the motor and pre-motor areas, but there is no generalised involvement of the cortex as in other types of virus encephalitis; the distribution of the lesions is thus quite distinctive.

Effects. The more acute changes usually pass off in a few days, but the infiltrate of lymphocytes and plasma cells may persist for some months. Many of the motor neurones which are only partially damaged recover; accordingly, considerable diminution in the amount of the paralysis may occur at a later stage. The destructive lesions in the cord are followed by absorption of the degenerated material and by proliferation of the neuroglial cells, with subsequent gliosis. Gradually the affected parts

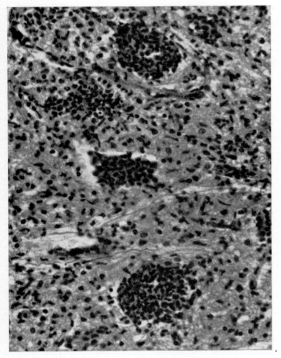

FIG. 20.37.—Ventral horn of lumbar cord in acute poliomyelitis (5th day). × 230.

Note nerve cell destruction with intense neuronophagia.

shrink, and if the lesion has been a severe one, a distinct difference between the two anterior horns may be distinguished, even with the naked eye; the anterior nerve roots also become wasted. Sharrard's work on the structure of the motor cell columns supplying the various muscles of the limbs has revealed a striking quantitative correlation between the length of the motor cell column and the chance of residual paralysis. Those muscles supplied by a short motor nucleus (e.g. tibialis anterior = 8 mm.) are much more often paralysed than paretic, whereas those with a long motor nucleus (e.g.

quadriceps femoris = 20 mm.) are more likely to be paretic than paralysed.

In view of the lesions described above, the effects on the peripheral nerves and muscles can be readily understood. There is a rapid onset of paralysis in the related muscles, though this, as already explained, may in part pass off. Wallerian degeneration occurs in the axons of the destroyed neurones and the anterior nerve roots become wasted and grey. The permanently affected muscle fibres soon give the reactions of degeneration and undergo rapid wasting, the classical histological feature being bundles of atrophied muscle fibres among fibres of normal size (Fig. 22.69, p. 808). Owing to the unopposed action of the unaffected muscles, deformities of the limbs, including various forms of club-foot, etc., are brought about. The bones in the affected limbs may show atrophy, being reduced both in thickness and in density (Fig. 1.32. p. 28).

In the cerebrospinal fluid there is usually at first a marked increase of cells, sometimes exceeding 500 per c.mm.; as a rule the majority are polymorphonuclears and the percentage of these may be very high. Later, there is a gradual fall in the number of cells, the polymorphonuclears usually disappearing rapidly, so that lymphocytes predominate. The protein at first is little changed, but afterwards there is a considerable increase to between 100 and 200 mg./100 ml. and there may be the formation of a fine fibrin web. The sugar remains normal throughout the disease (see Table, p. 652).

Zoster

This is a disease of adults, due to the same virus that causes varicella. During the illness there is often a rise in the antibody titre against the virus to levels above those commonly seen in varicella. Epidemiologically the diseases are related, for adults with zoster sometimes infect susceptible children, typical varicella resulting. The reverse, however, does not occur, and it is now believed that zoster is the result of recrudescence of a latent infection with varicella virus in a partially immune subject. In its ordinary form zoster results from an acute inflammatory lesion of a posterior root ganglion, especially those in relation to the nerves which supply white rami to the sympathetic ganglia; in one type of zoster the Gasserian ganglion is affected. Along the course of the nerve related to the affected ganglion, pain and hyperalgesia occur and are followed by erythema and the formation of vesicles which contain a serous fluid, sometimes with admixture of blood. The lesion of the posterior root ganglion is an acute inflammation, accompanied by infiltration of lymphocytes which may form dense aggregations, and by haemorrhage, while the nerve cells are injured in varying degree; inflammatory change is present also in the capsule of an affected ganglion (Fig. 20.38). Sometimes the lesion is mainly in one focus, usually towards the dorsal aspect of the ganglion, the substance of which may be largely destroyed; sometimes there are multiple small foci. Many of the nerve cells involved in the lesions undergo necrosis and are afterwards destroyed, whilst in other parts

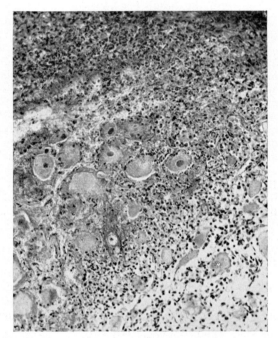

FIG. 20.38.—Section of posterior root ganglion in zoster, showing inflammatory infiltration and destruction of nerve cells. × 160.

they are practically unaffected. The inflammatory process may extend into the spinal cord at the level of the affected ganglion, and may be restricted to the same side of the cord. Central chromatolysis in anterior horn neurones is not uncommon.

As a result of the damage to the nerve cells, secondary degeneration shown by Marchi's method can be traced along the nerve fibres to their peripheral distribution, and also backwards through the posterior nerve roots and for a distance upwards in the posterior columns of the cord. At a later period secondary fibrosis occurs in the various structures which have been damaged. A zoster eruption of similar distribution is sometimes observed in chronic disease of the spinal cord, for example, tabes dorsalis or myelitis. It may be produced also by the spread of inflammatory change to a ganglion from a lesion in the neighbourhood, e.g. caries of a rib, and has been found to follow neoplastic invasion of a ganglion, leukaemia or Hodgkin's disease, all of which may act by stimulating a latent virus to renewed activity.

Rabies or hydrophobia

In this disease, changes like those in encephalitis lethargica but of less degree occur in the nervous system. The virus passes along the nerves from the primary lesion, usually a bite of a rabid dog or, in the West Indies, of a vampire bat, to the central nervous system. The histological changes, which are specially marked in the nuclei of the medulla, though occurring also in other parts, consist of capillary congestion with small haemorrhages, chromatolysis and other degenerative changes in the nerve cells, and a certain amount of perivascular lymphocytic infiltration. There is nothing characteristic in the histological picture and recognition of the nature of the disease rests largely upon the detection of peculiar structures called "Negri bodies" within the cytoplasm of nerve cells and their processes. Although found in all parts of the brain they are specially abundant in the cells of the hippocampus and in the Purkinje cells of the cerebellum, and can be readily found in histological sections or smear preparations from these areas. They vary greatly in size, measuring $0.5–25\mu$, and are rounded, oval or somewhat angular in form. They are composed of a homogeneous substance in which small round or oval bodies or granulations are present. In preparations stained by Giemsa's method or by eosin-methylene-blue, the bodies are coloured in varying tints but have on the whole an affinity for eosin. The nerve cells affected may otherwise appear comparatively healthy. Opinion still varies regarding the nature of the Negri bodies. One view is that they represent products of reaction or of degeneration around the virus within the nerve cells. Another is that they really consist of masses or aggregates of minute elementary bodies representing the virus. The important practical point is that they are specific to the "street" or fully virulent virus of rabies.

Herpes simplex encephalitis

This is a fulminating and often rapidly fatal type of encephalitis known also as *acute necrotising encephalitis* (ANE). There can be little doubt from serological studies that herpes simplex virus may also cause milder types of encephalitis but little is known about the pathology in such cases as they usually survive. The most characteristic feature of ANE is selective, bilateral but asymmetrical involvement of the temporal lobes. In a fatal acute case

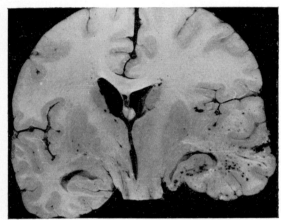

Fig. 20.39.—Acute necrotising encephalitis due to Herpes simplex virus. Within the swollen right temporal lobe there are many small haemorrhagic foci.

there is usually flattening of the convolutions and raised intracranial pressure, while the more severely affected temporal lobe is soft, swollen and often focally haemorrhagic (Fig. 20.39). There is often also an ipsilateral tentorial hernia (see p. 609). Necrosis usually occurs also in the insulae and in the cingulate gyri. Microscopic examination shows diffuse infiltration of the meninges and perivascular spaces by lymphocytes and plasma cells: where necrosis has occurred, plasma cells stream out from the perivascular spaces into the brain tissue. In the temporal lobes there is total necrosis of the cortex and the adjacent white matter and there are varying degrees of microglial hyperplasia. In the

cortex adjacent to the zones of necrosis, intranuclear inclusion bodies may be found within astrocytes in a proportion of cases. Neuronophagia is distributed widely throughout the brain and spinal cord. The diagnosis of herpes simplex encephalitis rests on the isolation of virus from brain tissue obtained either *post mortem* or from a brain biopsy taken through a burr-hole in the skull, or by demonstrating a rise in titre (at least fourfold) of complement-fixing antibodies to herpes simplex virus in the serum. Virus cannot usually be isolated from the cerebrospinal fluid. If the patient survives the acute phase, the necrotic tissue becomes shrunken and cystic.

Herpes simplex encephalitis may also occur in infants as part of an acute generalised infection.

Encephalitis lethargica

Between 1916 and 1926, this serious form of encephalitis, known also as epidemic encephalitis, occurred in various parts of the world, but it has since disappeared. The mode of infection was never established but its features were strongly suggestive of a virus origin.

Clinical features. The symptoms were those of a general affection of the brain—headache, pyrexia, drowsiness and delirium; there was usually a general weakness of muscular power, with marked disturbance of sleep rhythm and extreme lethargy by day, hence the name originally applied. In addition, there were local symptoms due to implication of the oculomotor, facial and other nerves, and sometimes there was nystagmus. The mortality varied in different epidemics, but averaged about 25 per cent. Amongst a high proportion of the non-fatal cases, however, a more or less permanent residual neurological syndrome occurred, including tremor, rigidity and loss of associated movements; this is described as of the Parkinsonian type because of its resemblance to *paralysis agitans* which was first described by Parkinson. Immobile facial expression, excessive salivation and emotional disturbances of various kinds occur and, especially in children, a loss of inhibitions with a tendency to violent actions.

Structural changes. *Post mortem*, in the acute stage, there is usually marked congestion of the leptomeninges, especially over the pons and medulla and the base of the brain, and occasionally minute haemorrhages are present. Intense congestion is found throughout the brain stem, basal ganglia and cortex, and minute haemorrhages and even points of softening may be present in the floor of the fourth ventricle. In some cases the naked-eye changes may be minimal, especially at a later period of the disease.

Microscopic examination shows the features typical of encephalitis. In severe acute cases, damage to vessels and nerve cells is the outstanding feature as shown by intense congestion, haemorrhages both into the perivascular sheaths and adjacent tissues, and sometimes by actual thrombosis: occasionally part of a vessel wall may appear swollen and hyaline. Many nerve cells show chromatolysis and other signs of acute degeneration, but neuronophagia is slight; nevertheless many nerve cells are destroyed. Perivascular cuffing by leukocytes, chiefly lymphocytes along with a few plasma cells, develops rapidly and becomes the most prominent

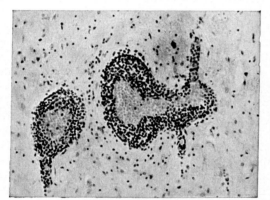

FIG. 20.40.—Section of posterior part of medulla in encephalitis lethargica, showing the extensive perivascular infiltration by lymphocytes and plasma cells. × 170.

feature in less acute cases (Fig. 20.40). Infiltration of similar cells occurs in the meninges. These abnormalities are usually most pronounced in the brain stem.

The cerebrospinal fluid may be quite normal but usually there is a lymphocytosis of 10–100 or even more cells per c.mm. This is not usually accompanied by any distinct change in the total protein or in the globulin—an example of the so-called cell-protein dissociation. The Lange colloidal gold test as a rule gives some reaction, usually a curve of the luetic type but sometimes of the paretic type (Greenfield) (see Table, p. 652).

The histological changes of *post-encephalitic Parkinsonism* are chiefly centred in the substantia nigra in the cerebral peduncles. A considerable proportion of the nerve cells have disappeared, with degenerative changes in some of those surviving; increase of astroglia with new formation of vessels and perivascular infiltration of leukocytes may be present. The changes suggest that they are not merely the result of damage done in the acute stage but that they are due to a persistence of the virus in the tissue of the brain. The lesions in the substantia nigra may interrupt fibres from the globus pallidus which pass directly or through other centres to the lower motor neurones in the spinal cord. The resulting loss of the inhibiting and controlling influence on movement causes the rigidity which is a characteristic feature of the late disease.

Encephalitis lethargica was the first pandemic encephalitis in modern times and its sudden appearance, rapid pandemic spread and subsequent disappearance are not its least mysterious features. It is generally accepted that it is a virus infection but proof is lacking, all attempts to transmit the disease to animals having failed. The few positive results reported appear to have been due to contamination with the virus of herpes simplex, which is a very common latent virus in man and is pathogenic for many lower animals. Herpetic encephalitis, however, presents different features (see p. 643).

Cytomegalic inclusion-body disease

Infants suffering from generalised infection acquired *in utero* with cytomegalovirus may show microcephaly. Cerebral involvement is common in infected infants, with lesions in the brain, chiefly ependymal and periventricular. In cases surviving the neonatal period such lesions may be responsible for some examples of hydrocephalus and cerebral calcification.

Subacute sclerosing panencephalitis

First described in children by Dawson in 1933, this variety of subacute encephalitis is known to be of world wide distribution: it is characterised by numerous large inclusion bodies within cortical nerve cells in addition to the usual cellular infiltrate of encephalitis. The subacute sclerosing leuko-encephalitis described by Van Bogaert is now generally accepted as a variant of the same disease.

The causal agent is the measles virus, and the titre of complement-fixing antibody to this virus is always high in the serum and usually in the CSF. Measles virus has recently been isolated from the brain in cases of the disease. The disease affects children and adolescents, has an insidious onset and is characterised by progressive mental deterioration proceeding to coma and death within weeks or months. A paretic colloidal gold curve has been observed in the CSF in most cases. *Post mortem* the brain may appear to be normal but is, in fact, the seat of extensive perivascular infiltration of lymphocytes in both grey and white matter. Degeneration of neurones, some of which may contain intranuclear inclusion bodies, and intense gliosis in the white matter in the absence of conspicuous demyelination, are characteristic features. The importance of establishing the diagnosis is that it is a cause of progressive mental deterioration in young people which is neither familial nor genetically determined.

Other virus diseases

Several other forms of encephalitis have been proved to be due to infection of the nervous system by viruses, some of which also cause infections in animals, from which they may be conveyed to man by insect vectors. Many of these present pathological features very similar to those of encephalitis lethargica. A brief mention of the chief of these disorders follows—

In *St. Louis encephalitis*, called after the place of its occurrence in 1933, the meningeal reaction is pronounced and inflammatory foci are abundant in the cortex and in the spinal cord with severe neuronal destruction. It has a high mortality, affecting chiefly adults but also children, and the latter on recovery may be mentally retarded and show hydrocephalus. It is readily transmissible to monkeys and to mice and is probably spread by mosquitoes in the late summer. The virus is distinct from that of other infections. *Eastern and Western equine encephalomyelitis, Murray Valley Fever and Japanese B encephalitis* are other forms of meningo-encephalitis which present similar pathological features, and the virus of the latter two may be identical. *Louping-ill* is a virus encephalitis of sheep transmitted by the tick, *Ixodes ricinus*: occasionally the virus infects man, chiefly laboratory workers handling infected materials, and it is related to that of *Russian Spring–Summer encephalitis*.

Acute viral meningitis. A number of viruses are capable of causing acute meningitis. In the United Kingdom, mumps virus and enteroviruses are most commonly responsible, less frequently other viruses, including that responsible for infectious mononucleosis (p. 458). In parts of Africa and America, the arboviruses are an important cause. The condition chiefly affects children and is usually mild. It is characterised by infiltration of the meninges, ependyma and choroid plexuses with lymphocytes, and there is mild encephalitis. There may be various symptoms of spinal irritation, such as nuchal rigidity; there may also be some pyrexia. The cerebrospinal fluid is under increased pressure and contains a greatly increased number of lymphocytes with slight increase of protein.

One type of acute virus meningitis, termed *lymphocytic chorio-meningitis*, is rare but of great interest. The infection has been transmitted to monkeys and mice and can be maintained in them indefinitely in series, the latter species being the natural host. Immunological reactions show that it is distinct from other virus infections. The mode of transmission to man is unknown. In infected colonies, the young mice harbour the virus, but develop neither antibodies nor the disease. If non-infected mice are placed in such a colony, or are inoculated with the virus, they develop lymphocytic chorio-meningitis and also antibodies and delayed hypersensitivity to the virus. These observations suggest that (1) mice infected with virus during fetal life develop immunological tolerance to it, and in this situation the virus is harmless; (2) in mice infected later in life, the disease follows the development of an immunological response to the virus. Further studies have lent strong support to these suggestions, and there is now good evidence that the chorio-meningitis is mediated by a delayed hypersensitivity reaction to the virus. There is evidence also that mice infected *in utero* may, in later life, gradually lose their tolerance: they then develop glomerular lesions due to deposition of virus-antibody complex, i.e. immune complex disease (see p. 697).

Other virus infections of the central nervous system (*q.v.*) and also leptospirosis may sometimes cause a similar form of meningitis.

Other forms of encephalitis

Toxoplasmosis. The protozoon *Toxoplasma gondii* (Fig. 20.41) is a not very rare cause of infection within the central nervous system of the newborn and occasionally of older children. Infection is acquired *in utero* and results in meningitis and a granulomatous encephalitis sometimes with actual necrosis (Fig. 20.42) and choroido-retinitis. Infants surviving the neonatal period may develop hydrocephalus, and some of the granulomas may heal with calcification. Serological tests indicate that toxoplasma infection may be a more common cause of blindness than has been generally realised.

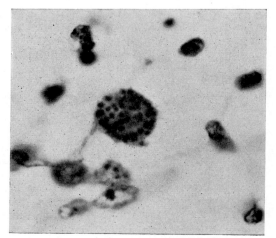

Fig. 20.41.—Congenital toxoplasmosis.

A large central pseudocyst containing many parasites: a few also in the cell below (from same case as 20.42). × 900.

Rickettsial encephalitis. In fatal cases of epidemic *typhus fever* and in scrub typhus, focal typhus nodules are usually present in the brain and are similar to those elsewhere in the body. They are commonest in the medulla and pons but are also widely distributed especially in the cortical grey matter, and are the result of the *Rickettsia* settling in the capillary endothelium. Thrombosis within the affected capillaries and endothelial proliferation then occur, while around there is an active enlargement and proliferation of the microglial cells. Polymorphonuclear leukocytes and other cells also take part in the reaction. The result is the formation of a minute tubercle-like, cellular nodule. Nerve cells in the vicinity may be involved and be destroyed by phagocytes. These focal lesions are often very numerous and no doubt play an important part in producing cerebral symptoms and in leading to death. A severe meningeal reaction with mononuclear cell exudate is often present.

Kuru. This is a subacute progressive, invariably fatal disease of the central nervous system restricted to the Fore-speaking people of the Eastern Highlands of New Guinea. The disease runs its course in about one year and is characterised clinically by progressive ataxia of gait, tremor and dysarthria, leading ultimately to complete paralysis. Histological examination shows loss of Purkinje and granule cells,

and reactive gliosis in the cerebellum; degenerative and reactive changes are seen also in the brain stem and spinal cord, particularly in the corticospinal and spinocerebellar tracts. There are also widespread changes in the cerebral hemispheres as shown by the occurrence of spongy (i.e. coarsely vacuolated) degeneration in the cortex and basal ganglia.

What is of particular interest about kuru is not only that it is restricted to a particular tribe but that a similar disease has been transmitted to the chimpanzee by injecting brain tissue from human cases. The incubation period in the chimpanzee is about two years. With serial passage to a second chimpanzee, the incubation period is reduced to about one year. Thus kuru appears to be caused by a transmissible replicating agent and is now classed as a *slow virus disease* of the central nervous system. There is, however, clearly also a genetic predisposition to kuru among the Fore people as the disease has not spread to adjacent tribes. Much remains to be learnt about kuru, but it has been suggested, in view of the epidemiological pattern, that cannibalism has contributed to the transmission of the replicating agent.

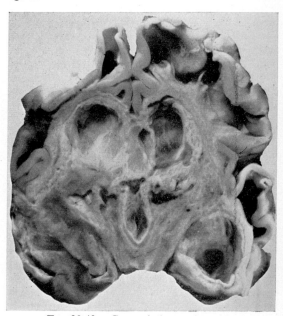

Fig. 20.42.—Congenital toxoplasmosis.

Coronal section of brain of a 2 months' old infant. Note enlarged ventricles with necrotic lining, and extensive cystic and gelatinous degeneration of hemispheres.

DEMYELINATING DISEASES

This is a convenient term to bring together a number of disorders characterised by loss of myelin unrelated to specific fibre systems or particular arterial territories. The group includes *acute* conditions associated with considerable cellular exudation, and *chronic* disorders, in which there is conspicuous fibrillary gliosis in the demyelinated areas, but forms intermediate in both clinical and pathological features are not very rare. Examples of the chronic type are *multiple* or *disseminated sclerosis*, where the lesions are focal and not specially perivascular, and *diffuse cerebral sclerosis* where the process is more generalised but may affect certain areas of the brain more severely than others. In the acute disorders the demyelination is usually strikingly perivascular and may develop with astonishing rapidity as in *acute disseminated encephalomyelitis*, which usually occurs as a complication of an acute virus infection, or in *acute haemorrhagic leukoencephalitis*, a condition in which the etiology is still completely unknown.

An acute demyelinating encephalomyelitis (experimental allergic encephalomyelitis, or EAE) is readily produced in animals by injection of homogenised neural tissue emulsified in Freund's adjuvant. The disease develops after a latent period of 10 days or more, and is believed to be due to the development of an immune response to neural tissue antigen in the inoculum and a subsequent immunological reaction with the animal's own neural tissue. EAE has been very extensively investigated in guinea pigs, rats, mice, rabbits and several other species. The antigen is a basic protein and is common to neural tissue of many species. The presence of antibody in the serum does not correlate well with the occurrence of the disease, and there is strong evidence to suggest that the lesions result from a delayed hypersensitivity reaction in which sensitised lymphocytes and possibly macrophages react directly with neural tissue. However, there is also evidence suggesting that early changes in the CNS precede the infiltration of lymphocytes and macrophages, and the pathogenic mechanism is not completely understood.

The changes of EAE vary somewhat depending on the experimental detail and the animal species. Typically, acute demyelination, inflammatory oedema and cell infiltration occur around venules in the brain and cord. In the guinea-pig, cellular infiltration is pronounced and demyelination slight. The changes in some experimental species are similar to acute demyelinating encephalomyelitis in man, and the normal incubation period of 10 days or so between the predisposing virus infection and the onset of neural changes suggests that an immunological process may be involved. Although EAE can be induced by one injection of antigen in Freund's adjuvant, its production in monkeys without use of Freund's adjuvant requires many injections, and it is very likely that the acute demyelinating encephalitis which occurs in man as a complication of vaccination against rabies is the equivalent of EAE and results from the repeated injection of the rabbit spinal cord preparation used for the prophylactic injections.

Acute disseminated encephalomyelitis

This disease, known also as *post-infectious encephalitis* or *acute perivascular myelinoclasis* because of the rapid occurrence of perivascular demyelination, occurs as a sequel to various acute virus diseases such as measles, rubella, or varicella, to certain presumably viral respiratory infections, or to primary vaccination (*post-vaccinial encephalitis*) or anti-rabic inoculation. The definitive pathological features of the disease were described by Turnbull and McIntosh in 1926 in a study of seven fatal cases of *post-vaccinial encephalitis* from one of which vaccinia virus was recovered, but it became apparent soon thereafter that similar pathological changes were present in the acute encephalitis complicating other virus diseases. Post-vaccinial encephalitis occurs mainly in older children and adults, about ten days after primary vaccination.

The focal lesions in the nervous system are mainly around small venules throughout the brain and spinal cord (Fig. 20.43) but often affecting the ventral half of the pons, the deeper layers of the cerebral cortex, the thalamus and the white matter of the cerebral hemispheres with particular severity. The characteristic histological features are a conspicuous excess of cells around venules (Fig. 20.44) comprised mainly of lymphocytes and macrophages in addition to occasional plasma cells, and perivenular loss of myelin (Fig. 20.45). This demyelination takes place with great rapidity, being sometimes almost complete within four days, and is in marked contrast to the much slower destruction of myelin occurring in Wallerian degeneration. Axons show only slight damage, nerve cells adjacent to the perivascular demyelination may show mild degenerative changes and there may be a slight increase of mononuclear cells in the leptomeninges. The lesions are therefore quite different, both in character and distribution, from those of acute viral encephalitis due to the presence of any known virus in the central nervous system.

The pathogenesis of the disease is not clear. The view that it is due to infection of the nervous system by the vaccinia virus is no longer tenable

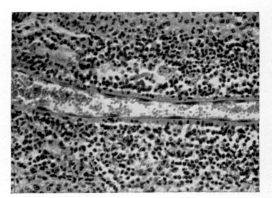

FIG. 20.44.—Acute disseminated encephalomyelitis following measles. Perivascular inflammatory and macrophage reaction. × 125.

lymphocytes, and possibly free antibody, react with the neural tissue to bring about the lesions.

Acute haemorrhagic leukoencephalitis

This relatively uncommon disease may also occur as a sequel to any one of several possible viral infections but it may have its onset during apparently perfect health. It frequently has a rapid, fulminating course, death occurring within a few days. *Post mortem* the brain is swollen and congested and there are numerous petechial haemorrhages restricted almost entirely to the white matter, the naked-eye appearances being very similar to those observed in cerebral fat embolism.

Histological examination shows varying degrees of necrosis of the walls of venules and arterioles, perivascular haemorrhage and de-

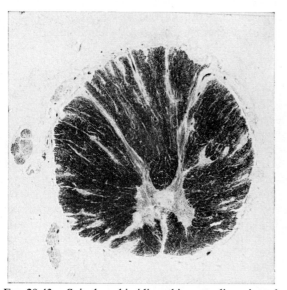

FIG. 20.43.—Spinal cord in idiopathic acute disseminated encephalomyelitis. There is pronounced perivascular demyelination. Around the vessels there was marked inflammatory cellular infiltration. × 7·5.

as precisely similar pathological changes occur after other virus infections. The suggestion that the disease might be caused by activation of some latent neurotropic virus has never been substantiated. It is now generally accepted that acute disseminated encephalomyelitis represents an immunological reaction in the CNS: from the similarity of experimental allergic encephalomyelitis (p. 647), it seems likely that the predisposing virus infection leads to the development of an immune response against neural tissue antigen, and that the resulting sensitised

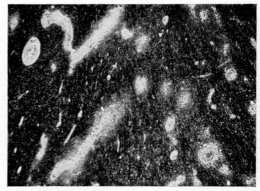

FIG. 20.45.—Acute disseminated encephalomyelitis following measles, showing widespread perivascular demyelination.
(Loyez method for myelin) × 15.

myelination often with an exudate first of polymorphonuclears and later of mononuclear cells, cerebral oedema and an inflammatory exudate in the leptomeninges. The grey matter is usually spared. The disease, therefore, has several features in common with acute disseminated encephalomyelitis but although some consider that acute haemorrhagic leukoencephalitis is simply a particularly acute form of this disease, the different distribution of the focal lesions suggests that the pathogenesis may not be the same.

Multiple or disseminated sclerosis

This disease is characterised by the presence of patches (usually referred to as *plaques*) of demyelination and gliosis in the central nervous system. It occurs most frequently in early adult life, though cases are encountered at an earlier and later period. The disease characteristically follows an episodic course, periods of partial remission alternating with acute exacerbations, but in the later stages it tends to become relentlessly progressive. Less frequently it is of steadily progressive character from its onset. A common early symptom is an acute unilateral optic neuritis which progresses to some degree of optic atrophy.

Structural changes. The abnormal plaques are scattered in an irregular manner throughout the spinal cord and brain. The plaques are typically grey and rather translucent in appearance, in marked contrast to the normal white matter from which they are usually sharply circumscribed. They vary in consistency, being sometimes firmer and sometimes less firm than the normal tissue. As there is little or no contraction, the configuration of the affected parts is well preserved. Smaller lesions are usually spherical or oval but larger plaques often have an irregular shape which may result either from the confluence of several small plaques or from extension of a previously smaller lesion. Recent lesions are often yellowish and rather soft, and in the more acute cases, may constitute a large proportion of the lesions. Plaques vary greatly in size and number in individual cases. They are usually most easily seen in the white matter of the cerebral hemispheres, particularly at the angles of the lateral ventricles and at the junction of the cortex with the white matter; but they

may be seen also within the cortex and central grey matter. They are also common in the brain stem, particularly around the aqueduct and adjacent to the fourth ventricle (Fig. 20.46), and in the spinal cord. If there is a history of retrobulbar neuritis, a plaque can usually be found in the optic nerve and they have been observed also in other cranial and spinal nerve roots.

In sections stained by the Weigert–Pal method, the most striking feature is the complete disappearance of myelin from the affected areas and the sharp line of demarcation from the adjacent healthy tissue; on one side of the line the myelin stains normally, on the other side it has quite disappeared (Fig. 20.47). In older

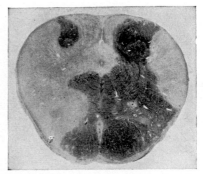

Fig. 20.46.—Multiple sclerosis. Section through lower part of medulla. × 3.

The demyelinated plaques appear pale. (Weigert–Pal method).

plaques there is a great increase in glial fibres and the vessel walls are thickened, but they often appear less cellular than the surrounding tissue owing to loss of oligodendrocytes. In contrast, recent plaques contain a great excess of cells; some are lipid-containing macrophages, others are perivascular lymphocytes and plasma cells. At this stage demyelination may be less sharply demarcated than in older lesions. Although the myelin sheaths are so extensively destroyed, many of the axis cylinders persist and continue to transmit impulses for a long period. Later, however, there may be much destruction of axis cylinders, especially in the spinal cord, with consequent Wallerian degeneration in the distal part of the axon. Nerve cells, in general, show little abnormality even when included in a plaque.

The *cerebrospinal fluid* in multiple sclerosis may at times contain a slight excess of lymphocytes, and there may also be increase of protein; but these changes are often absent. Lange's colloidal gold test gives a *"paretic" reaction* in about one third of cases, rather more give atypical curves. The Wassermann reaction, however, is negative. In the absence of spinal block, a paretic reaction in association with a negative Wassermann reaction is generally accepted as pathognomonic of multiple sclerosis (see Table, p. 652). The level of IgG in the CSF is usually raised, particularly when the disease is active.

Etiology and pathogenesis. It is generally accepted that the primary lesion is destruction of myelin and that microglial hypertrophy and phagocytosis of lipid in the early stages and overgrowth of the astroglia in the later stages, are

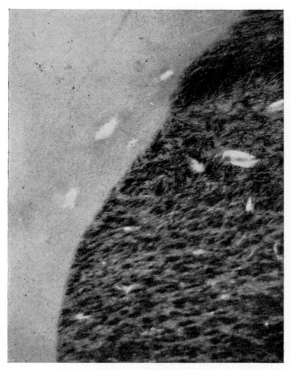

Fig. 20.47.—Margin of plaque in multiple sclerosis, showing the sharp interruption of the myelin sheaths at the margin, (normal tissue on right side). × 25. (Weigert–Pal method.)

secondary. Ischaemia and anoxia are probably not responsible because not all plaques are related to vessels and because neurones and axis cylinders survive. A virus causation also has been widely canvassed especially as demyelination is a feature of some virus diseases in animals, particularly in canine distemper, but so far neither has a virus been isolated, nor have

significant levels of antibodies to any known virus been demonstrated. The possibility that multiple sclerosis is a "slow-virus" disease is under active investigation. A delayed hypersensitivity reaction is suggested by the similarities between acute multiple sclerosis and some cases of acute disseminated encephalomyelitis, particularly those seen after the administration of anti-rabic vaccine. Epidemiological surveys point to some acquired or environmental factor to account for the observed correlation between the incidence of multiple sclerosis and the latitude of birth. In both the Northern and Southern Hemispheres, the disease is more prevalent in high latitudes than in low latitudes; yet, in low-incidence areas, the prevalence of the disease among immigrants is significantly higher in those of high incidence stock who have been born in high incidence areas. Present evidence seems to indicate that the environmental factor is acquired in the early years of life and that, as the disease is commonest between the ages of 20 and 40, the "incubation period" must be long.

The effects of the lesions on function vary greatly as the disease is so irregular in its distribution. In the early stages symptoms of focal lesions in the nervous system develop rapidly but are followed by a considerable degree of recovery. This is presumably due to the fact that the axons in an acute plaque, although not destroyed, are temporarily unable to transmit impulses. As the disease progresses, however, permanent disabilities due to the cumulative effects of the lesions become obvious and among these intention tremor, nystagmus, spasticity of the lower limbs and speech defects are prominent.

Neuromyelitis optica is the name given to a disease of adults characterised by rapid loss of vision and the occurrence of extensive demyelinating lesions in the optic nerves, cerebral white matter and especially in the spinal cord. The disease is commonly preceded by fever, it runs a more acute course than that of multiple sclerosis and the lesions are more severely destructive, but a proportion of cases recover.

In newborn lambs, the condition known as *swayback* is an acute demyelinating disorder which is usually fatal. It occurs in the offspring of ewes kept on pastures deficient in copper, and the administration of small amounts of copper to the ewes before lambing prevents the disorder.

Diffuse cerebral sclerosis

This comprises a group of diseases characterised by widespread demyelination in the white matter of the cerebral hemispheres and sometimes also in the cerebellum, brain stem and spinal cord. In the more rapidly fatal cases the affected white matter is softer than normal but if the illness is protracted, as is more common, the white matter becomes grey, translucent and firm because of a widespread diffuse reactive gliosis. Cases of diffuse cerebral sclerosis fall into two main groups, depending on the type of myelin disintegration that occurs. In one, myelin breakdown is similar to that seen in Wallerian degeneration, in infarction and in multiple sclerosis, with the formation of simple lipids which stain with ordinary fat stains, e.g. Sudan IV. This type is therefore known as *sudanophilic diffuse cerebral sclerosis*. In the other the myelin, which may be basically abnormal, breaks down to form substances which stain metachromatically with basic polychrome dyes, e.g. toluidin blue, and are positive with the periodic-acid-Schiff method. These substances are not stained by the Sudan dyes, and have been termed "pre-lipids". Accordingly this type is known as *metachromatic diffuse cerebral sclerosis*. Some cases of diffuse cerebral sclerosis are familial, being inherited apparently as Mendelian "recessives", and are appropriately termed *leukodystrophies*. Some sudanophilic and all metachromatic cases fall into this category. Diffuse cerebral sclerosis was formerly termed *Schilder's disease*, but if this term is to be used at all, it should be restricted to the non-familial sudanophilic type.

Sudanophilic cerebral sclerosis

This is the more common type and occurs both in childhood, when it may be familial, and in adult life. It is a progressive disease, characterised by mental deterioration, blindness and spastic paralysis. In subacute cases, death occurs within a few months, but more frequently the patient survives for one or two years. The brain exhibits widespread degeneration of the white matter notably in the occipital lobes (hence the common occurrence of visual impairment early in the disease), but any part of the cerebral hemispheres, cerebellum or brain stem may be affected. Typically, the subcortical arcuate fibres are spared and stand out as a conspicuous white band in the affected areas. In Weigert–Pal preparations, the demyelination is seen to be less sharply circumscribed than in disseminated sclerosis and shades off marginally into normally stained white matter. In the affected areas microglial cells stuffed with sudanophilic lipid are abundant while the degree of fibrous gliosis varies with the duration of the disease. Loss of axis cylinders is usually severe but, apart from occasional neurones showing central chromatolysis, the grey matter is normal.

Metachromatic cerebral sclerosis

This is a rare disease, occurring mainly in children between 2–5 years old, but not confined to this age group. Most cases are familial. The disease is progressive, tends to run a course of one or two years, and is characterised clinically by spasticity, ataxia, relentless mental deterioration and, as a late feature, visual impairment. The brain feels unusually firm and the white matter may be somewhat greyer and more translucent than normal; the subcortical arcuate fibres are not spared.

Histological examination demonstrates widespread demyelination in the white matter of the cerebral hemispheres, cerebellum, brain stem and spinal cord. The fibre systems which mature last are the most severely affected, hence the early onset of spasticity because of involvement of the corticospinal tract and the relative preservation of vision because of sparing of the optic radiation. The demyelinated areas contain large quantities of "pre-lipid", mostly extracellular, which stains metachromatically and is PAS positive. As the metachromatic granules are readily soluble in fat solvents, they can be demonstrated satisfactorily only in frozen sections. Axis cylinders tend to be preserved and there is a diffuse reactive fibrillary gliosis. Sudanophilic lipid is present only in small amounts in perivascular phagocytes. The same metachromatic lipid as is found in the degenerated white matter occurs in some neurones, in the Schwann cells of peripheral nerves, and also in the Kupffer cells and renal tubular epithelium. From this it might be inferred that metachromatic diffuse sclerosis should be classified as an inborn error of lipid metabolism, similar to the cerebral lipidoses. Biopsy of a peripheral nerve may be a useful diagnostic procedure.

The cerebral lipidoses

These diseases are inborn errors of metabolism, characterised by the accumulation within nerve cells of material having the staining properties of lipids more complex than neutral fat. The storage is usually associated with considerable swelling of the

	Normal	Acute Pyogenic Meningitis	Tuberculous Meningitis	Acute Virus Infection with Meningo-encephalitis
Pressure (horizontal posture)	60–150 mm. H$_2$O.	Increased—probably to 200 mm. or more	Increased to as much as 300 mm. or more	Increased sometimes to 250 mm.
Appearance	Clear and colourless	Turbid or frankly purulent	Clear or slightly opalescent. A fine fibrin coagulum may form	Clear or slightly opalescent
Cell content per c.mm.	0–4 leukocytes (all mononuclears)	Markedly raised 500–5000 polymorphs at first, mononuclears later	Increased up to 500 lymphocytes; some polymorphs at first	Increased 50–500 lymphocytes, some polymorphs at first
Protein mg./100 ml.	20–45	50–200 average; up to 1000 mg.	50–300 usually; if spinal block present, may rise to over 1000	50–200; 50–100 mg. in paralytic polio
Sugar mg./100 ml.	50–80	Absent or greatly reduced	Decreased to 20–30	Normal
Bacteriology	Sterile	Causative organisms present; type confirmed by culture	Tubercle bacilli in fibrin coagulum or in deposit. Positive cultures usually obtained	Sterile
Lange's colloidal gold test	Normal i.e. 0000000000	May be normal or meningitic i.e. 0012344320	Normal or meningitic	Normal or meningitic. Weak paretic or luetic in polio
Wassermann Reaction	Negative	Negative	Negative	Negative

cell body and is a widespread phenomenon in the various forms of amaurotic family idiocy, in most cases of Niemann–Pick's disease, in gargoylism and occasionally in infantile Gaucher's disease. The infantile form of amaurotic family idiocy (Tay–Sachs disease) is probably more common in Jews; it is inherited as a simple Mendelian recessive and is characterised by progressive mental deterioration, blindness and paralysis. On ophthalmoscopic examination the cherry-red spot at the macula is characteristic. The brain shows generalised atrophy, the surviving nerve cells are distended with abnormal lipids, mostly gangliosides; many neurones have disappeared and myelination of many fibres appears to have been arrested.

Other inborn errors of metabolism involving the nervous system

Phenylketonuria and galactosaemia are the most important of these because the ill effects can be prevented or mitigated by exclusion of the harmful substances from the diet.

In **phenylketonuria,** inherited as an autosomal recessive, absence of the active enzyme phenylalanine hydroxylase leads to accumulation of phenylalanine in the blood and excretion of phenylpyruvic acid in the urine. Epileptiform seizures, severe mental defect and some failure of myelination are the principal findings.

In **galactosaemia** there is hepato-splenomegaly, cataract and mental retardation associated with inability to metabolise galactose owing to absence of the enzyme galactose-1-phosphate uridyl transferase; consequently galactose-1-phosphate accumulates in toxic amounts and is excreted in the urine.

Despite the severe mental derangement no specific pathological abnormality has been recognised in the brain in these serious disorders.

The dementias

There is only poor correlation between organic changes in the nervous system and mental deterioration. Schizophrenia and the involutional psychoses show no constant pathological changes and in consequence are described as functional disorders. Other cases of dementia are secondary to certain organic brain diseases such as general paralysis of the insane, deeply-seated slowly-growing tumours, diffuse cerebral sclerosis and occlusive vascular disease. Of these the last is the commonest and in it the brain is small

AND IN CERTAIN DISEASES
LUMBAR PUNCTURE

General Paralysis of the Insane	Tabes Dorsalis	Multiple Sclerosis	Subarachnoid Haemorrhage	Complete spinal block (Froin's syndrome)
Normal	Normal	Normal	Raised, often to 300 mm. or more	Low: C.S.F. may have to be actively withdrawn
Normal	Normal	Normal	Frankly bloodstained: on centrifugalisation, supernatant is yellow	Yellow, opalescent and tends to clot
Up to 100 (lymphocytes)	Up to 50–100 (lymphocytes)	Slight increase to 20–100 (lymphocytes)	Many red cells	Slight increase of mononuclear cells
50–100	30–60	30–60	Normal in the early stages. Slight rise later	More than 500
Normal	Normal	Normal	Normal	Normal
Sterile	Sterile	Sterile	Sterile	Sterile
Paretic i.e. 5544321000	Luetic i.e. 123321000	Paretic, rarely luetic or may be normal	Normal	Meningitic
Positive	Positive in 80 per cent of cases	Negative	Negative	Negative

and the ventricles large, atheroma of the large and small arteries is widespread and severe, and numerous small infarcts can often be found.

There remains a group of primary organic dementias, usually relentlessly if slowly progressive, in which there are fairly specific pathological changes in the brain. Common to all is cortical atrophy, the gyri becoming rounder and firmer than normal and the sulci widened, and secondary hydrocephalus.

Alzheimer's disease and senile dementia. Alzheimer's disease is a pre-senile (onset before the age of 60) dementia in which the pathological findings resemble a gross exaggeration of those of the normal ageing processes in the brain. Death usually occurs a few years after the onset of the disease. Cortical atrophy is widespread but more conspicuous at the frontal and temporal poles. Histological examination reveals a generalised loss of neurones, reactive gliosis and vast numbers of senile (Alzheimer) plaques in the cortical grey matter. The plaques are composed of masses of small argyrophilic granules and filaments often with a core of amyloid material. In addition, there are tangles of coarse neurofibrils (Alzheimer's neurofibrillary change) in many of the larger nerve cells of the cerebral cortex.

Pick's disease is classed as a pre-senile dementia. Cortical atrophy from loss of neurones is particularly intense in the frontal and temporal lobes, giving the brain a distinctive naked-eye appearance. The consequent degeneration of axis cylinders probably accounts for the loss of myelin, reactive gliosis and considerable shrinkage of the underlying white matter. Some of the surviving neurones are greatly swollen by a globular mass of intracellular argyrophilic material.

Huntington's chorea. This disease of middle adult life is characterised by coarse choreiform movements, progressive mental deterioration and, in some cases, striatal rigidity. It is believed to be inherited by an autosomal dominant gene. In addition to widespread cortical atrophy, there is severe atrophy and loss of nerve cells in the caudate nucleus and the putamen.

II. THE SPINAL CORD

The tissue of the spinal cord is similar to that of the brain but the relative frequencies of various lesions are very different. Specific diseases of the spinal cord are described later but so-called *transverse lesions* and the consequent ascending and descending Wallerian degenerations within the cord will be dealt with first.

TRANSVERSE LESIONS

These occur when the full thickness of the cord is involved by gross intrinsic or extrinsic lesions. The effects may be produced slowly by pressure on the cord by extrinsic tumours in the extradural space, e.g. metastatic carcinoma (Fig. 20.48) or lymphoid neoplasm, or in the subdural space, e.g. meningioma (Fig. 20.67, p. 668) or Schwannoma. Intrinsic tumours, e.g. astrocytoma and ependymoma, are rare causes. Tuberculosis of the vertebral bodies although now uncommon in the British Isles is still frequently encountered in other parts of the world such as East Africa. It leads to angular curvature of the spine and tuberculous granuloma, both of which can cause pressure on the cord; this may be so severe that actual infarction of the cord may occur at this level. Syphilitic meningitis is now also an extremely rare cause of a transverse lesion in the British Isles. Acute transverse lesions may be due to *trauma*, usually a fracture-dislocation of the vertebrae, *infarction* when the circulation through the anterior spinal artery is impeded, *haemorrhage*, usually from a vascular malformation, *acute myelitis* (see below) or acute *demyelination* as in neuromyelitis optica (p. 650).

An inevitable consequence of a total or partial transverse lesion of the cord, besides the local damage, is the development of *ascending* and *descending* Wallerian degeneration in the respective tracts of the spinal cord. Degeneration occurs in those fibres that are separated from their cell bodies by the lesion and, when recent, is best demonstrated by the Marchi technique. The degenerating fibres appear black from about a week after onset (Fig. 20.49). The method is applicable until the degenerated myelin has disappeared—that is, for several months. In the case of long-standing lesions of the spinal cord, Weigert's method or one of its modifications, which stain the normal myelin black, should be used; accordingly, when the degenerated myelin has become absorbed, the affected tract appears as a pale area (Fig. 20.51).

Ascending degenerations

If we take as an example a comparatively recent lesion at the level of the lower dorsal region, the following ascending degenerations are found in a section taken a few segments above the lesion (Fig. 20.49). There is degeneration in the posterior columns (with the exception of a small area dorsal to the grey commissure

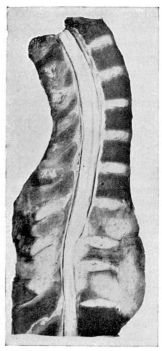

Fig. 20.48.—Sagittal section of the vertebral column in lower cervical–upper dorsal region, showing metastatic tumour pressing on the cord.

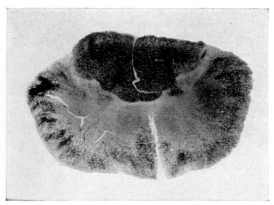

FIG. 20.49.—Immediately above the lesion. The whole of the posterior columns and antero-lateral ascending tracts are degenerating. × 7.

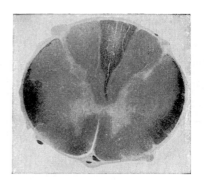

FIG. 20.50.—Cervical region. There are fewer degenerating fibres because of the inflow of fibres above the level of the lesion. × 4·5.

Figures 20.49 and 20.50.—**Ascending degeneration** above a recent transverse lesion in the lower dorsal region, stained by Marchi's method: the degenerating fibres appear black.

where there are chiefly commissural fibres) and in the spino-thalamic and spino-cerebellar tracts. At a higher level, however, in the cervical region, the degeneration in the posterior columns is practically confined to the gracile tract (Fig. 20.50) as the cuneate tract is composed mainly of ascending fibres that have joined the cord above the level of the lesion. Degeneration of the affected axons extends up to the nucleus cuneatus and nucleus gracilis in the medulla, from which a new set of healthy axons passes upwards to the lower part of the thalami chiefly in the medial lemniscus, where they decussate—the upper sensory decussation. Ascending degeneration in the posterior spino-cerebellar tract extends up to the inferior cerebellar peduncle and into the cerebellum, and in the anterior spino-cerebellar tract to the middle lobe of the cere-

bellum. In old lesions, loss of myelin (Figs. 20.51 and 20.52) and reactive gliosis are conspicuous only in the posterior columns as the inflow of normal myelinated fibres at higher levels masks the relatively small loss of myelin in the spino-cerebellar and spino-thalamic tracts.

Descending degenerations

These are encountered in two chief conditions, namely (*a*) when there is a transverse lesion in the cord, and (*b*) when the lesion is at a higher level. In a section taken from below a recent *transverse lesion* of the cord the most marked degeneration is in the crossed (lateral) and uncrossed (anterior) pyramidal tracts unless the lesion is low in the cord where the uncrossed tract

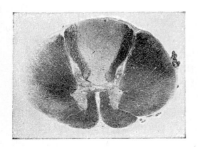

FIG. 20.51.—A short distance above the lesion.

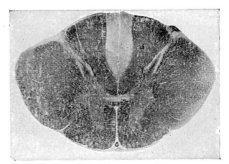

FIG. 20.52.—Cervical region. Degeneration appears to be confined to the gracile tract.

Figures 20.51 and 20.52.—**Ascending degeneration** above a long-standing transverse lesion in the dorsal region, stained by Weigert–Pal method. The degenerated fibres appear pale.

is no longer present. By Marchi's method there may be seen scattered degenerating fibres in the superficial parts in the lateral column in front of the crossed pyramidal tract, and also in the anterior column round to the median fissure. The former belong to the rubro-spinal tract, which comes from the red nucleus, and to minor bundles from medulla, corpora quadrigemina, and thalamus. In sections of the lesions at a late stage stained by Weigert's method, such degenerations are not recognisable, owing to the

is on the part of the mononuclears. These changes are grouped under the term "Froins' syndrome" (see Table, p. 652).

Prolapsed intervertebral disc

A very common cause of compression of the cord or of nerve roots is a prolapsed intervertebral disc (Fig. 20.55). The intervertebral disc consists of a central nodule of semifluid

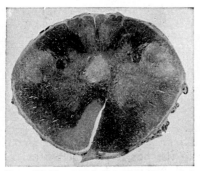

FIG. 20.53.—Medulla. The anterior pyramid on one side is degenerated.

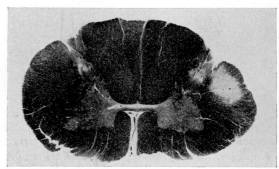

FIG. 20.54.—Thoracic region. The crossed pyramidal tract on one side is degenerated.

Figures 20.53 and 20.54.—**Descending degeneration.** Transverse sections through medulla and spinal cord showing descending degeneration from a long-standing lesion of one internal capsule. Stained by Weigert–Pal method: degenerated fibres appear pale.

scattered arrangement of the fibres, whereas the degenerated (unstained) pyramidal tracts can be clearly seen.

The commonest example due to a lesion at a higher level is destruction of the motor fibres in the internal capsule. In such a case there is degeneration of the crossed pyramidal tract on the opposite side (Fig. 20.53) and of the uncrossed pyramidal tract on the same side. In addition, there may be seen by Marchi's method some scattered degenerating fibres in the crossed pyramidal tract on the same side as the lesion, that is, in some motor fibres which have not crossed in the medulla. As the direct pyramidal tract does not usually extend lower than the first thoracic segment, degeneration in that site will not appear in sections below this level (Fig. 20.54).

When there is compression of the spinal cord by a gross lesion so as to block the subarachnoid space the cerebrospinal fluid below the block becomes altered. A great increase of protein occurs and the fluid shows massive coagulation on being removed from the body; it is often yellow (xanthochromia). The cells may or may not be increased; any increase

matrix of notochordal origin, the nucleus pulposus, surrounded by a circle of fibrous tissue and fibrocartilage, the annulus fibrosus. The posterior segment of the annulus is thinner and less firmly attached to bone and, following unusual stress, part of the matrix of the nucleus pulposus may herniate through it (Fig. 20.56). The lesion may occur, however, after slight injury and the symptoms produced depend on the direction taken by the material extruded from the nucleus pulposus. The herniated material usually tracks postero-laterally around the expansion of the posterior longitudinal ligament, appearing at one side and compressing spinal nerve roots in the intervertebral foramen. Clinically, disc protrusion in the lumbar spine is most common and L5–S1, L4–L5 and L3–L4 disc spaces are affected in that order of frequency, the cervical spine at the C5–6 and C6–7 level being less often involved. If the protrusion is slight, localised pain is produced by irritation of the posterior longitudinal ligament; if larger, there may be root pain due to pressure on nerves leaving the spinal canal giving rise to the clinical signs and symptoms of sciatica. A

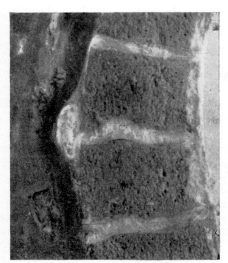

Fig. 20.55.—Sagittal section of vertebral column, showing ruptured disc protruding beneath the posterior longitudinal ligament. × 1.

single posterior disc protrusion may cause compression of the cord or obstruction of the anterior spinal artery, but this is only rarely severe enough to give rise to a transverse lesion. When there are several protrusions, as in cervical spondylosis, the resulting compression may impair the circulation and very variable degrees of ischaemia and spinal cord degeneration may result. There may be cavitation of the cord and loss of nerve cells in the severely affected areas, the condition being known as *spondylotic myelopathy.* Even in cervical spondylosis, however, nerve root compression is commoner than myelopathy.

The extruded disc material consists of fragments of cartilage amongst which there is sometimes notochordal tissue. Reactive changes with foreign body giant cells may occur and the mass may at first enlarge, but later it becomes fibrosed and shrunken. Disability may arise later from osteoarthritis of intervertebral joints.

Acute myelitis

This uncommon condition, by definition an acute inflammation of the cord, is more a clinical syndrome than a precise pathological entity. It is usually of acute or subacute onset and is characterised by flaccid paralysis and sensory loss, either of which may be total or partial, below the level of the lesion.

A considerable part of the cord may be affected—*diffuse myelitis*; or the lesion may be confined to one or two segments—*transverse myelitis.* The terms, however, tend to be used for any pathological process other than external pressure or tumour which causes intrinsic damage to the grey and white matter of the cord. There are various causes.

Etiology. It may be due to *bacterial infection* either by spread from an extradural abscess or in association with a generalised infection such as typhoid, puerperal fever, etc. Toxic action is probably of greater importance in the pathogenesis than secondary invasion by organisms. Small abscesses are very rare in the cord even in pyaemia and bacterial endocarditis. *Syphilis* was in the past a common cause, cord involvement being secondary to syphilitic leptomeningitis and obliterative changes in arteries. Myelitis may also be a consequence of infection by *viruses*, either as part of a generalised viral encephalitis or when there is particularly severe involvement of the cord in acute disseminated encephalomyelitis (see p. 647). (Anterior poliomyelitis is a specific myelitis of the *grey* matter.) Other causes are *demyelination*, as in neuromyelitis optica (p. 650) or in multiple sclerosis, or *infarction* which can occur when the anterior spinal artery is obstructed or in association with thrombophlebitis of spinal veins (subacute necrotic myelitis).

Structural changes. The appearances of the cord vary with the underlying pathological process. In general, however, the affected part of the cord is swollen and soft, the normal architectural markings are blurred and there may be foci of haemorrhage.

If the patient survives the acute stage, there may be considerable restoration of function. If, however, the cord has been too severely damaged to allow of resolution, the term *chronic myelitis* may be applied. This is characterised by shrinkage of the affected parts and varying degrees of gliosis, and ascending and descending degeneration in the white matter.

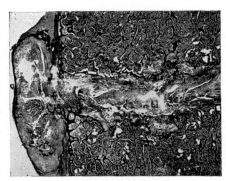

Fig. 20.56.—Histological section of other half of above lesion. × 2·5. (Dr. G. B. S. Roberts.)

LESIONS OF THE MOTOR NEURONES

The neuro-muscular system consists of upper and lower motor neurones and the muscles. Lesions which affect muscular action may be primarily either in the axons or in the nerve cells themselves. A primary wasting of the muscles is seen in the idiopathic muscular dystrophies (p. 809), while primary lesions of the axons of the lower neurones are seen in peripheral neuropathy, in the latter case along with sensory involvement; these will be described later. We have here to consider the diseases involving the spinal cord, and the distinction between the lower and upper neurones is of fundamental importance. Lesions of the former are characterised by paralysis attended by flaccidity and neurogenic atrophy of muscles. Conversely, in lesions of the upper neurones or of their axons, i.e. the pyramidal fibres, muscle weakness is accompanied by heightened irritability of the corresponding lower neurones—increase of the deep reflexes and tendency to spasm, but without neurogenic atrophy. The main acute motor affection, namely, *acute anterior poliomyelitis*, has already been considered (p. 639). There are also degenerative diseases involving the upper and lower motor neurones, and different names have been applied according to the main symptoms, namely, *progressive muscular atrophy*, *progressive bulbar palsy* and *amyotrophic lateral sclerosis*.

Chronic disease of the motor neurones

The motor neurones may be affected by system degenerations, insidious in origin and slow in progress. The lower and upper neurones are involved together in the great majority of cases, and then there is a combination of atrophic and spastic conditions, the term *amyotrophic lateral sclerosis* being applied. In a comparatively small group the changes are chiefly in the motor cells of the anterior horns, or in the cranial nerve nuclei though not confined to them; the conditions known as *progressive muscular atrophy* or *progressive bulbar palsy* then result. These three conditions should be regarded as variants of one disease, often known as *motor neurone disease*, which varies in its symptomatology according to the proportion in which the different neurones and their axons are involved, but noth-

ing definite is known regarding their etiology. They occur in middle and late adult life, much more frequently in men than in women, and whilst various conditions have been put forward as causal factors, none of these is regularly related to the origin of the disease.

Progressive muscular atrophy. In cases where atrophic changes are the outstanding feature, the lesion is mainly a progressive degeneration of the neurones in the anterior horns. It usually starts in the cervical enlargement in the neurones related to the small muscles of the hand. The affected muscles are the seat of fibrillar twitchings and, gradually, atrophy with corresponding weakness follows. Owing to the slow progress, the actual change in the muscles at any one time is not sufficient to give rise to the reaction of degeneration. The thenar and hypothenar eminences become markedly wasted, the interossei also become affected, and the hand assumes a characteristic claw-like form. Involvement then extends to the muscles of the arm and those of the shoulder girdle; as a terminal phenomenon the symptoms of bulbar paralysis may appear. In one type of the disease the wasting appears first in the muscles of the shoulder girdle. In the anterior horns corresponding to the wasting, the process is a progressive atrophy of the neurones. Some of them have disappeared, while many of those remaining show stages of atrophy; many have lost their processes and become irregular, or are somewhat oval in form; pigmentary changes are sometimes prominent. There is a certain amount of gliosis, but as a rule it is not a marked feature. The anterior spinal roots become wasted and appear grey and thin to the naked eye, while in the related muscles the atrophy corresponds to the loss of the neurones and is patchy in distribution (Fig. 1.31, p. 28).

Amyotrophic lateral sclerosis. In the cases classified as progressive muscular atrophy, there is to be seen in sections of the cord stained by Weigert's method a partial loss of myelinated fibres entering the anterior horns, and in the crossed pyramidal tracts; this indicates some involvement of the axons of the upper neurones. In cases, however, where spasticity is prominent and occurs early there is a much more extensive involvement of the upper neurones and this is designated amyotrophic lateral sclerosis. In addition to the atrophic changes in the anterior horns, there is widespread sclerosis and loss of myelin in the lateral and anterior white columns, most marked in, but not confined to, the pyramidal tracts (Fig. 20.57). The changes in the pyramidal fibres, as a rule, start first and are most marked at their lower extremities, the process then extending upwards. Atrophic changes, corresponding to those in the anterior horns, occur in the motor cells of the cerebral cortex and here also many disappear. The sclerosis of the pyramidal tracts may extend to a lower level in the cord than that at which the anterior horns are implicated. It would appear that the two sets of neurones are affected independently, one or other being involved first and to a greater degree.

Progressive bulbar paralysis. This variant of motor neurone disease may appear first, or may follow spinal involvement. It is characterised by progressive paralysis and wasting of the muscles of the

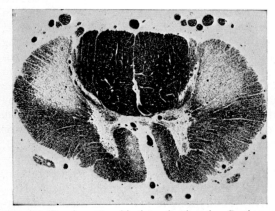

Fig. 20.57.—Amyotrophic lateral sclerosis. Section of spinal cord, showing degeneration in crossed pyramidal and direct pyramidal tracts.

(Weigert–Pal method.)

tongue, lips, jaws, larynx and pharynx; death often occurs by involvement of the respiratory centre, or by foreign matter entering the lungs through the paralysed larynx. The lesions are in the medulla and are essentially of the same nature as those in the cord. They are usually most marked in the hypoglossal and spinal accessory nuclei, but occur also in the nuclei of the vagus and seventh nerves, and in the nucleus of the motor part of the fifth. The oculomotor nuclei are rarely involved. There is, of course, wasting of the corresponding nerves, and degeneration occurs in the corresponding upper neurones and their axons. Along with the changes in the brain stem there is a varying involvement of the nerve cells in the anterior horns and in the pyramidal fibres. As stated above, nothing definite is known with regard to the etiology of motor neurone disease. There is also an acute form of bulbar paralysis in which the nuclei of the nerves mentioned are the seat of lesions produced by the virus of anterior poliomyelitis.

Motor neurone disease has in general an incidence of about 4 per 100,000 of population, but in the Mariana Islands of the Pacific, the aboriginal Chamorro people have the remarkably high in-

cidence of over 400 per 100,000. It is the commonest neurological disorder among the Chamorros and causes about 10 per cent of the adult deaths, usually from bulbar paralysis. There is some evidence that it may have a hereditary basis.

Friedreich's ataxia. This disease, in which there is atrophy in both motor and sensory tracts, often affects more than one member of a family, hence it is sometimes called *familial ataxia*; rarely it occurs in successive generations. Isolated cases of the disease are also encountered. It usually begins in the years before adolescence and the chief symptoms are ataxia with muscular weakness. Lateral curvature of the spine and talipes equinus are often present, and nystagmus and disturbances of speech also are common. In such cases, the spinal cord is found to be relatively thin and atrophy is present in the posterior and lateral columns (Fig. 20.58). The posterior roots show degeneration, especially the fibres within the cord, and involvement of the roots and posterior columns may be present in the cervical region as well as lower down; the cells in the posterior root ganglia, however, are little altered. In the lateral columns the pyramidal fibres are degenerate, the degeneration being most marked, below, and diminishing in an upward direction. The posterior spino-cerebellar tracts are similarly affected, and the cells of the thoracic nucleus show degenerative changes. There may be some degeneration also in the anterior spino-cerebellar and spino-thalamic tracts. The nature of the disease is obscure. Possibly the disease represents a condition of incomplete development, whereby certain systems of fibres

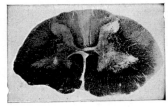

Fig. 20.58.—Section of cord in Friedreich's ataxia, showing degeneration in posterior and lateral columns.

(Weigert–Pal method.)

are in a sense shorter-lived than usual and undergo degeneration, which appears first in the distal parts of the long axons. Family studies have shown that Friedreich's ataxia and *Marie's hereditary cerebellar ataxia* are probably varieties of an essentially similar disorder; the two conditions sometimes overlap and intermediate forms occur, but each affected family presents its own variant. Friedreich's ataxia is frequently associated with a chronic progressive myocarditis, in which focal coagulative necrosis of the muscle fibres is followed by replacement fibrosis (Dorothy Russell).

Y

OTHER LESIONS OF THE SPINAL CORD

Subacute combined degeneration

Degeneration of the spinal cord, especially of the posterior and lateral columns, formerly occurred in a high proportion of cases of inadequately treated pernicious anaemia, but since highly effective purified preparations of cyanocobalamin have been available this complication is now much less common. Similar lesions have been found much more rarely in other chronic diseases, such as malabsorption syndromes, leukaemia, diabetes, and carcinoma. Subacute combined degeneration has been observed without the presence of anaemia, but gastrointestinal disturbance has been present in a considerable proportion of these, and detailed haematological examination will generally reveal megaloblastic erythropoiesis. The administration of vitamin B_{12} in adequate doses is completely effective in preventing the development of neural lesions, but folic acid not only fails to do so, but may aggravate the condition, ap-

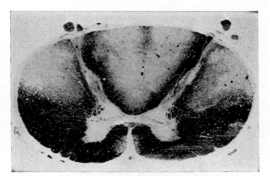

FIG. 20.59.—Subacute combined degeneration, showing marked lesions in both lateral and posterior columns.
(Weigert–Pal method.)

parently by diverting to the marrow any residual B_{12}. The favourable results following the administration of thiamine (vitamin B_1) come chiefly from improvement in the peripheral neuropathy which almost invariably accompanies the cord changes. The anatomical changes are of distinctive character, the long fibres in the cord being affected first in the thoracic region and both ascending and descending tracts are implicated (Fig. 20.59). The posterior columns may be diffusely degenerated, but there is no involvement of the nerve roots. The pyramidal tracts, both crossed and direct, may be affected, but the degeneration tends to spread beyond

them, especially in the thoracic region, where the disease is usually most extensive. In the involved segments the degenerate myelin is removed by phagocytes which migrate to the perivascular sheaths. In untreated cases there is practically no glial proliferation and the degenerated areas present an open spongy appearance. With long survival on B_{12} treatment, however, some gliosis eventually occurs. The degeneration in the motor tracts may ascend through the internal capsule and degenerative changes may be seen in the Betz cells of the cortex. The appearance, accordingly, is of damage especially to the long fibres, with, in addition, small foci of demyelination in the cerebral hemispheres. There is no evidence that anaemia in itself produces the lesions mentioned; in fact, it may be preceded by them. The symptoms depend on the tracts involved. If they are mainly the posterior columns, ataxic symptoms are prominent, whilst involvement of the lateral columns leads to spastic symptoms. In view of its progressive, disabling nature, and the arresting effects of B_{12} therapy, early diagnosis is of the utmost importance.

Syringomyelia

This term is applied to a space or spaces within the substance of the cord, containing fluid and enclosed by neuroglia. It has to be distinguished from *hydromyelia* which is a dilatation of the central canal: the space so formed is lined by ependyma but, when the enlargement is considerable, the morbid anatomical changes and the clinical features may closely resemble those of syringomyelia. Both conditions occur particularly in the cervical region; the pathogenesis of syringomyelia is not known but it has been suggested that cervical hydromyelia is due to CSF being propelled through a valve-like opening between the caudal extremity of the fourth ventricle and the central canal of the spinal cord.

In *syringomyelia* the cavity first appears behind the central canal, either in the white matter or in the base of one of the posterior grey horns. The cavity extends through several segments of the spinal cord (Figs. 20.60 and 20.61) and as it enlarges the cord becomes swollen and feels somewhat soft. On microscopic examination the tissue lining the cavity is composed of enlarged astrocytes and coarse astrocytic fibrils which are rarefied in the tissue around the central cavity. Syringomyelia rarely occurs in the lumbar region. Similar cavities may also occur in the lower brain stem (syringobulbia). Occasionally syringomyelia occurs in association with tumours affecting the spinal cord.

Effects. These are due principally to destruction of the structures in the cord by the enlarging cavity but pressure may also play a part. The first fibres to be affected are the decussating sensory fibres conveying the sensations of heat and pain: the resulting defect, known as dissociated anaesthesia, is a selective insensibility to heat and pain in the region corresponding to the involved segments of the spinal cord. Trophic disturbances affect the joints, bone and skin. A neuropathic arthritis occurs,

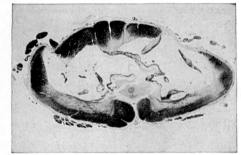

FIG. 20.60.—Syringomyelia: upper part of cervical enlargement.

(Weigert–Pal method.)

closely similar to that in tabes (p. 638), but, as syringomyelia is usually in the cervical region, it is the joints of the upper limbs which are chiefly involved. The trophic lesions of the skin are manifold, and the syndrome known as Morvan's disease, in which dissociated anaesthesia is associated with vesicles of the skin and painless whitlow, is one manifestation of syringomyelia. As the cavity enlarges it ultimately affects the lateral white columns leading to spastic paraplegia, the ventral grey horns leading to neurogenic atrophy of muscles, and the posterior white columns leading to even greater disturbances of sensation.

Dietary-induced disorders

In human nutritional disease, a pure deficiency of only one factor is very rarely encountered: variation in the clinical picture can then be explained by the presence of various deficiencies, one or more of which may be responsible for the most conspicuous abnormalities. *Pellagra*, for example, appears to be caused by deficiency of the B_2 complex but chiefly of nicotinic acid. Cutaneous lesions, glossitis, diarrhoea and mental changes make up the classical clinical picture, some cases show also a peripheral neuropathy very similar to that observed in beri-beri, and others exhibit a form of postero-lateral degeneration of the spinal cord which is not identical with that produced

by lack of B_{12}. In cases of chronic *ergotism* somewhat similar changes are observed in the spinal cord, and these are apparently the result of toxins produced by the fungus in rye. The term *lathyrism* is applied to a disease occurring especially in India amongst those of whose diet pulse forms an important part. It occurs sometimes in epidemics, chiefly in males in times of famine. The chief symptoms are spasticity affecting the extensor and adductor muscles of the lower limbs, but sensory symptoms also are present. Both lateral and posterior columns of the cord are affected, but the exact changes are not definitely known. Stockman attributed the disease to an alkaloid present in various species of *Lathyrus* and by feeding monkeys with the seeds of *Lathyrus sativus* he produced paralysis of muscles with changes both in the peripheral nerves and in the spinal cord.

A similar condition produced by a diet of chick peas (*cicerism*) is attributed to a toxic action of the pea protein; this can be prevented by choline or methionine (Diaz). The production of "hysteria" in dogs and ferrets by flour treated with nitrogen trichloride (agene) has been traced to the development of a toxic amino-acid derivative, methionine sulphoximine, from the gluten and gliadin of wheat and from the zein of maize. The significance of these observations in human pathology is not yet clear.

Caisson disease or Diver's palsy

Although the lesions are not restricted to the cord, this disease is considered here because, if unrelieved, the effects are like those of multiple focal lesions which result in numerous minute

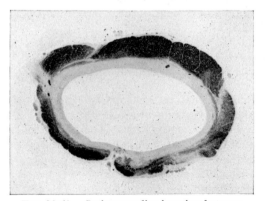

FIG. 20.61.—Syringomyelia: junction between cervical and thoracic portion.

(Weigert–Pal method.)

areas of softening irregularly distributed throughout the spinal cord. When divers, or other workers in compressed air, e.g. in caissons, are brought back too quickly to ordinary atmospheric pressure, they may suffer from weakness or paralysis, especially in the lower limbs; and sometimes actual paraplegia may be present. The symptoms usually pass off, but some permanent results may remain. During the exposure to the high atmospheric pressure, the gases of the air become dissolved in increased amount in the blood and then in the tissues, and it has been shown by Vernon that the nitrogen is specially soluble in fats, including the myelin of the nervous system. When decompression occurs the gases leave the tissues and are discharged by means of the blood stream, but if it is carried out too rapidly, bubbles of nitrogen may form in the substance of the spinal cord. These bubbles occur specially in the white matter (as can be seen in sections) apparently because it contains fewer capillaries than the grey matter, and also because it

absorbs more nitrogen. The bubbles produce symptoms by their pressure, which may disappear when they are ultimately absorbed. Sometimes, however, small foci of infarction result, and this is believed to be due to blocking of capillaries with bubbles, which will not only interfere with nutrition but also with absorption of the nitrogen. Occasionally there is fat embolism (Fig. 8.22, p. 172) not only in the renal glomeruli, but also in the cerebral capillaries. The short period of time during which the neural elements can withstand deprivation of blood is, of course, an important factor in bringing about the lesions. Changes may occur also in the bones (p. 67). The occurrence of caisson disease may be entirely prevented by carrying out the decompression in suitably graduated stages.

III. THE PERIPHERAL NERVES

Although the terms *neuritis* and *polyneuritis* have often been used in the past to describe virtually all disorders of the peripheral nerves, there is only rarely a true inflammatory process within the nerve. Thus the terms *neuropathy* or *polyneuropathy* are often more appropriate. The neuropathies fall into three major categories, viz. those with (a) primary degeneration of the nerve cell (parenchymatous neuropathy), (b) dysfunction of the Schwann cell, or (c) alterations in the blood supply to the nerve. A true, i.e. inflammatory, neuritis also occurs and is considered after the neuropathies.

Parenchymatous neuropathies

Parenchymatous neuropathies usually affect several nerves more or less symmetrically, i.e. they are polyneuropathies. The first manifestation of the primary abnormality in the nerve cell is degenerative change in the most distal part of the fibre as shown by dissolution of the axon and destruction of the myelin sheath. The myelin is broken up into globules, which undergo phagocytosis: these globules stain with Sudan dyes and are positive with the Marchi reaction (Fig. 20.62). This Wallerian-type degeneration then extends proximally—the so-called "dying-back" process. Ultimately, the most severely affected part of the nerve may become soft and develop a slightly yellow tint. In general the longest and

largest fibres are affected first with the result that the earliest neurological disturbance appears in the distal parts of the limbs: the most characteristic are paraesthesiae, muscle weakness, loss of vibration sense and diminished two-point discrimination. Histological examination of the proximal part of an affected nerve may show very few abnormal fibres although they may be very numerous in its distal part. In some cases where muscle weakness is considerable, abnormalities in the nerves may be restricted to the small

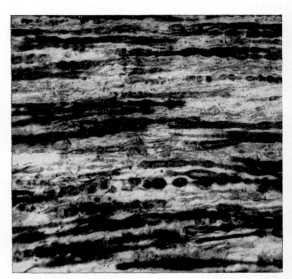

FIG. 20.62.—Longitudinal section of peripheral nerve in alcoholic neuropathy showing degeneration of myelin sheaths. (Marchi method). × about 400.

distal radicles actually within the muscle. As the motor fibres degenerate the muscle end-plates lose their innervation and the muscle fibres undergo neurogenic atrophy (see p. 808). If some healthy nerve fibres remain, attempted regenerative phenomena to reinnervate motor end plates are shown by the presence of collateral and ultraterminal axonal sprouting. As the degeneration extends proximally, central chromatolysis becomes apparent in the motor neurones in the ventral horns of the spinal cord and in the neurones in the dorsal root ganglia.

The causes of parenchymatous peripheral neuropathy are many and varied. Probably the commonest is *nutritional deficiency*, beri-beri being the most important disease in this group.

Beri-beri. In this disease the essential lesion is a polyneuropathy, which results from the absence or deficiency of vitamin B_1 (thiamine), and is usually caused by a diet consisting exclusively of over-milled cereals, especially rice. The disease, which is encountered principally amongst rice-eating populations, occurs in two forms. In one—the "dry" form—the peripheral nerves are chiefly affected. Degenerative changes are often prominent in the ventral horns of the spinal cord and in the dorsal ganglia. The levels of pyruvate in the blood and CSF are raised. In the other, or "wet" form, the disturbances are mainly cardiac; the heart becomes dilated, especially the right ventricle, there is general venous congestion, and oedema usually becomes a marked feature. Degenerative changes have been found in the vagi, in the phrenic nerves, and in the sympathetic system. It may be that the cardiac dilatation is secondary to the lesions in the nerves, but the possibility of a primary change in the cardiac muscle cannot be excluded.

Polyneuropathy can readily be produced in fowls and pigeons by feeding them with milled or polished rice; pigeons especially have been used in studying the distribution and metabolism of vitamin B_1. Polyneuropathy has been produced also in the rat by deprivation of vitamin B_1, but the changes are less constant and less marked. In the experimentally produced disease recovery takes place with great rapidity when the birds are fed with substances containing the necessary vitamin, and Peters has described the condition as a pure biochemical lesion. The essential pathogenesis is the failure of neural tissue to complete the oxidation of carbohydrate in the absence of co-carboxylase which normally

is produced by phosphorylation of thiamine. Consequently carbohydrate metabolism ceases at the pyruvate level and this substance accumulates in blood and tissue.

Since the body's requirements of thiamine are proportional to the amount of carbohydrate metabolised, the deficiency of thiamine is exaggerated by a predominantly carbohydrate diet, and the severity of the results on neural tissue are attributable to its dependence on carbohydrate oxidation. *In vitro* the metabolic defect of homogenised affected tissue is rectified very speedily by the addition of co-carboxylase, and *in vivo* by the administration of the precursor, vitamin B_1. These facts have been applied to the treatment of beri-beri. Substitution of under-milled for milled rice has caused beri-beri to disappear in many places and the etiological importance of vitamin B_1 is established. It has not, however, been established that beri-beri in man is due solely to the lack of thiamine, and deficiencies in other members of the vitamin B group may well contribute. Protein deficiency is thought to be partly responsible for the "wet" form of the disease.

Other metabolic disturbances. Deficiency of nicotinic acid or vitamin B_{12} are other causes of peripheral neuropathy, while a deficiency of various members of the vitamin B group is probably the principal cause of the peripheral neuropathy associated with chronic alcoholism. This is brought about partly by the restricted diet and partly by deficient absorption from the alimentary canal because of associated gastrointestinal disturbances.

Various intoxications may produce a parenchymatous polyneuropathy. Examples are various chemical substances such as *tri-orthocresyl phosphate*, dinitrobenzol and carbon disulphide or certain drugs such as isoniazid. Some metabolic or toxic derangement is probably the cause of carcinomatous neuropathy (see p. 665) while an endogenous metabolic defect is the cause of the neuropathy in acute porphyria.

In **acute porphyria,** there is usually a history of attacks of colicky abdominal pain followed by the onset of weakness in legs and arms and sometimes mental disturbances, an association of symptoms suggestive of lead poisoning. The essential lesion is a polyneuropathy, but in spite of paraesthesiae, there is little true sensory loss. In severe cases, paresis rapidly progresses to complete quadriplegia and death occurs in about 50 per cent. Some run a relapsing course, and others recover completely, though the metabolic abnormality may persist. The condition may be precipitated by drugs, especially allyl-barbiturates, but there is often a hereditary predisposition and the metabolic pigment abnormality may be present in healthy siblings; in some families, the disorder is transmitted as a Mendelian dominant. The diagnosis depends on the recognition of the abnormal chromogen, porphobilinogen, and other pigments in the urine, which darkens on exposure to light, uroporphyrin III being the usual pigment in idiopathic cases. Since these pigments are pharmacologically inert, the actual cause of the symptoms is still obscure. In chronic congenital porphyria, on the other hand, the pigment excreted is uroporphyrin I and photosensitisation is a prominent symptom. Recently a number of cases of the idiopathic disease with neurological symptoms have been recorded in which uroporphyrin I was excreted.

Schwann cell dysfunction

In neuropathies due to dysfunction of the Schwann cell, the characteristic abnormality is *segmental demyelination*, i.e. demyelination of an axon between two nodes of Ranvier. Many segments in a single fibre may be affected and there appears to be no predilection for their distal parts. Segmental demyelination affects nerve conduction but a particularly interesting feature is that remyelination may occur. The regenerated myelin, however, usually forms a thinner sheath than normal, while the formation of extra nodes means that the internodal distance becomes reduced. This type of nerve damage contributes to the neuropathy in individuals with diabetes mellitus, and occurs particularly in post-diphtheritic paralysis and in lead poisoning.

Vascular and ischaemic changes

These account for the third major group of neuropathies. In contrast to the types already described, the cause is usually local with the result that the distribution is not symmetrical although sometimes several nerves are affected. Probably the commonest cause is pressure such as in "crutch palsy" or "Saturday night paralysis". The duration of the disability depends on the degree of ischaemia produced by the pressure. Abnormalities in the vasa nervorum

account for the peripheral neuropathy commonly seen in polyarteritis nodosa (Fig. 20.63): the term *mononeuritis multiplex* is often used because of the presence of multiple individual lesions in various nerves. The ischaemia may be sufficient only to produce transient dysfunction but there may be frank infarction with subsequent Wallerian degeneration of the affected fibres. In peripheral vascular disease of the lower limbs, caused usually by atheroma, there may be a pronounced reduction in the number of nerve fibres and a progressive increase of fibrous tissue.

True peripheral neuritis

The peripheral nerves may also be affected by an inflammatory process—*true peripheral neuritis*—and as the interstitial tissue in the nerve is

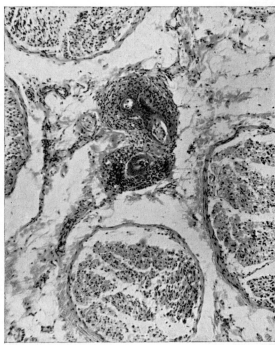

Fig. 20.63.—Transverse section of the sciatic nerve in polyarteritis nodosa, showing an acute arterial lesion × 170.

more severely affected than the nerve fibres themselves, the term *interstitial neuritis* is often appropriate. This type of neuritis may result from the extension of any type of local tissue inflammation, e.g. wounds, abscesses, bed-sores, arthritis, etc., into the nerve. The latter becomes swollen and congested and there is an interstitial inflammatory exudate. A similar though ill-understood process may be responsible for the neuritis that follows exposure to cold and wet as in *Bell's palsy* of the facial nerve.

Interstitial neuritis may also be *chronic* from the outset. A striking example of this is seen in *leprosy*, where the bacilli enter the supporting sheaths of the nerves, and give rise to interstitial proliferation of connective tissue followed by atrophy of nerve fibres, leading to paralytic and trophic disturbances. Interstitial neuritis may be produced also by syphilis, notably in the cranial nerves at the base of the brain. In any form of meningitis, the inflammatory change may spread to and affect the emerging nerves or roots. There is described also a senile form of chronic neuritis, in which there is sclerosis of the interstitial tissue with involvement of the nerve fibres. This is the result of advanced arterial disease, which interferes with the blood supply and causes fibrous atrophy.

Acute infective polyneuritis, often known as the Landry–Guillain–Barré syndrome, is the most important type of true neuritis. Its incidence is greatest in young adults and it usually follows a mild "non-specific" febrile illness. There is symmetrical progressive ascending paralysis usually commencing in the lower limbs and then spreading to the arms, the trunk, and the cranial nerves. Sensory disturbance is absent or only mild. Provided the patient can be tided over the acute phase, if necessary with the aid of artificial ventilation, a progressive slow recovery over a period of weeks or months is to be expected. Sudden death occurs in a proportion of cases and this is often attributable to a true myocarditis. In a fatal case the main *structural alterations* are seen in the proximal parts of spinal nerve roots where there is oedema of the nerve, infiltration by lymphocytes and plasma cells, and varying degree of damage to myelin and axons. The cerebrospinal fluid shows a highly characteristic dissociation of protein and cell count, the protein rising to as much as 800 mg. per 100 ml. while the cell count remains normal. This disease has been likened to the allergic neuritis that can be produced experimentally in animals by injecting homogenates or extracts of nerve tissue incorporated in Freund's adjuvant. This experimental disease has much in common with experimental allergic encephalo-myelitis (p. 647), and it may be that the human condition is an auto-immune disease of the delayed hypersensitivity type. The presence of antibody reactive with neural tissue has been detected in patient's serum early in the disease, but it did not react specifically with peripheral nerve.

Pathological changes in the nervous system in association with malignant tumours

The nervous system may be implicated by malignant tumours arising elsewhere by direct or metastatic invasion of the brain, cord and peripheral nerves, or by compression of the cord by extradural deposits. Recently, however, functional damage to the nervous system by some metabolic or toxic factors has been recognised in the absence of direct neoplastic infiltration. The commonest of these derangements is peripheral neuropathy which may be predominantly motor or sensory, or of mixed type. The most conspicuous histological abnormalities in the cases with sensory symptoms are loss of neurones in the dorsal root ganglia and degeneration of the dorsal roots, posterior columns and peripheral nerves. In predominantly motor neuropathies, histological changes are usually slight although there may be a varying degree of atrophy of muscle fibres. Other conditions in this group are a myasthenic syndrome, a diffuse encephalo-myelitis characterised by intense perivascular cuffing by lymphocytes, and subacute cerebellar atrophy characterised by an extensive loss of Purkinje cells, degeneration of the dentate nuclei and of the long tracts—motor and sensory—in the spinal cord. These changes are found most often in, but are not confined to, cases of bronchial carcinoma. The neurological symptoms not infrequently ante-date local ones caused by the tumour itself. In long-standing malignant reticuloses, and in widespread involvement of the reticulo-endothelial system by other conditions, e.g. carcinomatosis and sarcoidosis, the brain may show many irregularly disposed areas of demyelination and an unusually severe degree of astrocytic hyperplasia. The term *progressive multifocal leukoencephalopathy* is applied to this condition.

Congenital abnormalities of the brain and spinal cord

Brain. Defects of the brain are of considerable variety and the anatomical changes are often of a complicated nature; we can only summarise the main facts. *Anencephaly* is a condition in which there is deficiency of the cranial vault with absence of the brain, although there is often a small sac with remains of cerebral tissue on the exposed base of the cranial cavity, the base also being deficient in size. The condition, which is incompatible with life, is not infrequently associated with non-closure of the spinal canal or *rachischisis*.

Occasionally there is a deficiency in the cranial bones and a sac-like protrusion is present. This occurs in the line of a suture, is often median in position and as a rule occipital; or it may be lateral, e.g. at the side of an orbit or the nose. The sac is lined in some instances by the meninges and contains merely cerebrospinal fluid; the term *meningocele* is then applied. In other cases the sac is lined by neural tissue and sometimes when the defect is posterior, may contain a considerable part of the cerebrum; the condition is then known as *encephalocele*. The term *micrencephaly* means a congenital smallness of the brain. There is deficiency in the convolutions, and the sulci, especially the secondary, are imperfectly formed; the state is associated with a greater or lesser degree of idiocy. The whole brain may be abnormal, but as a rule the cerebellum and brain stem are less affected than the hemispheres. Sometimes again, there is a local defect in growth, often associated with a small size of the convolutions or *microgyria*. There is no doubt that micrencephaly is a primary defect in the growth of the brain, though its cause is not known, and it is not due to early closure of the sutures, as was once supposed. The term *porencephaly* is applied when part of the brain is replaced by a collection of fluid, covered by meninges and sometimes in communication with the ventricles. Two varieties of the condition are distinguished, namely, a primary or developmental form and a secondary. In the former, the defect is due to failure of growth or *agenesia*, and the edges of the space are usually smooth. Such a condition is occasionally bilateral and is sometimes associated with other abnormalities. In the secondary form, the lesion is supposed to be the result of encephalitis, e.g. toxoplasmosis, or of interference with the blood supply during intra-uterine life, and a somewhat similar condition may result from injury at the time of birth.

Spinal cord. A fairly common abnormality is non-closure of the spinal canal, or *rachischisis*, in which there is a local deficiency in the arches of the vertebrae, whilst the opening is covered posteriorly by soft tissues. The term *spina bifida* is applied to such a condition; a distinct rounded projection is usually present over the site of the defect, which is then known as *spina bifida cystica*. When there is no such projection the term *spina bifida occulta* is applied.

The commonest position of spina bifida is in the lumbo-sacral region, and in all cases the spinal cord extends to a lower level than the normal; in other words, it remains in the position it normally occupies only in the earlier stages of development. The cord and meninges are variously disposed in different cases. In the commonest form, the spinal cord is adherent to the posterior wall of the sac and the term *meningomyelocele* is applied. The dura mater is absent in the sac, and at the apex of the latter there is often an area where the skin is deficient. At this point there is a smooth membrane in which the spinal cord is incorporated, the cord being open posteriorly, and sometimes one or two small depressions are present, the latter indicating the upper and lower terminations of the central canal. The spinal nerves are spread out on the inner lining of the sac. In another rare form, the space containing the fluid is a distension of the central canal of the spinal cord and is lined by the epithelium of the ependyma. In this variety, which is called *myelocystocele* or *syringomyelocele*, the spinal cord has been closed in posteriorly, and thus the abnormality has arisen at a later period of development than the previous form. In a third variety, which is the least common, the sac is lined by a hernial protrusion of the arachnoid, whilst the spinal cord is in its normal position in relation to the vertebrae. This is called *meningocele*. In all three varieties the dura mater is absent locally. In spina bifida the sac contains cerebrospinal fluid. In the first variety, the fluid is in the subarachnoid space in front of the spinal cord; in the second, it is in the dilated canal of the cord, and in the third, it is in the subarachnoid space behind the cord.

The more severe forms of meningomyelocele are almost invariably associated with hydrocephalus and the Arnold–Chiari malformation (p. 613).

In *spina bifida occulta*, where there is no swelling to indicate the defect, the skin over the part usually shows abnormalities in appearance, and not infrequently there is excessive growth of hair on it. Here, also, the cord extends to a lower level in the spinal canal than normally. Abnormalities in connection with the central canal have already been described (see syringomyelia, p. 660).

Tuberous sclerosis. In this disorder multiple foci of hyperplasia of neuroglia and nerve cells occur in the cortex of the brain and in the subependymal tissue, in association with rhabdomyoma of the heart muscle (p. 325), adenoma sebaceum and other congenital abnormalities, the condition being known as tuberous sclerosis. In a few cases one or more of the glial foci give rise to a distinctive giant-celled type of astrocytoma.

TUMOURS OF BRAIN AND SPINAL CORD

Tumours of the central nervous system are comparatively common and of many types. They may originate from the meninges or nerve sheaths, or from the neural tissue proper of the brain and spinal cord: most tumours of neural tissue arise from the neuroglia.

Tumours of the meninges

The common tumour of this class is the *meningioma*, which takes origin from the arachnoid granulations (Fig. 20.64).

Meningiomas vary greatly in character, some being relatively hard or gritty, others less fibrous

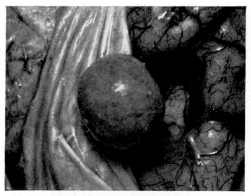

FIG. 20.65.—Meningioma attached to dura mater, showing the typical depression of the cerebral cortex from which the tumour is readily withdrawn. × 1.

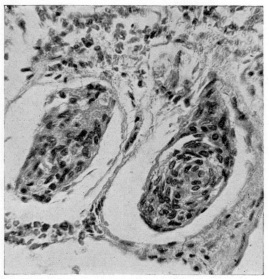

FIG. 20.64.—Two arachnoidal granulations lying in small dural veins.

and softer. In certain situations they may grow to a remarkable size before causing symptoms. They are solid lobulated tumours, well demarcated from the brain tissue in which they excavate a bed, and are, as a rule, firmly attached by a broad base to the dura. They are benign, and thus can sometimes be successfully removed surgically. They tend to be related to major venous sinuses and commonly arise parasagittally (Fig. 20.65) or on the base of the skull, where they may originate in the region of the olfactory groove and grow into the fissure between the frontal lobes (Fig. 20.66). Another common site is the sphenoidal ridge. Rarely a

meningioma may arise from the tela choroidea and appear as an intraventricular tumour. Frequently a meningioma infiltrates the overlying bone like a malignant tumour and gives rise to considerable thickening of the bone in relation to it. Metastases are very rare; most occur in the lungs when the tumour has spread into the soft tissues of the scalp after craniotomy, but a few have followed invasion of a venous sinus.

The *spinal meningiomas* correspond in their general characters, but, owing to their situation, are of smaller size (Fig. 20.67). They are intra-dural tumours which arise most frequently on the postero-lateral aspect of the cord, and the disturbances at first are chiefly sensory—pain, paraesthesia, etc. At a later period various effects up to complete paraplegia may result from pressure on the cord.

Microscopically the meningiomas show considerable variation in histological structure, the

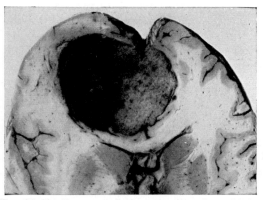

FIG. 20.66.—Large meningioma between frontal lobes.

most common variety being composed of a fibro-cellular tissue with a somewhat whorled appearance owing to the concentric arrangement of the cells (Fig. 20.68). In some the centres of the whorls contain small blood vessels, but others undergo hyaline change and become calcified, resulting in a hard gritty mass containing numerous spherical calcified particles—the *psam-*

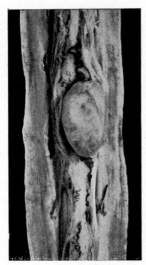

FIG. 20.67.—Spinal meningioma compressing cord. × ¾.

moma or *brain-sand tumour* (Fig. 20.69). In the more cellular varieties the whorls are composed of rather plump spindle-shaped cells resembling endothelium, but all degrees of transition to the fibrous type are encountered. The cellular type of tumour which invades the overlying bone, giving rise to hyperostosis, may subsequently spread into the surrounding tissues.

Sarcoma very occasionally arises from the meninges and extends widely over its surface. Some very highly cellular and rapidly growing meningiomas resemble spindle-celled sarcomas, but in children there are also rare pleomorphic sarcomas of uncertain origin. Occasionally a primary *melanoma* occurs as a diffusely spreading tumour in the meninges.

Tumours of vascular origin

Tumours of vascular origin are uncommon, forming about 2 per cent of cerebral tumours. They are divided into (1) *angiomatous malformations*, and (2) the *haemangioblastomas* or true neoplasms of blood-vessel elements. The former are not true tumours but are similar to vascular

hamartomas elsewhere. They may be chiefly capillary, venous, or arterio-venous, and their principal importance is as a cause of subarachnoid, intracerebral or intraventricular haemorrhage.

The true vascular tumours, which occur most frequently in the cerebellum, are composed of vascular channels or spaces (Fig. 20.70), between which there is a large accumulation of lipid-laden cells with a peculiar and abundant network of reticulin fibres between them. There is a marked tendency to cyst formation; transudation of fluid occurs into the tissue and forms a space or spaces containing fluid and lined with compressed neuroglia, the tumour being represented by a mural nodule. A peculiar syndrome in which one of the latter growths is present has

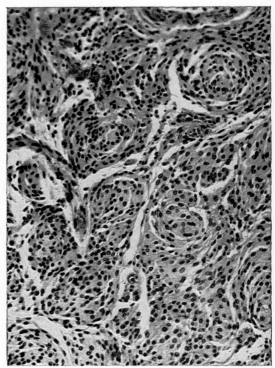

FIG. 20.68.—Section of meningioma of common cellular type showing the arrangement of cells and fibres in whorls. × 190.

been described by Lindau and is now known as Lindau's disease. In association with the growth there may be capillary angiomatosis in other parts of the nervous system and in the retina; there are also lesions which are not of vascular nature—cysts in the pancreas (p. 599) or kidneys, and adenomas in the kidneys or adrenals.

Tumours of neuro-ectodermal origin

The term is used in the strict sense to include all the tumours which arise from the primitive medullary epithelium. In the central nervous system these cells are represented firstly by the neuroglia, i.e. astrocytes, oligodendrocytes and

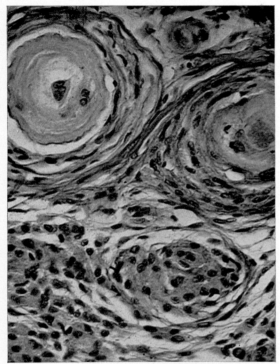

FIG. 20.69.—Meningioma, showing fibrocellular masses with concentric arrangement and formation of psammoma bodies × 350.

ependymal cells, and secondly by nerve cells. In their pioneer work, Bailey and Cushing classified neuroectodermal tumours on the basis of the similarity of the constituent cells to the different morphological stages observed in neuro-ectodermal cells in their embryogenesis, and most current classifications are based on this scheme. Opinion varies on certain points of nomenclature but one concept is that three main cell types take origin from the medullary epithelium, viz. (1) the primitive spongioblast, (2) an undifferentiated cell often referred to as the medulloblast, and (3) the neuroblast.

From the primitive spongioblast arise the cells of the astroglia which are formed through intermediate stages of apolar and polar spongioblasts and astroblasts, the adult cells being the

protoplasmic and fibrillary astrocytes (p. 607). The ependymal cell is derived from the medullary epithelial cells which remain attached to the internal limiting membrane of the neural tube and has as its immediate progenitor the ependymal spongioblast. They line the ventricles and the central canal of the spinal cord. The "medulloblast" gives origin to the cells of the oligodendroglia and probably also to astroblasts and neuroblasts (opinion varies on this point). The neuroblasts are at first apolar, and then pass through the stages of polar neuroblasts to form the adult nerve cells or neurones.

The gliomas

Nearly all neuroectodermal tumours are derived from the neuroglia and they are referred to collectively as the *gliomas*. Some are mature tumours composed of cells that have a fairly close resemblance to astrocytes, oligodendrocytes or ependymal cells, the respective tumours being called *astrocytoma, oligodendroglioma* and *ependymoma*. Secondly, there are tumours in which only a proportion of the cells are of this

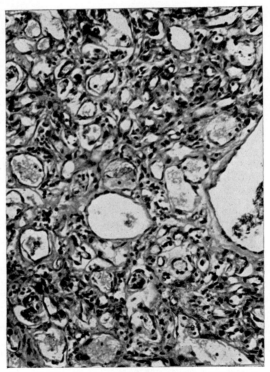

FIG. 20.70.—Haemangioblastoma of the cerebellum in a case of Lindau's disease. × 130.

type, the others being pleomorphic and less well differentiated: these are referred to as the *anaplastic* variants of these tumours. Finally there is a glioma where the cytological features are those of poor differentiation and anaplasia throughout, to which the term *glioblastoma multiforme* may be applied.

As in other tissues, the general rule usually applies that the more primitive or undiffer-

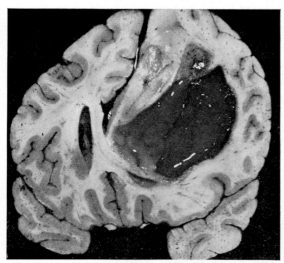

FIG. 20.71.—Cystic astrocytoma in right frontal lobe. Tumour tissue is identifiable adjacent to the upper pole of the cyst.

entiated the cells are, the more rapid is their growth, but in contrast to tumours in other systems the terms "benign" and "malignant" have a new connotation. All the tumours in this group, whether cytologically benign or malignant, infiltrate the adjacent brain tissue and are never truly sharply demarcated or encapsulated. Paradoxically the rapidly growing anaplastic forms appear to be the better demarcated, because they also compress and push aside surrounding tissues. Further, the intracranial neuro-ectodermal tumours *do not metastasise to other organs*, except in very rare cases, usually after craniotomy. They may however be disseminated by the cerebrospinal fluid to other parts of the nervous system. The terms "benign" and "malignant" therefore refer in this context purely to the degree of cellular differentiation and rate of growth.

The commonest gliomas are astrocytoma and glioblastoma multiforme.

Astrocytoma. This is a slowly growing whitish tumour, very badly defined at the margin where it merges with the surrounding nervous tissue. The consistency of the tumour varies with the number of glial fibres in it; if abundant, it is tough, almost rubbery; if scanty it is soft, often oedematous and then undergoes softening, cyst-like spaces thus resulting (Fig. 20.71). The cerebellar astrocytoma of childhood has a notable tendency to become grossly cystic.

In a fibrillary astrocytoma, microscopic examination shows unevenly distributed and often loosely arranged elongated cells separated by glial fibrils (Fig. 20.72). Even in the absence of gross cystic change there are often numerous microcysts. Sometimes the brain tissue is diffusely permeated by tumour astrocytes, often with remarkable preservation of nerve cells and fibres. The edge of this type of tumour often defies recognition with the naked eye. It is referred to as *diffuse astrocytoma* (formerly known as gliomatosis) and is a particularly common type of astrocytoma in the brain stem and spinal cord. Other rarer forms of astrocy-

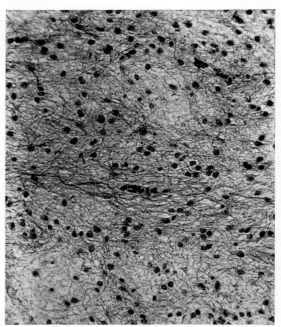

FIG. 20.72.—Astrocytoma of relatively low cellularity showing well formed glial fibrils. × 225. (PTAH).

toma are composed of protoplasmic astrocytes or swollen, so-called gemistocytic astrocytes.

All astrocytomas display a marked propensity to become anaplastic: this may be restricted to one part of the tumour or it may be multifocal.

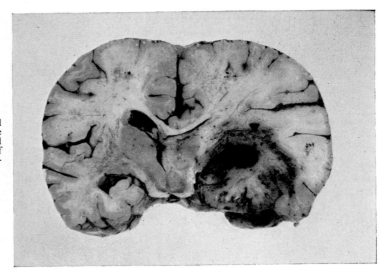

FIG. 20.73.—Glioblastoma multiforme of temporal lobe.

Note the well-defined margin and haemorrhagic areas within the tumour. There is a pronounced midline shift, virtual obliteration of the lateral ventricle and a supra-callosal hernia.

To the naked eye the anaplastic areas are haemorrhagic and necrotic and often appear to have a relatively well-defined edge. The microscopic features of these areas are similar to those seen in glioblastoma multiforme.

Glioblastoma multiforme. This is a tumour of adult life and occurs most frequently in the cerebral hemispheres forming a rapidly growing, apparently relatively well-defined mass with extensive necrosis and haemorrhage. It produces considerable distortion of the brain and often a rapid increase in intracranial pressure (Figs. 20.2, 20.73).

On microscopic examination the tumour is richly cellular in the areas that are not necrotic and there are great variations in cell type ranging from closely packed masses of small anaplastic cells to bizarre giant cells (Fig. 20.74). Mitoses are often frequent and glial fibrils extremely scanty. Small vessels in and around the tumour may show curious bud-like or "glomeruloid" endothelial proliferations (Fig. 20.75). Necrosis is pronounced within the tumour and frequently slightly elongated cells form a palisade around necrotic foci (Fig. 20.76).

As has been already mentioned, foci with appearances identical to glioblastoma multiforme may occur within an anaplastic astrocytoma.

Ependymoma. This not uncommon tumour is most frequently encountered in children, most often in the fourth ventricle but it may also occur in the other ventricles. The tumour cells often have a distinctly epithelial appearance and they are characteristically orientated around small blood vessels but are separated from them by an eosinophilic fibrillary band (Fig. 20.77). Less frequently columnar cells form small canaliculi (Fig. 20.78), and near the free edge of these cells there may be small rod-shaped blepharoplasts. Ependymomas may also become anaplastic as shown by the occurrence of cellular pleomorphism and poor differentiation, haemorrhage and necrosis: the term ependymoblastoma is sometimes applied. Closely related to the

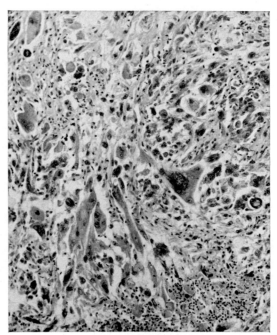

FIG. 20.74.—Glioblastoma multiforme showing many aberrant giant cells. × 95.

ependymoma is the *papillary tumour of the choroid plexus.* This is again most frequently seen in children when it forms a rounded bulky tumour usually in one lateral ventricle. The papillae have a vascular connective tissue core covered by columnar epithelium very similar in appearance to normal choroid plexus epithelium (Fig. 20.79). It frequently causes hydrocephalus.

There is also a curious type of tumour arising from the filum terminale, known as *myxopapillary ependymoma.* It is a slowly growing, markedly gelatinous tumour that occurs in adults,

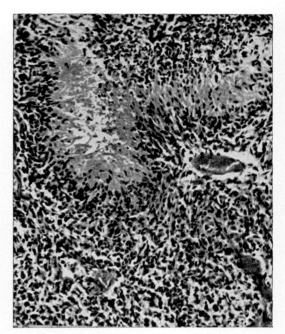

FIG. 20.76.—Glioblastoma multiforme, showing a common pattern of central necrosis with peripheral palisading of spindle-shaped cells. × 130.

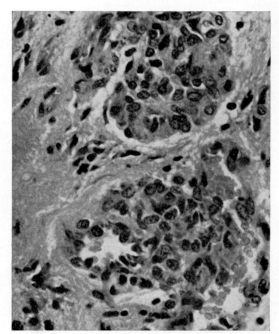

FIG. 20.75.—Glomeruloid endothelial proliferation in glioblastoma. × 390.

and gradually ensheathes the nerve roots of the cauda equina and the caudal part of the spinal cord. The stroma consists of a central vascular core surrounded by very mucoid connective tissue and covered in places by a cubical epithelium (Fig. 20.80); elsewhere the covering cells may form a network between the papillae. This tumour may cause pressure atrophy of the adjacent bones and may even invade them; it is then liable to be mistaken for chordoma (p. 788).

Oligodendroglioma. In our experience this glioma is rarer than ependymoma. It occurs in the cerebral hemispheres, is a slowly growing, rather gelatinous tumour, and commonly exhibits numerous small foci of calcification which

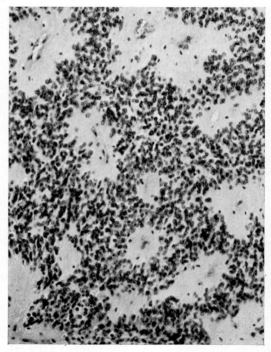

FIG. 20.77.—Ependymoma. Note the perivascular fibrillary halo that is particularly characteristic of ependymoma. × 125.

show on X-ray examination. The cells are uniform, small and rounded, like those of the oligodendroglia, with somewhat clear cytoplasm and distinct cell-membranes. Cell processes are small and difficult to demonstrate (Fig. 20.81). As with other gliomas, anaplastic change may occur in these tumours.

The principal characters of the commoner gliomas have now been described but many clearly defined variants have not been mentioned. It would be wrong to suggest that every glioma

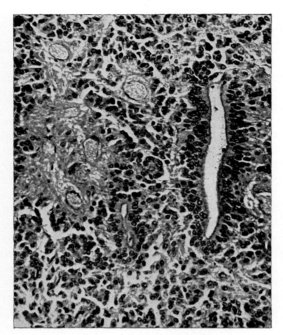

FIG. 20.78.—Ependymoma showing a canaliculus lined by columnar ciliated cells. × 180.

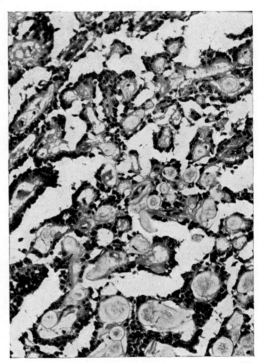

FIG. 20.80.—Myxopapillary ependymoma, a papillary structure with very gelatinous stroma, covered by a mainly cubical epithelium. × 115.

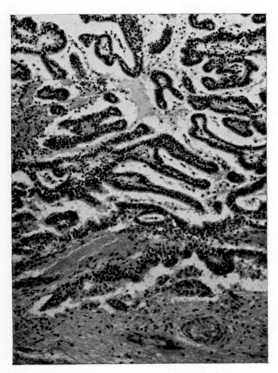

FIG. 20.79.—Papillary tumour of the choroid plexus, showing delicate papillary processes covered by cubical epithelium. × 100.

can be easily assigned to a specific category. Indeed a comprehensive microscopic examination of any glioma may result in the identification of various types of tumour and the name applied comes to depend on the most prominent element. Furthermore each main division tends to exist as a spectrum; at one end there is a mature well-differentiated tumour composed of cells similar to normal glial cells in many respects, while at the other there is a highly anaplastic and poorly differentiated tumour. As all gliomas infiltrate into the adjacent brain, particularly the better differentiated types, total surgical excision is rarely feasible: radiotherapy is also at best palliative and the ultimate prognosis for a patient with a glioma is usually poor.

Tumours of the neurone series

These include tumours composed of primitive cells, namely medulloblastoma, neuroblastoma and retinoblastoma and of mature ganglion cells —the ganglioneuroma, the last being an exceed-

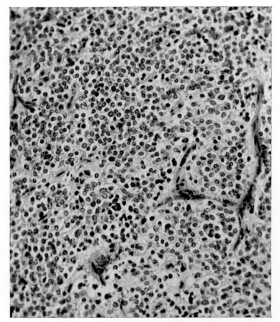

FIG. 20.81.—Oligodendroglioma. The tumour is very cellular, the cells being round or oval with distinct cell boundaries. × 115.

ingly rare finding in the central nervous system.

Medulloblastoma. This not uncommon tumour of childhood is composed of undifferentiated primitive cells. It is a rapidly growing cellular tumour, restricted to the cerebellum where it forms a soft greyish-white mass protruding into the fourth ventricle. Commonly it spreads over the surface of the cerebellum as a thin sheet that obscures the normal surface architecture. Seeding of tumour cells by the cerebrospinal fluid may result in diffuse implantation but sometimes only small secondary nodules develop on the nerve roots of the cauda equina.

Microscopically, its cells are either spherical with little cytoplasm and no fibrils, or somewhat triangular, like short carrots, and arranged

around blood vessels and also as circles and rosettes without a central cavity (Fig. 20.82).

Neuroblastoma and ganglioneuroma. It is convenient to consider these together; they are rare in the central nervous system and occur principally in the sympathetic chain and its derivatives.

Neuroblastoma and *sympathicoblastoma* are tumours of virtually identical cytological character. The more common sympathicoblastic peripheral tumour may occur in many situations but is seen most frequently in the adrenal medulla and sympathetic chain in infants and children. It forms a bulky soft cellular and haemorrhagic tumour with extensive necrosis, which destroys the adrenal, spreads rapidly to the upper abdominal lymph nodes, to the liver and notably to the skeleton, secondary tumours in the skull being especially frequent. Occasionally the tumour cells have in places undergone further differentiation to imperfectly formed ganglion cells so that some areas may have a ganglioneuromatous appearance.

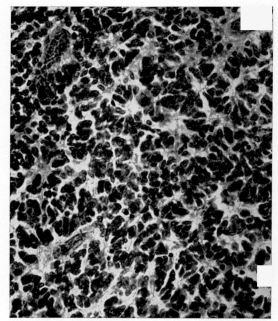

FIG. 20.82.—Medulloblastoma. The cells are small and closely packed, but form poorly defined rosettes. × 225.

On *microscopic examination*, the cells are small, round or oval, with little cytoplasm. In many parts they are irregularly arranged, while in places they may form small ball-like masses of cells which sometimes show further differentiation into rings or rosettes, the central part of the ring being occupied by a large number of fine fibrils which give, somewhat imperfectly, the staining reactions of nerve fibrils with silver impregnation. The cells surrounding such rosettes are radially arranged, tail-like prolongations of the cytoplasm projecting into the centre to form the fibrillary network (Fig. 20.83). These structures are closely similar to the clumps

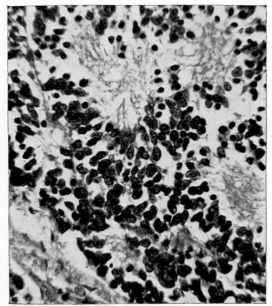

FIG. 20.83.—Sympathicoblastoma. Many of the cells are carrot-shaped and are arranged in well-defined rosettes, the centres of which contain the fine fibrils prolonged from the tapering cells. × 350.

of neuroblasts which grow out to form the sympathetic system, as can be well seen in the fetal adrenal when it is becoming invaded by neuroblasts to form the medulla of the gland. Rests of undifferentiated neuroblasts are occasionally found in the adrenal medulla in infancy (Fig. 20.84). We have also seen two tumours composed of neuroblasts and partially differentiated ganglion cells in the pineal region in infants (Fig. 20.85).

Tumours occur also in the adrenal medulla, the origin of which has been traced to the chromaffin cells; to such growths the term *paraganglioma* or *phaeochromocytoma* has been applied. These are usually benign but may cause severe symptoms by secreting catecholamines in excessive amounts. They are described in connection with the adrenal glands (p. 917).

Ganglioneuroma. Tumours of this nature are of rare occurrence, but numerous examples have been found in connection with the sympathetic system, in the abdomen, thorax, and cervical region, and in many instances have arisen from the adrenal medulla; a few have also been recorded in connection with peripheral nerves. Occasionally there occur in the cerebral hemispheres single or multiple nodules composed of neuroglia, in which a considerable number of nerve cells may be present, these apparently forming part of the tumour; such tumours, more accurately termed ganglioglioma, also may be regarded as a variety of ganglioneuroma. A ganglioneuroma in connection with the sympathetic system may form a large mass. It is usually firm, encapsulated like a simple tumour and of rounded or irregular outline. On microscopic examination, it is found to contain well-formed ganglionic nerve cells, irregularly arranged in a finely fibrillar stroma, and also smaller cells of various forms with nuclei of the characteristic type (Fig. 20.86). There are usually also a large number of nerve fibres both myelinated and non-myelinated, and some naked axis cylinders. The tumour is as a rule benign, but occasionally it is associated with a cellular malignant neuroblastoma. All types of tumour, from those composed of mature ganglion cells to those composed

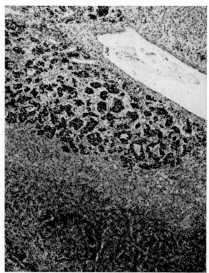

FIG. 20.84.—Adrenal medulla of an infant of 9 months, showing masses of undifferentiated neuroblasts. × 45.

of sympathogonia—the least differentiated type of sympathetic nerve cell—are encountered. The degree of malignancy varies with the stage of differentiation of the tumour cells.

The common embryological background of these various tumours derived from the sym-

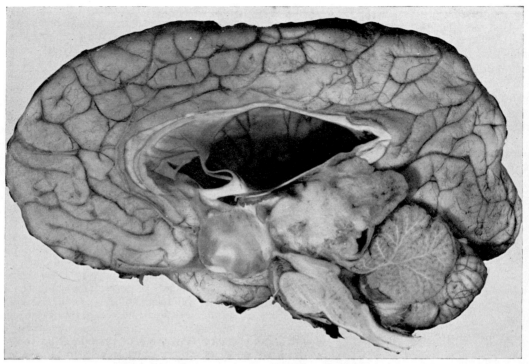

FIG. 20.85.—Neuroblastoma and ganglioneuroma of pineal region, causing pronounced dilatation of the third
and lateral ventricles.

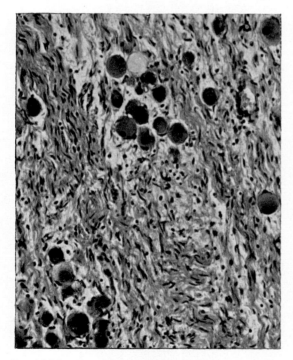

FIG. 20.86.—Ganglioneuroma of adrenal, showing abundant mature ganglion cells and non-myelinated nerve fibres.

pathetic rudiment is emphasised by the fact that certain neuroblastic and ganglionic tumours in infancy unconnected with the adrenals, e.g. in the thorax, may secrete pressor substances, notably dopamine and noradrenaline, causing severe hypertension. These are excreted in the urine respectively as homovanillic acid and vanillin mandelic acid (VMA).

Retinoblastoma. This is a very cellular tumour originating in the retina, usually in the first few years of life. It appears to be the result of a gene mutation, which subsequently behaves as a dominant. It not infrequently develops in both eyes (in 23 per cent of cases, according to Ewing), and tends to appear in more than one member of a family. Occasionally it has been associated with other congenital abnormalities in the eyes. It is composed of small rounded or oval cells with very little cytoplasm and of rather undifferentiated character. A characteristic feature is the presence of small rosettes formed by a circular arrangement of cells of short columnar epithelial type enclosing a lumen (Fig. 20.87), thus differing from the rosettes in neuroblastoma. Rosettes are present in only a proportion of cases, but even when they are absent, the arrangement of the cells is not uniform and traces of such structures may be seen. The tumour may extend through the eyeball to adjacent structures and lead to lymphatic infiltration; it may spread to the optic chiasm and to the other eye and also

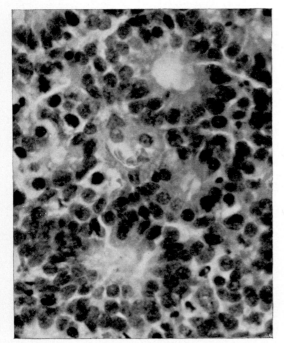

FIG. 20.87.—Retinoblastoma, showing round cells with formation of characteristic rosettes. × 750.

form secondary growths in other organs. On the whole, however, metastases occur late and only in a relatively small proportion of cases. The tumour is sometimes called "retinal neuro-epithelioma".

Tumours arising in developmental defects

Dermoid and epidermoid cysts are occasionally found in connection with the meninges, especially at the base of the brain. The epidermoid cyst is the commoner within the skull, but the dermoid is more frequent in the lower spinal cord region. An epidermoid tumour is well encapsulated, and its substance has a whitish and rather shining appearance (pearly tumour) and a somewhat crumbling character. The wall is thin and is composed of cells of squamous epithelial type from which keratinised squames are shed into the interior where they accumulate, together with crystals of cholesterol, and thus distend the cyst. There is little doubt that it is of epidermoid origin and represents a congenital abnormality. In dermoid cysts hairs and sebaceous glands are present. Inclusion epidermoid cysts in the region of the cauda equina can result from repeated lumbar puncture during childhood.

A somewhat similar tumour, partly cystic, partly solid, is found in children and adults in the region of the pituitary stalk, compressing the gland in the sella turcica and pressing upwards into the third ventricle. Probably these suprasellar growths arise from nests of epidermoid cells derived from the pars tuberalis and they are known as *suprasellar cysts* or *craniopharyngiomas*. Their lining epithelium is in part squamous, but in many there is a partial differentiation towards stellate reticulum resembling enamel organ (Fig. 20.88), and the name *adamantinoma* is sometimes applied. The wall is usually partially calcified. The chief clinical

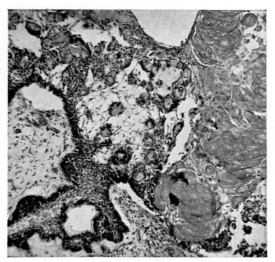

FIG. 20.88.—Craniopharyngioma, showing partly squamous, partly "adamantinomatous" structure.

Note the stellate reticulum within the epithelial bands. × 85.

features are disturbances of vision and of hypophyseal function (p. 883). True Rathke pouch cysts are intrasellar.

Teratomas are rare intracranial tumours, their chief site being the pineal, where, in boys, their occurrence is often associated with precocious sexual development. We have observed two examples of chorion-epithelioma in the pineal without other tissue elements; both were associated with sexual precocity.

Metastatic tumours

Metastatic tumours are very common in the brain and the possibility must be considered that a cerebral tumour which clinically appears to be primary may in fact be a secondary deposit. This occurs most commonly with bronchial carcinoma. Metastatic deposits are typically

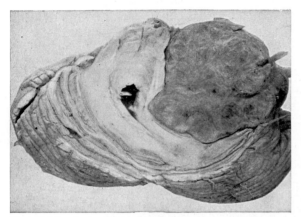

Fig. 20.89.—Large Schwannoma of the auditory nerve in the cerebello-pontine angle, which has caused great displacement of the adjacent structures. $\times \frac{2}{3}$.

multiple and are sharply circumscribed. The tumour cells have a tendency to spread along the perivascular spaces, so that vessels may be ensheathed by them. Not infrequently metastatic carcinoma spreads diffusely throughout the subarachnoid space, often producing the clinical features of a subacute meningitis. This is known as meningeal carcinomatosis, and in such cases it is usually possible to identify tumour cells in the CSF. The brain may also be infiltrated or compressed by tumours arising in the nasopharynx, e.g. lympho-epithelioma, or by a chordoma growing from the basisphenoid. Secondary tumours within the dura of the spinal cord are rare, but extradural spinal metastases are common.

Effects of tumours

Intracranial tumours produce local and general effects on the brain. The latter are due mainly to raised intracranial pressure and the characteristic features are headache, vomiting, papilloedema, and blunting of the intellect. The increase in pressure is brought about by the size of the tumour, by the frequent occurrence of

cerebral oedema around it, and, when the tumour is in a situation to block the free flow of cerebrospinal fluid, by hydrocephalus. The morphological changes brought about in the brain by any intracranial expanding lesion have been fully considered on p. 609. Local effects depend on the site of the tumour and include, for example, focal (Jacksonian) epilepsy, paralysis, and defects in the visual fields.

Tumours of nerve roots and peripheral nerves

These may be solitary or multiple, the latter being especially associated with von Recklinghausen's neurofibromatosis, a disorder inherited as an autosomal dominant. Some of these tumours have the general structure of a fibroma and both hard and soft varieties are seen. These are generally believed to originate from the cells

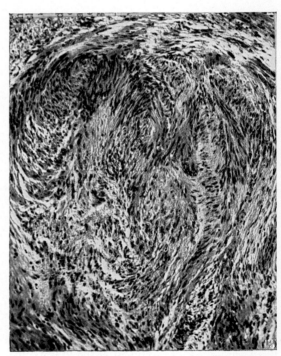

Fig. 20.90.—Schwannoma of acoustic nerve, showing whorling and palisading of cells. $\times$ 100.

of the endoneurium or perineurium and they may be referred to as *neurofibromas*. In others the cells are arranged in a distinctive pattern with their nuclei forming a palisade across the bundles of long spindle cells; these tumours are thought to arise from the neurilemma or Schwann cells and are therefore termed *Schwannomas*. There is, however, still much controversy as to the histogenesis of this group of tumours.

Schwannoma. This is typically a rounded or lobulated, often partly cystic, well circumscribed

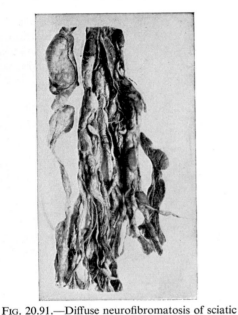

FIG. 20.91.—Diffuse neurofibromatosis of sciatic nerve and its branches.

Note the numerous nodules of various sizes and forms.

and encapsulated tumour arising in relation to a nerve; they may be intracranial, intraspinal or peripheral. Within the cranium the commonest site of origin is the vestibular portion of the auditory nerve, but they also occur in association with the trigeminal nerve. An acoustic Schwannoma ("acoustic neuroma") takes origin just within the internal auditory meatus, which it invariably expands; and the enlargement may be visible radiologically. The tumour fills the cerebello-pontine angle (Fig. 20.89) and produces severe distortion and displacement of the adjacent brain including some degree of hydrocephalus from compression of the fourth ventricle. When bilateral, they are usually associated with von Recklinghausen's disease. In the spinal canal, Schwannomas occur as intradural tumours on the dorsal nerve roots, mostly in the thoracic region. Their main effect is to compress the spinal cord, but they may extend through the intervertebral foramen to produce a much larger intrathoracic portion. On peripheral nerves they may occur as isolated single nodules or they may be multiple. The

nerve fibres tend to be spread over the surface, especially at one side, and are not incorporated in the tumour.

Microscopic examination shows the tumour to be composed of fibro-cellular bundles in a whorled pattern; within the fasciculi, the cells are closely arranged in parallel fashion with their rod-shaped nuclei forming a characteristic "palisade" (Fig. 20.90). In other areas the tumour may be of looser texture or even cystic and contain large numbers of fat-laden foamy cells between the fasciculi. The softer and more cellular tumours are prone to repeated local recurrence with progressive anaplasia, and may become frankly sarcomatous.

Neurofibroma. In some cases, a group of nerves, a plexus, or the sciatic and its branches, may be affected diffusely, and show numerous irregular thickenings with oval or beadlike swellings in their course (Fig. 20.91). There is

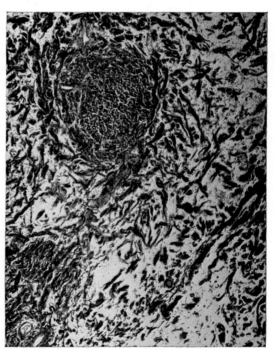

FIG. 20.92.—Plexiform neurofibroma showing nerve fibres surrounded by loosely arranged interlacing connective tissue bundles. × 100.

also the form known as the *plexiform* or *racemose* type, where the nerves of a region, usually the scalp or the neck, show irregular tortuous thickenings which often give rise to firm elevations with a somewhat convoluted appearance. Recently we have observed a remarkable example of this growth involving extensively the wall of the large bowel and rectum (Fig. 20.92). In *general neurofibromatosis* ("*von Recklinghausen's disease*"), nodules of various sizes, sometimes numbering hundreds, occur along small nerve branches, especially of the skin, but also in some cases along the visceral branches of the sympathetic. In this disease, tumours sometimes arise also on the spinal nerves and their roots, within the spinal canal, leading to compression of the spinal cord.

The connective tissue of the nodule varies in character but is often of dense hyaline nature; nerve fibres can be traced running through it. Neurofibromatosis is often associated with multiple pigmented patches in the skin.

Lastly, there is occasionally a localised general thickening of the tissues, with nodulation and folding of the skin—a sort of local elephantiasis, to which the name *elephantiasis neuromatosa* has been applied.

CHAPTER 21

URINARY SYSTEM

THE KIDNEYS

Fine structure and function

The kidneys are each composed of about one million nephrons, the major functions of which are to remove from the plasma various waste products of metabolism, and to maintain fluid and acid–base balances and normal levels of electrolytes. This is achieved by production of a very large volume of glomerular filtrate, which is subject to selective reabsorption as it passes down the tubules, urine representing what must be discarded for homoeostasis. Compared with most other organs, the blood flow of the kidneys is enormous; nearly all of this passes through the glomeruli, where 22 per cent of the plasma volume (550 ml./minute: 800 litres/day) is filtered off, giving a glomerular filtration rate (GFR) of 180 litres per day (125 ml./min.). The process of filtration is doubtless aided by the unusually high pressure in the glomerular capillaries. The capillary walls (Fig. 21.1) consist of the vascular endothelium, which is unusual in having cytoplasmic fenestrations where the capillary basement membrane is lined only by an extremely thin endothelial membrane. Outside the basement membrane is a layer of visceral epithelial cells, termed *podocytes*, cytoplasmic processes (*foot processes* or *pedicels*) of which are in contact with the basement membrane: in the spaces (*slit pores*) between the foot processes the epithelial lining (*slit membrane*) is also extremely thin. Each glomerulus is composed of several lobules, the structure of which is depicted in Fig. 21.2. The capillary loops lie at the periphery of the lobules, while the core is made up of *mesangial cells*, which are capable of collagen production: it contains also basement membrane-like material.

In its passage along the tubules, all but approximately 1·5 litres of the daily 180 litres of glomerular filtrate, and most of its contained solutes, are reabsorbed. This is a process in which the tubule cells exhibit a high degree of selectivity, and some of the fine structural features of the epithelial cells can be related to their special functions. The epithelial cells of the *proximal convoluted tubule* have a prominent brush border, which is seen by electron microscopy to consist of numerous fine, relatively long microvilli (Fig. 21.3): this feature provides a very large surface area for absorption, and four fifths of the fluid in the glomerular filtrate, together with most of its contained glucose, amino-acids, and much of its sodium, potassium and phosphate are reabsorbed here. Reabsorption of these solutes is an active process, requiring energy and this may account for the large number of mitochondria in the epithelial cells. A third feature of these cells is the presence of coiled microtubules, opening into the tubular lumen by pores between the bases of the microvilli: there is normally some leakage of plasma proteins into the glomerular filtrate, and this is apparently taken up into these microtubules, and presumably metabolised by lysosomal enzymes. When, owing to various glomerular lesions, there is increased leakage of protein into the glomerular filtrate, the cells of the proximal convoluted tubules come to contain protein-rich droplets— *hyaline droplets*, due to excessive protein absorption. Finally, the plasma membrane of the basal surface of the cells of the proximal convoluted tubule shows complicated infoldings which have the effect of increasing the surface area, and are probably important in the passage of reabsorbed fluid into the interstitial tissue, whence it enters the peritubular capillaries.

The cells of the descending limb of *Henle's*

loop, and of the thin part of the ascending limb, are relatively simple, and their role in reabsorption is probably largely passive, and dependent on the constitutions of the tubular and interstitial fluids. By contrast, the cells of the thick part of the ascending limb have abundant large mitochondria (Fig. 21.4), and it is probable that these cells actively remove sodium chloride from the tubular fluid and pass it into the interstitial fluid. This has two effects; firstly, it provides a hypertonic interstitial fluid in the renal medulla, and this allows passive reabsorption of water from the descending and thin ascending parts of Henle's limb; secondly, it renders the tubular fluid hypotonic and facilitates further concentration in the distal convoluted tubule. It is probable that aldosterone exerts its sodium-retaining effect by stimulating reabsorption of Na^+ by the cells of the thick part of the ascending limb of Henle's loop. There is evidence that, like sodium chloride, urea undergoes partial recirculation in this counter-current system, thus aiding in passive reabsorption of water. This ingenious

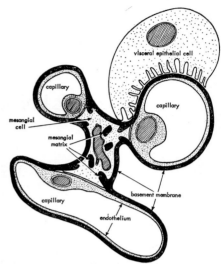

FIG. 21.2.—Diagram of a glomerular lobule in cross section. (The fenestrations in the endothelial cytoplasm are not shown.)

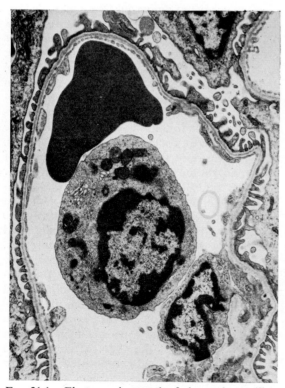

FIG. 21.1.—Electron micrograph of glomerular capillary containing a lymphocyte and red cell. Note, from within outwards, the endothelial cytoplasm with fenestrations, the continuous basement membrane, and the foot processes of the epithelium. × 12,000.

concentrating mechanism was suggested by Wirz (see Black, 1967) and has since received increasing support. The cells of the thick part of Henle's loop, and of the distal convoluted tubule, contain numerous microvesicles, and these may be related to their important functions of deaminating amino-acids to produce ammonia, and of providing free hydrogen ion: secretion of NH_4^+ into the lumen by these cells plays an important role in maintaining acid-base balance, and results in an acid urine. Fluid entering the distal convoluted tubule is hypotonic, and isotonicity is restored here by passive reabsorption of water. As the fluid passes through the medulla in the collecting tubules, passive reabsorption of more water is again possible because the concentrations of sodium chloride and urea in the medullary interstitial fluid are high (see above). It is probable that these final adjustments in concentration are mediated largely by antidiuretic hormone, which presumably renders the cells of the distal convoluted and collecting tubules more permeable to water.

In addition to these complex tubular functions, there is evidence that some substances are removed from the blood and actively secreted by the tubular epithelium. For example, creatinine and K^+ are reabsorbed in the proximal convoluted tubule, and the amounts appearing in the urine are dependent largely on their secretion, probably by the cells of the thick part of the ascending limb of Henle's loop and of the distal convoluted tubule. Excretion of administered diodone by the kidneys is dependent mainly on tubular secretion, and it may be used to assess tubular function.

In addition to their homoeostatic and secretory roles, the kidneys secrete renin, an enzyme which acts on a substrate in the plasma to produce angiotensin. The site of renin secretion is located in the granular cells of the afferent glomerular arterioles, which, together with the *macula densa* and the *lacis*, constitute the juxta-glomerular apparatus (Fig. 8.30, p. 186). Angiotensin has a direct effect on peripheral vascular resistance, and hence on blood pressure, and also stimulates the secretion of aldosterone by the adrenal cortex. These phenomena, and the fine structure of the juxtaglomerular apparatus, are described on pp. 185–7.

Another function of the kidneys, which is discussed in Chapter 16, is the production of *erythropoietin*, a factor stimulating the production of red cells.

Renal clearances. The renal clearance of a

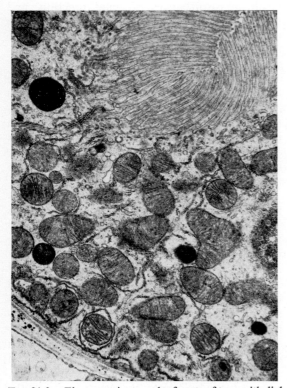

Fig. 21.3.—Electron micrograph of parts of two epithelial cells of the proximal convoluted tubule, showing the microvilli (upper right) and numerous mitochondria. The basal part of the epithelium rests on a thin basement membrane (lower left). × 16,000.

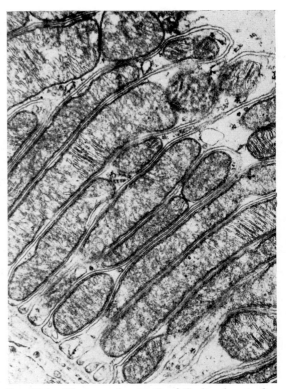

Fig. 21.4.—Electron micrograph of the basal part of an epithelial cell of the thick part of Henle's loop, showing the large, elongated mitochondria situated between infoldings of the basal cytoplasmic membrane (basal part of cell at lower left). × 20,000.

substance is an estimation of the volume of plasma completely cleared of that substance by the kidneys in one minute. It is calculated by measuring its concentration in the plasma (P), in the urine (U), and the volume of the urine (V) in ml. per minute, and applying the formula

$$\text{Clearance} = \frac{U \times V}{P} \text{ ml.}$$

In the case of a substance which passes freely into the glomerular filtrate, and which is neither reabsorbed nor secreted by the tubules, renal clearance is a measure of glomerular filtration rate. This is approximately the case for inulin, which may be administered for the purpose of measuring the renal clearance. Of endogenous substances, clearance of urea is commonly measured, but 30–50 per cent of the urea in the glomerular filtrate is normally reabsorbed, and accordingly the renal urea clearance (approx. 70 ml.) is appreciably below that of inulin (approx. 120 ml.). The clearance of creatinine is similar to that of inulin, but this results from a combination of reabsorption by the proximal tubule and secretion by the distal tubule, and is therefore not always a true indication of glomerular filtration rate in pathological states of the kidney.

Heterogeneity of nephrons. It has long been known that individual nephrons show morphological and circulatory differences—for example, in the length of Henle's loop. Recently, Thurau and his colleagues (see Horster and Thurau, 1968) have shown important functional differences between the majority of nephrons and the one fifth of nephrons originating in glomeruli close to the cortico-medullary junction. By an elaborate technique of micropuncture of individual tubules, they showed differences in glomerular filtration rates, and differences in responses to low and high sodium loading. These findings, based on work on rat kidneys, are likely to apply to the kidneys of other mammals, including man, in which case they will necessitate a reconsideration of various aspects of renal function, both normal and in pathological states, since our present views are based largely on the assumption of a functionally homogeneous population of nephrons.

Important renal diseases

The kidneys are subject to the various general pathological processes which are considered in the earlier chapters of this book. Some of these are without serious effect, e.g. chronic venous congestion or deposition of pigments. Others, such as atrophy and hypertrophy, are of importance, but can be understood from the preceding accounts, and do not require further comment. Some of the general conditions are of particular significance when they affect the kidneys, for example amyloid disease and the various grades of cellular degeneration resulting from injury: these are considered more fully in appropriate sections of this chapter. Inflammatory changes of the kidneys are also of great importance: they include some types of glomerulonephritis. These are of special interest not only because of their serious effects on renal function, but also because there is increasing evidence that antigen–antibody reactions are responsible for the glomerular injuries. Study of both the human diseases and experimental models is throwing new light on the inflammatory process. Bacterial-induced inflammation—pyelonephritis—is also a common and important condition, and

will be described in some detail. Because of their excretory and concentrating role, the kidneys are susceptible to various toxic chemicals, and the brunt of toxic injury usually falls on the tubular epithelium, necrosis of which is a potentially fatal, but often reversible condition. Renal tumours are relatively uncommon, but the commonest malignant tumour—clear-cell renal carcinoma—is important clinically, for early diagnosis and removal carry a fair chance of cure. Finally, renal homotransplantation, now practised widely, is meeting with a high success rate, at least for the first year or two following transplantation; one of the major hazards is immunological rejection of the transplanted kidney by the host, and a knowledge of its destructive effects on the transplant is important (p. 112).

Pathological physiology of renal disease

Many of the diseases described in this chapter result in disturbances of renal function, and these are considered in more detail later. The three major disturbances which are responsible for most of the clinical features of renal diseases are as follows.

(1) Impairment of blood flow through the kidneys can result in arterial hypertension (*secondary* or *renal hypertension*): this is encountered commonly in glomerular disease, but can result from extensive renal scarring from various causes, and also from an extra-renal lesion, e.g. narrowing of the main renal artery by an atheromatous patch in the aorta.

(2) *Renal failure* ("uraemia") with accumulation in the body of urea and other nitrogenous waste products, disturbances of water and acid/base balances and of electrolyte levels, can result from a reduced glomerular filtration rate, from tubular injury, or from a combination of both. Since lesions which impair renal blood flow reduce the glomerular filtration rate, it is not surprising that renal failure and hypertension are commonly associated.

(3) There are a number of diseases which injure the glomerular capillaries and render them abnormally permeable to plasma proteins; heavy and prolonged albuminuria results in fall of the level of plasma albumin, and this can set in motion a train of events leading to generalised oedema. The combination of proteinuria,

hypoalbuminaemia and oedema is known as the *nephrotic syndrome*.

Urinary casts. Increased leakage of plasma proteins into the glomerular filtrate results in proteinuria, most of the escaping protein being albumin. This is accompanied by the formation in the distal tubules of solid, cylindrical-shaped bodies, termed casts (Fig. 21.5), the presence of which in the urine indicates that the proteinuria is attributable to a renal lesion. When the proteinuria is unaccompanied by escape of cells in the urine, the casts are transparent and are termed *hyaline*, *colloid*, or *protein* casts; their solid component consists largely of a protein—*Tamm–Horsfall protein*—which is probably secreted normally by the epithelium of the distal convoluted tubule, and is precipitated to form casts by the presence of plasma albumin in the tubular fluid. When proteinuria is accompanied by escape of inflammatory cells into the tubular fluid, or desquamation of tubular epithelial cells, these become incorporated into the casts, giving *cellular casts* when the cells are largely intact and *granular* casts when the cells are disrupted. Similarly *blood casts* result from incorporation of red cells escaping into the glomerular filtrate or tubule, and *pigmented*

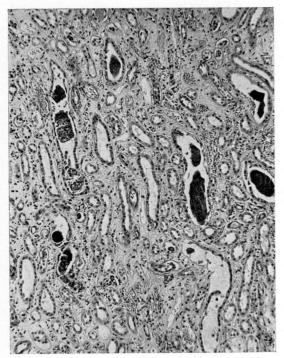

FIG. 21.5.—Casts in the distal and collecting tubules. × 90.

casts from incorporation of bilirubin when proteinuria accompanies regurgitative jaundice, or haemoglobin or myoglobin in conditions giving rise to haemolysis or breakdown of skeletal muscle respectively.

Renal changes in hypertension

The general features of hypertension and the associated vascular changes, namely arteriosclerosis and arteriolosclerosis, have already been described (pp. 270—3). The latter are usually more pronounced in the blood vessels of the kidneys than in other organs, and result in various grades of renal injury. In benign essential hypertension, the renal injury is generally slight, and renal failure does not usually occur, but quite commonly there is some scarring of the kidneys. By contrast, the renal vascular lesions in malignant essential hypertension are severe, and renal failure is a common termination unless the blood pressure can be reduced.

Chronic glomerulonephritis and certain other diseases of the kidneys can result in hypertension—secondary hypertension, and when this occurs further renal injury ensues, indistinguishable from that seen in benign or malignant essential (i.e. primary) hypertension. A complex picture results, and it is advantageous to consider first the pure lesions of essential hypertension before proceeding to the pathology of the various renal diseases which are complicated by secondary hypertension.

Benign essential hypertension

Pathological changes. The renal changes in this disease are attributable to ischaemia resulting from arteriosclerosis and arteriolosclerosis (p. 270).

The larger arteries in the kidneys, as elsewhere, become rigid and thickened, but their lumina are not seriously reduced, and may be enlarged. Similar changes occur in the arcuate arteries, but owing to their smaller calibre, thickening of the wall may result in reduction of the lumen: this is not uniform, and since the arcuates are, in effect, end arteries, ischaemia of patches of cortical tissue, seen as coarse depressed scars, may result. More commonly, ischaemia results from changes in the smaller vessels: the interlobular arteries become elongated and tortuous, with medial fibrosis and fibro-elastic thickening of the intima resulting in significant narrowing of the lumen. The afferent glomerular arterioles are also tortuous and show patchy hyaline thickening, the wall being converted to acellular, homogeneous, eosinophilic, rather transparent material, with various degrees of luminal narrowing (Fig. 21.6). Regarding the nature of hyaline arteriolar thickening, Lendrum (1969)

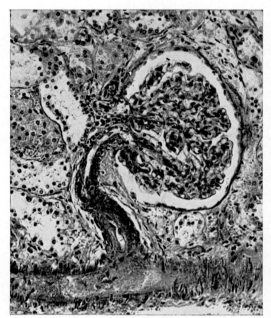

Fig. 21.6.—Benign essential hypertension, showing great hyaline thickening of an afferent arteriole. × 180.

has shown that at an early stage the hyaline material has the staining reactions of fibrin, and that as it ages the staining reactions come to resemble those of collagen. He has suggested that increased permeability of the vascular endothelium allows exudation of plasma constituents and that these form the hyaline material. He has termed the process *plasmatic vasculosis* and the older hyaline material *pseudocollagen*. This interpretation is now supported by histochemical, immunofluorescence, and electron microscopic studies, and provides a satisfactory explanation of the observed changes. These changes result in glomerular ischaemia, the glomerular tuft becoming shrunken and the capillaries gradually replaced by pale-staining homogeneous material, until eventually the whole tuft is converted to an acellular hyaline sphere (Fig. 21.7). This change is often accompanied by obliteration of the capsular space.

The related tubules become atrophic and inconspicuous, and fibrous tissue, often infiltrated by lymphocytes, develops between the affected tubules and glomeruli. These changes in the small vessels, and consequent loss of nephrons and scarring, are distributed randomly throughout the cortex of both kidneys. It is probable that the arteriolar changes are more important than those in the interlobular arteries, for the destruction of nephrons does not follow a

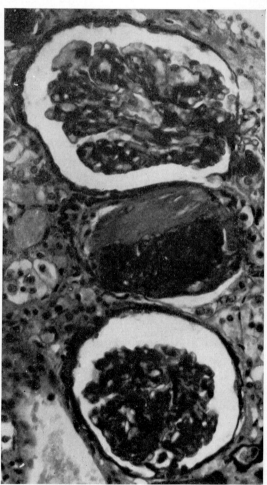

Fig. 21.7.—Kidney in benign essential hypertension. Of the three glomeruli, two show partial hyalinisation and collapse of the tuft. The third (middle) glomerulus is completely hyalinised and is seen as a solid pellet, composed partly of collagen (lighter area) and partly of collapsed, hyaline tuft (darker area). × 150.

lobular pattern, but affects single scattered nephrons, while those around may appear healthy.

The destruction of nephrons described above

proceeds very slowly, and at necropsy the kidneys may appear macroscopically normal apart from thickening of the arteries on the cut surface. However, enough nephrons are commonly lost to cause a slight reduction in size and slight diffuse thinning of the cortex: the capsule may be somewhat adherent, and the subcapsular surface diffusely and finely irregular (*granular*), contraction of scarred areas resulting in fine depressions (Fig. 21.8). In some longstanding cases, a sufficient number of nephrons may be lost to stimulate hypertrophy in those remaining, and the enlarged, hypertrophied tubules then contribute to the surface granularity (Fig. 21.9), but the kidneys are seldom greatly reduced in size, and renal function is not significantly impaired. In those patients who develop heart failure, the blood urea often rises, but this is attributable to inadequate renal blood flow, and is reversible if cardiac output again improves.

Malignant essential hypertension

This may arise *de novo*, usually at 35–45 years of age, or may supervene on benign essential hypertension. In the former case, the kidneys are of normal size, and the subcapsular surface is smooth and spotted with dark red areas due to patches of congestion and haemorrhage. The main renal, segmental and arcuate arteries show

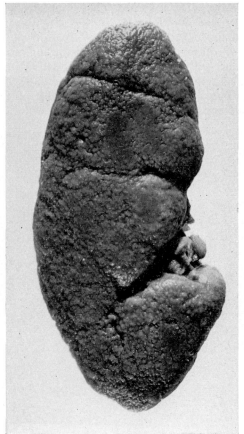

FIG. 21.8.—Kidney in longstanding benign essential hypertension. Note slight reduction in size, and the granularity of the subcapsular surface. × 1.

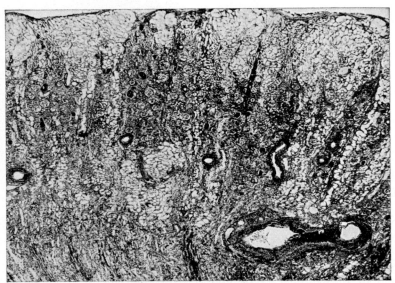

FIG. 21.9.—Kidney in benign essential hypertension, showing foci of fine cortical scarring, with enlargement of the tubules in the unaffected cortical areas. Note also the arterial thickening. × 12·5.

the usual arteriosclerotic changes of hypertension. The interlobular arteries display great intimal thickening, due to formation of fine concentric layers of connective tissue and smooth muscle cells, with very severe reduction of the lumen (Fig. 21.10). They may also show fibrinoid necrosis of the wall, especially at their distal end. The afferent arterioles show fibrinoid

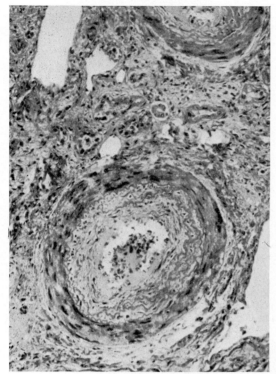

FIG. 21.10.—Interlobular artery in malignant hypertension, showing gross intimal fibro-cellular thickening. × 100.

necrosis, the wall being thickened, brightly eosinophilic, granular or homogeneous, and containing few or no living cells, but often pyknotic nuclei and red cells (Fig. 21.11): the necrotic material gives the staining reactions of fibrin, and the lumen is often completely obliterated, or occupied by thrombus which merges with the necrotic walls. The conspicuous fibrinoid necrosis may extend into the glomerulus, where it may involve parts or all of the tuft (Fig. 21.11, 21.12). Other glomeruli are less severely damaged, and show intense capillary dilatation and congestion. There is often blood or exudate in the capsular space, and here and there proliferation of the capsular epithelium (Fig. 21.12) to form crescents (p. 701). The

glomerular changes are the direct result of acute ischaemia resulting from fibrinoid necrosis of the afferent arterioles: this affects one arteriole after another, and even when death has resulted from renal failure, many are still unaffected and their corresponding glomeruli show little or no change. Some tubules show atrophy particularly of the proximal convoluted regions; others are of normal size or enlarged and hyaline droplets (p. 681) are conspicuous in the epithelial lining. Eosinophilic casts and sometimes red cells are seen throughout the length of some of the tubules.

Where malignant hypertension has supervened on benign essential hypertension, the changes corresponding to both conditions are seen in the kidneys. In recent years, the rapid downhill course of many patients with malignant hypertension has been arrested by antihypertensive drugs. Maintenance of the blood pressure below the very high levels of malignant hypertension prevents the severe lesions

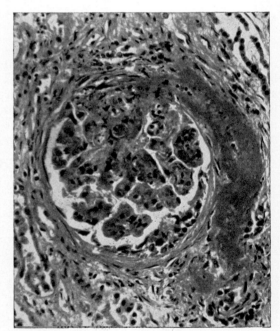

FIG. 21.11.—Malignant hypertension. Fibrinoid necrosis of the afferent arteriole to a glomerulus. × 230.

of the interlobular arteries, fibrinoid necrosis of the afferent arterioles, and the consequent rapid destruction of nephrons. Accordingly the prognosis has improved, particularly if treatment is begun before there is extensive renal damage. This suggests that fibrinoid necrosis of the arterioles is attributable to severe hypertension, and this is supported by various experimental observations; for example, partial clamping of one renal artery prevents fibrinoid necrosis in the clamped kidney in animals with severe hypertension (p. 274).

The vascular changes of malignant hypertension occur also in the other viscera, although the tensives, they occur also in some normotensive old people, and the kidneys present the same features as in benign essential hypertension. Here also, the changes do not seriously impair renal function.

Atheroma occurs in the main renal arteries and their segmental branches, but is much less common than in other arteries of comparable size,

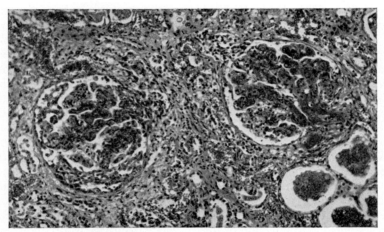

Fig. 21.12.—Kidney in malignant hypertension showing one glomerulus with an epithelial crescent (left) and one with fibrinoid necrosis and thrombosis. × 110.

effect is not usually so devastating as in the kidneys: an example of a lesion in the intestine is illustrated in Fig. 13.17, p. 273.

Secondary hypertension

As already indicated, the vascular changes and consequent renal injury observed in essential hypertension occur also in hypertension secondary to other conditions. Various grades of persistent hypertension result from certain renal diseases, and depending on the height of the blood pressure and the rate of rise, the renal changes described above for benign or malignant essential hypertension become superadded to those of the renal disease which has caused the hypertension. Such secondary hypertensive lesions are an important factor in hastening failure of the already damaged kidneys.

Other vascular diseases

Senile arteriosclerosis. Although arteriosclerosis and arteriolosclerosis, and their associated renal changes are seen particularly in hyper-

and, except in diabetes mellitus, is rarely severe enough to interfere with the renal circulation: superadded occlusion by thrombosis is also rare. Disturbances arise more commonly from involvement and narrowing of the origins of one or rarely both renal arteries by aortic atheromatous plaques. This can lead to hypertension, presumably from ischaemia of one or both kidneys. Compared with essential hypertension, this is a rarity, but it is important to diagnose, for in some cases relief of the stenosis by a by-pass operation, or removal of the ischaemic kidney, has resulted in cure of the hypertension. Such cases require careful investigation, including bilateral renal biopsy, for the non-ischaemic kidney may be damaged by hypertension or concomitant disease, e.g. pyelonephritis, and removing the ischaemic kidney may then do more harm than good. The mechanism of hypertension in renal artery stenosis is discussed on pp. 186, 274.

Fibromuscular dysplasia of the renal arteries. This term has been applied recently to several distinct abnormalities of the main renal arteries, affecting mostly the media, and including irregularities in thickness and in arrangement of the smooth muscle fibres, and irregular fibrosis. The changes are rare, and occur predominantly in women over a wide age range. They can give rise to renal artery stenosis or to dissecting or true aneurysms: we have observed a case in which an aneurysm of 3 cm. diameter com-pressed the renal pelvis and resulted in hydro-nephrosis.

The renal changes in *diabetes mellitus* are described on p. 718, and those of *polyarteritis nodosa* on p. 710.

GLOMERULONEPHRITIS

The essential fact established by Richard Bright, in his remarkable book of 1827, was that certain diseases characterised by albuminuria, and often accompanied by oedema, are due to renal lesions. Lack of knowledge of the micro-scopic changes in the lesions described by him precludes a satisfactory definition of *Bright's disease*, and use of the term should therefore be discontinued.

The term glomerulonephritis embraces a group of diseases in which the renal lesions are primarily glomerular, other changes in the kidneys resulting from the glomerular injury. It is necessary to add that in no type of glomeru-lonephritis is there a full understanding of the etiology, and that lesions due to infection of the kidneys are not included in this group. Hyper-tension develops as a consequence of various types of glomerulonephritis, and the renal changes of hypertension are thus commonly superadded to those of glomerulonephritis, resulting in a complex histological picture.

Classification of glomerulonephritis

The widespread practice of renal biopsy is now providing much information about the histological changes of glomerulonephritis and particularly about the early stages, while immunological studies, both clinical and experi-mental, are providing important etiological clues. However, there is still much to be learned, and classifications of glomerulonephritis must still be regarded as provisional, in the knowledge that modifications will be necessary in the coming years.

As regards the recognition of different types of glomerulonephritis, a major contribution was made by Volhard and Fahr (1914) and has since formed the basis of most classifications of this group of diseases. In the recent past the classi-fication proposed by Ellis in 1942 has been widely used. Without doubt, Ellis's contribu-tion was of major importance in distinguishing between two clinical syndromes accompanying glomerulonephritis, and relating them to the pathological changes in the kidneys. However, it has become increasingly apparent that his classification was an over-simplification and moreover it is now clear that the glomerular changes of his type I nephritis are sometimes associated with the clinical features of his type II. For these reasons, we consider that the Ellis classification has served its purpose, and that its continued use is likely to confuse the subject and retard further advances. In the classification of glomerulonephritis proposed opposite, we have selected, from the terms in common usage, those which seem to us to indicate best the major glomerular changes.

It must be emphasised that this classification is not intended to be comprehensive. Moreover, some of the types probably include more than one disease entity. Certain other conditions, e.g. systemic lupus erythematosus, diabetes mellitus and amyloidosis, can give rise to glomerular lesions resulting in clinical syndromes resemb-ling one or other types of glomerulonephritis, and it seems appropriate to discuss them together with glomerulonephritis.

There is danger of confusion over the term *chronic glomerulonephritis*. This presents typically as uraemia and hypertension, with polyuria and absence of generalised oedema: the kidneys are usually finely scarred and shrunken. It is the end-result of several types of glomerulonephri-tis, and in some patients the case history and renal changes indicate the course of events, but in many instances there is no history of preceding renal disease and the histological changes do not indicate how the disease has started.

Acute diffuse proliferative glomerulonephritis

General features. This relatively common type of glomerulonephritis occurs at all ages, but particularly in children and young adults. It affects males more often than females and usually follows an acute infection with Group A haemolytic streptococci—most often pharyngitis (including scarlet fever), but sometimes infections of the middle ear or skin. In many cases, the disease develops 1–4 weeks after the onset of the streptococcal infection, and very often this has settled down and there is a latent period of apparent well-being before glomerulonephritis becomes apparent.

reveals that larger protein molecules, e.g. IgG, are also usually present in appreciable amounts and the proteinuria is thus not a highly selective albuminuria. Microscopy of the urine shows many red cells, moderate or large numbers of neutrophil polymorphs, and protein casts (see p. 685) of hyaline, granular or cellular appearance.

Course of the disease. In most cases the clinical illness is mild and the kidney lesion reversible. The oedema, hypertension and raised blood urea

CLASSIFICATION OF GLOMERULONEPHRITIS

Recommended	Ellis	Alternatives
Acute diffuse pro-liferative	Acute type I	Acute post-streptococcal; acute; acute proliferative
Rapidly progressive	Rapidly progressive type I	Subacute; subacute azotaemic; subacute extracapillary
Lobular		
(a) Nephrotic stage	Type II	—
(b) Chronic stage		
Membranous	Type II	Idiopathic membranous
(a) Nephrotic stage	(a) Subacute stage	(a) Subacute; hydraemic stage; subacute intracapillary
(b) Chronic stage	(b) Chronic stage	(b) Chronic or azotaemic stage
Mixed membranous and proliferative	—	Mixed; unclassified
Minimal-change	Type II	Lipoid nephrosis
Focal		
Chronic	Chronic	Chronic azotaemic

The presenting clinical feature is usually puffiness of the face or discoloration of the urine. Puffiness is due to oedema and affects especially the lax tissues of the eyelids: it is most noticeable in the morning and tends to subside during the ambulatory day. Oedema may affect other parts of the body and in some cases is more severe and is then seen to be generalised. The blood pressure is commonly raised, and in most cases the rise is slight or moderate.

Biochemical changes. There is usually a mild or moderate rise in the level of blood urea. The urine is diminished in volume, of high specific gravity, and commonly brownish and turbid ("smoky") from the presence of altered red cells. There is moderate proteinuria and, as in all types of glomerulonephritis, the protein is mainly plasma albumin. Quantitative analysis

persist for only a week or two. Red cells and protein diminish in the urine, but may not disappear for several months or even a year or so.

In some instances the disease is more severe, and approximately 5 per cent of patients die from uraemia or from the effects of severe acute hypertension—acute heart failure or hypertensive encephalopathy. In some of these fatal cases, the glomerular lesion is atypical only in its severity: in others, additional features are present and the condition is then classified as *rapidly progressive glomerulonephritis* (p. 700). In a further 15 per cent or so of cases, the disease runs the usual short course, but although clinical recovery appears complete, proteinuria persists during a latent period varying from 2 to 20 years, when chronic glomerulonephritis becomes clinically apparent.

z

In the various published series of hospital cases, the prognosis of acute diffuse glomerulonephritis has been observed to be appreciably better in children than in adults. Approximately 5 per cent of children die in the acute stage or develop rapidly progressive glomerulonephritis, and no more than 10 per cent subsequently develop chronic glomerulonephritis. In adults, the comparable figures are of the order of 10 and 30 per cent respectively. Thus over 80 per cent of children and around 60 per cent of adults recover completely.

Pathological features

In acute diffuse glomerulonephritis the cortex is typically pale and distinctly enlarged due to oedema. In fatal cases (which cannot, of course, be regarded as typical), the cortex is up to twice the normal thickness, pale, and the glomeruli may be seen with a hand lens as light grey dots projecting from the cut surface.

Microscopically the most conspicuous changes

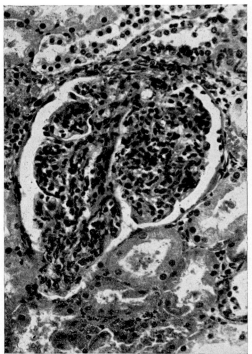

FIG. 21.14.—Glomerulus in acute diffuse proliferative glomerulonephritis, showing swelling and increased cellularity of the glomerular tuft, which has herniated into the proximal tubule. × 200.

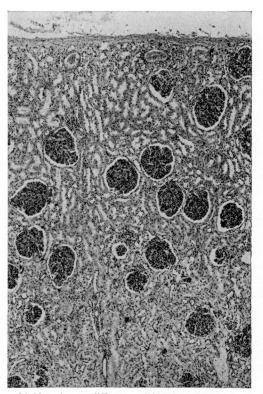

FIG. 21.13.—Acute diffuse proliferative glomerulonephritis. The glomeruli show diffuse enlargement and hypercellularity. × 38.

are diffuse enlargement and increased cellularity of the glomeruli (Fig. 21.13). The enlargement results in narrowing or obliteration of the capsular space (in the normal kidney the processes involved in embedding in paraffin and preparing sections result in glomerular shrinkage and the capsular spaces appear artefactually large). When a glomerulus happens to have been cut in the appropriate plane, part of the glomerular tuft can often be seen to have herniated into the lumen of the first part of the tubule (Fig. 21.14). The capillary lumina appear narrowed, the endothelial cells are swollen and probably increased in number, and there is also proliferation of mesangial cells. Neutrophil polymorphs add to the glomerular cellularity, particularly in the early stages, but they vary considerably in number from case to case.

An additional change in the glomerular tufts is an increase in the number of strands of basement membrane-like material demonstrable by electron microscopy in the mesangial regions. Little is known about these strands, but in cases which fail to resolve, the material apparently increases considerably and contributes to the hyaline appearance of the glomeruli in the chronic stage of glomerulonephritis.

The basement membrane of the glomerular capillaries shows no obvious thickening by light microscopy. Electron microscopy shows localised deposits of granular material, mostly projecting from the outer surface of the basement membrane (Fig. 21.15), while in some cases there are deposits also on the inner surface of the basement membrane. This feature provides an important clue to the nature of the glomerular injury and will be discussed further in the section on etiology.

The podocytes (p. 681) do not show widespread fusion of foot processes, although this

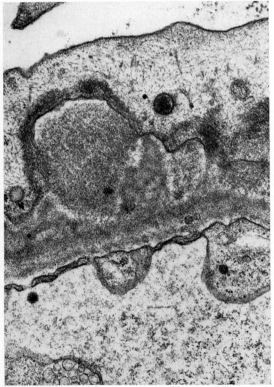

FIG. 21.15.—Electron micrograph of part of glomerular capillary wall in acute diffuse glomerulonephritis, showing a large granular sub-epithelial deposit. Note also fusion of the foot processes (lumen below, urinary space above). × 50,000.

may occur focally. Some proteinous debris, and occasionally red cells, may be seen in the narrowed capsular spaces. In most cases, the epithelium of Bowman's capsule appears normal, but here and there some proliferation may be seen. Epithelial crescents (p. 701) are not seen

in typical acute diffuse glomerulonephritis, although they are usually numerous and conspicuous in rapidly progressive glomerulonephritis.

Changes in the rest of the kidney are secondary to the glomerular lesion: there is diffuse oedema, seen as an increase in the loose interstitial tissue between the tubules, and often accompanied by a light scattering of polymorphs or mononuclear cells. The tubules contain proteinous and cellular casts, including red cells. The epithelial cells of the proximal convoluted tubules contain hyaline droplets (p. 681). Occasionally there are foci of disruption of tubular epithelial cells, possibly attributable to ischaemia secondary to the glomerular changes.

It must be emphasised that in the typical attack of acute glomerulonephritis, hypertension is not sufficiently severe or prolonged to produce changes in the heart and blood vessels, although the vascular changes of hypertension may be seen in the severe cases which persist for weeks or months as rapidly progressive glomerulonephritis.

With recovery from the disease, the glomeruli return to normal, although increased numbers of cells in the mesangial zones of the glomerular lobules may persist for months, and have been regarded as a retrospective diagnostic feature: there is evidence from serial biopsies that marked hypercellularity of the mesangial zones during and after acute glomerulonephritis indicates an increased likelihood of the subsequent development of chronic glomerulonephritis.

In fatal cases of acute glomerulonephritis, there may be fibrinoid necrosis of arterioles, thrombosis and necrosis of individual glomerular capillary loops, and glomerular haemorrhages. Other cases exhibit the features of rapidly progressive glomerulonephritis (p. 700).

Effects of renal changes

In acute glomerulonephritis, light and electron microscopy show narrowing of the glomerular capillary lumina attributable to increase in number and size of glomerular cells. Some impairment of blood flow through the kidneys might be expected, and indeed the renal plasma flow has been shown to be reduced in some cases, but is normal in others. However, the fraction of plasma filtered off by the glomeruli (the glomerular filtration fraction) is reduced, and hence the total *glomerular filtration rate* (GFR) is also less than normal. Rise in the blood urea level is attributable mainly to reduced GFR, although ischaemic injury of the tubular epithelium may play a part by impairing the functional selectivity of reabsorption.

The factors concerned in the production of oedema and oliguria in acute diffuse glomerulonephritis are not yet fully understood. The point is made several times in this chapter that the *volume* of urine produced, and its *concentration,*

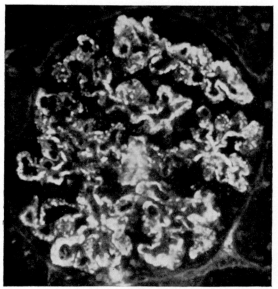

Fig. 21.16.—Renal biopsy in acute diffuse glomerulonephritis. Immunofluorescence technique, showing granular and ill-defined deposition of IgG in the glomerular capillary walls. × 250.

are dependent mainly on tubular reabsorption and not on the GFR. Two important factors in tubular reabsorption are, firstly the concentration of solutes remaining in the lumen (i.e. not reabsorbed)—a high concentration of solute, e.g. urea, produces an osmotic diuresis by interfering with reabsorption of water (p. 716); secondly, the pituitary antidiuretic hormone, which increases reabsorption of water. It is not clear what part these and other factors play in the oliguria and oedema of acute diffuse glomerulonephritis: the subject is discussed more fully on p. 183. The transient hypertension of this disease is presumed to result from decreased renal blood flow (p. 274).

Urine. It seems reasonable to assume that the

appearance of protein, red cells and leukocytes in the urine is attributable directly to the glomerular lesion. It must be admitted, however, that the severity of the glomerular changes does not correlate closely with the amount of protein or numbers of cells escaping in the urine. It is probable that the basement membrane is the main filter barrier in the glomerular capillary wall, in which case the glomerular lesion must result in increased permeability of the capillary basement membrane. The physico-chemical basis of the basement membrane change is not understood, but there is evidence that the primary change in the glomeruli is an immunological reaction involving the capillary basement membrane. The subject is discussed more fully in the next section.

In a small proportion of patients with the nephrotic syndrome, renal biopsy shows the histological changes of acute diffuse glomerulonephritis: the explanation of the very heavy proteinuria in such patients is not apparent, and at the other extreme are patients with the usual clinical and histological changes of acute diffuse glomerulonephritis but little or no proteinuria.

Etiology of acute diffuse glomerulonephritis

Two features which must be taken into account in considering the etiology of acute diffuse glomerulonephritis are the common preceding pharyngeal infection with Group A haemolytic streptococci and the latent period of 1–4 weeks (average 10 days or so) between the onset of infection and onset of glomerulonephritis. The type of streptococcus is of more importance than the site of infection, for streptococcal infection of the skin or middle ear may be followed by acute diffuse glomerulonephritis, and it has been shown quite clearly that infection with certain types of Group A streptococci (e.g. Griffith types 12, 4, 1, 25) are particularly liable to be followed by glomerulonephritis. Bacteriological examination of the kidneys and urine has failed to provide evidence of renal infection, and the onset after the disappearance of the febrile proteinuria which may accompany the preceding streptococcal infection suggests that the disease is not caused directly by streptococcal toxins. It is now widely held that the streptococcal infection provides an antigenic stimulus and that the resulting antibody response in some way brings about the glomerular injury. Evidence supporting this view will be presented below under the following headings: (1) evidence for an antigen–antibody reaction, (2) experimental immunological glomerular injury, and (3) interpretation of the findings in acute diffuse proliferative glomerulonephritis.

1. Evidence for an antigen–antibody reaction

(a) Serum complement levels. In most cases of acute diffuse glomerulonephritis the level of serum complement is abnormally low, but returns to normal with recovery. The most likely explanation is that an antigen–antibody reaction is taking place, and that complement is being fixed by the antigen–antibody complex: assay of the levels of individual complement components in acute glomerulonephritis has provided results consistent with this explanation.

(b) Immunohistological studies. The principles involved in immunofluorescence techniques have been described elsewhere (p. 80). In acute diffuse glomerulonephritis the method has been used to detect immunoglobulins fixed in the glomeruli by treating frozen sections of renal biopsy or post-mortem material with fluorescein-conjugated antibodies to human immunoglobulins. In most cases investigated, IgG has been shown to be deposited in the walls of glomerular capillaries: the deposits appear to be related to the capillary basement membrane, and usually have a granular appearance (Fig. 21.16), but in some cases there is also linear deposition. Immunofluorescence has also been applied using an antibody to β_{1C}-globulin, a component of complement, and complement has been shown to be present and to have the same distribution pattern as IgG, thus providing support for the view that the deposited IgG represents antibody in union with antigen. Deposits of other immunoglobulins, particularly IgM, have also been demonstrated, and immunoglobulins have been detected in other parts of the glomeruli, particularly in the mesangium, and in the tubules, but the close association of IgG and fixed complement is peculiar to the glomerular capillary basement membrane.

Immunological studies have also been made with the electron microscope, using the same principles as in immunofluorescence, but with antibodies labelled with ferritin (which has a characteristic electron-microscopic appearance) instead of fluorescent dyes. By this means, it has been confirmed that IgG is deposited mainly as nodules on the outer surface of the capillary basement membrane, and these deposits probably account for the "lumpy-bumpy" appearance of the membrane in electron micrographs (Fig. 21.15).

2. Experimental immunological glomerular injury

Glomerular injury has been produced experimentally by three distinct immunological procedures. These are as follows:

(a) Nephrotoxic antibody nephritis. This is commonly known as "Masugi-type" nephritis although it was described by Lindemann in 1900, long before Masugi's report in 1933. The disease is induced by injection of hetero-antibody to glomerular capillary basement membrane. The antibody is produced by administering immunising injections, containing kidney homogenate or more purified glomerular basement membrane, into an animal of another species. For example, ducks or rabbits may be immunised to produce antibodies to rat kidney and this antibody will induce acute glomerulonephritis when injected into rats. The features of the experimental disease vary considerably depending on the choice of species, the potency of the antibody, and the dose administered. In some circumstances, and particularly with high dosage of antibody, acute glomerulonephritis develops within a few hours, whereas under other conditions, and particularly with low dosage of antibody, the disease develops after a latent period of several days. The immediate type of injury results from the reaction of the foreign (heterologous) antibody with the glomerular capillary basement membrane, and the glomerular cellular changes are secondary to this (Fig. 21.17). In conditions in which there is no obvious immediate injury, two things happen. Firstly the hetero-antibody attaches to the glomerular capillary basement membrane, presumably in amounts too small to induce any significant injury, and secondly the injected heterologous IgG stimulates production of antibody in the recipient. After several days, this antibody appears in the serum and reacts with the heterologous antibody (IgG) already attached to the glomerular capillary basement membrane, and it is this event which leads to the glomerular injury developing several days after the injection (Fig. 21.17b). It has become customary to refer to the immediate injury as the *heterologous phase* of the disease and to the later lesion as the *autologous phase*. Since both phases result from the

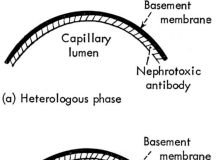

(a) Heterologous phase

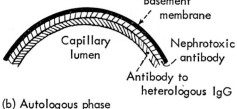

(b) Autologous phase

FIG. 21.17.—Diagrammatic representation of heterologous and autologous phases of nephrotoxic-antibody nephritis.

reaction of the hetero-antibody with a normal tissue constituent, they are to be regarded as type II hypersensitivity reactions (p. 102).

In many respects, nephrotoxic antibody nephritis resembles acute diffuse glomerulonephritis of man: the clinical features include rise in blood urea and blood pressure, and oedema. The glomerular changes are similar, and by varying the amount of antibody administered, disease of all grades of severity can be produced, and progressive or chronic renal injury can result. In the heterologous phase, the foreign IgG can be detected fixed to the glomerular capillary basement membrane, while in the autologous phase both foreign and autologous IgG are demonstrable here. In both phases, complement can be demonstrated in relation to the fixed IgG, and under suitable experimental conditions a fall in the level of serum complement can be shown to accompany both heterologous and autologous phase injury. An important difference from human acute diffuse glomerulonephritis lies in the linear distribution of fixed IgG and complement along the glomerular

capillary basement membrane (Fig. 21.18), whereas in the human disease the deposits are mainly granular (Fig. 21.16). Moreover electron microscopy has shown the linear deposits of the experimental disease to lie mainly on the inner side of the capillary basement membrane, whereas the granular deposits in human acute glomerulonephritis lie mainly on the outer side of the membrane.

The mechanism of injury by nephrotoxic antibody has not been established fully, but it has been shown that the heterologous phase of nephrotoxic antibody nephritis, produced in rabbits or rats by injection of sheep or rabbit anti-kidney antibodies respectively, is largely complement-dependent and is suppressed by depleting the recipient of complement before administering the antibody serum. Moreover, a major part of the complement-dependent glomerular injury has been shown to be due to chemotactic action of reacting complement upon circulating neutrophil polymorphs (p. 104): in other words, the reaction of complement results in infiltration of polymorphs which pass through the capillary endothelium and come to lie in contact with the basement membrane. Enzymic damage to the basement membrane is then brought about by disruption of the polymorph lysosomes and release of their multiple enzymes. Although this type of polymorph-induced

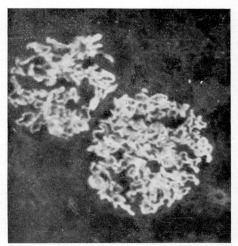

FIG. 21.18.—Nephrotoxic-antibody nephritis; linear deposition of heterologous nephrotoxic antibody in the glomerular capillary walls, demonstrated by the immunofluorescence technique. (Dr. R. Lannigan).

injury is of major importance in nephrotoxic antibody nephritis, recent work by Hawkins and Cochrane (1968) has produced evidence that injury to the glomerular capillary basement membrane may be brought about by nephrotoxic antibody *without* the participation of complement and polymorphs: the mechanism of this type of injury, which requires large amounts of nephrotoxic antibody, is not yet elucidated.

Although nephrotoxic antibody reacts *in vivo* with the basement membrane of capillaries throughout the body, a high proportion of it becomes attached to glomerular capillary basement membrane, and it persists longer here than in other tissues. This explains why the resulting injury is confined mainly to the glomeruli. Some of the antibody in nephrotoxic serum reacts with antigen present only in glomerular capillary basement membrane, but nephrotoxic antibody nephritis can be induced by antiserum prepared by immunising the donor animal with vascular tissues other than kidney, e.g. lung or placenta, and it is thus apparent that glomerular capillary basement membrane is more readily available to circulating antibody than is the basement membrane of other capillaries. The fenestrations in the glomerular capillary endothelium and the high pressure of blood in the glomerular capillaries may be important in this respect.

(b) Foreign-protein nephritis. In certain experimental conditions, the administration of single or multiple injections of foreign (heterologous) normal serum or normal serum protein leads after an interval to the development of a glomerulonephritis. This condition, which is also termed *immune-complex nephritis*, has been shown to result from the production of antibody to the injected heterologous protein, formation of circulating antigen–antibody complexes, and deposition of these on the glomerular capillary basement membrane. An acute glomerulonephritis of this nature can occur in man following injection of foreign IgG (e.g. antitoxins produced in horses) and forms part of the picture of serum sickness. In experimental animals the vascular lesions may be widespread, as in serum sickness; however, under certain experimental conditions the lesions are confined mainly to the glomeruli. Although the glomerular injury resembles that of nephrotoxic antibody nephritis insofar as both are attributable to antigen–antibody reactions, in foreign protein nephritis the complexes are formed in the circulation, and are deposited especially, for reasons not fully understood, on the glomerular capillary basement membrane (Fig. 21.19). The condition is thus a type III hypersensitivity reaction (p. 104). In nephrotoxic antibody nephritis, the antibody reacts specifically with the glomerular capillary basement membrane, i.e, type II hypersensitivity (p. 102).

Although foreign protein nephritis has been produced in several species by injection of various foreign proteins, and also by injection of antigen–antibody complexes, it has been studied most extensively in the rabbit, using foreign IgG or serum albumin as the foreign protein. A single injection results in an acute glomerulonephritis with proliferative changes, some polymorph infiltration and narrowing of the capillary lumina. Granular deposition of the foreign protein, host antibody and complement, is demonstrable in the glomerular capillary walls by immunofluorescence techniques (Fig. 21.20) and corresponding amorphous deposits may be detectable by electron microscopy in the outer part of the basement membrane (Fig. 21.21).

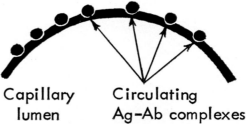

Capillary   Circulating
lumen   Ag–Ab complexes

FIG. 21.19.—Diagrammatic representation of deposition of antigen–antibody complexes in the outer part of the glomerular capillary basement membrane in foreign-protein nephritis.

These changes are accompanied by a fall in serum complement level, proteinuria, cellular and colloid casts, and a rise in the blood urea level. Lesions of various degrees of severity can be produced but, unless they are very severe, resolution without residual injury is the usual outcome. By administering repeated injections of foreign protein, progressive lesions can be produced in some rabbits, and include both diffuse thickening of the capillary basement membrane and proliferative changes.

As in other lesions resulting from formation of antigen–antibody complexes, foreign protein nephritis has been shown to develop while antigen is present in excess of antibody: the complexes formed in these circumstances are relatively small (Fig. 5.7, p. 105), are not readily phagocytosed, and tend particularly to deposit in the glomeruli. Thus the lesion develops approximately 7–10 days after a single injection of foreign protein, at which time free antigen is still present in the circulation, but is rapidly diminishing as it complexes with newly-produced antibody (Fig. 5.6, p. 105). Once antibody has appeared in excess (i.e. when free antibody is detectable in the serum) no further injury results. With multiple injections of foreign protein, the severity and duration will depend on the dosage of antigen and the amount of antibody produced, and the prolongation of glomerular injury depends on maintenance of excess of circulating antigen in rabbits which are producing sufficient antibody to provide pathogenic amounts of complexes. The mechanism of injury brought about by deposition of immune complexes in foreign-protein acute nephritis has not been fully worked out, but it is likely that it is similar to that for nephrotoxic antibody nephritis, and largely dependent on fixation of complement and polymorph enzymic activity (p. 696).

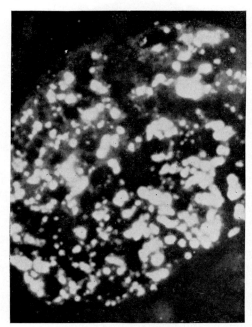

FIG. 21.20.—Experimental foreign-protein glomerulonephritis. Irregular deposition of immune complexes in the capillary walls, shown by fluorescent antibody to IgG. (Dr. R. Lannigan.)

Although the antigens participating in immune-complex nephritis are foreign proteins, it has been demonstrated recently that auto-immunisation against a normal body constituent can result in deposition of antigen–auto-antibody complexes on the glomerular capillary basement membrane, leading to the same range of pathological changes. For example, immunisation of rats by injection of a phospholipoprotein present in the apex of the epithelial cells of the proximal convoluted tubules (and also detectable normally in low concentration in the plasma) results in progressive lesions resembling human membranous glomerulonephritis (p. 703) and the experimental production in rabbits of antibody reactive with autologous thyroglobulin (which is also present in low concentration in the plasma), leads to an acute glomerulonephritis as a result of deposition of thyroglobulin–antithyroglobulin complexes in the glomeruli. These recent findings are mentioned here because they demonstrate that immune-complex nephritis may result from auto-immunisation, a phenomenon which is known to occur spontaneously in man (p. 110).

(c) **Experimental auto-immune glomerulonephritis.** The production of acute glomerulonephritis by experimental immunisation of animals against tubular epithelial antigen or thyroglobulin, referred to in the preceding section, are examples of auto-immune nephritis. In the present section, however, we are considering

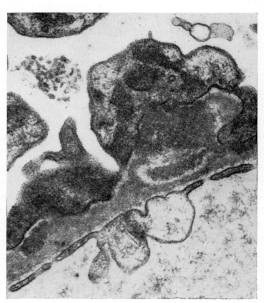

FIG. 21.21.—Electron micrograph of segment of glomerular capillary wall in experimental foreign-protein glomerulonephritis, showing dense nodular deposits in outer part of basement membrane (capillary lumen below; urinary space above). × 25,000.

glomerulonephritis resulting from the development of auto-antibodies reactive with the animal's own glomerular capillary basement membrane. To bring this about it is essential that the basement membrane material in the inoculum contains at least one antigenic determinant present also in the host's glomerular capillary basement membrane. This can be ensured by using autologous (the host's own) renal tissue (obtained by unilateral nephrectomy) to prepare the inoculum, or homologous kidney (obtained from another animal of the same species). Heterologous kidney can, however, be used for this purpose, as some glomerular basement membrane antigens are common to several mammalian species.

As might be expected, the production of nephrotoxic auto-antibody is less readily induced than hetero-antibody, and it has proved helpful to enhance the immune response by incorporating the antigen in Freund's adjuvant emulsion (p. 83). The incidence, severity, and morphology of the resulting condition depend upon the species of animal given the injections and the species of the kidney preparation injected. Sheep are highly susceptible, and develop an acute glomerulonephritis resembling rapidly progressive glomerulonephritis in man (p. 700): rabbits and other species are less susceptible. In general, injections of heterologous kidney are more effective than homologous or autologous kidney, but all three preparations are capable of inducing the disease.

As in nephrotoxic antibody nephritis, immunofluorescence studies show *linear* deposition of IgG and of complement along the glomerular capillary basement membrane. Antibody to glomerular capillary basement membrane has also been detected in the serum of animals with the disease, but usually in very low concentration, and its titre does not correlate with the severity of glomerular injury. This is probably because most of the auto-antibody released into the circulation is absorbed rapidly by glomerular capillary basement membrane: following bilateral nephrectomy of immunised animals the concentration of circulating antibody has been found to rise. It is of interest that the method long used to produce nephrotoxic rabbit hetero-antibody to rat kidney has been shown to be capable of inducing nephrotoxic auto-antibody and auto-immune nephritis in the rabbits receiving injections of rat kidney: the lesion is usually mild, and indeed its recognition is quite recent.

In summary, acute and chronic glomerular injury can be induced by nephrotoxic antibody reactive with the glomerular capillary basement membrane, or by deposition of circulating antigen–antibody complexes in the glomeruli. Nephrotoxic antibody is deposited in linear fashion, mainly on the inner side of the glomerular capillary basement membrane, while antigen–antibody complexes are deposited in a granular pattern mainly on the outer side of the basement membrane. In both types of disease, there is evidence that neutrophil polymorphs play an important pathogenic role by effecting enzymic injury to the glomerular capillary basement membrane, and that this action is dependent on chemotactic factors released during the reaction of complement with immune complexes in the glomerular capillary walls.

Both types of experimental nephritis described above can be induced by auto-immunisation, and there is no evidence that delayed hypersensitivity contributes to the lesions.

3. Interpretation of the findings in acute diffuse glomerulonephritis in man

The deposition of IgG and of complement on the glomerular capillary basement membrane, and the low levels of serum complement observed in this disease (p. 695) can now be discussed against the background of the experimental observations outlined above. One of the most important features to be taken into account is the pattern of fixed IgG and complement in the glomerular capillary walls. In acute diffuse glomerulonephritis, the granular deposits are related to the capillary basement membrane (Fig. 21.16), and probably correspond to the nodular deposits seen on the outer surface of the basement membrane on electron microscopy (Fig. 21.15): this is similar to the pattern observed in experimental foreign protein (immune-complex) nephritis (Figs. 21.20, 21.21), and is regarded as evidence that the deposits consist of antigen–antibody complexes which have formed in the circulation. The frequent association of the disease with a preceding streptococcal infection suggests that the antigen is of streptococcal origin, and that it is still present in appreciable amounts in the blood at the time of production of the corresponding antibody, with the result that antigen–antibody complexes are formed. So long as antigen is present in excess, the complexes are likely to be deposited in, and be injurious to, the glomeruli: once excess antibody has appeared, renal injury should cease.

This explanation of acute diffuse glomerulonephritis is an attractive one, but is by no means fully supported by the available evidence.

Firstly, it does not explain why certain types of Group A streptococci are nephritogenic while others are not. Secondly, there is no close correlation between the observed titres of various streptococcal antibodies and the occurrence of the disease. Most individuals infected with a nephritogenic strain of streptococcus do not develop the disease, and the spectrum of anti-streptococcal antibodies which they produce shows no characteristic difference from the antibody responses of individuals developing the disease. Thirdly, attempts to demonstrate streptococcal antigens deposited in the glomeruli (along with the fixed IgG and complement) have yielded conflicting results, and their deposition remains a doubtful possibility: this cannot, however, be regarded as strong evidence against the hypothesis, for difficulty has been experienced also in demonstrating deposited antigen in immune-complex nephritis induced experimentally by a single injection of foreign protein. Lastly, the hypothesis can explain the typical case of acute diffuse glomerulonephritis with recovery, and possibly also the progressive, fatal cases, in which the initial glomerular damage is very severe, but it does not readily explain those cases in which apparent recovery from the acute attack is followed, after some years without clinical recurrence, by chronic glomerulonephritis.

Despite these difficulties, the above theory, namely that acute diffuse glomerulonephritis is an immune-complex disease in which the antigen may be of streptococcal origin, seems to us to provide the best explanation so far advanced. The alternative possibility, that the disease results from development of auto-antibody reactive with the glomerular capillary basement membrane, appears less likely because in this case the deposition of IgG would be expected to be mainly linear and along the inner surface of the basement membrane, as in nephrotoxic antibody nephritis. Evidence has been advanced that nephritogenic types of streptococci possess an antigenic constituent similar to a component of the glomerular capillary basement membrane, and that antibody to the streptococcal antigen reacts with basement membrane, but various workers have failed to confirm these findings.

In conclusion, the demonstration of predominantly granular deposits of IgG in the glomerular capillary walls in acute diffuse proliferative glomerulonephritis suggests, by analogy with experimentally induced lesions, that deposition of antigen–antibody complexes is likely to play a major role in the human disease.

Rapidly progressive glomerulonephritis

This usually fatal condition may develop without known predisposing cause, or may follow a streptococcal infection. It can supervene also in patients with the focal glomerulonephritis associated with certain diseases (p. 709). It can occur at any age, and is commoner in males than females. The clinical features and urinary changes may be indistinguishable at first from those of acute diffuse glomerulonephritis (p. 691), but instead of regressing after a week or two, become progressively more severe, and death results from uraemia and hypertension after a period of a few months to a year or so. Rarely, proteinuria may be severe enough to give rise to the nephrotic syndrome. In other cases, there is severe oliguria or even anuria and death then results within a few weeks.

Rapidly progressive glomerulonephritis is much less common than acute diffuse glomerulonephritis, but because of its severity it makes an important contribution to the number of individuals dying of renal failure.

Pathological changes. The kidneys are normal in size, or enlarged due to oedema: on section the cortex is pale, but may show petechial haemorrhages (Fig. 21.23), and the glomeruli stand out conspicuously as grey dots, visible with a lens, on the cut surface. In most cases, there is little or no gross scarring and the surface of the kidneys is smooth.

Microscopy shows the most important changes to be glomerular. As in acute diffuse glomerulonephritis, there is proliferation of endothelial and possibly mesangial cells with narrowing of the capillary lumina, and variable polymorph infiltration of the tuft (Fig. 21.24). Although all the glomeruli are affected, some glomerular lobules may be more severely involved than others, and there may be necrosis and thrombosis of capillaries or lobules.

A surprising feature of the disease is the rapidity with which glomerular scarring may occur: thus in cases with a history of only 2 weeks or so, biopsy may reveal fibrous obliteration of lobules or whole glomeruli, and also fibrous adhesions between the tuft and Bowman's capsule (Fig. 21.25). There is thus a combination of glomerular proliferation, necrosis, thrombosis and scarring, amounting to very severe glomerular injury.

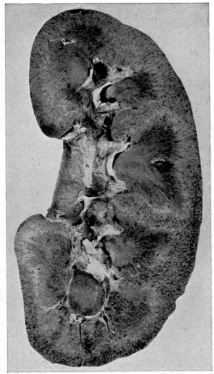

FIG. 21.23.—Enlarged kidney in rapidly progressive glomerulonephritis.

Numerous petechial haemorrhages are present in the cortex. × ¾.

A most characteristic histological feature is proliferation of the parietal epithelium of Bowman's capsule to form "*epithelial crescents*" (Figs. 21.24, 21.25, 21.26) which occupy the capsular space and surround the tufts. (This change used to be known as *extracapillary glomerulitis* to distinguish it from the *intracapillary* glomerular changes occurring in membranous glomerulonephritis, but these terms have largely lost their usefulness.) Formation of epithelial crescents occurs in other diseases, for example in subacute bacterial endocarditis, malignant hypertension, and in some cases of acute diffuse glomerulonephritis, but the crescents are neither so numerous nor so large as in rapidly progressive glomerulonephritis, in which they may fill and distend the capsular space of most glomeruli. Crescent formation appears to

be a reaction to haemorrhage or exudate in the capsular space. In time, the epithelial crescents are replaced by fibrous tissue, and appear as crescentic scars.

The tubules may be dilated (Fig. 21.24), and usually contain hyaline and cellular casts and red cells, and proteinous droplets are present in the cells of the proximal convoluted tubules. There may also be some irregular tubular atrophy and increase of intertubular connective tissue, presumably due to ischaemia resulting from the glomerular changes.

In some cases hypertension is severe, and the changes of malignant hypertension (p. 687) become superadded. There may also be left ventricular hypertrophy, and changes associated

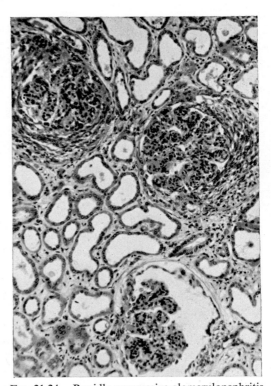

FIG. 21.24.—Rapidly progressive glomerulonephritis.

The three glomeruli show various degrees of damage and crescent formation. The tubules are dilated and lined with cubical epithelium. The interstitial tissue is oedematous and infiltrated by inflammatory cells. × 175.

with uraemia, e.g. fibrinous pericarditis, anaemia and superadded infections.

The glomerular changes result in severely impaired renal blood flow and consequent reduction in GFR: the clinical and biochemical changes are similar to those in acute diffuse glomerulonephritis, but becoming pro-gressively more severe.

Etiology. In a minority of cases of rapidly progressive glomerulonephritis, there is evidence of a preceding streptococcal infection, and the

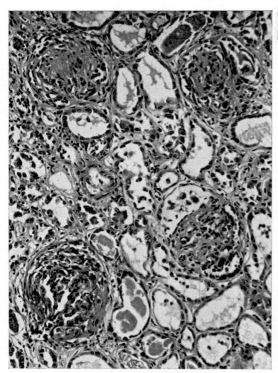

Fig. 21.25.—Rapidly progressive glomerulonephritis. The glomeruli are largely destroyed; there are also severe tubular destruction and casts in the lumina. × 110.

disease may therefore arise as a severe variant of acute diffuse glomerulonephritis. It arises also in certain diseases as a progression from focal glomerulonephritis (p. 709). Both of these associations raise the possibility of an immuno-logical pathogenesis, and indeed there are various reports of immunofluorescence studies in which IgG and complement have been de-tected in the walls of the glomerular capillaries, but usually the account of the pathological changes has been too sketchy to provide a convincing diagnosis of rapidly progressive glomerulonephritis. Recently, Lerner, Glassock and Dixon (1967) have described the detection of *linear deposition of IgG and complement* in the glomerular capillary walls, and have eluted from surgically excised kidneys antibody reacting with glomerular capillary basement membrane.

In one patient bilateral nephrectomy was performed prior to renal transplantation, and between the two operations antibody to glom-erular capillary basement membrane became detectable in the serum. This was shown to be nephrotoxic when injected into monkeys, and indeed glomerulonephritis developed subse-quently in the transplanted kidney. These observations suggest that rapidly progressive glomerulonephritis may, at least in some instances, be a nephrotoxic auto-antibody disease, but it must be emphasised that the findings are somewhat tentative. The signi-ficance of the findings is best considered in relation to the experimental types of glomerular injury described on pp. 695–9: the detection of nephrotoxic auto-antibody following bilateral nephrectomy may be of great significance, and supports the suggestion made elsewhere (Ander-son, Buchanan and Goudie, 1967) that failure to detect such antibody free in the serum of patients with various types of glomerulonephritis may well be due to its absorption *in vivo* onto glomerular capillary basement membrane.

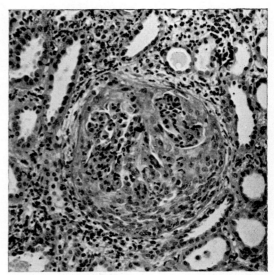

Fig. 21.26.—Glomerulus in rapidly progressive glom-erulonephritis, showing destruction and fibrosis of parts of the tuft, hypercellularity of the remainder, and formation of an epithelial crescent around the tuft. × 200.

Lobular glomerulonephritis

There is some doubt as to whether this uncommon condition is really a separate entity. It occurs mainly in young adults, and usually presents clinically as the nephrotic syndrome (p. 704), often accompanied by gross or microscopic haematuria and sometimes by chronic renal failure. In other cases, the nephrotic stage subsides and is followed, within a few years, by chronic renal failure. The prognosis is thus poor.

Pathological changes. In the nephrotic stage, the kidneys are enlarged or of normal size and the cortex may contain yellow deposits of lipid—the appearances are indistinguishable from those of minimal-change glomerulonephritis and from the nephrotic stage of membranous glomerulonephritis. At this stage, microscopy shows increased cellularity of the

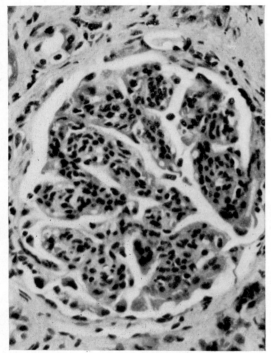

FIG. 21.27.—Lobular glomerulonephritis. The tuft is hypercellular and the lobular pattern is grossly exaggerated. × 350.

central parts of the lobules of all the glomeruli: the cells are probably endothelial and mesangial, and the hypercellularity is gradually replaced by centrilobular hyalinisation. The glomerular capillaries may show some patchy basement membrane thickening. The glomerular lobular pattern is accentuated, and in glomeruli sectioned through the hilum the lobules are seen as discrete and digitate (Fig. 21.27). The tubules and interstitial tissue show the changes associated with the nephrotic syndrome (p. 705).

In the stage of advanced renal failure, the changes are those of chronic glomerulonephritis. Centrilobular hyalinisation of the glomerular lobules extends to involve the glomerular capillaries, but although hyalinised, the lobules may still remain partly discrete, in contrast to the uniform solidity of hyalinised glomeruli in most cases of chronic glomerulonephritis. Also, all the glomeruli are affected, although some are more completely hyalinised than others. As usual in chronic glomerulonephritis, hypertension, sometimes malignant, supervenes.

Etiology. In approximately half the cases, lobular glomerulonephritis appears a few years after an attack of acute glomerulonephritis following a streptococcal infection, from which the patient has made a normal recovery apart from persistence of proteinuria. It is likely that the preceding glomerulonephritis is of the usual acute diffuse proliferative type, but as renal biopsy is not usually necessary in this acute disease, histological confirmation is lacking. In other cases, there is no preceding history of renal disease, and the etiology is quite unknown. Ellis's classification of lobular glomerulonephritis within "Type II", i.e. glomerulonephritis unrelated to haemolytic streptococcal infection, must now be regarded as incorrect in view of the undoubted association of some cases with a previous acute post-streptococcal glomerulonephritis.

Membranous glomerulonephritis

This condition develops insidiously and bears no obvious relation to the types of glomerulonephritis already described. The essential lesion is a diffuse thickening of the basement membrane of the glomerular capillaries, accompanied by increased permeability which results in heavy proteinuria and this in turn leads to hypoalbuminaemia and generalised oedema, i.e. *nephrotic syndrome* (p. 704). Eventually the lesion progresses to glomerulosclerosis, and the disease enters the *chronic* stage, characterised by the features of chronic renal failure, namely uraemia and hypertension.

Clinical features. The disease is commoner in males than females, and occurs over a wide age range, but more often in adults than in children. The presenting feature is oedema, usually developing gradually, often being first noticed in the face, and only partly influenced by gravity. The oedema eventually becomes severe and generalised, with free fluid in the pleural and pericardial cavities. Proteinuria is marked, and as a result the plasma albumin level falls, usually to below 1·6 g. per 100 ml. The urine often contains small numbers of red cells, and analysis of the protein reveals significant

quantities of globulins in addition to the high
concentration of albumin: the urine tends to be
concentrated and reduced in volume, but can
still vary considerably to accommodate fluid
intake.

The hypoalbuminaemia is an essential causal
factor in the generalised oedema seen in this
disease, and the train of events (albuminuria →
hypoalbuminaemia → generalised oedema) is
known as the *nephrotic syndrome*: it occurs in
other renal diseases where albuminuria is heavy,
and hypoalbuminaemia from other causes, e.g.
malnutrition or "protein-losing enteropathy",
also results in generalised oedema. Other
factors involved in the oedema are discussed on
p. 183. Hyperlipidaemia, with increased levels
of lipoproteins containing cholesterol and
phospholipids, is a common accompaniment of
the nephrotic syndrome regardless of the underlying renal pathology.

Before the widespread use of antibiotic drugs,
the nephrotic syndrome carried a high mortality
from superadded infections of the respiratory
tract, peritonitis and meningitis, and many
patients succumbed in the nephrotic stage of

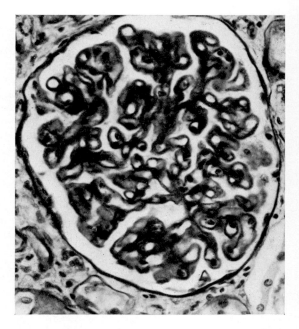

FIG. 21.28.—Membranous glomerulonephritis. The
capillary basement membrane is diffusely and uniformly thickened. × 350.

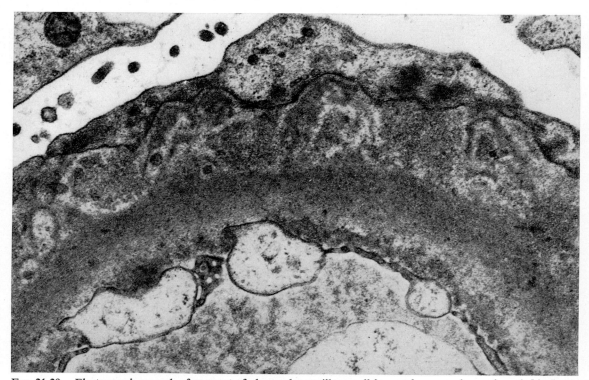

FIG. 21.29.—Electron micrograph of segment of glomerular capillary wall in membranous glomerulonephritis (lumen
below, urinary space above). The basement membrane is thickened and there are multiple, almost confluent
ill-defined deposits on its outer surface. × 50,000.

membranous glomerulonephritis. Nowadays, the nephrotic stage may fluctuate for months or years, eventually tending to subside and to be replaced by the chronic stage which presents as chronic renal failure (p. 714) and is clinically indistinguishable from other forms of chronic glomerulonephritis.

Pathological changes. The essential change is in the glomeruli, and consists of a diffuse hyaline thickening of the walls of all the glomerular capillaries. There is no obvious swelling or proliferation of endothelial or mesangial cells, and no leukocytic infiltration. By light microscopy the capillary walls appear thickened, eosinophilic and hyaline (Fig. 21.28) and

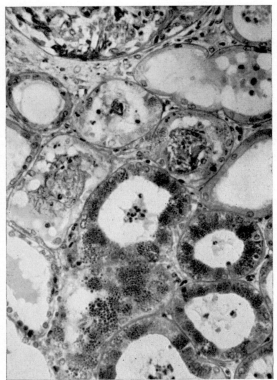

FIG. 21.30.—Hyaline droplets in renal tubular epithelium resulting from reabsorption of protein from the filtrate.

electron microscopy shows irregular deposition of dense amorphous material in the outer part of the capillary basement membrane, and thickening of the basement membrane between the deposits (Fig. 21.29). The foot processes of the epithelial cells are fused to form a continuous layer of cytoplasm over the basement membrane and the irregular deposits. Some reports describe

also deposits of dense material between the basement membrane and capillary endothelium, but this is not usually conspicuous and is often absent. At first, the glomerular capillary lumina do not appear to be narrowed, and ischaemic

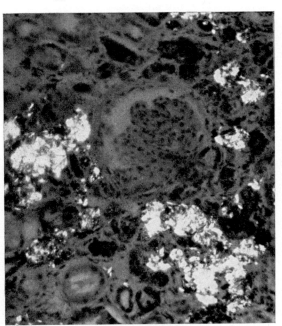

FIG. 21.31.—Kidney in nephrotic syndrome, showing abundant anisotropic lipid with some sudanophil neutral fat (dark) in the interstitial tissue and tubules. (Polarised light with crossed Nicol prisms.)

tubular changes are not seen. Eventually the electron-dense deposits are incorporated in the basement membrane which then shows considerable thickening. The other changes seen in the kidneys at this stage are common to the nephrotic syndrome from all causes: they include diffuse oedema, lipid-rich proteinous casts in the tubules, and albumin-rich droplets and globules of lipid in the cytoplasm of the proximal convoluted tubule cells (Fig. 21.30), attributable to reabsorption of protein and lipid from the lumen. Groups of lipid-rich foamy phagocytes are usually present in the interstitial tissue of the cortex (Fig. 21.31); this is related to the hyperlipidaemia, and probably results from uptake of lipids reabsorbed from the glomerular filtrate by the tubular epithelium. Crystals of cholesterol are sometimes deposited in the interstitial tissue, and induce a surrounding giant-cell granulomatous reaction.

If death occurs during the nephrotic stage, the kidneys are seen to be enlarged due to oedema, and lipid deposits may be visible as a radial yellow streaking of the cortex (Fig. 21.32): both these features are seen in nephrotic syndrome from any cause, and the diagnosis of the underlying disease cannot be made from macroscopic examination of the kidneys.

In the chronic stage of the disease, the thickening of the glomerular capillary walls results in narrowing of the lumina; renal blood flow and GFR are seriously diminished, and uraemia and hypertension develop. Proteinuria diminishes, polyuria often develops, and the oedema tends to subside and may disappear.

Microscopy of the kidneys at this stage shows gross diffuse thickening of glomerular capillary walls, some glomeruli being almost solid eosinophilic hyaline material, while others are less severely affected and still have some patent capillary lumina (Fig. 21.33). Tubular atrophy from ischaemia accompanies the glomerular hyalinisation, and interstitial fibrosis occurs. Lipid deposits often persist and may still be visible macroscopically. The kidneys may be slightly shrunken, and may show the superadded changes of hypertension. The pathological features of the chronic stage are compared with those of other forms of chronic glomerulonephritis on p. 714.

Etiology. There is no evidence that membranous glomerulonephritis is preceded by an infec-

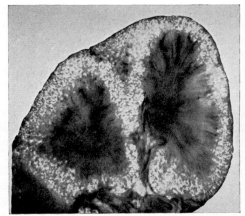

FIG. 21.32.—Kidney in nephrotic syndrome, showing abundant cortical deposits of neutral fat and anisotropic lipids. × ⅔.

tion, and in its typical form it appears quite distinct from diffuse proliferative glomerulonephritis. In fact, the changes are not of an inflammatory nature, and retention of the name is purely traditional. It should be added, however, that occasional patients with the nephrotic syndrome have been found to have a combination of the glomerular changes of membranous and proliferative glomerulonephritis.

Immunofluorescence studies of the kidneys in membranous glomerulonephritis have demonstrated IgG and complement deposited in rela-

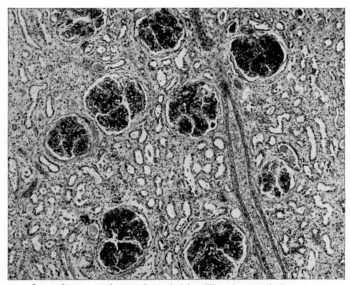

FIG. 21.33.—Late stage of membranous glomerulonephritis. The glomeruli show an extreme degree of hyaline sclerosis (black in the figure). The tubules are much altered and the interstitial tissue is increased. × 60.

From a 25-year-old man who died of uraemia. The kidneys together weighed 620 g. and the heart 420 g. The blood urea was 242 mg. per 100 ml.

tion to the basement membrane of the glomerular capillary walls. In some early cases, granular deposition has been observed (Fig. 21.34), and by analogy with experimental observations (p. 697) this suggests the deposition of circulating antigen–antibody complexes. However, by the time biopsy is performed and the diagnosis made, deposition of IgG is often too heavy to exhibit a distinct pattern. Electron-dense deposits are seen mainly on the epithelial side of the capillary basement membrane which is the site for deposition of immune complexes (p. 697). There is thus indirect evidence suggesting that membranous glomerulonephritis is an immune complex disease.

The disease is resistant to steroid therapy, and so far the use of immunosuppressive drugs has not been encouraging.

One feature of interest in membranous glomerulonephritis is the absence of proliferative change and of leukocytic infiltration of the glomeruli. In view of the deposition of IgG and complement, inflammatory changes might be expected (p. 696). Their absence remains unexplained, but it may be that antigen–antibody complexes are deposited very slowly over a long period, and that, although complement is fixed, the rate of fixation is too low to result in chemotaxis of polymorphs and inflammatory changes. Cases of a more acute type of **glomerulonephritis of mixed type**, i.e. showing a combination of membranous and inflammatory glomerular changes, are being recognised with increasing frequency, and in these it is likely that immune-complex deposition and complement fixation take place more rapidly than in pure membranous glomerulonephritis.

Minimal-change glomerulonephritis

While it is not altogether satisfactory to name a disease in this negative fashion, we have preferred the term "minimal change" glomerulonephritis to the more commonly used *lipoid nephrosis* because it indicates that the essential lesion is glomerular and that the structural changes are inconspicuous.

General features. The disease occurs especially in young children, the highest incidence in Glasgow being around the age of one year (Arneil, 1961), but it does occur also in older children and young adults and more rarely in

older people. It is by far the commonest cause of the nephrotic syndrome in children, and presents as gradually-developing oedema accompanied by, and consequent on, a heavy proteinuria. The oedema and proteinuria tend to fluctuate, spontaneous remission and recurrences being common. The blood pressure and blood urea are usually normal and tests of inulin clearance have confirmed that, in most cases, there is no detectable fall in glomerular filtration rate. As usual in the nephrotic syndrome (p. 704), there is a rise in the level of blood lipids, including cholesterol.

Formerly, there was a high mortality from superadded infections developing in the severely oedematous patient, but the outlook has been improved greatly by the use first of sulphon-

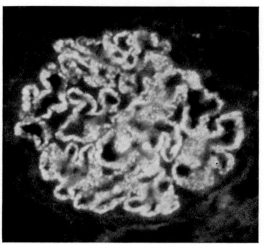

Fig. 21.34.—Renal biopsy in membranous glomerulonephritis. Immunofluorescence technique, showing granular deposition of IgG in the glomerular capillary walls. × 250.

amides and later of antibiotics. Glucocorticoid therapy has also improved the prognosis, for administration of cortisone and similar compounds cuts short the disease by suppressing the proteinuria. Steroid therapy usually takes 2–3 weeks to show an effect, and the mechanism is quite unknown: there is a risk of relapse on stopping therapy, and at present there is no way of predicting the cases in which this will occur. The progress of large series of cases has been observed for some years by Arneil and Lam (1967) and by others, and it appears that the prognosis is good, although a minority of patients eventually develop renal failure with uraemia and hypertension.

In spite of the almost normal appearance of the glomeruli, there is indirect evidence that the proteinuria is accounted for by increased glomerular leakage, and is not due to a defect of absorption of the protein which escapes normally into the glomerular filtrate. In many cases, the proteinuria is highly selective, albumin being accompanied by only very small amounts of the plasma proteins of larger molecular size, and this contrasts with the less highly selective

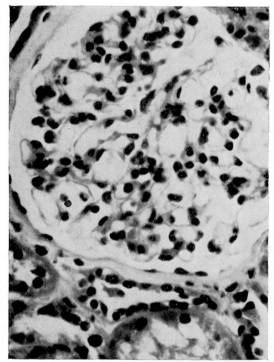

FIG. 21.35.—Minimal-change glomerulonephritis. The glomerulus shows no obvious abnormality apart from dilatation of many of the capillaries. × 560.

proteinuria observed in most other renal diseases, with or without the nephrotic syndrome. Usually there are no, or very few, red cells in the urine, and the spun deposit consists mainly of proteinous, lipid-rich casts.

Pathological changes. Some patients still die from infection supervening on the nephrotic syndrome and the kidneys are pale, particularly the cortex, and are enlarged by oedema. In some cases, yellow deposits of lipid may be seen, mainly in the cortex and showing a radial distribution: as already stated (p. 705) these changes are seen in the nephrotic syndrome from other causes, and are not diagnostic.

Microscopically, the glomeruli look normal

apart from an appearance of fixed dilatation of the capillaries; there is no thickening of the capillary walls and no increased cellularity of the glomerular tufts (Fig. 21.35). The most conspicuous glomerular change on electron microscopy is fusion of the foot processes of the epithelial cells, the basement membrane being covered externally by a layer of epithelial cell cytoplasm (Fig. 21.36): the epithelial cells also show increased vacuolation and in some cases the basement membrane is slightly thickened with loss of definition of the junction between its inner margin and the cytoplasm of the adjacent endothelial cells. Although fusion of the foot processes is the outstanding glomerular change, it is not necessarily the primary lesion, and indeed there is evidence that experimental production of proteinuria in animals *results in* fusion of the foot processes. It may be that a

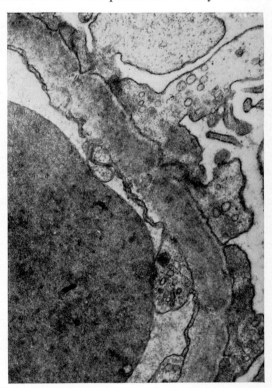

FIG. 21.36.—Electron micrograph of glomerular capillary wall in minimal change glomerulonephritis. The only abnormality is fusion of the foot processes. × 18,000.

reversible increase in the permeability of the capillary basement membrane, not reflected in any obvious structural change, is responsible for the heavy proteinuria and consequent changes in this disease.

Changes common to the nephrotic syndrome from any cause include protein casts in the tubules, proteinous and lipid droplets in the cells of the proximal convoluted tubules, and sometimes groups of foamy macrophages and cholesterol clefts in the interstitial tissue. These features are described more fully in relation to membranous glomerulonephritis on p. 705.

In the minority of patients who progress to uraemia, many of the glomeruli are hyalinised, with associated tubular atrophy and interstitial fibrosis, and the kidneys may show various degrees of shrinkage, cortical thinning and fine granularity (as in chronic glomerulonephritis of any type). It has been reported that, in these cases, hyalinisation occurs first in the juxta-medullary glomeruli and progressively involves those further out in the cortex. However, the number of such cases in which the diagnosis has been confirmed by earlier biopsy is small and further study is required to elucidate the progression, in a minority of cases, to renal failure.

Etiology. The nature of this disease remains unknown. It may follow immediately on a respiratory infection, but does not show a definite relationship to any particular micro-organism. Immunofluorescence studies have failed to demonstrate deposition of immuno-globulin or complement in the glomerular capillary walls, and the etiology is quite obscure, as is the mechanism of the beneficial effect of steroid therapy in curtailing the albuminuria.

Focal glomerulonephritis

This may be defined as a glomerulitis affecting only a proportion of the glomeruli. The lesions usually involve only part of the glomerular tuft, e.g. one or more lobules. The condition may occur in relation to acute respiratory infections, or as a feature of certain specific diseases; its best known association is with subacute bacterial endocarditis, in which the glomerular lesions may be embolic, and it occurs also in systemic lupus erythematosus, in anaphylactoid (Henoch–Schönlein) purpura, in the micro-angiopathic form of polyarteritis nodosa, and in the rare Goodpasture's syndrome. It must be emphasised that focal glomerulonephritis is not the only renal lesion which occurs in these conditions: rapidly progressive glomerulo-nephritis may develop in any of them, and is the

common lesion in Goodpasture's syndrome.

Haematuria is the usual presenting feature of focal glomerulonephritis, but in some patients it gives rise to heavy proteinuria and the nephrotic syndrome.

Pathological changes. The glomerular lesion consists of a cellular proliferation, probably of mesangial cells, affecting the peripheral part of one or more lobules (Fig. 21.37), and in some cases accompanied by fibrinoid necrosis of capillary loops: within the lesions, individual capillary lumina may be obliterated by eosino-philic thrombus which blends with the necrotic capillary wall. Red cells may be present in the

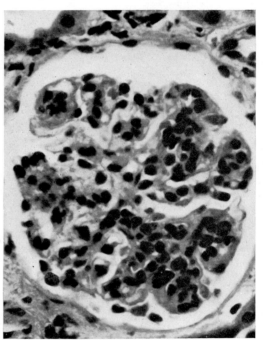

FIG. 21.37.—Focal glomerulonephritis: early lesion. Note the hypercellularity of the affected part of the tuft on the right. × 350.

capsular space and in the tubules, and there may also be some proliferation of the epithelium lining Bowman's capsule. Lesions may occur in only a small proportion of glomeruli, or may involve the majority. In patients with a long history, old scarred glomerular lesions are usually seen (Fig. 21.38), often adherent to the capsule. In cases developing the nephrotic syndrome, the renal changes consequent upon this condition (p. 705) may also be present.

While this account is concerned mainly with focal glomerulonephritis, opportunity is taken below to outline also the additional renal lesions which occur in the diseases giving rise to focal glomerulonephritis.

Idiopathic focal glomerulonephritis. When it occurs apart from specific diseases, focal glomerulonephritis is usually related to ill-defined respiratory infections, including pharyngitis, "colds" and "flu".

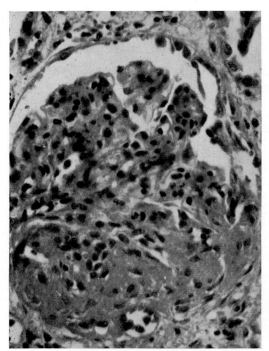

FIG. 21.38.—Focal glomerulonephritis: late lesion. The lower part of the tuft is scarred and adherent to the capsule. × 350.

In contrast to acute diffuse glomerulonephritis, there is no special relationship with Group A streptococcal infections, and the interval between the respiratory infection and the onset of renal disease is only a day or so. Haematuria is often the presenting feature and is usually of not more than a few days' duration. In most cases, there is only mild proteinuria and the illness subsides with no evidence of residual impairment of renal function. Some patients are subject to recurrences, each associated with a respiratory infection, and these may occur over many years: there is evidence that chronic renal failure eventually supervenes in a minority of cases. Patients presenting with the nephrotic syndrome have been observed to recover without evidence of residual impaired renal function. The condition is not common: it occurs particularly in children and young adults, more often males than females, and its etiology is unknown.

Subacute bacterial endocarditis. Renal lesions are commonly present in this condition, but in most cases they do not lead to serious impairment of renal function and their practical importance lies mainly in the resulting haematuria, either gross or microscopic, which is of diagnostic value.

As in other organs, infarcts are common in the kidneys in subacute bacterial endocarditis and are usually non-suppurative. Focal glomerulonephritis occurs in about 50 per cent of cases, and tends to develop after some months. Most of the cases have been caused by *Streptococcus viridans* or *Haemophilus influenzae*. Macroscopically, the kidneys are usually of normal size, and show petechial haemorrhages visible on the subcapsular surface and scattered throughout the cortex. Microscopically, a minority of the glomeruli are usually affected, and the focal lesions show capillary thrombosis, fibrinoid necrosis and proliferative changes (Fig. 21.39). Blood is often seen in the capsular space and tubules, and there may be epithelial crescents. Bacteria cannot usually be seen in the glomerular lesions, but have been recovered in some cases.

In a minority of patients with subacute bacterial endocarditis, diffuse proliferative glomerulonephritis develops, and may progress to renal failure.

Polyarteritis nodosa. The necrotising arteritis which is the essential lesion of this condition usually involves the larger arteries in the kidneys, with aneurysm formation and/or thrombosis, and renal

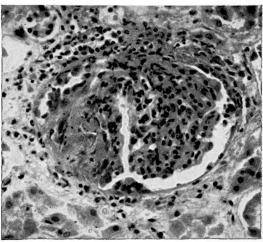

FIG. 21.39.—Glomerulus in subacute bacterial endocarditis, showing a large focal necrotic glomerular lesion, with inflammatory infiltration around. × 200.

infarcts are commonly present (Figs. 13.30, 13.31, p. 282). In about one third of cases, death results from renal failure with hypertension. In the *microangiopathic variant* of polyarteritis, the vascular lesions show the same features—fibrinoid necrosis and inflammatory changes—but involve mainly the interlobular arteries (Fig. 13.28, p. 281), afferent glomerular arterioles, and also the glomerular capillaries, giving rise to focal glomerulonephritis. As the disease progresses, most of the glomeruli may be involved and renal failure may develop, although hypertension is less common than in the classic form of the disease.

Anaphylactoid purpura occurs mainly in children, and gives rise to a skin rash, joint pains, and colic with bloody diarrhoea due to a haemorrhagic exudate into the gut. In some cases there is a focal glomerulonephritis, with haematuria and proteinuria, but renal failure is either absent or mild and transient, and there is little evidence to suggest permanent renal impairment, even after recurrent attacks. Rapidly progressive glomerulonephritis may, however, supervene.

Goodpasture's syndrome. In this rare condition, haemorrhage from the alveolar capillaries gives rise to haemoptysis, accompanied by haematuria and proteinuria attributable to focal glomerulonephritis. The outlook is poor: pulmonary haemorrhage may become increasingly severe and the renal lesion usually develops into rapidly progressive glomerulonephritis.

Systemic lupus erythematosus. Clinically apparent renal disease occurs in over 50 per cent of patients with this disease, and carries a poor prognosis. The nephrotic syndrome may develop when proteinuria is heavy, and uraemia, with or without hypertension, is an important cause of death. The essential changes are in the glomeruli, which show two distinct lesions, (*a*) focal glomerulonephritis, in which lobules or parts of lobules show proliferative changes and fibrinoid necrosis, and (*b*) thickening of the glomerular capillary basement membrane, which presents a refractile eosinophilic appearance; the change is usually patchy, but may be more diffuse, and is commonly termed the "*wire-loop*" appearance (Fig. 21.40). Electron microscopy has shown this to be due to irregular deposits of dense material, within and on both aspects of the basement membrane. Other changes include hyaline thrombosis of individual capillary loops, adhesions between affected glomerular lobules and Bowman's capsule, proliferation of the capsular epithelium, sometimes progressing to crescent formation, and focal or more extensive glomerular hyalinisation resulting presumably from scarring of the lesions of focal glomerulonephritis. As elsewhere in systemic lupus erythematosus, haematoxyphil bodies (p. 814) may be found in the glomerular lesions.

Etiology of focal glomerulonephritis. The widespread use of the term *focal embolic nephritis* for the focal glomerulonephritis of subacute bacterial endocarditis reflects the commonly held belief that the glomerular lesions are embolic. However, this is not firmly

established, and in other cases of focal glomerulonephritis there is no obvious source of emboli, particularly in the idiopathic form of the disease.

The available evidence suggests that the diseases which focal glomerulonephritis accompanies are attributable to abnormal immunological reactions. The evidence is strongest in the case of systemic lupus erythematosus, in which glomerular lesions have been shown to result from deposition of antigen–antibody complexes in the capillary walls (p. 111). Anaphylactoid purpura, as its name suggests, is widely regarded

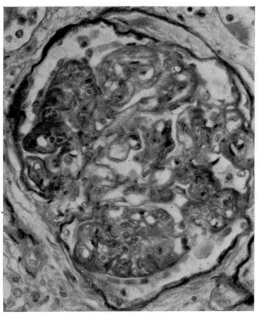

Fig. 21.40.—Glomerulus in systemic lupus erythematosus, showing the "wire-loop" appearance, most prominently of a capillary on the extreme left. × 350.

as a hypersensitivity disease, and the antigens which may be concerned include streptococci and certain foods. Lesions resembling those of polyarteritis nodosa occur in serum sickness, and fixed immunoglobulins have been observed in the vascular lesions of polyarteritis. Finally, in subacute bacterial endocarditis the prolonged infection provides a possible basis for immunological injury from circulating antigen–antibody complexes. Direct evidence for an immunological basis in focal glomerulonephritis is fragmentary. Antigen–antibody complexes have been demonstrated in the glomerular lesions of systemic lupus erythematosus and antibody to capillary basement membrane is demonstrable in

Goodpasture's syndrome (Fig. 21.41). In both conditions, however, the glomerular lesions are complex, and it is not clearly apparent that the immunological findings relate particularly to the focal glomerulonephritis. Deposition of IgG and of complement have been described in the

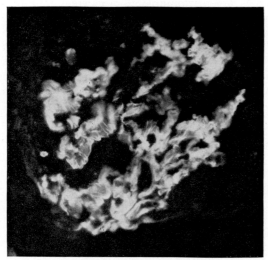

FIG. 21.41.—Antibody to glomerular capillary basement membrane showing the characteristic linear pattern of staining by the immunofluorescence technique. Necropsy specimen in Goodpasture's syndrome.

focal glomerular lesions of anaphylactoid purpura, but more extensive investigations are required.

While the above immunological findings suggest a possible common basis for focal glomerulonephritis, they do not explain the focal nature of the lesions.

Chronic glomerulonephritis

It is apparent, from the foregoing descriptions of the various types of glomerulonephritis, that an end-stage is commonly reached in which so many glomeruli are destroyed that chronic renal failure develops: this is characterised by uraemia and usually by hypertension. The time taken to reach this stage, and the rate of progression once it has developed, vary with the type of preceding glomerulonephritis, and also in individual cases. Hypertension often becomes of the malignant (accelerated) type; the resulting hypertensive vascular and glomerular lesions become superadded to the existing damage, leading, if untreated, to end-stage renal failure which progresses rapidly to death. In cases

where hypertension is absent or less severe, renal failure may progress more slowly, and the end-stage may last for several years.

In over 70 per cent of patients with chronic glomerulonephritis, there is no history to suggest preceding renal disease, and the renal lesions have progressed silently until chronic renal failure develops. In such cases, it is often not possible to decide, even by histological examination of the kidneys, what type of glomerulonephritis has led up to the chronic stage: in other cases, there may be evidence suggesting or indicating a previous acute diffuse proliferative glomerulonephritis, lobular glomerulonephritis, or membranous glomerulonephritis.

Pathological changes and pathogenesis. Both the kidneys are uniformly and equally reduced in size, sometimes only slightly so (Fig. 21.42), but often to about one third of normal. The capsule is often firmly adherent and the sub-capsular surface uniformly and finely irregular (often termed "granular"): surface granularity is most marked in severely shrunken kidneys. There

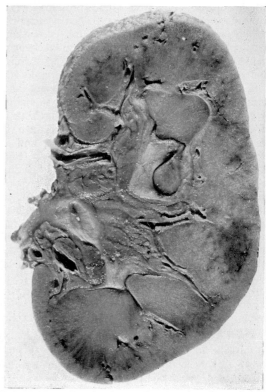

FIG. 21.42.—Chronic glomerulonephritis. Note the uniform thinning of the cortex and relatively normal medulla. In this case, the reduction in size of the kidney is only moderate. × 1·2.

is uniform thinning of the cortex, which accounts largely for the reduction in kidney size, while the medullary pyramids are also, although less markedly, shrunken. The amount of fatty tissue around the renal pelvis is not diminished, and often appears to be increased, so that the amount of surviving renal tissue is less than is suggested by the weight of the kidneys. In contrast to chronic pyelonephritis, the calyces and renal pelvis exhibit no special changes.

The renal arteries and their major branches show arteriosclerotic thickening, and in cases complicated by malignant hypertension the cortical mottling and haemorrhages of this condition are superimposed on the changes described above. The other organs and tissues show the changes of uraemia and hypertension.

Microscopically, the glomeruli show various degrees of scarring. Usually most of the glomeruli are destroyed and converted into shrunken dense hyaline scars of low cellularity (Fig. 21.43): the capsular space may be completely obliterated or may be broken up into epithelial-lined spaces by adhesions between the hyalinised glomerular tuft and Bowman's capsule. In some cases, the scarred remains of epithelial crescents may be discernible. A minority of glomeruli show lesser degrees of hyalinisation with some persisting capillaries and usually capsular adhesions, while it is common to find small numbers of glomeruli which show little or no evidence of injury and which, together with their associated tubules, have undergone compensatory hypertrophy (Fig. 21.44). The arcuate and interlobular arteries and the afferent arterioles show hypertensive changes which are likely, by causing ischaemia, to have contributed to the glomerular scarring. When malignant hypertension has supervened the changes typical of this condition are seen in those glomeruli which have not been destroyed already by the glomerulonephritic process. The tubules show extensive atrophy, many being completely lost, and there is an increase in the intertubular connective tissue and irregular interstitial aggregation of lymphocytes and usually smaller numbers of plasma cells. In most cases, a minority of tubules, connected to the less affected or hypertrophied glomeruli, are enlarged and conspicuous, and account for the elevations which give the sub-capsular surface its granular appearance. These surviving functioning tubules may show hyaline droplets in the epithelial cytoplasm, and frequently contain protein casts (p. 685), features which relate to the proteinuria: when malignant hypertension has supervened, there may be blood in the capsular spaces and in functioning tubules.

The above description relates to the findings in most cases of chronic glomerulonephritis. In a minority of these cases, there is good evidence of a *preceding acute glomerulonephritis* of poststreptococcal origin, often many years before, and separated from the chronic stage by a latent period of good health but with persistent pro-

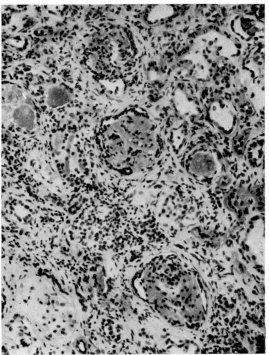

Fig. 21.43.—Chronic glomerulonephritis, showing hyalinisation of glomeruli; the tubular epithelium is atrophic and there is interstitial fibrosis. × 100.

teinuria. In most instances there is no history of acute glomerulonephritis and the type of glomerular disease which has led to the chronic stage remains unknown. It is difficult to accept that the variations in degrees of glomerular injury, ranging from complete hyalinisation to unaffected glomeruli, could have resulted from progression of the lesion of acute diffuse proliferative glomerulonephritis, which affects all the glomeruli in a rather uniform manner. It has been suggested that *focal glomerulonephritis* is a more likely cause of the typical changes of chronic glomerulonephritis, but there is at present no good evidence that the majority of cases have resulted from focal glomerulo-nephritis.

It has already been stated that patients who survive the nephrotic stage of *membranous glomerulonephritis* progress to a chronic stage with renal failure. In such cases there is usually a clear history of nephrotic syndrome, which may have subsided or may still persist when chronic renal failure supervenes: it is, of course, helpful if the diagnosis has been confirmed by previous renal biopsy. The renal changes of chronic membranous glomerulonephritis (p. 706) are somewhat different from those described above

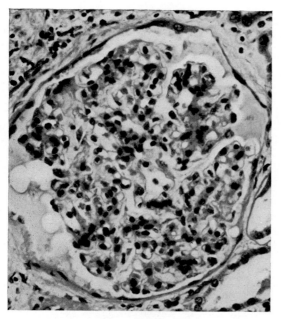

Fig. 21.44.—A relatively healthy, hypertrophied glomerulus in chronic glomerulonephritis. × 250.

for chronic glomerulonephritis: the kidneys may be enlarged, of normal size, or small: lipid deposits may still be visible in the cortex by the naked eye, and microscopy shows an advanced stage of diffuse hyaline thickening of the glomerular capillary walls, with obliteration of most of the lumina: many of the glomeruli are completely solid, but in those less severely affected the capillary wall changes can still be discerned. All the glomeruli are affected to some extent, and the tubular atrophy is accordingly more uniform, without prominent enlarged tubules: for this reason, the surface of the kidney is often smooth and does not exhibit the granularity usual in chronic glomerulonephritis.

A small proportion of cases of chronic glomerulonephritis result from *lobular glomerulonephritis*. The features of this condition, and its relationship to acute diffuse proliferative glomerulonephritis, have already been discussed (p. 703). In most cases, there is a history of nephrotic syndrome, and when chronic glomerulonephritis supervenes, the accentuation of the glomerular lobules may still be discernible, even in those which are completely hyalinised. Apart from the differences in glomerular changes, the kidneys show the same features as in chronic membranous glomerulonephritis.

Clinical features. Most patients developing chronic glomerulonephritis are between 10 and 50 years old. The clinical features and changes in other organs and tissues are those of *chronic renal failure* and are attributable to *uraemia*, usually accompanied by *hypertension*. Since chronic renal failure results also from various other diseases of the kidneys, a description common to all causes seems appropriate, and is given below.

CHRONIC RENAL FAILURE

Chronic renal failure results when the functions of the kidneys have been so reduced by a chronic disease process that there is retention of nitrogenous waste products normally excreted mainly in the urine, and loss of the capacity of the kidneys to maintain homoeostasis of fluid and electrolytes, and acid–base balance, in the face of the normal variations of fluid and dietary intake and of physical activity. In most cases, hypertension is superadded, and may be of the malignant type. Chronic pyelonephritis and

chronic glomerulonephritis account for the majority of cases, but there are many other causes, including essential (primary) malignant hypertension, polycystic disease of the kidneys, systemic lupus erythematosus, diabetes mellitus, amyloid disease, nephrocalcinosis, gout, irradiation injury, and heavy prolonged dosage of certain analgesics. The pathological changes characteristic of these diseases are described in the appropriate sections: in all of them, severe chronic renal injury may occur, but the resulting chronic renal failure presents biochemical, clinical and morphological changes which are sufficiently similar to warrant a common description.

Biochemical disturbances

In 1952, Robert Platt advanced the view that, in chronic renal failure, the renal deficiency was the result of loss of most of the two million nephrons, and that those remaining functioned normally, but were unable to maintain normal total renal function. This *intact nephron theory* is really another way of stating that destruction of any part of a nephron results in loss of function of the whole nephron. The pathological changes which result in renal failure in chronic pyelonephritis, in which the injury affects primarily the tubules, and in chronic glomerulonephritis, which affects primarily the glomeruli, provide support for the theory, for in both conditions most of the nephrons are virtually completely destroyed, while a minority escape serious injury and even become hypertrophic throughout. While the intact nephron theory has been widely accepted, and in general provides a good basis for explaining the observed functional disturbances, loss of function does not always occur at the same rate in all parts of the nephron. For example, in chronic pyelonephritis, glomerular injury lags behind tubular injury, and disturbance of tubular function is correspondingly more severe, particularly while the chronic inflammatory process is still active.

Non-protein nitrogen retention. Accepting that only a small proportion of functioning nephrons remains in patients with chronic renal failure, it follows that renal blood flow and total glomerular filtration rate (GFR) are considerably reduced. When GFR falls below normal, the amount of urea removed from the blood falls below the normal level of urea production, and the level in the blood rises. If kidney function remains steady, the blood urea will stabilise at a level at which the normal amount is removed in the glomerular filtrate. To give an example, the normal GFR may be taken as 120 ml. per minute, and the blood urea level as approximately 30 mg. per 100 ml. Since urea is very highly diffusible, the concentration in the glomerular filtrate will also be 30 mg. per 100 ml., and the total amount of urea filtered off

from the blood will thus be $120/100 \times 30$ mg., i.e. 36 mg. per minute. Some re-absorption of urea takes place from the tubule, and the amount excreted daily is about 25 mg. per minute (35 g. daily). Consider now the patient with chronic renal failure and sufficient functioning nephrons to provide a GFR of, say, 12 ml. per minute. Obviously, this will result in urea retention, which will be reflected in a high blood urea: when the level reaches 300 mg. per 100 ml., the 12 ml. of filtrate per minute will then contain 36 mg., i.e. the amount normally filtered, and provided that tubular reabsorption is not altered, the normal amount will be excreted. In fact, this is an over-simplification, for urea production varies with dietary protein intake, and there are also variations in the amount reabsorbed from the tubules. In chronic renal failure there is usually distinct polyuria and, as explained overleaf, less reabsorption occurs from the tubules. In spite of these complicating factors, the level of the blood urea gives useful information in chronic renal failure, and is easy to estimate: provided certain precautions are taken, changes in the level reflect changes in renal function. The level of blood creatinine is less influenced by dietary factors and tubular reabsorption and provides a better indication of renal function, but its estimation is less simple.

Urea itself has little or no toxicity, but its retention is an indication of retention of various other non-protein nitrogenous metabolites, some of which are toxic.

Excretion of water. In normal circumstances, the kidneys play the major role in adjusting water loss to suit intake. This is effected by varying the volume of urine from approximately 400 ml. to several litres daily. Within these limits, the excretion of urinary solutes is not affected significantly, and the specific gravity of the urine is inversely proportional to the volume, varying between 1·002 and 1·040. In chronic renal failure, the normal variability of urine volume is lost, and provided sufficient water is taken in, the kidneys excrete daily approximately 2·5 litres of dilute urine of specific gravity approximately 1·010. If water intake is inadequate in this condition, production of dilute urine continues and dehydration, with resultant fall in blood volume and blood pressure, results: renal blood flow and GFR are consequently diminished, the volume of urine falls and uraemia increases. If water intake is excessive, the urine volume is little affected, and the patient develops water intoxication and pulmonary oedema. The supervention of heart failure, a common complication of chronic renal failure with hypertension, results in further impairment of renal blood flow and fall in GFR, with consequent oliguria, increase in uraemia, and cardiac oedema.

The polyuria of chronic renal failure is at first sight surprising in view of the small amount of glomerular filtrate produced, but it will be recalled that in the healthy individual, the volume of urine is controlled mainly by the degree of concentration taking place in the tubules, and not by variations in the glomerular filtrate. Obviously, in chronic renal failure the polyuria results from failure of the tubules to effect the normal variations in concentration, and the most likely explanation is that the high concentration of urea in the glomerular filtrate exerts an osmotic diuretic effect similar to that which occurs when a large amount of urea is administered to a normal individual. The effect is not peculiar to urea, and can be induced by giving any substance which diffuses readily into the glomerular filtrate and which is largely unabsorbed in the tubules, e.g. inulin. Normally, 80 per cent of the volume of the glomerular filtrate is reabsorbed in the proximal part of the tubule, but the fluid remaining in the lumen does not exceed isotonicity. In chronic renal failure, the high concentration of urea in the glomerular filtrate results in isotonicity being reached when much less than 80 per cent of the volume has been reabsorbed, and further concentration cannot be achieved in this part of the nephron. In the distal part of the tubule and the collecting tubule, the "sodium pump" normally results in a high concentration of Na^+ in the adjacent medullary interstitial tissue, and this facilitates further concentration of the tubular fluid and production of a hypertonic urine. In chronic renal failure (and osmotic diuresis induced in a normal individual) failure to achieve the normal five-fold concentration in the proximal tubule results in a large volume of fluid passing into the distal tubule, and rapid absorption of water here dilutes the Na^+ in the interstitial fluid and so interferes with further urinary concentration.

Electrolyte disturbances. It is a remarkable fact that, in contrast to the blood urea, the plasma concentrations of sodium and potassium are virtually unaltered until the terminal stages of chronic renal failure. In the normal individual, the amounts of Na^+ and K^+ excreted in the urine vary considerably, depending on intake. In chronic renal failure, the range of excretion is limited, and extremes of intake are not well tolerated: nevertheless, considering that relatively few functioning nephrons remain, it is apparent that, to maintain homoeostasis, considerably more Na^+ and K^+ must be excreted per nephron than normally. This is brought about by the continuous state of osmotic diuresis, referred to above, which pertains in chronic renal failure, for diuresis is accompanied by decreased absorption of various solutes, including Na^+ and K^+. Deficiency of Na^+ is a common complication, for the urinary loss is somewhat inflexible, and deficiency may result from restricted intake of salt, or from vomiting and diarrhoea, attacks of which are common in uraemia. Na^+ deficiency in time leads to fall in plasma volume and blood pressure, and to oliguria: nitrogen retention increases and acidosis (see below) supervenes. In some cases of chronic renal failure due to pyelonephritis, sodium loss is severe, and the clinical features may be similar to those of adrenocortical insufficiency (Addison's disease). Correction of Na^+ deficiency in chronic renal failure must be carefully controlled, for administration of too much Na^+ and water can readily induce systemic or pulmonary oedema.

Potassium retention may arise in chronic renal failure from excessive intake or as a complication of dehydration and acidosis; in this state, dehydration results in oliguria and reduced K^+ excretion, while acidosis results in exchange of some intracellular K^+ for H^+; both effects raise the level of plasma K^+, and there is a risk of cardiac arrest. Potassium deficiency is uncommon in chronic renal failure, but can occur in certain cases of chronic pyelonephritis, where excessive loss of K^+ in the urine can result from secondary aldosteronism, attributable, in turn, to excessive Na^+ loss, and producing a picture like Conn's syndrome (p. 912).

To conserve the normal acid–base balance of the body, the kidneys must excrete 40–60 mEq of acid (H^+) daily. This is excreted in combination with urinary phosphate and organic acid radicles (e.g. creatinine), and by combination with ammonia as NH_4^+. For homoeostasis, therefore, the glomerular filtrate must provide sufficient dibasic phosphate and other available anions, and the cells of the distal convoluted tubules must produce and secrete an adequate amount of ammonia, which is normally derived by deamination of amino-acids. In chronic renal failure, the diminished volume of glomerular filtrate does not contain the normal amount of dibasic phosphate, but tubular re-absorption is also reduced as a result of the continuous osmotic diuresis, and the net amount available for excretion of acid is not very much less than normal until the late stages. Because relatively few functioning nephrons remain, total ammonia production and secretion into the tubules is reduced. There is also some loss of bicarbonate in the urine, whereas normally it is almost completely reabsorbed. As a result of these changes, the patient with chronic renal failure is prone to develop acidosis. In most cases, the plasma phosphate level is normal except in the late stages, but if lack of water or salt arises, either from deficient intake or from vomiting or diarrhoea, or if the glomerular filtration rate falls even further as a result of heart failure, phosphate excretion is diminished, the blood level rises and acidosis develops.

The level of plasma calcium tends to be slightly low in chronic renal failure, and is further depressed if the level of phosphate rises. In this state, however, acidosis is also likely, and this increases the proportion of plasma calcium in ionic form, with the result that frank tetany does not usually develop, although muscle twitching is common.

Hypertension

This develops in most cases of chronic renal failure, often before there is nitrogen retention, and is commonly of the malignant type. The renal changes resulting from hypertension cause further injury to the already damaged kidneys, and progress of renal failure is hastened. Life can be prolonged by amelioration of severe hypertension by antihypertensive drugs and this is now an important aspect of treatment.

The cause of hypertension in chronic renal failure (and indeed in renal disease in general) is not well understood: it is discussed on pp. 186 and 274.

Pathological changes

The disease processes most commonly responsible for chronic renal failure are listed on p. 714, and their pathological features are described in the appropriate sections. It remains to describe the pathological changes throughout the body which *result from* chronic renal failure, whatever the cause. These changes are neither constant nor specific. Fibrinous pericarditis, accompanied by little or no effusion, is common in the late stages, and also *"uraemic pneumonitis"*, consisting of a sero-fibrinous exudate into the alveolar spaces, sometimes fanning out from the hila, and giving a butterfly shadow on X-ray. The changes resemble those of neonatal hyaline membrane disease (p. 340), but there is often partial organisation of the exudate. Inflammatory changes occur also in the gastro-intestinal tract, including haemorrhagic ulceration and also a pseudomembranous enterocolitis. The cause of these various inflammatory lesions has not been established. Immunological depression, with a tendency to infections, is known to occur in uraemia, but the fibrinous pericarditis is usually sterile, and cannot be explained thus. In some cases, the fibrinoid necrosis of arterioles resulting from malignant hypertension may be responsible for some of the lesions (e.g. Fig. 13.17, p. 273). The cardiovascular features of hypertension are usually obvious in such cases, although cerebral haemorrhage is less common than in essential hypertension. The commonest lesion found in the brain at necropsy is cerebral oedema. Changes have also been described in the pancreas (p. 595).

Bone changes. Various bone changes may occur, and are termed collectively *uraemic osteodystrophy* (p. 764). In some cases, the plasma levels of ionised calcium and phosphate are sufficiently changed to induce increased function and hyperplasia of the parathyroid glands, with consequent bone changes (secondary hyperparathyroidism). In children, a condition bearing some resemblance to rickets, and termed *renal dwarfism* or *renal rickets*, may develop.

Haematological changes also occur in chronic renal failure, and are described more fully on p. 402. Briefly, there is a normochromic normocytic anaemia, the intensity of which bears a correlation to the degree of uraemia. It is due to depressed erythropoiesis, but increased red cell destruction can also occur, especially in the late stages (see p. 416).

Clinico-pathological correlations

Many of the clinical features of chronic renal failure can be surmised from the foregoing account of the biochemical and structural changes. Polyuria may be the presenting symptom, and is most noticeable at night when it replaces the low volume of concentrated urine normally produced. Any of the clinical features of severe hypertension may be present, including heart failure, visual disturbances due to retinal involvement, and convulsions followed by fatal coma from hypertensive encephalopathy. If heart failure supervenes, the volume of urine diminishes and oedema of cardiac type develops (p. 182).

Urea itself is without serious toxic properties, but the retention of other, ill-defined nitrogenous compounds in uraemia gives rise to toxic effects characterised by vomiting and anorexia and by mental dullness: coma often supervenes, but may be long delayed. As already explained, the impairment of renal function renders the patient liable to dehydration and acidosis, with their corresponding clinical features, and in this state there is also a danger of muscular irritability due to fall in plasma calcium, and of hyponatraemia and hyperkalaemia. Excessive fluid and sodium loss, e.g. from vomiting and diarrhoea, must be corrected with care to avoid these serious biochemical disturbances, but care must also be taken to avoid therapeutic overloading with sodium and water, as this leads rapidly to pulmonary oedema. When uraemia is advanced, severe anaemia is commonly present, and contributes to the clinical picture. Hypertensive encephalopathy may accompany uraemia, with generalised convulsions which are believed to result from cerebral ischaemia due to vascular spasm.

In most instances, the changes in the kidneys which have brought about chronic renal failure are irreversible, and the prognosis depends on the rate of progression and on the availability of, and suitability of the patient for, chronic dialysis or renal transplantation. In some cases of chronic pyelonephritis, however, renal function can improve, at least for a time, if the infection is active and can be suppressed, and while it is therefore important to search for evidence of chronic pyelonephritis, it is even more important that this condition should be detected and eliminated before it has caused sufficient renal injury to result in chronic renal failure.

MISCELLANEOUS RENAL DISEASES

Diabetes mellitus

Renal failure is an important complication of diabetes. It causes death in more than 10 per cent of all diabetics, and in over 50 per cent of these developing diabetes in childhood. The most important contribution to this high mortality is *diabetic glomerulosclerosis*, which can also give rise to the nephrotic syndrome. Hyaline thickening of the afferent glomerular arterioles is also very common in diabetes: it is similar to that already described in hypertensives and old people, but is more often very severe in diabetics, both with and without hypertension, and affects also the efferent arterioles much more severely than in non-diabetics (Fig. 21.45). Acute pyelonephritis is also unduly common in diabetics, and is particularly prone to be accompanied by papillary necrosis (p. 736).

Diabetic glomerulosclerosis. This consists of deposition of eosinophilic hyaline material in the mesangium of the glomerular lobules. The deposits may be discrete rounded nodules, sometimes laminated, situated near the tip of the lobule and therefore appearing peripheral in the glomerulus (Kimmelstiel–Wilson lesion). Such *nodular* deposition affects lobules and glomeruli unequally, and one or more nodules, of various sizes, may be seen in affected glomeruli (Fig. 21.46). The glomerular capillaries are seen around the margin of the nodules, and may long remain unaffected, but nodular glomerulosclerosis is usually accompanied by more diffuse deposition of hyaline material in the mesangium of all the glomerular lobules, with associated thickening of the glomerular capillary basement membranes (Fig. 21.45). This *diffuse* glomerulosclerosis may resemble membranous glomerulonephritis, but shows less uniform basement membrane thickening: it occurs together with the nodular lesion, and may eventually progress to obliteration of most of the capillaries and severe hyalinisation of the glomeruli. Ischaemic changes, including obliteration of the capsular space by collagen, and glomerular collapse, are also seen and are presumably related to hyaline thickening of the afferent arterioles. As

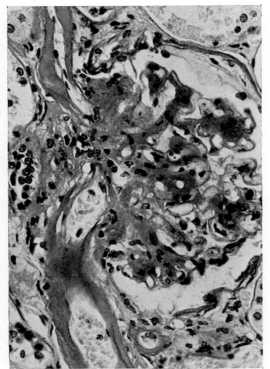

Fig. 21.45.—Hyaline change in the afferent and efferent glomerular arterioles in diabetes. Note also the diffuse glomerulosclerosis. × 250.

a result of glomerulosclerosis, secondary atrophy occurs in the tubules, and the kidneys may be reduced in size with thinning of the cortex and a granular surface.

The pathogenesis of diabetic glomerulosclerosis is not understood, and electron microscopy has so far not contributed much to its elucidation. The deposited hyaline material is PAS-positive and has an electron-microscopic appearance similar to basement membrane. At present, Lendrum's suggestion that the material originates from exudation of plasma constituents (p. 198) seems the most likely explanation, both for the glomerulosclerosis and for the hyaline material deposited in the glomerular arterioles. The observed differences in staining reactions of these two lesions may be due to differences in

their age. It has been suggested that glomerulosclerosis in diabetes may result from an immunological reaction. Beef insulin is antigenic to man, and most diabetics receiving it develop circulating antibody; there is thus the possibility of circulating insulin–antibody complexes and of immune-complex nephritis (p. 697). In support of this possibility, Berns *et al.* (1962) have reported immunofluorescence studies which suggest that beef insulin and antibody to beef insulin are deposited in the glomerular capillary walls. However, this cannot be the sole cause, for diabetic glomerulosclerosis occurs in some diabetics not treated with insulin, and was recognised before the introduction of treatment by insulin. The possibility remains of autoantibody, i.e. to autologous insulin, with consequent immune-complex deposition, but the evidence for this is not strong.

Diabetic glomerulosclerosis has been reported in 25–50 per cent of diabetics at necropsy. In most instances, the nodular and diffuse forms are combined, but in some the diffuse form occurs

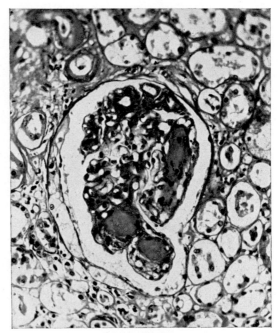

Fig. 21.46.—Nodular glomerulosclerosis in diabetes (Kimmelstiel–Wilson lesion). × 205.

alone. It is worth while distinguishing between the two forms, for while the nodular lesion is highly characteristic of diabetes, the diffuse lesion is related much more closely with disturbances of renal function. In many cases, diabetic glomerulosclerosis is unsuspected during life, and may be clinically silent. It is commonly associated with proteinuria, and when severe this may result in the nephrotic syndrome. It may also lead to chronic renal failure with the usual features of uraemia and hypertension. As already mentioned, glomerulosclerosis is especially common in early-onset diabetes; its incidence and severity increase with the duration of diabetes, and there is some evidence that poor control of the diabetic state is a contributory cause.

Other renal changes in diabetes. Atheroma is very common and often severe in diabetics. In non-diabetics the renal arteries rarely show severe narrowing from atheroma unless they are involved at their origins by aortic atheromatous plaques. In diabetes, however, severe atheroma does occur in the main renal arteries and their segmental branches: it has been suggested that diabetic glomerulosclerosis may be a conse-

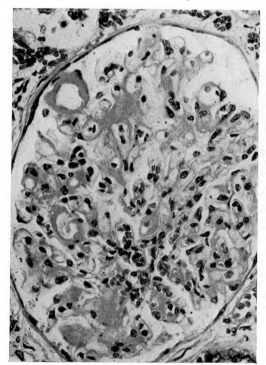

FIG. 21.47.—Deposition of amyloid in the glomerular capillaries at a relatively early stage as compared with Fig. 21.48. × 250.

quence of narrowing of the major arteries, and whether or not this is so, it is probable that severe atheroma of these vessels contributes towards the high incidence of hypertension in diabetes.

Other renal lesions occurring in diabetes have been referred to above, and include hyaline arteriolar thickening, pyelonephritis and papillary necrosis. The evidence for a high incidence of chronic pyelonephritis is not entirely convincing, but acute pyelonephritis, often with papillary necrosis, is common at necropsy in diabetics.

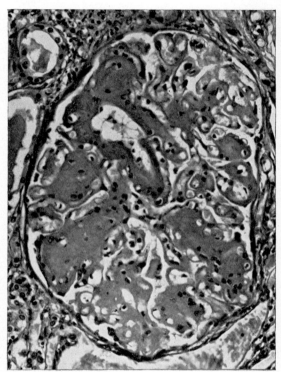

FIG. 21.48.—Glomerular amyloidosis, showing swelling and hyaline appearance of capillary walls. × 350.

Amyloid

The kidneys are involved in nearly all cases of amyloidosis secondary to chronic infections, rheumatoid arthritis, etc., and are also commonly affected in primary amyloidosis. The most important site of deposition is around the glomerular capillary basement membrane (Fig. 21.47): this is accompanied by increased permeability, and proteinuria may be sufficiently heavy to cause the nephrotic syndrome. As the deposits increase, capillary narrowing and obliteration ensue, and the glomeruli may be largely replaced by amyloid (Fig. 21.48). Secondary atrophy of the tubules and interstitial fibrosis result from the glomerular lesion, and chronic renal failure gradually supervenes. The kidneys are firm and pale (Fig. 21.49), may be of normal size, enlarged, or shrunken and granular, and the glomeruli are usually visible by naked eye after treating a slice of kidney with Lugol's iodine. In cases with the nephrotic syndrome, the usual accompanying features are seen in the kidneys (p. 705).

Amyloid is deposited also in the walls of the small blood vessels of the kidneys and upon the tubular basement membranes. The careful studies of Lendrum (1969) have revealed similarities in the pattern of amyloid deposition and hyaline change, e.g. in diabetes (p. 718), which have led him to suggest that amyloid may originate from an exudative process.

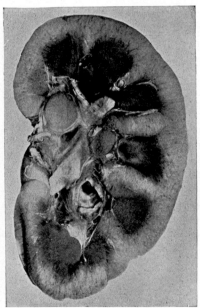

Fig. 21.49.—Amyloid kidney.
Note the marked pallor of the cortex. × ⅘.

There is a tendency to thrombosis of the intra-renal veins in renal amyloidosis, sometimes extending to the main renal veins, and causing acute renal failure.

Gout

The main features of gout are described on p. 799. The excretion of increased amounts of urates by the kidneys may result in crystal formation in the medulla. The crystals are deposited mainly in the collecting tubules where they cause local destruction of the tubular wall and become surrounded by a giant-cell reaction and eventually by fibrous tissue. They are usually at first needle-shaped, but tend to become amorphous. The destructive changes in the collecting tubules result in atrophy of the corresponding nephrons and the kidney may be reduced in size with a granular surface and scarring of the medulla. Urate stones may develop in the renal pelves and may cause renal colic, haematuria and obstruction.

A moderate degree of hypertension is common in gout and is accompanied by the usual renal changes. Features suggestive of chronic pyelonephritis are also common at necropsy; polymorphs are often seen in the tubules, but do not necessarily indicate an infection, for it has been shown experimentally that acute inflammation, including polymorph aggregates, can occur around injected urate crystals without super-added infection, and this happens around urate deposits in the acute attack of gout.

In spite of the high frequency and variety of renal changes in gout, renal failure supervenes in only a small proportion of cases.

Kidney lesions in pregnancy

There is no doubt that the incidence of renal disease is increased during pregnancy. A factor which contributes to this is the tendency to dilatation of the ureters, attributable to the relaxation of smooth muscle which is a feature of pregnancy, and also to pressure effects of the enlarged uterus: it is probably as a consequence of these effects that urinary infection, including pyelonephritis, is a common complication of pregnancy.

Secondly, acute tubular necrosis (p. 723), and rarely renal cortical necrosis (p. 727), are encountered as complications of pregnancy, particularly in cases of retroplacental haemorrhage, infected abortion, and post-partum haemorrhage.

Lastly, pregnancy increases the functional demands on the kidneys, and latent chronic renal disease (e.g. chronic glomerulonephritis) may first become clinically apparent during pregnancy. Essential hypertension may also be aggravated by pregnancy, during which the blood pressure may increase temporarily.

Toxaemia of pregnancy. Albuminuria is a common occurrence in pregnancy, particularly in the last trimester, and may be accompanied by some oedema of the ankles: these disturbances are not of serious significance unless there is also a rise in the blood pressure, when the combination of features is termed *pre-eclampsia* or *pre-eclamptic toxaemia*. This also may be mild, and the changes—oedema, proteinuria and hypertension—do not usually increase to alarming degrees, and subside usually within a few days after parturition. In other cases, the features become progressively more severe during late pregnancy, and impaired renal function is reflected in a rise in the levels of blood urea. In such cases, hypertensive convulsions may occur, the condition then being termed *eclampsia*. Death may result from uraemia or hypertensive encephalopathy, and considerable judgment is sometimes required to decide whether pregnancy should be allowed to continue to term.

In patients dying from eclampsia, the kidneys are of normal size or slightly enlarged due to oedema: the cortex is pale and the glomeruli may be visible with a hand lens as grey dots projecting from the cut surface. Microscopy (of biopsy or necropsy material) shows diffuse enlargement of all the glomeruli, but without obvious increase in cellularity. The glomerular capillaries contain very few red cells: their walls appear diffusely thickened, eosinophilic and refractile, and special staining techniques show the thickening to be due to enlargement of the endothelial cells. Electron microscopy shows the endothelial cell cytoplasm to be increased in amount and vacuolated: the capillary basement membrane is usually normal, but in severe cases may show some thickening. The epithelial cells may also be enlarged, but do not show fusion of foot processes.

The clinical and histological features of pre-eclampsia indicate impaired renal blood flow with narrowing of the glomerular capillary lumina. The hypertensive convulsions of eclampsia are probably attributable to cerebral vascular spasm (seen also in the retinal arteries) and there is evidence also of a reduced uterine blood flow in pre-eclampsia, probably due to arterial spasm, and sometimes resulting in retro-placental ischaemia. The causes of the glomerular changes, and of the vascular spasm, are not known, but the urinary output of aldosterone has been shown to be greatly increased.

Hypertension from any cause during pregnancy increases the risks of abortion, premature labour and retroplacental haemorrhage.

Interstitial nephritis

This term is of doubtful value, for in many acute and chronic renal diseases there are inflammatory changes in the interstitial tissue. *Pyelonephritis* is mainly an interstitial infection, and inflammatory cellular infiltration of the kidneys is sometimes observed in acute infections elsewhere in the body. *Hypersensitivity reactions* to certain drugs can result in peritubular inflammation and acute tubular injury. The renal lesions of irradiation, of analgesic abuse, and a form of chronic renal disease known as *Balkan nephritis* can all be described as interstitial nephritis, but there seems little advantage in lumping together an obviously heterogeneous group of conditions under this name.

Drugs, chemicals and renal disease

Many drugs are excreted predominantly in the urine, and in patients with impaired renal function conventional dosage may result in toxic levels being attained. It is therefore necessary to modify the dosage of many types of drug in patients with acute or chronic renal failure.

Various drugs can cause renal lesions, either by a direct cytotoxic effect, or because the patient has developed a hypersensitivity to the drug. The production of acute tubular necrosis by drugs and chemicals is dealt with on pp. 723–7. Chronic renal disease can result also from heavy and prolonged ingestion of certain popular analgesics, and also from lead poisoning.

Analgesic abuse. There are now many reports indicating that, in certain countries, a history of ingestion of large amounts of analgesic drugs over a period of years is unduly common in patients dying from a renal disease resembling chronic pyelonephritis. Commonly the analgesics are mixtures containing aspirin, phenacetin and codeine, but phenacetin appears to be most closely associated with renal disease. The association has been described particularly in Scandinavia and Switzerland and appears to be relatively rare in Great Britain and the U.S.A., the differences being unexplained.

The renal changes resemble those of chronic

pyelonephritis in that there is marked tubular atrophy and interstitial fibrosis and the glomeruli remain normal for a long time. However, the lesion is more diffuse than in typical chronic pyelonephritis and papillary necrosis is common, whereas in pyelonephritis it is unusual unless there is also diabetes or urinary tract obstruction. To complicate matters, typical lesions of pyelonephritis are often superadded to the diffuse "analgesic lesion" and there is still some doubt as to whether the whole picture is a modified form of chronic pyelonephritis or whether analgesics cause a specific lesion.

The clinical features are those of chronic renal failure, but some improvement may result from withdrawal of analgesics and treating active chronic pyelonephritis.

Lead poisoning is contracted most often in industry from inhalation of dust or fumes, or ingestion of lead compounds. In Queensland, Australia, lead paint was used up to 1930 for painting the wooden verandas of houses, and children playing on the verandas ingested paint powdered by the strong sunlight: acute lead poisoning was common, and follow-up studies have shown a high incidence of chronic renal failure, appearing often many years later and progressing very slowly. The kidneys are uniformly reduced in size with a finely granular surface

(Fig. 21.50), uniform cortical thinning, and hypertensive changes—in fact, closely similar to the changes in chronic glomerulonephritis. Microscopically, the lesion differs from glomerulonephritis; there is marked tubular atrophy with interstitial fibrosis, and the glomeruli are spared for a long time. However, as in granular contracted kidneys from any cause, the specific diagnosis is often difficult. Characteristic inclusion bodies are seen in the nuclei of the tubular and other cells.

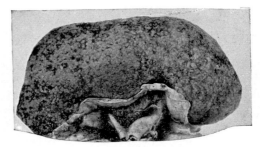

FIG. 21.50.—Granular contracted kidney in chronic lead poisoning. $\times \frac{2}{3}$.

The relationship to excessive intake of lead many years before is convincing in the Queensland studies, and the incidence has fallen considerably since the introduction of legislation against lead paints. The use of lead paint for cots and toys has also been responsible for lead poisoning in childhood.

ACUTE RENAL FAILURE

Renal function is impaired by any acute condition causing severe reduction in glomerular filtration. This occurs during the circulatory failure of shock following severe trauma and haemorrhage, and also as a result of marked dehydration (*pre-renal uraemia*). Renal failure may appear after recovery from the circulatory collapse, and is then usually accompanied by *acute tubular necrosis*, or rarely by *renal cortical necrosis*. Obstruction of both ureters or of the urethra also causes fatal acute renal failure unless relieved in time: this condition is termed *post-renal uraemia*. Impairment of renal blood flow and glomerular filtration occurs in some degree in most cases of acute diffuse proliferative glomerulonephritis; in some cases, acute renal failure is severe with virtual anuria, particularly in the rapidly progressive variant of the disease.

Output of urine is seriously impaired by acute injury of the renal tubules, and acute tubular necrosis is, in fact, the commonest renal lesion

associated with acute renal failure: it is described below in some detail. Acute renal failure occurs also with renal cortical necrosis, renal papillary necrosis, and hypersensitivity reactions to certain drugs, but these are comparatively rare.

The functional disturbances of acute renal failure are described in the section on the clinico-pathological correlations of acute tubular necrosis (p. 726).

Acute tubular necrosis

In this condition, which is by no means rare, injury to the tubular epithelium develops rapidly, and is usually accompanied by disturbances of electrolyte and fluid balance, and nearly always severe oliguria or anuria. The condition is thus one of acute renal failure, which may be fatal. If the patient can be kept alive during this *anuric phase*, by careful control of fluid and electrolyte intake and diet, supported if necessary by peritoneal or haemodialysis, tubular epithelial regeneration occurs, and in many cases renal function returns and recovery ensues. For some days or weeks, the recovering tubules do not regain fully their concentrating and selective absorptive functions, and during this *diuretic phase* death may result from excessive loss of electrolytes and fluid unless the urinary losses are replaced.

Causal factors

The mechanism of renal failure in acute tubular necrosis is not fully understood, and will be discussed later. At this point it is useful to note the main predisposing factors.

(a) Shock, trauma and haemorrhage. Any severe injury accompanied by shock is liable to be complicated, in a small proportion of instances, by acute tubular necrosis. Extensive surgical operations or severe burns are sometimes responsible, while unskilful abortion, retroplacental haemorrhage or post-partum haemorrhage carry a special risk. In the bombing of cities in the 1939–45 war, individuals were commonly trapped for some hours under fallen masonry and developed traumatic and ischaemic necrosis of skeletal muscle, particularly in crushed limbs. After rescue, myoglobin and other constituents of muscle from the areas of crush injury diffused into the blood, and myoglobinuria developed. The high incidence of acute tubular necrosis in such cases (*crush syndrome*), and also in the rare condition of acute paroxysmal myoglobinuria, suggests that products of muscle breakdown have a special predisposing effect. Acute haemolysis, as in transfusion of incompatible blood, is also followed, although much less commonly, by acute tubular necrosis. Operations on the liver and biliary tract are particularly likely to be complicated by acute tubular necrosis (*hepato-renal syndrome*), and although it is likely that shock, and fluid and electrolyte disturbances are at least partly responsible, there may be a special relationship between hepatic trauma and the renal lesion. The prognosis is appreciably worse in cases associated with severe trauma or surgery than in those following incompatible transfusion, complications of pregnancy or chemical poisoning.

(b) Various chemical compounds are either directly toxic to the tubular epithelium or are converted to toxic metabolites. Some of the more important examples include carbon tetrachloride, used extensively in the dry-cleaning of fabrics, trilene, ethylene glycol (antifreeze), carbolic acid (phenol), and organic mercurials used as diuretics. Metallic poisons are also important causes, including mercuric chloride and compounds of uranium, arsenic and chromium. Many other compounds have been implicated.

Pathological changes

In fatal cases, the kidneys are usually enlarged and the cut surface bulges, due to swelling of the damaged tubules and to interstitial oedema. The cortical vessels contain little blood, and the cortex appears pale, with blurring of the normal radial pattern, while the medulla is often dark and congested. Occasionally there are petechial haemorrhages in the cortex.

Microscopically, the glomerular tufts appear normal. Usually there is some granular debris in the capsular space and the parietal cells lining Bowman's capsule may be unduly prominent and cuboidal. The tubular changes are variable and depend on the severity and duration, and on the particular causal agents involved. In many cases, however, the causation is complex, and specific changes cannot readily be attributed to particular causal agents. Also, it is often difficult to identify, in histological sections, which parts of the tubules have been damaged, and the pathology of both human and experimental tubular necrosis has been elucidated by examination of dissected nephrons (Oliver *et al.*, 1951). At necropsy, the lesion is often obscured by terminal ischaemic changes and post-mortem autolysis.

In cases resulting from ischaemia, shock, crush injury, etc. (group (a) above) the changes are usually most marked in the distal convoluted tubules (hence the former term *lower nephron nephrosis*) although they occur also in the proximal convoluted tubule and in Henle's loop. It is unusual to see widespread epithelial necrosis, but foci of necrosis in individual tubules are sometimes detectable, and there is extensive exfoliation of scattered individual tubule cells. Rupture of the tubular basement membrane in relation to foci of epithelial necrosis was described in 1941 by Dunn, and has been confirmed by others: the overlying dead epithelial cells detach or disintegrate and there is then no barrier between the tubular lumen and the interstitial tissue. This lesion, known as *tubulorrhexis*, is seen most commonly in the distal convoluted tubule and the distal part of the proximal tubule, but can occur at all levels. It may be accompanied by a fibroblastic reaction

Distension of the intertubular connective tissue by oedema fluid is conspicuous in some cases, but almost absent in others. The vasa recta of the medulla usually contain groups of nucleated cells which appear to represent erythropoietic tissue, a feature which is sometimes seen in the hepatic sinusoids in liver cell necrosis.

The changes described above are seen in acute tubular necrosis resulting from shock, trauma,

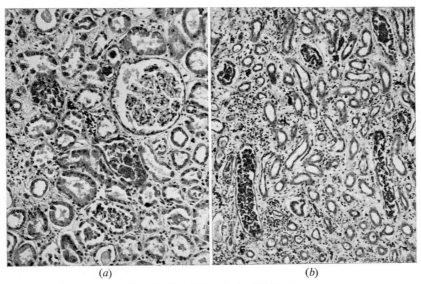

(*a*)   (*b*)

FIG. 21.51.—"Transfusion" kidney.

(*a*) The cortex shows debris and casts in the ascending limbs and distal convoluted tubules. × 130.
(*b*) The medulla shows oedema, cellular infiltration and casts. × 95.

with infiltration of inflammatory cells and in the event of recovery may lead to scarring with impaired function.

The distal convoluted tubules, and to a lesser extent the proximal tubules, are usually dilated and the lining epithelium is flattened, with basophilic cytoplasm and occasional mitotic figures: these changes, which are seen as early as three days after the onset of oliguria, are usually regarded as regenerative, and overgrowth of tubular epithelium may be seen, the proliferated cells growing around casts or forming syncytial masses projecting into the lumen.

From the ascending limb of Henle's loop onwards, the tubules contain proteinous and granular casts, and in cases associated with haemoglobinuria or myoglobinuria brown pigment casts and rounded granules of pigmented material are usually a marked feature (Fig. 21.51).

etc. They occur also in those cases resulting from administration of the nephrotoxic poisons listed above, but in the poisoning cases there is, in addition, more extensive necrosis (Fig. 21.52) affecting mainly the proximal convoluted tubule of all or most of the nephrons and resulting from the direct effect of the toxic compounds or their metabolites. This *nephrotoxic change* is often conspicuous but, unlike tubulorrhexis, it does not involve rupture of the tubular basement membrane, and provided the patient can be kept alive, it is often repaired by epithelial regeneration without leaving any residual damage or scarring.

Some variation is observed in the nephrotoxic lesions brought about by different chemicals. For example, mercuric chloride tends to affect the whole of the proximal convoluted tubule, and in some instances the necrotic part of the tubule rapidly becomes calcified, resulting in permanent injury. Carbon tetrachloride causes necrosis especially of the terminal part of the proximal tubule, and also centrilobular hepatic necrosis (p. 549); if ethylene glycol is ingested, a small proportion of it is converted into oxalate, crystals of which form in the tubular lumina, and in addition to tubular necrosis it may cause death from liver or brain injury or from acute heart failure.

Clinico-pathological correlations

The period of oliguria or anuria varies from a day or two to about 4 weeks, and is followed by a diuretic phase of roughly the same period. During the anuric

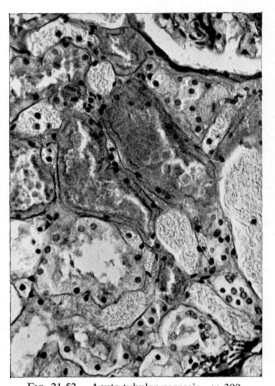

Fig. 21.52.—Acute tubular necrosis. × 300.

The tubule cells show extensive necrosis with nuclear pyknosis. From a case of methyl bromide poisoning. (Dr. G. Harvey Smith.)

phase, renal blood flow and GFR are reduced (see below). It must be appreciated that the absorption of fluid and electrolytes by the tubules is governed by homoeostatic mechanisms of great accuracy, and that there is normally no significant reabsorption of some waste products, while there is actual excretion of certain others. Even urea, a highly diffusible compound of small molecular weight, is normally concentrated sixty times or more in the tubules, less

than half being reabsorbed. In extensive tubular necrosis, these exacting functions are lost, and most of the glomerular filtrate, including its solutes, is reabsorbed unselectively from the damaged tubules. Consequently there is oliguria (defined as less than 400 ml. urine per day in adults) or anuria (less than 100 ml. daily), and the urine comes to resemble in composition a protein-poor filtrate of the plasma. There is thus a progressive rise in urea and other nitrogenous metabolites, and unless fluid and electrolyte intake is carefully regulated, death will result from a combination of uraemia, generalised and pulmonary oedema, and electrolyte disturbances. Acidosis may result from breakdown of endogenous fat and protein, particularly in the crush syndrome or other severe injury. Protein catabolism will aggravate the uraemia and accordingly the most appropriate diet is one which is low in protein and provides sufficient calories to avoid excessive endogenous protein catabolism. One of the most important electrolyte disturbances is retention of potassium, particularly in cases with severe injury and tissue breakdown, and dietary potassium should be carefully controlled. The level of plasma Na^+ is often low, usually due to its dilution by fluid retention, but the urine, even though markedly reduced in volume, may contain excess Na^+, and Na^+ administration may become necessary. The plasma level of phosphate tends to rise, with an associated fall of Ca^{++}, although this is rarely severe. Experience has shown that carefully controlled conservative therapy, including the use of osmotic diuretics such as mannitol, can prolong life in acute renal failure, and where the lesion is reversible, as in acute tubular necrosis, the prognosis has been greatly improved. However, in some cases peritoneal or haemo-dialysis is necessary.

A factor which has been suggested as contributing towards acute renal failure is leakage of tubular fluid into the interstitial tissue in tubulorrhexic lesions, with subsequent reabsorption into the blood. Obliteration of vessels by interstitial fluid is unlikely to be of importance, as oedema is sometimes minimal, and blockage of tubules by casts cannot always be a major factor, for casts are not always present. During the diuretic phase, tubular function is assumed to be only partially restored, and the main disturbance is then a failure to reabsorb fluid and electrolytes. Death can occur during this stage unless the excessive losses are made good. Renal homoeostatic mechanisms may continue to improve for over a year, but complete restoration does not always occur.

Etiology

Two factors are of known importance in the etiology of acute tubular necrosis. Firstly, the shock associated with trauma, incompatible transfusion, etc., and secondly, nephrotoxic chemicals. The part played by shock is by no means clearly defined: the most obvious possibility is ischaemic injury resulting from impaired renal blood flow, but experimental acute ischaemia of the kidney results in lesions particularly in the proximal convoluted tubules, whereas in those cases attributable mainly to trauma and shock the lesion in man (tubulorrhexis) is focal, and usually affects the distal convoluted tubules most severely. Because of this, and because tubulorrhexis is seen also in cases attributable to nephrotoxic chemicals, it may be that the lesion is produced by some endogenous mechanism which can be set in motion by various causal factors.

Although acute renal failure following the shock of severe injury, haemorrhage, or surgical operations, has long been attributed to tubular injury, there are unexplained discrepancies. For example, the extent of tubular necrosis does not correlate with the degree of renal failure; in some cases, renal failure is unaccompanied by obvious tubular cell changes, and in others there is no oliguria in spite of tubular necrosis (see Sevitt, 1959). Accordingly, it has been suggested that reduced glomerular filtration rate, attributable to diminished renal blood flow, is an important factor. There is no doubt that the renal blood flow is greatly diminished during the period of shock which precedes acute renal failure, but there is also evidence that the reduction in flow persists during the period of renal failure, and is largely responsible for it. Tubular injury, which is to be regarded as a consequence of the ischaemia of reduced renal blood flow, would thus be relegated to a secondary role in acute renal failure. These views have received increasing support in the past few years, and Lever and his co-workers (1969) have provided evidence favouring the possibility that the reduced renal blood flow of shock, haemolysis, etc., might result in over-secretion of renin by the juxtaglomerular apparatus and that this aggravates and prolongs the reduction in renal flow, thus bringing about acute renal failure. The recent observations on this subject support the earlier work of Trueta *et al.* (1947), who provided evidence that shock-producing stimuli could cause a virtual shut down of the arterioles to most of the glomeruli, while those adjacent to the medulla were less affected and continued to function (a situation which has been wrongly termed "renal shunt"), and it seems likely that reduction of renal blood flow persists in the renal failure following hypotensive shock. Nevertheless, it is reasonable to assume that tubular necrosis must severely impair renal function, and where the necrosis is extensive, as in chemically-induced acute renal failure, it is probable that it is of major importance.

The part played by haemoglobin and myoglobin in acute renal failure is also obscure. In experimental studies, haemoglobin has not been shown to be nephrotoxic in otherwise healthy animals, although it has been shown to cause injury in conditions of dehydration, acidosis and renal ischaemia. Myoglobinuria has been shown to be more prone than haemoglobinuria to be accompanied by acute tubular necrosis, particularly in crush injuries, and it may be that other products of muscle breakdown, in addition to myoglobin, are involved. The more extensive necrosis of the proximal tubules which occurs in cases attributable to various chemicals is more uniform, and is explicable as a direct toxic effect upon the tubular epithelium.

Renal cortical necrosis

This is an uncommon condition in which patchy or diffuse necrosis occurs in the cortex of both kidneys. When patchy, it usually spares the interpyramidal columns of the cortex, and even when complete the cortical tissue immediately beneath the capsule and that adjacent to the medulla is spared, and appears congested and haemorrhagic in contrast to the pale appearance of the necrotic tissue (Fig. 21.53). Microscopy shows necrosis of all the tissues in the affected areas, and when the lesion is patchy there is usually extensive necrosis of the epithelial cells of the proximal convoluted tubules in the unaffected areas. Except in patients dying very soon after development of the lesion, thrombus is usually present in the interlobular arteries, afferent arterioles and glomerular capillaries.

This condition occurs most commonly in pregnancy as a complication of retroplacental (concealed accidental) haemorrhage. It may also result from unskilful or infected abortion, or toxaemia of pregnancy. It also occurs rarely in children and non-pregnant adults, and may arise without obvious predisposing cause, or may follow an attack of diarrhoea or vomiting or severe infections, particularly peritonitis. Sheehan and Moore (1952) have studied a large series of cases, and have provided evidence that cortical necrosis results from vascular spasm, and that thrombosis is a secondary effect. The postulated vascular spasm remains unexplained.

Renal cortical necrosis develops acutely, and results in oliguria or anuria. It is usually fatal, but recovery has been reported in a few cases with patchy necrosis, and caution is therefore necessary in prognosticating upon a small biopsy specimen, even when virtually all the tissue withdrawn is necrotic.

The renal lesion of potassium deficiency

In conditions of potassium depletion and lowering of the plasma potassium level, the kidneys exhibit a striking morphological change consisting of intense hydropic vacuolation of the cells of the proximal tubules (Fig. 21.54), chiefly in the descending straight portion. The lesion is associated with marked loss of concentrating power, but only trivial albuminuria and absence of urea retention. Similar lesions had been previously observed in man in various states of severe prolonged alimentary fluid loss but their

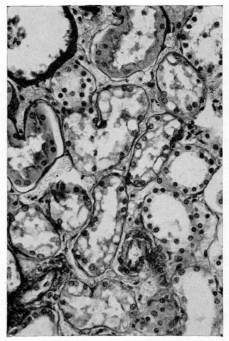

FIG. 21.54.—Kidney in severe potassium depletion following prolonged diarrhoea in ulcerative colitis. × 230.

dependence on potassium loss was revealed only by the study of experimental potassium depletion in animals. It is also observed in certain cases regarded as "potassium-losing nephritis" but Conn has shown that an essentially similar picture is brought about by excessive secretion of aldosterone by certain uncommon adrenal cortical tumours and that the diagnosis of potassium-losing nephritis cannot be sustained unless the presence of Conn's syndrome has been excluded (p. 912).

In man a significant degree of potassium depletion is encountered chiefly in states of severe intestinal fluid loss as a result of prolonged diarrhoea, e.g. in ulcerative colitis, or induced by excessive purgation. It is also seen in the stage of recovery from diabetic coma under insulin therapy, when the plasma potassium is lowered in the resynthesis and intracellular storage of glycogen. Serial biopsies of the kidney have shown the renal lesions to be completely reversible by restoration of normal potassium levels, and there is no evidence of permanent ill effects.

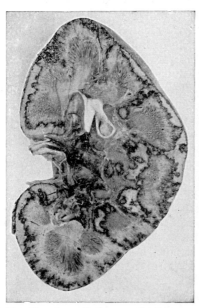

FIG. 21.53.—Renal cortical necrosis from a case of eclampsia; the pale necrotic areas with haemorrhagic margins are well shown. × ⅔.

PYELONEPHRITIS

Definition. Pyelonephritis is a bacterial-induced inflammation of the renal pelvis, the calyces, and the parenchyma of the kidney. There are acute and chronic forms and while either may occur without lower urinary tract obstruction, they are common in its presence. Pyelonephritis may be unilateral or bilateral and it is involvement of the kidneys that produces the serious sequelae. The condition is closely related to infection of the urinary tract, and the two are considered together in the following account.

Causal organisms. Initial acute episodes of pyelonephritis are usually caused by coliform bacilli, aerobacter, or the paracolon bacillus, any one of which is often obtained in the urine in pure culture. Patients with recurrent pyelonephritis, who have usually received previous antibiotic therapy and who may have been subjected to instrumentation of the lower urinary tract, generally have a mixed infection which may include coliforms, proteus and staphylococci simultaneously.

Bacteriuria. This is not synonymous with urinary tract infection, for the normal distal urethral mucosa is populated by bacteria such as coliform bacilli, proteus and staphylococci, and these may be washed off the mucosa by the stream of urine and thus be detectable in the collected sample; alternatively they may be carried into the bladder by a catheter or cystoscope and the "catheter specimen" of urine may similarly contain bacteria. In neither instance is there a urinary tract infection although bacterial cultures of the urine will be positive. It is therefore necessary to assess the importance of bacteriuric states. Experience has shown that bacterial counts of over 100,000 organisms per ml. of urine usually indicate urinary tract infection but that counts of less than this number can result from contamination. Significant bacteriuria can reflect inflammation at any level of the urinary tract and exact localisation is often clinically difficult. It is particularly important to determine whether or not bacterial inflammation has involved the renal parenchyma and two factors are often helpful in reaching such a conclusion. The first is the presence of a high titre of serum antibody to the bacterium cultured from the urine. If this is present renal involvement is highly probable.

The second is the presence of cellular casts in the urine: pus cells in the urine (*pyuria*) can result from infection anywhere in the urinary tract, but their aggregation into cylindrical casts can only have happened in the renal tubules, thus indicating pyelonephritis.

Asymptomatic bacteriuria. This term implies the presence of significant bacteriuria in the absence of symptoms referable to the urinary tract. This is most often encountered in pregnancy and in young females: some of these cases ultimately develop pyelonephritis.

Recurrent or persistent infection. The number of individuals who die from acute pyelonephritis in this country is very small, and the chief danger now is the recurrent or smouldering chronic types of infection, for these are often related to the development of chronic pyelonephritis with ultimate renal failure. It is not known whether the tendency for urinary tract infection to recur is due to a susceptibility of the individual to such infections, or to failure to eradicate the previous infection completely, with persistence of living bacteria and subsequent exacerbation. Bacteriological investigations in recurrent cases suggest that both factors may be concerned. There is no doubt that urinary tract infections are more liable to arise when there is obstruction of the urinary tract, and unless the obstruction can be relieved the infection is often difficult to eradicate and liable to recur. However, investigation of patients with recurrent urinary tract infection has failed to demonstrate an obstructive lesion in most of them.

Pathogenesis

Pyelonephritis may result from bacteria reaching the kidney either by the blood stream or by an ascending infection of the urinary tract.

Blood-borne infection occurs in acute pyaemia or septicaemia (Figs. 7.7, 7.8, p. 137), and this is seen as a complication of staphylococcal infections, e.g. boils and carbuncles. The bacteria normally present in the distal urethra can also gain entrance to the blood during surgical procedures upon the urethra: in these circumstances, the possibility of blood-borne infection of the kidneys is increased if the lesion which has required urethral surgery has also brought about urinary obstruction, e.g. urethral stricture or enlarged prostate (see below). Blood-borne infection is not, however, the cause of the majority of cases of pyelonephritis.

Ascending urinary tract infection. The commonest site of infection of the urinary tract is the bladder, and it is likely that cystitis is the predisposing factor in most cases of pyelonephritis. As already explained, most attacks of "spontaneous" cystitis are caused by *Esch. coli*, whereas cystitis following catheterisation is commonly a mixed infection. It has been shown in experimental animals that coliform bacilli and other bacteria die rapidly when placed on the surface of the bladder mucosa: the mechanism of this bactericidal effect is not known, nor is it known whether it is defective in patients

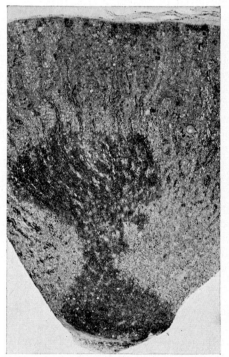

Fig. 21.55.—Acute papillitis in pyelonephritis showing severe inflammatory infiltration of the renal papilla extending to the boundary zone. × 5.

contracting urinary tract infections. In normal circumstances, the uretero-vesical valves are competent, and radiological studies have shown that reflux of urine from the bladder to the ureters is rare. However, there is evidence that cystitis may impair the competence of the valves, perhaps by inflammatory swelling and distortion

of the mucosa of the terminal parts of the ureters and adjacent parts of the bladder; in these circumstances reflux of urine from bladder to renal pelvis, during micturition, with consequent pyelitis, is not unusual. It is possible that bacteria may also spread throughout the urinary tract by passing along the interstitial tissue or lymphatics, but the evidence for this is not convincing.

When pyelitis has developed, the bacteria may spread into the kidney directly by the lumina of the collecting tubules, or by passing from the submucosa of the inflamed calyces into the interstitial tissue of the renal papillae. Here they proliferate, and an acute inflammatory response occurs, often with abscess formation, eventually involving the adjacent tubular lumina. From here, infection can spread peripherally to the cortex (Fig. 21.55) via both the tubular lumina and the intertubular connective tissue spaces. Thus there develop linear streaks of suppuration with considerable tubular destruction. Since there is haphazard spread of bacteria from variably infected calyces, the renal lesion is not uniform and diffuse, but irregular and patchy. This sequence of events can be produced in experimental animals and is almost certainly the mechanism in man.

Predisposing factors. *Urinary tract obstruction.* Patients with an obstruction of the urinary tract are particularly liable to develop pyelonephritis, and this is attributable to four factors. Firstly, stagnant urine, particularly that of females, provides a suitable culture medium for coliform and certain other bacteria which in normal circumstances would be washed out. Secondly, obstruction facilitates the upward spread of infection in the urinary tract by predisposing to vesico-ureteric reflux of urine: this can occur intermittently even without gross structural change in the ureters, but in prolonged partial obstruction the ureters become permanently thickened and dilated, allowing free reflux to occur. Thirdly, there is convincing evidence that obstruction impairs the capacity of the kidneys to resist infection. For example, if a ureter of an experimental animal is clamped and bacteria are injected intravenously, pyelonephritis is much more prone to occur in the obstructed than in the normal kidney. Lastly, chronic urinary obstruction may cause uraemia, and thus lower the resistance to infections in general (p. 717).

Structural abnormalities of the urinary tract without obstruction also appear to predispose to infection. In *diabetes mellitus*, there is a general susceptibility to infections, including cystitis, pyelitis and pyelonephritis, the exact mechanism being unknown (see p. 123).

Age and sex are also of importance in relation to pyelonephritis. At all ages, the incidence is higher in females than in males, possibly because of the shorter, wider urethra, and the turbulence of urethral flow, with peripheral eddying, in the female. Recurrent attacks of cystitis and pyelitis due to *Esch. coli* are common in young children, and in some cases lead to chronic pyelonephritis. In only a small proportion of cases (approx. 20 per cent) is there evidence of a structural abnormality of the urinary tract.

Pregnancy produces a degree of ureteric dilatation and urinary stasis by virtue of the effect of the hormonal climate upon the musculature of the urinary tract and latterly the mechanical pressure of the enlarged uterus. *Hypokalaemia*, *gout*, and the ingestion of excessive amounts of *analgesics* (usually a combination of aspirin, phenacetin and codeine—p. 722) over a long period can all produce renal histopathology similar to bacterial-induced chronic pyelonephritis, and these conditions should be kept in mind in the differential diagnosis of chronic pyelonephritis in renal biopsy material.

Incidence

Acute pyelonephritis is a not uncommon disease in young females, including children, and is especially liable to occur during pregnancy. It is less frequent in the male unless there is a pre-existing urinary tract obstruction. The frequency of chronic pyelonephritis is very difficult to assess. Incidences as high as 15 per cent have been reported in general hospital necropsies, but this usually includes cases in which a few cortical scars are present in otherwise normal kidneys. If the necropsy diagnosis is limited to those cases with severe chronic pyelonephritis, likely to have been of clinical significance, then the incidence is of the order of 1 per cent.

Acute pyelonephritis

This consists of acute suppurative inflammation of the pelvis, calyces, and parts of the kidney, with pale linear streaks of suppuration, bordered by a red rim of congestion, extending radially from the tips of the papillae to the

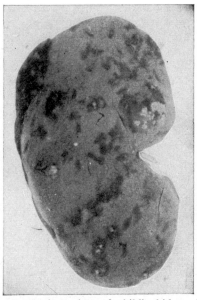

FIG. 21.56.—Surface view of child's kidney in acute pyelonephritis, showing small abscesses and areas of haemorrhage. × 1.

surface of the cortex (Figs. 21.56, 21.57) where adjacent lesions may fuse to produce extensive abscesses. Microscopically, all the features typical of acute inflammation are present in the pelvis, calyces and kidney. Within the kidney the suppurating lesions cause very extensive but focal tubular destruction. In the cortex there is remarkable sparing of glomeruli and large blood vessels, even when these structures are directly surrounded by intense acute interstitial inflammation (Fig. 21.59). All of these changes tend to be more florid and more extensive if there is obstruction in the lower urinary tract. Obstructed cases often, and very intensely inflamed non-obstructed cases sometimes, develop necrosis of the papillary tips due to circulatory impairment of these anatomical zones. In such cases the characteristic features of papillary necrosis (p. 736) will co-exist with those due to the primary inflammatory process.

Chronic pyelonephritis

The naked eye appearances of the kidney, calyces, and renal pelvis are of paramount importance in the differentiation of chronic pyelonephritic shrinkage from other varieties of scarred kidneys. The pelvic and calyceal walls are usually thickened and their mucosa may be either granular or atrophic: they are always distorted by scarring of the pyramids and the calyces are usually dilated. The kidney is reduced in size and shows irregular patchy contraction in which the pyelonephritic process has largely destroyed the parenchyma and led to

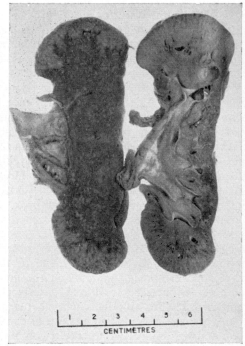

Fig. 21.58.—Chronic pyelonephritis associated with severe hypertension. Most of the kidney has been destroyed, and is scarred and shrunken. The tissue at the poles is relatively healthy. $\times \frac{2}{3}$

focal scarring and shrinkage. The intervening parenchyma may be normal or may show the changes of hypertension. The cortical surface is depressed over the contracted areas, and the cortex and medulla are both consistently narrowed (Fig. 21.58). The cortical surface depressions tend in most instances to be shallower than those produced by ischaemia but they may be very similar, and the single most important diagnostic feature of the pyelonephritic scar is its close relationship to a deformed calyx. Microscopically the pelvic and calyceal mucosa may be thickened by granulation tissue and infiltrated by lymphocytes, plasma cells and polymorphs; lymphoid follicles sometimes form and are often responsible for the surface granularity of the mucosa. When the inflammation is florid, the surface epithelium may be lost, the pelves and calyces then being lined by granulation tissue. In cases where the inflammation has subsided, the walls of the pelvis and calyces are atrophic with some scarring.

The scarred areas. There is extensive atrophy and loss of tubules, especially the proximal segments (Fig. 21.59), and this is a most impor-

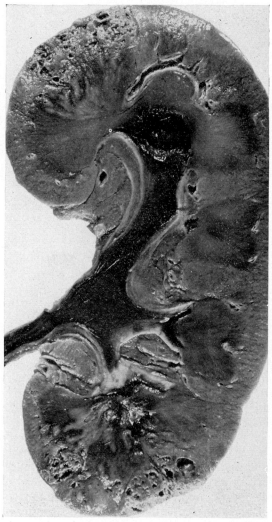

Fig. 21.57.—Acute pyelonephritis. In this case the lesions are at the upper and lower poles. Note the cortical abscesses and the streaks of suppuration in the medulla. $\times 1$.

tant histological feature of chronic pyelonephritis. Tubular atrophy is often accompanied by gross thickening of the tubular basement membranes, and there is increase in fibrous tissue between the tubules. Commonly partial

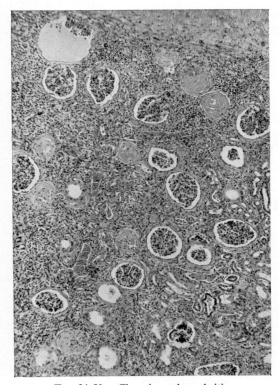

FIG. 21.59.—Chronic pyelonephritis.
The tubules are greatly atrophied, but most of the glomeruli are preserved. × 38.

destruction of tubules results in survival of isolated segments; these become distended with inspissated eosinophilic secretion (presumably produced by the lining epithelium), and the epithelium becomes flattened: these changes occur in groups of adjacent tubules which come to resemble superficially thyroid acini (Fig. 21.60). The interstitial tissue is densely packed with lymphocytes, plasma cells and sometimes neutrophil and eosinophil polymorphs: in the late stages of the disease the inflammatory cell infiltrate is replaced first by granulation tissue and finally by dense scar tissue. In such "burnt out" pyelonephritis, there may be little evidence of active inflammation. The glomeruli are preserved for a very long time but eventually a spectrum of glomerular abnormalities appears, the most specific of

which is concentric (pericapsular) fibrosis around a thickened Bowman's capsule (Fig. 21.61). Other changes include gradual replacement of the glomerulus by basement membrane and collagen, and in the late stages most of the glomeruli in the affected areas are converted into functionless solid spheres (Fig. 21.62): other glomeruli become collapsed and shrunken, often with formation of a thick layer of collagen between the tuft and Bowman's capsule, while at an earlier stage some capillary tufts may show irregular proliferation of endothelial and mesangial cells. Arteriolar and glomerular capillary necrosis occurs only if malignant hypertension has supervened. The arteries show variable degrees of medial and intimal fibrous thickening.

The non-scarred areas. The glomeruli may show compensatory hypertrophy. Other glomerular and vascular changes often develop as a result of arterial hypertension.

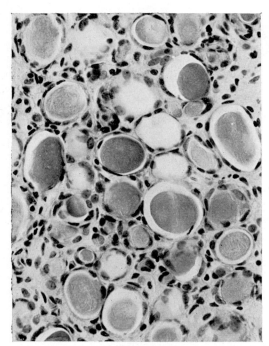

FIG. 21.60.—Chronic pyelonephritis. Inspissated colloid-like material in sequestrated portions of renal tubules, presenting an appearance resembling superficially that of thyroid tissue. × 250.

Hypertension in chronic pyelonephritis. Approximately 70 per cent of patients with extensive chronic pyelonephritis develop hypertension, and in 15–20 per cent of these the hypertension is of the malignant type. There has been some

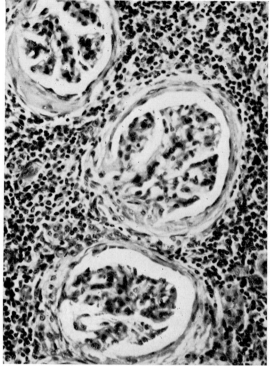

FIG. 21.61.—Chronic pyelonephritis. There is pericapsular fibrosis, a heavy chronic inflammatory infiltrate, and almost complete loss of tubules. × 150.

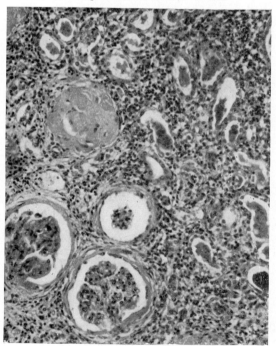

FIG. 21.62.—Chronic pyelonephritis, showing loss of tubules, and glomeruli in various stages of hyalinisation. × 85.

controversy over the nature of the relationship between the two conditions, and it has been suggested that the association might result from a predisposition of individuals with essential hypertension to develop pyelonephritis. We do not consider this a likely explanation, for it would not account for the occurrence of hypertension in young patients with chronic pyelonephritis. The obvious explanation is that chronic pyelonephritis, like other conditions giving rise to extensive scarring of the kidneys, commonly leads to hypertension of secondary (renal) type. Admittedly, the mechanism of production of the hypertension of chronic renal disease is not well understood (p. 274) but this seems to us no reason for doubting that it results from chronic pyelonephritis.

Tuberculous pyelonephritis

In acute miliary tuberculosis, minute grey tubercles develop in the kidneys, as elsewhere, but are not usually as numerous as in some of the other organs. Of more importance is the localised, progressive lesion—tuberculous pyelonephritis—produced presumably by deposition of a relatively small number of blood-borne mycobacteria in the kidney, and unaccompanied by miliary lesions. Other common sites of blood-borne metastatic tuberculous lesions in the genito-urinary tract are the epididymis in the male (p. 818) and the Fallopian tube in the female (p. 832), and spread from these sites can give rise to tuberculosis of the bladder, and ascending infection to involve the kidneys. Conversely, renal tuberculosis can spread to involve the ureters, bladder and other pelvic viscera.

Clinical features. Renal tuberculosis may produce vague illness, with weight loss and fever, or may present with local features such as lumbar pain, dysuria, haematuria or pyuria. *M. tuberculosis* can often be found in the urine, and pyelography may show distortion of one or more calyces. In most cases, there is neither evidence nor history of tuberculosis elsewhere in the body (although this must, of course, have been present), and even at necropsy active pulmonary tuberculosis is present in only a minority of cases. Renal tuberculosis occurs usually in adult life, and it may be that, as in the lungs, it can remain latent for many years and

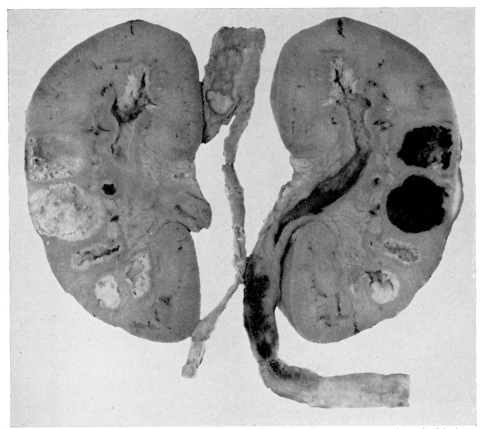

FIG. 21.63.—Tuberculosis of kidney, ureter and seminal vesicle. Two caseous renal cortical lesions are
excavated and there is early tuberculous pyelonephritis. The ureter is much thickened and caseous.

then flare up: this would account for its occurrence long after any primary lung lesion has healed.

The incidence of renal tuberculosis in Europe has declined along with tuberculosis in general, and it is now a rather uncommon condition: its main danger is the involvement of both kidneys to such an extent as to cause renal failure.

Pathological changes. The initial renal lesion results usually from blood-borne infection, a few mycobacteria becoming arrested in the cortex, with development of one or more tubercles: these enlarge, caseate and coalesce, while lymphatic and tubular spread leads to tubercles round about, and so the lesion grows as an enlarging patch of caseation. Spread through the adjacent papilla is common, and on reaching the renal pelvis the lesion may soften and discharge its contents, leaving a ragged cavity. Further tubercles develop in the walls of the renal pelvis and may caseate and ulcerate; from here infection spreads into other parts of the

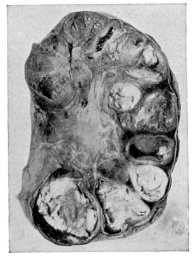

FIG. 21.64.—Old tuberculosis of kidney, which has been largely replaced by caseous lesions enclosed by fibrous tissue.

kidney, which may then develop multiple caseous lesions (Figs. 21.63, 21.64). The ureter or renal pelvis may become obstructed by tuberculous lesions in their walls, or by plugging with caseous material, and the urine (coming solely from the other kidney) may then be normal. Apart from this, renal pelvic involvement often results in haematuria and the renal lesions tend also to suppurate, giving pyuria.

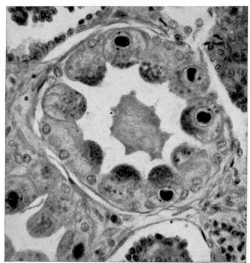

FIG. 21.65.—Renal tubules, showing intranuclear and cytoplasmic inclusion bodies in the lining cells in cytomegalic virus disease in an infant. × 400.

Cytomegalic virus disease of infants

In new-born infants dying with jaundice and erythroblastosis, and sometimes in older children dying from various causes, the renal tubule cells, and other epithelia, including that of the salivary glands, may contain large intranuclear and cytoplasmic inclusion bodies (Fig. 21.65) which are morphologically identical with those found in salivary gland virus disease of guinea-pigs, monkeys, etc. These lesions are due to the dissemination of a human strain of salivary gland virus, which may occur *in utero*. Involvement of the liver and bone marrow may bring about haematological changes similar to those of erythroblastosis fetalis. The disease appears to be rarer in Great Britain than in Europe or America. Recently it has been observed, as an opportunistic infection, in patients receiving immunosuppresive therapy, e.g. following renal transplantation.

Papillary necrosis

This consists of infarct-like lesions affecting the inner parts of some or all of the medullary pyramids. The necrotic papillae are yellowish-white, and the junction with living tissue may be congested. Microscopy shows complete tissue necrosis, with polymorph infiltration at the margin. The condition occurs in pyelonephritis, particularly if there is also obstruction of the urinary tract or diabetes: it is also a common feature of the renal changes of analgesic abuse (p. 722). The condition is usually reflected in rapid deterioration of renal function. In some cases, the necrotic papillae are sloughed off, and may be passed in the urine, leaving irregular enlarged calyces.

CONGENITAL LESIONS

Congenital cystic kidneys

This condition arises in the fetus, and the kidneys may be so large as to interfere with parturition, the individual cysts then being minute, and the normal lobular pattern of the kidney being absent. Death may occur in infancy or early childhood, but more commonly in the fourth or fifth decades from chronic renal failure with hypertension. The kidneys are greatly enlarged and occupied by numerous cysts of various sizes, while little kidney substance may be recognisable between the cysts. Prolonged survival presupposes, of course, the presence of enough functioning renal tissue, but as the cysts enlarge they compress, and impair the functional efficiency of the renal tissue, so that various ill-effects follow. Each kidney may weigh 1 kg. or even more (Fig. 21.66) and be easily palpable. The cysts may be of any size, up to 4–6 cm. diameter; they contain usually serous fluid, colourless or brownish, though it may be mucoid, especially in the smaller cysts. Occasionally the cystic change is practically restricted to one kidney. The condition is apparently the result of disturbance of normal development due to imperfect fusion between the kidney tubules proper and the collecting tubules, which grow up from the extremity of the ureter to meet them, but other embryological explanations have been proposed. There is a distinct familial predisposition, possibly determined by a single autosomal dominant factor, and there may be accompanying cystic change in the liver, although not sufficient to disturb hepatic function. Lesser degrees of cystic change are common in the kidneys, ranging from a few to many cysts, but with sufficient tissue remaining to avert renal failure. Occasionally a single cyst may reach such a size as to be palpable during life. The effects are merely mechanical.

The effects of cystic disease vary, of course, according to the amount of kidney substance which survives. In adults, cystic kidneys usually cause progressive hypertension, and death may be due to uraemia, heart failure, or less commonly cerebral haemorrhage. There is also an association with aneurysms of the cerebral arteries, and about 15 per cent of patients with polycystic kidneys die from subarachnoid haemorrhage.

Other congenital defects

These are comparatively common but unimportant. Occasionally one kidney, usually the left, is absent—*agenesia*—and there is generally an absence of the ureter also. In such cases, the surviving kidney undergoes compensatory hypertrophy, and its weight may sometimes double. *Hypoplasia* or imperfect development of one kidney is also observed, the kidney being sometimes an irregular atrophic structure around the upper end of its ureter. Here, also, hypertrophy develops in the other kidney. Hypoplasia of both kidneys may occur to such a degree as to be incompatible with life; minor degrees of the condition may possibly lead to renal dwarfism. Sometimes the two kidneys are fused, and this most frequently occurs at the lower pole, so that the "*horse-shoe kidney*" results; sometimes the union is merely a fibrous band. In such cases, the pelves are directed somewhat forward and the two ureters pass in front of the connecting bridge. In rarer forms the fusion of the kidneys is more complete and an oval or somewhat irregular kidney results, which varies in position. Occasionally

a kidney, more rarely both kidneys, may be displaced downwards to lie in front of the sacrum, in the pelvis; its ureter is correspondingly short and the arterial blood supply comes from the lower end of the aorta or an adjacent large branch. In these various renal abnormalities the position of the adrenals is usually quite normal. The kidney is originally composed of five lobules and ordinarily their fusion is complete. Sometimes slight grooves on the surface mark the original lobules and the term *fetal lobulation* is applied; the condition, which is of no importance, is not to be mistaken for a pathological change. It is more marked in the child than in the adult. The arrangement of the renal arteries is very variable and the so-called aberrant arteries are not accessory vessels but are the segmental renal arteries taking separate origin. Division of such an artery is likely to be followed by infarction of the tissue supplied by it.

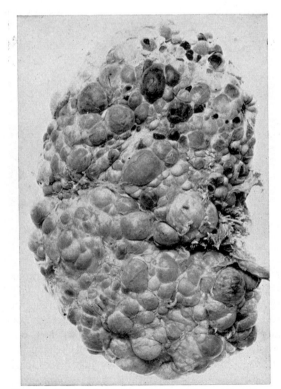

FIG. 21.66.—Surface view of congenital cystic kidney. The kidney weighed 1·5 kg.

TUMOURS

Benign tumours

These are not very rare, the commonest being a small *fibroma* in the medulla; it rarely reaches 1 cm. diameter. *Adenoma* occasionally occurs, usually in the cortex, and some have a characteristic appearance with narrow bands of stroma and papilliform ingrowths (Fig. 21.67).

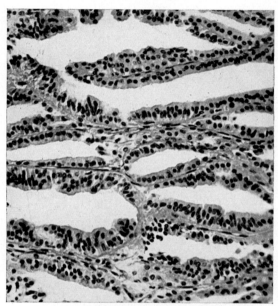

FIG. 21.67.—Papillary adenoma of kidney, showing the delicate stroma and the appearances of the epithelium. × 140.

It is usually benign, but carcinoma may supervene. In the renal pelvis *villous papillary tumours* are sometimes seen; they correspond to the papillary tumours of the bladder (p. 746) and are sometimes associated with them. *Angioma* is another uncommon benign tumour. It may occur in the pyramids or just underneath the lining of the pelvis, and, even when small, may lead to severe haematuria.

Malignant tumours

Malignant tumours are much less common in the kidneys than in several other organs, but two are of some importance—*renal carcinoma* and *nephroblastoma*.

Renal carcinoma

Clear-cell carcinoma is the commonest type. It was formerly called *Grawitz tumour* or *hypernephroma*. This last term was based on a superficial resemblance of this type of tumour to adrenal tissue, which led Grawitz to suggest that it arose from adrenocortical tissue misplaced within the kidneys. However, similar tumours do not arise in the adrenals, nor in other sites of misplaced adrenal tissue, and clear-cell renal carcinoma does not give rise to the hormonal effects associated with some adrenocortical tumours. It is now widely accepted that it originates from renal tubular epithelium, and accordingly the term hypernephroma is a misnomer.

Clear-cell carcinoma is often large, and may occasionally form an enormous mass. It may

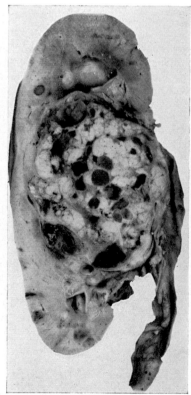

FIG. 21.68.—Clear-cell carcinoma of kidney, growing from the central part of the kidney and compressing the renal pelvis.

Note haemorrhagic and gelatinous areas and rounded nodules of whitish tumour.

occur in any part of the kidney and is not commoner, as was formerly believed, at the upper pole than elsewhere. On section, there are usually large areas of dull yellowish tissue (presenting a superficial resemblance to the adrenal cortex), interspersed with vascular,

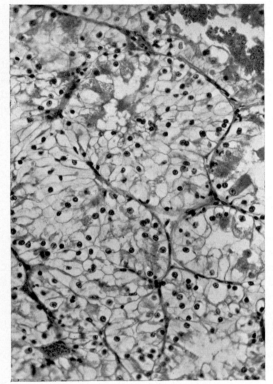

Fig. 21.69.—Clear-cell carcinoma of kidney. × 205.
Showing typical empty-looking cells with well-defined walls and delicate stroma.

haemorrhagic and necrotic areas, and also broad bands and patches of connective tissue, somewhat mucoid or translucent in appearance (Fig. 21.68). Although the tumour may often appear to be encapsulated, like a benign tumour, it shows distinctly malignant properties. It commonly grows into the tributaries of the renal vein and forms thrombus-like masses within them; metastases may follow, especially in the lungs and bones. It may also burst through the capsule of the kidney or into the pelvis. Haematuria is common and often a prominent symptom.

On microscopic examination, such a tumour has, as a rule, a distinctly acinous arrangement in many parts, the spaces being lined by tall columnar epithelial cells: a papilliform type of growth also is sometimes present, and in other parts the arrangement of the epithelium is in solid masses. The tumour cells are large, and often remarkably uniform, with abundant clear cytoplasm (Fig. 21.69) rich in glycogen and doubly-refracting lipid, and a relatively small round nucleus. There may, however, be greater variation in the cells, which may have an eosinophilic cytoplasm, or may be smaller and more anaplastic. As in other tumours, the prognosis depends on the degree of anaplasia, and invasion of the renal vein is not incompatible with long survival.

Tumours of purely adenocarcinomatous pattern occasionally occur in the kidney and papillary adenocarcinoma may arise both in the renal substance and in the pelvis, the two types being, however, quite distinct. We have encountered renal carcinomas in which the cytoplasm of the tumour cells contained large homogeneous acidophil inclusions of obscure nature.

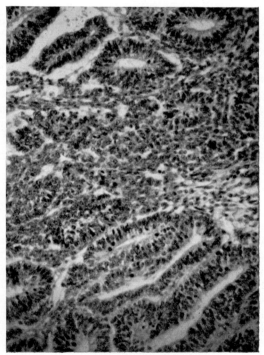

Fig. 21.70.—Nephroblastoma, showing cellular tissue with formation of acini by columnar cells. × 200.

Papillary cystadenocarcinoma. This is a rather uncommon type of renal carcinoma: it consists of numerous cysts containing papillary processes, the stroma of which is often packed with foamy macrophages filled with cholesterol fat.

It tends to invade the regional lymph nodes, and according to Thackray carries a prognosis similar to that of clear-celled carcinoma.

Nephroblastoma is an embryonic tumour, which has the general appearance of a rapidly growing sarcoma. It may reach a large size and, though fairly well enclosed within the kidney capsule, rapidly invades the blood stream and so produces metastases, chiefly in the lungs. It occurs especially in the first three years of life, and is known also as "embryoma", "mixed tumour" or "Wilms' tumour" of the kidney. Although rare, it is one of the commonest malignant tumours in childhood.

Microscopically, the tumour is composed of a spindle-celled tissue, with formation of acini and tubular structures, and apparent transitions may be seen between the spindle cells and those of epithelial type (Fig. 21.70). There may be also imperfect formation of glomeruli. The tumour was formerly described as adenosarcoma, but there is little doubt that it is derived from the cells of the kidney rudiment. In some instances it has a more complicated structure, striped muscle fibres being present, and the tumour may have originated from cells of the mesoderm before the differentiation of the myotomes.

Spindle-cell sarcoma is a rare renal tumour.

Secondary carcinoma in the kidneys is not uncommon, although metastases are neither as frequent nor as numerous as might be expected in view of the very large blood supply of the kidneys.

RENAL PELVES, URETERS AND BLADDER

The lesions of these structures are considered together, as they are so often involved in the same pathological process. Three main factors are concerned in the majority of these lesions, viz. (*a*) *obstruction to urinary flow*, (*b*) *infective inflammation*, and (*c*) the *formation of calculi*; and two or even all three of these may be present at the same time. We shall first consider the mechanical effects of obstruction.

Effects of obstruction

Serious mechanical obstruction to outflow of urine from the bladder is practically confined to the male sex, and is commonly produced by enlargement of the prostate or stricture of the urethra, occasionally by severe phimosis, tumour, or calculus. The chief effect on the bladder is the production of variable degrees of hypertrophy and dilatation. When the outstanding feature is hypertrophy, the muscular part of the wall is thickened and the bands of muscle, which have a reticulated arrangement under the mucosa, enlarge and form prominent ridges or bands with depressions between (Fig. 23.5, p. 821). Occasionally one of these depressions may become enlarged and form a large projecting diverticulum. When infection occurs, as is so often the case, purulent material may accumu- late in such a diverticulum, and ulceration and even perforation may follow. Obstruction to outflow from the bladder ultimately leads to dilatation of the ureters and pelves of the kidneys. The former may undergo considerable dilatation and their walls become somewhat thickened, and the pelves also become enlarged, so that there is a condition of bilateral hydronephrosis. The dilatation is sometimes more marked on one side than on the other.

Hydronephrosis

This means a dilatation of the renal pelvis and may occur on one or both sides.

Causation. In addition to obstruction at the outlet of the bladder, as just described, *bilateral* hydronephrosis is occasionally produced by a tumour, e.g. of the bladder or female pelvic organs, pressing on or implicating the lower ends of both ureters. Occasionally dilatation of the ureters and hydronephrosis are due to congenital abnormality in the posterior urethra, the mucosa of which forms valve-like folds; the resulting renal atrophy may be accompanied by renal dwarfism (p. 717). Another cause of hydroureters and bilateral hydronephrosis is neurogenic disturbance of bladder control due to lesions of the spinal cord. In all these conditions of bilateral hydronephrosis the dilatation of the ureters and pelves is usually moderate. The most striking degree of hydronephrosis occurs when the obstruction is *unilateral*, and this may be due to various causes. It may be due to a calculus impacted at the upper end of the ureter, at the level of the brim of the pelvis, or at the entrance to the bladder. It may be produced also by a scar, which sometimes follows ulceration due to the passage of a stone; or by a tumour of the ureter itself, or pressure of a tumour from outside. It occasionally results when the ureter is attached at an abnormally high level to the pelvis, so that it leaves it at an acute angle, and a valve-like obstruction results. This may cause intermittent accumulation of urine, and ultimately marked hydronephrosis may develop. Hydronephrosis may result when the ureter is kinked over an aberrant renal artery supplying the lower pole of the kidney. (Fig. 21.71). It is also encountered on rare occasions when the kidney has been in an abnormal position. In some cases there is pronounced stricture just below the uretero-pelvic junction, and while in

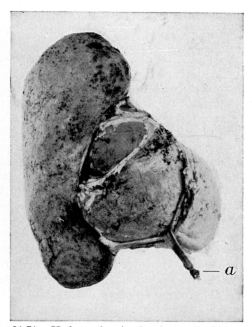

Fig. 21.71.—Hydronephrosis, showing ureter (*a*) hooked round renal artery.

a few this is related to an abnormal renal artery, in many no cause of the stricture is discoverable.

Structural changes. The effects of obstruction vary greatly. Sometimes a calculus may be

firmly impacted, and there may be obvious distension of the pelvis (Fig. 21.72), or the whole pelvis and calyces may be distended by a branching calculus, though this is more common when infection has been superadded (p. 745). In

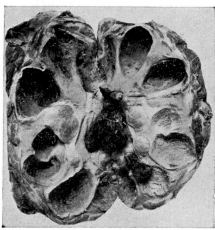

Fig. 21.72.—Impacted branched calculus in renal pelvis with resulting hydronephrosis and great fibrous thickening.

such cases, fibrosis and atrophy of the kidney follow. In other cases, the distension is so great that the dilated pelvis may become palpable. As the distension progresses, the calyces become flattened, the kidney substance becomes stretched over the dilated pelvis, and ultimately may form a mere rind; the surface of the kidney usually develops a lobulated appearance. Atrophy of the kidney substance may be regular or irregular, so that parts of considerable thickness may be left while the rest is much thinned; the latter result apparently depends on the degree to which the vascular supply is impaired, and the microscopic appearances resemble those resulting from major artery stenosis, i.e. the glomeruli are relatively spared, but the tubules are atrophied. Sometimes, however, the dilatation is mainly in the form of a sac projecting medial to the kidney and there is little effect on the appearance of the kidney—the *extra-renal* as contrasted with the *renal* type of hydronephrosis.

The results of experimental complete obstruction of a ureter vary somewhat; usually excretion of urine ceases and comparatively little dilatation follows, and the usual cause of severe hydronephrosis in man is intermittent obstruction. When the obstruction is relieved, e.g. by a calculus changing its position, there results a great flow of urine, and if the obstruction becomes partial again, this will lead to further expansion. It is easy to understand, therefore, how such an occurrence, often repeated, may bring about great distension. Occasionally, however, great hydronephrosis may be associated with complete obstruction and even obliteration of the ureter; in such a case obstruction may previously have been intermittent. When the kidney becomes greatly stretched and thinned, the tubules, and ultimately the glomeruli, become atrophied, and there ensues general overgrowth of the connective tissue. The contents of a dilated pelvis are, of course, at first urine; but, as the condition becomes chronic, the urinary constituents disappear, while proteins are added to the fluid by transudation from the wall of the sac.

Urinary tract infection

The commonest serious complication of urinary tract infection is extension to the kidneys, and accordingly the subject has already been discussed in the account of pyelonephritis (pp. 729–34). The main features of urinary tract infection are as follows:

(1) Normal urine is often contaminated by bacteria living in the lower urethra: normally, there are fewer than 10^5 bacteria per ml. of urine, and greater numbers are suggestive of infection.

(2) Infection is much commoner in females of all ages than in males, possibly due to the shorter, wide female urethra.

(3) Infection is especially common in pregnancy because of the hormonal relaxation of smooth muscle and the pressure of the uterus on the urinary tract.

(4) Most infections are caused by bacteria gaining entrance to the bladder via the urethra, and the renal pelves may be involved, spread being either intra-luminal or in the interstitial tissue of the urinary tract.

(5) In the presence of cystitis, reflux of urine from bladder to ureters is a common occurrence, and is likely to promote ascending infection.

(6) In patients without urinary tract obstruction, who have not been subjected to catheterisation or other instrumentation, urinary tract infections are usually caused by *Escherichia coli*. With obstruction or following instrumentation,

mixed infections, including coliform bacilli, proteus and staphylococci, are common.

(7) Urinary tract obstruction, including neurogenic disturbances of bladder control, is of major importance in predisposing to, enhancing, prolonging and spreading infection, especially when the obstruction is chronic and has resulted in ureteric dilatation.

(8) Once infection has involved the renal pelves and calyces (pyelitis), direct spread into the renal papillae can occur, leading to pyelonephritis.

(9) Chronic infection, especially with *Proteus* sp., predisposes to formation of phosphate deposits in the urinary tract, by splitting urea and thus rendering the urine alkaline, and these can both obstruct the flow of urine and enhance the infection.

In the early stages of an acute urinary infection, the urine may contain a heavy concentration of bacteria with few cells, but pus cells soon appear; in some instances, there may be sufficient haemorrhage from the inflamed mucosa to present clinically as haematuria.

The morbid anatomical changes in cystitis are usually classified as catarrhal, purulent, and pseudo-membranous. In pseudo-membranous, which is chiefly found when there is hypertrophy of the bladder, there occurs superficial necrosis of the mucosa with fibrinous exudate, especially over the muscular ridges, and the lining of the viscus becomes separated in gangrenous decomposing shreds. The most severe effects are usually observed where there is alkaline decomposition of the urine. Haemorrhages into the mucosa are common, and these may become greenish and almost black, while the surface is covered with pus and often a deposit of phosphates. Such an infection may ascend the dilated ureters, and produce a pyelitis with similar features, and the dilated pelvis may become ulcerated or filled with an accumulation of pus—*pyonephrosis*. Here also secondary deposit of phosphates may occur. Ultimately, the infection may extend to the kidneys and give rise to abscesses in their substance. Often only one pelvis is affected in this way, but both pelves may be involved, although in an unequal degree.

Pyonephrosis also arises when a hydronephrosis due to a calculus in the renal pelvis becomes infected. The presence of a renal calculus seems to predispose the pelvis to infection, and when this leads to alkaline decomposition of the urine, phosphates are precipitated in the dilated pelvis and calyces and particularly on the pre-existing calculus, which develops into an irregular branching mass with bulbous ends extending into the calyces, the whole forming a rough cast of the pyonephrotic sac. This is known as the *staghorn calculus.*

The urinary tract is not infrequently infected from the kidney by *typhoid bacilli* in the course of typhoid fever. Usually only a mild catarrhal inflammation is the result, and the condition may be almost a pure bacilluria. The bacilli may persist for an indefinite period of time, the patient being then termed a "urinary carrier" (p. 516); the establishment of the carrier state is facilitated by almost any anatomical abnormality in the urinary tract. In some cases of coliform infection also, there may be comparatively little inflammatory reaction. Cystitis may rarely be produced by the gonococcus in cases of *gonorrhoea*, and has usually the features of a purulent catarrh. It is to be noted that coliform bacilli and the gonococcus do not render the urine alkaline, but infection by proteus organisms is quickly followed by ammoniacal decomposition owing to splitting of urea.

Malakoplakia. This is a rare condition found in some cases of chronic cystitis, and is characterised by the formation of numerous soft rounded elevations or plaques in the bladder wall, varying up to 1–2 cm. They have a pale, sometimes yellowish appearance surrounded by vascular areas, and tend to ulcerate on the surface and be invaded by bacteria. They are essentially composed of cellular granulation tissue in which there are numerous large cells which contain droplets of various kinds and small hyaline spheres with concentric marking known as Michaelis–Gutmann bodies, also inclusions of red cells and leukocytes. The rounded structures may become free by disintegration of the cells. Calcium salts may be deposited in them and they have also an affinity for iron, as can be shown by the usual tests. The lesion is a granuloma of unknown cause.

Tuberculosis. Tuberculous disease of the bladder is, as a rule, the result of direct infection of its mucosa by the bacilli in the urine. It occurs most frequently in cases of renal tuberculosis, though also in tuberculosis of the genital tract. The bacilli invade the mucosa and give rise to tubercles which then undergo ulcera-

tion. In this way, multiple small ulcers are formed, especially at the base of the bladder, and sometimes the orifices of the ureters are specially involved. The ulcers increase in size and form large areas by confluence. Sometimes there is a considerable amount of caseous thickening of the lining. Secondary invasion by other organisms sometimes occurs, and more acute inflammatory change is superadded.

Schistosomiasis (bilharziasis). The bladder is the most frequent site of lesions in this condition, which is produced by *Schistosoma haematobium*. It is very common in many hot countries, notably in Egypt. The adult parasites lie in the veins of the bladder, and the eggs laid by the female pass into the surrounding tissues, where they are present in large numbers. The irritation produced results in the formation of abundant vascular granulation tissue which causes great thickening of the mucosa and submucosa. Nodular projections appear, and the interior of the bladder may be beset with rounded and somewhat pedunculated vascular polypi, which tend to become ulcerated. Haematuria is a common feature and the ova are readily found in the urine. Septic infections may become superadded, and carcinoma develops in a proportion of cases in Egyptians, but very rarely in infected Europeans. Schistosomal lesions sometimes occur also in the ureters and renal pelves.

Schistosoma haematobium is a dioecious trematode. The adult male is about 13 mm. long, the female about 20 mm.; the female is thinner, and lies enclosed in the gynaecophoric canal of the male. The eggs are oval in form, about 130μ in length, and the shell has a distinct terminal spine; the embyro is visible within. When the urine becomes diluted on being mixed with water, the investing shell swells and bursts and a ciliated embyro or miracidium escapes. This was shown by Leiper to penetrate the body of certain fresh-water snails of the genus *Bulinus* within which it passes to the liver and then develops into a sporocyst; ultimately free-swimming cercariae are developed: these enter the human host, chiefly through the skin but also through the mucous membrane of the mouth and pharynx. They pass by systemic veins to the lungs, through the pulmonary capillaries, and thence to the systemic arteries via the heart. Those reaching the liver mature into adult worms within the portal vessels. The young adults then pass against the blood stream to the portal radicles, especially those of the inferior mesenteric vein, and thence they reach the vesical plexus, where they settle and pair as described above. Occasionally the parasite remains in the liver and the eggs are discharged into the peri-portal connective tissue and give rise to hepatic fibrosis (p. 577). There are two other pathogenic species of schistosoma, *S. mansoni* and *S. japonicum*: they have similar life cycles to *S. haematobium*. The adult *S. mansoni* colonises the veins of the colon (p. 521), and *S. japonicum*, which occurs in the Far East, the veins of the small intestine. The ova of both species cause granulomatous reactions in the gut, with ulceration and melaena, and they may also colonise the liver, producing peri-portal fibrosis: the ova are found in the faeces. Several additional genera of snails have been found to act as vectors in various parts of the world.

Calculi

Urinary calculi are formed by precipitation of urinary constituents, a small amount of organic material also being incorporated. Deposition is favoured by a highly concentrated urine, and by secretion of excessive amounts of one or other constituents (oxalate, urate, etc.). Calculi occur in the renal pelvis or ureter, or in the bladder, although some of the latter originate in the kidneys, and subsequently enlarge in the bladder.

There are 3 main types of urinary calculus composed respectively of (*a*) a mixture of uric acid and urates—uric acid stones, (*b*) calcium oxalate; both (*a*) and (*b*) are laid down in acid urines and stones may contain a mixture of both substances; (*c*) calcium carbonate and phosphate combined in the complex forms of carbonate-apatite and hydroxyapatite; these are laid down in alkaline urines and often form an outer laminated deposit upon other stones.

The incidence of urinary calculi has fallen greatly in recent years in western Europe and the relative incidence of the various chemical types also appears to have changed. According to Prien and Frondel, amongst 600 calculi analysed chemically and by X-ray diffraction, etc., the commonest pure type of stone consists of calcium oxalate (36 per cent) whereas only 6 per cent are of uric acid. The majority of stones consist principally of the apatites. It has long been supposed that calculi begin as minute deposits in the collecting tubules of the kidney and then pass to the pelvis where further increase in size takes place. Randall has shown that some stones develop by enlargement of plaque-like deposits attached to the apices of the pyramids. Carr has modified and extended Randall's concept by very convincing radiographic evidence that the primary site of deposition is in the lymphatics

of the renal papillae that normally remove particulate matter from this region. If this mechanism is overloaded or if the lymphatic pathway is obstructed by inflammation of the papilla, microliths accumulate and are extruded through the lymphatic lining into the calyx where they grow into small concretions by further deposition of urinary solids. The part played by organic matter is uncertain, but Boyce and his co-workers have suggested that urinary mucoproteins attract and fix calcium ions which later, as a result of alterations of pH, are precipitated as crystalline salts to form the nuclei of stones: all the calcium-

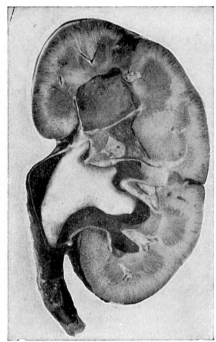

FIG. 21.73.—Large renal calculus, forming a cast of lower part of the pelvis and obstructing the ureter.

rich calculi except pure oxalate stones have a mucopolysaccharide binding agent. In the formation of calculi, excess of a particular substance is usually the important factor, as, for example, in hyperparathyroidism, where the increased excretion of calcium and phosphate in the urine very frequently leads to the formation of urinary calculi of the apatite variety.

Renal calculi. As stated above, early deposits may form in the collecting tubules of the kidney, or, according to Randall, on the apex of the pyramid, and then extend into the pelvis where further increase in size takes place. Within the pelvis multiple small stones may form, especially when it is dilated, and occasionally they may be present in enormous numbers, or a single calculus may form and develop into a branching mass filling the pelvis (Fig. 21.73). The degree of hydronephrosis produced varies greatly, as already described. A small calculus may pass along the ureter to the bladder, giving rise to renal colic with haematuria. It may be arrested temporarily, usually at the narrow lower end of the ureter. Permanent impaction, usually at the upper or lower ends of the ureter or at the level of the pelvic brim, produces hydro-nephrosis as already described, and when the

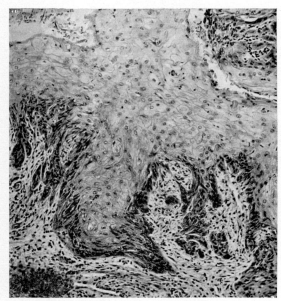

FIG. 21.74.—Section of lining of renal pelvis in nephro-lithiasis, showing metaplasia of epithelium to the strati-fied squamous type and early squamous carcinoma. × 65.

obstruction is intermittent, the hydronephrosis may be extreme. When the urine is infected with urea-splitting bacteria (e.g. proteus) am-moniacal decomposition of the urine follows and calculi or softer deposits composed of phosphates are precipitated in the inflamed pelvis. The condition may be accompanied by suppuration and ulceration. The large branch-ing "stag-horn" calculi arise in this way and are composed largely of triple phosphates, i.e. mag-nesium ammonium phosphate hexahydrate. A calculus in the renal pelvis, especially when it is movable, may give rise to metaplasia of the lining of the pelvis to stratified squamous epithelium. As a further result of the irritation, squamous

carcinoma has occasionally been found to arise, as is illustrated in Fig. 21.74.

With the advent of sulphonamide therapy it was soon found that precipitation of these drugs may occur in the renal tubules and pelvis unless the fluid intake is maintained at a high level to promote diuresis. If this is neglected, actual obstruction of tubules, pelves and ureters may result from masses of crystals of the drug or its acetylated form.

Bladder calculi

These may be single and reach a great size, or they may be multiple, sometimes numerous and like coarse sand. In many cases calculi form first in the renal pelvis, especially uric-acid and oxalate calculi, and they pass to the bladder, where they increase in size; in other cases they are formed locally. The larger calculi present great variations in composition and structure, but as a rule there is a nucleus or centre surrounded by concentric laminae. According to Kleinschmidt, the nucleus or primary stone is formed by the slow deposition of the par-ticular substance from a saturated solution in the urine, and has the same composition throughout. The *primary stones* formed in this way are composed of urates and uric acid, or of calcium oxalate or calcium phosphate, rarely of cystine or xanthine. The primary urate stone, seldom larger than a few mm., and often formed first in the renal pelvis, is round, hard and brown. The primary oxalate stone is small and very hard with irregular outline, and is often dark brown from altered blood pigment. The large oxalate calculus known as a "mulberry stone", a round hard stone with nodular surface (Fig. 21.75b), is usually a composite stone with a varying proportion of urates and oxalates in the outer layers. Primary phosphatic stones are whitish, often friable, but sometimes hard. They occur in hyper-parathyroidism and in experimental hyper-vitaminosis D (p. 765) and are mixtures of the apatites, chiefly hydroxyapatite. Any of these primary stones may have *secondary* deposits formed on their surface, and thus compound or laminated stones arise. The particular substance secondarily deposited, which need not be in a saturated state in the urine, depends not only on the composition of the urine but also on its reaction, urates especially being deposited when the reaction is acid (Fig. 21.75*a*), phosphates when it is alkaline. As the state of the urine varies from time to time, the great variations in the composition of stones can be readily understood. Thus a primary urate stone may be surrounded by laminae of mixed urates and oxalates (Fig. 21.75*b*), or of phosphates, etc. Vesical calculi

Tumours

Nearly all tumours of the urinary tract arise from the transitional epithelial lining. There is evidence that chemical carcinogenesis is of etiological importance, and, in accordance with this, it is not uncommon to encounter two or more tumours in the same individual, either simultaneously or over a period. It is not

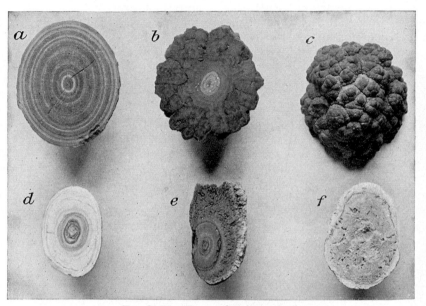

FIG. 21.75.—Types of vesical calculi.

a, uric-acid stone, showing characteristic lamination around the primary stone; *b*, oxalate or mulberry stone seen on section, and *c*, surface view of the same; *d*, laminated phosphate stone around a central nucleus; *e*, small laminated phosphatic stone with irregular incrustation deposit on the surface; *f*, non-laminated phosphatic stone. × ¾.

sometimes grow to measure several centimetres, and may weigh over 300 g.

These two kinds of stones, primary, and compound or laminated, may form without the presence of bacterial infection or inflammation, and lead to mechanical effects—pain and irritation with haematuria, intermittent obstruction, damage to the bladder mucosa with ulceration, etc. When, however, there is secondary bacterial invasion, and ammoniacal decomposition of the urine occurs, then triple phosphates and ammonium urate separate out, often in large amount, and form a further deposit on calculi already formed. Deposits of these substances may occur also in cases of purulent cystitis (p. 742) apart from the previous occurrence of calculi, and form primary inflammatory calculi or irregular deposits.

surprising that, having a relatively large surface area, the bladder should be a commoner site of tumours than the ureters or renal pelves, but the trigone appears to be particularly often involved.

It is difficult to adopt the usual classification of benign and malignant for urinary tract tumours, and the following classification takes into consideration the reported experience of the Institute of Urology of the University of London.

Benign papilloma. This is a pedunculated tumour, often less than 1 cm. in diameter, which projects into the lumen from a narrow stalk and is composed of fine branching fronds, each of which has a thin central core of vascular connective tissue and a lining which is 3–4 cells thick and resembles very closely the normal transitional epithelium of the urinary tract (Fig. 21.77). The cells are regular, and mitoses are few. Tumours showing this very high degree of differentiation are rare, and are benign.

Well-differentiated transitional cell carcinoma. These tumours may be papillary (Fig. 21.76) or solid, or may contain both types of structure. They comprise the majority of urinary tract tumours.

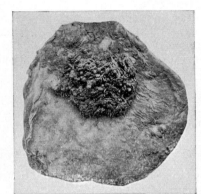

Fig. 21.76.—Papillary tumour of bladder. × ⅘.

(a) *Papillary.* Tumours of this type have a structure similar to the benign papilloma; they differ, however, in having a thicker epithelial lining composed of more layers of cells. Mitoses are more numerous, and the epithelial cell nuclei show variations in size, but tend to be larger and more deeply staining, giving the impression of crowding of cells. In spite of these appearances, the cells are sufficiently differentiated to be recognisably of transitional type. The base of the epithelium is not so regular as in the benign papilloma, and it extends more deeply into the underlying connective tissue. Careful search must be made for foci of invasion, and extension into lymphatics or venules. Even in the apparent absence of such changes, some of these tumours recur or behave as carcinomas, but the presence of invasion greatly worsens the prognosis.

(b) *Solid.* This has the appearance of a raised plaque attached to the surface by a broad base, and sometimes appearing lobulated or nodular. Microscopy shows solid sheets of epithelial cells with appearances similar to the cells of the papillary tumours (Fig. 21.78), but enclosed by bands of vascular connective tissue. The prognosis is similar to the papillary type, and the detection of invasion is again of great importance.

Some tumours are papillary in their superficial parts, but have a broad base of attachment and deeper solid elements.

Anaplastic carcinoma. This also presents as a plaque raised above the surface, but usually shows central necrosis and sloughing and thus appears as a sloughing ulcer with raised edges. The epithelium is in solid masses, and may have some resemblance to transitional cells, but with obvious cell aberration and numerous and abnormal mitoses (Fig. 21.79). Foci of poorly differentiated squamous epithelium are often present. There is frank invasion into the underlying muscle, and lymphatic and venous extensions are often apparent. The prognosis is poor.

Squamous carcinoma also occurs in the urinary tract: in some instances it arises from squamous

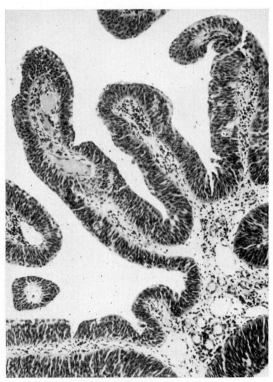

Fig. 21.77.—Papilloma of bladder. Part of the tumour, showing the frond-like processes. Where the epithelium has been cut perpendicularly, it is 3–4 cells thick: in other places, oblique section gives a false impression of more cell layers. × 85.

metaplasia attributable to the presence of calculi and chronic inflammation. In other cases, squamous cancer arises directly from transitional epithelium.

Adenocarcinoma is relatively uncommon. It

may arise from transitional epithelium and occurs particularly in congenital extroversion of the bladder, when the epithelium undergoes metaplasia to mucus-secreting type. Another possible origin is from remnants of the urachus around the apex of the bladder.

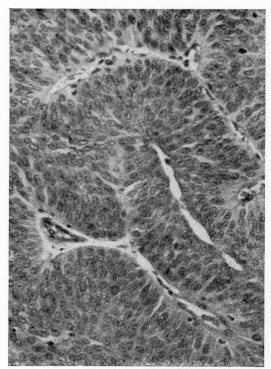

FIG. 21.78.—Well-differentiated transitional-cell carcinoma of the urinary bladder. × 350.

Clinical features. Both benign and malignant tumours of the urinary tract tend to bleed, and haematuria is the common complaint. In some instances, infection is superadded, and recurrent cystitis is not unusual, particularly with ulcerated malignant tumours. Symptoms may also arise from local invasion or distant metastases.

Etiology. Bladder tumours, and particularly the transitional cell types, are a well known industrial hazard in workers in the aniline dye industry, in which 2-naphthylamine has been incriminated (p. 215). There is also an increased incidence in workers in the rubber industry, and more recently there is evidence incriminating benzidine. The incidence is also increased in cigarette smokers. A high incidence of bladder tumours has been observed in Egypt, and is attributable to chronic schistosomiasis.

Other tumours. Myxoma and leiomyoma are occasionally encountered, and both leio- and rhabdomyosarcomas, the latter appearing as raised blunt processes.

Haematuria

This is so important a clinical sign that we may summarise with advantage the chief disorders that give rise to it. Apart from acute laceration of the kidney and injury to the bladder or urethra in fracture of the pelvis, the following are the major causes of haematuria. By far the most important causes in Great Britain are calculi and tumours.

(*a*) *Renal calculus.* Haematuria, of varying degree, accompanies an attack of renal colic due to the passage of a calculus along the ureter, but may occur even if the stone fails to leave the renal pelvis.

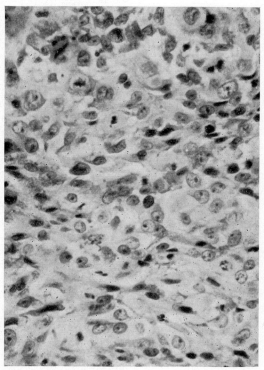

FIG. 21.79.—Anaplastic carcinoma of the urinary bladder. × 350.

The formation of crystals in collecting tubules and pelvis, e.g. calcium oxalate, or sulphonamide drugs, may be accompanied by renal colic and haematuria.

(*b*) *Tumours.* Haematuria is often a prominent feature of renal carcinoma and of tumours of the bladder. It is occasionally due to a papillary tumour of the pelvis, and profuse haemorrhage may be produced by a comparatively small angioma at the apex of a medullary pyramid.

(*c*) *Inflammatory conditions.* Red cells are present in the urine in the various forms of acute glomerulonephritis, and sometimes the presence of blood is clearly recognisable on naked-eye examination. It is often a marked feature of focal glomerulonephritis (p. 709). Haematuria may occur in suppurative infection, though it is usually slight; it may, however, be a marked feature in cases of renal tuberculosis.

(*d*) Infestation with *Schistosoma haematobium* is an important cause of haematuria in countries where the parasite is endemic, the presence of the eggs in the mucosa causing much injury and inflammatory reaction (p. 743).

(*e*) *Circulatory disturbances.* Red cells escape in the urine in chronic venous congestion, though usually the amount of blood is scanty; more marked haematuria occurs in renal infarction and in thrombosis of the renal vein. Occasionally it occurs temporarily after severe exercise.

(*f*) In certain *blood dyscrasias*, notably in the purpuras, haematuria may be a prominent symptom, and it is an indication of overdosage in patients on anticoagulant drugs, e.g. for coronary thrombosis.

The various renal conditions may, for practical purposes, be conveniently divided into those in which bleeding is unilateral and those in which it is bilateral. In some cases severe unilateral bleeding occasionally takes place without the presence of any of the above conditions, and when the kidney is excised, no change except the presence of blood in some of the tubules or pelvic mucosa is to be found. The nature of such cases is quite obscure.

Haematuria should not be confused with *haemoglobinuria*, i.e. the presence of free haemoglobin, but not red cells, producing a clear red urine. Haemoglobinuria results from intra-vascular haemolysis, the causes and features of which are described on pp. 203 and 404. *et seq.*

Congenital abnormalities

Abnormalities may affect the *pelves* and *ureters*. The ureter may be double in its upper part or in its whole length; in either case, a partial doubling of the pelvis is usually present. When the duplication is complete, the ureter from the upper part of the kidney opens separately into the bladder, or sometimes into the urethra or a seminal vesicle. Such a condition may be present on one or both sides. Congenital narrowing or *atresia* of a ureter may give rise to dilatation proximally; an abnormally high origin of the ureter from the pelvis may lead to hydronephrosis (p. 741). Such abnormalities appear to favour the occurrence of infection and also its persistence when established.

The most important abnormality of the *bladder* is a defect of its anterior wall, accompanied by a corresponding median defect of the abdominal wall, the condition being known as *extroversion* of the bladder. The posterior wall of the bladder is thus exposed, and appears as an area of vascular mucous membrane, on which the ureters open. The epithelium of the exposed mucosa undergoes metaplastic alteration, in part into squamous epithelium and in part into a columnar mucus-secreting epithelium resembling that of the intestine. In the male, the urethra remains open on its dorsal aspect, the condition being known as *epispadias*; in the female there is usually a split clitoris. The symphysis pubis is also usually deficient, though this may occur apart from extroversion of the bladder.

In the posterior urethra valve-like folds of the mucosa (Young's valves) may occur just below the urethral crest and give rise to obstruction to the passage of urine with consequent hypertrophy of the bladder and bilateral hydronephrosis.

CHAPTER 22

LOCOMOTOR SYSTEM

DISEASES OF BONE

Normal bone structure

Bone is a specialised form of connective tissue and certain fundamental concepts of its normal anatomy and physiology are essential to an understanding of its pathology. *Normal bone* consists of cells (osteocytes) lying in small spaces (lacunae) in a matrix formed of collagen fibres, amorphous ground substance and mineral complexes. The mineral consists of calcium and magnesium in combination with phosphate and carbonate, in the complex known as bone apatite.

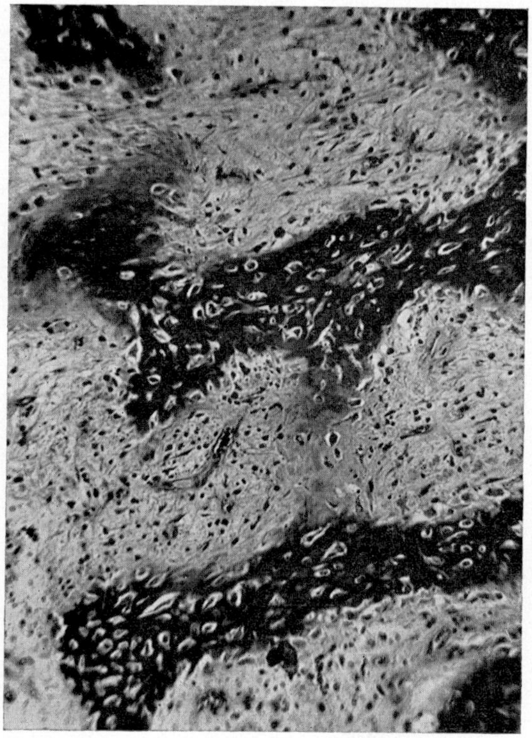

Bone formation and resorption. Bone may be formed through the intermediate stage of cartilage (endochondral ossification) or directly from collagen (membranous ossification) but in both these circumstances the production of bone is thought to occur in two stages. Firstly, an

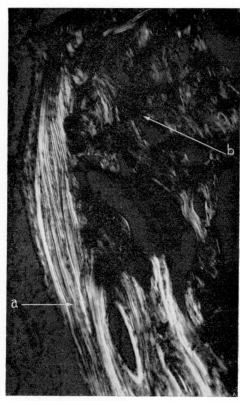

FIG. 22.2.—Lamellar bone in polarised light showing (*a*) the orderly orientation of the bone lamellae. On the surface are some new formed trabeculae of woven bone, (*b*) showing lack of lamellar orientation. × 190.

FIG. 22.1.—Woven bone, from provisional callus, showing large, closely packed lacunae. × 190.

uncalcified matrix, *osteoid*, is formed and secondly under normal conditions this is rapidly mineralised. The removal of bone (resorption) is generally believed to occur in one stage, mineral and matrix disappearing together. The terms decalcification and demineralisation are therefore to be avoided as they give a false picture of the process in living bone. At sites of bone resorption the bone surface has scalloped edges, *Howship's lacunae*, and these often contain multinucleated giant cells (osteoclasts). Bone is not a static tissue and throughout life the two processes of bone formation and bone resorption continue actively though at a slower rate in adult life than in childhood.

Types of bone. While all bone consists of cells, collagen fibres, ground substance and mineral, different types of bone may be formed depending on the arrangements of fibres and cells. Two main types are found in the human skeleton, woven fibre bone and lamellar bone.

Woven bone consists of coarse fibre bundles running in an irregular, interlacing pattern through a matrix rich in ground substance. The cells are large and closely packed (Fig. 22.1). It is formed whenever bone is rapidly laid down as in the embryonic skeleton, subperiosteally in a growing bone, in fracture callus, as reactive bone in relation to tumours, in Paget's disease, osteitis fibrosa and also in fibrous dysplasia. It is, however, an impermanent structure and, given time, is usually replaced by lamellar bone which is mechanically stronger.

Lamellar bone. The fibre bundles are fine and run in parallel sheets (Fig. 22.2), different sheets having different fibre directions and so giving the whole a stratified appearance. The cells are smaller and less numerous than in fibre bone and have more frequent and delicate processes. The histological differences are most clearly demonstrated either by silver stains or by viewing the sections in polarised light. Lamellar bone usually replaces pre-existing cartilage or woven bone.

PYOGENIC INFECTIONS OF BONE

Acute osteomyelitis

Different terms are applied to inflammations of bone according to the site—periostitis, osteitis proper, and osteomyelitis—but these should not be taken as indicating separate conditions; one may lead to another, and sometimes all three are present together. Acute osteomyelitis is seen most often in childhood though it occurs also in neonates and less frequently in adults. The metaphyses adjacent to the more actively growing epiphyses of long tubular bones, i.e. lower end of femur, upper end of tibia, upper end of humerus and lower end of radius, are the sites usually involved, though vertebrae, pubis, clavicle and indeed any bone may be affected.

Etiology

Bone infection may result from bacterial contamination of a compound fracture or, in the jaw, by direct spread from an adjacent focus of infection such as an apical tooth abscess, but in most cases it arises as a result of haematogenous spread of organisms and is initially an *osteomyelitis*, the organisms having settled first in haemopoietic marrow. Sometimes there is an obvious inflammatory lesion elsewhere such as a boil or paronychia, but frequently the path of entry cannot be traced and is probably some slight lesion of the skin or mucous membrane. While suppurative osteomyelitis may be produced by various organisms, by far the commonest cause is the *Staphylococcus aureus* (Fig. 22.3), β-*haemolytic streptococcus* and *pneumococcus* producing occasional infections especially in infants, while the other pyogenic organisms are uncommon as causal agents. In the tropics an attack of typhoid fever may be followed, sometimes many years later, by osteomyelitis, usually in the long bones or spine. Sickle cell anaemia in children and Gaucher's disease may be associated with salmonella osteomyelitis.

The pyogenic organisms may be recovered by blood culture at an early stage in the disease but treatment should not be delayed either for the result of the culture or for the appearance of radiological changes, lest fatal septicaemia or irreparable damage to the bone results.

Macroscopic appearances

From the vascular spongy bone of the metaphysis the suppuration may spread widely, so that the medullary cavity becomes largely occupied by pus (Fig. 22.4). In children, because of the presence of the epiphyseal cartilage plate, extension occurs more readily in a transverse direction than onwards into the epiphysis. The infection, after breaking through the thin metaphyseal cortex, may reach the periosteum which during growth is often only loosely attached to the underlying shaft though more firmly anchored at the epiphyseal plate. A

affected bone tissue is completely deprived of its blood supply and undergoes necrosis (Fig. 22.5). This is especially the case when, as may happen with a large accumulation of pus under the periosteum, the nutrient artery becomes involved and occluded by thrombus. In extreme cases, death of the whole diaphysis may result, and then the dead bone becomes separated from the epiphysis and forms a large *sequestrum* (Fig. 22.5). Towards its ends, the dead bone may become eroded by granulation tissue, and irregular resorption results; but the part actually bathed in pus undergoes little change and the surface remains smooth. As the process becomes less acute, new bone is usually produced under

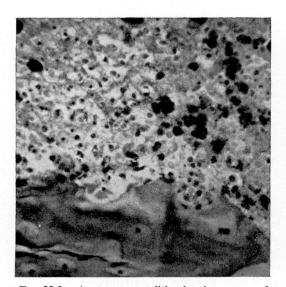

FIG. 22.3.—Acute osteomyelitis, showing masses of staphylococci. × 250.

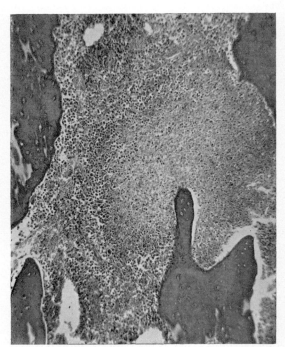

FIG. 22.4.—Acute osteomyelitis showing necrosis of bone and marrow and an intense polymorph reaction. × 95.

subperiosteal abscess thus forms which may spread extensively, bathing a large part or even the whole diaphysis in pus but usually sparing the epiphysis. The abscess may burst through the periosteum and lead to diffuse suppuration in the muscles and other soft tissues, and later, if the condition is not treated, may discharge externally. Suppuration leads to thrombosis in blood vessels, which in turn leads to bone necrosis. Suppurative periostitis by itself results in necrosis of only a superficial layer of bone owing to the anastomoses with the endosteal vessels, while in the case of medullary suppuration also, the resulting necrosis, though varying in degree according to the amount of vascular involvement, may be limited. If, however, both lesions are extensive at the same time, the

the periosteum (Fig. 22.6) and this may form an encasing sheath to the dead bone, known as an *involucrum* (Fig. 22.7). This new bone is irregular and is often perforated by openings or *cloacae* by which the pus may collect locally or may drain to the skin surface, forming a discharging sinus. The above description applies to the severer forms of the disease which are still commonly seen in tropical countries where delay in treatment and mixed bacterial infections

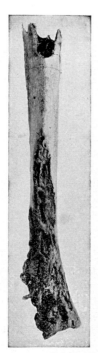

FIG. 22.5.—Sequestrum of shaft of tibia from a case of acute suppurative osteomyelitis.

Note the partial resorption of the bone at its ends.

tend to lead to large sequestra and sinus formation. In Great Britain however, good host resistance and the early administration of appropriate antibiotics have reduced the incidence both of large sequestra and of abscesses requiring drainage.

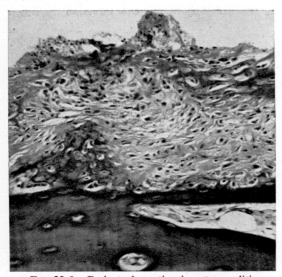

FIG. 22.6.—Periosteal reaction in osteomyelitis showing new bone formation. × 350.

Complications

Septicaemia or pyaemia. These complications are especially likely to arise in haematogenous osteomyelitis due to staphylococci, where, owing to the production of coagulase by these organisms, the delicate vascular channels in the marrow commonly become thrombosed and suppurative softening of the thrombi allows the organisms to invade the blood. Pyaemia with abscesses in the lungs, kidneys and myocardium and acute ulcerative endocarditis may be produced even when the osteomyelitis is not extensive or is at an early stage. The causal organisms are present in the blood and may be obtained from it by culture. Pyaemic abscesses are less frequent in infections with other bacteria.

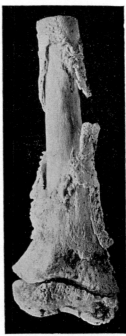

FIG. 22.7.—Femur from a case of long-standing suppurative osteomyelitis and periostitis, showing the irregular formation of an involucrum of new bone round the sequestrum.

Septic arthritis occurs more commonly when the metaphysis is within the joint capsule (see p. 790) and although rare in children is more frequent in infants especially when the osteomyelitis involves the femoral neck. Metastatic arthritis involving several joints may complicate infantile streptococcal or pneumococcal osteomyelitis (p. 754).

Alteration in growth rate. Growth is sometimes retarded especially in infants when the epiphyseal cartilage plate has been damaged, but occasionally is accelerated, probably due to increased vascularity of the metaphyseal side of the growth apparatus.

Chronic osteomyelitis. Acute osteomyelitis particularly in adults, may progress to a chronic state with recurrent exacerbations of infection, repeated formation of abscesses with discharging sinuses and increasing patchy bone sclerosis (Fig. 22.8). Long continuing osteomyelitis with the discharge of pus may be followed by *amyloid disease* or occasionally by the development of *squamous carcinoma* in the epithelial-lined wall of a sinus.

Neonatal osteomyelitis

Haematogenous osteomyelitis in the newborn presents a rather different picture from the disease in the older child. It may involve one bone only, often the maxilla, or many bones may be affected, so-called *generalised osteomyelitis of the newborn*. It arises sometimes in association with umbilical or other sepsis and is most commonly caused by *Staphylococcus*

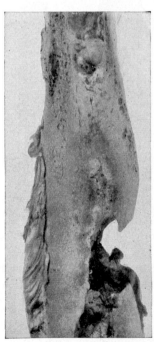

FIG. 22.8.—Chronic suppurative osteomyelitis of femur.
The lower part of the medullary cavity contains pus and granulation tissue; there is sclerosis of surrounding bone and the medullary cavity above is obliterated. Opening on right is surgical.

aureus, often of a penicillin-resistant strain and occasionally by β-*haemolytic streptococcus* or *pneumococcus*. In the more severe cases associated with septicaemia there may be accompanying symptoms of pneumonia or gastroenteritis and the infant is desperately ill. The osteomyelitis itself is characterised by the tendency to form a massive involucrum which may be completely resorbed after recovery, by damage to the epiphyseal cartilage causing growth retardation, and by septic arthritis. The involvement of the cartilaginous epiphysis and the joint may be facilitated by the vascular pattern in which metaphyseal vessels penetrate the epiphysis.

Osteomyelitis in the adult

This condition is relatively rare but may complicate injury or debilitating disease. There is a tendency for the diaphysis of the bone to be involved rather than the metaphysis or epiphysis. The periosteum in the adult is more fibrous and adheres more firmly to the bone; this tends to minimise the formation of subperiosteal abscesses, thereby retaining the cortical blood supply and preventing the separation of large sequestra. However, cortical erosion is common and chronic marrow infection almost invariable in the adult.

Subacute pyogenic infection

An increasing number of patients now seem to develop a subacute pyogenic infection often with an insidious onset and relatively little constitutional upset. This may give rise to localised abscess formation of which Brodie's is one type (see below). When the spine is involved, even if diagnosis is late, the prognosis is usually good since bone destruction is soon followed by sclerosis and bony bridging between affected vertebrae.

Brodie's abscess. This is a form of localised, subacute or chronic pyogenic osteomyelitis which arises insidiously without an acute attack and is usually situated in the metaphysis of a long bone, especially the upper end of the tibia. The central cavity contains pus, which may be sterile, is lined by granulation tissue and surrounded by reactive bone sclerosis.

Acute periostitis

Acute periostitis may occur as the result of trauma, there being inflammatory oedema with swelling and little accompanying leukocytic infiltration. Apart from this, it is produced by bacterial invasion and is sometimes suppurative. It may result from an external wound or from the spread of organisms from a skin ulcer, or, in the jaws, from a carious tooth. Haematogenous infection of the periosteum is rare but is a well-known complication of *typhoid fever*, when it may appear long after the primary illness has subsided.

TUBERCULOSIS OF BONE

With the virtual eradication of bovine infection in Britain, the human type of bacillus is the chief cause of tuberculosis of bone. This condition is decreasing in frequency but broadening its age incidence so that fewer children and an increasing proportion of adolescents and young adults are affected. The disease most commonly involves the vertebrae, the metaphyses and epiphyses of long bones such as femur and tibia (in which it is often accompanied by tuberculous arthritis (p. 791)) and the small tubular bones of the hands and feet. Infection usually arises as a result of haematogenous spread of bacilli from a tuberculous lesion in lung, lymph nodes or elsewhere; occasionally there is direct or lymphatic spread to bone from an adjacent focus, e.g. to ribs from pulmonary lesions, and, very rarely nowadays, to the petrous bone from the middle ear.

In some cases the onset of the disease in bones or joints appears to be related to local injury, and it has been shown experimentally that, when the bacilli have been introduced into the blood stream, trauma favours their settling at the site of injury and producing a lesion.

Structural changes. When tubercle bacilli settle in the spongy bone marrow, tuberculous follicles form and the disease process may then extend either as tuberculous granulation tissue with little caseation or form a frankly caseating mass. In both cases bone destruction results (Fig. 22.9). In contrast to pyogenic osteitis the disease is usually more slowly progressive and new bone formation is scanty in the active stage. The formation of large sequestra as the result of thrombotic infarction is rare although occasionally wedge-shaped areas of necrosis under the articular cartilage may result from interference with the blood supply, probably due to endarteritis. When healing does occur it is by fibrosis and at this stage some new bone formation may be seen. Tubercle bacilli may remain in these healed foci for a long time and the disease may later recrudesce.

Tuberculosis in different sites

Pott's disease of the spine. Tuberculosis of the spine is commonest in children and young adults. The dorsal, lumbar and cervical vertebrae are affected in that order of frequency.

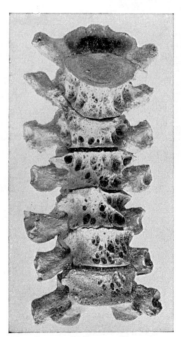

FIG. 22.9.—Involvement of several contiguous vertebrae by the destructive changes of tuberculosis (macerated and dried specimen).

Often more than one vertebra is involved; they are usually adjacent (Fig. 22.9) but occasionally widely separated. The disease most commonly arises near the intervertebral disc, the disc itself being involved early. When the infection arises in or spreads to the periosteum, the caseous

BB

material is invaded by polymorphonuclear leukocytes and converted into pus. This tends to accumulate to form a *paravertebral abscess* at the front and sides of the vertebra which may spread to infect other vertebrae. Later the pus sometimes penetrates the sheaths of muscles and extends in their substance (Fig. 22.10). In this way when the lumbar vertebrae are involved

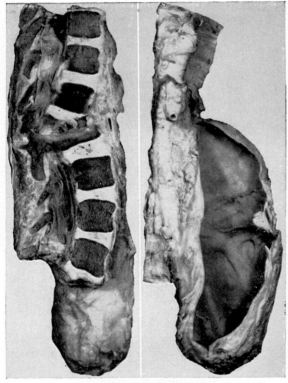

FIG. 22.10.—Tuberculosis of spine (Pott's disease). Loss of intervertebral disc and collapse of T.12 and L.1 with paraplegia and formation of psoas abscess.

a *psoas* or *lumbar "cold" abscess* may be produced, and the tuberculous pus tracks along the psoas sheath to point in the inner aspect of the thigh. When the cervical vertebrae are affected, a large collection of pus may form behind the pharynx—*retropharyngeal abscess*. The cold abscess may burst through the skin with the formation of a sinus which tends to become secondarily infected. Such patients are especially liable to develop *amyloid disease*. As the vertebral bodies are weakened by bone destruction they collapse anteriorly, and, especially when two adjacent vertebrae are involved, angulation of the spinal column results (Fig. 22.10).

Pott's paraplegia may supervene, either early in the disease, when it is usually the result of pressure on the cord in the canal by an abscess, granulation tissue, sequestrated bone or disc material; or sometimes late, when it results from bony pressure at the site of the vertebral collapse or from recrudescence of infection producing an inflammatory mass.

Tuberculous dactylitis may involve a single phalanx or rarely several phalanges of a hand or foot. The infection occurs in the medullary cavity and there is abundant formation of tuberculous granulation tissue which leads to resorption and also expansion of the bone, so that it may be reduced to a shell.

Tuberculous trochanteric bursitis. In this condition which usually arises in young adults the bursa is replaced by a mass of tuberculous granulation tissue and caseating material which ramifies in the surrounding tissue planes. This is usually associated with tuberculous disease of the trochanter but the hip joint is not involved.

OTHER BONE INFECTIONS

Syphilis of bone

Bone lesions may occur in both congenital and acquired syphilis but are now rare in Britain.

Congenital syphilis. The commonest form of bone disease in congenital syphilis is *osteochondritis*. The metaphyseal surface of the growth plate is marked by a broad irregular yellowish band which consists of a trellis of unresorbed, patchily calcified cartilage (Fig. 22.11*b*). Bone formation is inhibited and the marrow spaces of the adjacent metaphysis contain fibrous and granulation tissue. In severe cases there may be separation of the epiphysis due to fracture

through the delicate cartilage trellis at the metaphysis. Separation sometimes also occurs following gummatous softening which usually starts near the centre of the plate and may spread to the periphery (Fig. 22.11*a*). *Periostitis*, with the formation of subperiosteal new bone, is seen. *Dactylitis* in the hand and foot may involve several bones. *Saddle nose* results from perforation, destruction and collapse of the nasal septum.

Acquired syphilis. Transient periostitis involving especially the tibia and skull bones occurs occasionally in the secondary stage. The bone changes of tertiary syphilis are also seen in congenital syphilis in

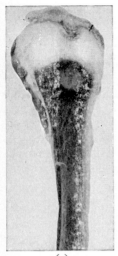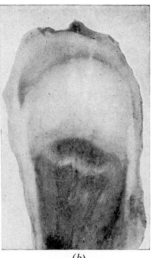

(a)   (b)

FIG. 22.11.—Lesions of bones in congenital syphilis. (a) shows gummatous epiphysitis and (b) shows the irregularity of the epiphyseal line at an earlier stage. (J. W. S. B.).

older children and adults. *Gummas* may form in the periosteum. The lesions may become adherent to the skin, ulcerate and discharge; secondary infection with pyogenic organisms follows with further destruction. The bone beneath the gumma may be resorbed producing a rough-floored depression with a raised irregular margin of reactive bone. *Periostitis*

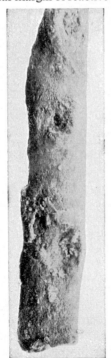

FIG. 22.12.—Syphilitic disease of periosteum of tibia, showing nodular thickenings and eroded areas in the bone.

is often associated with osteitis; the lesions may be multiple and widespread and great thickening and sclerosis of the bone may occur, the medullary cavity being reduced and the surface becoming extremely irregular (Fig. 22.12).

Periostitis may also be associated with actual necrosis with formation of sequestra; this is common when the lesions are extensive, and the vascular supply is interfered with. In the skull large areas of bone may die and sequestra separate, gummas may form both outside and inside the skull, giving rise to apertures with thickened and irregular bony margins (Fig. 22.13). These striking appearances are rarely seen nowadays outside museums. In the palate and nasal bones gummatous periostitis may be followed by ulceration, which penetrates deeply and leads to perforation of the nasal septum and hard palate.

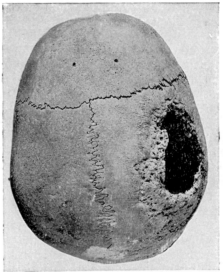

FIG. 22.13.—Syphilitic disease of skull. Note the large aperture with irregular margins resulting from a gumma.

Actinomycosis

The bones usually become involved as a result of extension of soft tissue suppuration (p. 151). The jaw may be affected by spread from an oral focus; the cervical vertebrae from a pharyngeal one; the ribs, sternum or dorsal vertebrae from pulmonary actinomycosis and the pelvis from an abdominal lesion. The infection is characterised by bone destruction and suppuration with little attempt at new bone formation. In *Madura disease*, which may be caused by an allied actinomycete the prominent feature is extensive destruction of the bones of the foot.

Brucellosis

Bone may be affected in this disease (p. 792).

EFFECTS OF RADIATION ON BONE

For a general description of the effects of radiation see pp. 22–7.

Radiation osteitis (Radiation osteodysplasia)

The term radiation osteitis was first used by Ewing to describe pathological changes in bone following external radiation, and later by Martland in his investigations of the bones of watch-dial painters who had ingested radium and mesothorium. While the condition is not inflammatory, the term is widely accepted. The radiation, whether external or internal, probably produces its effect by direct action on cartilage and bone cells as well as indirectly by its effect on blood vessels. A "safe" dosage cannot be stated with certainty as there is great variation in the individual response to radiation, but in general it is thought unlikely that bone damage will be caused in adults by doses of less than 3000 rads of external radiation though in children smaller doses may be incriminated. Some of the patients with internal radiation developed bone changes after quite small total body dosage; others with much larger dosage escaped injury.

External radiation

Growth. In children inclusion of the epiphyseal cartilage plate in the radiation field may result in retardation of growth due to cessation of division of the cartilage cells and their swelling and degeneration. Sometimes in severely damaged plates there is also premature closure of the epiphysis leading to further stunting of growth.

Aseptic bone necrosis may occur and is accompanied by necrosis and fibrosis of the bone marrow sometimes followed by calcification and the formation of abnormal, basophilic woven bone (Fig. 22.14). There may be some bone resorption and the radiological appearances are of patchy radiolucency and sclerosis.

Pathological fracture has been found in the femoral necks of women who were irradiated for carcinoma of the cervix or other pelvic organ malignancy and less frequently in the ribs or clavicle following postmastectomy irradiation. There is commonly a time interval of many years between irradiation and the fracture, which is often slow to heal.

Acute osteomyelitis. Any necrotic bone resulting from irradiation damage to the jaw is very susceptible to infection especially if the teeth are carious. The bone infection usually starts as a spreading periostitis. A rather similar picture of some historic interest was the jaw necrosis followed by osteomyelitis which used to be found in phosphorus poisoning of match workers—so-called *phossy jaw*.

Internal radiation

Radioactive fallout from the explosion of nuclear devices gives rise to increased ^{90}Sr in the

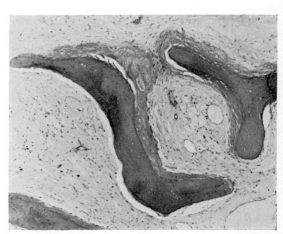

FIG. 22.14.—Following irradiation there has been formation of coarsely fibred woven bone on the trabecular surfaces. The marrow is oedematous and shows some fine fibrosis. × 40.

soil and vegetation. Cows eat the contaminated grass and excrete some of the radionuclide in their milk. The amount of ^{90}Sr in the human skeleton has risen in the last 20 years but although this has given rise to considerable concern the levels remain low. From animal experiments ^{90}Sr is also thought to be less toxic than radium.

Accidents at atomic reactors tend chiefly to involve contamination with the radioactive element plutonium. ^{239}Pu is concentrated mainly on endosteal surfaces of bone and in marrow macrophages. It, like radium, has a long half life, emits high energy α-rays and is found experimentally to produce bone tumours in animals and possibly, unlike radium, to have a leukaemogenic effect. Since, however, very little is known about the effect of these substances in man it is the effect of radium which is discussed below.

Bone damage has occurred both as a result of therapeutic administration of radium salts and of accidental intake as in the case of the watch-dial painters. Almost all radium salts which are not excreted are stored in bone, being initially deposited both diffusely and in a patchy manner in areas of active growth or bone remodelling where calcification is incomplete (*hot spots*). Later when bone resorption takes place the radioactive material may be laid down again in new sites of active bone formation. With large doses death of the patient is likely to occur at an early stage from blood dyscrasia and here the only bone abnormality is likely to be necrosis of the mandible with secondary sepsis. With smaller doses the bone marrow may be un-affected and the patient live long enough to develop aseptic bone necrosis with complicating pathological fractures or acute osteomyelitis in sites other than the jaw.

Neoplasia following irradiation

Leukaemia. External radiation of the skeleton tends to affect most severely the haemopoietic cells of the marrow. There is an increased incidence of myeloid leukaemia in the survivors of the atomic bombs, irradiated patients with ankylosing spondylitis and pioneer radiologists. Leukaemia, however, does not seem a common complication of ingested radium.

Bone sarcoma has occurred in as many as 20 per cent of survivors of those who ingested doses of radium or its salts, but is rare following external radiation. Dahlin reports 43 sarcomas of various histological types arising following therapeutic external radiation as compared with 750 similar tumours arising in non-irradiated bone. Where radioactive salts have been deposited in bone there is often recognisable radiation osteitis in the skeleton but it is rarely recognisable in association with the tumours produced by external radiation. It is now thought that injury and repair are not necessary accompaniments of sarcomatous change. The latent period before development of bone sarcomas is usually from 5–20 years and may be even longer following internal radiation. The tumours may be found anywhere in the skeleton and are sometimes multiple. They are usually osteosarcomas or fibrosarcomas and often rapidly fatal from pulmonary metastases.

Nasal carcinoma. A high incidence of carcinoma of the nose and nasal sinuses has been found up to 50 years after radium ingestion. This is thought to be due partly to the close proximity of the epithelium to the underlying bone and partly to an excess retention of radon in the air sinuses.

BONE CHANGES ASSOCIATED WITH VITAMIN DEFICIENCY OR EXCESS

Vitamin C deficiency

Scurvy

Scurvy results from vitamin C deficiency and is now a rare disease in Britain. It is characterised by a generalised defective deposition of fibrous proteins, including bone matrix, dentine and collagen, and results in abnormalities in growing bones and teeth. Also there is a tendency to haemorrhage because of capillary wall weakness and an impairment of healing of bone and soft tissues following injury. Scurvy is most common in infants and young children where bone and other connective tissues are being rapidly formed, but also occurs in old people taking a restricted diet (p. 446).

Bone changes in infants precede haemorrhage and are due to failure to lay down bony matrix, associated with the persistence of an unabsorbed calcified cartilage lattice. There is no failure of calcification (cf. rickets). The cartilage cells of the epiphyseal plate multiply and orientate themselves normally and the intervening matrix becomes calcified but osteoblasts fail to lay down osteoid and the calcified cartilaginous matrix is only slightly and patchily resorbed (*scorbutic lattice*) so that the epiphyseal plate becomes widened and irregular. Fracture of spicules of the calcified cartilage occurs and a very irregular, radiologically dense zone arises at the junction of epiphysis and shaft. The metaphysis itself is weak because of failure of bone deposition, the marrow spaces contain much loose fibrous tissue, and separation of the epiphysis through this site is not uncommon. The pre-existing bony trabeculae in the shaft are thin and delicate (osteoporosis) probably because of continuing normal resorption without bone deposition.

Haemorrhagic tendency. There is a tendency to bleed spontaneously or from trivial injury. The gums are spongy and bleed readily and the teeth may be loosened. There may be haemorrhage into the skin, mucous membranes, joints or subperiosteally.

Subperiosteal haemorrhages cause the severely affected child to lie immobile and to be apprehensive of movement which causes pain. Nothing may be seen radiologically until subperiosteal new bone is laid down on the surface of the haematoma. Bleeding into the kidney, orbit, brain or adrenals occasionally complicates the picture. The exact cause of capillary haemorrhage in scurvy is not clear even on electron-microscopy.

Failure of healing. In scorbutic patients, skin and flesh wounds and fractures either fail to heal or do so more slowly than normal, and occasionally there have been reports of old wounds breaking down. The administration of extra Vitamin C to non-scorbutic individuals does not however increase the rate of healing.

Anaemia. Hypochromic anaemia tends to occur probably as a result of the combination of blood loss, poor intestinal iron absorption and defective folic acid transformation (p. 423).

"Battered baby" syndrome

This syndrome may be confused clinically with scurvy and accordingly, although it does not arise from vitamin deficiency, is conveniently discussed here.

Subperiosteal haemorrhage with subsequent formation of an involucrum of new bone may be seen as a result of epiphyseal damage in the "battered baby" syndrome, where an infant has been repeatedly assaulted, usually by the parents. Several bones may be involved, the subperiosteal new bone formation being at different stages in different bones. The epiphyseal damage may be associated with multiple bruises, fractures of limb bones or more commonly of ribs or clavicle and with subdural haematoma or a head injury which may prove fatal. In this condition the bones are normal radiologically apart from the effects of trauma and there is no haemorrhagic tendency. It is important to make the diagnosis

since if the infant is returned to his home further assault, sometimes fatal, may occur.

Vitamin D deficiency

Osteomalacia and rickets

Definition. Dietary osteomalacia in adults and rickets in infants and children are due to a deficiency in Vitamin D which results in an increase in the amount of uncalcified bony matrix (*osteoid*) (Fig. 22.15) and in addition in rickets produces defective mineralisation of the epiphyseal cartilage. These appearances may have other causes than simple vitamin deficiency. It should be noted that the term osteomalacia is applied not only to a disease process but also to the abnormal bone structure.

Introduction. Vitamin D is the name applied to all the sterols with pronounced antirachitic properties. This fat-soluble vitamin exists in two

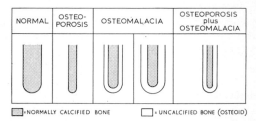

FIG. 22.15.—Diagram of bone changes.

main forms. Vitamin D_2 (calciferol) is produced by irradiation of ergosterol. Vitamin D_3 is present in fish oil and egg yolks, in much smaller amounts in butter and milk and may be synthesised by the action of ultraviolet light on 7-dehydrocholesterol in the human skin. The antirachitic effect of sunlight depends on its angle of incidence so that both latitude and season are important, as is the clarity of the atmosphere. Skin pigmentation may reduce the beneficial effects of ultraviolet rays. Children, particularly those of coloured immigrants, brought up in northern cities with their smoky atmosphere and few hours of winter sunshine are therefore especially liable to be dependent on their dietary intake of Vitamin D to prevent rickets. The preventive dose is about 400 international units/day for the fair-skinned infant but there is considerable individual variation both in requirements and in sensitivity to toxic effects of hypervitaminosis. (One international unit has been defined as being equivalent to 0·025 μg. of pure crystalline Vitamin D.) Since naturally occurring sources of Vitamin D are scanty, dried milk and cereals for infants and margarine are fortified either by added calciferol or by irradiation. The dietary requirement of the vitamin in adults is uncertain and probably less than 100 international units/day. It has recently been recognised that old people, often house-bound and living on restricted diets, are especially likely to develop osteomalacia.

Vitamin D in the presence of bile salts is incorporated in lipid-rich micelles in the gut and absorbed in this form by the mucosal epithelial cells in the upper part of the small intestine. It is then secreted into the mucosal lymphatics in the chylomicrons and is presumed to be stored in the liver and plasma. The store is relatively small.

The vitamin is essential for the absorption of calcium from the gut and also increases the absorption of phosphate. When Vitamin D is deficient intestinal excretion of both calcium and phosphorus is increased. There is a tendency towards a fall in blood levels leading, according to the classical myth, to a lowering of their product in mg. per 100 ml. below the critical level of 40 which permits the transfer and pre-cipitation of calcium and phosphate from the blood to bone and cartilage matrix. Whatever the cause, bone laid down after the onset of Vitamin D deficiency is poorly calcified and the remains of pre-morbid calcified trabeculae are covered by osteoid borders of varying thickness. Both osteomalacia and osteoporosis may give rise to bone weakness clinically and to decreased bone density radiologically and it is important to grasp the fundamental difference between them. In osteomalacia and rickets a normal or even excessive amount of matrix is produced but it is not calcified. In osteoporosis the matrix is diminished in amount but appears to be nor-mally calcified. Occasionally osteoporosis and osteomalacia may coexist (Fig. 22.15).

Osteomalacia

Nutritional osteomalacia in Britain is rare and is found chiefly amongst children, old people, and also occasionally in pregnancy, especi-ally in coloured immigrants. Associated with pregnancy there is in addition to lack of Vitamin D a loss of calcium to the fetus and in the breast milk. The condition is more frequent in India where Moslem women in purdah are particularly at risk. Osteomalacia (Vitamin D deficiency) may also arise following gastrectomy, in various forms of intestinal malabsorption and in obstructive jaundice. Excess osteoid may occur with some renal abnormalities (p. 764) and in patients on anticonvulsant drugs (p. 765).

Biochemical findings. Although Vitamin D deficiency gives rise to failure of calcium absorption, the plasma Ca is often normal rather than diminished and the plasma phosphate is low. It is thought that the initial tendency to hypocalcaemia stimulates the parathyroids which restore the normal serum level of calcium by release of the mineral from resorbed bone.

The plasma phosphate which may already be slightly lowered by decreased absorption is further lowered by the effect of parathyroid hormone in diminishing the renal tubular re-absorption of phosphate. Some support for this explanation of the biochemical findings is received both from the reports of clear cell hyperplasia of the parathyroids at necropsy in some patients with osteomalacia or rickets and from increased osteoclastic activity and marrow fibrosis in bone biopsies of some osteomalacic patients. The hyperparathyroidism is sometimes sufficiently marked for subperiosteal erosions to be recognisable radiologically (p. 767). When-ever the plasma calcium is low, tetany may occur. The explanation of the failure of the parathy-roids to respond to the hypocalcaemia in these cases may be that there is unusually complete coverage of the bone surfaces by osteoid which for some reason inhibits osteoclastic resorption.

The serum alkaline phosphatase is frequently raised, indicating increased osteoblastic activity.

Clinical and radiological features and structural changes. The patient commonly presents with muscular weakness especially noticeable on climbing stairs and with a waddling, penguin gait. Pain is usually vague, aching and poorly localised so that a diagnosis of "muscular rheumatism" may be suggested. Occasionally attention is first drawn to the condition by a fracture following minimal violence which fails to produce radiological evidence of callus formation although uncalcified callus may be present in abundance. An incomplete or green-stick fracture in an adult may also suggest the diagnosis. Sometimes *Looser's zones* or pseudo-fractures are seen and when present are almost pathognomonic. The radiological picture is of a linear zone of translucency, cutting across at right angles to and usually affecting only one cortex. Looser's zones are painless and are most often found in the pubic rami, ribs, inner scapular borders, neck of humerus and femur, sometimes being bilateral and symmetrical and probably representing bony remodelling at areas of stress. There may be a generalised decrease in bone density, especially noticeable in the peripheral skeleton compared with the spine (c.f. osteoporosis, p. 769). In the more severe cases deformity may occur in the absence of fracture, due to the weakening and softening of the bones. The pubic rami may be buckled and pushed forward into a beak (*triradiate pelvis*) with consequent narrowing of the pelvic outlet; the limb bones may be bowed and the spine kyphotic. These severe deformities are seldom seen nowadays and it must be emphasised that the skeletons of some patients with osteomalacia may show no recognisable radiological abnormality.

Microscopic appearances. The osteoid matrix (uncalcified bone) which is laid down after the onset of vitamin D deficiency fails to calcify (Fig. 22.16). The recognition of the osteoid borders covering the premorbid mineralised bone may be difficult in decalcified material and is best achieved by study of undecalcified sections stained by von Kossa's method (p. 207) in which calcified matrix is stained black and the osteoid remains unstained (Fig. 22.16). The diagnosis of osteomalacia can be made by bone biopsy and an area containing cancellous bone such as the iliac crest gives least technical difficulty. A word of caution is necessary in the diagnosis of minor degrees of osteomalacia. When bone is being rapidly formed for any reason in normal subjects, a thin border of osteoid may be present on the surface beneath the layer of osteoblasts and even in the slower process of bone turnover in the normal adult skeleton an occasional narrow border of osteoid may be recognisable. Osteomalacia is usually diagnosed either when more than half the trabecular surface is clothed by narrow osteoid seams bare of osteoblasts or, if osteoblasts are present, when osteoid seams are wide. In undecalcified sections of normal bone a haematoxyphilic line, the calcification front, can be seen in most places between calcified bone and any

osteoid present. This line tends to be deficient in osteomalacia. The amount of matrix formed in osteomalacia is very variable. It is sometimes markedly increased and the trabeculae are broader than normal probably partly due to an increased amount of formation but also to a decrease in bone resorption, the osteoid for some reason being less readily removed than normal calcified matrix. Occasionally, particularly in the elderly, the total amount of matrix is much diminished and the conditions of osteomalacia and osteoporosis exist together (see Fig. 22.15). Mild changes of osteitis fibrosa may be present (p. 767) with some marrow fibrosis and osteoclasis of bone not covered by osteoid.

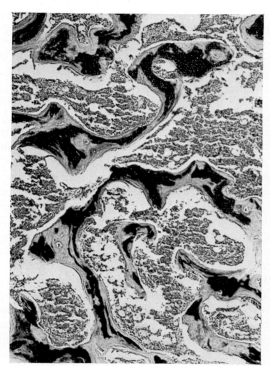

FIG. 22.16.—Severe osteomalacia. Undecalcified sections stained by von Kossa's method. Only the bone stained black is calcified. There are wide seams of unstained osteoid. No secondary osteitis fibrosa is seen here. × 40.

The diagnosis of dietary osteomalacia may be difficult sometimes on clinical, radiological or biochemical grounds. In any suspected case bone biopsy should be done and undecalcified sections examined. The diagnosis is very well worth making since the condition rapidly responds to Vitamin D administration in doses of 2,000–4,000 i.u. daily.

Rickets

Rickets in the infant or child is the equivalent of osteomalacia and also results from deficiency of Vitamin D. In addition to the failure of mineralisation of osteoid matrix as seen in osteomalacia there is failure of mineralisation of the cartilage of the epiphyseal growth plate.

The ends of the long bones are swollen (Fig. 22.18) and this may be particularly noticeable at the wrists. Radiological examination shows wide, irregular, fuzzy, cupped metaphyses, thin bony cortices and the late appearance of epiphyseal centres which are often indistinct. There may be greenstick fractures with apparent failure of callus formation. Sometimes Looser's

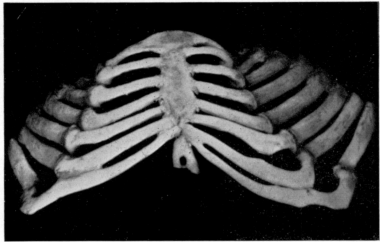

FIG. 22.17.—Rickets. Chest wall, showing the swellings at the costochondral junctions of the ribs—the so-called rickety rosary.

Dietary rickets is chiefly a disease of infancy, being commonest from 6 months to 2 years. Rickets is present at birth only in infants born to osteomalacic mothers. Prematurity predisposes to rickets since the skeleton is mineralised in the last three months of intra-uterine life and those born before then tend to be deficient in stored calcium. Prolonged breast feeding may also predispose since breast milk provides only about 20 units of vitamin D daily, i.e. about 5 per cent of the infant's requirements. A further group particularly at risk are infants in large low-income families who are weaned early from fortified dried milk to a share in the vitamin D-poor family diet.

Biochemical findings. As in osteomalacia, the serum calcium level is normal or slightly low, but the serum phosphate is usually between 1 and 3 mg. per 100 ml., i.e. markedly lower than the normal value for infants (4–7 mg. per 100 ml.). The plasma alkaline phosphatase is frequently raised.

Clinical and radiological features. There are muscular hypotonia, skeletal changes, sometimes anaemia and occasionally, in the early stages, tetany.

zones (pseudo-fractures) are seen (see p. 761). Deformity results from bending of the soft, poorly mineralised bone and anterolateral bowing of the femur and tibia is characteristic.

The costochondral junctions tend to be swollen ("rickety rosary") and "pigeon chest" due to indrawing of the ribs and protrusion of the sternum is sometimes seen (Fig. 22.17). Flattening of the pelvis with constriction of the outlet and scoliosis may occur. The skull appears square and box-like with bossing of the frontal bones and the closure of the fontanelles is delayed. Eruption of the teeth may be late.

Microscopic appearances. Under normal conditions proliferation of cartilage cells at the epiphyseal plate is followed by mineralisation of the matrix, hypertrophy of the chondrocytes, vascularisation of the lacunae of these hypertrophic cells by metaphyseal vessels, laying down of osteoid on the surface of the mineralised cartilage and finally brisk calcification of the osteoid followed by metaphyseal remodelling. The primary change at the epiphyseal growth plate in rickets is failure of the normal mineralisation of the cartilage matrix. As a result the hypertrophic cartilage cells persist for an abnormally long time and as proliferation continues at the usual rate the epiphyseal plate becomes thicker. Patchy calcification leads to some irregular ingrowth of blood vessels but long tongues of cartilage remain projecting far down into the metaphysis (Fig. 22.19). The osteoid matrix which is laid down on the surface of the cartilage is not calcified and since osteoid is less readily resorbed by osteoclasts metaphyseal remodelling is also deficient. These micro-

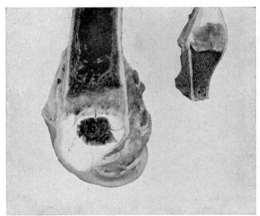

Fig. 22.18.—Rickets. Section through lower end of femur and rib at costochondral junction.

scopic changes account for the gross and radiological appearances of a wide, irregular growth plate with flared metaphyses. It must be emphasised that if for any reason the infant has ceased to grow the changes in the epiphyseal plate will not be seen though there will of course be osteomalacic change in the bone as in the adult. Osteoid matrix formed by intramembranous bone deposition also fails to calcify.

Administration of vitamin D leads to resumption of calcification which in the epiphyseal plate occurs first in the region of those cartilage cells which have most recently become hypertrophic. Since the amount of osteoid laid down is not usually diminished in rickets and its removal is impaired, the bones may become heavier than normal when calcification does occur. Deformities may become less marked but tend to persist to some extent so that the child with healed rickets may have permanently bent long bones with bow legs, knock knees or other abnormalities.

Non-dietary causes of osteomalacia and rickets

It is unusual nowadays in Great Britain to see dietary rickets or osteomalacia but failure of mineralisation, alone or associated with other bone abnormalities, may accompany a variety of conditions. The structural changes are not different from those described above except that they tend to be less severe and may be modified by other co-existent bone disorders. The more important conditions are as follows.

A. Malabsorption syndromes. The association of rickets and osteomalacia with steatorrhea has been recognised for some time and was assumed to be due to simple failure of absorption of the fat-soluble vitamin D. Osteomalacia has also occasionally been described following gastrectomy and in congenital biliary atresia and it is now considered due both to malabsorption of the vitamin and to some resistance to its effect. There is sometimes an associated osteoporosis.

B. Uraemic osteodystrophy, renal rickets. Bone changes which, in mild degree, are very common, may result from any renal disease which gives rise to prolonged uraemia, e.g. congenital hypoplasia of the kidneys, valvular obstruction to the urethra with pyelonephritis in infants, and chronic nephritis or pyelonephritis in adults. Bone disease is not found in the nephrotic syndrome.

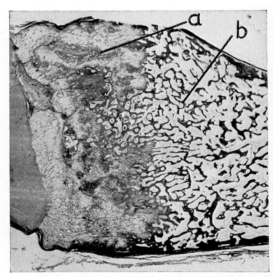

Fig. 22.19.—Costochondral junction of rib in rickets.
a. The cartilage of plate is thickened and irregular. *b.* The spongy bone is partly uncalcified. × 6·5.

In uraemic osteodystrophy the bones may show rickets (osteomalacia) and osteitis fibrosa (p. 767), alone or together and in any degree of severity. The changes of secondary hyperparathyroidism may be very striking (Fig. 22.22) and associated with a diffuse chief-cell or clear-cell hyperplasia of all the parathyroid glands. *In children* growth may be stunted and bony deformities of the rachitic type develop. The changes in the epiphyseal cartilage plates are rachitic but in addition there is often severe osteitis fibrosa, especially in the metaphyses. *In adults* there is usually no deformity though bone pain, decreased skeletal radiodensity, subperiosteal erosions and other abnormalities may be present. Occasionally osteosclerosis may be seen in some bones especially the vertebrae, due to an increase of apparently normal bone or, more commonly, associated with osteitis fibrosa. When osteitis fibrosa is severe, metastatic calcification may occur.

Patients on chronic renal dialysis may develop bone changes of hyperparathyroidism but with marked lack of osteoblast activity. Osteomalacia is sometimes seen.

Biochemical changes. The serum phosphate is almost always raised, the serum calcium low or normal and if bone disease is marked the alkaline phosphatase is raised.

The mechanism of production of the osteomalacia is not known but may possibly be an acquired insensitivity to vitamin D and the secondary hyperparathyroidism may result from acidosis increasing the excretion of calcium as a fixed base. Improvement may be brought about by massive doses of vitamin D, sometimes as much as 200 times the dose given to cure dietary osteomalacia.

C. Renal tubular osteodystrophy. 1. *Vitamin D resistant rickets.* This condition, which is now known to be inherited by a sex-linked dominant gene, is found chiefly in children and is associated with a tubular reabsorption defect of phosphate (and sometimes also glucose) with consequent hypophosphatemia. The condition may be indistinguishable from dietary rickets, leading to stunting and deformity, though muscle weakness is not usually marked. It is relieved by phosphorus supplements with massive doses of vitamin D. It may regress spontaneously but there is a tendency for recurrence in middle age. Renal failure does not occur.

2. *Fanconi syndrome.* This disease occurs mostly in children, is due to a recessive gene defect and is associated with impaired tubular reabsorption of phosphate, glucose, various amino-acids and sometimes potassium. There may also be inability to form an acid urine and sometimes a metabolic defect of cystine metabolism (Lignac–Fanconi syndrome) and patients with these additional defects tend to develop uraemia. Microdissection of the kidney has shown a long thin segment at the glomerulo-tubular junction associated with a short proximal tubule. The bone changes, which are initially rachitic and osteomalacic, may later, especially in the uraemic cases, become complicated by osteitis fibrosa.

3. *Renal tubular acidosis* is another cause of osteomalacia and rickets. This condition can occur at any age and is not usually hereditary. The primary defect is an inability to form an acid urine and the chronic hyperchloraemic acidosis leads to an increased urinary excretion of phosphate and of fixed bases such as calcium and potassium. If treatment with alkali is given there may be little renal damage, but if untreated nephrocalcinosis and progressive renal failure result. Secondary hyperparathyroidism may occur.

D. Anticonvulsant drugs. Long-continued high dosage of several anticonvulsant drugs may lead to osteomalacia, probably by stimulating production of liver iso-enzymes which destroy vitamin D abnormally rapidly.

Hypophosphatasia

In 1948 a disorder of infancy of rachitic type associated with deficiency in the activity of serum alkaline phosphatase was described. Later it was found also to be accompanied by the presence of phosphotidyl-ethanolamine in the serum and its excretion in the urine, an observation that is probably significant because this substance can act as a substrate for alkaline phosphatase. The disease is thought to be inherited as an autosomal recessive, the parents being clinically normal but having either or both of the biochemical abnormalities in lesser degree. While the bone changes are similar to rickets in some respects there is greater severity of defects of intramembranous ossification of skull bones so that the head may become shaped like a water-filled balloon. Vitamin D even in large doses usually fails to improve the condition and when clinical improvement does occur spontaneously, it is commonly not accompanied by any alteration in the serum alkaline phosphatase or the excretion of phosphotidyl-ethanolamine. At this stage the whole of the cranial suture lines may undergo premature ossification so that further growth is prevented and craniostenosis may result. The bone changes of osteitis fibrosa do not occur.

Vitamin D excess

Hypervitaminosis D

If doses of vitamin D several thousand times the usual therapeutic dose are administered there is an increase in the blood calcium. Increased excretion of calcium and phosphorus in the urine occurs and renal calculi may form. In addition, provided that there is sufficient calcium in the diet, there is often widespread metastatic calcification in the arteries, myocardium, kidney and stomach. If, along with the excess of vitamin D, there is insufficient calcium in the food, hypercalcaemia is maintained by increasing bone resorption, particularly in cancellous bone. The effects of hypervitaminosis D on bone to some extent resemble those due to hyperparathyroidism, but the action is direct and not through the parathyroids.

Infantile hypercalcaemia

The relatively mild form of this condition is the result of vitamin D poisoning and was relatively common in Britain in the 1950s due to high fortification of many infant foods and of cod liver oil.

Individual susceptibility to the toxic effects of the vitamin is a factor since some infants are poisoned by doses which are harmless to others. Although the amount of vitamin D in fortified foods is now reduced occasional sensitive babies are still affected. Infantile hypercalcaemia is characterised by a raised blood calcium, sometimes over 14 mg. per 100 ml., by anorexia, vomiting and failure to thrive. Deposition of calcium in the renal parenchyma (*nephrocalcinosis*), may lead to scarring and uraemia. Radiological examination sometimes shows dense epiphyses. In the severe form of the condition the pathogenesis is not understood and the babies may develop the additional features of mental retardation, goblin facies and osteosclerosis.

BONE CHANGES IN ENDOCRINE DISORDERS

Primary hyperparathyroidism

This results usually from an adenoma of one of the parathyroid glands (Fig. 24.20, p. 905); occasionally an adenoma may be present in two or more glands and very rarely hyperparathyroidism results from parathyroid carcinoma. Primary hyperplasia of the glands is also a cause of primary hyperparathyroidism but is much less common than an adenoma. Excess hormone may be produced intermittently. It has a direct action on bone, stimulating resorption as well as increasing the excretion of urinary phosphate and probably also increasing calcium absorption from the gut. The effect of the hormone is to mobilise calcium and raise the blood calcium from the normal level of 10 mg/100 ml. to 12 mg/100 ml. or more. The blood phosphorus falls to 2 mg/100 ml. or less and the alkaline phosphatase is increased. A rise in the urinary excretion of calcium follows so that these patients tend to develop *renal calculi* (p. 744). Sometimes when the bones are severely affected *metastatic calcification* of the walls of blood vessels, soft tissues, the renal substance and other sites may occur.

Bone changes. It is puzzling that a proportion of patients with clinical and biochemical evidence of hyperparathyroidism fail to develop demonstrable bone changes. In the majority of patients, however, there is evidence of increased bone resorption, osteoclasts and Howship's lacunae are prominent on the surface of the trabeculae which become surrounded by delicate, fibrillar fibrous tissue. There may also be "dissecting resorption" of trabeculae, the

central parts being replaced by fibrous tissue. The picture is often one of great activity (Fig. 22.20), with an increase also in osteoblasts; resorption and new bone formation may be seen

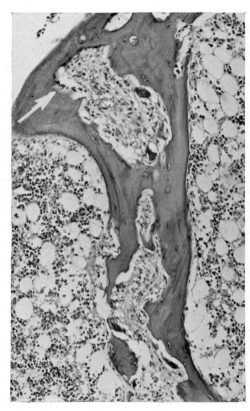

FIG. 22.20.—Osteitis fibrosa of hyperparathyroidism. There is osteoclastic resorption of the central part of a bone trabecula with fibrous tissue replacement, so-called dissecting resorption. Some osteoblasts are also seen (arrow). × 100.

on opposite sides of the same trabecula. At this stage radiology may demonstrate subperiosteal erosion of the phalanges and of other bones due to patchy replacement of subperiosteal bone of the cortex by fibrous tissue. A helpful radiological sign may be the disappearance of the bone

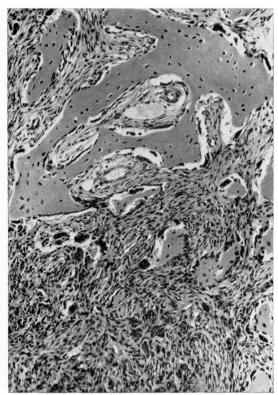

FIG. 22.21.—Bone in hyperparathyroidism. Numerous multinucleated giant cells and spindle cells from a "brown tumour". Newly formed bone is seen in the upper part of the photograph. × 120.

surrounding the roots of the teeth (lamina dura). As the condition increases in severity the marrow spaces become filled with fibrous tissue— hence the term *osteitis fibrosa*—and the normal structure of bone in both cortex and medulla is replaced by a meshwork of fine, irregular and delicate trabeculae. These consist chiefly of normally calcified bone; narrow osteoid borders may be present beneath a row of plump osteoblasts as is sometimes observed in fracture callus and indicate only the rapidity of bone formation rather than a real deficiency of mineralisation. Radiology now shows loss of definition between cortex and medullary cavity, the whole bone having a fuzzy, mottled appearance, and because of the loss of normal structure it is more liable to

fracture. The loose fibrous tissue is vascular and secondary changes may occur in it as a result of degeneration or haemorrhage. Cystic spaces may form and in areas of haemorrhage the resulting haemosiderin and the large numbers of multinucleated giant cells give rise to the "*brown tumour of hyperparathyroidism*" (Fig. 22.21). The differentiation of this lesion from giant-cell tumour of bone may give considerable difficulty and the possibility of brown tumour should always be considered especially in a site unusual for giant-cell tumour such as jaw or skull and above all when the lesions are multiple.

Effect of removal of the parathyroid tumour. Excision of the parathyroid tumour, which may be in the neck or, in some instances, behind the sternum, leads to a fall in the serum calcium level, and within a week bone biopsy may show

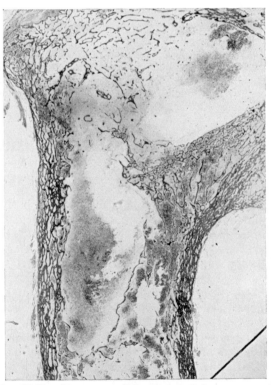

FIG. 22.22.—Upper part of femoral shaft from a case of hyperparathyroidism secondary to chronic renal failure. There is osteitis fibrosa and osteoporosis, with severe cancellisation of the cortex. × 1·5.

diminution of osteoclast activity, the bone structure slowly returning to a more normal appearance. Failure of improvement after operative removal may indicate the presence of a second tumour. In some instances tetany has followed immediately after removal of the affected para-thyroid, but function of the remaining parathy-roid glands, apparently suppressed by the tumour, soon returns to normal.

Secondary hyperparathyroidism

In dietary rickets, osteomalacia, pregnancy, chronic uraemia and some other conditions, there is a tendency to a fall in serum calcium levels and there may be a compensatory increase in parathyroid activity leading to enlargement of the glands. Of these conditions chronic uraemia especially may give rise to bony changes, slight or severe, exactly mimicking those of primary hyperparathyroidism Fig. 22.22).

Excess of growth hormone after puberty (acromegaly)

Bone enlargement occurs and is due partly to subperiosteal proliferation but possibly also to re-establishment of endochondral ossification of the articular cartilage and vertebral end plates. The bones of the hands and feet and the jaw are most strikingly affected. Osteoporosis may occur.

Excess of corticosteroids (Cushing's syndrome)

Cushing's syndrome is associated with osteoporosis (Fig. 22.24) and has the usual clinical and morbid anatomical features, the spine and pelvis being especially affected (p. 769). The porosis is thought to be the result of both a reduced rate of bone formation and an increased rate of resorption though osteoclasts are not prominent in histological material. Identical skeletal changes may occur with prolonged cortisone therapy.

Thyroid deficiency in infants (cretinism)

Longstanding hypothyroidism in early life results in severe dwarfing. There is slowing of normal endo-chondral growth, late appearance of centres of ossi-fication and sometimes delay in closure of epiphyses. The epiphyses may also be irregular, deformed, and radiologically stippled. The bones may become thickened with broad cortices and wide medullary trabeculae.

Excess of thyroid hormone (thyrotoxicosis)

Prolonged hyperthyroidism may cause osteo-porosis. There is thought to be an increase of both resorption and bone formation but resorption exceeds formation.

MISCELLANEOUS BONE CONDITIONS

Osteoporosis

In osteoporosis there is a decrease in the amount of bone tissue but the matrix is normally mineralised, at least as judged by histological methods and inorganic analysis (Fig. 22.15). It may result from decreased bone formation, increased bone resorption or a combination of both. Osteoporosis arises in a localised and a generalised form following various unrelated disorders.

Disuse atrophy (immobilisation osteoporosis, disuse osteoporosis, localised osteoporosis). Dis-use atrophy is found in immobilised or paralysed limbs, e.g. following poliomyelitis. It may be recognisable within weeks and seems to be associated both with loss of muscle action and with loss of weight bearing. It is striking that in even the most severely affected bones cancellous trabeculae remain prominent along lines of stress. The bones become increasingly radio-lucent; the trabeculae of spongy bone are scantier and more slender; the cortical bone

becomes thinner due chiefly to opening up of Haversian spaces on the endosteal surface, so-called *cancellisation*. The changes of osteo-porosis may be patchy in distribution and are usually first recognised in cancellous bone especially that in the metaphysis and subchon-dral articular regions, probably because bone turnover is more rapid in these sites. Focal radiological bone changes due to osteoporosis may be mistaken for other localised osteolytic processes such as tuberculosis.

An initial increase in resorption is thought to cause the porosis (Fig. 22.23) but later bone deposition and resorption may return to equili-brium. Once muscle activity is resumed there is an increase in bone production and the bone slowly returns to normal. Occasionally perma-nent deformity results from *premature epiphyseal fusion* in children. Generalised immobilisation may be complicated in the early stages by hyper-calcaemia and the formation of renal calculi. Similar osteoporosis is said to have been found in the first astronauts, probably due partly to the enforced relative inactivity within the space capsule and partly to the weightless state.

Generalised osteoporosis. Only a small proportion of people with thin bones suffer from known endocrine abnormalities such as Cushing's syndrome (p. 912) or thyrotoxicosis. (p. 892). There is a much larger group of postmenopausal women and elderly males who have

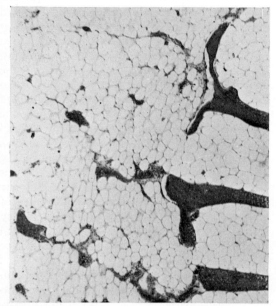

FIG. 22.23.—Immobilisation osteoporosis. The articular surface is beyond the left hand border of the picture. The subchondral trabeculae to the left have almost completely disappeared and there is active osteoclasis spreading to involve the normal sized trabeculae on the right. × 45.

thin bones, vertebral collapse and a tendency to fracture and there is controversy as to whether these patients suffer from a pathological process as distinct from a "normal" loss of bone with ageing. It is known that skeletal mass decreases after the age of 35 in both men and women, probably as a result of increased bone resorption. There is evidence to suggest that the average amount and rate of skeletal loss is the same in everybody. It thus appears that elderly people with thin bones and a tendency to fracture have probably neither lost more bone than normal nor have they lost it more quickly than normal. Those who have the thinnest bones in their age group probably had the thinnest bones during young adult life. While it is certainly true that the group with a propensity to fracture tend to have thinner than average bones for their age

group there are others with bones as thin or thinner, who do not suffer fractures. Neither oestrogens nor calcium supplements in the diet appear capable of increasing the amount of bone in elderly patients' skeletons though they may give some symptomatic improvement.

The structural changes associated with thin bones, whether they arise in association with known endocrine disorders or with ageing, are essentially the same. Vertebral changes (Fig. 22.24) may be particularly striking with bulging of the intervertebral disc through the weakened end plate (Schmorl's nodes), increased concavity of the vertebrae (codfish vertebrae), collapse with wedging, or less commonly equal flattening (vertebra plana). These changes give rise to a decrease in stature, development of a thoracic hump or lumbar lordosis and the compression fractures are frequently accompanied by pain.

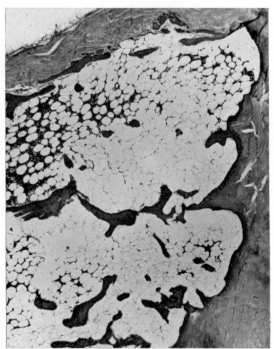

FIG. 22.24.—Osteoporosis of a vertebral body in Cushing's syndrome. Note thin bony trabeculae and loss of cortical bone. × 30.
(Cortex at top, disc on right.)

There is also a tendency to fracture of long bones from trivial trauma, especially at the femoral neck, wrist and ankle and for the production of cough fractures in the ribs. The blood calcium and phosphate levels are usually normal. It is essential to exclude, if necessary by bone biopsy, osteomalacia, osteitis fibrosa, myelomatosis or carcinomatosis before attributing radiological decreased vertebral density or collapse to osteoporosis.

Paget's disease of bone (Osteitis deformans)

This condition was first described by Sir James Paget in 1877. It was for many years confused with the osteitis fibrosa of hyperparathyroidism.

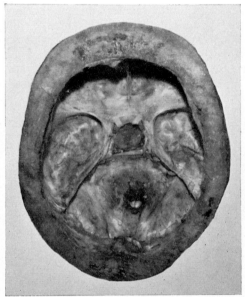

FIG. 22.25.—Paget's disease of the skull, showing enormous thickening of the calvarium. The sella turcica is much enlarged owing to the fortuitous presence of a chromophobe adenoma of the pituitary. × ⅔.

Paget's disease, however, is not thought to be a generalised metabolic disorder but a chronic bone dystrophy of unknown etiology and the blood biochemistry is usually normal apart from a raised alkaline phosphatase level, indicating increased osteoblastic activity. The condition is commoner in males than females and usually appears after the age of 40.

Sites of occurrence. The lumbar vertebrae and sacrum, skull and pelvis are the most frequently affected bones, though limb bones may also be involved. In about 10 per cent of cases a single bone, often a vertebra, or even a part of a bone, is the only area involved. The condition may be widespread but is always multifocal and not diffuse (cf. osteitis fibrosa).

Incidence. Necropsy series show Paget's disease in about 3 per cent of patients over 40 years of age, but in only about a third of these has the disease given rise to symptoms such as bone pain, tenderness, bowing of the lower limbs or increase in skull size.

Macroscopic appearances. In the long bones, the shafts become thickened both subperiosteally and endosteally, so that the bone, as a whole, is enlarged and the medullary cavity is diminished. The femur and the tibia often show forward bowing and the neck of the femur becomes set more nearly at a right angle to the shaft (coxa vara). Cysts and stress fractures may be present. The skull enlarges and the thickness of the calvarium may be three or four times the normal (Fig. 22.25). The distinction between diploë and the tables is gradually lost (Fig. 22.26), and the whole bone becomes fairly uniformly porous and so soft that it may be cut with a knife. (The form of localised rarefaction and softening of the skull known as *osteoporosis circumscripta* is probably a variant of Paget's disease.) Similar less severe changes may be present in the bones of the face. When the vertebrae are involved they tend to collapse anteriorly so that a dorsal kyphus forms and the patient may come to have a crouching attitude.

Microscopic appearances. There is simultaneous and irregular resorption and regeneration of bone with cellular fibrosis and greatly increased vascularity of the intertrabecular marrow. The picture is often, especially in the early stages, one of intense activity, both osteoclasts and osteoblasts being abundant. To begin with, bone resorption is most marked and the bone is lighter than normal with a consequent tendency to fracture and bowing deformities. Later resorption decreases and the trabeculae are often thickened with the formation of a *mosaic pattern* of irregular cement lines indicating numerous previous phases of resorption and reconstruction (Fig. 22.27). At this stage the bone may be heavier than normal but because of the destruction of the cortical Haversian systems it remains structurally weaker.

Complications. (1) The weakened bones are liable to *fracture*, which in the long bones is often transverse and due to stress. There may occasionally be sequelae such as cord compression due either to vertebral collapse which is rare or more often to bony overgrowth narrowing the vertebral canal. Occasionally cranial nerves may be compressed.

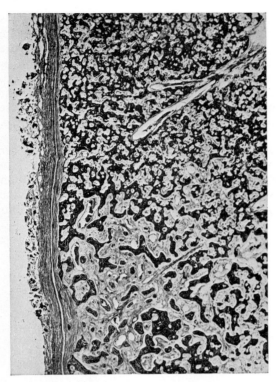

FIG. 22.26.—Paget's disease of the skull, showing loss of distinction between the table and the diploë and the variable density of the bone. The marrow is fibrous and highly vascular. × 7·5.

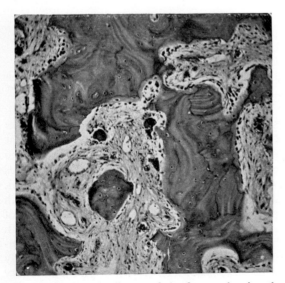

FIG. 22.27.—Paget's disease of the femur, showing the typical mosaic structure of the bone, with both active osteoclastic resorption and osteoblastic formation. (Professor J. B. Gibson.) × 90.

(2) *Osteoarthritis* (p. 796) may result from the bony deformities throwing unusual stress on joints.

(3) *High output cardiac failure* may stem from the greatly increased bone vascularity which leads to some degree of arteriovenous shunt.

(4) *Paget's sarcoma*, sometimes involving multiple bones, occurs in 3 per cent of severe cases. The tumours are almost invariably osteolytic and may be osteosarcomas, fibrosarcomas or occasionally chondrosarcomas, often very pleomorphic and with numerous tumour giant cells. The prognosis is very bad because of early pulmonary metastases. It is interesting that a bone affected with Paget's disease is a common site of *metastatic carcinoma*, probably because of its increased vascularity.

Leontiasis ossea

In this condition, known also as "craniosclerosis", there is a marked enlargement and increase of density of the bones of the skull and face. Swellings occur both subperiosteally and endosteally, the cavities become encroached on and the foramina are narrowed, with resulting pressure on the nerves. The cranium becomes greatly increased in thickness. While some of these cases are clearly the result of chronic osteomyelitis leontiasis ossea may be due to a variety of conditions including Paget's disease, fibrous dysplasia and renal osteodystrophy.

Fibrous dysplasia

Fibrous dysplasia is a benign fibro-osseous abnormality of bone of unknown etiology. It is sometimes monostotic, less commonly polyostotic and rarely the polyostotic form is associated with patchy skin pigmentation and precocious sexual development (*Albright's syndrome*). In monostotic cases the lesions are commonly found in a rib (often symptomless), jaw bone, femur or tibia, though any bone may be involved. In polyostotic cases the femur and tibia are most frequently affected along with various other bones and often the condition is almost but not entirely unilateral. Attention is often drawn to the lesions in childhood and new foci may continue to appear even after puberty. When many bones are affected early in life the condition tends to progress with increasing deformity and multiple fractures. Malignant change to fibrosarcoma is very rare indeed.

Macroscopic appearances. The normal bone is sharply demarcated from the whitish, gritty fibrous tissue, often containing cysts and small nodules of cartilage, which expands the bone. The epiphyses of long bones tend to be spared. The typical focus of fibrous dysplasia shows a ground-glass, finely mottled appearance on X-ray and can sometimes be cut with a knife, but lesions in the skull and jaw tend to be more densely bony and indeed often appear radiologically as areas of increased density.

Microscopic appearances. There is a loose, small spindle-celled fibrous stroma in which curving and lobster-claw trabeculae of non-lamellar woven bone (Fig. 22.28), apparently devoid of osteoblasts, are found irregularly scattered. These trabeculae are characteristic and repeated biopsy has shown that they fail to mature to lamellar bone. Groups of osteoclasts and occasional nodules of cartilage may be present.

Hand–Schüller–Christian disease

This condition, which usually occurs in children, is characterised by the formation of multiple osteolytic lesions, often affecting the skull and consisting of lipid (predominantly cholesterol) filled histiocytes with neutrophil and eosinophil polymorphs, plasma cells and lymphocytes and sometimes small multinucleated cells. As the age of the lesion increases there is a tendency to fibrosis and formation of cholesterol clefts with foreign body giant-cell reaction. Its other features are described on p. 456.

Eosinophil granuloma of bone is usually solitary but sometimes multiple, and affects most often the skull, vertebrae and long bones in children and young adults. The histological picture is that of a granuloma with a preponderance of eosinophils, lipid-containing macrophages and some small multinucleated giant cells. It usually heals but is thought occasionally to progress to a more generalised granulomatosis of the Hand–Schüller–Christian type (see p. 456).

Digital clubbing and hypertrophic osteoarthropathy

Clubbing of the distal phalanges of the fingers and less commonly the toes may be found in association with various chronic lung diseases, e.g. bronchiectasis, fibroid tuberculosis, emphysema, bronchial carcinoma and, more rarely, with other abnormalities such as congenital heart disease and cirrhosis of the liver. The phalanges are widened and thickened, whilst the nails are raised, curved, and often fibrous in texture. The clubbing is the result of thickening and fibrosis of the soft tissues particularly under the nailbed, and is thought to be associated with vascular engorgement. Occasionally there is an increase in subperiosteal bone of the terminal phalanges.

Patients with hypertrophic pulmonary osteoarthropathy develop, in addition to finger clubbing, a periostitis and sometimes also synovitis. Subperiosteal new bone formation starts in the distal thirds of the shafts of the bones of the forearms and lower legs and later

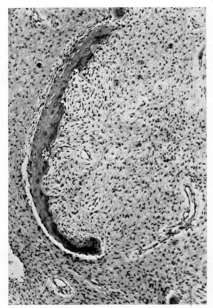

Fig. 22.28.—Fibrous dysplasia of bone. Delicately cellular fibrous tissue containing many thin sheets of woven bone. × 75.

sometimes spreads to involve the remainder of these bones and the femora and humeri. The new bone may be in several distinct layers and eventually leads to much thickening of the cortex without encroaching on the medullary canal. The condition is associated most frequently with pleural mesothelioma, bronchial carcinoma of acinar or squamous pattern, sometimes with metastatic lung tumours, rarely with non-neoplastic lung disease and very infrequently with other disorders. Hypertrophic pulmonary osteoarthropathy may appear early in the course of the pulmonary disease and disappear after surgical resection of the diseased lung. It is thought that a neurovascular reflex mediated through the vagus nerve may be important in the pathogenesis but much remains unknown.

Fluorosis

Low concentrations of fluoride help to prevent dental caries, but excessive amounts may give rise to sclerotic changes in the bones and lesions in the teeth. In *animals* there is hypoplasia of the teeth with mottling of the enamel and the teeth show abnormal wear; the mandible and other bones become thickened by deposition of layers of new periosteal bone so that the bone when macerated shows a chalky irregular porous surface. In *man* dental hypoplasia with mottled enamel is the commonest manifestation and has long been known. In more severe degrees of chronic fluoride intoxication there is much new bone formation by the periosteum and endosteum so that the medullary cavities are narrowed and the bone everywhere is of increased density. Osteophytic outgrowths occur and later extensive calcification of tendons and ligaments, so that the vertebral column becomes fixed and immobile. These changes are found in men exposed over many years to fluoride by inhalation of dust and fumes in industrial processes. They also occur naturally in man and animals in districts where the water supply is very hard and contains fluoride in excessive amounts or where water and soil have been contaminated by recent volcanic eruptions.

Increased radiological density of bones is also seen in osteopetrosis, idiopathic hypercalcaemia and cretinism in infants (p. 889), in certain heavy-metal poisonings (lead, bismuth), and rarely in the skull, vertebrae and hands in chronic uraemia. Bones affected by rickets and osteomalacia may also exhibit increased bone density after healing.

GENERALISED DEVELOPMENTAL ABNORMALITIES OF BONE

Osteopetrosis, marble-bone disease (*Albers-Schönberg*). This disorder is characterised by excessive density of all the bones with obliteration of the marrow cavities and the development of osteosclerotic anaemia. It is associated with failure of resorption of the cartilaginous spongiosa. Involvement of the skull leads to narrowing of the foramina with deafness and impairment of vision. In spite of the increased density the bones are brittle and fractures occur from slight violence. The disease is a hereditary one, and is transmitted in young severely affected patients as an autosomal recessive character and in its relatively benign form as an autosomal dominant.

Osteogenesis imperfecta. Osteogenesis imperfecta is a hereditary disease characterised by generalised osteoporosis with slender bones and increased fragility. The condition may develop during intra-uterine life (*osteogenesis imperfecta congenita*) and is then generally fatal or in later childhood or adult life (*osteogenesis imperfecta tarda*) when the severity varies greatly.

The long bones are thin with narrow, poorly formed cortices. Spontaneous fractures may be numerous and result in short, bowed, deformed bones especially in the lower limbs. Fracture and callus formation may occur *in utero*. Fractures usually heal without trouble but pseudarthrosis sometimes occurs and occasionally callus is very hyperplastic, forming tumour-like masses which may be difficult to distinguish microscopically from osteosarcoma. Severe spinal *osteoporosis* may give rise to markedly biconcave ("codfish") vertebral bodies, to collapse or to scoliosis. Narrowing of the pelvic outlet may occur. Membrane bones are also poorly formed. The skull is thin, bulging, particularly over the ears and with a mosaic pattern due to numerous Wormian bones. It forms little protection to the brain during birth and many affected infants die of intracranial haemorrhage.

Microscopically in bones formed by endochondral ossification there seems to be no defect in the epiphyseal cartilage and invasion of regularly arranged cartilage columns by capillaries is normal but little bone is laid down (Fig. 22.29) probably due to a functional abnormality in the osteoblasts. The bone which is formed, whether by endochondral or membranous ossification, consists of a spongy, open network of small delicate trabeculae with little production of cortical bone. The bone is thought to show abnormalities of both mineral distribution and fibre pattern with failure of maturation to lamellar bone. There seems to be a generalised defect in collagen formation beyond the stage of reticulin-like fibres and this may cause other associated abnormalities. The sclerae appear blue because they are so thin that the pigmented choroid shines through and the dentine of the teeth may be poorly formed. Herniae, thin translucent skin and joint hypermobility with lax ligaments may also be present. Patients may become deaf due to defective bone conduction.

Osteogenesis imperfecta is usually inherited as an autosomal dominant but it is likely that an autosomal recessive form exists, usually giving rise to the congenital type of disease.

Achondroplasia. This remarkable condition, which is known also as *chondrodystrophia fetalis*, is brought about by failure of endochondral ossification. It is present at birth and may be diagnosed radiologically *in utero*. The head appears large, the forehead

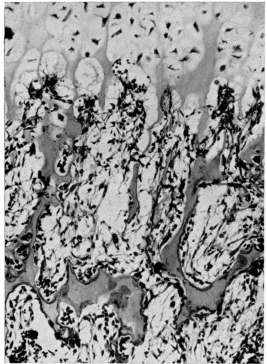

FIG. 22.29.—Osteogenesis imperfecta showing poor formation of bone at the epiphyseal line. × 115.

studies have been few it appears that the characteristic changes depend on the failure of the process of bone formation in cartilage. At the epiphyseal line, the cartilage cells form only short rows, or are irregularly arranged, and there is only a little or no ossification, hence the failure of growth. The cartilaginous epiphysis is sometimes considerably broadened, and with the small shaft presents a mushroom-like appearance; there may be also areas of softening in the cartilage. The indrawing of the nose results from a shortening of the base of the skull, and this also is due to imperfect ossification, which is sometimes accompanied by premature union of the basi-sphenoidal and sphenoidal sutures. In fact, all the bones ossified from cartilage are small, whilst intramembranous ossification proceeds normally. There are varying degrees of the condition, and 80 per cent of affected children die within the first year of life usually of neurological complications such as hydrocephalus due to undue smallness of the skull base and posterior fossa. The less severely affected child may survive to adult life as a dwarf with short thick limbs, but with no other important change. Achondroplasia is due to a dominant gene with a very high mutation rate; thus most cases are the result of a mutation in one or other parent, whose chance of producing a second affected child is no greater than that of other normal persons. Achondroplastic dwarfs who survive to adult life may produce normal and affected children in equal numbers when mated with normal persons.

bulging and the root of the nose is indrawn or sunken; the limbs are short and stumpy, sometimes curved, and as there is more growth of the soft tissues than of the bones, the skin of the limbs is in folds. Obesity is common, and sometimes there is some oedema. The hands are broad with fingers of equal length (trident hands). While pathological

Multiple osteocartilaginous exostoses (*diaphyseal aclasis*) and **multiple enchondromatosis** (*Ollier's disease*) are discussed with benign cartilage tumours (pp. 780, 781).

TUMOURS IN BONE

Metastatic tumours in bone

Frequency. Metastatic tumours in bone are commoner than primary bone tumours and probably occur in as many as 70 per cent of cases of disseminated malignant disease. Bone, along with lungs and liver, is the most frequent site of secondary spread. An accurate assessment of frequency depends on meticulous post-mortem study. The true incidence of vertebral secondaries, for instance, is higher than suspected from radiological examination, as about one-third of the thickness of a vertebra must be destroyed before any change is evident radiologically.

Sites of occurrence. If metastases are present anywhere in the skeleton the vertebral column will almost certainly be affected, especially the thoracic or lumbar regions. Bony secondaries are commonly found in areas where haemopoietic marrow is normally present, i.e. the axial skeleton and the proximal ends of humerus and femur. Skeletal metastases are uncommon below the knee and very uncommon below the elbow. Tumour usually reaches the bone by arterial emboli but it has been suggested that retrograde spread along the vertebral venous plexus may account for the frequent involvement of lumbar vertebrae by tumours of the pelvic organs.

Common primary sites. Tumours which most often give rise to secondaries in bone are carcinomas of breast, prostate, lung, thyroid, kidney, melanomas and in young children neuro-blastomas.

Types of secondary tumours. Bone secondaries are commonly *osteolytic* or destructive, the bone trabeculae being resorbed and pathological fracture often resulting. If the destruction is widespread there may be hypercalcaemia.

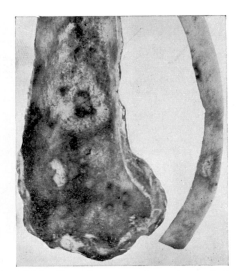

Fig. 22.30.—Secondary prostatic carcinoma in lower end of femur and rib.

The section of rib shows that the medulla has been replaced by dense sclerotic bone; the femur contains similar irregular small areas.

Sometimes infiltration of the marrow by carcinoma stimulates marked laying down of new bone by osteoblasts, a process similar to the stimulation of collagen production in a breast carcinoma. In these patients especially the serum alkaline phosphatase may be raised due to the increased osteoblastic activity. These *osteoplastic or osteosclerotic* secondaries arise most commonly in association with prostatic carcinoma (Fig. 22.30) but carcinoma of breast, lung, stomach and various other sites may infrequently give rise to the same picture. Sometimes both osteosclerotic and osteolytic secondaries are present in the same patient. Where much of the bone marrow is encroached on by new bone formation (Fig. 22.31), osteosclerotic anaemia may result. This is often leuko-erythroblastic and is associated with splenomegaly due to myeloid transformation (p. 430).

Occasionally there is widespread diffuse marrow replacement with little bony change.

Solitary secondaries. Metastatic tumours in bone sometimes present as solitary lesions and,

while this is usually rapidly followed by the appearance of further secondaries, in a very occasional case of renal or thyroid carcinoma, the bony focus may remain the sole metastasis. Only very rarely is surgical resection of both primary and secondary followed by worthwhile remission or by cure.

Primary tumours of bone

The precise diagnosis of certain bone tumours is so difficult that it is essential for the clinical and radiological features to be considered along with the naked-eye and microscopic appearances before a final decision is reached. Classification also is not easy, for in some the histogenesis is obscure and in others the very nature of the lesion is uncertain (see Table on p. 776).

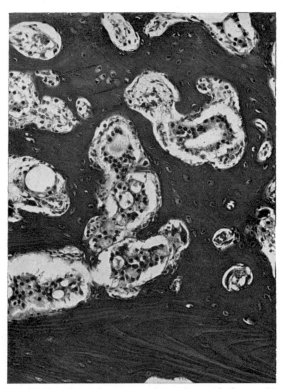

Fig. 22.31.—Secondary prostatic carcinoma in bone with reactive new bone formation causing osteosclerosis. × 130.

Classification. *Firstly*, it may be difficult to decide whether one is dealing with a true tumour or a developmental abnormality, e.g. multiple osteocartilaginous exostoses is clearly a hereditary condition and possibly solitary exostosis is

CLASSIFICATION OF BONE TUMOURS

Derivation or type of tumour	Benign	Malignant
Fibrous tissue	Non-ossifying fibroma Desmoplastic fibroma	Fibrosarcoma
Cartilage	Osteocartilaginous exostosis ⟶ Enchondroma ⟶ Benign chondroblastoma Chondromyxoid fibroma	Chondrosarcoma
Bone	Osteoma Osteoid osteoma Benign osteoblastoma	Osteosarcoma (including some Paget's and post-irradiation sarcomas) Parosteal osteosarcoma
Unknown	Giant-cell tumour ⟶	Giant-cell tumour
Vascular tissue	Haemangioma Glomus tumour	Haemangioendothelioma Angiosarcoma
Fat cells	Lipoma	Liposarcoma
Plasma cell precursors	Solitary plasmacytoma ⟶	Myelomatosis
Marrow stroma		Reticulum cell sarcoma "Ewing's tumour"
Neural tissue	Schwannoma Neurofibromatosis ⟶ Ganglioneuroma	Neurofibrosarcoma
Notochordal tissue		Chordoma

The arrows indicate that the benign lesions may progress to malignancy

a *forme fruste* of this, but, since exostoses, whether single or multiple, may progress to malignancy, they are discussed in this section. Similarly, non-ossifying fibroma may or may not arise from a metaphyseal fibrous defect. *Secondly*, in many cases, although the tumour has a distinctive histological appearance, its histogenesis is uncertain; even osteosarcoma is best regarded as a tumour which produces bone or osteoid rather than one which arises from osteoblasts. The number of malignant mesenchymal tissues which may be found in an osteosarcoma points to its origin from a more primitive cell and serves as a reminder that the mesenchymal cell is capable of differentiation in different directions. In spite of these difficulties a classification is worthwhile because when it can be applied to a given tumour it allows a useful prediction of its behaviour.

In this section certain lesions are not discussed but they have been included in the table for the sake of completeness. Lesions of doubtful origin and non-neoplastic lesions simulating bone tumours have been mentioned in relation to the tumours with which they may be confused.

Osteoma

The term "osteoma" is now almost entirely restricted to bony outgrowths of skull bones which sometimes protrude into the orbit or paranasal sinuses. These lesions may be formed of osteoblastic connective tissue and spongy bone trabeculae or of extremely dense compact bone or a mixture of these components. They are benign but may cause pressure symptoms.

Osteoid osteoma

This is a benign osteoblastic lesion which is usually less than 1 cm. in diameter. It occurs chiefly in the long bones of the lower limbs of adolescents or young adults although any bone and age may be affected. The clinical history is of increasingly severe and unusually well-localised pain and tenderness, the pain often relieved by salicylates. Radiology shows the lesion itself as a rounded zone of radiolucency. If cortical, there is often massive sclerosis of adjacent bone whereas in cancellous bone sclerosis may be minimal. Macroscopically the osteoid osteoma is usually red and cherry-like and microscopic examination shows a very vascular nidus of osteoblastic tissue with a disorderly mass of irregular small trabeculae of osteoid or bone undergoing active remodelling (Figs. 22.32, 22.33). Sometimes the central part of the nidus is more solid. If incompletely removed, symptoms may recur.

Osteosarcoma (osteogenic sarcoma)

Osteosarcoma is a malignant tumour in which osteoid or bone is formed directly by sarcoma cells and is thought to arise from cells of the primitive bone-forming mesenchyme. It is probably the commonest primary malignant bone tumour and occurs more frequently in males than females.

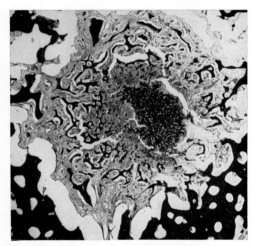

FIG. 22.32.—Osteoid osteoma, showing the characteristic central focus with trabecular bone in radiate arrangement, the whole surrounded by sclerotic reactive bone. × 12.

Age incidence. Osteosarcoma is rare under the age of 5 years and about 75 per cent of patients are between 10 and 25 years old. In older patients the tumour is often associated with Paget's disease of bone.

Sites of occurrence. The commonest site of osteosarcoma is in the metaphysis of long bones and about half the cases occur around the knee but also frequently at the upper end of femur and humerus. It is sometimes found in vertebrae,

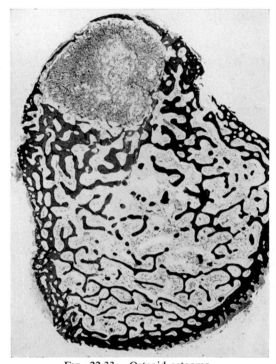

FIG. 22.33.—Osteoid osteoma.
A transverse section of the fibula shows a lesion in the cortical bone with only slight surrounding sclerosis. × 6.

pelvis and skull, especially when associated with Paget's disease. Osteosarcoma is very uncommon in the small bones of the hands and feet. Multicentric tumours are occasionally reported usually in association with Paget's disease.

Clinical features. Patients often give a fairly short history of increasingly severe pain, worse at night, and this may be followed by swelling, oedema, increase in local heat and dilated subcutaneous veins. Pathological fracture is relatively rare. The patients are usually in good general health; if they are not the presence of metastases should be suspected.

Radiological and macroscopic appearances. Osteosarcoma usually arises in the medullary bone in the region of the metaphysis or diaphysis. The epiphyseal cartilage plate may act as a barrier for a while but when this is perforated, the tumour spreads to the epiphysis. The joint cavity is seldom involved. Osteosarcoma may spread quite rapidly through the bony cortex without either perforating or markedly expanding it and form a subperiosteal mass (Fig. 22.34) which, in its turn, may burst through the periosteum and infiltrate muscles. When the peri-

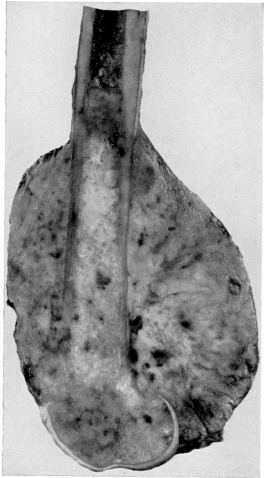

FIG. 22.34.—Osteosarcoma of lower end of femur. The medullary tumour has permeated and partly destroyed the cortex, spreading outwards to form a large subperiosteal mass.

osteum is raised spicules of new bone are laid down at right angles to the bone shaft (Fig. 22.35) giving rise radiologically to sunray spiculation. At the junction between raised and normal periosteum, Codman's triangle of reactive bone develops. Neither of these appearances is present in all cases of osteosarcoma, nor when present are they specific signs of osteosarcoma; the same appearances may be seen in metastatic carcinoma or even sometimes in infections. Biopsy material should not be

taken from an area where reactive bone formation is active as this may greatly increase the difficulty of diagnosis. Apart from spread outside the bone there may be medullary extension of the tumour and this is sometimes greater than is suspected radiologically. The gross appearances of the tumour vary according to the amount of tumour osteoid and bone which has been formed. Some tumours contain little bony matrix (*osteolytic*) and these tend to be soft, friable, vascular destructive lesions with areas of haemorrhage and necrosis. Others may contain much tumour bone (*osteosclerotic*)

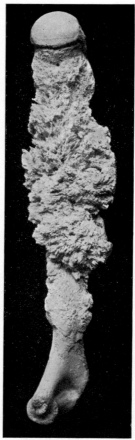

FIG. 22.35.—Osteosarcoma of humerus. Macerated specimen to show the characteristic spiculation on the surface of the bone.

especially in their central areas, and are dense and of turnip-like consistence in their soft parts. The amount of ossification is not related to the age of the tumour nor does it appear to affect the prognosis.

Microscopic appearances. Though the essential criteria for the diagnosis of osteosarcoma are the presence of a frankly sarcomatous stroma and the direct formation of tumour osteoid or bone from this malignant connective tissue, the histological pattern of osteosarcoma is very variable. In addition to tumour bone, some osteosarcomas contain a large amount of cartilage

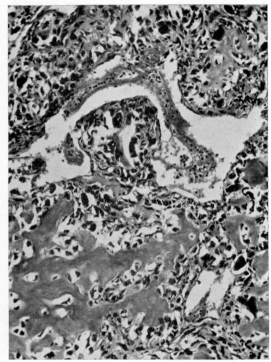

FIG. 22.36.—Osteosarcoma. A highly vascular, cellular tumour with osteoid formation. × 200.

and others much malignant spindle-celled tissue of fibrosarcomatous type. In the osteolytic type of osteosarcoma the bulk of the tumour is often made up of pleomorphic and giant tumour cells with many aberrant mitoses and irregular vascular channels lined by tumour cells (Fig. 22.36). In the osteosclerotic type, on the other hand, such a mass of tumour bone may be laid down on and between pre-existing trabeculae that malignant cells between the matrix are small and scanty except at the growing edge. Osteosarcomas in Paget's disease are almost invariably of the osteolytic type (Fig. 22.37) and are characterised by their extreme pleomorphism and by large numbers of tumour giant cells.

Metastatic spread. As in most sarcomas spread of the tumour is almost invariably by the bloodstream to the lungs and sometimes to

other bones and viscera, lymph node metastases being rare. Pulmonary metastases occur early and are often thought to have arisen before the patient appears for treatment although at that time they may not be visible radiologically. The prognosis in osteosarcoma is therefore poor and a five-year survival rate of only 5–20 per cent is reported. In some series the outlook is better in tumours of the distal skeleton. Osteosarcomas arising in Paget's disease may be multicentric and have an even worse prognosis than those arising in normal bone. Local recurrence or seeding of the tumour in the wound is unusual, in contrast with chondrosarcoma (p. 782).

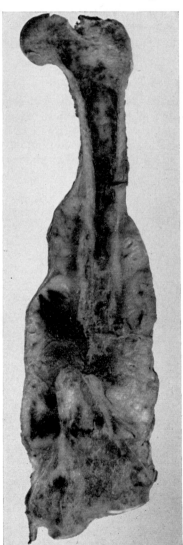

FIG. 22.37.—Paget's disease of femur showing osteolytic sarcoma with pathological fracture.

Parosteal (juxtacortical) osteosarcoma. This is a rare tumour but worth distinguishing since it has a much better prognosis than medullary osteosarcoma. In most of the reported cases the tumour has arisen at the metaphysis of the lower end of femur, tibia or humerus. It forms a broad-based swelling arising initially on the surface of the bone and sometimes coming to encircle the shaft, cortical penetration and medullary infiltration being late. Microscopically the tumour usually consists of well-formed bony trabeculae separated by atypical spindle cells; sometimes near the surface the bone is less well formed and there may also be islands of cartilage. The tumour grows slowly and tends to occur in a wider age group than osteosarcoma. If the lesion is inadequately dealt with it may recur or become frankly malignant and metastasise, sometimes within two years, sometimes not for 20 years. If it is treated by radical surgery initially the outlook is usually good.

Benign cartilage tumours

Osteocartilaginous exostosis (osteochondroma, ecchondroma) is the commonest benign tumour of bone and consists of a bony excrescence. Its outer shell and medulla are continuous with that of the bone from which it arises and it is covered

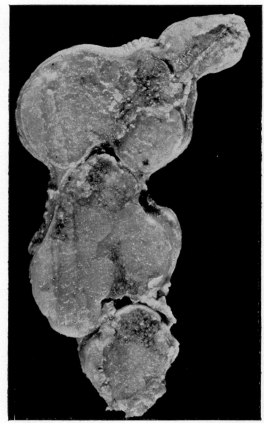

FIG. 22.39.—Benign enchondromas of finger. The finger has been amputated just proximal to the metacarpal head. While the joint spaces remain intact each phalanx is replaced by a mass of hyaline cartilage. The cortices have disappeared but periosteum still surrounds the cartilage.

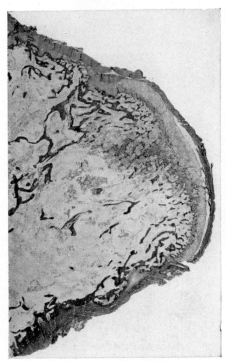

FIG. 22.38.—Osteocartilaginous exostosis of humerus consisting of cancellous bone covered by cartilage and perichondrium. Endochondral ossification is occurring. × 7.

by a cartilage cap from the undersurface of which endochondral ossification occurs (Fig. 22.38). The lesion may be single or multiple; when multiple the condition is familial and may be associated with some failure of bone remodelling (*hereditary multiple exostoses, diaphyseal aclasis*). Exostoses may arise in any bone formed by endochondral ossification but the metaphyses of long bones, especially the femur, humerus and tibia, are the commonest sites. The lesions are usually first noticed in childhood and adolescence and growth commonly ceases in adult life, the cartilaginous cap sometimes completely disappearing. Malignant change is rare in solitary exostoses but between 10–20 per cent of patients with multiple lesions develop chondrosarcoma, usually in adult life. Exostoses of the axial skeleton or proximal limb bones are much more likely to become malignant than those in the peripheral skeleton (see chondrosarcoma for discussion). So-called *subungual exostosis* is not an exactly comparable lesion. It arises as a cartilage-capped outgrowth of the terminal part of a distal phalanx, often of the great toe, and gives rise to pain.

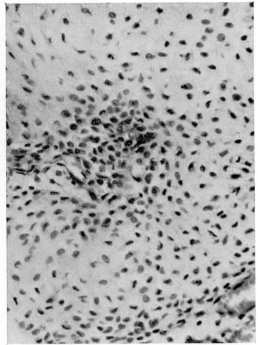

FIG. 22.40.—Benign enchondroma from finger in multiple enchondromatosis. The cartilage is highly cellular but the cells are mononuclear and fairly uniform in size. × 250.

Enchondroma is a benign cartilage tumour arising within the medullary cavity most commonly of the small bones of the hands and feet (Fig. 22.39). The cartilage tumours may be single or multiple and when multiple are thought to arise as a failure of normal endochondral ossification (*multiple enchondromatosis*). In multiple enchondromatosis the hands are almost invariably involved but there may also be lesions in long tubular bones associated with bowing and deformity, especially of the forearm. When the enchondromas are predominantly unilateral the condition is sometimes referred to as *Ollier's disease*. Solitary benign enchondroma may also be found in long tubular bones, particularly the humerus and femur. The tumour arises initially in the metaphysis and may spread into the shaft or occasionally into the epiphysis if the cartilage plate is fused. Radiologically the lesions are radiolucent, sometimes with spotty calcification and naked-eye examination of an enchondroma shows the usual appearance of cartilage though often more gelatinous than normal. Microscopic examination of the benign lesion shows small uniform cells with small and few double nuclei (Fig. 22.40). The lesions of the phalanges and metacarpals, especially in multiple enchondromas, may be unusually cellular without there being any sinister prognostic significance. The common clinical complaints, particularly in the phalangeal lesions, are of swelling or pathological fracture. Malignant transformation in cases of solitary enchondroma is probably rare but the risk is appreciable in patients with multiple enchondromatosis, some authors giving figures as high as 50 per cent. Pain unassociated with fracture, or the onset of enlargement in an enchondroma of the axial skeleton or long tubular bones in an adult, should immediately raise the suspicion of malignant change.

Chondrosarcoma

Chondrosarcoma is a malignant cartilage tumour and may arise *de novo* or from a pre-existing benign cartilage tumour. It may be situated within the bone (central) or outwith it (peripheral). The tumour is, in our experience, only slightly less common than osteosarcoma and is twice as common in males as in females. In contrast to osteosarcoma, which may contain a substantial cartilage component, true chondrosarcoma is rare under the age of 30 years and most cases are in the 40–70 age group.

Sites of occurrence. About half the lesions arise in the pelvic girdle (Fig. 22.42) and ribs; the proximal femur is another common site. A careful watch, therefore, should be kept on cartilage tumours of the axial skeleton, particularly in adults and increase in size and pain should arouse the suspicion of malignancy. The incidence of malignant change decreases in the distal part of the skeleton and is very rare in the bones of the hands and feet except for the os calcis and talus.

Macroscopic appearances. *Central tumours.* A central cartilage tumour usually causes bone expansion and in slowly growing tumours there is often buttressing of the cortex in response to endosteal erosion. Not uncommonly, however, the cortex is broken through and the tumour is found growing in the adjacent soft tissue. Sometimes, especially in large tumours which are especially prone to arise in pelvis and ribs, the exact site of origin becomes difficult to identify and the lobulated tumour is

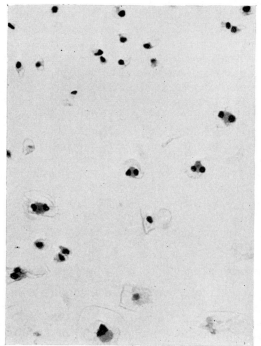

FIG. 22.41.—This recurrent low grade chondrosarcoma killed the patient by local spread without metastases. The cartilage matrix is well formed and the tumour is not very cellular but there are numerous foci of chondrocytes with double nuclei. × 250.

soft, slimy and cystic due to mucoid degeneration of the matrix. Spotty calcification may be present and sometimes is extensive, an aid in the radiological diagnosis of these tumours.

Peripheral tumours may arise *de novo* or from previously existing osteocartilaginous exostoses; the cartilage caps are then much thickened and in the early stages the normally smooth surface may be covered with little nodules of proliferating cartilage. Later these tumours may become very large and undergo heavy calcification or myxoid degeneration.

Microscopic appearances. Chondrosarcoma has been more consistently under-diagnosed by pathologists than almost any other tumour. If the cells in a cartilage tumour are pleomorphic with vesicular nuclei and there are abundant multinucleated tumour cells and moderate numbers of mitotic figures, the recognition of malignancy is easy (Fig. 22.43). In slowly growing

tumours, however, it may be difficult and the indications of malignancy are given by only very subtle changes from the normal, by increase in plumpness of nuclei, by increase in the number of binucleate cells and the occasional presence of a multinucleated cartilage cell (Fig. 22.41). The absence of mitotic figures does not necessarily indicate that the tumour is benign. The best opportunity of arriving at a correct assessment of the tumour's potentialities is in studying material from the growing edge and every scrap of biopsy tissue must be examined microscopically. Biopsies from heavily calcified or degenerate cartilage are useless. Because of variations in histological malignancy in different parts of the same tumour a microscopic diagnosis of chondroma should be viewed with suspicion if clinical and radiological features suggest malignant change. It is particularly important in this tumour that the pathologist should be aware of the *age* of the

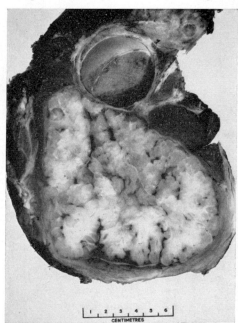

FIG. 22.42.—Low-grade chondrosarcoma of pelvis showing the large cartilaginous tumour destroying the ilium.

patient and the *site* of the tumour. Minor changes from normality which would be alarming in cartilage tumours of the axial skeleton may be, from experience, discounted to a large extent in growing cartilage tumours in children and often in lesions of the small tubular bones of the hands and feet.

Implantation. Cartilage cells have low biologic requirements and probably because of this these tumours have a special tendency to implantation and growth in soft tissues. This has great practical importance to the surgeon as it means that the site of biopsy must be carefully planned in a

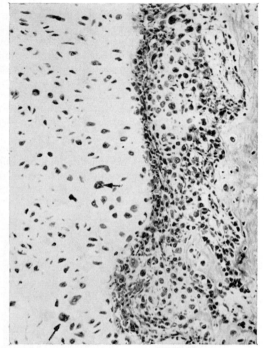

FIG. 22.43.—Metastasising chondrosarcoma of ilium. The cartilage cells vary greatly in size and there are several mitoses, two of which are arrowed. × 100.

suspected case so that the whole of the tissue planes opened up may be excised at the time of definitive treatment. This characteristic also results in a very marked tendency to local recurrence after excision even when the original operation appeared to be clear of the tumour. In order to prevent this in areas where eradication of a recurrent tumour would be difficult such as chest wall or pelvis, a radical operation is often necessary in the first instance.

Course of the disease and prognosis. Chondrosarcoma runs, in contrast to osteosarcoma, a more prolonged course. The patients have often some years' history when they first come to hospital. The slowly growing tumours may continue with repeated local recurrences for more than twenty years before the patient is finally killed by involvement of some vital structure from local spread rather than by pulmonary metastases. These are the tumours which respond most successfully to radical treatment in

the first instance where this is surgically feasible. More malignant rapidly-growing and metastasising chondrosarcomas may lead to death within a few years but even they may persist for a surprisingly long time. We have seen one patient who survived six years after the development of pulmonary metastases. In adolescence primary chondrosarcomas are rare and usually rapidly fatal. Chondrosarcoma metastasises by blood spread, frequently to the lungs and has a tendency to direct retrograde spread along veins. Lymph node metastases are rare. In the past the prognosis has been poor partly as a result of the pathologist's under-diagnosis of the lesion and partly from inadequate initial treatment.

A better prognosis can be anticipated in the light of a fuller understanding of the clinical and pathological features of this tumour.

Chondromyxoid fibroma of bone

This is a rare benign tumour of bone important only because of its tendency to be misdiagnosed as chondrosarcoma. It occurs chiefly in the metaphyses of long bones of adolescents or young adults especially in the lower limb. It usually gives rise to a sharply defined, eccentric, osteolytic defect which bulges the periosteum. The tumour is commonly rather firm and rubbery and lacks on naked-eye examination the gelatinous, slimy features that one would expect from the histology. Microscopy shows relatively poorly cellular tissue separated into pseudo-lobules by curving strands or trabeculae of aggregated cells (Fig. 22.44). The cells of the lobules are spindle-shaped or stellate and lie in a myxomatous vacuolated matrix. The trabecular cells are similar but may show some hyperchromatism, pleomorphism and occasional mitotic figures—features which may lead to misdiagnosis of malignancy. Small multinucleated giant cells may also be seen. Sometimes the tumour becomes collagenised, areas more like hyaline cartilage appear and there is a tendency to lose the lobular pattern. The tumour is benign, and though it may recur, usually responds to simple curettage.

Fibrosarcoma

This is a rare malignant tumour which may arise within the medullary cavity (endosteal) or beneath the periosteum (periosteal), usually in adults. Endosteal fibrosarcoma, though other sites are not exempt, affects especially the bones around the knee joint and in long bones commonly involves the metaphysis and sometimes the shaft. While the tumour in general is osteolytic, destructive and may break through the cortex and into the soft tissues, it tends, in some places at least, to infiltrate between pre-existing medullary bone trabeculae without destroying them. This gives rise radiologically to a peculiarly

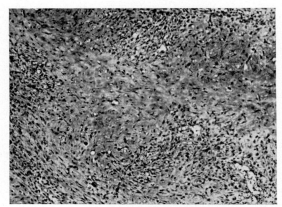

FIG. 22.44.—Chondromyxoid fibroma of bone, showing the loose spindle-celled tissue with imperfectly formed cartilage. × 60.

moth-eaten appearance of the bone and because of it the extent of radiological destruction may not indicate the true extent of tumour spread in the medulla. Microscopically fibrosarcoma varies from a fasciculated spindle-celled tumour producing collagen in its more mature parts, to a highly pleomorphic tumour with little recognisable fibrous tissue. Such variations when present in the same tumour can be misleading.

In general it is stated that the degree of differentiation is a good indication of the prognosis, that tumours producing much collagen tend to recur locally and be late in metastasising while pleomorphic tumours metastasise early. In our experience this is true of periosteal tumours but endosteal fibrosarcomas have a poor prognosis regardless of their histological type. Multiple bones may be involved when the patient is first examined.

Ewing's tumour

In 1921 Ewing described a tumour of bone under the name of diffuse endothelioma and while the endothelial origin has not been accepted there is little doubt that this is a specific variety of tumour. The histogenesis remains unknown and accordingly we prefer to retain the eponymous title.

Age and sex incidence. Ewing's tumour occurs chiefly in young persons, it is rare over the age of 30, and most common between the ages of 5 and 20 years; it is very rare in the first two years of life. Males are slightly more often affected.

Sites of occurrence. The long tubular bones are most frequently involved, e.g. femur, tibia, humerus and fibula but the pelvis and ribs are also affected.

Naked-eye appearances. The tumour appears to originate within the medullary cavity and in long bones may involve the metaphysis and shaft. It is usually osteolytic and perforation of the cortex with raising of the periosteum may occur early. This subperiosteal elevation may give rise to parallel layers of reactive new bone (onion skin appearance) and less frequently to strands of bone forming at right angles to the cortex (sunray spiculation).

The tumour is usually whitish; some may be rather firm while others are very soft, almost puriform. It is not of very rapid growth, as compared with many other tumours of childhood.

Microscopic appearances. Ewing's tumour is composed of fairly uniform rounded, or polyhedral cells, often with pale nuclei due to the fine dispersion of chromatin. The cell boundaries are indistinct and the cells are arranged in syncytial sheets (Fig. 22.45)

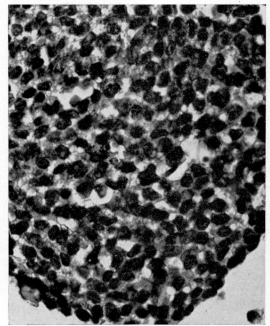

FIG. 22.45.—Ewing's tumour of femur showing syncytial structure and uniform cell type. × 450.

without a lobular pattern but divided by broad strands of collagen. Reticulin is scanty and there is often much necrosis. Intracellular glycogen may be demonstrated. Here and there the cells may be arranged in clusters resembling rosettes but without clearly defined central fibrils. This very inconstant feature is probably the result of degeneration.

Clinical features. Ewing's tumour usually presents with pain and swelling often of some months' duration. Sometimes fever, anaemia and leukocytosis suggest low-grade osteomyelitis and the patients with these systemic symptoms have the worst prognosis. The tumour is at first radiosensitive, but frequently later recurrence takes place and secondaries appear in other bones, especially the skull, and in the lungs. The liver is less often involved and lymph nodes only rarely.

Differential diagnosis. Willis has pointed out that many alleged examples of Ewing's tumour are metastases from an unrevealed neuroblastoma of the adrenal or elsewhere. There is no doubt that this differential diagnosis must be made but the absence of cases in the first two years of life and the paucity of lymph-node and hepatic metastases are features different from those of neuroblastoma. The increased urinary excretion of vanillin mandelic acid, homovanillic acid and other catecholamine derivatives in many cases of neuroblastoma and their normal values in patients with Ewing's tumour helps to distinguish between these tumours. The lack of clearly distinctive histological features sometimes requires the consideration of leukaemic deposits, lymphoid neoplasms, myelomatosis and secondary carcinoma in the differential diagnosis and occasionally the true diagnosis only becomes apparent at necropsy.

While some pathologists have ascribed the origin of Ewing's tumour to the reticulum cells of the bone marrow and do not distinguish between primary reticulum-cell sarcoma of bone and Ewing's tumour, others do not accept this view.

Reticulum-cell sarcoma

Bone, in contrast to lymph nodes and other parts, is a relatively uncommon site of primary reticulum-cell sarcoma but its true incidence is uncertain because of the difficulty in diagnosis of malignant round cell tumours of bone.

Age and sex incidence, and sites. Reticulum-cell sarcoma is encountered chiefly in adult life, with fewer examples in childhood or early adolescence than Ewing's tumour. It is twice as common in males and affects both the metaphysis and the shaft of long bones; flat bones and the axial skeleton may be involved.

Clinical features. Reticulum-cell sarcoma of bone presents with pain and swelling but fever is rare. X-ray often shows a fairly widespread, diffuse, moth-eaten area of patchy rarefaction. Periosteal new bone formation is not usually conspicuous but there may be patchy reactive bone sclerosis in the medulla. The radiological appearances may suggest a chronic osteomyelitis and in small biopsies with much necrosis and secondary inflammatory cell infiltrate considerable difficulty may also arise in making this histological differentiation. The tumour is radio-

sensitive, the bone after treatment often becoming somewhat sclerosed. The prognosis after radio-therapy or amputation is distinctly more favourable than that in Ewing's tumour, one to two-thirds of cases are said to survive for five years. Involvement of regional lymph nodes may occur early or late and may be followed by more extensive infiltration in spleen, liver and lungs. Occasionally leukaemia develops.

Macroscopic appearances. The sarcoma tends to affect chiefly the metaphyseal region and adjacent shaft, and it is osteolytic so that the bony cortex becomes mottled and rarefied. The tumour penetrates the cortex usually without eliciting any new reactive periosteal bone, and spreads into the adjacent tissues.

Microscopic appearances. The tumour is composed of round or polyhedral cells often discretely arranged and with large round, oval or reniform nuclei. Between the cells there is sometimes a rich reticulin network, a feature conspicuously absent in Ewing's tumour. Intracellular glycogen is usually absent.

We believe that reticulum-cell sarcoma is probably a condition different from Ewing's tumour but the distinction may be difficult or even impossible on the initial, often inadequate, biopsy. When, however, a group of such cases is surveyed retrospectively with the clinical course, radiological and pathological features fully available, it seems that they can often be separated into the two categories.

Giant-cell tumour of bone (osteoclastoma)

Giant-cell tumour is an osteolytic, eccentrically placed tumour arising most commonly in the end of a long bone of an adult.

Age. The lesion frequently arises in the 20–40 age group. The diagnosis should be regarded with suspicion under the age of 15 as there are several benign lesions in children and adolescents which to some extent simulate giant-cell tumour. Some of these are discussed below.

Site of occurrence. Half of all the tumours occur at the knee (Fig. 22.46), in the lower end of femur or upper tibia. The upper end of femur and the lower end of radius are other common sites. Although flat bones may be involved giant-cell tumour is rare in the jaw and in the vertebral column. When giant-cell tumour occurs in a long bone it arises almost invariably in the bone end and the metaphysis is involved only later. Because of this situation symptoms tend to be referable to the joint.

Macroscopic appearances. Giant-cell tumour

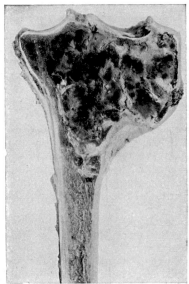

FIG. 22.46.—Section of giant-cell tumour of upper end of tibia showing eccentric expansion of the bone end and much haemorrhage within the tumour.

is usually located eccentrically in the epiphysis and often causes marked expansion of the bone end (Fig. 22.46). It is covered, at least initially, by a thin shell of newly-formed subperiosteal bone (Fig. 22.47) which may be renewed on the surface as expansion goes on but through which it may later break into the soft tissues. Invasion of the joint through the articular cartilage is uncommon. The tumour is entirely destructive and its cells do not form bone. There is none of the subperiosteal sunray bony spiculation seen in an osteosarcoma. As a result of its osteolytic propensities patients often present with a pathological fracture. The tumour is usually reddish-grey and commonly shows areas of haemorrhage and necrosis. If fracture or previous treatment has taken place the picture may be complicated by callus formation, fibrosis and cystic degeneration.

Microscopic appearances. Giant-cell tumour consists of plump spindle or ovoid mononuclear cells abundantly interspersed with giant cells containing many nuclei, sometimes as many as 100 (Fig. 22.48). Fibrous tissue is usually scanty unless the tumour has previously fractured or been treated. There is virtually no formation of bone or cartilage in the tumour. Areas of necrosis, haemorrhage, lipid-containing macrophages and cholesterol are sometimes seen.

Prognosis. About half the tumours respond to thorough local removal, about a third recur

and the remaining 15–20 per cent are liable to be malignant from the beginning or after recurrence and metastasise to the lungs. The tumour may recur as a fibrosarcoma. Some help in assessing the prognosis is given by the histology in that tumours which look frankly sarcomatous usually behave badly; however very rarely tumours which appear microscopically benign later metastasise.

Lesions likely to be confused with giant-cell tumour

Besides the differentiation of true giant-cell tumour from the benign lesions principally of childhood and adolescence described below, the lesion must be distinguished from brown tumour of hyperparathyroidism (p. 767). Since this may not be possible on histological grounds the blood chemistry should be investigated and a radiological search for subperiosteal erosions made especially if the apparent giant-cell tumour is in the skull or jaw.

Aneurysmal bone cyst. This is probably not a true tumour but has been confused with giant-cell tumour. It is commonest in the long bone *metaphyses* or vertebrae of children or young adults and gives rise to an extremely eccentric osteolytic lesion which may balloon out the periosteum and sometimes involves contiguous bones. On penetrating the thin bony shell the "cyst" is found to consist of cavernous bloodfilled spaces separated by a brownish spongy meshwork of trabeculae. These are formed of vascular fibrous tissue, the larger ones reinforced by osteoid or bony strands. Giant cells are smaller and less evenly distributed than in giant-cell tumour (Fig. 22.49). The lesion is benign and we can vouch for the fact that it is cured by surgery, sometimes

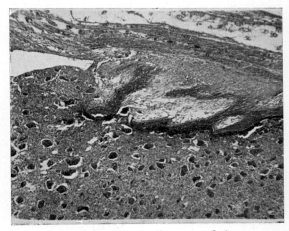

FIG. 22.47.—Giant-cell tumour of ulna.

Note the layer of new-formed periosteal bone on the surface of the giant-cell tumour. × 30.

even when removal has been incomplete. If untreated it may progressively increase in size, but sometimes appears to be self-limiting.

Benign chondroblastoma. This rare benign bone tumour of uncertain histogenesis is important because it may be mistaken for a malignant giant-cell tumour or occasionally a chondro- or osteosarcoma. Benign chondroblastoma occurs most often in adolescents and is usually located in the epiphysis of long bones, especially around the knee or in the upper humerus. Radiologically there is a well-defined radiolucent area sometimes with mottling due to spotty calcification in the tumour. The tumour may spread across the epiphyseal plate into the metaphysis and rarely into the adjacent joint. Microscopically the lesion consists of fairly uniform small rounded or polygonal cells with a moderate sprinkling of multinucleated giant cells. A charac-

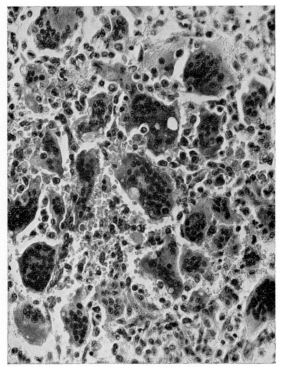

Fig. 22.48.—Giant-cell tumour. The mononuclear tumour cells have the same characteristics as the scattered multinucleated cells. × 240.

teristic lacy pattern of intercellular calcification may be seen and this is thought to be followed by cellular necrosis and later transformation of necrotic areas to plaques of hyaline chondroid or osteoid-like material. The tumour, while liable to recurrence, is benign and curable by curettage.

Non-ossifying fibroma (non-osteogenic fibroma). This doubtfully neoplastic lesion was once thought to be a healing variant of giant-cell tumour. It

CC

sometimes appears to arise from a metaphyseal fibrous defect, a developmental lesion which is readily diagnosable radiologically as a small scalloped radiolucent area with a sclerotic edge hugging the metaphyseal cortex in the long bones, particularly

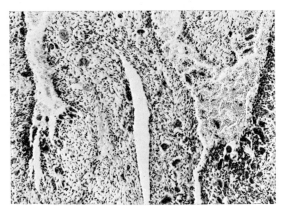

Fig. 22.49.—Aneurysmal bone cyst. Vascular spaces lined by fibrous and osteoid tissue with giant cells. × 54.

the femur, of young children. These developmental abnormalities have the same naked-eye and microscopic appearances as do larger lesions involving the medullary cavity, which are described as non-ossifying fibromas and it seems possible that the larger ones may be derived from the smaller. Macroscopically the tissue is usually bright orange-yellow and microscopically shows whorled fibrous tissue with moderate numbers of small giant cells, haemosiderin and in some cases large zones of lipid-containing macrophages. These lesions, whatever their derivation, are benign and heal after curettage.

Simple bone cyst. This is a benign non-neoplastic unilocular cystic lesion, probably related to some local disturbance of bone growth and commonly arising in the upper humeral or femoral metaphyses in children and adolescents. As the bone grows the cyst appears to migrate down the shaft away from the epiphyseal line. It is commoner in males. Attention is frequently drawn to the lesion by pathological fracture and occasionally, following this, the cyst fills in. The appearances are of a smooth walled cavity containing clear fluid and usually slightly expanding and markedly thinning the cortices. The lining consists of a meagre layer of rather acellular collagen. When fracture has occurred the fluid may be bloody and the lining transformed to a thick layer of granulation or fibrous tissue with areas of haemorrhage, cholesterol clefts, calcification, new bone formation and osteoclast aggregates which sometimes have given rise to confusion with giant-cell tumour. The cysts, while perfectly benign, have a strong tendency to recur, particularly if they are near the epiphyseal plate when initially treated.

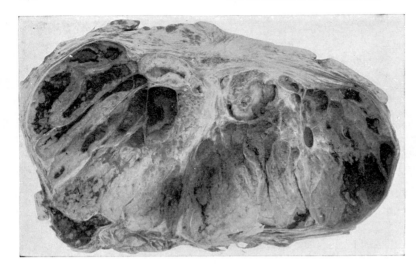

FIG. 22.50.—Section of sacral chordoma.

Note strands and islets of translucent chordal tissue separated by haemorrhagic areas. × ¾.

Chordoma

This tumour arises from notochordal remnants, and usually develops within or in close proximity to the axial skeleton. In post-natal life the notochord persists in the nucleus pulposus of the intervertebral discs. In addition, small remnants are found in the hollow of the sacrum and coccyx and as little gelatinous nodules in the region of the spheno-occipital synchondrosis (*ecchordosis physaliphora*); the latter are, of course, observed as merely incidental findings at necropsy.

Sites of occurrence. Chordoma usually comes to notice in adult life and most commonly involves the sacrococcygeal region (Fig. 22.50) and the spheno-occipital part of the skull base. Cervical, dorsal and lumbar vertebral tumours are much rarer. They, and possibly all chordomas, are thought to arise from ectopic notochordal remnants rather than from the nuclei pulposi, for the tumour begins in the bone, the discs at first being spared.

Clinical features. Chordomas are very slow-growing and commonly give rise to pressure on adjacent structures, so that in the sacral region they may attain a large size, causing pressure on the rectum; in the spheno-occipital site the symptoms are chiefly referable to encroachment on cranial nerves or nerve roots but pituitary dysfunction may occur. The latter group are inevitably more quickly fatal. Radiological examination usually shows a lytic bone lesion with soft tissue shadow and sometimes some patchy calcification. Death usually occurs from local extension of tumour rather than metastasis.

Macroscopic appearances. The chordoma usually appears well circumscribed in its soft tissue mass but irregularly infiltrates adjacent bone. It is often firm and elastic, lobulated, greyish, semi-translucent and gelatinous with areas of haemorrhage and softening.

Microscopic appearances. The tumour tissue consists of lobules of rounded or polyhedral cells often arranged in alveoli or cords: some of these cells contain numerous intracytoplasmic vacuoles of mucin, "*physaliphorous cells*". Syncytial strands of cells with poorly defined borders may also be present in a sea of extracellular mucin (Fig. 22.51). The differentiation between chordoma and chondrosarcoma or even mucin-secreting carcinoma may be difficult.

A characteristic pattern is that in which long tapering strands of chordoma cells extend radially from the lobular margin, the central core and space between the radii being filled with gelatinous mucin, which is stained by the PAS method like the connective tissue mucins and gives a very strongly metachromatic reaction with toluidine blue, etc. Staining reactions are, however, of less significance in recognition than careful assessment of the architecture and morphology of the tumour.

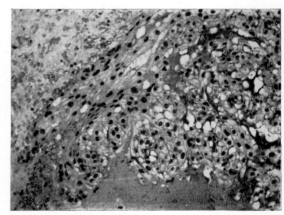

FIG. 22.51.—Chordoma from sacro-coccygeal region, showing masses of cells in alveoli with mucoid secretion in places. × 154.

DISEASES OF JOINTS

Normal joint structure

Joints may be categorised as those without a joint cavity, the non-synovial *synarthroses* and those with a joint cavity, the synovial *diarthroses*. In a diarthrosis the bone ends are almost invariably covered by hyaline articular cartilage and the surfaces lubricated by synovial fluid produced by the synovial membrane which is supported by the fibrous joint capsule.

Articular cartilage. Normal articular cartilage forms a smooth, glistening, slightly elastic covering to the bone ends. It is bluish and translucent in the young, averaging 2–4 mm. in thickness; in the old it becomes yellower, more opaque, loses some of its elasticity and is thinner. The matrix consists partly of fine collagen fibres which run parallel to the surface in the superficial layer, form a meshwork around the cells and elsewhere run as coarse fibres in tight spirals. The interfibrillar material contains much of the mucopolysaccharide, chondroitin sulphate, which gives cartilage its metachromatic staining.

The chondrocytes lie in lacunae in the matrix and have branching processes which extend into it. Those cells near the surface are flattened and horizontal, the deeper ones are arranged in columns. A wavy basophilic line marks the junction between the uncalcified cartilage and the small layer of calcified cartilage which is adjacent to the subchondral bone.

Articular cartilage is avascular and has a low rate of metabolism. Its nourishment is derived from the synovial fluid and probably also, especially in growing animals, from blood vessels of the subchondral marrow. Exchange between the synovial fluid and cartilage is thought to be promoted by the varying intra-articular pressures associated with joint movement. Hyaline cartilage has some power of regeneration and the amount varies with age and species.

Synovial membrane forms synovial fluid: it lines tendon sheaths, bursae and it covers all the surfaces of joints except articular cartilage and menisci. The synovium may be smooth or folded and especially at the joint margins may form small villi. It is lined by a single layer of spindle cells or by one or more layers of ovoid or polygonal cells. These intimal cells are not separated by a basement membrane from the underlying tissues which may be areolar, dense fibrous or fatty in different parts of the joint. Two types of intimal cells are distinguished on electron microscopy. It is thought that Type A, the more numerous, is concerned with absorption while Type B synthesises mucopolysaccharides such as hyaluronate.

The synovial membrane has a rich network of blood vessels, many of which run close to the surface. It is able to regenerate after synovectomy and a lining indistinguishable from synovium may form in adventitious bursae and pseudarthroses, presumably by metaplasia.

Synovial fluid is a dialysate of blood plasma with the addition of hyaluronic acid which gives the fluid its viscous property. The proportion of hyaluronic acid and hence the viscosity is said to diminish with age. Under normal circumstances human joints contain less than 1 millilitre of synovial fluid. It is thought that in healthy human joints there are 50–400 nucleated cells per c.mm. with few polymorphs, about 25 per cent lymphocytes, a few synovial cells and a majority of mononuclear phagocytes, perhaps derived from synovial histiocytes. There may be some red cells from the haemorrhage associated with the aspiration. In animals and probably in man the number of cells varies in one individual from one joint to another.

Albumin and globulin are present in lower concentration in the fluid than in plasma with a preponderance of albumin in the ratio of about 4:1. Glucose levels are normally much less than those found in the blood.

JOINT INFLAMMATION OF KNOWN ETIOLOGY

Acute infective arthritis

Acute arthritis formerly sometimes accompanied a generalised infection and occasionally progressed to suppuration, but this is now rare, probably on account of early response to specific chemotherapy. If adequately treated, infection by gonococci, pneumococci or typhoid bacilli seldom causes more than a transient non-suppurative arthritis which leaves little joint damage, at the most some synovial thickening and fibrosis. Accordingly infection by "pyogenic" organisms does not necessarily lead to suppuration. As an example of suppurative arthritis *acute staphylococcal or streptococcal arthritis* will be described. The disease is commonest in the hip and knee of children and young adults. In children, pneumococci occasionally give rise to a suppurative arthritis.

Path of infection. Acute infective arthritis arises chiefly as a result of haematogenous spread and sometimes a focus of infection such as a staphylococcal boil is identifiable. It may also result from spread from adjacent osteitis especially when the affected metaphysis is within the joint cavity, i.e. upper humeral, upper and lower femoral and all the metaphyses at the elbow. Rarely the organisms gain entrance directly through a penetrating wound or a compound intra-articular fracture.

Clinical features. There are the usual signs of acute inflammation, i.e. local redness, heat, pain, tenderness, oedema, joint effusion and limitation of movement and, associated with this, often pyrexia and a raised white cell count and erythrocyte sedimentation rate. Difficulty in diagnosis may arise when a pyogenic infection complicates pre-existing joint disease such as rheumatoid arthritis.

Early non-suppurative stage. The joint effusion contains a large increase of cells, mostly polymorphs, but may be sterile, bacteria only reaching the fluid if the synovial lining is ulcerated. Synovial fluid and blood cultures should immediately be obtained in a suspected pyogenic arthritis and antibiotics administered thereafter without delay. The synovium at this stage is intensely red and congested and flecked with yellowish fibrin. Microscopically it shows the features of acute inflammation. If the disease is arrested at

this stage the condition resolves with little residual joint damage.

Suppurative stage. If, however, suppuration ensues, within a few days there is, particularly over contact points, extensive cartilage destruction due in part to digestion by proteolytic enzymes in the pus. The exposed bone also undergoes necrosis (Fig. 22.52). An acute suppurative arthritis is entirely destructive but once the condition subsides into a subacute or chronic stage there is proliferation of granulation tissue within the joint, which is followed by ossification and bony ankylosis. Bony ankylosis occurs more commonly in suppurative arthritis than in tuberculous or rheumatoid disease.

Gonococcal arthritis. In pre-antibiotic days gonococcal arthritis was a relatively common complication of gonorrhoea, especially in males and often resulted in long-continuing chronic synovitis and in permanent joint damage. Now-

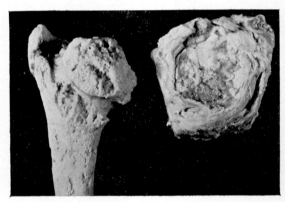

Fig. 22.52.—Suppurative arthritis of hip joint. The articular cartilage of both the femoral head and the acetabulum is destroyed and there is erosion of the underlying bone.

adays however it appears to be less common, probably affecting about 1 per cent of patients with gonorrhoea, is seen chiefly in females, responds to systemic penicillin therapy and even when septic arthritis has occurred seldom gives rise to serious joint destruction though occasionally some stiffness may remain. In the more acute form pain, tenderness and soft tissue swelling often affects many joints, especially the knee, wrist, and elbow within a few days of infection. The joint symptoms may be accompanied by chills and fever and by a gonococcaemic skin eruption, but meningitis, bacterial endocarditis and pericarditis are now rare. Tenosynovitis may occur especially around the wrist. Blood cultures are often positive in these patients though the synovial fluid may be sterile, perhaps related to the relatively short period after infection available for bacterial proliferation.

Sometimes joint symptoms appear relatively late after the original venereal infection; they may then involve only one joint and the infection is usually not septic.

Tuberculous arthritis

Joint tuberculosis is decreasing in incidence. While no age is exempt, the emphasis has slowly changed from children to the elderly: the hip and knee joints are the commonest sites. Since pasteurisation of milk became widespread the disease is usually the result of infection by the human and not the bovine strain of bacillus. Infection occurs almost invariably by blood-spread from a primary or reactivated tuberculous focus elsewhere in the body, especially in the lungs or lymph nodes. The synovium is frequently primarily involved but in some cases there may be secondary involvement by spread directly or *via* the periosteum from small or large tuberculous foci in bone.

Macroscopic appearances. There is often a moderate joint effusion, usually of clear or slightly turbid fluid, with "melon-seed bodies" (see p. 800) and only in the exceptional very late case is there "tuberculous pus". The synovial membrane is oedematous, hyperplastic and congested and may be studded by small greyish tubercles with yellowish caseating centres. There may also be an abundant growth of soft gelatinous granulation tissue arising from the synovial membrane and this may grow in from the periphery of the joint to form a *pannus* (Fig. 22.53) creeping over and replacing the articular cartilage where the joint surfaces are not in contact. In addition the articular cartilage may be destroyed by the ingrowth of sub-chondral granulation tissue which separates it in large flakes from the underlying bone. The cartilage may float free in the joint fluid or retain a tenuous attachment to bone. The exposed bone has an irregular surface with necrosis and exudation. Occasionally caseous foci with suppurative softening form in the capsule of the

joint and in the soft tissues outside, and pus may break through the skin surface giving rise to sinuses and allowing secondary infection to occur. Tuberculous arthritis heals by fibrosis, but the fibrous adhesions which form across the joint surfaces may later, if secondary infection occurs, become ossified with complete obliteration of the joint space and the burial in this bony mass of any remaining caseous material.

Microscopic appearances. The histological diagnosis of tuberculosis from synovial biopsy may be made most readily if the synovium is studded with discrete tubercles showing the usual microscopic features of foci of Langhans type giant cells, epithelioid cells and lymphocytes and sometimes caseation. When the synovium is replaced by gelatinous granulation tissue, however, the condition may appear to be a

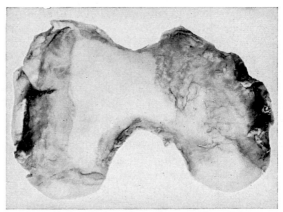

FIG. 22.53.—Tuberculous disease of knee-joint.
Note the spread of vascular tissue with tubercles over the surface of the cartilage.

non-specific inflammation with only a diffuse infiltrate of lymphocytes and plasma cells unless very careful search is made for the scanty and often ill-defined epithelioid follicles. The pannus on the surface of the cartilage and the subchondral granulations are even less fruitful sites for diagnostic examination. The thorough examination of 15 μ thick Ziehl-Neelsen stained tissue sections reveals acid-fast bacilli in rather more than half the cases and bacteriological culture of synovial tissue is positive in about the same number. When bone is also involved the marrow spaces may contain tubercle follicles with caseation and there may be some resorption and necrosis of bone.

The synovial fluid has a raised cell count and half or more of the cells may be lymphocytes.

Melon-seed bodies and flakes of articular cartilage may also be present, the melon-seed bodies
being formed usually of fibrin and sometimes
of necrotic synovial fronds.

In patients with an undiagnosed monarthritis
it is advisable to examine a synovial biopsy
histologically in order to exclude tuberculosis
rather than to rely on synovial fluid culture
alone.

Course of the disease. The earlier diagnosis
and prompt treatment of tuberculous arthritis
with antibiotics leads not infrequently to the
disease remaining confined to the synovium and
good function returns to the joint. When
articular cartilage and bone are involved, function is inevitably impaired and operative arthrodesis may be required. It is unusual in Great
Britain now to see cases of joint tuberculosis
proceeding to massive joint destruction with
discharging sinuses and final spontaneous
ankylosis, although these conditions may be
seen in countries where tuberculosis is unchecked
by specific therapy.

Senile tuberculosis. A low grade, slowly progressive form of tuberculosis is sometimes found
in elderly patients, the commonest site of the
disease being the shoulder joint. It was once
known as *tuberculosis sicca*.

Tuberculous tenosynovitis. Tuberculosis may
also affect the tendon sheaths, especially of the
flexor tendons at the wrist. There is, as in joint
tuberculosis, effusion of fluid into the sheath,
the formation of melon-seed bodies and sometimes proliferation of exuberant granulation
tissue within the sheath.

Syphilitic arthritis

In contrast to tuberculosis, syphilis comparatively
seldom gives rise to important joint lesions.

Acquired syphilis. In the *secondary* stage there
may be transient pain and stiffness of joints sometimes accompanied by effusion. Involvement, often
bilateral, of the knee joint or of the sternoclavicular
joint may be seen.

In *tertiary* syphilis, chronic interstitial inflammation and gumma of the joint capsule may occur. The
first may give rise to a mild form of inflammatory
arthritis, the latter, whether it arises in the synovium
or discharges from intracapsular bone, results in a
granulomatous synovitis, which may form a pannus
over the articular surfaces. Fibrosis followed by
bony ankylosis may result. Patients with tabes
dorsalis sometimes develop neuropathic arthritis
(p. 798).

Congenital syphilis. There may be joint pain and
swelling in infants and young children in association
with syphilitic epiphysitis. In older children there is
a condition known as *Clutton's joints*, often affecting
both knees, characterised by painless effusion with
synovial thickening and sometimes associated with
interstitial keratitis. It is transient and does not
progress to severe joint damage.

Brucellosis

Joint symptoms are the presenting feature of about
25 per cent of cases of undulant fever, the joints
being involved in the course of the septicaemia. The
arthritis is transient and of non-specific inflammatory
pattern. Sometimes granulomas similar to those
of sarcoidosis are seen (p. 152).

JOINT INFLAMMATION OF UNKNOWN ETIOLOGY

Arthritis associated with rheumatic fever

Rheumatic fever is a disease of uncertain
etiology characterised by pancarditis, fever and
transient arthritis. It is not thought to be related
to rheumatoid arthritis. The large joints are
usually affected, i.e. knees, ankles and wrists,
and as the condition subsides in some joints
others become affected.

In the acute stage there is usually a sterile joint
effusion with a high cell count around
10,000/c.mm (normal up to 400/c.mm), most of
these being polymorphs. The synovium is
congested and oedematous and the surface may

show fibrinous exudate and some polymorph
infiltrate.

As the condition subsides the polymorphs
diminish in the synovial fluid and lymphocytes
become prominent. A diffuse chronic inflammatory cell infiltrate may be seen in the synovium
but it lacks both the intensity and the accompanying proliferative changes seen in rheumatoid arthritis. Small granulomas resembling
Aschoff bodies (p. 311) may be present in the
synovium. The joint usually returns to normal,
the inflammatory cell infiltrate disappears and
the granulomas fibrose. Occasionally, especially
when the capsule has been involved, there may

be some residual pain and stiffness with persistent chronic inflammation and synovial thickening. In children small subcutaneous nodules the size of a split pea may be found in groups at sites of trauma such as around the olecranon and ulnar border of the forearm and about the patella. These granulomas usually consist of small areas of degenerate collagen with histiocytes, chronic inflammatory cells and some proliferation of fibroblasts and capillaries. They become fibrotic and disappear within a few months. (For a discussion of the etiology of rheumatic fever and its other manifestations see Chapter 14.)

Rheumatoid arthritis

Rheumatoid arthritis is one of the connective tissue diseases (p. 812), and is characterised by a subacute or chronic non-suppurative arthritis usually affecting several joints and its course is punctuated by spontaneous remissions.

Age and sex incidence. The disease usually begins in the years between 25 and 55 but may affect both older and younger ages. *Still's disease* in children consists of rheumatoid arthritis with associated splenomegaly, lymphadenopathy and occasionally pericarditis. Rheumatoid arthritis is more than twice as common in females as in males.

Sites of occurrence. Any synovial joint may be affected but the joints of the hands and feet are most often involved, the disease often being bilateral and sometimes symmetrical. Temporomandibular, crico-arytenoid joints and those of the cervical spine are occasionally involved. Neurological complications may follow spinal disease.

Course of the disease. The onset is often insidious but sometimes acute. The condition may abate after a single attack but more commonly there are repeated recrudescences and remissions, the joint each time suffering further damage. Involvement of tendons, soft tissue swelling, muscle atrophy, ligamentous and capsular laxity, all contribute to increasing deformity. Sometimes the disease progresses to fibrous, occasionally to bony, ankylosis. The tendency is for the rheumatoid disease eventually to burn itself out but even then the joint disability may increase due to further damage from secondary osteoarthritis. During the active phase tests for rheumatoid factor are usually positive (p. 795).

Clinical and macroscopic appearances. In the early acute stage or during exacerbations, the joints are hot, swollen and tender; the usual appearances of an acute inflammation. There is often general constitutional upset, the ESR is raised, there is a leukocytosis and sometimes a normocytic, normochromic anaemia. The swelling, which often gives the finger joints a spindle appearance, is partly due to synovial effusion which may be turbid but is sterile. There is an

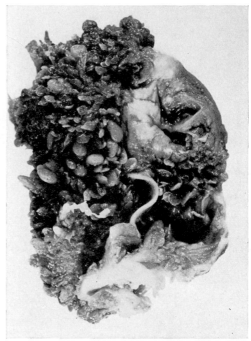

FIG. 22.54(*a*).—Synovium from a rheumatoid knee joint. The synovial surface is markedly frondose and some of the villi are tipped with white fibrin.

increase in cells sometimes up to 50,000/c.mm. with about 75 per cent polymorphs and fibrin flakes may be present. The primary changes are in the synovium which is red and congested, oedematous, markedly frondose and frequently patchily covered by fibrinous exudate (Fig. 22.54*a*). After the early stages it may be heavily pigmented with haemosiderin.

Microscopic appearances. In the florid case there is marked villous hypertrophy of the synovium with synovial cell proliferation, fibrinous and polymorph exudate on the surface, lymphocytes in dense focal aggregates, sometimes with germinal centres, accompanied by a heavy and more diffuse plasma cell infiltrate (Fig. 22.54*b*). These appearances may persist for an indefinite period after an acute attack. When these features are all present in a marked degree, the diagnosis of rheumatoid arthritis may be suggested with fair, though not with absolute certainty. However, the synovium has only a limited range of response to different stimuli and less severe degrees of these changes

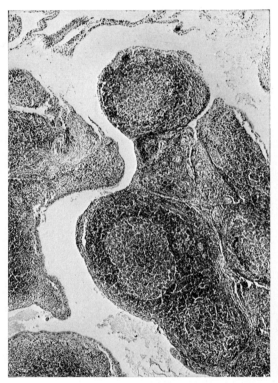

FIG. 22.54(*b*).—Synovial membrane in chronic rheumatoid arthritis.

The synovium shows villous hypertrophy and is extensively infiltrated with lymphocytes, amongst which occur poorly defined germinal centres. Plasma cells also are abundant. × 38.

may be seen in a wide variety of conditions, e.g. following trauma, in joints adjacent to tumours, in psoriatic arthritis, in various non-specific arthritides and occasionally even in osteoarthritis. Rarely a typical "rheumatoid nodule" (see below) may be seen in the subsynovial tissue and clinch the diagnosis.

While the changes in rheumatoid arthritis are confined to the synovium, the functional disability is reversible, but this is often followed by secondary irreversible changes in other joint structures. While the synovial changes described above persist, subchondral erosions form at the joint margin and a thin layer of vascular

granulation tissue (*pannus*) grows over, erodes and destroys the joint cartilage. If the underlying bone is exposed it may become pocketed by chronic granulations. In the later stage this granulation tissue may eventually become fibrosed with resultant adhesions across the joint space and later ossification sometimes converts fibrous to bony ankylosis, especially in the small joints of the carpus and tarsus.

While these changes are going on in the joint, *the bone* at an early stage may become markedly porotic probably partly as a result of disuse. *The muscles* become atrophic and there is wasting and weakness especially of the interossei and sometimes also of the hand flexors. *Tendons* may also become infiltrated by rheumatoid granulation tissue and this leads to pain and disability and sometimes to rupture of the tendon with further deformity. As a result of muscle atrophy and tendon destruction, ligamentous and capsular laxity, the hand in particular comes to be greatly deformed with marked ulnar deviation, subluxation and dislocation of joints.

Non-orthopaedic features of rheumatoid disease. Rheumatoid nodules consisting of a central area of fibrinoid necrosis of collagen surrounded

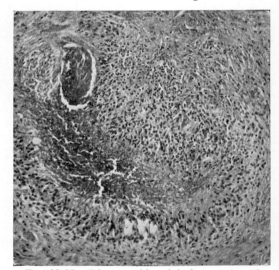

FIG. 22.55.—Rheumatoid nodule from region of elbow-joint. × 90.

by palisaded fibroblasts (Fig. 22.55) occur in the subcutaneous tissues over pressure sites in about 20 per cent of cases. These nodules persist throughout life and are a helpful clinical and histological diagnostic aid. They tend to occur in more severely affected patients and to be associated with a worse prognosis.

Similar nodules may be found at other sites, not only in the lungs of coalminers with rheumatoid disease (Caplan's syndrome, p. 372) but also in the pleura, the heart and pericardium, the eye and elsewhere.

Inflammation of arteries and veins may occur and when severe gives rise to skin ulceration and occasionally gangrene, bowel perforation and myocardial infarction. Peripheral neuropathy may also result. The skin is often atrophic, thin and papery.

Reactive and hyperplastic changes occur in lymph nodes and spleen (see p. 814). About 20 per cent of cases of chronic rheumatoid arthritis coming to necropsy have some evidence of amyloid disease affecting the spleen, liver and kidney, although clinically symptoms attributable to amyloid are rare. Sjøgren's syndrome (p. 477) may accompany rheumatoid disease.

Serum factors. The serum of most patients with rheumatoid arthritis contains *rheumatoid factor*, a 19S-macroglobulin (IgM) which behaves like an antibody and reacts with 7S-γ-globulin (IgG), including the patient's own IgG. The factor is best demonstrated by using as "antigen" IgG which has been altered by heating or by combination with inert particles, e.g. erythrocytes or latex. In the *Rose–Waaler* test, dilutions of the patient's heat-inactivated serum are tested with sheep erythrocytes sensitised with rabbit IgG. Agglutination in a significantly higher serum dilution than occurs with unsensitised sheep erythrocytes indicates a positive result. The rheumatoid factor may be present at an early stage or appear only later in the disease. Its absence is, in general, associated with a less severe case, although there are many exceptions. The factor is usually absent in cases of polyarthritis associated with psoriasis.

Recent work has demonstrated the complicated nature and heterogeneity of rheumatoid factors. Two factors may be present, one reacting with both rabbit and human IgG, the other only with human IgG. Moreover, rheumatoid factors which react specifically with genetically determined human IgG iso-antigens (termed Gm factors), have been detected, and in some instances the patient's serum has contained such a factor which reacts with an iso-antigen absent from his own IgG. Because of this observation, and the fact that rheumatoid factors react more strongly with altered than with native IgG, it is doubtful whether or not rheumatoid factor should be regarded as an auto-antibody. Although rheumatoid factor has not been implicated as a pathogenic agent, an immunological dyscrasia is suggested by raised incidences of antinuclear factors (p. 814) and of chronic thyroiditis and thyroid antibodies which have been demonstrated in rheumatoid arthritis.

Ankylosing spondylitis

Ankylosing spondylitis is a polyarthritis leading to bony ankylosis of the sacroiliac, intervertebral, and costovertebral joints with ossification of spinal ligaments and the borders of

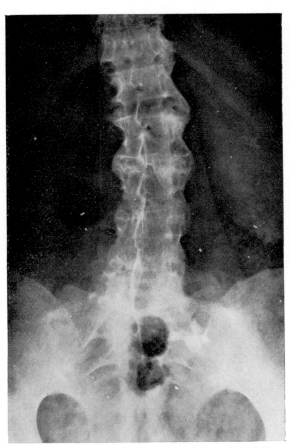

FIG. 22.56.—Radiograph of spine and sacro-iliac joints in late ankylosing spondylitis of the annulus fibrosus, producing the typical appearance of "bamboo" spine. The sacro-iliac joint spaces are obliterated. (Dr. W. Watson Buchanan.)

intervertebral discs and it results in rigidity of the spine. Sometimes the sternoclavicular and hip joints are similarly involved. The disease is much commoner in males than females and usually the onset is in adolescence or early adult life. It is sometimes familial.

Course of the disease. There is usually an insidious onset of stiffness in the back with clinical and radiological evidence of inflammation of the sacroiliac joints. The condition may be self-limiting but often progresses with exacerbations and remissions until the patient is left with an absolutely rigid back showing the radiological appearances of *bamboo spine* (Fig. 22.56). When the cervical spine is involved there is danger of atlanto-axial dislocation or vertebral fracture and care must be taken in the handling of the anaesthetised patient. During exacerbations the ESR is commonly raised. The hips may be involved transiently, or chronically with final bony ankylosis in the most severely affected patients. Respiratory complications may result from diminished thoracic excursion.

Etiology. The etiology is unknown but it has been suggested that the disease may be related to rheumatoid arthritis on the grounds that the histology of the synovium resembles that of rheumatoid arthritis and also that a proportion of patients have clinical rheumatoid changes in proximal limb joints. The sex incidence, the vertebral involvement, the extra-articular ossification, the lack of rheumatoid nodules, arteritis and peripheral neuropathy are all, however, points against this suggestion. Furthermore serological tests for rheumatoid arthritis are usually negative in ankylosing spondylitis.

Aortic lesions. A few patients with longstanding ankylosing spondylitis may develop aortic valvular incompetence due to changes in the aorta indistinguishable from those of syphilis, but limited to the immediate vicinity of the aortic valve and sinuses of Valsalva. Serological tests for syphilis have been consistently negative and this appears to be a non-syphilitic lesion associated specifically with ankylosing spondylitis.

Leukaemia. Irradiation of the spine in ankylosing spondylitis includes a large volume of the haemopoietic marrow and this predisposes to the subsequent development of leukaemia; one in 400 patients treated develops leukaemia within five years, a number greatly in excess of the incidence of the disease in the general population, and the added risk continues indefinitely, probably for life.

Psoriatic arthritis

Patients with psoriasis, especially those with involvement of the nails, have a tendency to develop a remittent arthritis which has a predilection for the distal joints of the hands and feet. While the microscopic appearances of the synovium show much the same non-specific picture of hyperplasia with lymphocytic and plasma cell infiltrate as is seen in the less florid cases of rheumatoid arthritis, the clinical and radiographic features and the negative test for rheumatoid factor serve to make the distinction. While deformities of the hands and feet may result, the condition is usually less disabling than rheumatoid arthritis.

Reiter's syndrome

This is of unknown etiology and consists of abacterial urethritis, conjunctivitis and arthritis sometimes following diarrhoea and most frequently affecting adult males. The knee, ankle, spine and small joints of the hands and feet are involved in a transient polyarthritis which in contrast to gonococcal arthritis may not respond to penicillin therapy. While often there is no permanent disability there may be recurrences with a tendency to destructive changes in the feet and sacroiliac joints. The mouth may be involved and skin lesions affect especially the soles and palms.

DEGENERATIVE ARTHROPATHIES

Osteoarthritis or degenerative arthritis

Osteoarthritis is the commonest form of chronic joint disease and is characterised clinically by the insidious but progressive onset of pain and joint stiffness. In spite of the name it is not an inflammatory or systematic disease but results from slow destructive and degenerative changes in the articular cartilage of joints. In children the articular cartilage is bluish, translucent, resilient and has regenerative powers, but in adults the cartilage tends to become yellowish and opaque and to lose its reparative powers. This is the probable cause of the articular damage seen to some degree in almost all adults over the age of 40, though in most cases minor and symptomless (Fig. 22.57). Osteoarthritic joint changes may be looked on as an exaggeration of the alterations of joint structure associated with ageing.

Age incidence. Osteoarthritis is chiefly found in the elderly. Degenerative joint changes may be hastened by a variety of lesions which predispose to cartilage injury or lay unusual stress on the joint.

Predisposing causes. These may be *intra-articular* such as fractures involving the joint surface, or conditions which damage the joint cartilage such as rheumatoid arthritis, gout, ochronosis, haemophilia or loose bodies (Fig. 22.61, see p. 800). Amongst the *extra-articular*

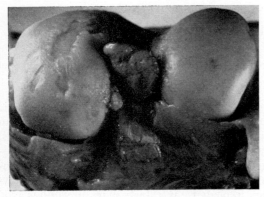

FIG. 22.57.—Knee joint from middle-aged patient with no symptoms, showing early destruction of cartilage.

causes are obesity or deformities which lead to malalignment of the joint such as knock-knee, scoliosis, the lower limb bowing associated with rickets or Paget's disease, or fractures healed in bad position.

When osteoarthritis occurs in the young some predisposing factor is usually clearly apparent.

Sites of occurrence. The large joints are chiefly affected especially the weight-bearing ones, e.g. the hip, knee or spinal joints; those with a large range of movement, e.g. the shoulder joint; and those especially susceptible to misuse, e.g. the metatarso-phalangeal joint of the first toe.

Structural changes. *Articular cartilage.* The first change in the articular cartilage is that it loses its smooth surface and becomes slightly irregular due to loss by tangential flaking. This is associated with loss of mucopolysaccharide (chondroitin sulphate) in the superficial layers. Later there is perpendicular fibrillation of the matrix and gradual thinning of the cartilage which may eventually be completely lost over large or small areas. At this stage there is likely to be radiological evidence of loss of joint space. Vascularisation of the cartilage from below also may occur early with resumption of endochondral ossification.

Bone. While these changes are occurring in the articular cartilage there is much active remodelling of bone at the osteochondral junction and the subchondral bone trabeculae become greatly thickened (Fig. 22.58b). When this dense bone is exposed it becomes polished and eburnated, sometimes grooved in the direction of joint movement (Figs. 22.58a, 22.61). The bone forming the actual joint surface is usually necrotic. Fibrocartilaginous metaplasia tends to occur in any exposed marrow spaces.

One of the results of the marked bone remodelling is change in the shape of the joint surface. This is particularly obvious in the flattening and mushrooming of the weight bearing surface of the femoral head in osteoarthritis of the hip joint (Fig. 22.58a, b). Another result is the formation of radiological "cysts" in the subchondral bone. These are areas devoid of bone but filled by fatty marrow or loose rather degenerate fibrous tissue and sometimes surrounded by new bony trabeculae. At the joint margins small excrescences form, giving first an appearance of beading and later of lipping of the joint. These osteophytic outgrowths form by proliferation of cartilage, followed by endochondral ossification (Fig. 22.58b), but the stimulus to cartilage production is not fully understood. The osteophytes may give rise to deformity and limitation of movement. Spontaneous ankylosis does not occur in uncomplicated osteoarthritis.

Synovium. In the early stages the synovium is normal but when disintegration of the joint surface takes place there is absorption of abraded fragments of cartilage and bone, associated with some synovial hyperplasia and villous hypertrophy and followed by subsynovial fibrosis. Chronic inflammatory cell infiltrate is usually minimal. Sometimes fatty villi are prominent in obese patients and occasionally, particularly in the knee joint and sometimes in the elbow, *lipoma arborescens* may be present. In this condition very large numbers of fatty synovial covered polypi project into the joint. It is thought, however, that these predispose to osteoarthritis rather than result from it.

Synovial fluid. In a small proportion of cases there is synovial effusion and the fluid is thick.

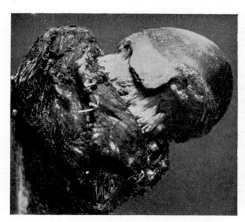

FIG. 22.58(a).—Osteoarthritis of the femoral head. There is eburnation and grooving of the articular surface. The irregular growth of bone and cartilage at the margins forms osteophytes.

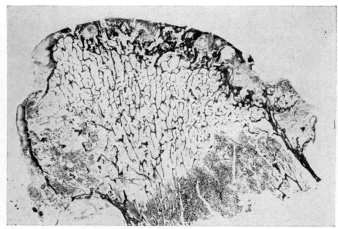

FIG. 22.58(b).—Osteoarthritis of hip joint.

The weight-bearing surface of the femoral head is flattened and mushroomed and the articular cartilage has largely disappeared. The exposed bone is dense, small osteoarthritic cysts are present and there are peripheral osteophytes.

The cell count is only slightly raised and only about 15 per cent of cells are polymorphs.

Heberden's nodes. These are small bony elevations on the terminal phalanges of the fingers near the joint line. They may give rise to some deformity and limitation of movement. Some are the result of osteoarthritis; others result from post-traumatic ossification of para-articular tissues.

Primary generalised osteoarthritis sometimes has a familial incidence, affects multiple joints often in relatively young patients and is almost invariably associated with Heberden's nodes.

Chondromalacia patellae is a condition arising in young people and giving rise to pain, effusion, loss of movement and crepitus of the knee joint. A history of trauma to the patella is often given. The naked-eye and microscopic appearances of excised patellae are of localised degenerative changes in the articular cartilage.

Neuropathic arthritis (Charcot's joint)

Neuropathic arthritis is a degenerative arthritis resulting from the progressive disorganisation of an insensitive joint when subjected to trauma. It was first described by Charcot as occurring in tabes dorsalis and has since been found in a wide variety of other neurological conditions. In syphilis the joints commonly affected are the hip, knee, ankle, tarsus, vertebrae and shoulder and in syringomyelia the joints of the upper limb, especially shoulder and elbow. The commonest cause nowadays is probably diabetic neuropathy. Cases have also been described in leprosy, spina bifida, peripheral nerve injuries, transverse myelitis, subacute combined degeneration of the cord, in the rare condition of congenital universal indifference to pain and following repeated intra-articular injections of cortisone.

While Charcot held the view that the bone changes resulted from the removal of the "trophic" influence of the nervous system over bones and joints, the condition is explicable on other grounds. A cycle of events may occur in, for instance, the knee joint in a case of tabes dorsalis. The ataxia leads readily to some minor or major trauma to the joint which results in effusion, the swelling and muscular hypotonia increase the instability of the joint and its liability to further damage. Because the joint is painless the patient fails to guard it and continued use leads to repetition of the cycle. The condition can therefore be attributed to continued use of an analgesic joint with associated proprioceptive loss without invoking the loss of so-called trophic influences. The morbid anatomical changes in this condition are basically those of an extremely severe osteoarthritis. The cartilage is destroyed, the bone ends grossly distorted (Fig. 22.59) partly by remodelling and partly by the early formation of very large osteophytic outgrowths which may fracture and cause further damage. Fracture may also occur in the condylar region and the pathology of neuroarthropathy may be complicated by hyperplastic callus formation.

Arthritis associated with gout

Gout is a disease with a hereditary tendency, associated with an incompletely understood disorder of purine metabolism and results in repeated attacks of acute arthritis which may be followed by chronic degenerative joint changes. Most patients with gout have hyperuricaemia,

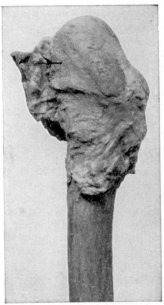

FIG. 22.59.—Upper end of femur in neuropathic arthritis of the hip joint in a patient with tabes.

Note the irregular absorption of the head and the new formation of bone below.

i.e. a blood uric acid level of more than 6·5 mg. per 100 ml. Hyperuricaemia is much commoner than clinical gout and the symptomless relatives of patients with gout may have raised blood uric acid levels.

So-called *secondary gout* may arise in patients with leukaemia or polycythaemia vera especially in the course of treatment with some cytotoxic drugs when hyperuricaemia results from the increased nucleoprotein breakdown. Occasionally secondary gout complicates uraemia, the decreased renal secretion leading to a raised blood uric acid level.

Age, sex and site incidence. The first attack usually occurs over the age of 40, and the disease is much commoner in males. In about half the cases the metatarsophalangeal joint of the great toe is the first area affected, but the knee, elbow and other toe and finger joints may be involved.

The acute attack. In the susceptible subject an acute attack of gout may be precipitated by a wide variety of factors such as trauma, alcoholic or dietary excess, certain diuretics and purgation. Some of the drugs given to gouty patients to promote urinary excretion of uric acid may produce an acute attack since they free some of the acid which is bound to plasma proteins and so increase the amount of diffusible uric acid. Acute gout is sometimes ushered in by pyrexia, leukocytosis and a raised erythrocyte sedimentation rate. The onset is sudden, may be nocturnal and there is excruciating pain in the affected joint, often the great toe (*podagra*) or its associated bursa, which shows all the signs of an acute inflammation. This stage is associated with the deposition of microcrystals in the tissues. These strongly negative birefringent crystals may be recognised in the synovial fluid, often within polymorphs (c.f. pseudo-gout, p. 800). Cells in the synovial fluid may increase to 14,000/c.mm. with 70 per cent or more polymorphs. The attack lasts usually for a few days or weeks and is followed by remission. The prompt beneficial effect of colchicine may be used as a therapeutic test of acute gout.

Chronic gout is associated with the formation of crystalline deposits of sodium biurate often with cholesterol and calcium salts in relatively avascular collagen, fibro- and hyaline cartilage. These are known as tophi and may be found in the fibrocartilages of the ear, in bursal walls, especially the olecranon and prepatellar bursae and in the articular cartilage of joints (Fig. 22.60). Tophi are not significantly radioopaque.

Microscopic examination of alcohol-fixed material from a tophus shows sheaves of biurate crystals, with a surrounding very marked foreign-body giant cell and granulomatous reaction.

In joints the urate deposition occurs first in the superficial articular cartilage where it can be seen as opaque white spots like paint. The crystalline deposits are accompanied by degenerative changes in the articular cartilages which may cause some of the disability of chronic gouty arthritis. Later urates may be precipitated

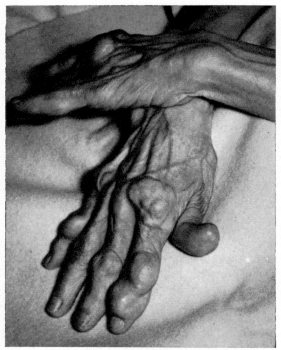

FIG. 22.60.—Tophi in the hands of a gouty patient.

in the subchondral and subperiosteal bone giving rise to bone destruction and punched out defects which are radiologically diagnosable. Tophi may occur in relation to synovium or para-articular tissues and these may sometimes reach great size and destroy cartilage, bone, synovium and capsule, leaving a totally disorganised joint. (For discussion of renal changes in gout see p. 721 and of etiology and purine metabolism p. 209.)

Articular chondrocalcinosis (pseudo-gout)

In recent years a condition with only a slight male preponderance has been described chiefly in the middle-aged and elderly. It is characterised clinically by episodes of acute or subacute inflammation of one or more large joints, especially the knees. Involvement of the big toe is rare. During the acute stage crystals of *calcium pyrophosphate* may be identified in the synovial fluid, mostly within polymorphs. During the process of the disease calcification may appear in the menisci of the knee, the articular disc of the distal radio-ulnar joint, the annulus fibrosus of the intervertebral discs, the symphysis pubis and also in articular cartilages, ligaments, tendons and joint capsules. Chronic degenerative joint disease may follow. While about a third of patients have hyperuricaemia and an occasional one has clinical gout the condition should be distinguished from true gout by the involvement of large joints, the distinctive radiological findings and the characteristic crystals which exhibit a faint positive birefringence in polarised light.

Haemophilic arthritis

Acute haemarthrosis especially in the knee is a common finding in haemophilia and the joint may become greatly distended by blood which is gradually resorbed. The synovium becomes deeply pigmented with haemosiderin. After repeated haemarthroses there is often some destruction of the articular cartilage, probably partly the result of subchondral haemorrhages and in addition organisation of intraosseous haemorrhage may lead to bone resorption and the formation of bone "cysts". Where damage to cartilage has occurred osteoarthritic changes may supervene.

MISCELLANEOUS JOINT CONDITIONS

Intra-articular loose bodies

Multiple soft loose bodies are sometimes known as "*rice or melon-seed*" bodies. They are usually formed from fibrin or necrotic synovial tissue and are found in tuberculosis and rheumatoid arthritis. Symptoms are those of the accompanying arthritis.

Hard loose bodies may be caused by:

(1) *Osteochondritis dissecans*. Here the loose body is derived from part of the articular cartilage and underlying bone which for some reason undergoes necrosis and separates. When com-

pletely separated, the cartilaginous part of the body remains viable, the bone dies. Usually one, occasionally several, loose bodies may be present.

(2) *Osteoarthritis*. The fracturing of marginal osteophytes is a rare occurrence. This is said to occur more commonly in the severe osteoarthritis associated with neuroarthropathy.

(3) *Fracture of the articular margins*. Occasionally fracture of the articular margins results in one of the fragments of the fracture entering the joint and acting as a loose body, i.e. in fractures of the lower end of the humerus the medial epicondyle may, in spite of its muscle

attachments, form a loose body in the elbow joint.

(4) *Synovial chondromatosis or osteochondromatosis.* In this condition the synovial membrane shows cartilaginous metaplasia. These very numerous cartilaginous nodules may then ossify.

Clinically hard loose bodies may give rise to episodes of locking of the joint. Damage to the articular cartilage may result in osteoarthritis (Fig. 22.61).

Pigmented villonodular synovitis

Pigmented villonodular synovitis is an uncommon condition of unknown etiology, thought to be reactive rather than neoplastic and which may affect joints, bursae or tendon sheaths in a localised or in a diffuse form. Males between the ages of 20–50 years are most commonly affected and the knee or hip joint are often involved. The synovitis gives rise to pain, serosanguineous effusion and sometimes to locking of the joint.

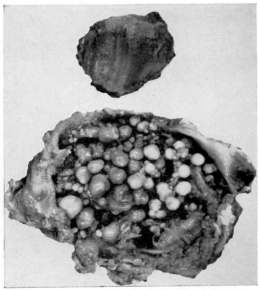

FIG. 22.61.—Chondromatosis of synovium of the knee joint. Osteoarthritis of patella.

Macroscopic appearances. The diffuse form has a most striking appearance. In the early stages the synovium looks like a tangled reddish brown beard; matting together of the hyperplastic, pigmented villi later gives rise to a spongy orange and brown pad of great complexity.

There may also be firm nodules, sessile or pedunculated and one or several of these may be present in the localised form of the disease. Occasionally adjacent bone is infiltrated by the pigmented tissue and the extra-articular soft tissue may be involved. Regional lymph nodes may become pigmented with haemosiderin.

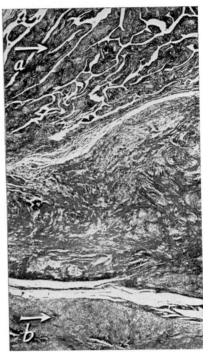

FIG. 22.62.—At (*a*) there is diffuse pigmented villonodular synovitis while at (*b*) a solid mass containing abundant lipid macrophages and haemosiderin has developed. × 10.

Microscopic appearances. The villi are enlarged, the synovial lining cells increased and prominent, macrophages and chronic inflammatory cells and sometimes small multinucleated giant cells are abundant (Fig. 22.62). Much haemosiderin is present partly in macrophages and synovial lining cells and also lying free in the tissue. There may also be xanthomatous areas with foamy lipid-laden macrophages. When the villi become matted together clefts lined by synovial cells are seen and may give an appearance alarmingly similar to synovial sarcoma. The nodular projections often are more hyalinised with dense collagen, little pigment and many giant cells and bear a striking resemblance to so-called benign giant-cell tumour of tendon sheath (Fig. 22.63).

Prognosis. This condition in its diffuse form

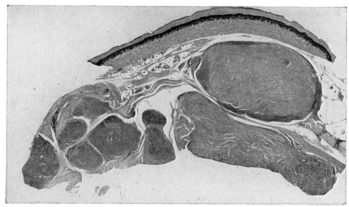

Fig. 22.63.—Pigmented villonodular synovitis of tendon sheath. Multiple nodules of pigmented giant-cell tissue are loosely attached to the flexor tendon of the ring finger. × 5·5.

is difficult to eradicate completely and there is a tendency to recurrence. In spite of recurrence, its occasional involvement of bone, its liability to spread into extra-articular tissue and its sometimes alarming histological appearance, no carefully documented case has been known to metastasise and the differentiation between this lesion and synovial sarcoma is of the first importance if needless amputation is to be avoided.

Bursae. The popliteal bursa is the most frequently involved. A tumour-like mass forms, and the gross and histological appearances are the same as in joints.

Tendon sheaths. Very rarely there is diffuse involvement of a tendon sheath but the common finding is of solitary or multiple rounded nodules on the extensor tendons of the hands (Fig. 22.63). The histological appearance of these nodules is identical with those of the sessile or pedunculated lumps sometimes seen as part of the diffuse form of the disease. These have formerly been described as benign giant-cell tumours of tendon sheath, and while the etiology and nature of pigmented villonodular synovitis is still under discussion it is probably immaterial which label is used.

Synovial tumours

Benign giant-cell tumour of tendon sheath

This condition is considered to be analogous to pigmented villonodular synovitis and is discussed above.

Synovial sarcoma (malignant synovioma)

Synovial sarcoma is a rare and highly malignant tumour usually found adjacent to but outside a joint and most often occurring in young adults. The most common site is the popliteal fossa and the tumour is four times as common in the lower as in the upper limb.

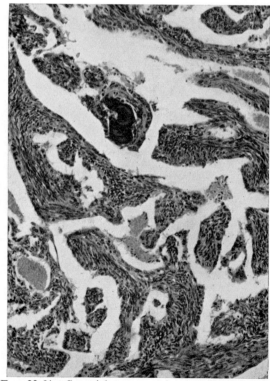

Fig. 22.64.—Synovial sarcoma showing fibrosarcoma-like spindle cells and clefts lined by cubical cells. There is a focus of calcification. This tumour metastasised. × 115.

Macroscopic appearances. This malignant tumour often has, as do many soft tissue sarcomas, a falsely reassuring appearance of encapsulation due to compression of surrounding tissue. It may be white or pinkish-grey, sometimes with areas of haemorrhage and frequently with spotty calcification which may be sufficient to be seen radiologically.

Microscopic appearances. The well-differentiated tumour consists of fibrosarcomatous and pseudo-epithelial elements. In the fibrosarcomatous tissue there are clefts or gland-like spaces sometimes containing mucin and lined by cuboidal cells without a basement membrane (Fig. 22.64). The latter point sometimes helps in the occasional case where there is difficulty in differentiating between synovial sarcoma and secondary carcinoma. Invasion of blood vessels is sometimes seen.

Prognosis. Metastases develop in lungs, lymph nodes and other organs. The mortality figures are high, there being only a few 5-year survivors. An increasing awareness of the serious nature of this tumour and more prompt and radical treatment are expected to lead to some improvement in prognosis.

MISCELLANEOUS DISORDERS OF THE PARA-ARTICULAR TISSUES

Ganglion. Ganglia occur in the soft tissue around joints or tendon sheaths. The commonest site is the dorsum of the wrist, but they may also be found on the palmar aspect and around the knee. They usually develop by myxoid change and cystic softening of the fibrous tissue of the joint capsule or tendon sheath and occasionally have a direct connection with a joint cavity. Rarely they are found within nerve sheaths and may give rise to symptoms of nerve compression. They consist commonly of a thin, fibrous-walled sac, often rather gelatinous due to the patchy mucoid change, and not lined by synovium. A ganglion contains clear glairy fluid.

Similar lesions occasionally arise in the periosteum particularly of the tibia and also sometimes within bone, beneath a normal articular surface.

Cyst of semilunar cartilage. The cyst arises in relation to the external semilunar cartilage (lateral meniscus) and has naked-eye and histological features identical with those of a ganglion. It appears to arise in the loose fibrous tissue adjacent to, rather than actually within, the fibrocartilage of the meniscus.

Bursitis. A bursa is a synovial-lined sac and is found chiefly over bony prominences. It may communicate with a joint and is subject to many of the same disorders. Inflammation may arise as a result of repeated trauma as, for instance, in prepatellar bursitis (*housemaid's knee*). The bursa becomes distended with fluid, often with much fibrin and the synovial lining may show villous hyperplasia or may be replaced by granulation and later by fibrous tissue. Loose bodies of the melon-seed type may form. *Baker's cyst* arises in the popliteal space by herniation of the synovial membrane through the joint capsule. The connection to the articular cavity may be closed by scarring.

Tumoral calcinosis. In tumoral calcinosis radio-opaque calcium phosphate forms small discrete nodules or larger masses around joints, especially the hip, or in soft tissues. Young Africans are particularly likely to be affected. The condition is usually initially painless though later there may be pressure on nerves. The overlying skin may ulcerate and chalky fluid or granular white material be discharged. Microscopically the deposits of calcium

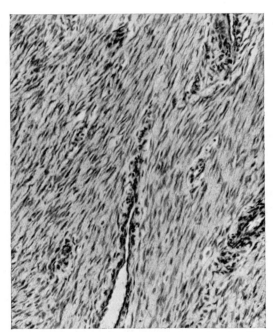

FIG. 22.65.—Dupuytren's contracture, showing the highly cellular fascial tissue. × 130.

are often surrounded by macrophages, foreign-body giant cells and dense collagen. Plaques of degenerate collagen may be seen near the deposits. The patients are usually healthy and the blood biochemical changes are inconstant. The etiology remains uncertain. It has been suggested that the deposits may be the result of traumatic fat necrosis or of an abnormality of phosphate metabolism.

Dupuytren's contracture is a painless hereditary condition involving the palmar fascia and resulting in flexion contracture of the fingers. It occurs most commonly in middle-aged males and is often bilateral. The fifth, fourth and third fingers tend to be affected in that order of frequency. The fascia becomes thickened, contracted and sometimes nodular. Microscopy shows, in the active phase, a whorled pattern of very marked fibroblastic proliferation which may give rise to alarm on account of its cellularity (Fig. 22.65). It progresses, however, to extremely dense hyalinised collagen and is entirely benign. Usually a mixture of fibroblastic and hyalinised areas are seen. A similar condition (*plantar fibromatosis*) may be present in the sole of the foot, causing nodules in the plantar fascia without contracture. This also is benign though often locally recurrent and difficult to eradicate surgically.

Fibrositis and panniculitis. The clinical syndrome of muscular pain, localised tenderness and sometimes stiffness more pronounced on waking may be accounted for by a variety of conditions from cervical spondylosis to Coxsackie virus infection. There is some doubt as to whether "fibrositis" itself exists though tender fibrofatty nodules have been described associated with oedema, a mild chronic inflammatory cell infiltrate and followed by fibrosis. Acute pain of sudden onset may sometimes be due to herniation of a fatty lobule through a small aperture in the investing fibrous tissue and this is termed panniculitis. When associated with obesity the condition may be designated *adiposis dolorosa* or *Dercum's disease*.

Relapsing febrile nodular panniculitis (Weber–Christian syndrome). In this condition successive attacks of weakness and muscular pains are followed by bouts of fever in which tender nodules appear in the subcutaneous and other adipose tissues. These consist of foci of subacute inflammation with areas of secondary fat necrosis and granulomatous reaction. Rarely suppuration may occur and ulceration of the skin then follows, but micro-organisms have not been found in the lesions. The cause is unknown, but it may be associated with focal streptococcal lesions elsewhere, e.g. in the tonsils.

DISEASES OF SKELETAL MUSCLE

Normal muscle structure

A muscle consists of bundles of muscle fibres bound together by fibrous tissue, the epimysium. This fibrous sheath penetrates between the muscle bundles as the perimysium and each muscle fibre is surrounded by a delicate tenuous sheath of endomysium. Fat cells normally may lie between the muscle bundles but not within them. The muscle or sarcolemmal nuclei in the human lie at the periphery of the fibre under the cell membrane or sarcolemma except in the ocular muscles and at tendinous insertions. Cross-striation, which is recognisable under the light microscope, results from the parallel arrangement of myofibrils with alternating series of interdigitating myosin (thick) and actin (thin) protein filaments. During contraction these filaments are thought to slide into one another.

Each muscle fibre is a single, elongated, multinucleated cell, varying in length and diameter both within a muscle and from one muscle to another. Each fibre has one neuromuscular junction or motor end plate which lies at the midpoint. A motor unit consists of all the muscle fibres which are innervated by a single anterior horn cell and in the human nearly all the fibres in a muscle bundle are included. The number of muscle fibres in a motor unit varies. The more delicate the function to be performed the fewer the fibres in the unit and the smaller the individual fibre diameter.

Sensory organs in muscle are numerous, the most common type being the muscle spindle, though other varieties concerned chiefly with stretch and pressure are found in the tendinous insertions. The muscle spindle consists of a long ovoid fibrous capsule containing several thin striated muscle fibres with numerous nuclei in their centre. Sensory endings connected with cells in the posterior root ganglia are present and the fibres receive their motor supply from small cells in the anterior horn. About a third to a half of myelinated fibres in nerves supplying muscle are of sensory origin.

Muscle biopsy. Artefacts produced in the processing of muscle biopsies are common, sometimes confusing and may be minimised by allowing the biopsy to lie unfixed for a minute or two on a piece of card, to which it readily adheres, and then dropping it into fixative. Both longitudinal and cross-sectional blocks should be taken when fixation is complete.

Muscle diseases. Most lesions in skeletal muscle fall into the following main groups: (a) traumatic and circulatory disturbances, (b) inflammatory, (c) atrophy secondary to degeneration of the lower motor neurone (*neurogenic atrophy*) and systematised primary diseases of muscle of unknown etiology such as the (d) *muscular dystrophies* and (e) *polymyositis*.

A. Traumatic and circulatory disturbances

Anterior tibial syndrome, traumatic necrosis of anterior tibial muscle. In this condition, the patient, usually a young adult male, experiences pain, swelling and a degree of paralysis of the anterior tibial muscle group, sometimes associated with constitutional upset, following unaccustomed exercise. It seems probable that the exercise results in excessive production of metabolites, leading to swelling, and because of the unyielding nature of the muscle compartment formed posteriorly by tibia, fibula and interosseus membrane and anteriorly by the anterior crural fascia, the increased pressure, if unrelieved, results in ischaemic muscle necrosis and later fibrosis.

Microscopic examination shows necrosis of muscle with loss of sarcolemmal nuclei, increased eosinophilia and sometimes either loss or prominence of cross-striations. At the periphery of the dead muscle there is usually polymorph infiltration, phagocytosis of clumps of eosinophilic sarcoplasm and production of cellular fibrous tissue which grows into and replaces the dead muscle, later becoming more densely collagenous. Abortive muscle regeneration may be seen and is characterised by thin muscle fibres with increased sarcolemmal nuclei, sometimes terminating in regressing multinucleated muscle buds. Adjacent groups of atrophic muscle fibres are the result of involvement of nerve bundles in the necrosis (p. 808).

Volkmann's ischaemic contracture. Occasionally, displaced supracondylar fractures of the humerus, dislocation of the elbow or fractures of the forearm are followed by acute ischaemia of arterial origin and lead to massive infarction of

forearm muscles and also to involvement of the median and less commonly of the ulnar nerves. A characteristic deformity results. This consists of slight flexion of the wrist and clawing of the fingers with hyperextension of the metacarpophalangeal joints. There are associated sensory changes. In the fully developed lesion there is an ellipsoid of necrotic forearm muscles, soft and greenish-yellow surrounded by an area of fibrous replacement. If a major nerve runs through the centre of an area of complete necrosis it may also be dull, yellowish and avascular, or if

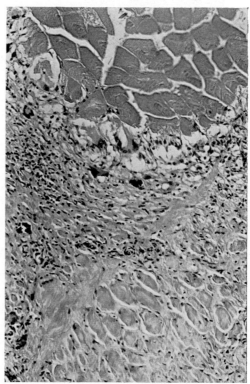

FIG. 22.66.—Volkmann's ischaemic contracture. Dead muscle fibres undergoing phagocytosis are seen at the top. In the lower part muscle tubes have been colonised by fibroblasts, and the sarcoplasm replaced by collagen. × 100.

nearer the periphery, shrunken and fibrosed. The microscopic appearances are similar to those in the anterior tibial syndrome (Fig. 22.66). Much of the muscle may come to be replaced by dense collagen and, in addition, as a result of the nerve damage, surviving muscle may suffer severe neural atrophy (p. 808).

Massive ischaemic necrosis of muscle is seen in cases of "crush syndrome" where compression of a limb has resulted in prolonged arterial obstruction. On release of pressure and re-establishment of the circulation, large portions of muscle may fail to recover. From these necrotic muscles the myoglobin and other substances are absorbed and excreted in the urine and acute renal tubular necrosis may result

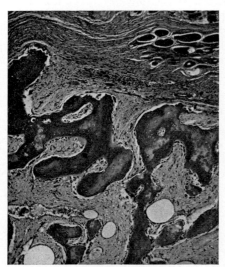

FIG. 22.67.—Bone formation in the wall of a calcifying haematoma in muscle. × 40.

(p. 724). The affected muscles become pale and soft—so-called fish-flesh appearance—and if the patient recovers, they undergo fibrous replacement.

Congenital torticollis. This is a condition of fibrosis and contraction of the sternomastoid muscle which develops in the early years of life. It is alleged to be the result of an ischaemic birth injury (whether venous or arterial is uncertain) with necrosis of the distal part of the muscle, in which a tender spindle-shaped swelling, the *sternomastoid tumour of infancy* develops soon after birth. It is said to consist of intense venous engorgement, oedema and haemorrhage, followed by phagocytosis of the remnants of the original muscle fibres and formation of granulation tissue, which becomes collagenous. While this etiology is not proved, contracture of the muscle occurs, the head tends to be inclined to the affected side, and asymmetry of the face and skull may result, probably from the abnormal tension during the period of bone growth.

Traumatic myositis ossificans is a localised benign lesion and may result from either a single injury or repeated minor trauma. A well-known example of this is the development of

bone in the adductor muscles of the thighs in horsemen. A corresponding condition is seen in the deltoid of soldiers, produced by the recoil of the rifle in firing, and in the biceps and brachialis muscles in fencers. The initial injury is to muscle and soft tissue and is associated with a variable amount of haemorrhage. There is fibroblastic proliferation of intramuscular tissue in which metaplastic woven bone may arise directly (Fig. 22.67) or as a result of ossification of islands of cartilage. The muscle fibres are not primarily involved but may become compressed and surrounded by osseous tissue. When adjacent bone and periosteum are injured the area of ossification often forms in continuity with the periosteum and may be difficult to distinguish from parosteal osteosarcoma. A similar condition of unknown pathogenesis involving both muscles and the pararticular tissues (*heterotopic ossification*) of paraplegics is also described. It affects particularly the hip or knee joint, the joints sometimes being completely fixed by bridges of bone.

Progressive myositis ossificans is a very rare disease of unknown etiology, not hereditary but sometimes associated with congenital abnormalities, in which there is progressive ossification of various muscles in the body, in some cases almost the whole skeleton being immobilised by the newly-formed bone. The affection starts in early life, usually in infancy, and involves the neck, back and shoulders; the disease then extends to other muscles, those of mastication not infrequently being involved. The first indication of the disease is the formation of doughy and sometimes painful swellings in the muscles, and when the swellings subside ossification takes place in the areas of fibrosis. In this way strands and plates of bone of an irregular form are produced in the muscles. The disease advances by a series of attacks rather than by steady progression, and the exacerbations are sometimes accompanied by fever.

B. Inflammatory diseases of muscle

Skeletal muscle becomes secondarily implicated by acute and chronic inflammation of the interstitial tissue. The changes vary according to the nature of the inflammatory lesion. Thus in acute inflammation, oedema and necrosis of the muscle followed by phagocytosis are prominent features, whilst in chronic inflammation there is fibrosis with atrophy and disappearance of the muscle fibres.

Acute myositis also occurs in Weil's disease.

Bacterial myositis

Gas gangrene is an important acute lesion of muscles lacerated by severe trauma and contaminated by soil and often by foreign bodies such as fragments of clothing. If there is sufficient deprivation of oxygen in the wound, the muscles are invaded by anaerobic organisms, the commonest of these being *Clostridium welchii*, which spreads within the sarcous sheath, causing oedema and necrosis of the fibres throughout their length and in all the tissues adjacent to the wound through the effects of its α-toxin. The muscle fibres show coagulative necrosis and vacuolation and contain, as do the interstitial tissues, large numbers of Gram-positive bacilli (Fig. 22.68). At the margins of the infection, oedema, haemorrhage and vascular damage are seen, and there is some leukocytic infiltrate which, owing to the leukocidins produced, is abundant only in mild infections and the less severely damaged areas (see p. 139).

Suppuration in muscle is usually the result of direct extension from other suppurative lesions, especially of joints and bones. The metastatic type, due to haematogenous infection associated with *Staphylococcus aureus*, is very uncommon in Great Britain and occurs in the tropics, and particularly in West Africa, when it may have an association with filarial infection.

Zenker's degeneration (pp. 68, 516), a form of focal coagulative necrosis, is sometimes seen in the abdominal muscles in typhoid fever, and occasionally in epidemic influenza. The affected muscles may sometimes be recognised by the naked eye from their pale hyaline appearance.

Viral myositis

Epidemic myalgia (pleurodynia, Bornholm disease) is an acute transient febrile illness due to Coxsackie B virus and involving the muscles in the costal region, back and shoulders. The affected muscles are tender and painful on movement and in some cases biopsy has shown acute myositis. In the CSF there is pleocytosis and a raised globulin level.

Parasitic myositis

Trichinosis. This affection is produced in the human subject usually by the ingestion of uncooked pork containing the embyros of *Trichinella* or *Trichina spiralis*. It is rare in this country, except for an occasional epidemic. When an infested muscle, e.g. a portion of trichinous "measly" pork, is examined, whitish oval specks may be seen with the naked eye. On microscopic examination, it is found that these represent small oval cysts, containing embryonic trichinellae. A number of the cysts may be calcified, and when the parasites die, they also

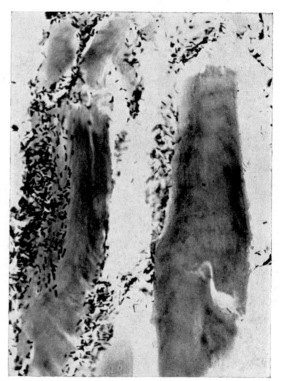

FIG. 22.68.—Gas gangrene, showing necrosis and oedema of muscle with numerous *Cl. welchii* but virtually no leukocytes. × 400.

become calcified. When infested muscle is eaten by another animal, the cyst walls become dissolved by the gastric juice and the embyros are set free. In the bowel they reach full sexual maturity, and the impregnated females bore their way into the wall of the small intestine. The young trichinellae are discharged and migrate by lymphatics to the thoracic duct and circulating blood, from which they penetrate the muscles, especially those of the abdominal and thoracic walls, the diaphragm, muscles of the pharynx, tongue and eye, though the heart and limb muscles may also be affected. The larvae encyst probably in the interfascicular fibrous tissue and the adjacent muscle fibres become swollen, lose their striations and are destroyed.

The symptoms which occur during the passage of the young parasites from the intestine to the muscle vary in intensity according to the number of the parasites; when the infestation is heavy there may be fever, muscle pains, difficulty in swallowing and breathing. Oedema of the face, especially around the eyes, is a common symptom. Death occasionally follows due to myocarditis or involvement of respiratory muscles, with bronchopneumonia. There is marked eosinophilia in the acute phase of invasion.

C. Secondary neural atrophy of muscle

Generalised progressive muscular weakness is usually due to neurogenic atrophy, muscular dystrophy or polymyositis. The differentiation between the various types may sometimes be fairly straightforward but in others the correct diagnosis can be reached only after careful clinical, neurophysiological and biochemical studies and histochemical, histological and ultrastructural examination of muscle. As this is an extremely complex field, only the salient facts will be considered in the accounts that follow. The histological changes in the muscle follow a similar pattern in all conditions of neural atrophy with variations dependent to some extent on the type of onset and rapidity of progression. Following acute nerve section histological changes may be seen in about six weeks, but in a slowly progressive condition clinical weakness may be present for many months before any abnormality in the muscle is diagnosable. Only those fibres atrophy which have lost their nerve supply and this leads to small or large groups of atrophic fibres lying adjacent to groups of normal unaffected fibres (Fig. 22.69), though occasionally, e.g. in poliomyelitis, a whole muscle may be atrophied. The atrophied muscle fibres may be 5–10 μ in diameter and there is an apparent increase in sarcolemmal nuclei due to shrinkage of sarcoplasm, which, however, retains its cross-striations and normal staining reactions. Sometimes the sarcolemmal sheaths are empty but there is little interstitial cellular infiltrate. Later there may be fibrous tissue proliferation around atrophic muscle groups, and a considerable increase in fat. The unaffected muscle fibres usually show little if any compensatory hypertrophy.

Anterior poliomyelitis is a good example of an acute neural atrophy and here it is common to find, within an atrophic motor unit, between one atrophic unit and another and even in different muscles, that muscle fibres are in much the same stage of atrophy. In diseases of less acute onset, such as motor neurone disease (p. 658) and in the various types of polyneuropathy (p. 662), the fibres show a greater variation of size within the motor unit as though all did not undergo atrophy at the same pace. A particularly characteristic feature in progressive neurogenic atrophy is the occurrence of collateral and ultraterminal axonal sprouting and the formation of new

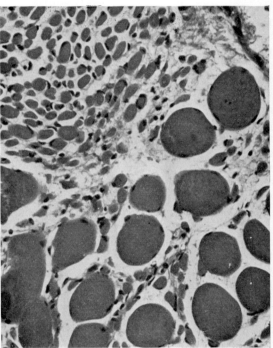

FIG. 22.69.—Muscle following neural atrophy. A group of small atrophic fibres in the upper left hand corner is seen adjacent to normally sized fibres. × 320. (Dr. A. McQueen.)

motor end plates (p. 663). Later, groups of muscle fibres may become more uniform in size but there is still variation from one group to another and it is only in longstanding disease that uniform atrophy is seen.

Peroneal muscular atrophy of Charcot-Marie-Tooth. This is a hereditary disease, commoner in boys and usually developing in children or young adults. Weakness and atrophy, often symmetrical, first develop in the extensor and abductor muscles of the feet, giving rise to pes cavus; later all muscles below the middle of the thigh and sometimes the hand and forearm muscles may be involved. The muscular atrophy is thought to be secondary to degeneration of the lower motor neurons, but there may also be changes in the spinal cord similar to those seen in Friedreich's ataxia (see p. 659).

D. Muscular dystrophies

The muscular dystrophies are hereditary conditions, usually of insidious onset, characterised by progressive muscular weakness and wasting and due to an intrinsic defect in the muscle itself.

While muscular dystrophy comprises many different clinical syndromes the histological appearances have a basic similarity. Each muscle fibre is affected as an individual unit and this leads to a very intimate admixture of muscle fibres of all sizes, a few of normal size, many in varying stages of atrophy and some of increased diameter. The atrophying fibres lose their polygonal shape on cross-section and become rounded and may be further diminished in size by longitudinal splitting. Degenerative changes such as increased eosinophilia, loss of cross-striation, flocculation and phagocytosis of sarcoplasm are seen, often associated with an interstitial cellular infiltrate (Fig. 22.70). Transverse sections of muscle sometimes show that nuclei, instead of being confined as normally to the peripheral sheath, are present within the sarcoplasm—*central nuclei*. Infiltration of fat between individual fibres may be notable and endomysial rather than perimysial fibrosis occurs.

Pseudohypertrophic muscular dystrophy (Duchenne type of muscle dystrophy). This form of muscular dystrophy is inherited as a sex-linked recessive, is almost exclusively found in males and usually arises insidiously about the age of 5 years, though occasionally older patients are affected. The wasting and loss of power begin symmetrically in the thighs and pelvic girdle, the calf muscles may be enlarged and the shoulder girdle is sometimes later involved. The child waddles, has difficulty in standing up, rising from sitting and climbing stairs. Tendon reflexes are reduced. The disease progresses inexorably without remission and the patient often dies in adolescence from intercurrent infection. The affected muscles, including the "hypertrophic" calves, in the terminal stage of the disease are almost entirely replaced by fat, only a few scattered muscle fibres remaining though the muscle spindles are unaffected.

Facio-scapulo-humeral dystrophy. The disease, which usually begins in adolescence, may arise earlier or later, the more delayed the onset the better the prognosis. Both males and females are affected and there is often a family history. The initial stage is insidious and asymmetric involvement of the muscles of the shoulder girdle, arms, trunk and face sometimes progresses later to affect the lower limbs. Pseudohypertrophy is not seen. The dystrophy is very chronic, slowly progressive but with long remissions, and seldom gives rise to total disablement. In the later stages there is often some fatty

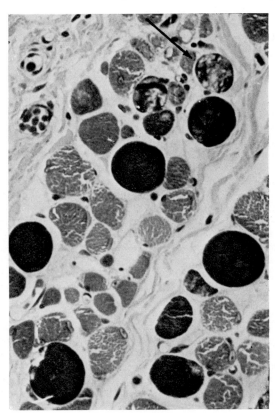

Fig. 22.70.—Muscular dystrophy. Muscle fibres of all sizes are intermixed. Enlarged fibres are conspicuous. A group of fibres in the upper right corner (arrowed) are undergoing floccular degeneration. × 200. (Dr. A. McQueen.)

infiltration but not to the same extent as in pseudohypertrophic muscular dystrophy and endomysial fibrosis may be marked.

Dystrophia myotonica. This muscle dystrophy, which occurs in both sexes, usually in adult life, is inherited as a Mendelian dominant. It is associated with premature cataract, gonadal atrophy and sometimes other endocrine disturbances, and is accompanied by myotonia. When a voluntary movement is performed by a patient with myotonia, especially when cold and tired, the muscular contractions take place more slowly and last longer than normal. A similar prolongation of contraction occurs following mechanical or electrical stimulation. The muscles commonly affected by myotonia are those of the tongue, giving rise to dysarthria, and of the hand and forearm resulting in difficulty in releasing any object held in the hand. There is also muscle weakness followed by atrophy of the distal muscles of the upper limb, the face and sternomastoids and sometimes later of the distal muscles of the lower limb. The disease is progressive and disabling, death usually occurring in late middle age.

Microscopically a striking feature may be the presence of long rows of central nuclei.

E. Polymyositis and dermatomyositis

These conditions are regarded as acute degenerative muscle diseases of unknown etiology which sometimes are difficult to differentiate from the dystrophies. In *dermatomyositis* in addition to muscle involvement the skin shows a diffuse erythema with oedema and sometimes also, in the arteriolar walls, multiple foci of fibrinoid degeneration resembling those lesions found in disseminated lupus erythematosus and other connective tissue diseases (p. 812). *Polymyositis* and *dermatomyositis* usually begin in adult life and run an acute course resulting in death, remission or arrest within a year. Muscular weakness, sometimes with tenderness, is an early feature, the proximal muscles being most often affected and in contrast to the dystrophic pattern the bulbar musculature is not infrequently involved with consequent dysarthria and dysphagia. Muscle wasting with diminished tendon jerks follows. The disease may be rapidly fatal due to involvement of the heart or respiratory muscles and in these cases myoglobinuria may result from severe muscle destruction. In less severe cases spontaneous remission may occur at any stage, but is not uncommonly followed by further exacerbation leading to increasing muscle weakness and disability. Occasionally the disease runs a chronic course from the outset.

Microscopic appearances are those of an acute degeneration of muscle fibres with increased eosinophilia, increase in sarcolemmal nuclei, patchy loss of cross-striation and floccular change. In the interstitial tissue a diffuse or focal infiltrate of chronic inflammatory cells, macrophages, neutrophil and eosinophil polymorphs occurs. The muscle fibres show varying degrees of atrophy and some are hypertrophied. There may be attempted muscle regeneration as shown by the presence of thin basophilic muscle fibres sometimes with sarcolemmal giant cells. Even in the later stages endomysial fibrosis is seldom marked. The histological differentiation

between dystrophy and polymyositis becomes increasingly difficult the less acute the lesion and in the later stages or in the chronic form of polymyositis may be almost impossible.

Miscellaneous disorders of muscle

Muscle weakness associated with carcinoma

Muscle weakness and wasting in patients with carcinoma may be due to nutritional factors, to neural atrophy which is sometimes attributable to suitably placed metastases, but sometimes to carcinomatous neuropathy (p. 665), and also possibly to a primary affection of the muscle. In the latter group the weakness, occasionally associated with myasthenia, usually involves the proximal muscles. The condition is most commonly associated with bronchial and pancreatic carcinoma and one of the striking features is that the severity of the myopathy does not parallel the extent of the malignant disease. The myopathy may be striking many months before the carcinoma is diagnosable clinically, or may remit when the patient is dying from the neoplasm.

Histological changes in the muscle may be non-specific, being those of simple atrophy with an increase of sarcolemmal nuclei. A clear understanding of this condition has not yet been achieved. In other cases the changes resemble those in polymyositis, with flocculation and vacuolation of the sarcous substance and pronounced cellular infiltration between the fibres, some of which show longitudinal splitting (Fig. 22.71).

Myasthenia gravis

Definition. This is a disease in which excessive weakness of voluntary muscles develops during prolonged or repeated use, apparently as a result of impaired neuromuscular transmission of motor stimuli.

Neurophysiological considerations. The arrival of a nerve impulse at a neuromuscular junction normally releases acetylcholine, and causes depolarisation of the adjacent, specially modified surface of the muscle fibre: when depolarisation exceeds 15–20 mV, contraction is stimulated. In normal subjects the amount of acetylcholine released is much greater than is required to achieve this degree of depolarisation.

The defect in myasthenia gravis has not been fully elucidated, but the available evidence suggests that there is an inadequate liberation of acetylcholine.

Clinical features. Usually myasthenia gravis begins during adolescence or early adult life and principally affects females. Less often, it presents in middle age and is then commoner in males, rarely it occurs in the babies of myasthe-

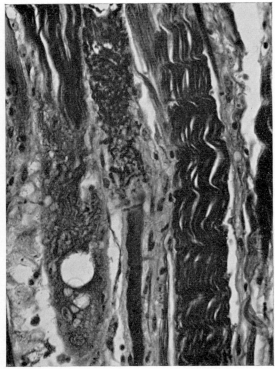

Fig. 22.71.—Carcinomatous myopathy showing splitting of muscle fibres, flocculation and loss of striation. × 400.

nic women—"neonatal myasthenia". The external ocular muscles and those of the head and neck are most frequently affected, the arm muscles less frequently, and those of the leg and trunk least often. Muscle function may be normal early in the day but with use symptoms develop which are, at least partly, reversed by rest or anticholinesterase drugs. The severity of the disease varies considerably and fluctuations occur in the intensity of the muscle weakness in individual cases. Dramatic accentuation of the myasthenic state—myasthenic crisis—is common, and is sometimes precipitated by infection or trauma. Death may result from weakness of

respiratory muscles. Overdosage with anticholinesterase drugs produces a "cholinergic crisis" due to persisting depolarisation of the motor end plates.

Clinically, myasthenia gravis is frequently associated with various types of thyroid disease, notably thyrotoxicosis.

Pathological features. *Muscles.* Histologically the voluntary muscles are involved in an irregular and patchy fashion. Three distinct types of lesion may occur: (1) patchy coagulative necrosis of individual muscle fibres with an associated inflammatory infiltrate; (2) lymphorrhages, in which there is focal atrophy of a muscle fibre with infiltration of lymphocytes around it; (3) simple atrophy without reactive changes affecting single muscle fibres or groups of fibres.

None of these changes is specific for myasthenia gravis. Lymphorrhages occur in Addison's disease, rheumatoid arthritis and Hashimoto's disease, while focal necrosis is seen in various types of myositis, and atrophy in many conditions.

Motor end plates. The motor end plates are elongated and distorted in myasthenia gravis and there is proliferation of subterminal nerve fibres, but it is not clear whether these are primary or compensatory changes. Descriptions of the ultrastructural appearances are somewhat contradictory.

Thymus. Ninety per cent of patients with myasthenia gravis have thymic changes and these are of two kinds: (*a*) Numerous large lymphoid follicles with germinal centres develop in the thymic medulla in over 80 per cent of patients who do not have a thymic tumour and also commonly in the residual thymus gland in patients with a thymoma. In addition to the large germinal centres the glands often show failure of age involution of the cortex. This type of lesion is found predominantly amongst young female patients. (*b*) Thymic tumours are present in myasthenia gravis in 10 per cent of patients, most of whom are middle-aged and male. The tumour is usually of mixed epithelial and lymphocytic cells, the proportion of the two cell types varying between tumours and in different areas of the same tumour. The epithelial cells are usually plump and rounded. The tumours are locally invasive; they frequently become adherent to the mediastinal blood vessels and may invade the lungs though distant metastases are uncommon. Rarely, myasthenia gravis may develop after removal of a thymic tumour which has presented with other symptoms.

The likelihood of improvement or cure following thymectomy depends on the type of thymic change. In general, response is best in young patients without a thymic tumour, particularly if the symptoms are of short duration, however, there is considerable individual variation and the response in any particular case is not predictable. Removal of a neoplastic thymus is not usually followed by dramatic improvement.

Immunological aspects. It is known that the serum of most normal subjects contains antibodies to the I bands of skeletal muscle. In myasthenia, especially in subjects who have thymic tumours, the titre tends to be higher, and is likely to be a result of muscle damage rather than its cause. Some myasthenic patients with a thymic tumour have antibodies to the A bands of skeletal muscle. There is a significant increase in the incidence of auto-antibodies to thyroid tissue antigens in myasthenic subjects.

Etiology. Since the thymus is now known to play a major role in immunological responsiveness, the presence of thymic changes in myasthenia gravis, and the response to thymectomy in some cases suggest the possibility that immunological factors might play a part in the etiology though this still remains obscure. The occurrence of transient neonatal myasthenia raises the possibility of a humoral causal factor but none has been isolated and there is no correlation between neonatal myasthenia and the titre of maternal antibody to muscle. Recently Goldstein has suggested, from immunological studies in guinea-pigs, that the thymus is damaged by an auto-immune reaction and that this leads to the liberation of increased amounts of a substance, "thymin", which inhibits neuromuscular transmission. Other workers have so far failed to confirm his findings.

Periodic paralysis

Muscular activity requires that the intracellular potassium concentration be maintained at normal levels but if the plasma potassium is depleted, as in gastro-intestinal fluid loss, in certain renal disturbances, and on recovery from diabetic coma, weakness of the voluntary muscles and cardiac irregularity may develop and the former may amount to temporary muscular paralysis. The rare familial disorder known as *periodic paralysis*, inherited as an autosomal dominant, is associated with intermittently low levels in the plasma potassium concentration and attacks of muscle weakness may be precipitated by rest following exercise, and by the ingestion of large amounts of carbohydrate. The cardiac irregularity is curiously slight in contrast to the findings in other states of potassium depletion.

Myotonia congenita (Thomsen's disease)

This rare congenital and hereditary disease was described by Thomsen who suffered from it himself. It is commoner in males and first appears in childhood, muscular contraction either voluntary or on electrical stimulation being delayed in onset and slower in performance than is normal. Myotonia may be localised or widespread and the affected muscles are hypertrophied and more powerful than normal. The tendon reflexes are not abnormal. The myotonia may diminish with advancing age and in any case life is not shortened. Occasionally involved muscles may eventually become somewhat atrophic. Histologically the muscle fibres may be enlarged with some central nuclei, and striation is poorly marked.

THE CONNECTIVE TISSUE DISEASES

The concept that the connective tissues of the body comprise a system, subject to its own specific diseases, led Klemperer and his colleagues to introduce the term *diffuse collagen disease*. It has subsequently become apparent that in most types of disease affecting the connective tissues, collagen is not solely nor primarily involved, and accordingly the term *connective tissue disease* is to be preferred. The diseases most commonly included under this heading are rheumatoid arthritis (RA), systemic lupus erythematosus (SLE), rheumatic fever, progressive systemic sclerosis, scleroderma, polyarteritis nodosa and dermatomyositis. The group of diseases is also referred to, somewhat loosely, as the *rheumatic diseases*. They are now classed together not because they are clear-cut examples of diseases affecting primarily the cells or matrix of the connective tissues (which is doubtful), but because they present associations with one another, suggesting common etiological and pathogenic factors. Many other conditions—mostly rare and of unknown etiology—could be regarded as connective tissue diseases, but this simply increases the size and heterogeneity of the group.

General features. Little is known of the etiology of the connective tissue diseases. There are, however, certain features which are generally applicable to the group: these are as follows:

(1) *Sex incidence.* As a group, these diseases affect females more often than males.

(2) *Overlap between diseases.* Although readily distinguishable from one another in typical cases, the connective tissue diseases show considerable overlap. For example, patients presenting mixed features of systemic lupus erythematosus (SLE) and rheumatoid arthritis are not uncommon, while polyarteritis nodosa may complicate either of these conditions and develops also in some patients with progressive systemic sclerosis.

(3) *Hereditary factors.* Epidemiological studies suggest that rheumatoid arthritis tends to occur with undue frequency among the blood relatives of cases. However, this familial tendency is not strong, and moreover it is not known whether it is dependent on genetic predisposition, environmental factors (e.g. a transmissible agent), or both. There is some evidence also that the other diseases tend to occur with undue frequency in the relatives of individuals with rheumatoid arthritis.

(4) *Immunological features.* The serum level of IgG is commonly raised in patients with SLE, less commonly in rheumatoid arthritis and the other diseases. Of more interest is the presence in the serum of various auto-antibodies. The best known of these are rheumatoid factor and antibodies to deoxyribonucleoprotein and other constituents of cell nuclei. Rheumatoid factor (p. 795) is present in a high proportion of patients with RA, and a high titre is usually associated with this condition. However, it is by no means always present in RA, and low titres are quite common in apparently healthy individuals. The incidence and titres of rheumatoid factor are increased in the other connective tissue diseases. Antinuclear antibodies (p. 111), particularly antibody to deoxyribonucleoprotein, are virtually always present in the serum of patients with active SLE, and are frequently demonstrable in the other diseases. Like rheumatoid factor, antibody to deoxyribonucleoprotein is not uncommon in low titre in apparently normal individuals. Various other auto-antibodies to cellular constituents have been described in the serum of patients with connective tissue diseases: like antinuclear antibodies, they react with antigens common to a wide variety of cells and are not "organ-specific".

(5) *Pathological changes.* The lesions of the connective tissue diseases vary considerably in appearance, and the differences are due to the occurrence, in various combinations, of fibrinoid change, necrosis, acute and chronic inflammation and dense fibrosis. The changes occur focally in the connective tissues in various parts of the body, and also in the walls of small blood vessels. Vascular involvement is of particular importance, because it leads to ischaemia and thus to secondary changes, not only in the connective tissues, but also in the parenchyma of various organs and in the skin. Since none of these pathological changes is specific, morphological diagnosis of the connective tissue diseases depends upon the appearance and site of the individual lesions, e.g. the polyarthritis of RA, the glomerular and skin lesions of SLE, and the necrotising inflammatory arterial lesions of polyarteritis nodosa. The major pathological features of the individual diseases are described in the appropriate systematic chapters, and the following brief accounts are intended simply to summarise the various manifestations of each disease.

Rheumatoid arthritis. This disease is described on pp. 793–5. In addition to the characteristic polyarthritis and lesions in other tissues, it may accompany overt SLE, and may also be complicated by the incomplete picture of SLE, e.g. a positive LE-cell test (see below). Anaemia is common in RA; usually it is of dyshaemopoietic nature, but occasionally auto-immune haemolytic anaemia develops.

Polyarthritis resembling RA, but usually relatively mild, complicates some cases of psoriasis, and typical RA is a common feature of Sjögren's syndrome (p. 477). Pain in the joints, usually without progressive structural changes, is common in rheumatic fever, progressive systemic sclerosis, and polyarteritis nodosa.

The etiology of rheumatoid arthritis remains unknown. Features suggesting an immunological disturbance include (1) enlargement of the lymph nodes, which show microscopically a marked hyperplasia of the cortical germinal centres, suggestive of an antibody response; (2) the common occurrence of rheumatoid factor and antinuclear antibodies, and (3) the heavy lymphocytic and plasma-cell infiltration of the synovia of affected joints. These features, together with the occurrence of acute arthritis in such hypersensitivity states as serum sickness, suggest that the disease is due to a hypersensitivity reaction, but the nature of the hypothetical antigenic stimulus has not been established.

Systemic lupus erythematosus. This is an uncommon condition, affecting mostly adolescent females and young women. It may run an acute course with fever, and if untreated is often fatal in months or years, the commonest cause of death being renal failure. The clinical features and pathological changes show great individual variation. The tissues most often involved are the skin (p. 933), the kidneys (p. 711), the endocardium (p. 320), and the serous membranes, but any organ may be affected. There may be arthritic pain, pleurisy, albuminuria, haematuria and the nephrotic syndrome. Fibrinoid change is seen in the small vessels—arterioles, capillaries and venules—in the various tissues. This may have important effects by causing ischaemia, but fibrinoid change occurs also in avascular connective tissue, e.g. in the heart valves. Necrosis, a granulomatous reaction and fibrosis are also common features.

Patients with SLE have a strong tendency to develop hypersensitivity to various drugs. Haematological features include leukopenia, sometimes thrombocytopenia, and less commonly auto-immune haemolytic anaemia. These are probably all due to immunological reactions. Auto-antibodies to nuclear and other cellular constituents occur with greater frequency in SLE than in the other connective tissue diseases. In the LE-cell test, examination of the patient's leukocytes following incubation of whole blood at 37°C shows phagocytosis of homogeneous basophilic material by neutrophil polymorphs (Fig. 22.72). These so-called LE cells result from

the reaction of auto-antibody to deoxyribonucleoprotein with the nuclei of degenerate leukocytes, with subsequent fixation of complement and phagocytosis of the altered nuclear material. The test is positive in patients with a high plasma level of antibody to deoxyribonucleoprotein ("LE-cell factor"). It is not positive in all cases of SLE, and is positive in a small proportion of patients with RA or other connective tissue diseases. The lesions of SLE

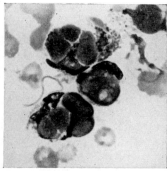

Fig. 22.72.—LE cells from a case of disseminated lupus erythematosus. × 600.

Three cells are shown with the characteristic ingested masses of altered nuclear material.
(From a preparation kindly lent by Dr. J. M. Robertson.)

commonly exhibit patchy basophilia, the so-called haematoxyphil bodies, due to deposition of deoxyribonucleoprotein complexed with antibody. Serological tests for syphilis, e.g. the Wassermann reaction, are commonly positive in SLE, and are due to auto-antibodies which cross-react with antigenic constituents of cardiolipin.

There is now good evidence that the glomerular lesions are due to a type III hypersensitivity reaction (p. 711) resulting from deposition of immune complexes composed of auto-antibodies and the corresponding auto-antigens, in the glomerular capillary walls. Fibrinoid lesions in the skin and elsewhere may be of similar nature. The cause of the predisposition to develop auto-antibodies and hypersensitivity to drugs is, however, not known. Investigations on NZB/NZW mice, which develop spontaneously a disease resembling SLE (p. 111) suggest the possibility that virus infection may play a pathogenic role, but virological studies in SLE have so far been inconclusive.

Progressive systemic sclerosis. The main features of this rare chronic disease are intimal thickening of small arteries and arterioles, patchy loss of specialised tissue, and replacement fibrosis. In addition to the skin lesion (p. 934), the gastro-intestinal tract, heart, skeletal muscles, kidneys and lungs are most often affected. Clinical features include dysphagia from fibrosis and loss of smooth muscle of the oesophagus, respiratory insufficiency and repeated infections resulting from progressive pulmonary fibrosis, and disturbances of the gastro-intestinal tract. The interlobular renal arteries are narrowed by severe concentric intimal fibrosis resembling closely that of malignant hypertension: patchy renal ischaemia results, and there may be associated hypertension. Vascular involvement and shrinkage of the skin bring about ischaemia of the extremities, often with Raynaud's phenomenon (p. 283), and sometimes progressing to ulceration and gangrene. There may also be subcutaneous calcification. Cardiac function may be impaired by myocardial fibrosis, hypertension and lung involvement.

The etiology of progressive systemic sclerosis is quite unknown. Antinuclear auto-antibodies may be present in the serum, and the condition may be accompanied by rheumatoid arthritis or lesions suggestive of SLE.

The major features of *scleroderma* (p. 933), *polyarteritis nodosa* (p. 280) and *dermatomyositis* (p. 810) are described in the appropriate systematic chapters.

Rheumatic fever (p. 309) is characterised by severe joint disease, myocardial injury, focal fibrinoid and inflammatory lesions of the connective tissues of the endocardium and of the myocardium, a fibrinous pericarditis and lesions of small vessels. It differs from the other connective tissue diseases in being a complication of a specific infection, namely a pharyngitis due to β-haemolytic streptococci. The pathogenesis is not fully understood, although the cross-reaction of streptococcal antibodies with myocardium, and the demonstration of such antibody attached to myocardium (p. 310) provide strong evidence for the participation of a cytotoxic (type II) immunological reaction (p. 102).

There is little association between the connective tissue diseases and the organ-specific auto-immune diseases (p. 110) except in Sjögren's disease, in which features of both groups are commonly demonstrable.

CHAPTER 23

REPRODUCTIVE SYSTEM

I. MALE

The following account includes little on the relationships between the various endocrine glands and the male reproductive system. This subject is considered in Chapter 24.

INFLAMMATORY CONDITIONS

Acute inflammations of the male genital tract are due to two main causes, gonorrhoea, and septic infections usually secondary to cystitis. Metastatic infection by the blood stream also may occur, but it is less common.

Gonorrhoea

This is acquired by coitus. It is an acute catarrhal inflammation which ascends from the urethral meatus to the anterior part of the urethra. The discharge, at first thick and glairy, soon becomes purulent, and in it gonococci, mainly in neutrophil polymorphs, are usually numerous. If untreated the disease, after running a course of several weeks, often resolves without residual effects, but not infrequently infection may spread to the posterior urethra and a chronic urethritis is established.

Infection of the prostate may be accompanied by acute inflammatory swelling, while in the chronic stage gonococci often persist in the tubules of the gland and maintain the infection. The organisms may also ascend by the vas deferens and set up acute suppuration, which at first is restricted to the epididymis—*gonorrhoeal epididymitis*, but may occasionally extend to the body of the testis, leading to scarring and atrophy. Infection of the bladder by gonococci occasionally causes cystitis. Two other serious complications may occur: firstly, ulceration of the posterior urethra, leading to stricture, dilatation and hypertrophy of the bladder, secondary infection by other organisms and septic cystitis; and secondly, the organisms may be distributed by the blood stream and give rise to inflammation in other parts of the body. The commonest of these are in the joints and sheaths of tendons, but occasionally other conditions, such as pleurisy, endocarditis and even septicaemia may develop. Gonococcal infections are usually highly susceptible to treatment with penicillin or the sulphonamide drugs and all these complications have become in consequence much less frequent. However, drug-resistance and changes in social behaviour are probably responsible for the increase in gonorrhoea and its complications observed in recent years.

Non-bacterial urethritis

Acute non-bacterial urethritis in males is commonly of venereal origin. The causal agent is unknown, but there is some evidence implicating an organism of the Bedsonia group, apparently identical with the TRIC agent (TR for trachoma and IC for inclusion conjunctivitis of neonates). This form of urethritis, known as Reiter's syndrome (p. 796), is sometimes accompanied by conjunctivitis and followed by arthritis. There is indirect evidence that the same agent may cause infection of the cervix uteri in women and conjunctivitis with inclusion bodies in the newborn.

The testis

Orchitis

As mentioned above, epididymitis and orchitis may result from spread of gonococci or coliform bacilli along the vasa deferentia as a complication of gonococcal urethritis or coliform cystitis respectively. The inflammation may progress to suppuration, and result in fibrosis and obliteration of the testicular tubules.

Of infections by the blood-stream, the commonest is that which occurs in mumps, this complication being comparatively common in adults but rare in children. The lesion is a diffuse non-suppurative inflammation of the testis itself, which may give rise to fibrosis with atrophy and secondary infertility. Orchitis may complicate smallpox and other viral diseases and occasionally also various pyogenic infections by staphylococci, streptococci, pneumococci, etc.

Strangulation of the testis as a result of acute torsion of the spermatic cord leads to infarction of the organ, which may be intensely haemorrhagic. Clinically, it may resemble acute orchitis.

Chronic orchitis. This may be the result of the acute conditions already described, or it may be chronic throughout—*primary fibrosis* of the testis, which may be localised or diffuse. In many instances the etiology of interstitial fibrosis is obscure, but the possibility of tertiary syphilis must be investigated. There is also a condition of *chronic granulomatous orchitis* which presents clinically as a unilateral painful swelling of the testis; after a few weeks this subsides leaving an indurated organ of diminished sensitivity to pressure. The etiology is obscure. The lesion is characterised by interstitial inflammatory infiltration of lymphocytes, plasma cells and sometimes eosinophils, together with atrophy of the germinal epithelium and replacement by inflammatory cells including many giant cells. The lesion bears a superficial resemblance to tuberculosis because the outlines of the replaced tubules confer a follicular appearance on the lesion, but caseation is absent and tubercle bacilli have not been demonstrated. It is regarded by some as a low-grade infection by coliform bacilli; others have suggested, with little supporting evidence, an auto-immune pathogenesis.

Prostatitis

Acute inflammation of the prostate is usually produced by spread of organisms from the urethra, in either gonorrhoea or septic cystitis. The gonococcus produces an acute catarrhal inflammation in the prostate with swelling of the surrounding tissue and increased secretion. Gonococcal prostatitis may pass into a chronic state in which the organisms persist for a long time in the tubules, the secretion of which remains infective. In cases of septic cystitis, acute inflammation of the prostate is often followed by multiple foci of suppuration, or a large abscess may form and the prostate may be extensively destroyed. Similar changes may occur also in the seminal vesicles in the conditions mentioned above.

Chronic interstitial prostatitis or *prostatic fibrosis* is a condition in which there is a diffuse scarring of the gland, leading to diminution in size. Like prostatic hypertrophy, it may lead to urethral obstruction. Its etiology is unknown but probably it is the result of a mild infection. A granulomatous prostatitis, with eosinophils, endothelioid cells and giant cells like that in the testis, has also been observed.

Tuberculosis

Tuberculosis of the male genital tract is less common than formerly; it is usually of haematogenous origin, being secondary to a tuberculous lesion elsewhere; in some instances it results from the spread of bacilli along the vas deferens from the base of the bladder. In nearly all cases the epididymis is first affected. Tubercles form in some part and undergo caseation, and ultimately the tissue of the epididymis may be entirely destroyed. The epididymis becomes enlarged and firm, and forms a sausage-shaped structure attached to the testis (Fig. 23.1). On section, large caseous and softened areas are seen. Later the tunica vaginalis may become infected with obliteration by fibrous adhesions or the development of caseous tubercles; the disease then sometimes extends into the substance of the testis. In untreated cases there may be involvement of the skin, and ulceration with formation of a sinus may follow. The vas deferens usually becomes affected, and may contain tuberculous pus and be focally obliterated. The disease ultimately reaches the seminal vesicles and may involve also the prostate and the base of the bladder. As already mentioned, it occasionally spreads in the reverse direction, i.e. upwards from the bladder to the epididymis in cases of urinary tuberculosis. In children we have occasionally seen tuberculosis affect the body of the testis without involvement of the epididymis, but this is rare.

Tuberculosis of the *prostate* is occasionally blood-borne, but in most cases results from secondary spread of infection, either by the vas deferens from the epididymis or from tuberculosis of the bladder. It usually caseates and may destroy the gland. When septic cystitis supervenes in tuberculosis, suppurative prostatitis may also result. Tuberculosis of the seminal vesicles is common in the conditions mentioned, and the lesions are often extensive. The vesicles become greatly enlarged and tense, and may be entirely replaced by caseous softened material in the central parts; some surgical authorities regard this as the commonest initial focus of infection in the genital tract and consider that it spreads from there to epididymis and prostate.

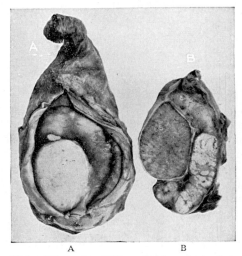

FIG. 23.1.—Bilateral epididymal tuberculosis: in A, the irregularly swollen epididymis is seen above the testis; in B, caseation in the other epididymis is shown on section. × ⅔.

Syphilis

Apart from the primary sore, which has been described already (p. 148), the commonest site of syphilis in the genital tract is the testis, where

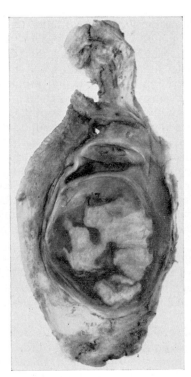

FIG. 23.2.—Gumma of testis, showing large irregular necrotic areas. × ⅘.

gumma and diffuse interstitial inflammation are often combined. Gumma starts almost invariably in the body of the testis, causing painless enlargement and induration. Extensive dull yellowish necrotic areas develop with an irregular outline of more translucent granulation tissue which forms a contrast to the rest of the tissue (Fig. 23.2). Syphilitic orchitis without gummatous change is characterised by growth of cellular connective tissue which afterwards becomes fibrosed, while the tubules become atrophied and disappear.

MISCELLANEOUS DISORDERS OF THE MALE REPRODUCTIVE ORGANS

Atrophy of the testis

This may follow any form of orchitis, and may be of any degree from total destruction to localised scarring. Trauma or vascular obstruction may have similar effects. There are also more selective types of atrophy affecting especially the seminiferous epithelium: this may be produced by X-rays, by treatment with oestrogens, or as a result of pituitary hypofunction. It may also appear as a congenital defect of the germinal cells. In the del Castillo type of atrophy there is a total lack of germ cells, apparently congenital, in all or most of the tubules, which are lined only by Sertoli cells but are otherwise normal.

Sex chromatin. Only one X chromosome is functionally active in the normal cell, and if a second X chromosome is present, it is visible microscopically in most types of cell as a small nodule of chromatin (Barr body) within the nucleus (Fig. 23.3). In neutrophil polymorphs, the chromatin body is seen in a small proportion of cells as a small racquet-like nuclear projection into the cytoplasm (Fig. 23.4).

Klinefelter's syndrome

Properly speaking, this term embraces all cases of major tubular atrophy not involving the Leydig cells: because the tubules are small the Leydig cells appear

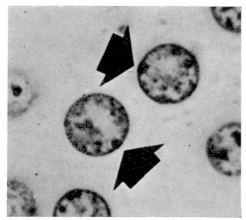

FIG. 23.3.—Nuclear sex chromatin, resembling that of normal females, in the Leydig cells of a case of XXY Klinefelter's syndrome. Testicular biopsy. × 1500.

more prominent than normally, but there is actually no true hyperplasia. All such cases are sterile, gonadotrophic hormone is raised, and there is a tendency to eunuchoidism and gynaecomastia. The del Castillo type of atrophy mentioned above produces a mild form of Klinefelter's syndrome, but

DD

the most interesting variety, to which the name is often restricted, is due to a chromosomal defect. In its most typical form this is XXY—i.e. there is an extra X chromosome in addition to the normal male set. They develop as males, but the extra X is responsible for the features noted above, a very severe

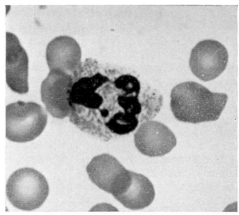

FIG. 23.4.—Polymorphonuclear leukocyte showing typical female sex-chromatin drumstick. × 1500.

degree of tubular atrophy, which results in very small testes, and for the presence, in some cases, of mental defect. The extra X chromosome is also responsible for the appearance, in most of the cells of the body, of the nuclear sex chromatin, recognition of which makes it possible to diagnose the condition with considerable confidence from a biopsy (Fig. 23.3), a smear of buccal epithelium, or a blood film (Fig. 23.4) without doing a complete chromosome count. A male who is chromatin-positive is much more likely to be a case of chromosomal Klinefelter's syndrome than anything else. The condition is far from rare, 1 in 400 male births and 1 in 100 male mental defectives having the XXY chromosome abnormality. The presence of mental defect in other conditions in which an extra chromosome is present, e.g. Down's syndrome (trisomy-21) and the XXX syndrome, indicate that this follows from the chromosomal disorder. In addition to the usual XXY, cases of mosaics (e.g. a mixture of XXY and XY cells) and of grosser disorders such as XXXY and XXXXY occur: in the latter severe additional congenital defects appear.

Sterility in the male

Total failure to produce spermatozoa (azoospermia) or their production in inadequate numbers (oligospermia) may be due to any of the causes of testicular atrophy mentioned above. There are two major additional forms: *obstruction* in any part of the outflow tract, usually the epididymis or the vas, or a condition known as *maturation arrest*, in which, for reasons not understood, germ cells present in normal numbers, and capable of active division through the earlier stages of spermatogenesis, are yet incapable of producing mature sperm.

Hermaphroditism

This term is properly confined to the rare individuals who possess both testis and ovary: there may be an ovary on one side and a testis on the other, or various mixtures of the two. Intermediate forms of sexual development are a natural consequence: most often the external genitalia are predominantly male at birth and internal genitalia correspond to the gonad nearest to them. Breast development or other signs of feminisation appear at puberty. In most cases the cause is obscure, but some are true mosaics, mixtures of XY and XX cells. There is strong evidence that this can result from double fertilisation, and can be regarded almost as an extreme case of Siamese twinning, with total fusion at the cellular level. These XX/XY mosaics should not be confused with XX/XY blood cell chimeras, in which exchange of blood occurs between twins of unlike sex *in utero*: the chimerism in these cases is limited to the blood-forming tissues, and has interesting effects on the blood groups but none on sexual development.

Intersexes

The term intersex is applied to individuals who are not indisputably of one sex or the other.

States of intersex are not restricted to cases of true hermaphroditism. Both XXY Klinefelter's syndrome (see above) and XO Turner's syndrome (p. 857) can be regarded as intersexes at the chromosome level. Two particularly important and relatively common forms of intersex are:

(a) Adrenal virilism (p. 914) in which a defect of steroid hormone synthesis leads to virilisation of the external genitalia in females: the condition is of special importance because, if recognised early, it can be treated effectively.

(b) Male pseudo-hermaphroditism in which, presumably as a result of temporary failure of testosterone output from the testis *in utero*, male external genitalia are imperfectly developed.

A child of doubtful sex at birth is usually one or other of these two: the sex chromatin (p. 819) distinguishes them reliably.

(c) Testicular feminisation is an interesting though rarer form of intersex in which there is also apparently a defect of male hormone metabolism which affects target organs rather than Leydig cells: the effect is one of usually complete feminisation, though the patients are XY and possess (undescended) testes. The condition results from a defect of a gene of the X chromosome, heterozygous females acting as asymptomatic carriers.

Hypospadias

In this minor maldevelopment of the male external genitalia the urethra opens on the ventral (inferior) surface of the penis. In its greater degrees, with the urethra widely open or opening on the perineum, it merges into the intersexes described above.

Maldescent of the testis

This is another condition which, in its major degrees (with both testes in the abdomen), may be regarded as shading into the intersexes. Most often, however, the condition is unilateral and the affected testis is partly descended: in such cases the opposite testis is usually normal. An undescended testis is usually smaller than normal and to some extent malformed: most show a deficiency of germ cells and many have none at all. This defect is, at least in many cases, present in early infancy. In most cases it is probably usually the defect of the testis that is responsible for the maldescent rather than the reverse. It is well established that the risk of development of tumour (usually seminoma) in an undescended testis is substantially increased, though the size of the risk is disputed.

Hyperplasia of the prostate

This is a common condition after the age of about fifty, the incidence rising in each later decade, and enlargement is sometimes marked. The lateral lobes of the gland may be symmetrically or unequally enlarged, and the surface may be comparatively smooth or may be nodular. Such enlargement leads to lateral compression of the urethra. These changes are due to nodular overgrowth chiefly of the inner peri-urethral group of prostatic glands and their fibromuscular stroma, and as the masses enlarge, the outer portion of the gland is compressed into a pseudo-capsule. There may be also enlargement of the so-called median lobe of the gland which comes to form a rounded swelling, growing up at the inner end of the prostatic urethra (Fig. 23.5). This so-called lobe is hardly present normally as a distinct structure, but is represented by collections of glands under the prostatic urethra behind the urethral crest. These may undergo great enlargement along with enlargement of the rest of the gland, but they may be proportionately much greater, and

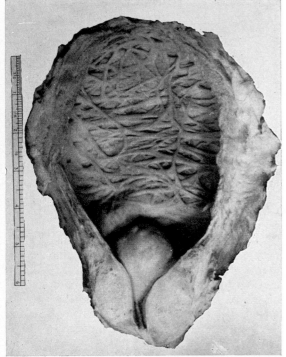

FIG. 23.5.—Hyperplasia of prostate, involving both lateral lobes and the so-called middle lobe. The bladder wall shows marked trabeculation owing to great hypertrophy of the muscle bundles. $\times \frac{5}{12}$.

are often the chief cause of obstruction. A hyperplastic prostate varies in consistency, but is usually firm; the cut surface may have a fairly uniform appearance or adenomatous nodules may be present.

Effects. The urethra may be lengthened, compressed laterally, curved, etc., depending on the form of the prostatic enlargement. The resulting chronic obstruction is followed by hypertrophy and dilatation of the bladder, dilatation of ureters (hydroureter) and renal pelves (hydronephrosis). If unrelieved, these changes may impair renal function and chronic uraemia may result; a fall in the blood urea usually occurs after drainage of the bladder. Pyogenic infection of the urinary tract, including pyelonephritis, is often superadded

(p. 730) and spread to the prostate may precipitate acute retention, as may also partial infarction of the enlarged gland.

Microscopically there is usually increase both of the glandular elements and the stroma (Fig. 23.6). The glands are arranged chiefly in acini lined by columnar cells, and not infrequently show small papilliform ingrowths into the lumina (Fig. 23.7). Often some of the acini are dilated and occasionally small cysts are formed; small concentric concretions or "corpora amylacea" are common. The connective tissue stroma usually contains a substantial proportion of smooth muscle fibres. While the gland acini are usually lined by a single epithelial layer, there may be small foci of more active hyperplasia

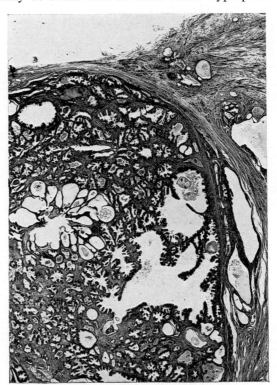

FIG. 23.6.—Simple prostatic enlargement. There is fibromuscular and glandular hyperplasia and some of the gland spaces are dilated. $\times 10$.

with the formation of masses of cells, and a cribriform pattern may develop. Cell aberration may rarely appear and, just as in the breast, all transitions to carcinoma may be observed. Prostatic enlargement is sometimes due chiefly to increase of muscle, but this is rare. The possible relationship between prostatic hyperplasia and carcinoma is considered on p. 827.

The cause of prostatic enlargement is not clearly understood. It is common in middle-aged and elderly men, and may be due to androgen/oestrogen imbalance. There is also some resemblance to the histological changes of cystic disease of the breast. The injection of oestrogens and allied compounds in male mice leads to prostatic enlargement along with other hyperplastic and metaplastic changes in the urinary tract, but the changes do not closely resemble those found in man. The prostate is normally dependent on androgen, and following castration it becomes atrophic. This can be prevented by administering testosterone, and can be delayed by oestrogen. It is apparent, therefore, that the male and female sex hormones are not simply antagonistic in their effects on the prostate. It has been suggested by Franks that the "inner mass" of the prostate, consisting approximately of the peri-urethral part of the

gland, is oestrogen-dependent, and that the "outer mass", consisting of the sub-capsular prostatic tissue, is androgen-dependent. Prostatic hyperplasia affects mainly the inner mass, and might be attributable to relative preponderance of oestrogen as androgen production declines in old age.

Cysts

These occur mainly in relation to the testis. The commonest is *hydrocele*, in which the tunica vaginalis is distended with clear serous fluid. It may result from chronic inflammatory conditions of the testis or from trauma, but often the cause is obscure. Along with the accumulation of fluid, there is dense fibrous thickening of the tunica; inflammatory change is sometimes superadded. If there is haemorrhage as the result of trauma, the term "haematocele" is applied. Clotting of the blood may take place, and the organisation which follows may lead to great thickening of the tunica vaginalis, which may raise suspicion of a testicular tumour. *Encysted hydrocele* or *hydrocele of the cord* is due to a distension with fluid of the non-obliterated remains of the processus vaginalis, the original communication between the tunica vaginalis and the peritoneum. Sometimes the processus is obliterated only at its lower end, and there is an elongated space containing fluid in communication with the peritoneal cavity. Cysts of the body of the testis are rare, but are not uncommon in relation to the *epididymis*. They are usually multiple and small, but occasionally a single large cyst may displace the testis. Cysts in this position contain a clear or turbid fluid, and sometimes spermatozoa, often in a degenerate condition; the cyst is then known as a *spermatocele*. Occasionally rupture into the tunica vaginalis may take place. Cysts of the epididymis are believed to arise by obstruction following infection, especially of the vasa aberrantia, though some may be of congenital origin. A cyst may form also from dilatation of the hydatid of Morgagni.

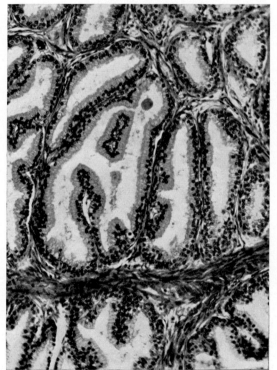

Fig. 23.7.—Section of enlarged prostate, showing hyperplasia of the glandular epithelium. × 130.

TUMOURS

Tumours are much less common than they are in the female genital tract. The following is a summary of the chief types:—

Penis

Papilloma gives rise to sessile or pedunculated reddish lesions of considerable size covering the coronal sulcus and prepuce. These are condylomata acuminata, similar to the commoner vulval growths, and caused by a virus; they are reactive lesions, probably not true tumours (if such a distinction is still tenable) and may involute rapidly under treatment. Giant forms may occur; these are only rarely malignant, but have sometimes been misdiagnosed as squamous carcinoma. The penis is a site of certain precancerous lesions, e.g. leukoplakia and Bowen's disease. A rare variety of epithelial irregularity limited to the penis is that known as *Queyrat's erythroplasia*, an irregular hyperkeratotic overgrowth with much chronic inflammatory infiltration of the dermis. The commonest malignant growth is *squamous carcinoma*, which usually originates from the glans or prepuce; as in other sites it varies from an indurated fissured ulcerating nodule to a massive fungating cauliflower type of growth. It is an uncommon tumour, occurring mainly in non-circumcised men. Among peoples practising ritual circumcision within a few days of birth, penile carcinoma is virtually unknown, but when circumcision is delayed until about puberty, as in Moslems, the incidence of penile carcinoma is only slightly reduced. The smegma which accumulates beneath the prepuce is probably an important carcinogenic factor in this disease. Pigmented naevi and malignant melanomas also occur on penile skin; they present the usual features (p. 942).

Scrotum

In certain occupations, the rugose scrotal skin is prone to retain dirt, and if this is carcinogenic, pre-cancerous papillomas and ultimately squamous carcinoma are apt to develop. Examples were formerly encountered in the classical chimney sweeps' cancer of the scrotum (Fig. 10.2, p. 214), in the scrotal cancer of machine-tool operators, gas-retort workers and men handling arsenic. Precautions to prevent soiling of the scrotal skin with carcinogenic chemicals have greatly reduced the incidence of the condition, but it still occurs. A few years ago we observed a case in a worker in an arsenic-containing weed-killer factory who had neglected to wear protective clothing. The tumour progresses to a fungating ulcer and microscopically is usually a fairly well differentiated squamous carcinoma. The typical naked-eye and microscopic appearances are seen in Figs. 23.8 and 23.9.

Testis

The most important tumours are (*a*) seminoma, (*b*) teratoma, (*c*) papillary adenocarcinoma, and (*d*) orchioblastoma.

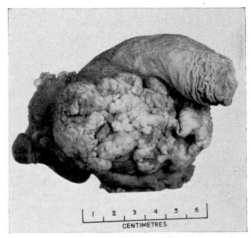

FIG. 23.8.—Squamous carcinoma of the scrotum showing papilliform growth and also extensive ulceration.

(a) Seminoma

This is the commonest malignant tumour of the testis. It occurs particularly in young men, mostly below 30 years of age, and although in most cases there is no known predisposing cause, an undescended testis carries an increased risk of seminoma. The tumour is rounded, has often destroyed the whole testis by the time of removal, and has a white, homogeneous, "potato-like" cut surface (Fig. 23.11*a*). It is composed of rounded

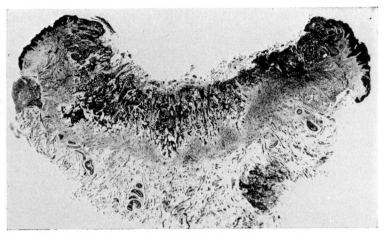

Fig. 23.9.—Squamous carcinoma of scrotum in a worker exposed to arsenic (sheep-dip).
A typical ulcerating squamous carcinoma showing the raised margins and early invasion of the underlying tissues. × 4.

cells, usually large, which are arranged in sheets with comparatively little stroma, or in smaller groups separated by stroma: the cells may have indistinct margins or may appear to be separate from one another due to a shrinkage artefact. In most cases, the tumour is infiltrated with lymphocytes: these tend to aggregate in foci (Fig. 23.10) but may be more diffuse. There is some evidence that heavy lymphocytic infiltration improves the prognosis. Another common feature is a granulomatous sarcoid-like reaction within the tumour. A seminoma forms a large cellular mass, displacing the surviving parenchyma and distending the tunica. It grows along the spermatic cord, and metastases frequently occur in the para-aortic lymph nodes. Nevertheless, the cells are highly sensitive to radiotherapy and therefore long survival occurs in about 90 per cent of cases without obvious spread beyond the testis, and in over 50 per cent of patients with lymphatic and/or blood spread. Dissemination by the veins resulting in pulmonary metastases was present in most of our patients who died within two years.

Seminoma arises from the germinal epithelium. It may arise from a teratoma, and as the prognosis is then much worse, it is important to search carefully for teratomatous elements in a seminomatous testis.

(b) Teratoma of testis

This tumour is less common than seminoma and on average occurs at an earlier age. Some are relatively solid but in others tiny cysts are present; part or whole of the testis may be replaced by the tumour. Although teratoma may be of congenital origin (see p. 258) it does not produce testicular enlargement until adult life. Sometimes there is a history of trauma preceding the development of the tumour.

Some teratomas are less complex and contain

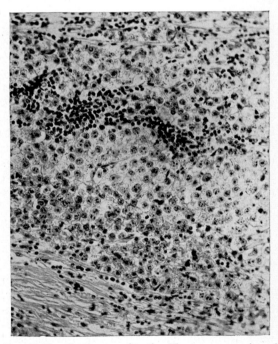

Fig. 23.10.—Seminoma of testis. The tumour consists of large round cells with vesicular nuclei. Note also the lymphocytic infiltration of the stroma. × 210.

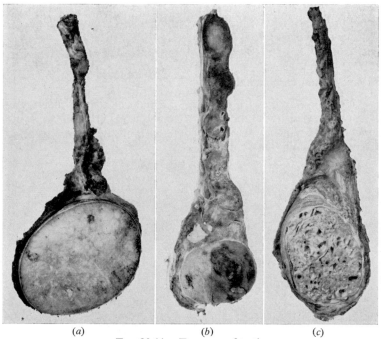

FIG. 23.11.—Tumours of testis.

(*a*) Seminoma testis. × ⅔.   (*b*) Papillary adenocarcinoma. × ¼.   (*c*) Teratoma. × ½.

much cartilage (Fig. 23.12*b*), and the epithelial structures undergo cystic change to produce the distinctive naked-eye appearance which led to the former application of the term "fibrocystic disease" (Fig. 23.11*c*). Very rarely has a testicular teratoma the characters of the common ovarian dermoid cyst.

The most important prognostic feature is that malignancy very frequently supervenes so that undifferentiated or papillary adenocarcinoma (Fig. 23.12*a*) or primitive neuro-epithelial elements are conspicuous (Fig. 23.12*c*). Not infrequently choriocarcinoma may develop. Tests for chorionic gonadotrophin in the urine then become positive in high titres. A positive test at lower titre may also less commonly be associated with other testicular tumours, e.g. seminoma or adenocarcinoma. It is of interest that folic-acid antagonists, which have been shown to have some effect on the growth of post-conceptional choriocarcinoma, are without effect on the growth of teratomatous choriocarcinoma. The prognosis is bad; metastases are common and secondary tumours may be carcinomatous, sarcomatous or even teratomatous. Spread is both by lymphatics and blood stream and retroperitoneal lymph nodes, lungs, liver and other organs may be involved.

(c) Papillary adenocarcinoma

This is a highly malignant tumour of adults, giving rise to a nodular and haemorrhagic mass from which multiple nodules extend along the lymphatic drainage of the cord (Fig. 23.11*b*).

Microscopically it is highly anaplastic, often syncytial and may present areas resembling cyto- and syncytio-trophoblast. The prognosis is extremely bad, none of our cases having survived more than two years.

The relationship between the three chief varieties of malignant testicular tumour is not clear. Most writers accept seminoma as a distinctive tumour, and the prognosis is much better. In an analysis, undertaken some years ago, of our material over the previous 30 years, 50 per cent of cases are alive and well; indeed after adequate therapy it appeared that recurrence either developed within two years or failed to occur at all. With papillary adenocarcinoma and teratoma, the prognosis was uniformly bad, and a noteworthy feature of the teratomas was recurrence and distant metastasis at irregular intervals, sometimes as long as ten years after removal of the primary tumour. Improvement in the prognosis of both types of tumour has been substantial in recent years. Seminoma is extremely radiosensitive, and with adequate early treatment the cure rate is probably now over 90 per cent.

(d) Orchioblastoma (embryonal carcinoma of infancy)

This name has been applied to a uniform cellular whitish tumour that replaces the testicular body in infants, displacing the rete and epididymis, which may be well preserved.

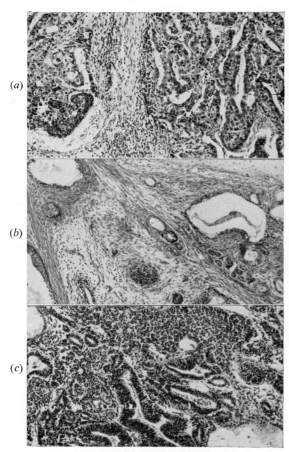

FIG. 23.12.—(*a*) Papillary adenocarcinoma with invasion of venule on left. × 70.

(*b*) Teratoma of testis showing cartilage above and various types of glandular epithelium. × 45.

(*c*) Teratoma of testis, showing highly cellular tissue, probably neuro-epithelial in type. × 60.

Microscopically it shows areas of solid trabecular carcinoma with numerous microscopic cysts, and in places a papilliform architecture (Fig. 23.13). At the margin immature testicular tubules are seen and these may be incorporated

in the growth. This tumour is less highly malignant than the adult papillary adenocarcinoma.

Other tumours

Unless as a constituent of a teratoma, sarcoma of the testis is rare. A small-round-cell tumour resembling lymphosarcoma is occasionally seen

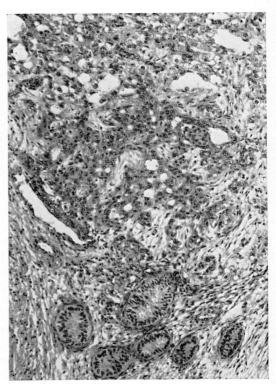

FIG. 23.13.—Orchioblastoma (embryonal carcinoma) of the testis of an infant. × 115.

in the body of the testis, and is highly malignant. Tumours of the interstitial cells of Leydig form yellowish-brown nodules in the body of the testis: in childhood they may cause precocious sexual development by secreting androgens.

Epididymis

Tumours are rare. The commonest is slow-growing and benign and is termed the *adenomatoid tumour*. It consists of flattened or cuboidal cells lining small spaces and embedded in a connective tissue stroma.

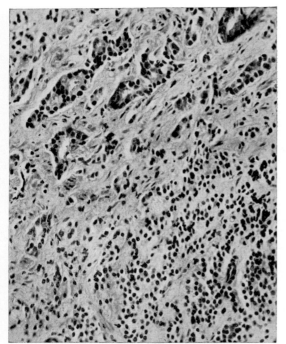

Fig. 23.14.—Carcinoma of prostate gland. The growth is of scirrhous type, consisting of poorly formed micro-acini with transitions to a fine permeation of the tissue by rows of small darkly stained cells. × 225.

Prostate

Carcinoma of the prostate is one of the commoner cancers in older men; sometimes it arises in a hyperplastic prostate, but as some degree of hyperplasia is very common in old men, the significance of the association is doubtful. Moreover, carcinoma arises most often in the posterior lobe which is not usually involved in hyperplasia. The tumour causes urethral obstruction and often pain: it produces general induration of the gland without enlargement, together with adhesions between the gland and its capsule. At first confined to the prostate, the tumour later extends into the neighbouring tissues. It is often not possible to be certain of the diagnosis till microscopic examination is made, but difficulty in removing the gland at operation in one continuous mass is highly suggestive of malignancy. The growth may be of scirrhous micro-acinar carcinoma (Fig. 23.14) or a more cellular florid adenocarcinoma. Carcinoma of the prostate has a tendency to give rise to multiple secondary tumours in the bones, often with considerable bony thickening around them—*osteosclerosis* (p. 775), and accompanied by a marked rise in the acid phosphatase in the blood. These osseous metastases may occur without the presence of secondary tumours in the lungs or other organs, and may be due in part to retrograde venous spread along the veins of Batson, which join the prostatic plexus to the vertebral venous system. Prostatic cancer can often be suppressed by oestrogen therapy for a considerable time: such treatment commonly induces squamous metaplasia of the tumour cells and prostatic glands.

Small foci of subcapsular epithelial overgrowth presenting all the histological features of cancer, including local perineural lymphatic invasion, are found with increasing frequency as age advances; they are present in about 20 per cent of otherwise normal prostates in men over the age of 50 years. The incidence is somewhat lower in glands removed because of benign enlargement, perhaps because the compressed peripheral portion is often left behind in surgical enucleation. The significance of these foci is uncertain, but it is quite apparent from their frequency, and from the relative infrequency of more extensive prostatic cancer, that these small focal "cancers" are in a latent state, and seldom extend sufficiently to cause symptoms or death. Their presence in a surgically-removed hypertrophic prostate poses a problem to pathologist and surgeon, but for clinical purposes it is probably correct to regard as carcinoma only those tumours which have invaded the capsule of the gland.

Adenomatous nodules—single or multiple—occur in the prostate but are usually part of the picture of prostatic hypertrophy. *Sarcoma* of the prostate is rare but is occasionally observed in children; we have personally studied three examples, each of which proved to be a rhabdomyosarcoma.

II. FEMALE REPRODUCTIVE SYSTEM

Few regions of the body are so prone to undergo pathological change as the female genital tract. For detailed information textbooks of gynaecological pathology should be consulted.

For convenience we shall consider the subject under the three main headings of infections, tumours and lesions associated with pregnancy.

INFLAMMATORY CHANGES

Apart from gonorrhoea, acute pyogenic inflammations of the female reproductive organs are rare except for those which follow pregnancy and parturition, abortion and surgical operations. In most cases the organisms enter by the uterine cavity, and spread to other parts, though in certain infections, notably in tuberculosis, infection may occur by the blood stream.

Acute endometritis

This is due to bacterial infection following abortion or parturition. In the absence of products of conception, acute endometritis is very rare, but it occurs occasionally in infective fevers. In the *puerperal state* the retention of portions of placenta or decidua, along with lacerations of the cervix, gives an opportunity for invasion by pathogenic organisms. In addition to the usual pyococci, various bacilli of the coliform and proteus types and even clostridia, e.g. *Cl. welchii*, may be present. In some cases the changes are chiefly within the uterus, and the inflammatory process may be severe and may be accompanied by putrefaction of any retained material.

Gonorrhoea leads especially to a *cervical endometritis*, though the condition may spread to the body of the uterus and thence to the tubes. Gonococcal infection is often accompanied by a superficial interstitial metritis, and is apt to become chronic. The endometrium is, however, somewhat resistant to infections, as there is normally free drainage and the regeneration after menstrual shedding facilitates recovery.

Macroscopic appearances. There is swelling and congestion of the mucosa, desquamation of the surface epithelium, sometimes with haemorrhages, and increased secretion from the glands, mucoid from the cervix and more serous from the body. Later the discharge becomes purulent. In severe cases after abortion or parturition with retained gestational fragments, the uterus is bulky and flabby, and there is a fibrinous exudate on the surface of the mucosa, with some superficial necrosis which may be followed by ulceration. In some cases there is a spreading lymphangitis, much inflammatory oedema, and suppuration; spread to the peritoneum readily occurs and peritonitis follows. Acute endometritis may become chronic, and persist until all gestational products have been removed.

Complications. Inflammatory conditions within the uterus are apt to extend into the uterine wall—*myometritis*—and may spread by the lymphatics to the pelvic connective tissue, with diffuse inflammatory infiltration or *parametritis* as a result; the inflammatory exudate may be serous, fibrinous, or even purulent. Certain organisms, notably the gonococcus, may spread along the Fallopian tubes, causing salpingitis and sometimes peritonitis and oöphoritis.

Infection of the placental site, especially by *Staphylococcus aureus*, may lead to septic thrombosis of the veins locally, and from these, thrombosis may spread to the iliac veins, resulting in *phlegmasia alba dolens* or "white leg". The thrombi may undergo suppurative softening, and the liberation of septic emboli may cause pyaemia. In cases of infection with haemolytic streptococci, fatal septicaemia may occur. Less acute cases with spreading thrombosis may be caused by anaerobic streptococci. These various infections were formerly very common and were combined in various ways; they are accompanied by symptoms which constitute "puerperal fever". After recovery, permanent residual effects were common—thickening of the pelvic connective tissue, peritoneal adhesions, chronic endometritis, subinvolution and displacements of the uterus.

Chronic endometritis

The term "chronic endometritis" is now limited to a condition in which there is indisputable evidence of a chronic inflammatory process in the endometrium; this is less easily defined than in most organs owing to the variable structure resulting from normal cyclical changes and also those following disordered endocrine control. In some cases it follows on an acute attack. In many others, however, it is chronic from the onset, the result of mild infection either following pregnancy or gonorrhoea. It is apt to occur along with subinvolution of the uterus after parturition, the size of the uterine cavity being then increased.

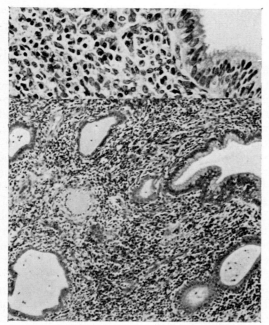

Fig. 23.15.—Chronic endometritis. The glands are irregular and there is increased cellularity of the stroma. × 100. The upper strip shows plasma cell infiltration of the stroma. × 250.

True chronic endometritis is characterised by thickening and infiltration of the stroma by chronic inflammatory cells along with failure of the glands to respond to hormonal stimulation (Fig. 23.15). The normal cyclical changes fail to develop and are less advanced than the dates of the menstrual cycle indicate. The presence of numerous plasma cells in the endometrium is diagnostic, as these cells do not normally occur at any stage of the cycle, whereas polymorpho-nuclear leukocytes are invariably present in the early menstrual breakdown of the endometrium and foci of lymphocytes may also occur normally. In severe and longstanding cases the endometrial stroma may become spindle-celled and almost fibrous, and the glands are then much atrophied. In all such cases the tissue removed by curettage should be carefully examined for products of conception such as degenerate chorionic villi, and the possibility of endometrial tuberculosis should also be borne in mind, as this infection is still commoner than is generally realised.

Pyometra

The cervical canal may be obstructed by a tumour or polyp or by cicatricial stenosis following treatment of cervical cancer by irradiation, or occasionally occurring spontaneously in elderly women. Retention of fluid and infection may then result in the accumulation of pus, *pyometra*. Pyometra is present in 4 per cent of cases of cervical carcinoma, and 70 per cent of cases of pyometra are associated with uterine malignancy.

Macroscopic appearance. The uterus is usually much dilated and the wall is correspondingly thin; the cavity is distended with pus, which is usually confined to the uterus, and does not involve the Fallopian tubes. In longstanding cases the cavity is lined by a rough pyogenic membrane which may simulate extensive carcinoma. In cases of tuberculous endometritis with cervical stenosis the cavity may be filled with caseous pus.

Microscopically the appearances depend on the duration and extent of the process. There may be marked leukocytic infiltration with atrophy of the mucosa, or even loss and replacement by granulation tissue.

Complications. The condition can be remarkably silent, but eventually rupture may occur, either externally, or rarely into the peritoneum which is likely to be fatal. Secondary involvement of the tubes, producing pyosalpinx, is uncommon.

Inflammations of the cervix uteri

Endocervicitis. The mucosa of the endocervix and its associated glands are lined by a single layer of tall columnar mucus-secreting epithelium, which at the external os changes abruptly to a stratified squamous type. Acute endocervicitis may result from gonorrhoea, or from infection by other pyogenic organisms. After childbirth it frequently results also from lacerations of the cervix and subsequent pyogenic infection. The condition often becomes very chronic with failure of lacerations to heal, and gives rise to a mucopurulent discharge (*leukorrhoea*). Changes in the surface epithelium and also obstruction of glands with formation of small cysts may follow. Chronic endocervicitis is the common lesion in persisting gonococcal infection in the female.

Inclusion conjunctivitis in the newborn results from infection of the mother's cervix and vagina with the TRIC agent, acquired usually by coitus with a male suffering from non-gonococcal urethritis.

Cervical erosions. This term is applied to red raw-looking areas which occur on the vaginal portion of the cervix around the external *os uteri* due to its becoming lined by columnar glandular mucosa; they are not, in fact, true erosions. Their surface may be granular or smooth. The red velvety appearance of erosion may result from persistence of the columnar epithelium that covers the ectocervix in infancy—the so-called *congenital erosion* seen in young nulliparous women, or it may result from the extension of columnar epithelium from the endocervix or glands in the healing of cervicitis or cervical abrasions, and subsequently glands may develop. Later in the process of healing, the columnar epithelium may be replaced by squamous epithelium which may also extend into and replace the epithelium of the cervical glands, producing an appearance of *epidermidisation* which has sometimes been mistaken for early carcinomatous change. A common result of catarrhal inflammation of the cervix is obstruction of glands causing the formation of small cysts around the os, known as *Nabothian follicles*. They rarely are more than 5–7 mm. in diameter, and are filled with tenacious mucus. They may be associated with erosions and small papillomatous growths, and there are aggregations of lymphocytes and plasma cells.

Ectropion. This is an eversion of a portion of the cervical mucosa towards the vagina as the result of a fissure of the cervix caused by laceration at parturition. The everted mucosa is naturally exposed to bacterial invasion from the vagina and to irritation, and its columnar epithelium may change to the squamous type. There is persistent mucopurulent discharge, which may give rise to vulvar pruritus.

Salpingitis

Classification. Infections of the Fallopian tubes may be classified as:

(*a*) *Endosalpingitis*, when infection occurs by direct surface spread from the endometrial cavity, as in gonorrhoea, or more rarely from the peritoneum via the abdominal ostia in acute peritonitis.

(*b*) *Interstitial salpingitis*, when infection spreads from the uterine wall via the lymphatics and blood vessels as in post-abortal and puerperal myometritis.

Tuberculosis of the Fallopian tubes is blood-borne and is discussed later.

Endosalpingitis. In acute gonorrhoea the mucosal surface is primarily involved by gonococci spreading upwards and a catarrhal and purulent condition, commonly bilateral, results. The tubes are only slightly swollen but greatly congested, and purulent exudate may escape from the fimbrial end; occasionally there is some fibrinous exudate on the fimbrial and peritoneal surface. The inflammation is initially catarrhal, the epithelium is denuded in patches from the surface of the plicae, the stroma of which is engorged and infiltrated with polymorphonuclear leukocytes, while the lumen is filled with exudate.

Interstitial salpingitis. The acute stage is mainly the result of spread of pyogenic infection from the uterine wall after inexpert abortion or less commonly other forms of instrumentation. The chief feature is gross enlargement of the tubes due to inflammatory oedema and cellular infiltration of the interstitial tissue of the whole wall and adjacent mesosalpinx, while the mucosal surface may show little involvement.

Both forms of infection can result in chronic salpingitis but interstitial salpingitis is more likely to resolve without serious permanent effects.

Chronic salpingitis. Unless adequately treated, salpingitis may pass into a chronic stage in which the mucosal folds that have lost their epithelium in the acute stage adhere to one another and to the tubal wall. They become permanently joined together by growth of the epithelium over them in the process of healing (Fig. 23.16). The plicae thus come to form numerous pockets and depressions which predispose to arrest of the fertilised ovum, and so to tubal pregnancy. The mucosal folds are often heavily infiltrated with lymphocytes and plasma cells and their ends are bulbous (Fig. 23.17). The lumen is irregularly

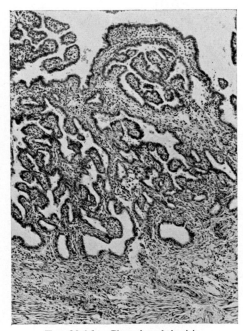

FIG. 23.16.—Chronic salpingitis.
The plicae have fused together extensively, producing many pockets and crypt-like spaces in the mucosa. × 110.

narrowed especially towards the isthmus, where the epithelium grows outwards among the muscle bundles, producing small nodules and crypts beneath the serous coat. The appearances are reminiscent of those in chronic cholecystitis with Aschoff–Rokitansky sinuses. The condition is distinguished from tubal adenomyosis by the absence of endometrial stroma around the gland-like spaces.

Pyosalpinx is the name given to a Fallopian tube distended with pus. It occurs when salpingitis leads to obstruction of the ends of the tube by indrawing and fusion of the fimbriae together with adhesions to adjacent structures. The lumen of the cornual end is only about 0·5 mm. diameter and even mild inflammation of the wall is enough to occlude it.

Macroscopic appearances. Progressive accumulation of pus within the tube leads to great dilatation and a spindle- or sausage-shaped structure results, often bent on itself and distorted by adhesions. The pus may become inspissated and calcified, while the wall may undergo great thickening, simulating tuberculosis. The organisms found in the pus are usually gonococci or the other pyococci. In a large proportion of chronic cases the pus is sterile, a finding very suggestive of gonococcal infection.

Microscopical appearances. The wall of the tube shows the usual features of chronic pyogenic infection, together with stretching, and flattening of the plicae.

Hydrosalpinx. This is normally the end result of a pyosalpinx in which infection has died out and the pus has been absorbed. Distension is more marked at the ampulla as the muscle is thinner there and the secretory epithelium is more extensive. The hydrosalpinx is thus usually retort-shaped with a smooth bulbous end that may be fused with the ovary; the wall is thin

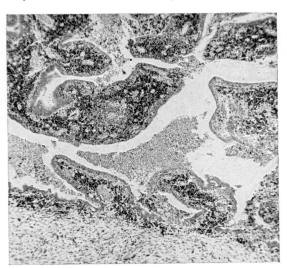

FIG. 23.17.—Chronic gonococcal salpingitis. There is pus in the lumen, and the dark staining of the mucosal folds is due to the presence of numerous plasma cells. × 50.

and semitranslucent and the lining may be as smooth as a serous membrane with only an occasional fold representing the remains of the plicae. The fluid may be discharged into the uterus but may reaccumulate later.

A hydrosalpinx may become twisted, causing some degree of strangulation and consequent haemorrhage into the tube—*haematosalpinx*, but a grossly haemorrhagic tube is more often the result of tubal pregnancy.

Oöphoritis

Acute inflammation of the ovaries is rare and is most frequently the result of secondary infection from the Fallopian tube by gonococci or other pyogenic organisms (p. 830). The inflamed end of the tube readily becomes adherent to the ovary, and thus organisms spread into the substance of the ovary, giving rise to a tubo-ovarian abscess. Infection may occur also from the peritoneal cavity in cases of peritonitis due to appendicitis and other conditions. Occasionally the whole of an ovary may be destroyed by suppuration, and the abscess may reach a large size, and be accompanied by at least local peritonitis.

Chronic oöphoritis may follow on acute pyogenic inflammation, sometimes gonococcal.

Tuberculosis

Tuberculosis of the female reproductive organs usually starts as a haematogenous infection of a *Fallopian tube*, secondary to some tuberculous lesion elsewhere; in this respect the tube is analogous to the epididymis in the male. The tube may become infected also through the ostium in tuberculosis of the peritoneum, though spread in the reverse direction is commoner. Tubercles form in the interstitial tissue of the tubal mucosa, and these soon lead to ulceration and destruction of the mucosa, so that the lumen becomes filled with caseous material, while the wall is greatly thickened. Commonly, the lumen is closed at the ends, the tube becoming greatly distended with caseous pus—*tuberculous pyosalpinx* (Fig. 23.18*a* and *b*). Both tubes may be affected in this way; adhesions form and the tubes may be grotesquely distorted. The tuberculous infection may pass by the ostium to the peritoneum, but it may extend also through the wall of the tube, the surface of which may be studded with tubercles. In rare instances tuberculous salpingitis in young children is due to a direct spread of infection from the vagina.

Talc granuloma of the Fallopian tubes. We have seen a number of examples of chronic salpingitis associated with sterility, in which the mucosa of the thickened tubes exhibited numerous tubercle-like follicles devoid of caseation, but with giant cells in

which minute doubly-refracting crystals believed to be talc were present. The talc had probably entered the tubes from the peritoneum, into which it had been accidentally introduced at a previous laparotomy. The condition is easily mistaken for chronic tuberculosis.

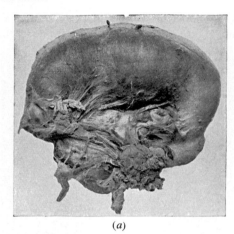

(*a*)

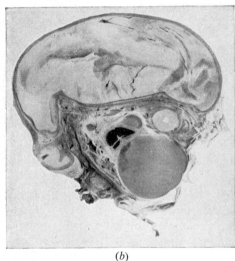

(*b*)

FIG. 23.18.—Tuberculous pyosalpinx. (*a*) Surface view of tube, showing adhesions. (*b*) View of section: above, caseous material distending the tube; below, the ovary (containing cysts). × ⅔.

Tuberculosis of the *uterus* is usually a descending infection from a tube, and is a not uncommon complication. The bacilli settle in the tissue of the mucosa, giving rise to tubercles which are often difficult to distinguish with the naked eye. The recognition of the tubercles in the endometrium removed by curettage in cases of sterility reveals that the disease is commoner than has been supposed. It is usually accompanied by non-specific changes such as polymorphonuclear leukocytes in the gland acini and plasma cells in the stroma. *Caseating endometritis* may follow. Occasionally obstruction of the lumen may occur, and an accumulation of caseous pus may then form. Rarely infection may spread from the uterus to the vagina, and ulcers may be produced in its wall. Tuberculosis of the cervix, which is much rarer than that of the body, may be accompanied by papillary outgrowths. Haematogenous infection of the endometrium occurs in acute miliary tuberculosis.

Tuberculosis of the *ovaries* is relatively uncommon. Infection is usually secondary to tuberculosis of the tube and adhesions are often present; less frequently infection occurs from the peritoneum. Infection by the blood stream is exceptional.

Syphilis

The primary chancre occurs mostly on the labia but may appear on the cervix uteri; secondary lesions may occur on the portio vaginalis, along with condylomas on the perineum. Apart from these, syphilitic lesions are not common. Gummas and chronic interstitial inflammation in the female genital tract are rare.

Actinomycosis

A few cases of this disease in the female genital tract have been recorded; in an example involving the ovaries the lesions were of the usual multilocular suppurative character.

TUMOURS

(1). Vulva

The cutaneous tissues of the vulva are comparable to the sex skin of the higher primates and are subject to the influence of steroid hormones. The only benign epithelial tumour commonly seen on the vulva is the papilloma or condyloma acuminatum—p. 823. Hidradenomas are occasionally found on the labia, and present special characteristics (p. 940).

Malignant tumours are relatively rare; most are squamous carcinomas but adenocarcinoma of Bartholin's gland, basal cell carcinoma, melanoma and sarcoma also occur. Metastatic deposits in the vulva occur infrequently from endometrial carcinoma and choriocarcinoma.

Carcinoma of the vulva occurs most commonly in women of the sixth and later decades and therefore arises in atrophic tissues. In over 60 per cent of cases the changes of senile keratosis are present in the vulvar skin. "Leukoplakia" of the vulva is poorly defined and the term should not be employed as a pathological diagnosis; as used clinically, it includes a variety of conditions of unrelated etiology, their common feature being the presence of white plaques on the vulvar skin. Vulvar carcinoma may arise also in association with hypertrophic skin lesions and this has led to the unwarranted suspicion clinically that eventual malignant transformation may occur in any white area of the vulva. In the vulval region, however, any of the chronic dermatoses can be associated with white areas, e.g. neurodermatitis, monilial infection, *lichen sclerosus et atrophicus*, as well as senile keratosis. In primary atrophy of the vulva the microscopic picture reveals thinning of the epidermis with loss of the rete pegs, hyalinisation of the superficial dermis, and absence of elastic tissue. This histological picture resembles that of lichen sclerosus et atrophicus but in the latter there is hyperkeratosis. Monilial infection is more common in women using contraceptive steroids and in pregnancy.

In hypertrophic white lesions of the vulva, hyperkeratosis, parakeratosis and acanthosis in association with hyalinisation of the superficial dermis and evidence of chronic inflammation are seen (Fig. 23.19). Areas of epidermal dedifferentiation may occur in hypertrophic lesions and atypical features are present in the basal layer, such as the presence of keratinised cells (dyskeratosis). Some authors restrict the use of the term leukoplakia to this pre-malignant condition. Between this picture and that of invasive carcinoma is the microscopic pattern of carcinoma in situ.

Squamous carcinoma of the vulva

Most vulval cancers start on the muco-cutaneous surface of the anterior half of the labia. Naked-eye examination reveals an ulcer with a sloughing surface and a deeply indurated base; less commonly it will appear as a flat plaque or a fungating papillomatous growth.

The microscopic appearances are those of a typical squamous cell carcinoma (see Fig. 11.22, p. 239). It is usually moderately well differentiated with keratinisation and cell nests. In about one-third of cases the tumour is anaplastic and very malignant.

with supporting connective tissue, which may be abundant—it is thus often incorrectly called a fibromyoma or a "fibroid". Uterine myomas are among the commonest of tumours, being said to occur in more than 15 per cent of women over 35, but they often remain quite small.

Macroscopic appearances. The tumours may be single or multiple, and one is often much larger than the others. A myoma usually starts

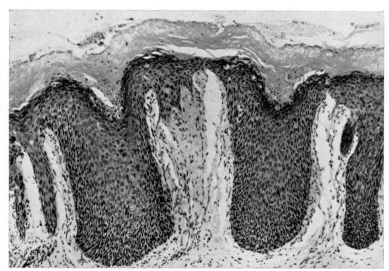

Fig. 23.19.—So-called leukoplakia of the vulva, showing hypertrophied rete pegs and hyperkeratosis of the epithelium. × 95.

The superficial and deep inguinal lymph nodes are involved at an early stage and often on both sides because of the bilateral lymphatic drainage. A feature of vulval cancer is that it may appear to be multifocal, as a result of deep-seated lymphatic extensions of the primary tumour giving rise to surface growths that may appear independent.

(2). Uterus

Tumours of the uterus, both benign and malignant, are common and of great clinical importance. Of the benign tumours, myoma is the most frequent, but adenomyoma and glandular polyps also occur. Carcinoma is the commonest malignant growth.

(a) Benign uterine tumours

Myoma (leiomyoma). This tumour forms a circumscribed growth of smooth muscle along

in the substance of the wall—it is then described as *interstitial* or *intramural*. But as enlargement takes place it expands either into the cavity of the uterus—*submucous* type—or outwards under the peritoneum—*subserous* type. It may also originate in either of these sites. A submucous myoma expands the uterine cavity, and may project through the os as a pedunculated mass (Fig. 23.20); occasionally it becomes expelled by the hypertrophied uterus. It tends to become infected and ulcerated: severe haemorrhage is a common result, and if the tumour is not removed, marked anaemia may follow. A subserous myoma passes outwards as it grows, and often comes to have a distinct pedicle. It may reach 10 kg. in weight, and may cause great abdominal distension. Also, a superficial myoma may pass between, and open out, the layers of the broad ligament.

A myoma is usually of firm and somewhat elastic consistency, with a regular and well-defined outline; the cut surface is, as a rule, paler than the uterine wall and shows a peculiar concentric or whorled marking produced by the bundles of muscle fibres (Fig. 12.13, p. 249). Occasionally the tumour is composed of a number of foci and has a nodular outline. Sometimes a myoma becomes soft and oedematous; or it may become myxomatous in parts (Fig. 23.21). It may

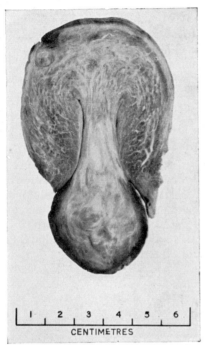

FIG. 23.20.—Large submucous myoma of uterus projecting through the cervix. × ¾.

thus become fluctuant and clinically may simulate an ovarian cyst. Infarction also may take place from thrombosis of vessels or from twisting of the pedicle, and softening of the tissue may follow; this may be accompanied by haemorrhage into its substance—the so-called *red degeneration*, which is commoner during pregnancy. At the menopause, uterine myomas usually cease to grow, and undergo a process of fibrosis and shrinkage. The muscle cells atrophy and many disappear, while the stroma becomes increased and hyaline. Deposition of calcium salts often occurs in the hyaline stroma and ultimately the tumour may be changed into a hard stony mass or "womb-stone", in which the characteristic concentric markings may be distinguished. Occasionally, in a myoma a marked development of wide vessels occurs—*telangiectatic* form, or more rarely, wide lymphatic spaces are formed.

Microscopic appearances. These have already been described (p. 249) but all degrees of cellularity are encountered between tumours composed almost entirely of interlacing bundles of smooth muscle and others in which a high proportion of fibrous stroma is present. Rarely sarcomatous change may arise in a myoma, and the presence of numerous mitotic figures in a myoma should be regarded with suspicion.

(b) Malignant tumours of uterus

Carcinoma of the uterus is very common and causes widespread destructive changes. Two forms are to be distinguished according to the sites of origin; namely, *carcinoma of the cervix*, which may originate from the ectocervical or endocervical epithelium, and *carcinoma of the endometrium*.

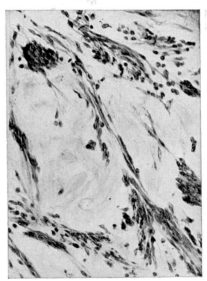

FIG. 23.21.—Myoma of uterus undergoing mucoid change.

Note the clear matrix which has accumulated between the muscle cells. × 250.

Cervical carcinoma

Carcinoma of the cervix constitutes 10 per cent of malignant tumours in the female and accounts for 60 per cent of genital cancer. It has long been evident that the percentage of successfully treated cases of cervical carcinoma parallels the percentage of early cases in any reported series and as a result a vast amount of attention is now paid to the early diagnosis of this condition. Clinically-obvious cervical cancer is all too often incurable.

Classification. Cancer of the cervix may arise from the epithelium of the ectocervix or the mucous membrane of the cervical canal and it is

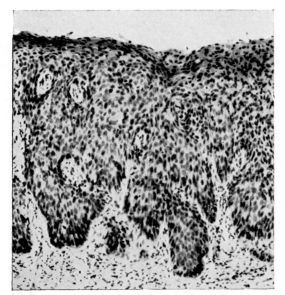

FIG. 23.22.—Carcinoma in situ of uterine cervix, showing the typical thickening and alteration of cell type. There is virtually no differentiation into layers, the cells near the surface being similar to those at the base × 120.

often impossible to prove the site of origin due to the marked tendency of the cervical epithelium to undergo metaplasia. Cervicitis, epidermidisation of endocervical glands, or squamous metaplasia are commonly observed on microscopic examination of the endocervix. Most carcinomas of the cervix are of the squamous-cell type and only about 5 per cent are adenocarcinomas (Fig. 23.25). The former usually arises in the region of the squamo-columnar junction but 20 per cent arise in the endocervical canal.

The invasive stage of carcinoma of the cervix may be preceded for a considerable time, sometimes for many years, by a pre-invasive stage. The squamous surface epithelium undergoes cytological changes suggestive of malignancy but without invasion. To this condition the name *carcinoma in situ* is given (Fig. 23.22) and its recognition and treatment in the pre-invasive stage may reduce the mortality of the disease.

Etiology. Early marriage, early coitus and multiparity appear to be important etiological factors. Carcinoma of the cervix is rare in patients who have had diathermy conisation of the cervix for chronic cervicitis. Both *carcinoma in situ* and *invasive carcinoma* of the cervix are rare in Jewish women but whether the relative immunity among Jewesses is due to an hereditary factor, to careful personal hygiene, or to early ritual male circumcision, is not known.

Macroscopic appearances. Malignant change can be confirmed or excluded only by histological examination. For example in cases of *carcinoma in situ* the cervix may appear normal, while a lacerated and chronically infected parous cervix, near the site of malignancy, may appear suspicious.

Invasive carcinoma is suggested by an irregular induration of the cervix followed by ulceration (Fig. 23.23). It commonly arises in one or other lip of the cervix and may eventually form a huge mass with a nodular surface. The largest tumours are infected, ulcerated, and have a greyish-green necrotic surface. As the tumour enlarges, it invades the adjacent cervical tissue and upper vagina.

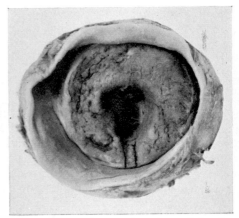

FIG. 23.23.—Carcinoma of cervix uteri showing ulceration. × ¾.

Lymphatic spread is usually early and the regional lymph nodes and parametrial tissues are soon involved, so that partial or complete obstruction of the ureters may follow and death from renal failure is common. The tumour may extend into the bladder or rectum resulting in fistulous communications. Extra-pelvic metastases are rare until later and in fact over 67 per cent of patients who die have the disease localised to the pelvis.

Microscopic appearances. In *carcinoma in situ* the cytological changes which characterise malignancy are present without invasive growth as shown by lack of penetration of the lamina propria (Fig. 23.22). The cells show variation in size and shape of nuclei, increase in nuclear–cytoplasmic ratio and hyperchromatism. There is lack of differentiation from the basal to surface layer, with increased numbers of mitoses at all levels. Extension into endocervical glands does

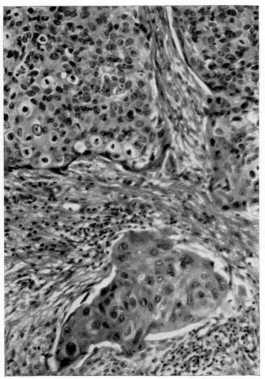

Fig. 23.24.—Carcinoma of cervix uteri, showing infiltrating masses of epithelial cells without formation of cell-nests. × 165.

Note the very numerous mitotic figures.

not imply invasive carcinoma as long as the basement membrane of the glands is intact. It is important to distinguish carcinoma in situ from squamous metaplasia, epidermidisation and atypical hyperplasia but with squamous differentiation in the upper layers, none of which have the cytological features of malignancy. Furthermore, it is essential to examine numerous blocks of biopsy material to rule out microscopic invasion since 10 per cent of cases diagnosed as pre-invasive on single biopsy have evidence of invasive carcinoma on further study, and this

profoundly influences prognosis. When the cells penetrate the stroma their staining properties change, which make the recognition of micro-invasion fairly simple.

In invasive squamous carcinoma large branching solid epithelial masses penetrate the fibro-muscular stroma of the cervix (Fig. 23.24). The peripheral cells are cubical and the central cells tend to be polygonal, but cell nests and keratinisation are seldom features of cervical carcinoma as the tumour is rarely well enough differentiated. Accordingly it is usually relatively sensitive to radiation therapy, which is the most common method of treatment.

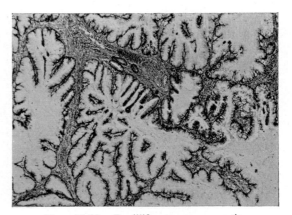

Fig. 23.25.—Papilliform mucus-secreting adenocarcinoma of the cervix uteri. × 60.

(Dr. M. A. Head.)

Vaginal and cervical cytology. It is now well established that malignant cells from uterine cancers are exfoliated into the vagina; Papanicolaou first realised the potentialities of exfoliative cytology in the early diagnosis of cervical cancer. Aspiration of the vaginal contents and staining by Papanicolaou's technique will detect 70 per cent of endometrial cancers and approximately 80 per cent of cervical cancers. Examination of scrapings from the squamo-columnar junction of the cervix will pick up 90 per cent of early cervical cancers and if carried out in conjunction with aspiration of the endocervical mucus will result in a presumptive diagnosis in almost 95 per cent of cases. Cytological studies are not fully diagnostic but they are a strong indication of the necessity for an adequate biopsy. The importance of cytology in preventive medicine is well illustrated by the British Columbia study where in a 12-year period approximately one third of the female populace over the age of 20 years had regular cervical cytological examination, and a reduction of clinically invasive squamous cell cancer has been reported.

Endometrial carcinoma

Cancer arising from the endometrium is usually an adenocarcinoma but in about 20 per cent squamous metaplasia is also present; in such cases the tumour is termed an adeno-acanthoma, but its behaviour is similar to that of endometrial carcinoma in general.

Etiology. There is increasing evidence that nulliparous women with hypertension, obesity, diabetes and abnormal bleeding at the menopause are more prone to develop endometrial cancer. This condition has been reported with undue frequency in patients who have received prolonged oestrogen stimulation either therapeutically or from a feminising ovarian tumour, and this suggests that endocrine dysfunction may play a part in the etiology of endometrial cancer in general. The presence of focal atypical adenomatous hyperplasia in the endometrium in relation to frank carcinoma also supports this view, and while the evidence is inconclusive, focal adenomatous hyperplasia in a diagnostic curettage should be regarded with suspicion. Endometrial carcinoma is infrequent in women under the age of 45 years and when it occurs in the younger patient some endocrine disturbance has commonly been present over a period; in about 20 per cent of cases the ovaries have a smooth fibrotic surface beneath which multiple small follicular cysts are present—the so-called Stein–Leventhal ovaries.

Macroscopic appearances. Cancer of the endometrium may be a localised sessile tumour with a broad base, which may become polypoidal, or a diffuse growth involving a large area of the endometrial cavity (Fig. 23.26). The uterus is frequently enlarged but the contour of the organ is preserved. The tumour invades the uterine muscle and ulceration and infection are inevitable in the later stages. Necrosis and infection in the presence of cervical obstruction results in pyometra. The tumour may extend to the cervix or ovaries. Vaginal metastases occur by lymphatic or venous dissemination. Lymphatic spread via the broad ligament to the para-aortic lymph nodes, or via the lymphatic channels in the round ligaments to the inguinal nodes, occurs in advanced cases.

Microscopic appearances. Cancer of the endometrium is usually a moderately well differentiated adenocarcinoma but more solid areas and a cribriform gland pattern are frequently seen, or the structure may be papillary. An extremely aberrant type of growth is not uncommon, with many enormous multinucleated cells and multipolar mitoses. In *adeno-acanthoma*, the adenocarcinoma is well differentiated and the superimposed squamous elements can be readily distinguished (Fig. 23.27), sometimes intimately mingled with the main tumour, sometimes as separate foci of development; this feature does not influence prognosis or treatment. Carcinoma

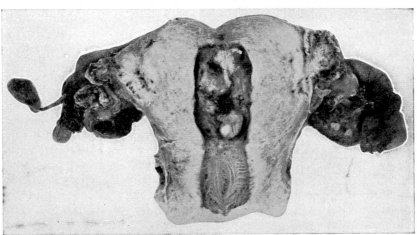

FIG. 23.26.—Carcinoma of body of uterus.
Note the irregular and ulcerating mass occupying the cavity of the body. $\times \frac{3}{4}$.

of the endometrium is not highly sensitive to radiation, and treatment consequently is by total hysterectomy.

Sarcoma

Sarcoma of the uterus is uncommon. It may originate from the endometrial stroma or from the uterine muscle, probably from a myoma. It is then usually of the spindle-celled variety but polygonal cell and mixed mesodermal tumours occur, especially in sarcomas arising in the endometrial stroma. *Stromal sarcoma* forms an enormously thick layer around the cavity, the muscle being well preserved. *Rhabdomyosarcoma* occurs in infants as a rare polypoid tumour which projects from the os and cervix as a cluster of blunt, clubbed processes—the so-called *sarcoma botryoides*.

Choriocarcinoma is described below (p. 853).

(3). The Fallopian tubes

Benign tumours—fibroma, myoma, adenoma —and small cysts sometimes arise from the tubes, and malignant tumours, both carcinoma and sarcoma, are occasionally seen, watery discharge being a diagnostic feature. Choriocarcinoma has been recorded as a sequel to tubal pregnancy. All forms of tumour, however, are extremely rare.

(4). The ovaries

Tumours of the ovaries are of considerable variety and some present features of special interest and importance. Both solid and cystic types occur, the latter more frequently.

Benign ovarian tumours and cysts

In the interpretation of small simple cysts of the ovary, due regard must be paid to the wide variation in appearances produced within the physiological ovulatory cycle. *Endometriosis* with the formation of cysts and haemorrhage into them is described on p. 848.

Non-neoplastic cysts

Cysts of the ovaries form an important group of abnormalities. Some are non-neoplastic, and derived from dilatation of follicles or corpora lutea. Others are cystic tumours. The following are the main types.

Cysts are formed by the dilatation of atretic Graafian follicles, and sometimes from corpora lutea—*true follicular cysts* and *corpus luteum cysts* respectively. The former are usually multiple, and the surface of the ovaries may be beset with them. Usually they are small, but occasionally a cyst may reach 5–7 cm. in diameter; they are generally bilateral and may lead to atrophy of the ovarian tissues. They are

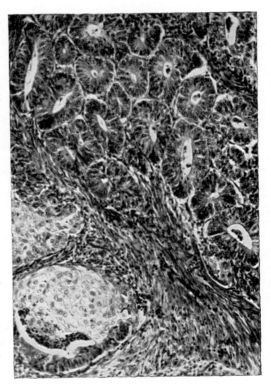

Fig. 23.27.—Adenocarcinoma of body of uterus, showing squamous foci (adeno-acanthoma). × 130.

unilocular, but adjacent cysts may become confluent; they have ordinarily clear serous contents, though sometimes fresh or altered blood may be present and such cysts must be distinguished from endometriosis. Occasionally considerable haemorrhage takes place into a large cyst, and this haematoma may burst into the peritoneal cavity. Follicular cysts have a smooth wall lined by one or more layers of cubical or columnar epithelium; sometimes, however, the epithelial lining is lost. Follicular cysts are commonly associated with endometrial hyperplasia. *Corpus luteum cysts* are formed by haemorrhage or exudation of fluid into corpora lutea, and their appearances vary according to the stage of formation of the latter. The wall is often fibrous or hyaline without a distinct epithelial lining, and sometimes lutein cells

into the lumen of the adherent tube and a *tubo-ovarian cyst* thus result.

Ovarian haematomas. These may be formed in two ways; firstly by haemorrhage into a follicular cyst or corpus luteum cyst, forming a haematoma. The blood then becomes altered in colour. Secondly, "tarry cysts" or "chocolate cysts" result from menstrual haemorrhage in foci of ovarian endometriosis (p. 848).

Parovarian cysts. These cysts, which are fairly

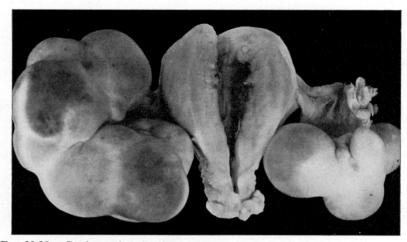

FIG. 23.28.—Cystic ovaries, showing large theca-lutein cysts. The patient also had a hydatidiform mole. $\times \frac{1}{2}$.

derived from the membrana granulosa are abundant and form a yellowish layer, usually thicker at one side; the term *lutein cyst* is then applied. Lutein cells are comparatively large, rounded or polyhedral, and contain abundant lipid and also a yellowish pigment. They may form a broad zone which is surrounded and partly invaded by connective tissue. Lutein cells may be present in considerable number also around true follicular cysts, and are derived from the theca interna, not from the membrana granulosa—*theca-lutein cysts.* Occasionally such cysts are numerous and give rise to polycystic ovaries with enlargement (Fig. 23.28). They represent atretic follicles with luteinisation and have been found chiefly in cases of chorio-carcinoma and hydatidiform mole, under the influence of chorionic gonadotrophin formed by the trophoblastic epithelium.

Novak states that true "retention" cysts show degeneration of the granulosa cells and loss of hormonal activity. The origin of the cysts is, however, often obscure, as is also their relation to functional disturbance. A cyst may rupture

frequent, are derived from the epoöphoron or anterior part of the parovarium or Wolffian body, which lies in the broad ligament between the ovary and the tube, the cysts having a corresponding position. They are usually single, spherical and unilocular. Their contents are a clear watery fluid containing little or no albumin and no mucin. They are usually lined by a ciliated columnar epithelium, though in places the layer may be of the cubical type. As the cyst increases in size, it separates the layers of the broad ligament, and is thus covered by an outer layer of peritoneum. The tube is stretched over the surface; the ovary lies at the other side and may undergo atrophy. Usually there is no distinct pedicle, but if the cyst is very large it may derive a thick pedicle from the broad ligament.

Multilocular ovarian cystadenoma

This tumour is of great importance because it constitutes rather more than 50 per cent of all ovarian tumours, and also because, unless removed, it becomes very large, may rupture, and may become malignant.

Macroscopic appearances. It is usually unilateral, and may become enormous. If not removed surgically such cystic tumours may weigh 25 kg. or more. It is usually rounded and comparatively smooth on the surface, and though it contains numerous cysts, there is usually one of specially large size. At one side of this there is a more solid-looking mass

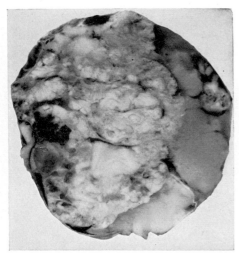

FIG. 23.29.—Multilocular cystadenoma of ovary, showing numerous cysts of various sizes, filled with gelatinous mucroid secretion. × ½.

which is composed of innumerable smaller cysts, some quite minute (Fig. 23.29). The contents of the cysts are always mucoid, and often glairy or ropy, sometimes almost semi-solid, so that on section the contained material does not readily run out.

Microscopic examination shows the cysts to be lined with a layer of tall columnar epithelium; the nuclei of the cells are basally placed, while the cytoplasm generally is clear and mucin-containing (Fig. 23.30). The lining of the spaces is thrown into folds, and papillary ingrowths are numerous (Fig. 11.7, p. 232). The stroma between the smaller cysts and in the papillae is scanty and may form merely a thin line. The cysts contain mucoid glyco-protein material, along with desquamated cells and granular debris.

Complications. An ovarian cyst, as it increases in size, rises from the pelvis, and may distend the whole abdomen. It then has a distinct pedicle,

in which the blood vessels run, and the anatomical relations of the ovary are essentially maintained. Occasionally the pedicle is twisted, obstructing the venous return, and then the cyst wall becomes dark red from diffuse haemorrhage —a condition of strangulation; blood may escape also into the peritoneal cavity. Occasionally a cyst may rupture, and its mucoid contents escape into the peritoneal cavity, being continually augmented by secretion from the tumour and from epithelial cells seeded on to the peritoneal surfaces. The mucoid material acts as a mild irritant, and it is invaded by connective tissue cells and young capillaries as in the process of organisation. The result is that adhesions form between the coils of intestine and other structures, while the mucoid material still persists. The term *pseudo-myxoma peritonei* has been applied to this rare condition.

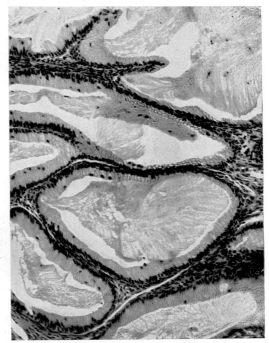

FIG. 23.30.—Multilocular cystadenoma of ovary, showing acini filled with mucoid secretion, lined by a tall columnar epithelium. × 130.

Although not truly malignant, the prognosis is grave. More often adenocarcinoma supervenes in a multilocular cystadenoma and may disseminate throughout the peritoneal cavity.

Papillary cystadenoma

This form of tumour, known also as *serous cystadenoma*, is less common than the multi-locular cystadenoma, but it is by no means rare and is usually bilateral (Fig. 23.31). It may reach 10 cm. in diameter, though it is usually considerably smaller. The tumour consists of a

removal of the primary tumours, the peritoneal seedlings may undergo atrophy, but usually they continue to grow. Sometimes the surfaces of both ovaries are covered with papillary growths, and there may also be a single cyst or several small cysts in the ovaries. True carcinoma develops in a papillary cyst much more commonly than in a multilocular cyst.

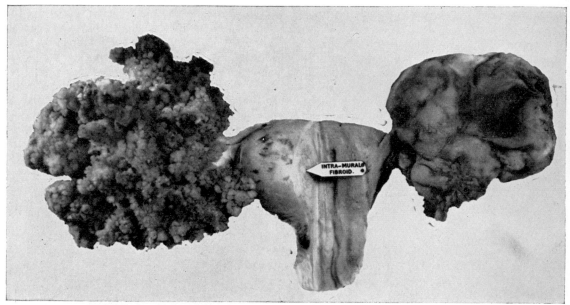

FIG. 23.31.—Bilateral papillary cystic tumours of ovary, also an intramural fibroid. × ½.
The numerous wart-like growths on the external surface of the cyst shown on the left indicate malignant change.

single main cyst, but along with this there may be some small cysts; the contents are usually a clear, serous fluid. The characteristic feature is the presence on the inner surface of the cyst wall of small wart-like or fairly large papilliform excrescences, the surface of which is broken up into numerous projections, somewhat resembling a cauliflower (Fig. 23.31). These ingrowths are covered by columnar or cubical epithelium which is often ciliated (Fig. 23.32), but the cells do not form mucin as in the multilocular cystadenoma, and their nuclei are less basally placed (Fig. 23.32). Such cysts grow relatively slowly, and never reach the great size of the multilocular cyst. Not infrequently, however, the cyst wall ruptures, and the contents along with papillary fragments escape into the peritoneal cavity, and are distributed by the intestinal movements over the peritoneal surface on which they may form numerous outgrowths, usually accompanied by marked ascites. After operative

Histogenesis. There is still doubt regarding the exact origin of the cystadenomas of the ovary. The view which has now most support is that the multilocular cystadenoma is of teratomatous nature, with a special growth of one of its component tissues, namely a tall mucin-forming endodermal epithelium. Teratoma and mucinous cystadenoma may co-exist in the ovary. The origin of the papillary cystadenoma is ascribed to the germinal epithelium of the surface of the ovary.

Teratomas

(a) Cystic. The commonest is the tumour known as *dermoid cyst*, which is usually one large cyst with occasionally a few much smaller compartments, the contents of which may be different. The term is applied because the main cyst is lined by squamous epithelium, usually with well-developed skin appendages, but the tumour is really a cystic teratoma. The tumour is usually single, but occasionally bilateral and rarely more than one have been present in an ovary. It often forms a rounded swelling which may reach 10 cm. diameter, but is usually

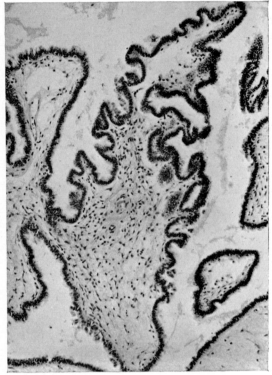

FIG. 23.32.—Papillary cystadenoma of ovary, showing the papillae covered by columnar epithelium. × 100.

smaller. The contents are fatty material, which is fluid at the temperature of the body, but becomes semi-solid on cooling. Mixed with it are hairs and desquamated epithelium. The lining is a stratified epithelium, and the skin structures—hairs, sebaceous and sweat glands—are abundant. At one side there is often a hard protuberance, and on the inner surface several teeth, irregularly arranged, may be present (Fig. 23.33). On section this projection may contain bone and other tissues—cartilage, smooth muscle, various glandular structures representing alimentary and respiratory systems and even nervous tissue. There may be mammary tissue but, in common with teratomas in general, gonadal tissue has not been observed. Cystic teratomas vary much in complexity and

epidermal structures usually preponderate; occasionally they are composed wholly of thyroid —*struma ovarii.*

(b) Solid teratomas. Less common than this cystic form is the more solid teratoma, which usually forms an irregular rounded mass, in which an even greater variety of tissues may be found, and these may give rise to an enormous number of small cysts. In the testis, on the contrary, the solid type is the more frequent. The structure and derivation of these tumours is discussed on p. 258. Malignant change rarely occurs in cystic teratomas, but so often develops in teratomas of the solid type that they should be regarded as essentially malignant. The change is usually carcinomatous, less often sarcomatous; choriocarcinoma is, however, very much rarer than in testicular teratomas.

Malignant ovarian tumours

The malignant tumours of the ovary present a considerable variety, and are often partly

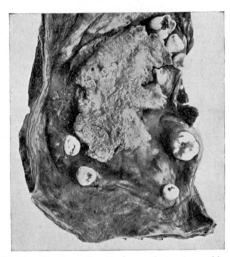

FIG. 23.33.—Portion of wall of a cystic teratoma (dermoid cyst) of ovary, showing irregular growth of teeth from inner surface of cyst. × ⅚.

cystic. Carcinoma is more frequent than sarcoma. Carcinoma sometimes becomes superadded to a cystic tumour, either of the mucinous or papillary variety, more frequently the latter, but it is often uncertain whether a tumour has been malignant from the start.

Carcinoma in the ovaries may occur comparatively early in adult life. It is often bilateral but one is often considerably larger than the other. It presents the usual invasive features, but varies in type, being sometimes hard and nodular, sometimes soft and leading to great enlargement. It may burst through the capsule and produce secondary growths in the peritoneum, as well as metastases in the regional nodes and in other organs. Histologically, considerable variations in structure are observed. The cells may be arranged in solid masses as in carcinoma of the breast, they may have an

coma combined with carcinoma have been described; these may, however, represent mixed mesodermal tumours.

Primary ovarian tumours with special features

Other forms of ovarian tumour are distinguished and two of these, the granulosa-cell tumour and the arrhenoblastoma, are specially interesting in view of their hormonal effects.

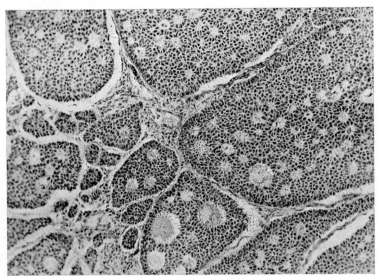

FIG. 23.34.—Granulosa-cell tumour of ovary, showing characteristic masses of cells with tendency to follicle formation. × 150.

irregular acinous formation, or, in the softer varieties, a more diffuse type of growth may be present, with great aberration in appearance of the cells. The criteria for the diagnosis of malignancy in a cystic ovarian tumour are: (*a*) the presence of nodules on the exterior of the cyst; (*b*) multiplication and heaping up of the epithelial cells into several layers; (*c*) invasion of the supporting stroma; (*d*) cellular dedifferentiation with many mitoses. A tendency to rupture during removal is often suspicious.

Sarcoma is much less common than carcinoma. Like the latter, it sometimes affects both ovaries and may occur in association with cysts; the tumour may be large. Usually it is of the spindle-cell type and has a fasciculated appearance on section; forms intermediate between fibroma and sarcoma are observed. Round-cell and pleomorphic varieties also occur. Angiosarcoma, rhabdomyosarcoma and sar-

Granulosa-cell tumour

Formerly also known as *folliculoma* or *carcinoma folliculoides*, this tumour is generally believed to arise from groups of granulosa cells which have not developed into Graafian follicles.

Macroscopic appearances. Granulosa-cell tumours are usually unilateral, solid and encapsulated. They vary from a few millimetres to 50 cm. or more in diameter, and are composed of moderately firm and fairly cellular yellowish tissue, in which cysts, usually small, may be present.

Microscopic appearances. These vary considerably. The cells are often rounded or polyhedral with clear pale-staining cytoplasm, often containing lipids. They are arranged in solid, well-defined trabeculae like a carcinoma; sometimes, however, they are more cubical or columnar and have an acinar or follicle-like arrangement (Fig. 23.34). In some specimens the growth resembles sarcoma, though in places evidence of the characteristic arrangement of cells is usually to be found. The histological appearances may vary much in different parts of the same tumour. As a rule, they are of rather low malignancy. Sometimes the cells resemble thecal or luteal cells and the tumours are then called *thecomas* or *luteomas* respectively.

Age distribution and effects. Granulosa-cell tumour is observed most frequently after the menopause, but occurs at other ages. At all ages, the tumour produces a distinct hormonal effect by secretion of oestrogenic hormones in excess. After the menopause the effects are hyperplasia of the endometrium and enlargement of the uterus, with irregular uterine bleeding—post-menopausal bleeding. During the

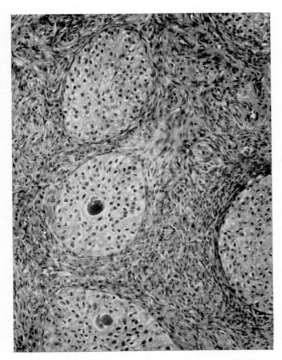

FIG. 23.35.—Brenner tumour of ovary. × 150.

child-bearing period the effects are similar. In the few cases observed in young girls the effects are striking, there being precocious growth, establishment of menstruation and development of the secondary female sex characters. Ovulation does not occur, but bone age is advanced, and premature epiphyseal closure leads ultimately to dwarfism and skeletal

disproportion. These endocrine effects disappear when the tumour is removed.

In a small proportion of cases the granulosa cells may undergo a transformation into lutein cells; accordingly a sharp distinction between granulosa-cell tumours, theca-cell tumours and lutein-cell tumours is not possible.

Fibroma of the ovary

Benign fibroma is one of the commonest solid ovarian tumours. They are usually small and nodular but may become large, and are hard, dense growths. The cut surface is whitish with the characteristic whorled watered-silk appearance, but when large, the pedicle may undergo torsion, leading to strangulation. In some, there is an admixture of smooth muscle fibres and rarely of other mesenchymal elements. Large fibromas of the ovary are sometimes accompanied by wasting, ascites and right-sided hydrothorax (Meig's syndrome); these disappear when the tumour is removed. It is difficult to distinguish a fibroma from a Brenner tumour or thecoma without microscopic examination.

Brenner tumour

This ovarian tumour is much less common than the granulosa-cell tumour. It was called by Brenner *oöphoroma folliculare*. It varies greatly in size and it is firm, sometimes resembling a fibroma. Microscopic examination shows an abundant and dense fibrous stroma in which are scattered islands or nests of epithelial cells. These islands may be solid collections, but very often show a circular central space (Fig. 23.35). The cells are rounded or polyhedral and are comparatively uniform and inactive in appearance. The nuclei may show characteristic longitudinal folding. Sometimes the cells lining the space become columnar resembling those in a mucinous cystadenoma, mucoid secretion accumulates and a tumour composed of the two types of epithelium results. The tumour is slowly growing and benign. According to Meyer it takes origin from collections of indifferent cells, known as *Walthard's rests*, which are found most readily in the superficial parts of the ovaries in infants, but Schiller attributes it to urogenital epithelium of Wolffian origin. Unlike the granulosa-cell tumour, the Brenner tumour only rarely shows evidence of endocrine activity.

Arrhenoblastoma

This rare tumour, which occurs chiefly in young women, is supposed to arise from "male-directed" cells in the region of the rete ovarii, persisting from an early period of gonadogenesis. It may be of an adenomatous type (Fig. 23.36), but the structure may be more like that of a sarcoma. Leydig type cells may be present, and the hormonal effect, which has been more pronounced in atypical growths, is like that of some adenomas of the adrenal cortex,

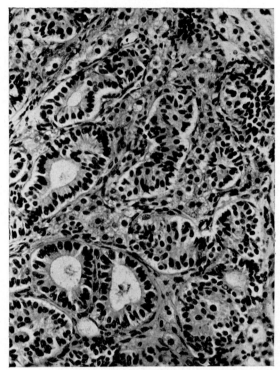

FIG. 23.36.—Arrhenoblastoma of the ovary, showing tubular structures and interstitial cells. × 205.

namely, loss of feminine characters and virilism. In a previously healthy woman there may be atrophy of the uterus and breasts, amenorrhoea, enlargement of the clitoris, growth of facial hair and the appearance of the male secondary sex characters. Removal of the tumour has been followed by the disappearance or modification of these abnormalities and even by subsequent pregnancy. Its malignancy is usually low grade, but it may become large.

Dysgerminoma

This is another rare form of ovarian tumour. Histologically it corresponds closely to the seminoma and it has been called *seminoma ovarii* by French writers. It is supposed to arise from undifferentiated sex cells and does not exert hormonal influence; that is, does not accentuate masculine or feminine characters. It may develop at a relatively early age, often about the time of puberty, and has accordingly

been called *carcinoma puellarum*. In many cases it has been associated with retardation of sexual development or with pseudo-hermaphroditism. Its removal, however, has no effect on these abnormalities. In our experience the prognosis is bad and extensive metastases are likely to occur.

Secondary carcinoma of the ovaries

Metastasis to the ovaries is comparatively frequent in carcinoma of the stomach and colon, and though nodules may also be present over the peritoneum, this is not invariably the case. The secondary growths sometimes reach a large size. It would seem that ovarian tissue is a specially favourable nidus for growth, and that a few cancer cells gaining access to the peritoneum have a marked tendency to settle and multiply in the ovaries. In a similar way carcinoma cells may pass from one ovary to another without

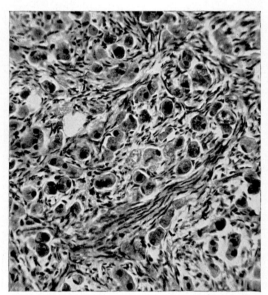

FIG. 23.37.—Krukenberg tumour of ovary, secondary to a primary carcinoma of stomach.
Note the abundant spindle cell stroma and the large round mucin-containing carcinoma cells. × 215.

producing nodules in the peritoneum. Ovarian metastases are not uncommon from cancer of the breast; the manner of spread is doubtful—possibly either by the peritoneal cavity or by lymphatics.

Krukenberg described a bilateral tumour of the ovaries under the term "*fibrosarcoma mucocellulare carcinomatodes*"; it now bears his name.

There is a very cellular sarcoma-like stroma in which cancer cells are scattered or occur in masses (Fig. 23.37). Many of the cells contain mucin which has pushed the nucleus to one side, giving a signet-ring appearance. Such tumours have been found to be almost invariably secondary to a primary carcinoma elsewhere, usually in the stomach, less often in the colon or breast.

DISORDERS OF THE ENDOMETRIUM

The morphological changes in the endometrial cycle

The changes which occur in the endometrium during the normal menstrual cycle are of great importance in the study of menstrual disorders. It is essential to be familiar with the morphological appearances in the different phases of the normal cycle; accurate details of the clinical history and menstrual dates are important in assessing the microscopic appearances.

The endometrial cycle consists of three phases —menstrual, proliferative and secretory. Following menstruation, a new Graafian follicle develops and its granulosa cells produce oestrogens which stimulate regeneration of the endometrium producing first a thin surface epithelium, short straight glands and a compact stroma of spindle cells lying parallel to the surface (Fig. 23.38). The proliferative phase continues to develop until ovulation occurs about the 12–14th day, the surface epithelium becomes columnar and the glands tortuous (Fig. 23.39). The secretory phase begins after ovulation and is brought about by the combined action of oestrogenic and progestational hormones produced by the corpus luteum. It is recognised first by basal vacuolation in the gland cells and increasing glandular tortuosity; later, secretion appears in the lumina, the interstitial cells show a predecidual reaction and polymorph leukocytes appear in the surface layers. The endometrium can now be divided into three layers, the superficial *stratum compactum*, the intermediate *stratum spongiosum*, and the deepest *stratum basale* (Fig. 23.40). When menstruation ensues the compact and spongy layers disintegrate and the deeper basal layer remains to give rise to the regenerative phase of the next cycle.

Oral contraceptives. The use of oral contraceptive pills, consisting usually of mixtures of oestrogenic and progestational steroids, less commonly of the latter alone, interrupts the menstrual cycle and leads to unusual histological appearances in the endometrium. The glands are commonly small and poorly developed (microtubular), and the stroma abundant, but various other bizarre pictures are observed, and in some instances there is a well-developed decidual reaction, a reflection of the induced state of "pseudo-pregnancy".

Endometrial hyperplasia

Definition. A pathological condition of the endometrium associated with irregular uterine haemorrhage resulting from disordered endocrine control. It is known clinically as *metropathia haemorrhagica*.

Conditions of occurrence. It may occur at any time in child-bearing life but its maximum incidence is about the age of forty; it is also the condition found in the menorrhagia of the pubertal period before ovulation is fully established, and it occasionally occurs in the postmenopausal period in association with an oestrogen-secreting ovarian tumour. It may also be produced by prolonged oestrogen therapy.

Macroscopic appearances. The hyperplastic endometrium forms a thick, soft and vascular layer; its surface often shows elevations and polypoid elevations. Its thickness in exceptional cases may exceed 10 mm.

Microscopic appearances. In the deeper parts there is a general hyperplasia of the uterine glands and at a higher level many of these show dilatation with a tendency to cyst formation and epithelial ingrowths (Fig. 23.41). In the superficial parts there are patches of degeneration and necrosis, along with hyaline thromboses in thin-walled vessels and haemorrhage. The interstitial tissue generally is cellular, vascular and oedematous and there may be haemorrhages. At the junction of myometrium and endometrium adenomyosis is commonly present.

Etiology. These changes in the endometrium are the result of ovarian dysfunction. Usually a single follicular cyst or several cysts are present in one or both ovaries, and as a rule corpora lutea are absent. The essential factor is failure of ovulation and the series of changes is explicable in view of the known effects of the ovarian hormones. If ovulation does not occur the proliferative changes due to oestrogens persist, as there is no corpus luteum formed and no progesterone to complete the cycle; normal disintegration of the endometrium then fails to occur and there is a period of amenorrhoea. If

raise the suspicion that this tumour is present, provided that the patient is not on oestrogen therapy.

Membranous dysmenorrhoea

In this disorder, menstruation is painful, and is followed by the passing of membrane-like material in shreds or as a partial cast of the

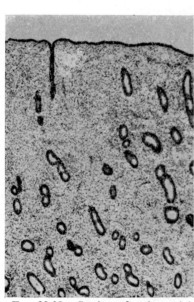

FIG. 23.38.—Section of endometrial curetting on 10th day of the cycle. Proliferative phase. The glands are relatively small. × 50.

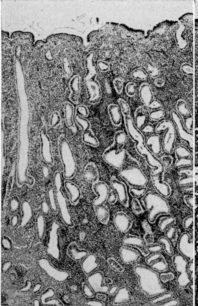

FIG. 23.39.—Fifteenth day of cycle. The glands have increased in size and basal vacuolation of glandular epithelium is apparent. × 50.

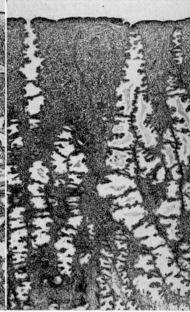

FIG. 23.40.—Twenty-fifth day of cycle, showing the secretory or lutein phase. × 50.

the persisting Graafian follicle becomes cystic it continues to secrete oestrogens which, in turn, induce further endometrial growth; the hyperplastic condition of the endometrium is thus the result of uninterrupted action of oestrogens. When the cystic or abnormal follicle involutes and the supply of oestrogen ceases, areas of localised necrosis and breakdown are responsible for the irregular bleeding so common in this disorder. In some cases the cessation of oestrogenic stimulus is followed by severe bleeding due to oestrogen withdrawal. It is significant that the same changes in the endometrium are brought about also by a granulosa-cell tumour of the ovaries, which produces oestrogens in excess. In fact, when this endometrial lesion with bleeding occurs after the menopause it should

uterus. The membrane consists of the superficial part of the uterine mucosa, the interstitial cells of which are usually considerably swollen with a marked decidual reaction; sometimes much fibrin is present. It is clear that the normal piecemeal disintegration of the superficial part of the mucosa, which should occur at menstruation, does not take place and that the tissue separates as a layer like a decidual cast. Although various theories have been put forward, the cause of this rare abnormality is not known.

Endometriosis
Pelvic endometriosis

Endometriosis may be defined as the presence of functioning endometrial tissue in areas other than the uterine mucosa. The usual sites of pelvic endometriosis are the ovaries, peritoneum and the pouch of Douglas, uterosacral ligaments and serosa of the rectosigmoid region. Endometriosis is also found in the appendix (Fig. 23.42), ileum, rectum, bladder, umbilicus, laparotomy scars, lower genital tract. A few cases are recorded where endometrial tissue was found in such sites as the lung, pleura, breast, arm and thigh.

phatic spread must have occurred. Meyer suggested that the coelomic epithelium is capable of undergoing metaplasia into functioning endometrium in different sites. The observation that in extra-uterine pregnancy the pelvic mesenchymal tissues may exhibit a pronounced decidual reaction supports this.

Endometriosis is easily induced by implantation of endometrium in a laparotomy wound at Caesarean section or other operation on the

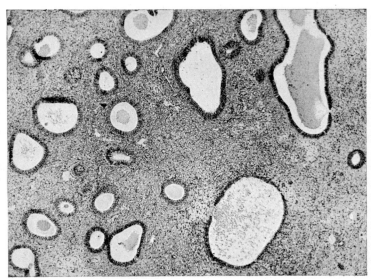

FIG. 23.41.—Cystic hyperplasia of the endometrium, showing dilatation of glands and early cyst formation. (A. C. L.)

A feature of endometriosis is that its continued growth depends on oestrogen. It also has the rare characteristic of benign invasion of the supporting tissues.

Etiology. The histogenesis of endometriosis is unsettled and because of the widely separated sites on which it has been noted, no simple explanation will cover all varieties. It is significant, however, that endometriosis has never been recorded in women with congenital absence of the uterus.

Sampson elaborated the theory that during menstruation endometrial fragments are transported via the Fallopian tubes to the pelvic peritoneum and the ovaries with subsequent implantation. There is good evidence that at least some of the desquamated endometrium at menstruation is viable and capable of growth.

To explain areas of endometriosis in the lungs, pleura, pelvic lymph nodes, arm and thigh it has been postulated that haematogenous or lym-

uterus where the endometrial cavity has been opened, a fact which supports the transplantation theory.

Macroscopic appearances. In the pelvis, small puckered, bluish nodules may be found on the serosa of the bowel, uterosacral ligaments, pelvic peritoneum, or ovarian surfaces. Commonly the ovaries are grossly enlarged by cysts containing dark brown "tarry" material due to haemorrhage at the time of menstruation. These cysts are at first smooth walled and brownish-blue and they are liable to bring about adherence of the ovary to the broad ligament or distal colon. Later they become much distorted by dense fibrosis resulting from organisation of the extravasated blood.

Microscopic appearances. Endometrial glands and stroma are usually evident at first but haemorrhage and resultant pressure atrophy may obscure the ectopic endometrium. The repeatedly shed blood is broken down to haemosiderin and lipids which accumulate in macrophages having a superficial resemblance to lutein cells; recognition of these may be enough to give a presumptive diagnosis of endometriosis.

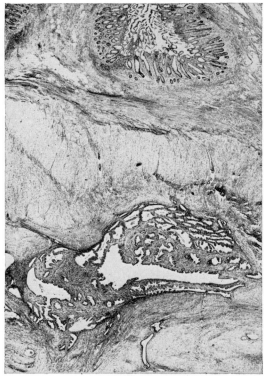

Fig. 23.42.—Endometriosis of the appendix and caecum. A focus of endometrial glands and stroma showing cyclical changes is present in the muscular coat of the caecum close to the appendix. × 12.

Clinical features. Endometriosis occurs only after the menarche and is rarely seen in women with anovulatory cycles. The condition improves during pregnancy and during amenorrhoea induced by progestational steroids. Frequent pregnancies, if initiated from an early age, appear to prevent the development of endometriosis.

The most characteristic symptom is progressive pelvic pain beginning with or just before menstruation, but in 20 per cent of cases there are no symptoms that can be ascribed to pelvic endometriosis.

Adenomyoma or uterine endometriosis

This is a condition in which there is associated growth of endometrial glands and stroma together with non-striped muscle, within the wall of the uterus.

Macroscopic appearances. Adenomyoma may be diffuse or circumscribed. Neither type is a true neoplasm. The *diffuse type* occurs chiefly in the inner part of the myometrium, sometimes in one part, sometimes all round the cavity, the whole uterus being enlarged. The lesion presents a somewhat nodular appearance with whorling as in a myoma, and in the muscular masses there are small translucent areas and spaces which represent the glandular tissue. The outer part of the uterine wall is usually unaffected, but the line of the demarcation is not so sharp as in the case of an ordinary myoma. In the *circumscribed type* multiple nodular masses form submucous or subperitoneal projections, especially from the posterior wall. The nodules may become large and develop cystic spaces containing altered blood, due to cyclical changes

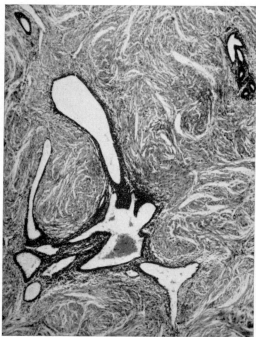

Fig. 23.43.—Adenomyoma of uterus, showing multiple foci of endometrial glands and stroma deep in the uterine wall. × 40.

and menstrual bleeding of the ectopic endometrial tissue. Usually, however, the endometrium is of the basal pattern and fails to undergo cyclical changes. The diffuse type is the commoner and has been called "adenomyosis", though it appears to be of similar nature to the circumscribed type.

Microscopic appearances. The glandular tissue is seen to be composed of branching slits with tubular and acinar structures, lined with columnar epithelium, and usually surrounded by a cellular tissue like endometrial stroma (Fig. 23.43). The continuity of the glandular tissue with the lining epithelium of the uterus has been established by means of serial sections. The condition is accordingly now often known as an *endometriosis of the uterus* and is regarded as an acquired heterotopia.

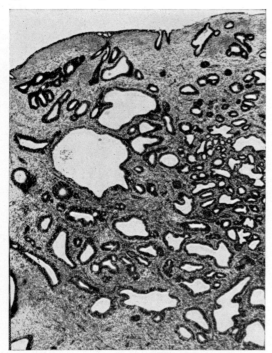

FIG. 23.44.—Benign endometrial polyp showing numerous glands, some of which are dilated, in a fibro-cellular stroma. × 25.

During pregnancy, decidual cells have been observed to have developed in the stroma around the acini.

Uterine polyp

This, the commonest benign proliferation of epithelial origin, may be regarded as a local outgrowth of the mucosa. Masses of this nature grow from either the body or the cervix. In the former situation they are blunt or rounded projections, though sometimes pedunculated; in the latter, they are often pear-shaped and project through the os uteri, being then especially prone to cause irregular bleeding. The surface is usually relatively smooth, sometimes it is papillomatous, and sometimes cysts are present. They are small, rarely exceeding 3 cm. diameter, and they may be either single or multiple. In addition to bleeding, they may become infected or necrotic. A polyp consists of a vascular core or base, covered by a mucous membrane with glands which correspond to those of the corpus or cervix, though they are more irregular in their arrangement and often contain retained secretion. Some polyps consist mainly of glands, with relatively little stroma, and are termed adenomatous polyps or pedunculated adenomas (Fig. 23.44). The connective tissue core may be cellular and vascular, or relatively fibrous. A cervical polyp may be covered in whole or in part by stratified squamous epithelium. Polyps may develop in association with inflammatory conditions or with hyperplasia of the mucosa, but occur apart from any such conditions.

ABNORMALITIES RELATED TO PREGNANCY

The pathology of pregnancy is too large a subject to be considered in detail here. We shall therefore give an account of only some of the more important abnormalities. The trophoblast possesses the property of invading the maternal tissues to achieve nidation, normally without producing any "homograft reaction". In normal pregnancy, fragments of chorionic villi are commonly transported to the lungs, and trophoblastic cells can be demonstrated in the blood of the uterine veins. The factors controlling trophoblastic growth and invasion are as

EE

yet poorly understood, but greater knowledge of the immunological relationships between the fetal tissues and the maternal host may eventually throw light on this problem.

Hydatidiform mole

In this condition the embryo dies but early abortion fails to occur and the terminal branches of the chorionic villi enlarge to form discrete, translucent, tense, grape-like vesicles of 3–

15 mm. diameter (Fig. 23.45). A true hydatidiform mole occurs in the middle trimester of pregnancy and usually no trace of the fetus is seen. Evidence of hydropic degeneration of the chorionic villi in focal areas is found in 50 per cent of cases of spontaneous abortion where the

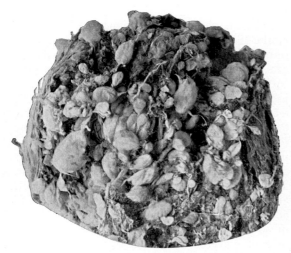

Fig. 23.45.—Part of a hydatidiform mole, showing the enlarged grape-like chorionic villi.

fetus is abnormal, but there are too few cases intermediate between ordinary abortion and hydatidiform mole to accept a continuous spectrum of transition. The occurrence of cases in which an imperfectly developed embryo in its sac, with a partly formed placenta in which hydatidiform villi are embedded, is distinctly uncommon.

Etiology and pathogenesis. The true cause of hydatidiform mole is unknown but the condition occurs more frequently in mothers under 18 and over 40 years of age. Twin pregnancies have been recorded in which a mole was present along with a normal fetus and placenta, an indication that the defect is in the zygote. It is not yet agreed whether the defect lies primarily in the death of the embryo or in some abnormality of the trophoblast. The pathological criteria for the diagnosis of hydatidiform mole are (*a*) trophoblastic proliferation of both Langhans layer and syncytium, (*b*) hydropic degeneration of the stroma of the villi, (*c*) virtual absence of fetal blood vessels in the villi. The extent and degree of trophoblastic hyperplasia varies greatly whereas the hydropic change in the villi is remarkably constant, the villi merely growing larger with age.

On microscopic examination, the substance of the villi is seen to be myxomatous tissue showing extreme oedema. The almost complete absence of capillary blood vessels is striking. On the surface the chorionic epithelium shows proliferation. There are several layers of Langhans cells, and the syncytium is correspondingly prominent (Fig. 23.46); the surface in places may, however, be denuded of epithelium. Usually the mole is constituted mainly by altered villi, and there is no trace of fetus or normal placenta; the villi in such cases penetrate and destroy the decidual layer in an irregular manner. Hydatidiform moles may sometimes reach a weight of 1–1·5 kg., and their presence often causes an abnormally rapid increase in the size of the uterus. They lead to abortion, which

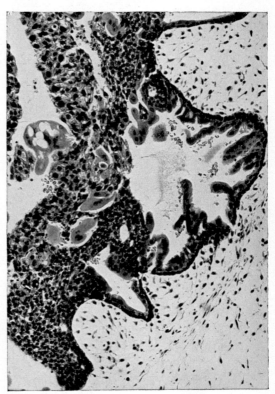

Fig. 23.46.—Hydatidiform mole, showing the oedematous avascular villi, covered by hyperplastic Langhans cells and syncytiotrophoblast.

is often preceded by haemorrhage, sometimes severe; the blood may be retained and form a firm clot which results in the so-called "fleshy mole".

Penetrating mole. There are also cases in which the villi of the hydatidiform mole show much more extensive penetration, extending into and destroying the uterine wall (Fig. 23.47), simulating the behaviour of a malignant tumour —the so-called "invasive mole", to which the unsuitable name *chorio-adenoma destruens* has

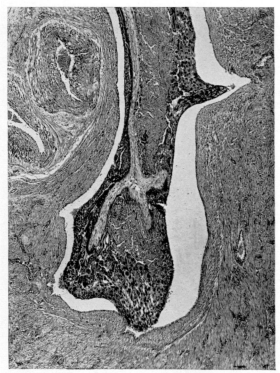

FIG. 23.47.—Penetrating mole, showing deep penetration of the uterine wall by degenerate villi covered with hyperplastic trophoblast. × 32.

been applied by Ewing. Occasionally "metastases" of both trophoblast and villi have occurred but the condition is rarely truly malignant and involution of the "metastases" follows hysterectomy.

Lastly, the chorionic epithelium of the altered villi may become frankly malignant, the tumour then constituting a choriocarcinoma, but, as Park has emphasised, it is not possible to predict on morphological grounds which hydatidiform mole will develop frank malignancy in its trophoblastic epithelium. The hydatidiform mole, like choriocarcinoma, is often associated with theca-lutein cysts in the ovary (Fig. 23.28, p. 840), which appear to arise from the effects of the abundant chorionic gonadotrophin produced by the trophoblastic cells. Chorionic gonadotrophin is usually present in large amounts in the urine, and its

detection is of diagnostic value in these conditions.

Choriocarcinoma

This is a malignant tumour of trophoblastic epithelial type. The tumour cells differentiate into recognisable cyto- and syncytio-trophoblast. It is of special interest as representing an invasion of the maternal tissues by fetal cells (p. 260). In half the cases it is a sequel to a hydatidiform mole and, as has been stated, the infiltrating mole is a transitional form. About 25 per cent of cases of choriocarcinoma follow an abortion, and some of these may have been due to unrecognised hydatidiform degeneration of the chorion. The remainder, excluding those that originate in a teratoma, follow a normal pregnancy, and give rise to symptoms some time, even several years, after delivery: no doubt they arise from portions of retained placenta. We have seen it after 50 years of age, the menopause having occurred only the previous year, and the date of the last pregnancy being uncertain. Very occasionally choriocarcinoma may develop during a pregnancy and give rise to abortion or premature delivery.

Macroscopic appearances. The tumour appears as a soft mass within the uterus, often of crumbling texture and dark red owing to haemorrhages (Fig. 23.48) which result from erosion of the blood vessels by the syncytial cells. It invades and destroys the uterine wall, and may penetrate to the peritoneal coat. Dissemination occurs early, mainly by the blood stream, but also by lymphatics, and metastases are seen most commonly in the lungs, vaginal wall and vulva, lymph nodes, liver and brain. The secondary growths have the same general characters as the primary, and are usually very haemorrhagic and necrotic. Occasionally a secondary nodule in the lungs may undergo complete necrosis, and may become enclosed in fibrous tissue, so that a process of local healing takes place.

Very rarely, choriocarcinoma has been observed to originate in a Fallopian tube or an ovary, and in such cases it apparently develops from an ectopic pregnancy.

Microscopic appearances. The tumour is composed of the two elements of the chorionic epithelium. The Langhans cells, which are rounded or polyhedral with clearly defined margins, often form large masses, on the surface of which are the syncytial cells. The latter present a great variety of shapes, and often have long trailing processes; their cytoplasm is finely granular and more eosinophil than that of the Langhans cells (Fig. 23.49). In reaching a diagnosis of choriocarcinoma on histological

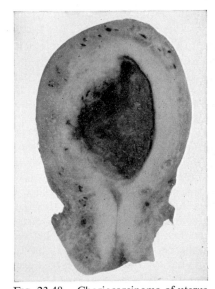

Fig. 23.48.—Choriocarcinoma of uterus.

The tumour is a large haemorrhagic mass in the interior of the uterus. $\times \frac{2}{3}$.

grounds, it must be appreciated that syncytial cells normally penetrate deeply into the myometrium and may persist there for long periods if a portion of placenta is retained. These appearances are best seen in the younger and actively growing parts of the tumour, but in other parts the arrangement is more irregular, the two kinds of cells being mixed together. There is little stroma, and the growth has no blood vessels of its own; areas of necrosis and extravasated blood are usually present, even in small metastatic nodules.

Hormonal changes. In choriocarcinoma and hydatidiform mole the urine usually contains abundant chorionic gonadotrophin, which is often present in much greater concentration than in a normal pregnancy. The level falls to normal if the tumour is completely removed. Failure to become negative, or the return of a positive rest, indicates the presence of active trophoblastic elements, and the presence of neoplastic chorionic epithelium can be deduced from the hormone titre in the urine. In a considerable proportion of cases of choriocarcinoma or hydatidiform mole the ovaries have been found to be replaced by large cysts of the theca-lutein type (p. 840), as a result of this hormonal influence.

Etiology. The factors that bring about the malignant transformation of the trophoblastic cells are unknown, except that it is commoner late in reproductive life and that age appears to be more important than multiparity. The disease is world-wide in its distribution but has a very much higher incidence in Chinese and other Far Eastern women.

Cells closely resembling chorionic epithelium may be present in teratomas, e.g. of the testis,

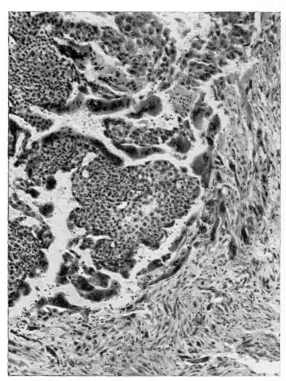

Fig. 23.49.—Choriocarcinoma, consisting of masses of Langhans cells and syncytiotrophoblast deep in the uterine wall. $\times$ 100.

mediastinum, pineal, etc., and choriocarcinoma may arise from them. This can be understood in view of the fact that nearly every fetal tissue may be represented in teratomas. As with fetal-derived choriocarcinoma, the urine usually contains a high concentration of chorionic gonadotrophin.

Ectopic pregnancy

This condition arises when the fertilised ovum becomes implanted and develops before it reaches the uterus. It may occur (*a*) in the Fallopian tube (*tubal pregnancy*), (*b*) between the fimbrial end of the tube and the ovary, when these are adherent (*tubo-ovarian*), (*c*) in the ovary itself (*ovarian*), or (*d*) in the peritoneal cavity (*abdominal*). All these forms, with the exception of the tubal, are rare. Abdominal pregnancy is usually secondary to rupture of a tubal pregnancy, the placenta then becoming attached to the peritoneal surface; but a primary form also is recognised. The commonest site in the tube is the ampullary portion, but *interstitial pregnancy* also occurs, i.e. in the intra-uterine end of the tube. Tubal pregnancy is in most instances the result of some abnormality of the tube—usually chronic inflammatory change. This is probably due in part to loss of the ciliated epithelium, but also to adhesions between the plicae, which have resulted in the formation of pockets or depressions in which the ovum tends to lodge. Within the tube the ovum passes through the mucosa and develops underneath it or in the muscular layers. The fetal structures develop in the usual way and there is great enlargement of blood vessels (Fig. 23.50), but the formation of decidua is only imperfect. The surrounding structures are invaded by the chorionic villi and stretched by the growing pregnancy. Rupture of the blood vessels is common at a comparatively early stage, and the haemorrhage tends to separate the pregnancy from the surrounding tissues. Rupture into the peritoneum, which is common, is usually accompanied by severe haemorrhage, even at a quite early stage of the pregnancy, and without transfusion this may prove fatal. Occasionally the placenta becomes separated from the ruptured tube and then attached to the peritoneum. The fetus may then reach various stages of development, secondary abdominal pregnancy resulting. The fetus may die, become encapsulated, and eventually heavily calcified (*lithopaedion*). In many instances a live child has been removed by operation from the peritoneal cavity. In extra-uterine pregnancy decidua forms within the uterine cavity. This is an important diagnostic finding in curettage of the uterus in cases of ectopic pregnancy. It may become separated and passed as a uterine cast. It is important to bear in mind that the use of oral contraceptive pills may induce a decidual reaction in endometrium, and that this may be misleading when encountered in uterine curettings in a suspected case of ectopic pregnancy.

Inflammation of the placenta

Syphilis. Important changes are produced in the placenta by syphilis, but it is often impossible to say whether a particular lesion is syphilitic or not. In many undoubted cases of syphilis the placenta is paler, denser and heavier in proportion to the child than normally. The connective tissue of the villi is increased and many villi are fused. This change leads to a diminution in the blood supply and thus of the nourishment of the child. Even when the internal organs of the fetus are swarming with the spirochaetes, it may not be possible to find any in the placenta, and in any given case the presence of syphilis is much more likely to be detected by an examination of the fetus than of the placenta.

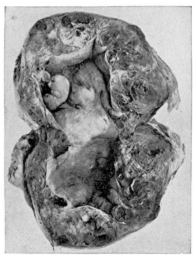

Fig. 23.50.—Section through tubal pregnancy, showing the very vascular wall; the embyro is seen in the upper part. × $\frac{2}{3}$.

The presence of necrotic areas or *infarcts of the placenta* must not be taken as evidence of syphilis. These may be numerous and large, irregular yellowish-white or pale red, and of dull necrotic appearance. Such infarcts occur in various conditions, and the smaller ones are not uncommon in normal pregnancy.

Tuberculosis of the placenta. This is rare, and may result from spread of tuberculous endo-

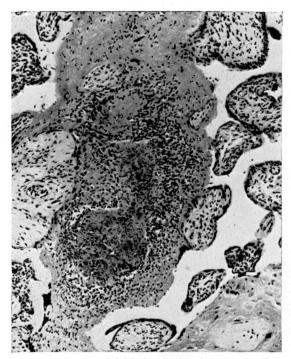

FIG. 23.51.—Vaccinial lesion in the placenta, showing necrosis and cellular reaction in the villi. × 112.

metritis, or it may occur in acute miliary tuberculosis of the mother. In the latter case, the bacilli settle on the epithelial covering of the villi and then penetrate their substance and give rise to tubercles. Infection of the fetus may follow, and thus a congenital form of tuberculosis, usually of miliary type with marked involvement of the liver, is produced. It is very uncommon.

Vaccinia. Vaccination during pregnancy should be avoided if possible on account of the risk of viraemia, leading to infection of the placenta and fetus. Intra-uterine death is apt to occur, resulting in the birth of a macerated fetus with pock-like lesions on the skin and foci of necrosis and cellular reaction in the placenta (Fig. 23.51).

The placenta in haemolytic disease of the newborn

Enlargement, pallor and oedema of the placenta occur in cases of *hydrops fetalis* (p. 412), and when a severely macerated fetus is born, the placenta may indicate the nature of the condition. Microscopically the villi are greatly swollen, fibrous and oedematous (Fig. 23.52), the Langhans cell layer persists on their surface and there is usually evidence of erythroblastosis in the vessels and stroma of the villi. In less severe haemolytic disease, e.g. icterus gravis, the placental changes are usually less conspicuous and the organ may look normal but the cord is often bile-stained.

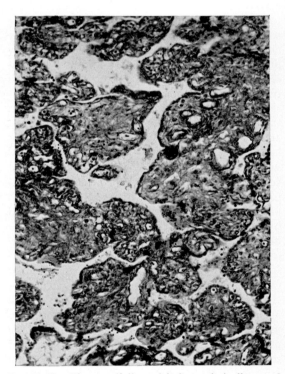

FIG. 23.52.—Placenta (full term) in haemolytic disease of the newborn, showing thickening and fibrosis of the villi. × 100.

CONGENITAL ABNORMALITIES

These are of considerable variety due to failure in the normal fusion of parts, to incomplete development or absence of certain structures, to pathological closure or atresia of openings, etc.; there is also the important group of abnormalities due to displacements of cells or portions of tissue, from which certain tumours arise, especially in the ovaries.

Uterus. Certain abnormalities arise from variations in the fusion of the lower parts of the ducts of

Müller, the upper portions of which constitute the two Fallopian tubes, while the lower portions coalesce to form the uterus and upper vagina. From imperfect fusion there arises duplication of structures which are normally single, and various degrees of this occur. Thus there may be a double uterus and vagina, a double uterus and single vagina (uterus bicornis duplex), or the uterus may be doubled only in its upper part (uterus bicornis unicollis); then again there are variations according to the degree in which the walls of the doubled cavities are fused. In the mildest degree of this type of abnormality the uterus has two short cornua and the outline of the fundus is concave upwards instead of convex, the condition being known as *uterus arcuatus*. Occasionally the ducts of Müller have split in their upper part, so that there are two Fallopian tubes on each side; or the splitting may be only partial, but this is a rare abnormality.

Deficiency of growth or *aplasia* is likewise of variable degree. Absence of the uterus and tubes is the extreme example, but is very rare, and in such cases it is necessary to determine the true sex of the subject first by examining a buccal smear for sex chromatin followed by chromosome analysis if doubt exists. Absence of uterus or of its lower part is occasionally observed while the tubes are present. Then again the uterus may be well formed, while there is occlusion or atresia of the os, less frequently of the isthmus; such lesions may lead to accumulation of the menstrual blood. Occasionally one duct of Müller has failed to develop, and then there is an absence of one tube, and the uterus is asymmetrical —*uterus unicornis*. In other cases asymmetry is due to a rudimentary cornu on one side, which is sometimes cut off from the uterine cavity. There are also other variations in which a tube or part of a tube is absent. Portions of the Wolffian ducts may fail to undergo the usual obliteration and may persist in the wall of the vagina; they may there give rise to cysts or tumour growths. The normal division of the cloaca with formation of the septum may be in-complete, and thus there remains a communication between the vestibulum and the lower end of the rectum—vestibulo-rectal fistula. This condition may be associated with imperforate anus (p. 537).

General *hypoplasia* of the uterus is observed in ovarian defect and may be accompanied by other abnormalities, e.g. pseudo-hermaphroditism, sometimes associated with hyperplasia of the adrenal cortex (p. 914). Hypoplasia, or rather the persistence after puberty of the infantile type or uterus, is seen in conditions of infantilism, for example that resulting from deficiency of the thyroid or of the anterior pituitary lobe secretions.

Ovaries. As already indicated, the most important abnormalities are those affecting the disposition of the germinal epithelium and the formation of the Graafian follicles; the various cystic tumours of the ovaries probably arise in this way. Small congenital cysts are occasionally encountered, and may be associated with a certain amount of fibrosis. True doubling of the ovaries has been recorded, but is extremely rare; aberrant portions of ovarian tissue are occasionally observed, and one or both ovaries may be in an abnormal situation, for example, one may be present in a patent inguinal canal. The ovaries are sometimes abnormally small, and there is then usually hypoplasia of other parts of the genital system; occasionally pseudo-hermaphroditism is present.

Gonadal agenesis (Turner's syndrome). This remarkable condition is the result of a chromosome anomaly, usually XO—i.e. the presence of only one X chromosome and no Y, with only 45 chromosomes in all. The affected individuals are females of normal intelligence, but with ovaries represented only by fibrous streaks and a total lack of sexual development at puberty; they are of very short stature and present a number of other lesser defects of which webbing of the neck is particularly characteristic. There are a number of variants depending chiefly upon varying degrees of partial retention of the second sex chromosome.

THE BREAST

Inflammations

Acute infections

Acute inflammatory conditions of the female breast may be non-suppurative or suppurative, and these have widely different results.

(a) Acute non-suppurative "mastitis". The commonest type occurs in connection with lactation, and is thus a form of puerperal mastitis. Al-though accompanied by some pyrexia, it is mainly a condition of congestive swelling and oedema, and is essentially hormonal in origin from failure to establish satisfactory lactation, very commonly as a result of early termination of suckling.

(b) Acute pyogenic mastitis. The most important form of suppurative mastitis is also related to lactation and is the result of infection by the ducts or through some abrasion of the nipple. It is usually caused by staphylococci acquired in hospital from the mouth of the suckling infant which has been colonised by the prevalent strain of *Staphylococcus aureus*. In

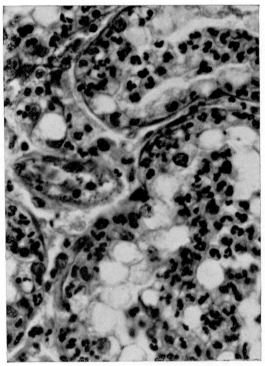

FIG. 23.53.—Acute puerperal mastitis showing the secreting mammary acini, heavily infiltrated with polymorph leukocytes. × 500.

staphylococcal mastitis multiple foci of suppuration may become confluent and form a loculated *intramammary* abscess; sometimes suppuration occurs more superficially by lymphatic extension from the nipple—*premammary* abscess, and occasionally infection extends between the breast and pectoral fascia—*retromammary* abscess. Much destruction of the breast may result, or multiple small abscesses may become encapsulated by fibrous tissue resulting in irregular induration. Infection by pyogenic streptococci is occasionally responsible for puerperal mastitis (Fig. 23.53) and a spreading cellulitis may result. In pregnancy and the puerperal period, a form of diffuse mammary carcinoma may present as a hot, swollen and tender breast and biopsy may be necessary to establish the diagnosis (p. 867).

Chronic inflammatory mastitis

A group of hyperplastic and cystic conditions of the breast was formerly termed "chronic mastitis"; these conditions are probably of hormonal nature, and not inflammatory; they are described under mastopathy (p. 860). Chronic inflammatory mastitis, in the strict sense, is a localised lesion which usually follows acute mastitis or difficult lactation, when there has been some infection, e.g. from cracked nipples, resulting in chronic low grade infection and granulomatous reaction.

Mammary duct ectasia

This condition of progressive dilatation of the mammary ducts commences in the subareolar lactiferous sinuses and extends peripherally to the parenchymal ducts. Neutral fat and cellular debris accumulate in the ectatic ducts leading to a coloured nipple discharge which may be confused clinically with that from a duct papilloma, from which it may be distinguished by cytological examination; in simple duct ectasia only foamy macrophages are present whereas in duct papilloma red blood cells and tumour cells are usually to be seen.

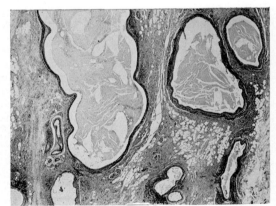

FIG. 23.54.—Mammary duct ectasia. The ducts are dilated and filled with fatty material. Their walls show hyperplasia of the elastic tissue. × 12.

Microscopic examination. The dilated ducts show marked elastic hyperplasia with thickening of their walls (Fig. 23.54); there are often many lymphocytes and plasma cells around the ducts. Fibrosis of the ducts may lead to retraction of the nipple and arouse suspicion of malignancy.

Low grade infection within the ducts leads to ulceration of the lining and liberation of lipids into the surrounding tissue resulting in a chronic inflammatory and granulomatous reaction (Fig. 23.55) with many giant cells and tubercle-like follicles on which an erroneous diagnosis of tuberculosis may be made. These changes may

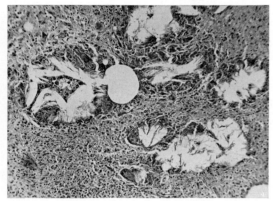

FIG. 23.55.—Granulomatous reaction due to duct ectasia. Foreign-body giant cell reaction around fatty material, giving rise to a hard mass. × 50.

be accompanied by a marked plasma cell reaction (*plasma-cell mastitis*) suggesting that some immune response is going on.

Recurrent areolar infection

Some women suffer repeated inflammation, scarring and fistulous formation in the subareolar and juxta-areolar tissues; this may be associated with mammary duct ectasia. Sometimes a fistula lined by granulation tissue communicates with a subareolar duct in which squamous metaplasia has occurred. This is called a *mammillary fistula*.

Traumatic fat necrosis

This lesion in the fatty tissue of an obese and pendulous breast is caused by trauma (often forgotten by the patient). It gives rise to a localised firm or even hard mass which may underlie and be adherent to the skin and has not infrequently been mistaken for carcinoma. The appearances vary at different stages but there is often a central cavity containing brown oily fluid. This is surrounded by a broad zone of dull yellowish-white tissue with scattered areas of similar appearance in the outer part. At the periphery there is a fibrous capsule.

Microscopic examination shows the presence of rounded foamy cells containing small fatty globules and multinucleated giant cells which may form large collections (Fig. 23.56). Many of the giant cells contain crystals of fatty acid and at places a number of them may be arranged around masses of crystals. There is usually comparatively little doubly refracting fat. Macrophages containing iron pigment are usually also present. The lesion represents the result of traumatic rupture of fat cells followed by a slow lipolysis along with phagocytosis and other reactive changes. Similar appearances are sometimes seen after minor surgical operations on the breast.

Tuberculosis

Tuberculosis of the breast is now rare. It may be the result of haematogenous infection, or it may be due to lymphatic or direct spread from caseous axillary lymph nodes or tuberculosis of the pleura or ribs. The bacilli settle in the interstitial tissue, invade the lobules, and cause the formation of tubercles which may spread to the subepithelial connective

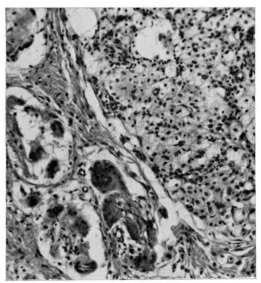

FIG. 23.56.—Traumatic fat necrosis of breast, showing lipophages and foreign body giant cells. × 150.

tissue of the ducts and acini. Ulceration may then occur into them and the bacilli may be spread by the ducts. Sometimes the condition may be localised and lead to a large caseous swelling which may simulate tumour; in other cases, the lesion is a more diffuse infiltration with nodular thickenings, a form of true chronic interstitial mastitis. In untreated cases, the caseous change may spread to the surface of the breast and ulceration with formation of a sinus may result. In view of the histological similarity of various non-tuberculous lesions (e.g. duct ectasia; fat necrosis), the diagnosis of mammary tuberculosis should not be made without proof that tubercle bacilli are present in the lesion.

Syphilis

When wet nursing was common practice a primary sore might develop on the nipple of the wet nurse suckling a child affected by congenital syphilis. Infection may also be conveyed from an individual with the highly infective oral lesions of the secondary stage, by kissing the nipple or breast. Gumma of the breast is now rare. As in gumma elsewhere, the structural outlines of the tissue are long retained, and gross scarring may result.

Actinomycosis

Multilocular abscesses of this nature are rare, but the infection may extend to the breast through the chest wall from the pleura.

Mastopathy

Generalised cystic mastopathy

It is difficult to find a comprehensive term to cover the various pathological changes commonly seen in the breasts that are neither inflammatory nor truly neoplastic. The changes include hyperplasia, metaplasia and cyst formation, and either inflammation or neoplasia may subsequently complicate the picture. The non-committal term "mastopathy" is a convenient one for that succession of mammary changes that are probably the result of hormonal imbalance though precise quantitative hormonal studies in support of this view are not available.

Conditions of occurrence. Generalised mastopathy is commoner in nulliparae and is sometimes associated with menstrual irregularity. The incidence increases towards the menopause, but it may occur in severe form early in the third decade. Although the changes may at first be local they tend to extend progressively and eventually affect much of the parenchyma of one or both breasts.

Structural changes. These are of considerable variety and complexity, but can best be considered under the headings, (a) fibrosis, (b) cyst formation, (c) adenosis and (d) epitheliosis. The breast tissue tends to be firmer and more nodular than usual and the lobules may be visible as groups of small elongated yellowish-brown foci in the white rubbery collagenous stroma. Cysts of 2–10 mm. diameter frequently occur in clusters: less commonly one or more larger cysts of bluish appearance, containing a thin mucoid or dark brownish fluid, are present.

Microscopic examination reveals a great variety of structural changes. When the changes are limited to fibrosis, adenosis, sclerosing adenosis and cyst formation, the name *simple cystic disease* is applied; but when epithelial hyperplasia (epitheliosis) is marked in ducts and acini the condition is better termed *hyperplastic cystic disease*. This distinction is important since only in the latter condition is there evidence of transition to neoplasia.

Fibrosis. Some fibrosis accompanies most cases of mastopathy but is difficult to assess; the normally fibrous breast of young women persists even after the menopause in those of spare build, whereas in obese women the fibrous tissue of the breast may be extensively infiltrated with fat, and as age advances the fibrous mammary stroma becomes hyaline and relatively acellular while the epithelial elements atrophy. It is this collagenisation of pre-existing stroma rather than renewed fibroblastic activity that leads to fibrosis of the breast. Occasionally in heavy pendulous breasts this process leads to the appearance of an indurated mass in the upper outer quadrant.

Cyst formation may begin in ducts, terminal ductules or acini, presumably from increased secretion by the epithelial lining cells accompanied by some degree of narrowing of the excretory passages. Generalised dilatation of the ducts with disordered secretion constitutes mammary duct ectasia which has already been described. Some cysts show metaplasia of the epithelial lining cells; these become large, columnar and eosinophilic with a feathery outline and at their apices may contain granules resembling those seen normally in apocrine gland epithelium. Cyst formation is more frequent at about the time of the menopause or thereafter and tends to affect both breasts. It is probably an involutional effect related to changes in hormone production.

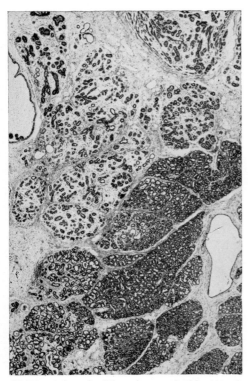

FIG. 23.57.—Adenosis. There is a marked increase in the size and number of the lobules. Cystic dilatation of occasional ductules is present. × 22.

Adenosis. This is the name applied to the new formation of breast lobules and/or to enlargement of pre-existing lobules: these retain their usual histological pattern (Fig. 23.57) and there is no intraluminal proliferation of cells to fill the acini, as occurs in pregnancy. A mild degree of adenosis occurs in the second half of each normal menstrual cycle, and the mammary hyperplasia of pregnancy begins as adenosis; during lactation secretory phenomena are superadded.

Adenosis is a feature of some mastopathies, and there it almost certainly results from hormonal stimulation. Adenosis plays no part in the development of carcinoma of the breast but may be prominent in the breast parenchyma around fibroadenomas.

Sclerosing adenosis. This is a perversion of simple adenosis which may occur as an isolated phenomenon producing a palpable rubbery greyish mass in the breasts of young women. Commonly it follows incomplete involution after an interrupted pregnancy or lactational failure. Sclerosing adenosis also occurs in microscopic foci in the breasts of women of widely different age groups and may be present along with epithelial proliferative lesions, e.g. papilloma. As in simple adenosis the changes are always lobular but lack the simple acinar pattern seen in adenosis. Sclerosing adenosis proceeds through a sequence of changes beginning with an early florid, confused picture of proliferation of both epithelial and myo-epithelial elements (Fig.

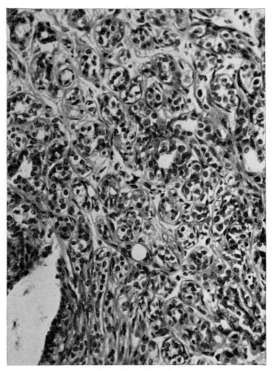

FIG. 23.58.—Sclerosing adenosis in the florid phase; many small acini and solid cords of cells with much myo-epithelial hyperplasia. × 200.

23.58). Mitotic activity may be high at this stage. Later the true epithelial elements atrophy and the myo-epithelial cells produce a corded appearance which simulates infiltrative carcinoma. Eventually the myo-epithelial elements undergo collagenisation which increases the resemblance to scirrhous carcinoma. Sclerosing adenosis has no significance as a precursor of carcinoma; its importance lies in the possibility of misdiagnosis as cancer, especially on immediate section in the operating theatre. Such errors are best avoided by careful low-power examination which reveals the typical *lobular* nature of the change.

Epitheliosis. This term was coined by Mrs. E. K. Dawson to describe the condition in which hyperplasia of the epithelium of ducts and acini results in the heaping up of lining cells which may eventually fill the lumina of ducts and acini more or less completely (Fig. 23.59). This hyperplasia may take three forms (*a*) a solid type in which the ducts are solidly filled, (*b*) a cribriform variety in which there is a tendency to acinar arrangement without stroma formation, and (*c*) a papillary arrangement in which the exuberant epithelial ingrowths are usually less well provided with fibrovascular cores than are true papillomas. Epitheliosis is an important condition and, unlike adenosis and sclerosing adenosis, may be associated with the development of carcinoma, although many patients with epitheliosis escape this change. The presence of epitheliosis is the essential feature that distinguishes hyperplastic cystic disease from simple cystic mastopathy.

Localised hyperplastic cystic disease

While all the changes enumerated above may occur in generalised mastopathy it is probable that local areas of epitheliosis more often give rise to a clinically detectable lesion. Localised hyperplastic disease begins during the reproductive period and leads to an irregular induration or discrete swelling of the breast which demands surgical excision for exclusion of malignancy. Pain is not usually a feature and consequently hyperplastic disease often escapes notice. Necropsy studies have shown significant epithelial hyperplasia in a considerable proportion of unselected women. In a proportion of breasts presenting with carcinoma, hyperplastic cystic disease is found to coexist with and almost certainly to have preceded the tumour. In this localised form of disease cyst formation is often slight or absent. The epitheliosis present may be severe and in any combination of patterns, affecting few or many ducts or duct and acinar

systems. From examination of a large number of amputated breasts a picture of progressive dedifferentiation of the proliferative cells is built up. Even within the same breast an evolutionary sequence from obviously benign to obviously malignant cells may be traced within the ducts and may, although less frequently, extend to the acini. Ultimately the ducts and acini are filled partially or completely by masses of cells with

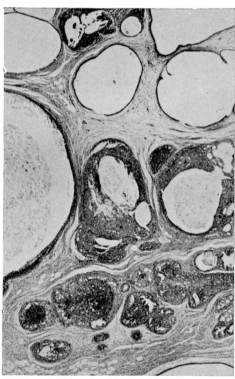

FIG. 23.59.—Epitheliosis of breast. Some of the ducts are filled with masses of epithelial cells and others are dilated with granular secretion. × 22.

hyperchromatic and aberrant nuclei to which the terms *intraduct carcinoma*, and *intra-acinar carcinoma* are suitably applied. From either lesion malignant cells may break through the investing basement membrane and invade the surrounding stroma as an ordinary infiltrative carcinoma.

Etiology. The cause of hyperplastic cystic disease and its significant component of epitheliosis has not yet been fully elucidated. It can be categorically stated that inflammation plays no part and that the commonly used synonym "chronic mastitis" is quite unjustified. These changes clearly seem to represent an endocrine effect, either from excess of oestrogen, which in certain species has been shown to bring about mammary hyperplasia and neoplasia, or from failure to achieve the normal balanced action of the sex hormones. Therapeutically administration of hormones has not, however, clarified the nature of the presumed imbalance.

"Hypertrophy" of the female breast

This form of enlargement must not be confused with the gross mammary adiposity observed in some obese middle-aged women. So-called hypertrophy usually develops soon after puberty although occasionally it may follow pregnancy. The breasts enlarge progressively and may eventually weigh several kilograms. The condition is usually but not invariably bilateral but development may be unequal. The term hypertrophy is not always apt since the breast enlargement may result from increase in soft oedematous connective tissue, and sometimes also of adipose tissue. Glandular elements may not be increased and, indeed, often appear scanty. Sometimes superficial inflammatory change occurs in the pendulous portions of the enlarged breasts. The cause of hypertrophy is quite unknown but is presumed to be hormonal; occasionally hypothalamic disorder is implicated. We have observed an exceptional case of pathological mammary enlargement resembling the so-called virginal hypertrophy described above, in which breasts weighing 7 kg. were removed surgically, but in which the increase in size was due to multiple enormous benign fibroadenomas.

TUMOURS OF THE BREAST

Benign Tumours

Fibroadenoma

This is by far the commonest simple tumour of the breast and arises from the whole anatomical unit of the lobule. Both stromal and epithelial elements participate in the neoplasm, which occurs chiefly in young women. Sometimes in young girls the fibrous component is inconspicuous and the tumour is then termed a simple *adenoma*. Fibroadenomas are small, well-circumscribed, elastic, round or ovoid masses which may occasionally attain a diameter of up to 7 cm. They are apparently encapsulated and although they may readily be removed from the surrounding breast tissue by the surgeon's finger, they should not be so treated since satellite portions of the tumour may be left behind from which recurrence takes place.

Two forms of fibroadenoma are usually distinguished but such a division is artificial since many tumours show both types of structure in different areas (Fig. 23.60). In young adults the so-called *pericanalicular type* occurs, in which the epithelial arrangement corresponds roughly to that in the normal breast lobule with an investment of loosely fibrillary connective tissue. The predominantly *intracanalicular* type seen usually in older women shows numerous curved and branching clefts lined by epithelium but indented by the growth of blunt rounded projections of fibrocellular tissue into the lumina of ducts and acini. Growth of the lining epithelium merely keeps pace with that of the stroma and the characteristic clefting is produced.

The site of origin of fibroadenoma is within the ductal elastic tissue; usually this is not obvious on cursory examination but occasional tumours present as intraduct lesions reminiscent of intraduct papilloma. In such cases bleeding from the nipple may occur. Multiple small fibroadenomatous areas sometimes occur in association with cystic disease suggesting an intermediate phenomenon between hyperplasia and neoplasia. Fibroadenomas grow not only by proliferation of the actual tumour but also by incorporating at their periphery altered lobular units showing such fibroadenomatous change. Some intracanalicular tumours contain large amounts of smooth muscle in their stroma; while it is tempting to assume that this is derived from myo-epithelium we have seen no convincing evidence of this and in some cases the smooth muscle appears to be derived from vein walls.

Giant intracanalicular fibroadenomas. In older women certain large fibroadenomas tend to recur after operative removal (especially if "shelled out") and the recurrent tumour may show a highly cellular and often a distinctly

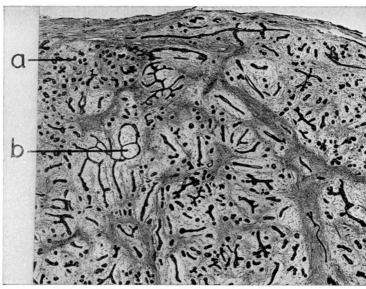

FIG. 23.60.—Fibroadenoma of breast, showing the loose periacinar stroma. In places the tumour has a pericanalicular structure (*a*), at other parts an intracanalicular arrangement (*b*). Transitions are seen between the two types.　× 16.

myxoid stroma. In some cases, especially after repeated recurrence, stromal proliferation is so marked that the epithelial elements may be quite inconspicuous and the tumour merits the designation of myxosarcoma. The term *Brodie's serocystic sarcoma* was sometimes applied to such tumours (Fig. 23.61), and simple mastectomy or very wide local excision is the treatment of choice. They should not be designated as sarcoma unless unequivocal malignant changes in the stromal cells have occurred; the development of frankly sarcomatous change is discussed further below.

Papillary cystadenoma

This simple tumour is much less common than fibroadenoma. Cysts of varying size are present and within these there is epithelial proliferation. Often these epithelial tumours have a somewhat papilliform pattern but they are composed of acini and do not show the investment of fibrovascular cores by epithelium in the way characteristic of papilloma. Papillary cystadenoma may become large and, if not removed, may ulcerate through the skin and present as papillary masses on the breast surface. Most are simple tumours but occasionally cystadenocarcinoma supervenes; it is, however, usually of low malignancy.

Papilloma

Duct papilloma occurs most often as a rounded pedunculated tumour which forms within and eventually distends a lactiferous sinus, in or close to the nipple (Figs. 11.4, p. 230; 23.62). A papilloma comprises a branching fibrovascular stromal core clothed by a double-

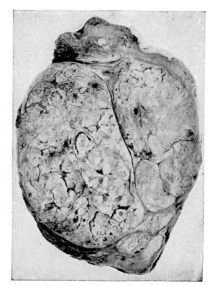

FIG. 23.61.—Giant intracanalicular fibroadenoma of the breast; the stroma was very cellular and showed sarcomatous change.　× ⅓.

layered cuboidal or columnar epithelium (Fig. 23.63). The tumour may be solitary and attain a size of more than 10 mm. but sometimes multiple tumours are present throughout the duct system of the breast. The larger tumours are often accompanied by nipple discharge and those in the lactiferous sinus may present with frank bleeding from the nipple. Microscopic examination of such discharges usually shows red blood cells and tumour epithelial cells and often permits distinction from the coloured discharges present in mammary duct ectasia. There is a distinct resemblance between certain papillomas of the lactiferous sinuses and papillary hidradenoma of the vulva, the lesion that has been described as *naevus syringo-cystadenomatosus papilliferus*. The nipple contains no sweat glands and the resemblance may be related to the developmental similarity of the breast to a sweat gland. Epithelium of apocrine-like appearance is not uncommon in intraduct papilloma.

Papillary forms of epitheliosis occur in hyperplastic cystic disease and it is difficult to draw a clear line between papillary epitheliosis and papillomatosis; the presence of well-formed

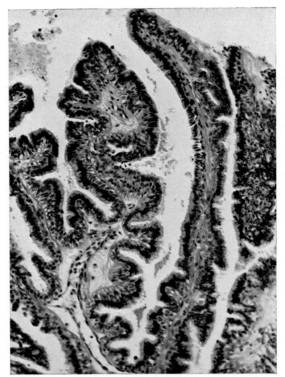

FIG. 23.63.—Duct papilloma of breast, showing branching papilliform processes covered by epithelium mainly of columnar type. × 130.

fibrovascular stromal cores is in favour of multiple neoplasms. When such small papillomas are present in large numbers multicentric carcinoma may occasionally develop. Carcinomatous change is rare in solitary papilloma.

Other benign tumours

These are uncommon but fibroma, myxoma, lipoma, angioma and chondroma are recorded. Granular cell myoblastoma (p. 473) occasionally occurs in the breast and clinically may simulate carcinoma.

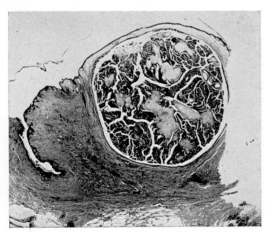

FIG. 23.62.—A rounded duct papilloma distending a lactiferous sinus within the nipple. × 6·5.

Malignant Tumours

Carcinoma

Mammary cancer is one of the commonest malignant neoplasms that affect mankind, as revealed by morbidity and mortality statistics. While it occurs more often in later adult life it is by no means rare in the third and fourth decades:

for this reason all lumps in the breast, whatever the age of the patient, must be regarded clinically as possibly malignant until proved otherwise by histological examination. Immediate histological examination of fresh sections at the time of operation is of value in enabling the surgeon to decide upon the type of treatment required.

Carcinoma of the breast is at least two hundred times more common in the female than in the male; it is more common in nulliparous than in multiparous women and several successful lactations appear to decrease the risk that it will develop. These observations suggest that endocrine factors may be important in the etiology of breast cancer.

Several types of breast carcinoma are described but this should not obscure the important fact that they are all manifestations of one disease process.

Endocrine dependence. In 1896 Beatson in Glasgow first showed that bilateral oophorectomy was followed by prolonged remission in some cases of advanced breast cancer and he postulated that such mammary cancers required for their continuing growth some influence from the ovaries. This original idea has been developed in the light of modern surgery and endocrinology into the concept of hormone-dependent (i.e. oestrogen-dependent) tumours. Some post-menopausal women with breast cancer continue to secrete oestrogens and in an attempt to deprive such patients of all sources of oestrogen, removal of the ovaries was undertaken, followed by adrenalectomy and hypophysectomy when cortisone became available for maintenance treatment.

In a small proportion of cases such procedures are successful in relieving symptoms, notably pain from skeletal metastases, but after a variable period the malignant cells resume their uncontrolled growth, i.e. the tumour becomes *hormone-independent*. No histological differences have been demonstrated by which hormone-dependent tumours can be recognised under the microscope and at present it is impossible except by therapeutic trial to determine which cases will respond to endocrine ablation. It is not known whether hormones other than oestrogen are implicated and it has been suggested that progesterone, androgens and mammatrophic prolactin may play a part. Large-scale prospective studies are being carried out which may throw light on this problem.

Despite the clinical remission obtained in cases of hormone-dependent cancer by such procedures there is only minimal evidence of tumour-cell destruction in most instances and only temporary arrest of tumour growth, but the relief of pain has made these drastic surgical procedures an accepted form of therapy.

Macroscopic varieties of breast cancer

Scirrhous carcinoma. This is the commonest form of breast cancer; it produces an indurated mass of indefinite outline and the resulting fibrosis of the stroma causes contraction and shrinkage rather than obvious enlargement of the breast (Fig. 23.64). Fibrosis is most marked in the atrophic scirrhus where the tumour may

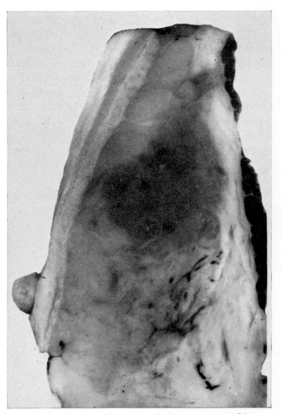

FIG. 23.64.—Section through scirrhous cancer of breast, which appears as a darker, poorly defined mass in the upper part. $\times \frac{1}{2}$.

remain less than 1 cm. diameter. When cut with a knife a scirrhous cancer gives a creaking sensation and the cut surface shows small yellow areas due to degeneration of tumour cells; this "unripe pear" appearance is very characteristic of a scirrhous cancer. In the late stages distortion or retraction of the nipple or puckering and indrawing of the skin may occur depending on the site of the tumour, which may be in any part of the breast, including the axillary tail, but is most frequent in the upper outer portion. Microscopy shows groups and cords of spheroidal carcinoma cells (Fig. 11.15, p. 236) between bands of fibrous tissue which are more hyaline at the centre while at the periphery this change is less advanced.

The scirrhous carcinoma of the breast was recognised as early as Hippocratic times and the appearances of a central tumour mass with infiltrating prongs (Fig. 23.65) gave rise to the words *cancer* and *carcinoma* (i.e. crab-like).

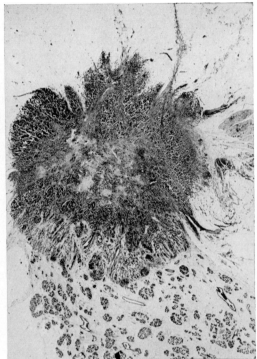

FIG. 23.65.—Small scirrhous cancer of breast. The tumour has originated at the periphery and is invading both the breast tissue and the surrounding fat. Note the claw-like extensions along lymphatic channels. × 5·5.

Encephaloid carcinoma. This tumour is less common than the scirrhous variety; it forms a large soft mass or masses, with a consistency likened to that of brain, and with ill-defined margins and extensive areas of necrosis and haemorrhage. Sometimes necrosis and ulceration through the skin occurs. Microscopically a comparatively scanty and cellular stroma, often containing many lymphocytes, separates large collections of spheroidal tumour cells amongst which cellular aberration and frequent, often multipolar mitoses are seen (Fig. 11.16, p. 237). The heavy lymphocytic infiltration seen in some tumours may represent an immune reaction directed against the tumour cells, and surveys have demonstrated that such *medullary carcinomas* carry a high rate of five-year survival.

Mammary carcinoma in pregnancy and lactation. A distinct variety of mammary cancer is the acute cancer of pregnancy and lactation in which rapid growth may be accompanied by hyperaemia, warmth and sometimes pain. Pyrexia may also be a feature and the whole picture suggests inflammation, although the tumour is highly malignant in every respect. This variety of breast cancer is sometimes very diffusely infiltrative, so that the whole breast is swollen, hard and hyperaemic with no discrete lump; consequently it looks more like a cellulitis than a malignant tumour.

Histological appearances of breast carcinoma

In most scirrhous and encephaloid carcinomas the cells are quite anaplastic, spheroidal and arranged in irregular clumps (Fig. 11.13, p. 235). Less commonly the cells retain a certain polarity and a recognisably adenocarcinomatous pattern results. Such adenocarcinomas are said on statistical evidence to have a slightly better prognosis than anaplastic spheroidal cell tumours. Rarely breast carcinomas are composed of masses of closely applied cells between which there are small circular spaces, sometimes containing mucoid material: this is termed *cribriform carcinoma* (Fig. 23.66), and although most typically seen within the ducts the pattern may persist when the tissues are infiltrated. More often, however, when infiltration supervenes the cribriform pattern is lost and the structure of the infiltrating tumour is of the usual anaplastic spheroidal-cell type. These observations are of importance in tracing the evolutionary sequences from epitheliosis through intraduct cancer to anaplastic infiltrative tumour.

Other histological types of breast cancer

Mucoid carcinoma. Mucoid or "colloid" cancers are uncommon although microscopy of apparently ordinary breast carcinomas sometimes show small areas of mucoid change. Further, a small proportion of apparently ordinary spheroidal-cell cancers may be seen to produce mucin when appropriately stained. When mucoid change is generalised the tumour is usually bulky, translucent and slimy. Microscopy shows islands of surviving carcinoma cells floating in a sea of mucin. Such carcinomas are sometimes, but not always, less malignant than the commoner varieties, with delay in nodal metastasis. Sometimes the stroma of a cancer undergoes myxoid or mucoid degeneration, the so-called *carcinoma myxomatodes*.

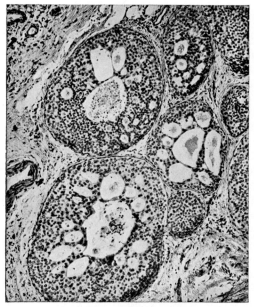

Fig. 23.66.—"Cribriform carcinoma", showing masses of carcinoma cells among which are small circular spaces. The growth is still contained within ducts. × 75.

Squamous carcinoma. Areas of squamous metaplasia sometimes occur in anaplastic carcinoma; the two histological variants may infiltrate together through the breast tissue and metastasise to lymph nodes. Occasional carcinomas are apparently entirely of squamous type. A further interesting variant is the fibrosarcoma-like squamous carcinoma in which the bulk of the tumour is spindle-celled; only careful search reveals that these cells are undoubtedly derived from squamous carcinoma which is recognisable in occasional areas. Such tumours are sometimes misdiagnosed as carcino-sarcoma.

Spread of infiltrative carcinoma

The axillary lymph nodes are involved at an early stage by lymphatic dissemination and in many cases the internal mammary lymph nodes are also affected. Later the local skin lymphatics may be permeated leading to either focal nodularity or wider-spread involvement (known as *cancer-en-cuirasse*). If the skin lymphatics are blocked, lymph-drainage is impaired and the skin becomes oedematous and swollen except where it is tacked down by hair-follicles; this produces the characteristic *peau d'orange* appearance of advanced breast cancer. Further lymphatic spread occurs through the connective tissues to the pectoral fascia and muscles and thence to the pleural cavities. In all of these situations microscopy may be required to reveal collections of malignant cells along the lymphatic pathways. It is upon these observations that the operation of radical mastectomy is based; unfortunately at the time of operation often there is already further spread by lymphatics (and possibly by the blood-stream) to other sites. Viscera and the dorso-lumbar spine are frequently affected, the latter possibly by retrograde venous spread. Modern surgical treatments, e.g. oöphorectomy, adrenalectomy and hypophysectomy have also revealed microscopic metastases in these organs. Metastatic spread to the opposite breast is not uncommon and may sometimes be distinguished from a cancer in the second breast by the absence of intraduct carcinoma, which we believe to be nearly always present in primary breast cancers (see below). Lymphatic dissemination of tumour occurs as rapidly in the atrophic scirrhous as in the fast-growing encephaloid variety.

Intraduct carcinoma and its relationship to infiltrative tumour

Intraduct carcinoma is a malignant proliferation of epithelial cells still confined within the ducts of the breasts, i.e. it is a pre-invasive neoplasm which has not yet broken through the walls of the duct system (Fig. 23.67). In the larger ducts intraduct carcinoma can be recognised macroscopically and is readily seen with a hand-lens. The ducts are filled with cylindrical masses of cells and degenerate fatty material which can sometimes be expressed like toothpaste from a tube; this is termed *comedo carcinoma*. Sometimes calcification occurs in the central necrotic material. Intraduct cancer may be relatively localised to one area or may affect the duct system extensively. There may be some periductal fibrosis and elastosis, with increased firmness of the affected part.

Microscopic examination shows rounded or polyhedral cells with a vesicular and often hyperchromatic nucleus, packed closely together or arranged in a cribriform pattern (Fig. 23.66). Both cells and nuclei may show considerable aberration. The condition spreads slowly along

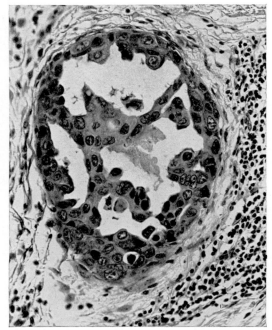

FIG. 23.67.—Section of intraduct carcinoma of breast, showing collections of carcinoma cells of characteristic appearance in a duct. × 250.

the ducts towards the nipple and also deeply into the acini, and there may be a long period during which the neoplastic cells remain confined within the basement membranes. Local obliterative changes with fibrosis and elastosis sometimes occur with local healing of the lesion but this sclerosing process is never generalised.

A corresponding change may occur in which the acini become filled with malignant cells; this is called *lobular* or *intra-acinar carcinoma* (Fig. 23.68). This may co-exist with intraduct carcinoma but pure intra-acinar is less common than intraduct change. The appearances must not be confused with those of lobular adenosis (see p. 861). As in intraduct carcinoma there may be a long period during which neoplasia is confined to the acini. This long pre-invasive period probably explains why intraduct carcinoma tends to be found in rather younger

women than those with infiltrative cancer. When infiltration supervenes the subsequent behaviour is that of ordinary cancer. If, however, the intraduct neoplasm primarily affects or later reaches the ducts of the nipple, extension to and spread within the epidermis may lead to *Paget's disease of the nipple*. If the breast is not then removed breakthrough may occur and ordinary infiltrative carcinoma will supervene, although this may be a very slow process.

Muir made extensive studies of the evolution of breast carcinoma and showed that in most cases of infiltrative carcinoma intraduct cancer could also be detected and he concluded that intraduct carcinoma was a precursor of the infiltrative tumour. He was unable to detect epitheliosis (pre-neoplastic hyperplasia) in most cases; it is therefore possible that intraduct carcinoma may arise *de novo*, or that supervention of neoplasia may destroy evidence of previous epitheliosis. In a small proportion of cases, however, an evolutionary sequence from epitheliosis to infiltrative carcinoma can be detected in ducts or acini or in both. In such cases

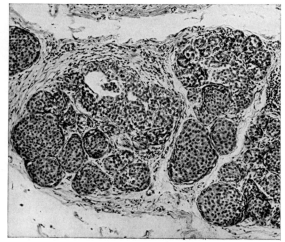

FIG. 23.68.—Lobular or intra-acinar carcinoma, showing groups of acini filled with anaplastic carcinoma cells without any break-through into tissue spaces. × 75.

multicentric origin of neoplasia is common; this suggests a gradual process affecting cell groups in a diffuse manner. This is well seen in intra-acinar carcinoma. Muir believed that these changes imply that neoplasia is the final result of some growth stimulating agent (possibly hormonal) acting progressively and that there is no evidence of a dual causation, i.e. of one agent leading to epitheliosis and of a second factor (such as a virus) acting locally and causing malignant transformation.

Paget's disease of nipple

In this condition, first described clinically by Sir James Paget in 1874, the surface of the nipple, either in whole or in part, becomes reddened, excoriated and has a florid eczematous appearance with oozing of clear fluid. The tissues of the

flattened between them (Fig. 23.70). Usually many Paget cells undergo degeneration, i.e. their nuclei become irregular and pyknotic and their cytoplasm has a rather shrivelled appearance. When many of the cells show this change their nature may not be clear. Paget cells may take up melanin from adjacent melanoblasts and sometimes they contain a small amount of mucin. The epidermal cells around groups of Paget cells undergo compression atrophy, and may appear to form a dense capsule-like structure. Paget cells never grow down into the underlying

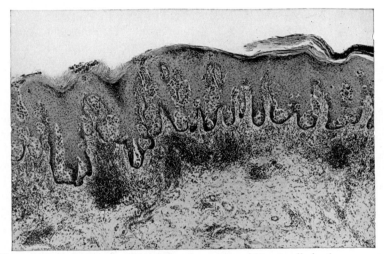

FIG. 23.69.—Skin of nipple in Paget's disease, showing scattered Paget cells in deeper part of epidermis. Note marked lymphocytic infiltration of dermis. × 35.

nipple are often firmer than normal. Paget observed that this state might persist for years but that eventually cancer commonly developed. This cancer might be present deep in the breast parenchyma and separated from the nipple by an interval of apparently normal tissue.

Microscopic examination reveals *Paget cells* within the affected epidermis. There has been much debate concerning the nature of these cells, which occur singly or in groups and often most abundantly in the deeper epidermal layers where they may form blunt processes projecting down into the dermis (Fig. 23.69). Paget cells in their active period of growth are large round or oval cells with pale cytoplasm and vesicular, often hyperchromatic nuclei, with prominent nucleoli. Mitotic figures are sometimes seen. The appearance of the cells is reminiscent of those of an undifferentiated carcinoma of glandular origin. They infiltrate and displace the cells of the Malpighian layer which become drawn out or

dermis but the latter shows reactive changes, e.g. plasma cell infiltration, formation of new capillaries, hyperaemia and serous exudation. It is these changes in the dermis which cause the characteristic *clinical* appearances of the condition.

Paget's disease is always accompanied by intraduct carcinoma in the ducts of the nipple (Fig. 23.71) and frequently direct continuity may be traced between the cells in the ducts and those in the epidermis. Statements that Paget's disease is the result of a field change of neoplasia independently but concomitantly affecting the nipple epidermis and the ductal epithelium are not well substantiated. Obviously intraduct carcinoma may be complicated by Paget's disease of nipple or by infiltrative carcinoma of the breast parenchyma depending on the site of origin of the intraduct carcinoma. The clinician must appreciate that the diagnosis of Paget's disease indicates the presence of carcinoma within the nipple ducts, that similar changes may be present deeper in the parenchymal ducts and that infiltrative carcinoma may therefore supervene. Simple mastectomy is therefore essential. Whether intraduct carcinoma is followed by Paget's disease or by ordinary infiltrative carcinoma depends upon whether the affected ducts are in the nipple or breast parenchyma. If

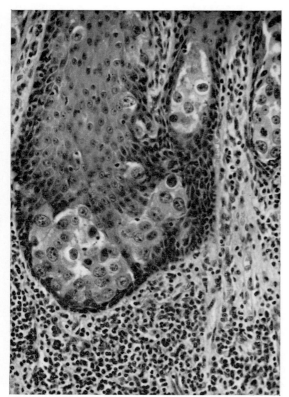

FIG. 23.70.—Paget's disease of nipple. Epidermal rete ridge invaded by cancer cells—"Paget cells". The cells are specially well preserved and show a marked contrast to the epidermal cells which are being stretched and atrophied. × 240.

Paget's disease appears mastectomy is usually performed before infiltration occurs; similarly when infiltrating carcinoma is detected mastectomy follows and there is no time for the intraduct neoplasia to reach the nipple and lead to Paget's disease. Occasional mastectomy specimens show on examination of the apparently normal nipple that Paget's disease is commencing or that intraduct neoplasm is nearing the epidermis.

Occasional primary intra-epithelial tumours of the nipple epidermis occur. Bowen's disease of skin and malignant lentigo of the nipple

may also produce widespread intra-epithelial growth, but in neither case is there intraduct carcinoma. Squamous carcinoma of the nipple is rare.

Sarcoma of the breast

This is much less common than carcinoma. It may supervene in giant intracanalicular fibroadenoma of middle-aged or elderly women especially after inadequate resection. Carcinomatous change is extremely rare in such circumstances. Primary sarcoma is usually of spindle-celled type (Fig. 23.72) but may be markedly myxomatous or highly pleomorphic. Cellular aberration and mitotic activity are related to the degree of malignancy. Some sarcomas show metaplasia with formation of chondroid and

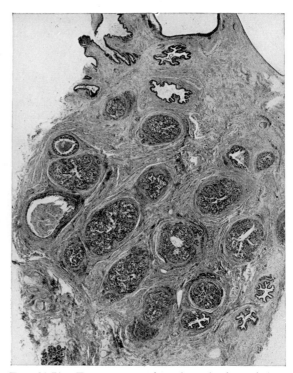

FIG. 23.71.—Transverse section through ducts below nipple in Paget's disease, showing malignant proliferation of epithelium within ducts—intraduct carcinoma. × 12.5.

osteoid and may resemble osteosarcoma or giant cell tumour of bone. In these cases the prognosis is bad and death from pulmonary metastases is the rule. Malignant haemangioendothelioma, which is a rare neoplasm, shows an unusual predilection for the breast as the primary site and we have seen several cases terminating with very widespread metastases.

Secondary carcinoma in breast

Spread to the contralateral breast may occur from a primary breast cancer. Carcinomas in other organs, e.g. bronchus, may also occasionally metastasise to the breast.

Malignant reticuloses

Hodgkin's disease, lymphosarcoma, reticulosarcoma and the leukaemias may all affect the breast. We have seen massive enlargement of the breasts by chloromatous tumours in acute leukaemia, and rarely, enlargement of one or both breasts may be the presenting symptom in leukaemia or Hodgkin's disease. As the axillary lymph nodes are likely also to be affected the clinical diagnosis may be difficult.

Congenital abnormalities. The absence of one or both of the breasts—*amazia*—is rare; in some instances it has been associated with a corresponding defect of one or both of the ovaries. *Athelia*, or con-

genital absence of the nipple, is less uncommon; it usually occurs on both sides. Hypoplasia of the breasts occurs in association with a similar condition of the ovaries and other parts of the genital system. The term *polymastia* is applied to a condition where there are multiple masses of glandular tissue. Such an accessory mass may or may not possess a nipple; in the former case it is usually rudimentary but sometimes milk is secreted through it. Supernumerary mammary structures occur most frequently below the breasts, although sometimes in the axillae or elsewhere along the mammary line. The term *polythelia* signifies the presence of multiple nipples.

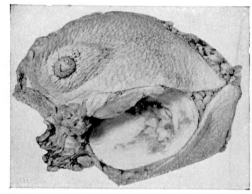

FIG. 23.72.—Sarcoma of breast cut across. × ½.

THE MALE BREAST

Hypertrophy of male breast. The male breast is essentially similar to that of the female until the onset of the secondary sex characters at puberty; in some adolescent males one or both breasts may then enlarge. This is known as *pubertal hypertrophy* and is rarely marked, although there may be some pain or discomfort. The condition tends to regress and operative removal is rarely necessary.

Enlargement of the male breast (gynaecomastia) may be associated with pathological changes in other organs and also with malnutrition, for example, in cirrhosis or prolonged chronic venous congestion of the liver. This enlargement is due to failure of the liver to metabolise and break down oestrogens. Hypertrophy also follows prolonged administration of di-ethyl stilboestrol in the treatment of prostatic cancer. Occasionally hypertrophy results from an underlying endocrine disease such as a feminising tumour of the adrenal cortex. Less

often testicular injury is causal. In chromatin-positive *Klinefelter's syndrome* (p. 819) the enlarged breasts show lobules comparable with those of the normal female breast. Lobule formation is excessively rare in other forms of enlargement, which are due mainly to increase in the fibrous stroma of the male breast and of the ducts, the epithelium of which may be hyperplastic and surrounded by a zone of oedematous fibrillary connective tissue.

Tumours of the male breast are rare. Carcinoma may be of anaplastic spheroidal-cell type or may show an adenocarcinomatous pattern. Prognosis is often poor because of early spread to lymph nodes and to the chest wall. Paget's disease of the male breast is very rare. Metastatic carcinoma, e.g. from bronchus, occasionally occurs and the male breast, like that of the female, may be involved in generalised lymphoid neoplasms and the leukaemias.

CHAPTER 24

THE ENDOCRINE GLANDS

Introduction

Knowledge of the intimate relationships of abnormal endocrine states to conditions of disease is still incomplete. In many instances, the secretion of an endocrine gland has a widespread influence on various parts of the body, and thus a disturbance of the functions of the gland may produce a complicated picture. The chief changes in disease now recognised are the result mainly of *hyperfunction* due to increased secretion, or conversely of *hypofunction* due to deficiency of secretion. There is also the possibility that alteration in the quality of a secretion—*hormonal dysfunction*—may occur, a notable example being the profound effects on the sexual functions brought about by congenital enzymatic failure to elaborate the normal spectrum of adrenal 17-hydroxysteroids, as a result of which the adrenal cortex comes to produce an excess of androgenic hormones (p. 914). In the case of glands which secrete a number of hormones with separate physiological effects, e.g. the anterior lobe of the pituitary and adrenals, quantitative differences in the secretion of the various fractions produce the effects of dysfunction. Further, certain endocrine glands exert a restraining or antagonistic action on one another, and the normal state results from a balance of their activities—a "feed-back" mechanism well exemplified in the reciprocal relationships between the pituitary gland and the thyroid, adrenals and gonads. For example, *growth and development* are controlled by the anterior pituitary, the thyroid and the gonads; and marked abnormality occurs when the secretion of any of these is deficient or absent. Overgrowth resulting from hyperfunction is less frequently seen, but a striking example is presented by giantism and acromegaly produced by hyperactivity of the anterior lobe of the pituitary.

The *reproductive function* is dependent on the production of the various steroids which are vital to the development, maintenance and function of the reproductive organs. These sex steroids are produced mainly by the gonads and adrenal cortex which are under the control of the appropriate trophic hormones of the anterior pituitary. As a regulator of *general metabolic processes* the thyroid is an outstanding example of an endocrine gland of profound importance to the tissues of the body in general: hyperfunction raises the normal basal metabolism, whilst deficiency reduces it. In the *metabolism of carbohydrates*, the secretion of insulin by the pancreatic islets is essential for the storage and utilisation of sugar, and deficiency leads to hyperglycaemia and glycosuria, that is, to diabetes. Conversely, the secretions of the thyroid, of the chromaffin system, of the anterior pituitary and of the adrenal cortex act in mobilising sugar, and accordingly *excess* of their secretions leads to glycosuria. In this respect the action of the pancreas opposes that of other endocrine glands.

Calcium metabolism is controlled by the internal secretion of the parathyroids, removal of which is followed by a fall in the amount of calcium present in the blood and by decreased excretion. Conversely, parathyroid hyperfunction, usually due to a parathyroid adenoma, leads to resorption of bone with calcium release, and hypercalcaemia results. Injection of parathyroid hormone has a like effect.

The nervous system may influence endocrine activity; for example thyrotoxicosis may be precipitated or aggravated by mental strain, while emotional states influence the secretion of various hormones, and particularly catecholamines by the adrenal medulla. Conversely, hormones can influence the nervous system; thus in hyperthyroidism, irritability and excitability are the rule, whereas in hypothyroidism the individual becomes sluggish. Presumably these changes illustrate the effect of thyroid hormone upon the metabolism of tissues in general.

In the following account we shall deal with the chief disorders of endocrine function and structure relating to human disease, and the experimental results referred to will be mainly those bearing directly upon the pathological states under consideration.

The pituitary will be considered first as it is the gland exercising the greatest control over the endocrine system by reason of its nervous connections with the nuclei at the base of the brain, the number of hormones produced by it with their specific trophic effects, and the fact that removal of the pituitary produces atrophic changes in many of the other endocrine glands. The feed-back mechanism of the various glands on the pituitary is also very important, and in disease several glands may be affected together, so that the disease appears to be "polyglandular"; in such cases it may sometimes be impossible to say whether there is a primary lesion in one, or whether several are affected by a similar process.

THE PITUITARY

The Anterior Lobe (Adenohypophysis)

Introduction

The name "pituitary" reminds us of the ancient belief that the pituitary gland secreted the nasal mucus; it remained for Pierre Marie to show, in 1886, that the disorder called by him "acromegaly" was associated with enlargement of the pituitary gland. Since this pioneer observation, extensive pathological studies and experimental work have clearly shown that the pituitary is an endocrine gland producing many hormones that exercise control over other endocrine organs, and its several distinctly different cell types provide the basis for such diverse functional activities.

The blood supply is peculiar in that there is no direct arterial inflow, the arteries breaking up into capillaries in the pituitary stalk and adjacent hypothalamus, from which the blood passes in the hypophyseal portal system of vessels to the pars distalis where they open out into the sinusoids of the anterior lobe. This vascular arrangement enables the hypothalamus to control the composition of the blood entering the anterior lobe and thus perhaps to influence its activity. It also renders the anterior pituitary liable to deprivation of blood supply by injury to the stalk and by the circulatory collapse of severe shock. We have to deal not only with anterior and posterior lobes and pars intermedia, but also with the different kinds of cell which compose them. Thus in the anterior lobe we have cells which by simple stains appear to be devoid of granules, i.e. chromophobe cells, which constitute fully 50 per cent of the total number, and also chromophil cells, the latter being of two types, namely, eosinophil cells and basophil cells; both types consist of heavily granular cells together with a smaller number of lightly granular elements which may represent the most actively functioning cells. The basophil cells usually number a little more than 13 per cent; the eosinophil cells, which lie mainly in the lateral portions of the gland, occupy an intermediate position with a percentage a little under 37. By Pearse's tri-PAS stain, however, all the basophil cells, some of the eosinophil cells and some of the chromophobes contain mucoid granules, some being heavily stained and others only lightly. These sparsely granulated cells are now regarded as the actively secreting cells of the gland and have been designated *gamma* cells; they probably comprise elements from the eosinophil (*alpha*) cells and from the basophil cells but during the active secretory phase their function may not be clearly recognisable. The basophil cells are again subdivided into *beta* and *delta* types on the basis of certain tinctorial differences, and probably also by reason of the nature of their secretion. The heavily granulated cells of all types are now regarded as cells in a phase of storage of secretion, in contrast to the sparsely granulated elements in the phase of active secretion. Exact correlation of the staining reactions of the cells with hormone production has not yet been fully achieved and certain abnormal forms appear in pathological states.

Not all the pituitary hormones have as yet been obtained in a pure form; some are protein in nature, but others are polypeptides. The chief varieties are: (1) a growth-stimulating hormone, *somatotrophin*, a globular protein of molecular weight about 44,000, now isolated in crystalline form, (2) *gonadotrophic hormones*, thought to be glycoproteins, (3) a *thyrotrophic hormone*— also a glycoprotein, (4) an *adrenocorticotrophic hormone*, a polypeptide, (5) a *lactogenic hormone*, prolactin, also a globular protein, and (6) a *melanocyte-stimulating hormone*, a polypeptide. Probably all of these are implicated in human disease, and the adrenocorticotrophic hormone is probably concerned in the resistance of the body to unfavourable environmental conditions. These are products of the anterior lobe; the eosinophil cells give rise to somatotrophin and lactogenic hormone, the *beta*-basophil cells give rise to thyrotrophin, and the *delta*-basophils to adrenocorticotrophin and the gonadotrophins. An important general principle appears to be that while the pituitary stimulates the other endocrine glands through its trophic hormones, the amount of these trophic hormones liberated is in turn controlled by the blood level of the individual endocrine secretions, i.e. by the feedback mechanism. Thus the secretion of gonadotrophic hormone (FSH) can be inhibited by an excess of oestrogens in the blood, and the output of thyrotrophic and adrenocorticotrophic hormones is similarly influenced by the blood level of thyroid and cortical hormones respectively. There is evidence that the feed-back mechanism is at least in part governed by uptake and storage within the hypothalamus of the individual endocrine secretions circulating in the plasma. The hypothalamus in turn releases from the median eminence into the hypophyseal-portal blood stream polypeptides which affect the release of the corresponding pituitary trophic hormones, that for ACTH being known as corticotrophin-releasing factor (CRF).

Growth-stimulating hormone. This hormone is essential for normal growth and development and requires for its effective action the presence of both thyroid hormone and insulin. Extirpation of the anterior lobe, along with the posterior lobe, produces infantilism in puppies,

the animals remain small owing to interference with osseous growth, the sexual glands fail to develop, and there may be marked adiposity, now believed to be due to injury to the tuber cinereum or adjacent parts. In adult animals extirpation causes corresponding effects and atrophy of the sexual glands, and hypophysectomy is now extensively used as a method of investigation.

The functions of the pituitary have been studied also by the injection of extracts of the lobes of the gland, both in normal and in hypophysectomised animals, i.e. by substitution therapy. Attempts to promote growth by anterior lobe extracts have been rather unsuccessful in man because heterologous somatotrophin, being of protein nature, is antigenic and the effectiveness of the extract is of brief duration. In rats, extracts of the anterior lobe of the ox produced marked increase of the bony skeleton and soft tissues, in adult rats as well as in young animals, but in the former the characteristic changes of acromegaly did not occur in the skeleton—only giantism, because in the rat the epiphyseal lines of the bones do not become ossified. In certain breeds of dog, however, some of the features of acromegaly have been reproduced by injections of anterior lobe extract.

Gonadotrophic hormones. These almost certainly arise from the *delta*-basophil mucoid cells, increase in the number of which appears to indicate more active formation of the hormones. The pituitary is responsible for two gonadal functions, namely, (*a*) the establishment of sexual maturity and (*b*) the reproductive cycle. Excision of the anterior lobe has a depressing effect on the gonads, inhibits gonadal development in young animals and produces atrophic changes in adults. The opposite effect, that of stimulation, is obtained by transplantation of anterior lobe tissue to immature rats and mice, the action directly on the gonads leading to precocious sexual maturity. Similar results have been obtained by anterior lobe extracts.

The basophil cells produce two glycoproteins with action on the ovaries, follicle-stimulating hormone (FSH) and luteinising or interstitial-cell stimulating hormone (LH or ICSH). FSH regulates the growth of the Graafian follicle and ovulation, and the follicle in its turn produces oestrogenic hormones which stimulate the reparative changes in the endometrium after menstruation (p. 847). ICSH controls lutein formation, the corpus luteum in its turn producing a hormone, progesterone, which brings about the secretory changes in the endometrium and also inhibition of ovulation. Both of these hormones are required in optimum proportion for the proper growth and maturation of the ovarian follicles and for the secretion of the follicular hormones, and prolactin is also concerned in the continued secretion of progesterone. FSH also stimulates male germ cells to complete spermatogenesis while the luteinising hormone acts on the interstitial cells of the testis to induce the secretion of testosterone.

There is a remarkable interdependence of the pituitary and reproductive organs. Rare cases of infertility in both men and women result from gonadotrophin deficiencies. Excessive production of LH may also give rise to the syndrome of polycystic ovaries and infertility. It is possible that certain abnormalities of the breasts, such as cystic change, may depend upon pituitary abnormality.

Adrenocorticotrophic hormone (ACTH). This hormone is thought to be formed by those mucoid basophil cells classified as of *delta* type; it has now been prepared in pure form and appears to be a polypeptide containing 39 amino-acid residues; accordingly it is not antigenic and can be administered repeatedly without loss of effect. The precise configuration of human ACTH has not yet been fully worked out but the three types isolated so far from sheep, ox and pig differ only in the arrangement of amino-acids in the middle part of the chain. The purified substance is assayed by its potency in depleting the adrenal ascorbic acid in hypophysectomised rats. ACTH is essential for the maintenance of the adrenal cortex and governs the secretion of certain adrenal cortical steroids, especially corticosterone and the 17-hydroxy-steroids, hydrocortisone and cortisone, by means of the reciprocal feed-back mechanism already described and the release of the appropriate CRF from the median eminence of the hypothalamus into the hypophyseal-portal vessels. In conditions of emergency and stress, the outpouring of adrenaline from the adrenal medulla brings about rapid release of ACTH from the pituitary but does not appear to stimulate its further production by the pituitary cells (Dixon).

Administration of purified ACTH causes hypertrophy of the adrenal cortex, and increases the output of glucocorticoid hormones which bring about gluconeogenesis, atrophy of the thymus and lymph nodes and lymphopenia. The secretion of the adrenal cortical hormone most active in controlling sodium and potassium —aldosterone—does not appear to be under anterior pituitary control; the factors controlling its release are not fully understood, but one of them is renin, produced by the granular cells of the juxta-glomerular apparatus (p. 185).

The importance of ACTH has been emphasised by the therapeutic effects of certain adrenal cortical hormones, in various diseases, notably those attributable to hypersensitivity reactions (Chapter 5), and certain others of unknown etiology.

Thyrotrophic hormone (TSH) is secreted by the mucoid *beta*-basophil cells and is a specific glycoprotein. It promotes the breakdown of thyroglobulin, and the release of thyroxine into the plasma, so that the colloid content of the thyroid is diminished: at the same time it increases the synthesis of thyroxine and brings about hyperplasia of the thyroid acinar epithelium, and increased trapping of iodine from the plasma. The output of TSH is depressed by thyroxine and stimulated by lack of thyroxine in the plasma, i.e. there is reciprocal action analogous to that between the adrenals and ACTH, and here, too, there is evidence that this interaction is partly a direct one on the pituitary, and partly an indirect one in which the hypothalamus participates through selective uptake of thyroid hormones from the blood stream.

Lactogenic hormone (Prolactin) is a protein hormone secreted by the acidophil cells, but whether it is by the same cells as secrete somatotrophin is uncertain. It is concerned in the initiation and maintenance of lactation in the mammary gland suitably developed by oestrogen and progesterone, and it appears also to act synergistically with these two hormones in the full maturation of the ovarian follicles. Prolactin may be the mammotrophic hormone found in the urine of many post-menopausal women, and may be chiefly concerned in so-called hormone-dependent mammary tumours, but this is not fully established.

The melanocyte-stimulating hormone (MSH, Intermedin) is secreted by the pars intermedia in lower animals, but in man apparently by the basophils of *delta* type. It is a polypeptide structurally similar to the first part of the ACTH molecule, and exists in two forms.

When the adrenals are destroyed by disease, the output of MSH in the urine is increased, because increased pituitary secretion results from lack of inhibition by adrenal hormones. This is probably responsible for the increased pigmentation in Addison's disease (q.v.), and also in chloasma of pregnancy.

We shall give an account of the conditions depending upon excess and deficiency of secretion respectively, but some of the views expressed are of necessity speculative. The interpretation of the lesions and symptoms of pituitary disease is particularly difficult; owing to the anatomical relation of the gland to the bone, enlargement of one cellular element may lead to compression of others, and thus hyperactivity of one cell type may be associated with hypoactivity of the others. A state of hyperactivity of one secretory element may be succeeded by one of hypoactivity, as will be illustrated below. Furthermore, a pituitary tumour may affect the hypothalamic region, and conversely a suprasellar lesion may produce pressure effects on the pituitary. The problem presented is often one of great complexity.

Pituitary Hyperfunction

Acromegaly

The term, originally applied by Marie, means enlargement of the extremities, and the condition is due to hyperactivity of the anterior lobe with excessive somatotrophin secretion either from hyperplasia or tumour of the eosinophil cells (Fig. 24.1); in the late stages, hypoactivity usually appears and leads to secondary deficiency effects.

Clinical features. The hands and feet are increased in size, especially in width, and the hands have been described as spade-like; the increase is mainly of the soft tissues, though thickening of bone is present later, notably outgrowths from the heads of the phalanges. The face is enlarged, especially the nose, which is widened, and the lower jaw is lengthened and its angle is widened, so that the teeth project beyond those of the upper jaw. The lips become thickened and there is enlargement of the tongue. The skin is thickened and sometimes warty, and the hair coarse and wiry. In the skeleton generally there tends to be an increase of the bony prominences, and there may be roughening of the surface of the bones. Kyphosis is often present from irregular vertebral atrophy and hypertrophy. The sternum is increased in size and the thoracic cavity is enlarged. Although the changes occur after normal ossification is completed, a slight increase in height has been noticed in some cases. The effects of the growth-promoting hormone are seen also in the internal organs, there being enlargement of the liver, kidneys, etc.—a condition of visceral splanchnomegaly. Hyperplastic changes have been found also in the thyroid, parathyroids and adrenal cortex.

After an initial period of increased muscular strength, general lassitude, muscular weakness and slowness of speech appear, and these increase during the progress of the disease. At first diminished sugar tolerance may be noted, sometimes glycosuria with blood sugar curves indistinguishable from those of diabetes, but later increased sugar tolerance is present. In early stages there may be increased libido, but this is followed later by impotence in the male, and amenorrhoea in the female. Galactorrhoea, due to excessive prolactin secretion, has been observed in acromegalic women and has been found to abate after destruction of the pituitary tumour. Symptoms may be produced by mechanical pressure of the causative pituitary tumour, e.g. implication of the inner halves of the optic nerves with blindness in the nasal half of each retina, i.e. bitemporal hemianopia. Papillodoema and other signs of intracranial pressure may be produced when the hypophyseal growth is large, and occasionally total blindness results. Although acromegaly in its fully developed form is rare, slighter degrees of the condition are more frequent, and may accompany adenomas apparently of chromophobe type. The mortality rate in active acromegaly is almost double that of the population: premature death may result from diabetes mellitus, hypertension, or cardio-respiratory disease.

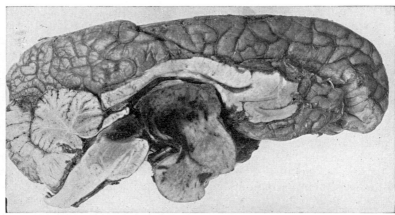

FIG. 24.1—Brain and pituitary tumour from a case of acromegaly.

Giantism

Hyperactivity of the anterior lobe, before ossification is completed, is now recognised as one cause of giantism. There is excessive growth at the epiphyseal lines and this may be prolonged beyond the normal period. The growth is precocious and of proportionate character: ultimately a height of over eight feet may be reached. In some cases, the effects of hyperactivity persist after the period of normal growth and some of the features of acromegaly may be superadded. At an early stage there may be abnormally great muscular power and energy, which are usually attended by precocious sexual development and libido; but at a later stage these are replaced by muscular feebleness, impotence, etc., along with mental impairment. There is often glycosuria at first, but later increased sugar tolerance may develop.

Structural changes. In both giantism and acromegaly, there is an irregular overgrowth both of bone and the soft tissues. Acromegaly is usually due to a tumour of the anterior lobe, described as an adenoma, though occasionally it may show aberrant characters. The tumour may reach a considerable size, giving rise to enlargement of the sella, as can be seen on X-ray examination, and also growing upwards and leading to pressure on the optic chiasma and overlying parts of the brain. Sometimes the adenoma undergoes cystic degeneration, and its functional activity decreases. The pituitary adenoma associated with acromegaly is composed of cells of the eosinophil type, both fully granular and lightly granular cells being involved. In giantism, the lesion is more frequently hyperplasia of eosinophil cells than actual adenoma. The effects on the sexual functions, at first hyperactivity then hypoactivity, may be due to an initial stimulating effect of the secretion on the basophil cells followed by their destruction from pressure. The close association between stimulation of growth and stimulation of gonads is, however, noteworthy. In most cases of acromegaly the tumour is a pure eosinophil adenoma of considerable size, but small eosinophil adenomas may be found fortuitously without the occurrence of acromegaly.

Cushing's syndrome (Pituitary basophilism)

Cushing described a remarkable clinical picture which he attributed to the presence of a small basophil adenoma of the anterior pituitary. It is now known that the condition is brought about by excessive secretion of hydrocortisone and cortisone by the adrenal glands, hyperplasia or neoplasia of which is invariably present, whereas a basophil adenoma is present in less than 10 per cent of cases. Adrenal hyperplasia (with or without a basophil adenoma) accounts for 85 per cent of adult cases, and only 15 per cent are due to tumour of the adrenals (Symington). In some cases without evidence of a pituitary tumour, cure has resulted from pituitary ablation. In children, however, adrenal tumour is much the commoner (p. 913). In the absence of basophil adenoma the syndrome may be associated with bronchial carcinoma, a tumour of the thymus, pancreas or ovary, and in such cases there may be no increase in the number of basophil cells in the pituitary. In Cushing's syndrome, Crooke found that there was invariably present a peculiar hyaline change in the basophil cells scattered around the periphery of the anterior lobe (Fig. 24.2); this was the only pituitary lesion common to the conditions mentioned above. The change is probably brought about by the presence of excess adrenal cortical hormones, since it occurs not only in cases of adrenal hyperplasia, but also in cases of autonomously secreting adrenocortical tumours and after prolonged therapeutic administration of ACTH or cortisone. In a large number of other conditions in which the syndrome was absent, the change was found in only a few, and in them it was slight. Crooke's results have been confirmed by others. In adrenal virilism without the specific features of Cushing's syndrome (p. 914) hyalinisation of the basophils is absent. It is therefore associated with glucocorticoids circulating in excess, but may represent temporary suppression of ACTH secretion; its exact significance is not yet known.

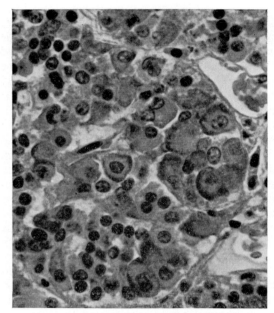

FIG. 24.2.—Anterior pituitary in Cushing's syndrome, showing cytoplasmic hyaline change in the basophils. × 500.

Pituitary Hypofunction

This may occur at any age. The features are mainly those resulting from deficiency of the growth and gonadotrophic hormones. The pituitary defect *per se* is often complicated by the effects of lesions in the hypothalamic region, e.g. in one type (*Fröhlich's syndrome*) adiposity is present in addition (p. 880), whereas in others there is no such tendency to accumulation of fat. The hormonal deficiency may be brought about either by a lesion within the pituitary itself, tumour or destructive lesion, or by pressure from a lesion outside. Various syndromes have been described but in many the underlying structural change has not been determined.

In progressive pituitary failure, secretion of growth hormone and gonadotrophins is first affected, followed by ACTH and TSH. However, any individual hormone may be deficient singly without obvious consequences; such deficiencies are most likely due to defects in the hypothalamic centres, or to inhibitory factors.

Simmonds' disease (Sheehan's syndrome)

This is the commonest and most important example of anterior lobe hypofunction. Simmonds described the lesion as being a necrosis produced by vascular disturbance, and he observed such a lesion as a post-partum condition. Later a similar syndrome was described in cases of fibrosis, and more rarely of tumours and cysts involving the anterior lobe. Occasionally the pituitary is destroyed by a granulomatous lesion of unknown etiology containing many giant cells and in some cases similar granulomas are present in the adrenals and other organs. The histological findings are suggestive of an auto-immune process, but confirmatory evidence is lacking.

Clinical features. Sheehan has described both pathological and clinical features. Contrary to Simmonds' view, marked wasting is not a feature, and the most conspicuous external change is the total loss of pubic and axillary hair together with atrophy of the gonads. During the puerperium there is absence of lactation and this is succeeded by amenorrhoea, absence of libido, atrophy of the ovaries, mammary parenchyma and uterus. The basal metabolic rate and blood pressure tend to be lowered and there is often hypochromic anaemia. The patients show lassitude, asthenia and sensitivity to cold. Extreme hypersensitivity to insulin is present and this may be helpful in diagnosis, but the test is not without risk. There are also atrophic changes in the adrenal cortex and thyroid. Later, symptoms of hypothyroidism develop and gradually become more and more prominent; these do not respond well to administration of thyroid extract, a form of therapy known to be dangerous because it promotes the excretion of sodium chloride and may thus precipitate acute symptoms of adrenal insufficiency.

Structural changes. Sheehan demonstrated that the original lesion is necrosis of varying extent in the anterior lobe, occurring especially when labour has been complicated by collapse or shock, notably when accompanied by haemorrhage. The necrosis is the result of ischaemia, to which the anterior lobe is especially liable by reason of the swelling resulting from the significant increase in volume and weight that occurs in pregnancy, and because of its encasement within the rigid sella. The curious vascular arrangement of indirect arterial supply through the hypophyseal portal vessels inevitably leads to sinusoidal perfusion at low pressure and may prove inadequate in conditions of circulatory collapse, particularly if arterial spasm is followed by stasis and actual thrombosis of the stalk vessels analogous to the sequence of events in renal cortical necrosis. Necrosis is followed by organisation of the necrotic tissue and by fibrosis, with consequent shrinkage. It is probable that cases with fibrosis recorded by others have been produced in this way.

Simmonds' disease is therefore a striking example of the diminution of function of the anterior lobe, which Sheehan's work has related to a definite lesion of known etiology. A number of the symptoms described may be present along with great wasting in conditions apart from a pituitary lesion, especially in *anorexia nervosa*, which is of psychoneurotic origin, and from which complete recovery may take place.

Fröhlich's syndrome

The condition thus named was described by Fröhlich in 1901 as *dystrophia adiposo-genitalis*.

Clinical features. Children affected by this dystrophy are small, of infantile appearance and abnormally fat, and the sexual glands remain undeveloped. Boys develop some of the female characters, the hips are wide and there is an accumulation of fat in the breasts and over the buttocks. Basal metabolism is lowered and the temperature tends to be subnormal; there is also increased sugar tolerance.

Pathological findings. The results of operations and post-mortem examinations have shown that while occasionally a chromophobe adenoma has been present, in most cases the lesion has been a tumour or cyst overlying and compressing the pituitary. Clearly such a suprasellar tumour may compress both the pituitary below and the hypothalamus above, and experiments have shown that hypophysectomy alone does not lead to such changes and that injury to the anterior tuberal part of the hypothalamus is the essential element in the production of the obesity, which is accompanied by voracious appetite. Of the tumours bringing about this result the commonest is the congenital craniopharyngioma (Fig. 20.88, p. 677). These contain epithelial elements, are solid or cystic, and not infrequently calcified, occasionally with bone formation, especially in their periphery; thus they can often be seen on X-ray examination. In some instances the growth has been a meningioma or a glioma, and the Fröhlich syndrome has been observed to result also from severe internal hydrocephalus.

Cases with features resembling Fröhlich's syndrome occur also in adults and may be the result of lesions in the tuberal region occurring after growth has ceased. Here also there is great accumulation of fat with impotence in the male, and amenorrhoea and sterility in the female; there is also increased sugar tolerance. In the male the disposition of the surplus fat may lead to a female appearance. Women are more frequently affected and the increase of fat is sometimes great, especially over the trunk where it may be somewhat irregularly distributed; the adipose tissue is often tender or even painful. Cases of the latter type are often spoken of as *adiposis dolorosa* or Dercum's disease, but probably different conditions have been included under this term. It cannot be said at present whether all such cases are due to hypothalamic damage with or without hypophyseal deficiency, but in many cases of the kind carefully examined, the lesion present has been an adenoma of the chromophobe type, which evidently produces anterior lobe deficiency by obliterating the chromophil cells; it may also cause effects from pressure on the hypothalamic region. The mechanical results of such an adenoma are the same as those in acromegaly, viz. headache, restriction of the field of vision, bitemporal hemianopia and sometimes blindness.

Pituitary dwarfism and infantilism

Cases also are recorded of interference with osseous growth and the development of the sexual glands, but without accumulation of surplus fat. In such cases the normal proportions of the body are maintained. Skeletal growth is diminished, and the bones are slender and sometimes fragile; intelligence is usually im-

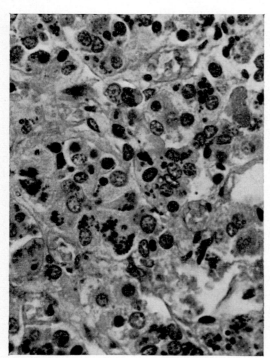

FIG. 24.3.—Anterior pituitary in primary myxoedema. The PAS-positive inclusions in the basophil cells show up here as black spheres. × 500.

paired. In extreme examples a condition of dwarfism results, now usually known as the *Lorain–Lévi syndrome*, or *nanosomia pituitaria*. Probably the anterior lobe alone is involved, and when deficiency in growth is associated with accumulation of fat, as in Fröhlich's syndrome, some injury to the hypothalamus is likely to be present. In many cases of pituitary dwarfism no evidence of tumour has been found on X-ray examination, and in the early diagnosis blood assay of growth hormone may be of great value.

Other examples of dwarfism attributed to pituitary dysfunction have been described, but until the underlying lesions have been defined we have little knowledge of the real meaning of the syndromes. In the *Lawrence–Moon–Biedl syndrome*, there is evidence that a genetic influence is concerned, the dwarfism being accompanied by *retinitis pigmentosa* and *polydactyly*. In the Lorain–Lévi syndrome, there are few necropsy reports, but in a Lorain–Lévi dwarf examined in this department there was a Rathke-type cyst and a chromophobe adenoma in a hypoplastic pituitary.

Changes in the anterior pituitary in other diseases

Changes in the pars anterior have been noted in various conditions. In *myxoedema* there are conspicuous large and sparsely granulated cells which presumably are secreting TSH, and contain PAS-positive inclusions (Fig. 24.3). Other mucoid cells are vacuolated. The alpha cells also show reduction in granulation and number; this may be apparent even on macroscopic examination of stained sections. Acidophil granularity is restored by administration of L-thyroxine. In *Addison's disease* acidophil cells are poorly granulated and may disappear. Mucoid cells are much degranulated and numerous transitional forms are seen representing active ACTH secretion. In *pregnancy* the pituitary is much enlarged and therefore susceptible to vascular changes as in Sheehan's syndrome. Mucoid cells are increased and so also are partly degranulated acidophils which are presumably secreting prolactin. In *rheumatoid arthritis* an increase in polar bigranulated mucoid cells has been reported but this is by no means invariable.

The Posterior Pituitary or Pars Nervosa

This is made up of irregular fusiform cells, probably of astrocytic origin, known as pituicytes. In the adult increasing numbers of basophil mucoid cells appear in the *pars nervosa* and lipofuscin-containing phagocytes also accumulate with advancing age. The *pars intermedia* is represented in man by a row of colloid-containing vesicles. The microscopic architecture does not suggest an endocrine function. Nevertheless early experimental results showed that an extract of the *posterior lobe*, pituitrin, when injected into normal animals causes certain effects. There are, in fact, two hormones in the *pars nervosa*; one, *vasopressin* or *antidiuretic hormone* (ADH), plays a physiological role in the resorption of water from the renal collecting tubules (p. 682). In large dose, it causes a rise in blood pressure, but it is doubtful if enough is ever secreted to produce this effect naturally. Deficiency of ADH is an essential feature in diabetes insipidus. The other hormone, *oxytocin*, has a stimulating effect on the uterine muscle and may be concerned in physiological stimulation of uterine contraction at the end of pregnancy; it also assists in expulsion of milk during lactation. Removal of the posterior lobe, however, leads to no permanent ill effects provided that the hypothalamic region and the anterior lobe are not injured. This finding has been explained by the discovery that the source of the posterior lobe hormones lies in the neurones of the supra-optic, paraventricular and tuberal nuclei which elaborate the specific hormones and transmit them along the axons of the hypothalamic-hypophyseal tract to the posterior lobe where they are stored, probably in combination with a carrier substance, as hyaline bodies. Vasopressin is derived chiefly from the supraoptic nuclei and oxytocin from the paraventricular and tuberal nuclei. The hormones are relatively simple peptides consisting of 8 amino-acid residues and both have now been synthesised: they are characterised by a very high content of cysteine which has

enabled the distribution of the neuro-secretory material to be studied by histochemical methods. A functional state depending on excessive formation of posterior lobe hormones has not been recognised, but the effects of interruption of the hypothalamic-hypophyseal tract or destruction of the hypothalamic nuclei are seen in the syndrome of diabetes insipidus. The action of vasopressin on the kidneys is to control the facultative reabsorption of water in the distal renal tubules, and because of this effect it is now commonly known as anti-diuretic hormone (ADH); the effects are normally closely integrated with those of aldosterone which plays a large part in the control of electrolyte and water balance.

Diabetes insipidus

This is characterised by persistent failure to concentrate urine and thus by polyuria of low specific gravity, also by polydipsia and some emaciation. The underlying lesion is usually in the hypothalamic region and is of varying nature—tumour, inflammatory, injury, etc.; in some cases it has been post-encephalitic. Persistent polyuria has been produced by bilateral experimental lesions in the supra-optic nuclei or in the fibres of the supraoptic-hypophyseal tracts. A lesion in the nucleus, or interruption of all the fibres by incision or by clamping, results in diabetes insipidus and this, like the disease in the human subject, is relieved by injections of vasopressin. Total extirpation or radioactive destruction of the pituitary does not produce the condition nor does it usually occur when only the posterior lobe is destroyed by tumour. Low stalk section usually spares a sufficient number of fibres from the active nuclei to prevent the occurrence of diabetes insipidus. It has been found, too, that the presence of a certain amount of functioning anterior lobe is necessary for permanent polyuria.

Pituitary Tumours

These are of considerable variety; minute tumours are not uncommon as an incidental necropsy finding but clinically significant tumours are rare. Enlargement of the hypophysis may be due to an adenoma. and this may be composed mainly of one of the three types of cells in the anterior lobe—*chromophobe, eosinophil, basophil*. The frequency of occurrence of the corresponding adenomas large enough to cause physical signs is in this order. Occasionally an adenoma shows cellular pleomorphism and is locally aggressive with a high mitotic rate, but malignancy is rare, as judged by the formation of metastases.

Chromophobe adenomas do not lead to specific symptoms or evidence of hyperfunction but to anterior lobe deficiency. They may also cause effects by pressing on the hypothalamic region. Such tumours are, however, rare before adult life, and the results of anterior lobe deficiency in early life are usually produced by the pressure of a growth, e.g. a suprasellar cyst, outside the pituitary. *A chromophobe adenoma* is composed of masses of round cells of rather nondescript appearance enclosed by fibrous stroma. Prolonged injection of oestrone in mice produces hyperplasia of the chromophobe or degranulated cells and sometimes an actual adenoma, in which eosinophil and basophil cells are very scanty. This is a very interesting example of the action on the pituitary of the hormone of another endocrine gland.

Chromophil adenomas. *Eosinophil adenomas.*

When small these may be asymptomatic but larger tumours quite clearly show hyperfunction which leads to acromegaly or to giantism, and also effects on the gonads. Both chromophobe and eosinophil adenomas may reach a considerable size, causing expansion of the sella with erosion of bone and bitemporal hemianopia from pressure on the optic chiasma. *Basophil adenomas* are the rarest type of tumour and are usually small; occasionally they are associated with Cushing's syndrome and adrenal hyperplasia.

The commonest tumour outside the pituitary and producing anterior lobe deficiency by pressure is the **craniopharyngioma**, of congenital origin and derived from ectodermal cells of the craniopharyngeal upgrowth, from which the hypophysis is developed; it is usually suprasellar in position and is often cystic (Fig. 20.88, p. 677). Cystic tumours or cysts occasionally arise also from the pars intermedia and may contain ciliated epithelium. These are true Rathke pouch tumours and they may cause atrophy of the rest of the gland. Metastatic deposits from carcinoma of the breast or bronchus are not uncommon, and pericapsular deposits occur in some cases of leukaemia. Extra-pituitary tumours in the suprasellar region may involve the nuclei of the hypothalamus and lead to disturbances of fat metabolism or to polyuria. Sarcoma in this site is very rare. Spheno-occipital chordoma may cause pressure effects in this region.

Pineal Body

Knowledge of the function and lesions of this organ is restricted mainly to the appearance and behaviour of tumours arising from it. These are rare, of various types, the least uncommon being teratoma, choriocarcinoma, and ganglioneuroma (Fig. 20.85, p. 676). According to Dorothy Russell, some of the so-called pinealomas are also teratoid, their structure resembling that of seminoma or dysgerminoma, but true pineal parenchymal tumours do occur, though rarely. All of these occur especially in early life. Effects are produced by pressure on neighbouring structures; thus hydrocephalus, ocular paralyses and deafness from implication of the corpora quadrigemina, also cerebellar effects, giddiness, etc., may result. In young boys the phenomenon of *pubertas praecox* may accompany a pineal tumour of any

type, there being an excessive growth of the body and premature development of the sexual organs accompanied by hirsuties and sometimes obesity. In other cases of pineal tumour such effect have been absent, and a similar group of changes has been observed in other lesions in the neighbourhood, such as tumour in the floor of the third ventricle, hydrocephalus, etc. The syndrome is probably not a pineal effect but rather the result of disturbance of nerve tracts possibly related to the pituitary. The pineal and adjacent diencephalon have been thought to elaborate substances concerned in the control of aldosterone secretion, but in man ACTH, renin and plasma levels of sodium and potassium ions are the principal regulators of aldosterone secretion.

FF

THE THYROID GLAND

The thyroid gland produces three hormones, thyroxine, triiodothyronine and calcitonin. The last is a polypeptide which lowers the concentration of calcium in the blood by causing increased deposition of bone crystal, but its physiological and pathological importance is still uncertain. In animals, and probably in man, calcitonin is secreted by specialised epithelial cells (interstitial or C cells) which do not form part of the lining of the thyroid vesicles.

Thyroxine (tetraiodothyronine, or T_4) and triiodothyronine (T_3) are iodinated amino-acids with a hormonal effect of influencing heat production in the tissues of the body by uncoupling oxidative phosphorylation, i.e. increasing oxygen utilisation relative to the rate of formation of high energy phosphate bonds, two processes which are closely linked in the economy of the cell. T_3 and T_4 are essential in normal physical and mental development and in the metabolism of protein, carbohydrate and fat. Excessive secretion of these thyroid hormones causes the serious disorder known as *thyrotoxicosis* or *hyperthyroidism* while inadequate secretion results in *hypothyroidism* which can have severe pathological consequences. Important physiological mechanisms have evolved to ensure that the amounts of T_3 and T_4 released into the circulation are appropriate to the varying bodily requirements in differing circumstances (e.g. environmental temperature), and, within limits, to compensate for suboptimal intake of dietary iodine.

Iodine metabolism in the thyroid gland. Iodide ions are concentrated in thyroid cells by a special concentrating or *trapping mechanism* which can be inhibited by perchlorate or thiocyanate ions. Iodide within thyroid epithelium is rapidly *oxidised*, probably by a thyroidal peroxidase, to an active form which readily enters *organic combination* with the tyrosine present in the glycoprotein, thyroglobulin, which has been synthesised by thyroid epithelium and stored extracellularly in the colloid within the vesicles. The organic binding of oxidised iodine results in the formation of mono- and diiodotyrosine within the thyroglobulin molecule and the synthesis of the iodothyronine is accomplished by *coupling* of two appropriate iodotyrosines to give T_3 or T_4. (Both the antithyroid drugs thiouracil and carbimazole inhibit the organic binding of iodine and the coupling reaction.) The hormones, still part of the thyroglobulin molecule, are stored within the colloid until required in the circulation. Thyroglobulin is then digested by a cathepsin, T_3 and T_4 are released as free amino-acids and transported through the epithelial cells lining the vesicles to the vessels within the stroma of the gland. Hormonally inactive iodotyrosines which have not taken part in iodothyronine formation are also released from digested thyroglobulin but these are deiodinated by a *dehalogenase* enzyme and the released iodide is available for reoxidation and organification.

Due to inborn errors of metabolism one or other of these steps is sometimes defective and this leads to the condition of *dyshormonogenesis*. Thus failure of the iodide-trapping mechanism, defective organification of iodide, impaired coupling of iodotyrosines, secretion of abnormal iodoprotein, and dehalogenase deficiency each constitute a different form of dyshormonogenesis and result in a tendency to hypothyroidism.

Control of thyroid secretion. The secretion of thyroid hormone from the thyroid is mainly controlled by thyrotrophin (TSH), a hormone produced by the mucoid cells of the adenohypophysis. Inadequate plasma levels of T_3 and T_4 cause release of TSH from the pituitary by a feedback mechanism and this stimulates all the processes of thyroid hormone formation and release described above. The stimulation is associated with important structural changes in the gland, in particular a change of the epithelium from cubical to columnar, proliferation of epithelial cells to form new follicles, and diminution of the volume and eosinophilia of the colloid stored within the vesicles. If the TSH stimulation is marked and prolonged, *goitre*, i.e. enlargement of the thyroid, develops. When the plasma level of thyroid hormone exceeds the physiological requirements of the body, the production of TSH by the pituitary is suppressed and the thyroid reverts to its resting state with diminished hormone production, diminished secretion and increased storage of hormone within the eosinophilic colloid which accumulates within the vesicles.

Hypothyroidism. The effects of subnormal secretion of T_4 and T_3 vary depending upon the severity of thyroid hormone deficiency and the age of onset of the disorder. Infantile hypothyroidism is called *cretinism* and is described on p. 889.

metabolic rate is lowered and the patient feels cold. Hypothermia and coma may develop.

Biochemical abnormalities include raised serum cholesterol level due to reduced rate of catabolism, but most significant is the low thyroid secretion rate of T_4 and T_3 most conveniently assessed in current routine clinical practice as a low serum protein-bound iodine concentration.

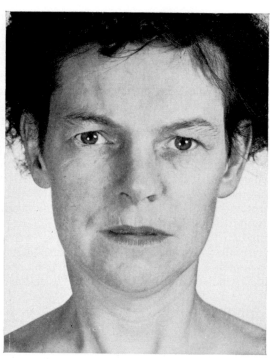

FIG. 24.4.—Myxoedema: left, before treatment: right, the effects of administration of thyroxin.

In the adult the syndrome is called *myxoedema*. In severe cases there is lethargy, slowing of speech and impaired intellectual function sometimes associated with frank psychosis. The hair, brittle and lustreless, tends to fall out. Hydrophilic mucoprotein ground substance accumulates in the dermal connective tissue causing coarsening of the features (Fig. 24.4) and firm non-pitting oedema of the supraclavicular fossae and dorsum of the hands. Similar mucinous deposits around nerves may impair peripheral nerve function and cause, for example, carpal tunnel syndrome or deafness, while involvement of tongue and larynx cause a characteristically slurred croaking voice. Despite a poor appetite and constipation the patient gains weight. The pulse is slow, the basal

In most cases the secretion of TSH is increased and this is reflected in the mucoid cells of the anterior pituitary which contain only a few prominent storage granules (vesiculate mucoid cells—Fig. 24.3). There is diminished sexual function and menorrhagia is common due to failure of ovulation and continued endometrial proliferation. All of the above changes, except the low thyroid hormone secretion rate, are reversed by therapy with T_4 or T_3.

In clinical practice, by far the most common cause of hypothyroidism is primary myxoedema (the atrophic form of auto-immune thyroiditis) but hypothyroidism with goitre is found in Hashimoto's disease, dyshormonogenesis, severe iodine deficiency and as a result of drugs with antithyroid effects. Extensive surgical resection of the thyroid, therapy with radioiodine and hypopituitarism with diminished TSH secretion are other causes.

Hyperthyroidism (syn. **thyrotoxicosis**) results from excessive secretion of thyroid hormone and causes clinical features which are almost the opposite of those found in hypothyroidism. The patient though weak is restless, hyperkinetic and emotionally unstable. The appetite is increased but the patient loses weight. There is increased nitrogen excretion, and sometimes impaired glucose tolerance and glycosuria. The skin is warm and sweating, the pulse rapid and bounding and the cardiac output is increased. Cardiac arrhythmia, particularly atrial fibrillation, may occur, especially in older patients and cardiac failure may be the presenting feature. Osteoporosis affecting cancellous bone may be present, associated with increased calcium excretion in urine and faeces. Many of the above features are attributable to the raised basal metabolic rate which is in turn due to the effects of excessive amounts of T_3 and T_4 on the tissues. The serum protein-bound iodine concentration is raised. Pituitary TSH secretion appears to be inhibited. In the common clinical form of hyperthyroidism, *Graves' disease*, there is unexplained prominence of the eyes (exophthalmos) (Fig. 24.5) which cannot be attributed to the action of T_3 and T_4.

Most cases of thyrotoxicosis appear to be due to an abnormal thyroid stimulator in the blood. Less often autonomous hyperfunctioning thyroid nodules are responsible, while in very rare cases, hyperthyroidism is the result of excessive pituitary TSH production in acromegaly.

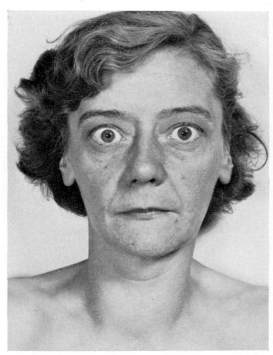

Fig. 24.5.—Thyrotoxicosis. Note the prominence of the eyes and the diffuse thyroid enlargement.

Nontoxic Goitre (Simple Goitre)

Nontoxic goitre refers to various non-inflammatory conditions which result in enlargement of the thyroid gland without hyperthyroidism. All forms of nontoxic goitre are probably preceded and for a time accompanied by a phase of impaired thyroid hormone synthesis due to inadequate supply of iodide or to impaired thyroid enzyme activity, the result of genetic defect or exogenous toxic substances. To counteract the diminished secretion of thyroid hormone in these circumstances more TSH is produced and there is increased activity of the thyroid epithelium which becomes hyperplastic. These compensatory changes may increase T_4 and T_3 secretion enough to prevent hypothyroidism, but the defect may be so severe that goitrous hypothyroidism results, a condition which some authors would not include under the heading of simple or nontoxic goitre.

Anatomically the following varieties of nontoxic goitre are recognised: (*a*) *parenchymatous goitre*, showing hyperplasia of the type illustrated in Fig. 24.6 with little colloid storage; (*b*) *colloid goitre*, in which there is marked accumulation of colloid in the vesicles. These varieties may occur in a diffuse form in which the gland is generally involved or in a nodular form in which increase occurs in scattered rounded nodules of varying size.

Epidemiology. Goitre may occur sporadically in any locality. Before the introduction of iodised salt, goitre was unduly common in certain districts (*endemic goitre*), notably in the valleys of Switzerland, the Pyrenees, the

Himalayas and in New Zealand; in Great Britain in Derbyshire; in parts of Southern Ireland, and in America in the region of the Great Lakes. Where deficiency of iodine was great, as in the mountainous regions, e.g. the Alps, the goitre was usually parenchymatous, diffuse at first and becoming nodular later. Thyroid deficiency and cretinism were common, especially where the disease was very prevalent and of severe type.

ide. In goitrous districts the disease also affects rats, sheep and other animals. When iodine deficiency is severe goitre appears in childhood; when it is moderate, goitre is not only less common but also appears later, occurring especially at puberty and in pregnancy and lactation, when there is a drain on the iodine supply. Males are affected less frequently than females. In the early stages especially treatment by iodine may

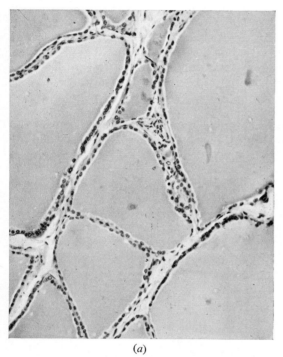
(a)

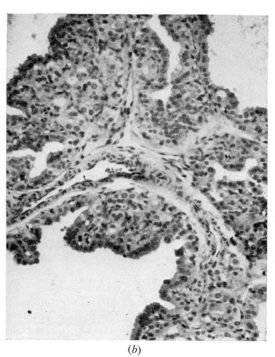
(b)

FIG. 24.6.—Normal thyroid tissue (a) and thyroid showing the effects of chronic stimulation with TSH (b): note the hypertrophy and hyperplasia of the thyroid epithelium and diminished colloid storage. × 185.

In goitrous districts in Switzerland the average weight of the thyroid at birth was often double the normal and occasionally a congenital parenchymatous goitre was present. In America, goitre was usually of the colloid type, either diffuse or nodular.

Etiology. The causation of endemic goitre is not fully understood, but it is known that deficiency of iodine is the chief factor in its production. In remote communities where little food is imported, lack of iodine in the soil, water, and in locally produced food is the basic defect. There may be contributory factors which render unavailable any iodine present, such as pollution of water supplies by sulphur-containing organic matter or the presence of much calcium or fluor-

arrest the thyroid enlargement or cause it to regress. In the region of the Great Lakes and in Switzerland, the administration of small quantities of iodine to school children has resulted in remarkable diminution in the incidence of goitre. In New Zealand and certain other districts the results have been less striking, perhaps because of the presence of iodine inhibitors.

Sporadic nontoxic goitre, i.e. that occurring in areas where goitre is not endemic, appears to have three main causes: (1) iodine deficiency due to improper dietary habits; (2) dyshormonogenesis due to one of a group of inherited defects of the process of thyroid hormone synthesis or secretion (see pp. 884, 889); (3) the action of substances which interfere with thyroid hormone synthesis. In practice, and excluding antithyroid drugs used in treating thyrotoxicosis, perhaps the most important of these is large

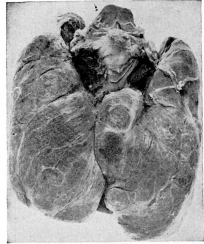

FIG. 24.7.—Diffuse colloid goitre with general enlargement of the gland. × ½.

doses of iodine given in the form of iodopyrine, or less commonly simply as iodide as expectorants in asthma or chronic bronchitis. In idiosyncratic subjects this inhibits coupling of iodine with tyrosine; there is a fall in thyroid hormone release, and patients with "iodide goitre" frequently become hypothyroid. Resorcinol, *para*-aminosalicylic acid and sulphonylureas are other drugs which occasionally cause nontoxic goitre.

Parenchymatous goitre. The initial changes are enlargement of the acinar cells to columnar type and new formation of many small colloid-deficient vesicles. The enlarged gland lacks normal thyroid translucency and resembles pancreas to the naked eye. The changes are at first diffuse, affecting the entire gland, but if the iodine lack persists, foci of excessive activity in iodine uptake appear, while other parts of the gland become refractory and fail to take up and store iodine as has been shown by autoradiography of thyroids excised after a dose of radioactive iodine. The hyperactive foci enlarge and compress the adjacent parenchyma so that the gland becomes nodular.

In the nodular type of goitre a great variety of structure may be encountered. There may be only one or two nodular masses, or the gland may be studded with them, the parenchyma

between becoming atrophied. It is probable that a degree of diffuse parenchymatous hyperplasia invariably occurs in the early stages, and the subsequent development seems to depend on the severity of the continuing iodine deficiency, however brought about.

Colloid goitre. In diffuse colloid goitre the whole gland may be affected (Fig. 24.7), or one lobe may be chiefly involved. The gland substance is tense and firm, and on section presents a translucent brownish appearance due to the accumulation of colloid, which is usually fairly firm. There is a honeycomb-like structure representing the stroma, and colloid-filled spaces of considerable size may be present. Dark red or brown areas due to haemorrhage may be seen, and in places there may be fibrosis, sometimes with calcification of the stroma. On microscopic examination, the acini are large and distended with deeply-staining colloid, and the epithelium may be flattened (Fig. 24.8). Cysts may be formed by the confluence of acini. Colloid goitre is much commoner in women than in men, usually appears first at puberty or in pregnancy, and may be dependent on a less severe degree of iodine lack than that associated with

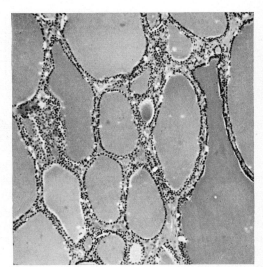

FIG. 24.8.—Colloid goitre, showing accumulation of colloid in vesicles with flattened epithelium. × 40.

the parenchymatous type of goitre. This seems to hold generally with regard to the disease in low-lying countries.

Effects. Goitre is often not associated with distinct functional effects or constitutional symptoms, though minor disturbances are not so rare as was once supposed. The enlarged gland may rarely bring about important results by pressure on a recurrent laryngeal nerve, the oesophagus, or on the trachea, which may become much narrowed, and death by suffocation may follow. In mountainous regions the thyroid enlargement in children, usually of the nodular type, may be associated with cretinism, the result of severe deficiency of the thyroid hormone. In America colloid goitre has been associated with some degree of thyrotoxicosis.

Despite much study, it is uncertain whether nontoxic goitre predisposes to the development of carcinoma.

Cretinism

Severe hypothyroidism beginning in infancy is called *cretinism.* Cretins usually seem normal at birth, having received maternal thyroid hormone while *in utero,* but within a few weeks or months it becomes apparent that mental and physical development is retarded. The characteristic cretin is a dwarf with severe mental defect, disproportionately short limbs, coarse dry skin, deficient hair and teeth, a large protruding tongue and pot belly with umbilical hernia (Fig. 24.9). The skeletal changes of cretinism are mentioned on p. 768. Unless replacement therapy with T_3 or T_4 commences early, the changes, especially the mental defects, become irreversible, though there may be some improvement in physical appearance.

Endemic cretinism occurred almost exclusively in mountainous districts such as Switzerland, where iodine deficiency was severe and endemic goitre common. It is said rarely to appear in a goitrous family until the second or third generation, and cretins of this type are nearly always the offspring of goitrous mothers. Unexplained deaf-mutism is very often present as an additional condition.

The thyroid. In most cases of endemic cretinism a goitre is present, although in some instances the thyroid is atrophic and fibrous. The goitre is nearly always nodular, the gland being occupied by nodules between which the rest of the parenchyma is compressed and atrophic. The appearances are similar to those seen in the nodular goitres of long-standing iodine deficiency.

Sporadic cretinism. This condition, due to congenital absence or hypoplasia of the thyroid tissue, is encountered from time to time in all localities and the causation is unknown. In some cases no trace of thyroid may be found, although in some instances small nodules of atrophied thyroid tissue have been found near the foramen caecum at the root of the tongue. In other cases the thyroid is small and shrunken, sometimes containing cysts. The thymus is usually atrophic, but the parathyroids are not affected and occupy their usual position.

Dyshormonogenesis. Goitre in sporadic cretinism is very rare, but it occurs as a familial recessive abnormality manifested by congenital absence of some essential enzyme system. In one variety, studied by McGirr and Hutchison in a family of Scottish tinkers, absence of the dehalogenase enzyme, which normally removes iodine

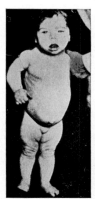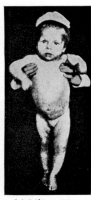

FIG. 24.9(*a*).—Child with sporadic cretinism, showing the characteristic features.

FIG. 24.9(*b*).—The same child after 2 months' treatment with thyroid extract.

(The figure is on a somewhat smaller scale than Fig. 24.9(*a*).)

from iodotyrosine, allows mono- and diiodotyrosine to escape from the thyroid into the blood, from which they are excreted in the urine, thus leading to gross iodine deficiency. In another type the condensation of diiodotyrosine to thyroxine is impaired and hormone synthesis is therefore incomplete. In a third type iodide accumulates in the gland but there is enzymatic failure to oxidise iodide to free iodine which is therefore not available in the thyroid to combine with tyrosine. Accordingly iodinated hormone synthesis fails. In some of these congenital goitrous cretins deaf-mutism is present, an interesting finding in view of its unexplained frequency in endemic goitrous cretinism.

The thyroid is often greatly enlarged and nodular, and on microscopic examination the epithelial hyperplasia of parenchymatous goitre is found.

Auto-immune Thyroiditis

In this condition there is infiltration of the thyroid by lymphocytes and plasma cells associated with abnormalities of the thyroid epithelium and, in many cases, thyroid-specific auto-antibodies in the serum.

Three main variants are encountered: (1) *Hashimoto's disease* (lymphadenoid goitre)—a diffuse and massive lesion causing goitre; (2) *primary myxoedema*, in which the thyroid is shrunken and the epithelium atrophic; (3) *focal thyroiditis* in which patchy lesions occur in an otherwise normal or hyperplastic gland.

Gross appearance. Areas of thyroid affected by auto-immune thyroiditis appear solid and white or peach coloured, lacking the translucent appearance normally presented by colloid stored in the vesicles. In Hashimoto's disease the gland is firm and there is enlargement, usually symmetrical and of moderate degree; the cut surface has a solid lobulated appearance resembling pancreas on section, and in most cases the cap-

sule is not adherent to surrounding tissues. The shrunken thyroid of primary myxoedema is firm and white while in focal auto-immune thyroiditis ill-defined white patches of about 1 mm. in diameter are seen on the cut surface of the gland.

Microscopic appearance (Fig. 24.10). The basic lesion common to all forms is the presence of small follicles lined by large cubical epithelial cells with granular cytoplasm and large nuclei which are frequently bizarre in shape. These cells, known variously as Askanazy cells, Hürthle cells, oxyphil cells or oncocytes, owe their eosinophilic (pale pink to bright red) cytoplasmic granularity to the presence of numerous large mitochondria.

The colloid is densely eosinophilic and may contain macrophages or multinucleated giant cells. Surrounding the abnormal follicles, and sometimes invading them, is an infiltrate of plasma cells and/or lymphocytes, accompanied by a variable amount of fibrous tissue.

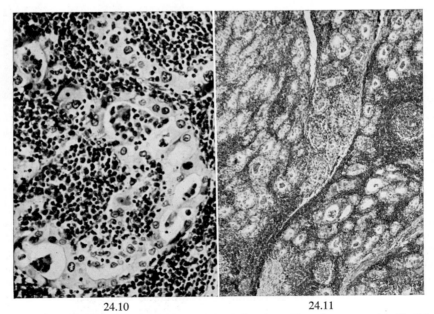

24.10   24.11

Thyroid in Hashimoto's disease, showing extensive infiltration of lymphocytes and epithelial changes in acini, the lining cells of which are of Askanazy cell type.
Note germ centre at right side of Fig. 24.11. × 200 and 48.

In Hashimoto's disease (Fig. 24.11) the epithelium is all abnormal and increased in amount. The lymphoid infiltrate is massive and true germinal centres may be present. Mitotic figures are very infrequent. The amount of fibrous tissue is variable. Most of the gland in primary myxoedema consists of fibrous tissue (Fig. 24.12)

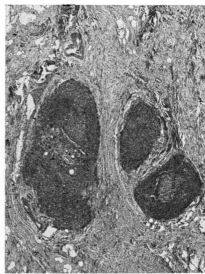

FIG. 24.12.—Thyroid in primary myxoedema. Most of the parenchyma has been lost, and there is extensive fibrosis. The dark patches contain surviving thyroid tissue showing severe chronic thyroditis. × 17.

containing sparse clusters of small follicles lined by Askanazy cells and islets or cysts of epithelium with a squamous appearance (a feature also seen occasionally in Hashimoto's disease). The lymphocytic and plasma cell infiltration is usually slight and situated mainly around the surviving epithelium. Focal auto-immune thyroiditis (Fig. 24.13) differs from both these conditions by the presence of greater or smaller areas of normal or hyperplastic epithelium free of lymphoid infiltrate. The more severe examples, however, approach Hashimoto's disease in extent.

Clinical features. In Hashimoto's disease the patient, usually a middle-aged female, has a firm goitre of moderate size. Hypothyroidism is present in about half the cases, and is the rule if partial thyroidectomy is undertaken. The thyroidal uptake of iodine is reduced and organification is impaired. An abnormal iodinated thyroprotein, which differs from serum protein-bound T_4 in being insoluble in butanol, is sometimes found in the serum.

Primary myxoedema is characterised by hypothyroidism in the absence of goitre. Chronic focal thyroiditis is usually asymptomatic, but if partial thyroidectomy is performed hypothyroidism may develop in the more severe cases.

Etiology. Auto-antibodies against thyroglobulin and/or against a lipoprotein of the smooth-surfaced vesicles of the endoplasmic reticulum ("microsomes") of thyroid epithelial cells are found in high titre in the serum of most, but not all, patients with Hashimoto's disease. The frequency and titre of such antibodies is lower in primary myxoedema and lower again in focal thyroiditis. There is evidence that most of the auto-antibody is formed by the plasma cells which are usually a conspicuous feature of the inflammatory infiltrate of the gland.

Experimental auto-immune thyroiditis can be produced in various animals, including primates,

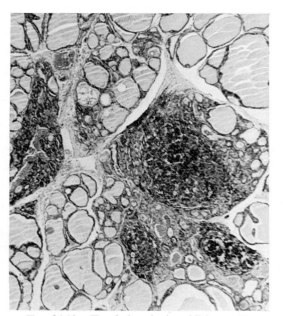

FIG. 24.13.—Focal chronic thyroiditis. × 20.

by injecting thyroglobulin in Freund's adjuvant emulsion (p. 83) which enhances immunological responsiveness, particularly the development of delayed hypersensitivity. The experimental thyroid lesions closely parallel the development of delayed hypersensitivity and transfer of the disease to normal animals has been accomplished only with lymphoid cells. It is thought that delayed hypersensitivity is likely to be more important than cytotoxic antibody in the pathogenesis of human auto-immune thyroiditis.

Patients with auto-immune thyroiditis are unduly prone to have in addition auto-immune gastritis (p. 490) (sometimes accompanied by pernicious anaemia), or auto-immune adrenalitis (idiopathic Addison's disease, p. 909) and this suggests that the predisposition to organ specific auto-immunity is due to a disorder of the lymphoid tissue rather than to primary abnormalities in these various organs. Further-more, the occurrence of all these diseases within certain families suggests that the basic predisposition is inherited.

It remains to be discovered what event triggers the auto-immune process, why the disease occurs mainly in females, and what factors determine whether the lesion is focal or diffuse and whether the epithelium becomes hyperplastic as in Hashimoto's disease or atrophic as in primary myxoedema.

Other Forms of Thyroiditis

Thyroiditis due to causes other than auto-immunity is very rare in Britain. Multiple small abscesses may be found in the thyroid in pyaemia and acute thyroiditis is said sometimes to complicate influenza and typhoid fever. Occasionally the thyroid is affected by tuberculosis, either as a large caseous mass resulting from lymphatic spread from an adjacent cervical lymph node, or from haematogenous spread, or as minute foci in miliary tuberculosis. Fibrosis and gumma formation have been encountered in congenital and acquired syphilis.

Giant cell thyroiditis (de Quervain's thyroiditis). This variety of subacute thyroiditis begins with the distinctive features of fever and pain in the neck with tenderness. There is a neutrophil leukocytosis and a raised ESR. Elevation of the protein-bound iodine with reduced thyroid iodine uptake is said to be pathognomonic of the disorder. Microscopically there is polymorphonuclear infiltration followed by lymphocytes and plasma cells; destruction of acini with formation of epithelioid cells and giant cells give a pseudotuberculous appearance. Israeli workers have recovered a virus having the characters of mumps virus from two cases and have shown the presence of neutralising and complement-fixing antibodies to mumps virus in others.

Riedel's disease. This very rare disease is characterised by enlargement of the thyroid by fibrous tissue of extremely hard consistency; the condition usually affects only one lobe and involves adjacent muscles. Microscopically the fibrous tissue may be more or less cellular, and in the affected part the vesicles become atrophic and disappear. Hypothyroidism is unusual. The nature of the disease is unknown; a few cases have been associated with retroperitoneal fibrosis; other supposed cases may be more properly classified as sclerotic thyroid adenomas or as fibrous variants of Hashimoto's disease.

Hyperthyroidism

When there is excessive secretion of the thyroid hormones thyroxine and triiodothyronine the condition is described as hyperthyroidism or thyrotoxicosis. Three clinicopathological varieties are recognised. (1) Graves' disease, the most common, is characterised by diffuse thyroid hyperplasia apparently due to the presence of an inappropriate thyroid stimulator in the blood. Protrusion of the eyeballs (exophthalmos) and certain other features of the disease cannot be ascribed to thyroid hormone excess alone. (2) Toxic adenoma, is a relatively uncommon condition, in which an autonomous thyroid tumour produces thyroid hormone in excess of the requirements of the body. (3) Toxic nodular goitre, in which excessive hormone is produced in multiple discrete foci within the thyroid, occurs in older patients who already have a simple nodular goitre. The main features of hyperthyroidism have already been outlined on p. 886.

Graves' disease (exophthalmic goitre)

In this disease **the thyroid** shows hyperplasia which is characteristically diffuse though sometimes one lobe is larger than the other. On section the parenchyma is less brown and less translucent than normal owing to diminished colloid storage and the gland resembles salivary tissue, being dull greyish-pink in colour and lobulated. However, even in untreated cases some parts may contain a considerable amount of colloid and the surface may be slightly nodular. The gland is moderately firm and succulent, though if thyroiditis is marked there may be a certain amount of fibrosis. The surface veins and arteries may be enlarged but the organ as a whole does not look specially vascular after surgical removal or at necropsy. The appearances may be much modified by treatment.

The alterations described are usually fairly uniform throughout the gland but in places there may be quiescent acini which contain a considerable amount of colloid, especially when, at a later period, the acute symptoms are beginning to subside. The picture may thus be one of hyperplasia and subsequent involution irregularly distributed, even with fibrosis in places.

The administration of iodine induces retro-

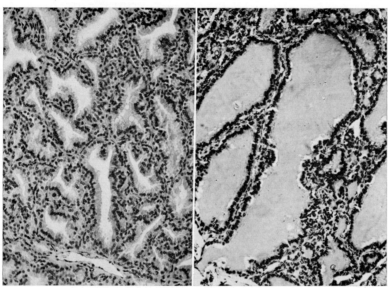

Thyroid gland in exophthalmic goitre.
24.14. Before treatment, showing epithelial hyperplasia and disappearance of colloid.
24.15. After iodine treatment for 10 days, the gland shows reaccumulation of colloid. × 110.

On microscopic examination, hyperplasia of the epithelium and diminution in the amount of the colloid stored are constant (Fig. 24.14). The epithelial cells of the acini are increased in size and more columnar in type. Numerous small acini are formed, while in the larger ones papilliform ingrowths are often present: both of these factors lead to a great increase in the epithelial surface area. What colloid remains stains less deeply and appears more watery. These changes reflect increased formation of secretion, which is, however, not retained but passed on to the blood-stream. In many cases there is focal autoimmune thyroiditis with lymphocytic infiltration (Fig. 24.13), and sometimes the formation of lymphoid follicles. When such infiltration is widespread, the lesion comes to resemble Hashimoto's disease (p. 890), and in such cases hypothyroidism commonly follows partial thyroidectomy.

gression of the hyperplastic changes in the thyroid; the epithelium becomes more cubical, and colloid accumulates in the acini (Fig. 24.15). These retrogressive changes after iodine therapy bring about only temporary improvement in the symptoms, and the mode of action of iodine is uncertain. The antithyroid drugs derived from thiourea used in the treatment of hyperthyroidism prevent the synthesis of thyroxine and this leads to a striking reduction in the thyrotoxicosis although the epithelial hyperplasia is undiminished or even exaggerated. The histological effects of iodine and of thiouracil on the thyroid are thus antagonistic and when both are administered before thyroidectomy the histological picture in the excised gland is complex.

Other organs. The thymus shows distinct enlargement in three-quarters of the cases, and the thymic lymphoid tissue (which contains medullary lymphoid follicles) is increased in amount. There may also be some enlargement of the lymph nodes. Some observers consider that such changes are in proportion to the severity of the disease; they may reflect the auto-immune response concerned in the focal thyroiditis which is present in many cases, or may be due to lowered adrenal cortical function resulting from the accelerated inactivation of cortisol found in thyrotoxicosis. Hypertrophy of the heart occurs in most cases of exophthalmic goitre. There may be neutropenia with relative lymphocytosis. Occasionally, however, there is an absolute lymphocytosis, and this is thought by some to occur in the more severe cases.

Occasionally bilateral patches of myxoedematous thickening appear on the anterior (pretibial) aspects of the lower leg, even while thyrotoxicosis is active. In former times, before operative removal became relatively safe owing to premedication with antithyroid drugs, it was recognised that in a few cases thyroid involution might culminate in hypothyroidism.

Orbital changes. Exophthalmos in mild cases is attributable to fatty infiltration of the extrinsic muscles of the eye. When proptosis is severe there is, in addition, increase in amount and oedema of the orbital tissue, and marked lymphocytic infiltration of the extrinsic eye muscles and perivascular connective tissue.

Etiology. The disease is most common in females, particularly during the reproductive period, and sometimes runs in families, especially in those in which there is an abnormally high incidence of tissue-specific auto-immune diseases, e.g. Hashimoto's disease and pernicious anaemia.

The cause of Graves' disease is uncertain. The diffuse nature of the thyroid hyperplasia and the fact that children born to mothers with Graves' disease show transient evidence of the disorder (congenital thyrotoxicosis) points to the presence of a thyroid stimulator in the blood. In about two-thirds of cases an abnormal thyroid stimulator has been found by a laborious assay procedure in which the patient's serum is injected into guinea pigs or mice and the release of hormone from the animal thyroid is measured (as radioactive iodine): Graves' disease serum, in contrast to specimens containing pituitary TSH cause a protracted release of iodine, and the active principle, LATS (long acting thyroid stimulator), has been shown to be the immunoglobulin IgG, to be independent of pituitary TSH and to be formed in some site other than the pituitary. Consideration of the frequent coexistence of thyrotoxicosis with focal auto-immune thyroiditis and the less common but significant associations with auto-immune gastritis has led to the view that LATS is a thyroid auto-antibody which excites a stimulatory cytotoxic effect on thyroid epithelium and is thus the proximate cause of thyrotoxicosis. Consistent with this view is the failure to demonstrate TSH in the serum of patients with Graves' disease, and the failure of administered T_3 to suppress thyroid activity in these patients, findings which indicate that pituitary TSH production in Graves' disease is fully suppressed by the inappropriately high blood levels of thyroid hormone. Further support is obtained from the correlation between the presence of LATS and the occurrence of congenital thyrotoxicosis, pretibial myxoedema, and, to some extent, with severe exophthalmos. The apparent absence of LATS in a third of patients with Graves' disease and the imperfect correlation between LATS and exophthalmos are against the hypothesis that Graves' disease is an auto-immune disease due to LATS, but it is possible that these objections will be overcome with improved assay systems for LATS and further knowledge of its mode of action.

Toxic adenoma

Approximately one per cent of simple thyroid adenomas give rise to hyperthyroidism, usually of mild degree and not accompanied by exophthalmos or demonstrable LATS in the serum.

The tumours are usually single adenomas more than 3 cm. in diameter and are composed of small vesicles resembling those seen in Graves' disease. Towards the centre of the adenoma stromal oedema and fibrosis may separate the vesicles. Haemorrhage may occur into the tumour and destroy so much of the epithelium that the hyperthyroidism is cured.

Scanning of the neck following administration of radioiodine shows marked radioiodine uptake by the tumour, and, because of the autonomous nature of the growth, this cannot be suppressed by T_3. The remainder of the gland does not concentrate iodine since the hormone produced by the tumour results in diminished secretion of TSH by the pituitary.

Toxic nodular goitre

This disorder usually affects patients over fifty years of age who have had nontoxic goitre for many years. The thyrotoxicosis which subsequently develops is usually mild as judged by thyroidal iodine uptake studies and hormone levels in the blood. Cardiac arrhythmias and failure may be the presenting symptom. Exophthalmos is uncommon.

The macroscopic and histological features are similar to those described in nontoxic nodular goitre (p. 886). Autoradiography shows in some cases one or two hyperfunctioning nodules (in effect, and perhaps in fact, toxic adenomas) with complete suppression of radioiodine uptake by the remainder of the goitre. In other cases multiple small groups of hyperplastic follicles concentrate radioactive iodine though much of the gland is inactive, the appearances suggesting the effect of some extrinsic thyroid stimulator on a gland part of whose tissue is refractory. Thyroid microsomal antibody is found in the serum of such cases with the same frequency as in Graves' disease, but it remains to be seen whether LATS is also demonstrable.

Degenerative Changes

Excluding changes in nodular goitre and tumours, degenerative changes in the thyroid are comparatively rare and of little importance. Evidence of damage produced by toxins is found in infections, and there may be actual necrosis of the epithelium. Amyloid degeneration sometimes occurs as an isolated finding or as part of widespread amyloidosis. When well marked, it causes thyroid enlargement (*amyloid goitre*). Amyloid is found in the stroma of medullary carcinoma of the thyroid (p. 897). Hyaline change, calcification, etc., are often present in the stroma of chronic goitres.

Tumours of the Thyroid

Thyroid adenomas are comparatively common. They are enclosed by a fibrous capsule, compress the surrounding gland, are more often multiple than single, and present varying appearances depending on the extent of degenerative change and the type of acini formed. Thus they may be haemorrhagic or cystic, and in the absence of degeneration, they may have the brown honeycomb appearance of colloid goitre on section or be composed of pale, fawn, soft, fleshy tissue. Microscopically some are composed of strands and cylinders of epithelium without acinar structure, others consist of very small acini containing little colloid—such tumours have been called "*fetal adenomas*", but they do not seem to be due to developmental errors (Fig. 24.16). In yet others there may be considerable colloid storage. *It is not possible to draw a line between circumscribed hyperplastic changes constituting the nodules in nodular goitres and true adenomatous tumours.* Thyroid adenomata usually present clinically merely as localised swellings in the gland; those of the more cellular type are sometimes associated with hyperthyroidism. Adenomas are believed by some occasionally to become malignant in the later years of life. A point of importance is the clinical difficulty of distinguishing benign adenoma from carcinoma in the absence of metastases; solitary tumours in the thyroids of children and young adults should be regarded with suspicion.

Adenoma of parathyroid origin is occasionally observed in the substance of the thyroid. Simple connective tissue tumours such as fibromas and osteochondromas are rare.

Malignant tumours

Carcinoma of thyroid causes about 0·5 per cent of all deaths from malignancy. Its chief effect is invasion of surrounding structures including the trachea and recurrent laryngeal nerves and death is commonly due to asphyxia. Its incidence is said to be higher in regions with endemic goitre but this is doubtful, and it has been found frequently following X-irradiation of the neck in childhood for such simple conditions as haemangioma or supposed thymic enlargement. Some of the better differentiated human carcinomas may be TSH-dependent for there are records of rapid growth of metastases following total thyroidectomy or the administration of antithyroid drugs; and treatment with thyroxine, which suppresses TSH production, seems to have resulted in regression of established meta-

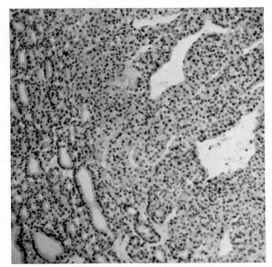

Fig. 24.16.—Adenoma of thyroid, showing two types of growth—acinar type on left side of field and more solid type of growth on right. × 120.

stases in some cases and is thought to have prevented metastases in others. A noteworthy feature of well-differentiated thyroid carcinomas, especially in young patients, is the prolonged survival and well-being of the patient despite the presence of metastases.

Papillary adenocarcinoma is the form most commonly encountered and is sometimes seen in children and young adults. The tumour is not well encapsulated, is sometimes only a few millimetres in diameter, and despite its relatively innocuous microscopical appearance it frequently spreads to the cervical lymph nodes, particularly of the side affected (Fig. 24.17). Indeed all papillary tumours of the thyroid should be regarded as potentially malignant. It was previously erroneously thought that cervical lymph-node metastases of this tumour were "lateral aberrant thyroids". Pulmonary and skeletal metastases are rarely found.

Follicular adenocarcinoma. Certain encapsulated tumours, with the gross appearance of adenomas, are carcinomas composed of glandular acini. The best differentiated examples

closely resemble normal thyroid but more often there are mitotic figures and aberrant cells; in many cases solid sheets of tumour cells are also present, sometimes of eosinophilic "Hürthle" type. Malignancy is recognised by invasion of the fibrous capsule and blood vessels, and metastasis is particularly common in bone and lung. Some of these tumours take up ^{131}I, which can be used therapeutically.

Occasionally squamous carcinoma is seen, possibly arising from the thyroglossal duct.

Anaplastic tumours. Anaplastic tumours of various types—round-cell, spindle-cell and pleomorphic—are relatively common and the majority are probably anaplastic cancers rather than sarcomas. They cause respiratory obstruction from rapid enlargement of the gland. Tumours having the general appearance of reticulo-sarcoma are sometimes difficult to distinguish

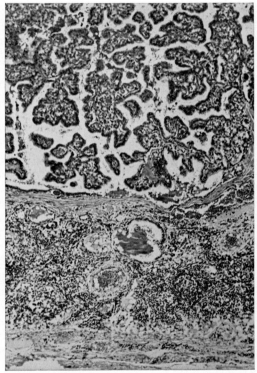

Fig. 24.17.—Papillary cystadenocarcinoma of the thyroid in the cervical lymph nodes—so-called lateral aberrant thyroid. × 65.

from the more extreme examples of Hashimoto's disease, a difficulty accentuated by the fact that some have responded to radiotherapy and have not recurred, whereas others, histologically indistinguishable, behave as unequivocal malignant tumours. Brewer and Orr propose the term *struma reticulosa* for this group and they call attention to the frequency of multiple growths of similar structure in the lymphoid tissue of the small intestine.

Medullary carcinoma. This tumour, which arises from the cells producing calcitonin, forms solid masses of cells set in a hyaline stroma which in places contains amyloid and is sometimes calcified. Despite its rather anaplastic appearance the mitotic rate is usually low and survival for many years is common. No clinical syndrome of calcitonin excess has been recognised in patients with this tumour but some have diarrhoea, possibly due to the production of prostaglandins by the tumour.

Congenital abnormalities. The isthmus of the thyroid is formed by a downgrowth of a tube of epithelium from the base of the tongue (foramen caecum). The upper portion of this tube above the hyoid bone is lined by squamous epithelium. If this persists and if the buccal end is obstructed, it may give rise to a "lingual dermoid". The lower part of the duct below the hyoid bone is lined by columnar ciliated epithelium. Thyroglossal cysts may take origin from this part when it does not undergo involution. Such a cyst may rupture on the skin surface, forming a median cervical fistula. In the walls of these cysts portions of thyroid tissue are sometimes found. Occasionally a mass of thyroid tissue is found in the base of the tongue, the so-called "lingual thyroid", and the thyroid may be then absent from its normal site. Congenital absence and hypoplasia of the thyroid are among the causes of sporadic cretinism.

THE PANCREATIC ISLETS

The lesions of the exocrine pancreas have already been described (p. 595), and we have to consider here only its function as an endocrine organ concerned with carbohydrate metabolism. The hormone *insulin* formed by the islets of Langerhans of the pancreas is essential for the utilisation of sugar; when it is absent or markedly deficient, diabetes results. We shall first give an account of the main features of diabetes and then discuss its relationship to the pancreas; we shall afterwards refer to other conditions where glycosuria is present.

Diabetes mellitus

In diabetes there is a failure in varying degree to store and metabolise carbohydrate, with consequent hyperglycaemia and glycosuria. The failure to store glucose in diabetes is shown by the diminution of the amount of glycogen in the muscles and the inability to catabolise glucose is shown by its increase in the blood and its excretion in the urine. Normally, the blood contains 80–100 mg. of glucose per 100 ml., this figure rising following ingestion of carbohydrates. If the amount rises to about 180 mg., glucose is excreted by the kidneys in amounts readily detectable by simple chemical tests. In diabetes there is always hyperglycaemia after ingestion of carbohydrate, the glucose sometimes reaching 400 mg. per 100 ml. or more, and the glycosuria is a secondary result; the fasting blood sugar may, however, be within the normal range.

Clinical and biochemical changes

Thirst and polydipsia are constant features. They are due to the polyuria, which in turn results from osmotic diuresis in the renal tubules owing to the glucose present; accordingly the urine is pale and of high specific gravity. In severe cases of diabetes, owing to the failure to utilise glucose, proteins and fats are metabolised in increased amount and the glucose derived from protein is excreted in the urine. Thus, when carbohydrates are excluded from the diet the urine may still contain a considerable amount of glucose derived from proteins, and the relationship between the amounts of glucose and of nitrogen excreted may correspond to that in pure protein metabolism. Further, as energy has to be derived chiefly from the oxidation of proteins and fats, there is a marked fall in the respiratory quotient to 0·8 or even lower. Owing to the increased metabolism of proteins and fats for the supply of energy, and also as a result of the fact that neutral fats are no longer formed from carbohydrates, marked emaciation occurs. The abnormal metabolism necessarily leads also to muscular weakness.

In cases of diabetes, serum has often a turbid appearance due to hyperlipidaemia, and when the blood is allowed to stand, a white film composed of fatty globules gathers on the surface. The β-lipoprotein, and therefore cholesterol content of the blood is usually increased, and not infrequently there is a deposit of cholesterol esters in the skin, resulting in yellow patches of xanthelasma (p. 592). Accumulation of lipids may occur in the reticulo-endothelial cells of the spleen, and occasionally this is said to result in clinical enlargement of the organ. Although synthesis of neutral fats from carbohydrates is greatly reduced, the synthesis of cholesterol from acetate proceeds normally. Pronounced fatty change in the kidneys is fairly common, and is frequently accompanied by accumulation of glycogen in Henle's tubules, representing a reabsorption from the glomerular filtrate.

Ketosis. An important phenomenon in uncontrolled diabetes is the appearance of *acetone bodies* in the urine (*ketonuria*), these comprising acetone, aceto-acetic acid, and β-hydroxybutyric acid. The last, which is the least highly oxidised of the three, becomes most abundant in severe cases of the disease, hence its level in the blood is of importance: the amount of hydroxybutyric acid in the urine may reach 50 g. per day or more, whilst the amount of aceto-acetic acid and acetone together rarely exceeds 5 g. The utilisation of carbohydrates by the tissues is essential for the proper oxidation of fats, which at the 2C atom stage are incorporated into the tricarboxylic acid cycle; in the absence of carbohydrates, acetone bodies are formed as the result of the failure to complete the oxidation of the higher fatty acids. This is aggravated by the wastage of carbohydrate and consequent increased catabolism of fats, which above a certain level becomes inefficient and incomplete, with resultant accumulation of ketone bodies in the plasma and hence in the urine; in severe ketosis excretion of acetone in the expired air imparts a sweetish odour to the breath. This occurs, for example, in starvation, or when carbohydrates are excluded from the food, while in diabetes inability of the tissues to utilise glucose leads to the same result. The amount of the acetone bodies in the urine thus supplies an index of the severity of this important biochemical disturbance.

Accumulation in the blood of aceto-acetic and hydroxybutyric acids produces a state of *acidosis*. The term does not mean that there is a marked change in the hydrogen-ion concentration of the blood, but simply that acids are constantly being added to it, and alkalis constantly required for their neutralisation. This is at first effected by the fixed alkalis, but there is also an increased formation of ammonia from deamination of amino-acids in the kidney, especially glutamine, and the ammonia participates in neutralising the acids. Along with the acidosis in diabetes, there is thus an increased amount of ammonia nitrogen in the urine. As has been already indicated, there are different degrees in the disturbance of carbohydrate metabolism, and many diabetics can utilise sugar to limited extent.

Diabetic coma. In untreated cases of diabetes death results from acidotic coma. The onset is usually indicated by air hunger and deep respiration. The venous blood is redder than the normal, and contains a diminished amount of carbon dioxide owing to occupation of fixed base by organic acids so that the plasma bicarbonate is reduced. These changes are due to the fact that while the Na^+ is conserved to a considerable extent by the production of ammonia, as explained above, the amount available becomes diminished because Na^+ is diverted to neutralising the acids in the blood, and thus the CO_2-combining power is lowered. The lack of available sodium would require excretion of chloride but there is usually considerable loss of chloride by vomiting, which is common in diabetic ketosis, and chlorides may be absent from the urine in consequence. The combined loss results in secondary dehydration with a fall in the blood volume and haemoconcentration (p. 179). Along with this, phosphates and potassium are excreted in excess and this may bring about a serious loss of muscular power. The respiratory centre and tissues generally suffer from a degree of hypoxia. This is probably not the whole explanation of diabetic coma, but it is increasingly recognised that dehydration and disturbance of the intracellular electrolyte balance are of the highest significance. It is probable that the condition of ketosis leads to actual damage to the nerve cells.

Other features. Another important change in diabetes is a greatly increased susceptibility to bacterial and fungal infections (p. 123). Boils and carbuncles and urinary tract infections, including pyelonephritis and renal papillary necrosis, are of frequent occurrence and tend to precipitate coma. Occasionally there follows a systemic infection with secondary abscesses in internal organs. Diabetics have an increased incidence of tuberculosis especially of the lungs, and the disease tends to run a rapid course. Again, inflammatory conditions may assume a specially severe type; for example, pneumonia may progress to gangrene of the lung. Peripheral neuropathy is another complication, and trophic disturbances, such as perforating ulcer of the foot, may result. Marked atheroma, apparently related to hyperlipidaemia, is often present and arterial thrombosis commonly results. Thus gangrene of part of a limb is one of the recognised complications of diabetes (p. 140); coronary artery thrombosis is another. The ocular fundi show a characteristic pattern of hard white exudates, and micro-aneurysms on the retinal arteries. In the kidneys diabetic glomerulosclerosis presents characteristic features described on p. 718. Diabetic mothers show an increased liability to pre-eclamptic toxaemia and pregnancy aggravates the diabetic state. The babies of diabetic mothers are usually much above normal weight and are flabby and oedematous with a degree of erythroblastosis. Many are stillborn, and those who survive usually grow tall and show an increased tendency to become diabetic. A succession of unduly large children, especially if stillborn, is strongly suggestive that the mother is diabetic or will later become so.

Glucose tolerance tests. When 50 g. of glucose is given to a fasting normal person there soon occurs a distinct rise of the blood sugar, the maximum level of about 150 mg. per 100 ml. being reached in about half an hour. In spite of continuing absorption from the gut, a comparatively rapid fall then occurs and the blood sugar reaches a normal level again within two hours. The rapid fall is due to stimulation of the β-cells of the pancreatic islets by the rise in the level of glucose; secretion of insulin is increased, and this enhances the utilisation of glucose in fatty acid synthesis in adipose tissue cells, and also its conversion into glycogen in skeletal muscle cells. Oxidative breakdown of glucose in the tissue cells in general may also be increased.

The blood sugar curve of a diabetic patient after 50 g. of glucose is quite different. It is absorbed normally from the gut and the blood level rises rapidly as before, and continues to do so for three or four hours, though the curve becomes less steep, and then there is a gradual fall which may go on for some hours. This shows that there is a deficiency in the normal metabolism of glucose. When the blood sugar rises above 180 mg. per 100 ml. or thereabouts, glycosuria occurs, but in established cases the renal threshold is raised and glycosuria does not occur until the blood sugar is substantially above the level at which spill-over into the urine normally occurs. Glucose tolerance tests are not required for diagnosis in frank diabetes, but are of great service in the diagnosis of doubtful cases, where slight or transient glycosuria is found on routine examination in the absence of overt symptoms. Diabetes is excluded by a normal rise followed by the normal fall. In some such cases, the glycosuria is due to the kidney threshold value being lower than normal, e.g. about 130 mg. per 100 ml., so that when glucose or much carbohydrate is administered and the blood sugar rises above this level, glucose is excreted by the kidneys. Such a condition is usually known as *renal glycosuria*. The condition is without serious effects. The result of a glucose tolerance test in which the 30–60 min. specimen shows marked elevation of the blood sugar, often with glycosuria but with a normal 2-hour value, the so-called *lag curve* is usually due to over-rapid absorption of glucose from the intestine without impairment of ability to metabolise glucose. Occasionally this type of curve is seen in persons who show a mild degree of impairment of glucose metabolism, and a few come to give a diabetic type of curve even in the continued absence of symptoms —the *pre-diabetic state*.

Relation of diabetes to the pancreas. It was shown in 1890 by v. Mering and Minkowski that the experimental removal of the pancreas in dogs produces a rapidly fatal form of diabetes in which all the essential phenomena of the disease, as above described, are present—hyperglycaemia and glycosuria, disturbed metabolism, wasting, acidosis, excretion of acetone bodies in the urine, etc.; death, usually preceded by coma, occurs within three or four weeks. The symptoms of disease did not develop when about a fifth of the pancreas was left in the body, and later it was found by Houssay that hypophysectomy ameliorates the symptoms. That the diabetes is not due to loss of the pancreatic juice supplied to the intestine was shown by the fact that, when the duct is brought to the skin surface so that the juice is discharged externally through the fistula, diabetes does not follow. It thus became clear that the diabetes resulted from the loss of a hormone supplied by the pancreas.

Complete obstruction of the pancreatic duct leads to atrophy and secondary fibrosis of the acini of the pancreas, and ultimately the exocrine tissue may largely disappear and be replaced by fibrous and adipose tissue; the islets of Langerhans, however, persist practically unchanged (Fig. 24.18). MacCallum excised half a pancreas and by ligaturing the duct produced in the other half the atrophic changes described. Diabetes did not result, but when the atrophied pancreatic tissue containing the islets

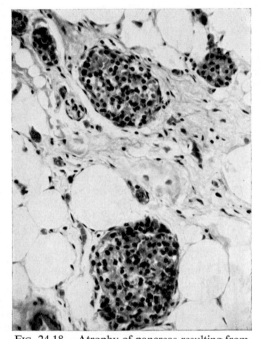

FIG. 24.18.—Atrophy of pancreas resulting from obstruction of the duct. × 190.
The exocrine tissue has been replaced by fat while the islets of Langerhans are unaffected.

was removed, severe diabetes developed. These observations led Banting to the discovery of *insulin* as the active agent concerned in diabetes. In collaboration with Best he tested the action of an extract prepared from a pancreas degenerated in this way, and found that injection of the extract markedly diminished the hyperglycaemia and the glycosuria in depancreatised dogs. The active principle concerned has since been known as *insulin*. Insulins of similar potency, but different chemical structure, can be extracted from the pancreas of fish and of mammals, and, indeed, two somewhat different insulins can be extracted from the pancreas of the rat and possibly of man. The precise mechanism of the effect of insulin metabolism is not fully understood, but an important, and possibly its chief, effect is to facilitate the transport of glucose into cells.

The administration of insulin to a diabetic patient is ordinarily followed by the disappearance of all the important biochemical abnormalities of the disease. The blood sugar falls, glycosuria and ketonuria disappear, the storage of glycogen in the liver and muscles again occurs and the normal metabolism of fats is regained. There is also a rise in the respiratory quotient owing to the restored oxidation of carbohydrates. In the normal animal the injection of insulin causes increased carbohydrate metabolism with hypoglycaemia, and particularly the utilisation of glucose in lipogenesis. Whenever the blood sugar falls below about 50 mg. per 100 ml., nervous symptoms develop, ultimately ending in convulsions, coma and respiratory failure. This may occur not only in the normal animal when insulin is given in excess, but also in the diabetic patient, and it may also result from an islet cell tumour secreting excess of insulin. Mann and Magath showed that acute symptoms following removal of the liver are due to hypoglycaemia. The symptoms are promptly relieved by administration of glucose and, by taking advantage of this fact, they were able to prolong the lives of dogs after hepatectomy.

Etiology of diabetes

(1) **Structural changes.** In the human subject the structural basis of diabetes is obscure. While lesions of the pancreas are fairly common there is no one lesion characteristic of the disease. In some the pancreas is merely reduced in size (35–40 g. instead of 90–100 g.) and the islets show little beyond diminution in number; in a minority of cases chronic interstitial pancreatitis with fibrosis is found and, as Opie has pointed out, interacinous and intralobular pancreatitis can lead to fibrosis and destruction of the islets and consequently to diabetes. Occasionally calculus or carcinoma may be the underlying cause of the pancreatitis and, rarely, acute or chronic pancreatitis (p. 900) may be followed by diabetes. The islets may be extensively replaced by bands of hyaline refractile material (Fig. 24.19), but such hyalinisation of the islets is conspicuous in only a minority of cases. In acute diabetes in young subjects islet cells are swollen and pale (hydropic degeneration), apparently from accumulation of glycogen in them.

(2) **Early- and late-onset types.** Early-onset diabetes presents a distinct hereditary tendency (Harris) and inheritance appears to be multifactorial and rather complex. It is generally severe but also highly responsive to insulin, the nature of the defect being inability of the β-cells to respond normally to the blood glucose level. Late-onset diabetes (developing at over 40 years of age) occurs particularly in obese, hypertensive subjects. Such cases show a female preponderance: the diabetes is usually not severe, but is often relatively resistant to insulin. Himsworth has emphasised the close correlation between the amount of fat consumed in the national diet and the prevalence of late-onset diabetes but the total

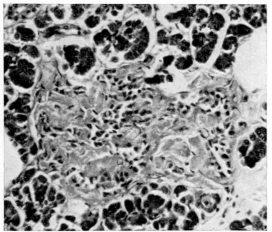

FIG. 24.19.—Islet of Langerhans showing hyaline degeneration in a case of diabetes. × 240.

caloric intake may be more important than the amount of fat. The significance of obesity is thought to lie in failure of the obese to transform carbohydrate rapidly into storable fat once the fat depots are filled (Lawrence), consequently there is hyperglycaemia leading to excessive functional demands on the β-cells. Elderly obese diabetics may, however, be cured of their diabetes if their obesity can be reduced by strict dieting, and the striking fall in the incidence of late diabetes under war-time rationing of food is probably attributable largely to the prevention of obesity in the elderly.

The islets of Langerhans are composed of cells of three types—α-cells, β-cells and δ-cells. The α-cells secrete the glycogenolytic hyperglycaemic factor "glucagon" which is present in many samples of insulin as a contaminant and

so reduces their activity. The granules of the β-cells correspond in their solubility to insulin and the evidence points to functional inhibition of insulin or destruction of these cells as the essential cause of diabetes.

Recently the assay of insulin in the plasma has shown that the diabetic state is not merely one of simple insulin lack. Some diabetics, especially of early-onset type who require insulin, have attached to the plasma albumin one or more insulin antagonists which neutralise its action. The nature and source of these substances is not yet known; glucagon does not seem to be implicated, but the anterior pituitary growth hormone is known to antagonise insulin under experimental conditions, and the adrenal cortex also appears to be concerned.

The presence of these antagonistic substances leads to a constant overproduction of insulin and, consequently, first to hypertrophy of the islets and then to hydropic degeneration and hyalinisation. The hereditary tendency to diabetes may, perhaps, reside in the production of anti-insulins, and the variability of expression may merely indicate the degree to which the islets can cope with the excessive demand for insulin.

(3) **Experimental observations.** In partially pancreatectomised animals diabetes may be prevented by a diet mainly of protein and fat, whereas a high carbohydrate diet may precipitate the diabetic state; in the latter animals hydropic changes in the β-cells are present. Timely administration of insulin, by reducing the functional load on the β-cells, allows recovery to take place and restores the granules, the loss of which probably represents a state of functional depletion following oversecretion, but if the hydropic degranulated state of the cells persists it may be followed by destruction and hyalinisation of β-cells and the diabetic state becomes permanent.

Diabetes can also be produced experimentally in certain animal species, e.g. in dogs and cats, by repeated administration of certain adrenocortical steroids (e.g. cortisone, 17-hydroxycorticosterone) and also of certain anterior pituitary extracts. In the latter method the diabetic condition exists at first only during the period of injection (*idio-hypophyseal diabetes*) and during this time it is unresponsive to insulin; after a prolonged course of injections, however, a permanently diabetic state is established which persists after cessation of treatment with anterior pituitary extract (*meta-hypophyseal diabetes*). The islets at first show loss of granules from the β-cells and later complete hyalinisation, indicating that the development of such experimental diabetes is attributable to destruction of the insulin-secreting β-cells of the islets. Metabolic studies indicate that anterior pituitary extracts interfere with glucose metabolism by inhibiting the enzyme hexokinase which catalyses the conversion of glucose to glucose-6-phosphoric acid, this being an essential step in the utilisation of sugar by the tissues. Accordingly the degranulation of the islet cells is probably the morphological expression of functional overactivity in response to the diabetogenic effect of pituitary hormones. It is probable that growth hormone, ACTH and TSH and possibly other hormones, all contribute to the diabetogenic effect of pituitary extracts.

Repeated intraperitoneal injections of glucose in cats cause sustained hyperglycaemia which can *per se* lead to functional exhaustion of the islet cells with the characteristic hydropic degeneration and permanent diabetes. In man, diabetes resistant to insulin occurs in Cushing's syndrome, as the result of overproduction of glucocorticoids by the hyperplastic or neoplastic adrenal, and adrenal glucocorticoid secretion in response to stress may also determine the worsening of the diabetic state by infections.

Alloxan diabetes. The functional significance of the β-cells was confirmed by Shaw Dunn's discovery in 1942 of the diabetogenic properties of alloxan. This substance causes a highly selective necrosis of the β-cells, which then liberate insulin so that death in hypoglycaemic coma results. If the animals are kept alive by administration of glucose, the hypoglycaemia is later succeeded by hyperglycaemia and a permanent state of diabetes is produced. This remarkable discovery provided a new experimental approach to diabetes. Alloxan appears to work through attacking certain sulphydryl compounds and a rapid fall in the glutathione content of the blood follows. Injection of glutathione or cysteine before the injection of alloxan prevents the selective necrosis of islet cells, owing to rapid oxidation of alloxan to dialuric acid, a substance closely related to uric acid. The possibility is thus opened up that an abnormality of purine metabolism might lead to the production of an alloxan-like substance with a selective action on the islet cells and the well-known association between diabetes and gout lends indirect support to such a hypothesis.

In summary, all these diverse experimental methods of producing diabetes appear to exert their diabetogenic effect through a common site of action upon the β-cells of the islets of Langerhans. Indeed there may be only a single ultimate site of interference with the processes of carbohydrate metabolism, namely inability to metabolise glucose either because of inhibition of the enzyme hexokinase or because of failure to transfer glucose across the cell membrane so that it is not available to the hexokinase.

In diabetes we have an excellent example of disturbance of the balanced action of endocrine glands. In one sense diabetes is the result of insulin deficiency, but in another sense it is due to the unopposed action of the pituitary and adrenal cortex. How the disease is induced in man is still obscure but disturbance of this balanced endocrine control appears, in the light of present knowledge, invariably to be concerned.

The opposite condition to insulin deficiency is exemplified by the increased production of insulin and the resulting hypoglycaemia which has been observed in some cases of tumours of the islets of Langerhans (p. 600).

Other causes of glycosuria

As already explained, excretion of glucose in the urine occurs when the amount in the blood rises above the renal threshold, either as the result of hyperglycaemia or because the threshold is abnormally low. Hyperglycaemia may be produced by excessive formation of glucose from glycogen in the liver and in the muscles, and may be brought about either through the nervous system or by means of the secretion of the endocrine glands; both of these factors may be involved. For example, increased formation of glucose and hyperglycaemia may be produced by stimulation of the sympathetic fibres going to the liver, and adrenaline appparently acts in this indirect way. The best known example of glycosuria resulting from a nervous lesion is the glycosuria due to puncture of the floor of the fourth ventricle, discovered by Claude Bernard. This is the result of increased formation of glucose by the liver with consequent hyperglycaemia, and it does not occur when the store of glycogen in the liver is exhausted. The action on the liver takes place through the sympathetic fibres. It has been stated by some that this form of glycosuria is produced through the medium of adrenaline, but Stewart and Rogoff have shown that the puncture or "piqûre" glycosuria occurs when the action of adrenaline is artificially excluded, just as it does in normal animals. Glycosuria sometimes resulting from various lesions in the brain is apparently of the same nature. Glycosuria due to excessive endocrine secretion is seen in thyrotoxicosis (p. 886), Cushing's syndrome (p. 914), and occasionally also in acromegaly (p. 877). The glycosuria which may result from narcosis, morphia and nitrites, is apparently of nervous origin, and it has been shown, at least in the case of ether glycosuria, that adrenaline is not concerned. In all these forms of glycosuria the increase of glucose is prevented or reversed by the administration of insulin.

As already stated, glycosuria in man is sometimes due not to hyperglycaemia, but simply to a lowering of the threshold value for sugar so that it escapes more readily by the kidneys—*renal glycosuria* (p. 899).

Phloridzin diabetes. In this condition, produced experimentally by administration of the glucoside phloridzin, the glycosuria is due to a lowering of the renal threshold for sugar owing to poisoning of the phosphorylating enzyme by means of which the glucose of the glomerular filtrate is reabsorbed in the tubules; the amount of sugar in the blood thus falls below normal.

Glycosuria occurs throughout the normal range of blood sugar and continues till the amount may fall even below 100 mg. per 100 ml.; the sugar thus drains away. If this form of glycosuria is produced in a starving animal, the available carbohydrate soon becomes used up and then there is an increased breakdown of protein for the supply of energy as in ordinary diabetes, while sugar formed from protein appears in the urine.

THE PARATHYROIDS

Experimental observations. The endocrine secretion of the parathyroids is essential to life; it is designated *parathormone* and is a protein of molecular weight about 9,500. Even the purest preparations both mobilise calcium from the bones and increase the excretion of phosphate by the kidney. Their secretory activity is regulated chiefly by the levels of ionised calcium and phosphate in the blood, and there is no evidence of overriding pituitary control by means of a trophic hormone. Thus a fall in the calcium level or a rise in the inorganic phosphate leads to increased parathormone secretion, and increased excretion of phosphates in the urine. Mobilisation of calcium from the skeleton tends to correct the biochemical abnormalities in the blood. Extracts prepared by weak hydrolysis of ox parathyroids are shown to contain parathormone by their efficacy in removing tetany and hypocalcaemia after parathyroidectomy. At the same time a fall in the inorganic phosphorus of the blood occurs and also an increased excretion of both phosphate and calcium in the urine. The parathyroids have, therefore, an intimate relation to phosphorus as well as to calcium metabolism; in fact one of the primary actions of parathor-mone is to raise the excretion of phosphate and lower the plasma level with consequent rise in the level of the ionised calcium in the blood. In addition parathormone mobilises calcium even in nephrectomised animals. Corresponding results are obtained in normal individuals, the blood phosphorus being reduced and the blood calcium being raised by administration of parathormone.

Persistent rise in the level of blood phosphate, or fall in blood calcium, as in chronic renal failure, leads to hyperplasia of the parathyroid glands.

Parathyroidectomy is followed by a group of relatively acute symptoms constituting a form of tetany—*tetania parathyroideopriva*; these vary somewhat in different animals, but they include general depression, fibrillar twitchings and jerking movements, spasms especially of extensor muscles, sometimes disturbance of the balance of the body, convulsions and emaciation; death usually follows within a few days. The nervous phenomena depend essentially on hyperexcitability of the lower motor neurones. There is also increased electrical excitability of the neuromuscular junctions of the motor nerves to galvanic stimulation. After parathyroidectomy there is a marked fall in the level of calcium in the blood; this produces an increased excitability of the nerves, and the administration of calcium relieves the nervous symptoms.

Partial removal of the parathyroids gives rise to *latent tetany*, in which obvious symptoms may be absent, but there is the characteristic increased excitability of the nerves. Partial parathyroidectomy in rats causes deficient formation of enamel and dentine in the incisor teeth, which are apt to break. Ossification also is impaired and while osteoid tissue is laid down, it is only partially calcified: fractures heal imperfectly in such animals, with the formation of soft callus. These changes are apparently the direct result of the calcium deficiency in the blood, which results from parathyroidectomy.

When parathormone is given in excess to dogs it causes toxic symptoms, vomiting and diarrhoea, which may be followed by death. Parathormone acts on calcium essentially as a mobiliser, removing it from the bones. When administered to animals for some time in fairly large doses the hypercalcaemia is followed by metastatic calcification in the arteries, kidneys, stomach, etc., very much in the same way as has been described in the case of vitamin D (p. 208). Calculi of calcium phosphate type—hydroxyapatite—may form in the bladder. The mode of production of the hypercalcaemia is, however, quite different in the two cases. The essential changes of osteitis fibrosa have been found by Jaffé and Bodansky to follow the injections of parathormone in young dogs and guinea-pigs. Since parathormone is a protein, continued injection of the heterologous hormone leads to antibody formation and ineffectiveness.

Human hypoparathyroidism and tetany

Tetany results from lowering of the plasma ionic calcium, and this may be brought about in several different ways. Firstly, parathyroid hypofunction may be responsible, and this is due almost always to removal of, or damage to, the parathyroids during thyroidectomy—*post-operative tetany*. Secondly, tetany used to be not uncommon in children with rickets, in which there is deficient absorption of calcium from the intestine, although in many cases a compensatory hyperplasia and over-activity of the para-

thyroids is observed and may prevent tetany. Calcium deficiency may also result from the increased loss during pregnancy and lactation and this may lead to tetany. Thirdly, alkalosis may lower the level of ionic calcium in the plasma, and tetany is thus seen occasionally in patients with pyloric stenosis and repeated vomiting of acid gastric juice; indeed, even the alkalosis induced by hyperventilation may bring about or aggravate tetany.

Naturally the acuteness, duration and severity of the symptoms vary with the cause of the calcium depression, and cases of *latent tetany* occur in which there is increased excitability of the nerves to electrical and mechanical stimulation, but without naturally-occurring muscular spasms. In *overt tetany* the muscle spasms are usually paroxysmal, but may be persistent, and fibrillary contractions are also observed. The muscles of the limbs are specially affected, but others may be involved, for example those of the larynx and pharynx.

Idiopathic hypoparathyroidism. There is a rare acquired form of idiopathic hypoparathyroidism; it is commoner in women than men, and in many cases antibody to a cytoplasmic constituent of parathyroid epithelium is demonstrable in the serum by the immunofluorescence technique. The condition is probably an organ-specific auto-immune disorder (p. 111), and other disorders of this group, notably primary adrenocortical atrophy, pernicious anaemia, chronic thyroiditis or thyrotoxicosis, occur with undue frequency in patients with the parathyroid disorder. Another association is with moniliasis of the fingers and toes.

Pseudo-hypoparathyroidism. A familial hereditary disorder, with the clinical and biochemical features of hypoparathyroidism, skeletal defects and metastatic ossification, has been described and given the above title because the abnormalities are not responsive to parathormone, and the parathyroids are actually hyperplastic. The disorder is therefore not due to lack of secretion but to failure to respond to it.

Parathyroid hyperfunction

This is seen in a chronic form in cases of generalised osteitis fibrosa due usually to a parathyroid adenoma but occasionally to primary hyperplasia affecting all four glands, the cells being increased in number and size and of the "water-clear" type. The bone changes in this disease have already been described (p. 766), but it may be recalled that they are essentially the result of osteoclastic resorption of the cortex and spongiosa of bones under the influence of excess of parathormone, and it has never been established that there is loss of bone mineral without loss of bone matrix. The hypercal-

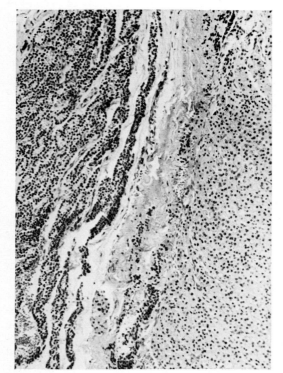

FIG. 24.20.—Parathyroid adenoma, showing parathyroid tissue (left) separated by a thin capsule from the adenoma (right). × 100.

caemia, increased excretion of calcium and phosphate, and sometimes metastatic calcification are the results of this greatly increased bone turnover. Nephrocalcinosis and the formation of calcium phosphate stones in the renal pelvis and urinary bladder are not uncommon. Parathyroid adenoma is the usual cause and removal of the tumour is followed by striking results. Usually there is a single oval tumour of yellowish tint, and variable size; it may reach more than 5 cm. in length but is usually smaller (Fig. 24.20); the severity of the symptoms has no relation to the size of the tumour. The removal of such adenomas has demonstrated clearly that the metabolic disturbance is the result of parathyroid hyperfunction. The level of calcium in the blood falls at once and the excretion of calcium and phosphate in the urine diminishes

unless there happens to be a second adenoma in another parathyroid. In about 6 per cent of cases there is more than one adenoma. The removal of an adenoma may be followed by a fall of the blood calcium to an abnormally low level and sometimes tetany appears; it may be corrected by administration of calcium and by means of parathormone but occasionally it is intractable and may lead to death by exhaustion. The occurrence of such an untoward result suggests that the remaining parathyroids are not functioning fully, as removal of a single parathyroid does not usually lead to serious effects. It may, however, depend on too rapid deposition of calcium in the skeleton, and according to Albright may fail to respond to parathormone because of changes in the structure of the bones;

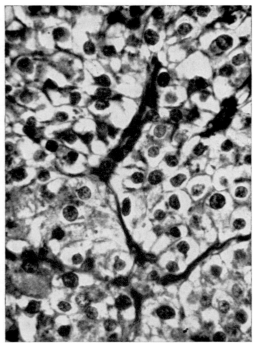

FIG. 24.21.—Adenoma of parathyroid from a case of generalised osteitis fibrosa. Both pale oxyphil and water-clear cells are present. × 500.

dietary phosphorus should be kept as low as possible at first in order to delay depletion of the blood calcium by deposition in the skeleton. In cases of parathyroid adenoma where excision of the growth restores normal calcium metabolism, reversal of the changes in bones follows but it is slow.

Tumours

The commonest form of tumour is the adenoma, and in a considerable proportion of cases this has been associated with hyperfunction as described above. Microscopic examination shows that the cells of the tumour are similar to those of the normal gland—chief or principal cells, and different forms of oxyphil cells (Fig. 24.21). The proportions in which the different types occur vary, and correlation of the cell type with the blood chemistry indicates that the dark oxyphil cells do not secrete parathormone. The cells are often larger than the normal cells and their nuclei may be very large in parts of the tumour; this does not indicate any tendency to malignancy. Their cytoplasm often contains a considerable quantity of glycogen. A stretched rim of normal parathyroid is often seen at the periphery of the adenoma, a feature that is absent in parathyroid hyperplasia. Cells of columnar form may occur and a papillary type of growth may be present in an adenoma, which may be incorporated in the substance of the thyroid. Carcinoma may arise in a parathyroid but is very rare; as a rule the presence of hyperparathyroidism is necessary as a criterion of the parathyroid origin owing to the fallibility of histological appearances. We have seen three examples of parathyroid carcinoma that satisfied these criteria.

THE ADRENALS

Introduction. In the pathology of the adrenals the double constitution of the glands is of great importance. The essentially different structures and developmental origins of cortex and medulla are well-recognised; they are functionally interrelated, for adrenal medullary hormones can bring about release of ACTH in conditions of stress.

The adrenocortical hormones. From the adrenal cortex many physiologically active and many inactive substances have been obtained in small amounts in crystalline form, but it is probable that the normal functions of the adrenal cortex are dependent on three crystallisable hormones, together with which many precursor and intermediate substances are present. The cortical hormones are all steroids and fall into three main physiological groups: (1) **mineralocorticoids**, concerned with the water and electrolyte content of the tissues and blood; (2) **glucocorticoids**, acting on carbohydrate metabolism and on the blood and lymphoid tissues; and (3) those influencing the gonads and sexual functions. The first two groups are C21 steroids; the androgenic group are C19 steroids which lack the alpha-ketol side chain on C17, and there are also C18 steroids which are oestrogenic.

The first group may be conveniently described as mineralocorticoids; the most active of these is aldosterone, of which about 80–100 μg. is secreted daily, principally by the zona glomerulosa. The second group is represented by corticosterone and hydrocortisone (cortisol), the latter being the most active physiologically, of which about 20–30 mg. are secreted daily. These are known as glucocorticoids from their action on carbohydrate metabolism; in large doses they also have some effect on electrolytes and water balance. The third group consists of substances chemically related to the sex hormones, some showing androgenic and others oestrogenic activity, but the significance of these in the normal adrenal is uncertain, as they are quantitatively less active biologically than the true gonadal hormones; they are especially important in neoplasms and hyperplasias of the cortex when their overproduction may result in abnormalities of sexual function and changes in the secondary sex characters.

Since the glucocorticoid output of the adrenal cortex is controlled by the secretion of adrenocorticotrophic hormone (ACTH) from the anterior pituitary, hypophysectomy leads to adrenal cortical atrophy although atrophy has been found to be slow in onset after pituitary ablation by radioactive implants. The zona glomerulosa is much less affected than the inner zones and death from electrolyte imbalance does not follow, because the secretion of aldosterone by the glomerular zone is not under pituitary control, but appears to be governed by the plasma volume and the plasma sodium and potassium levels, by renin secreted by the kidneys, and possibly by a secretion from the pineal region of the diencephalon. The fact that administration of ACTH stimulates predominantly the output of glucocorticoids indicates their origin from the inner zones, from which also the adrenal androgens and oestrogens are believed to arise. Symington states that the zona reticularis is probably the chief site of formation and that the zona fasciculata is devoted chiefly to storage of hormone precursors, which are quickly depleted under the influence of ACTH.

Symington and Currie have studied the changes in the adrenals in man following trauma and acute conditions of stress and have tried to correlate their adrenal findings with the ACTH content of the pituitary. They found that stress brings about depletion of the lipid content of the cells of the zona fasciculata, which become compact and rich in ribonucleic acid and enzymes, indicating increased functional activity. In severe cases complete loss of lipid in the inner zones may result in appearances incorrectly described as exhaustion of the cells. The pituitaries showed an increase in the lightly granulated basophil cells (mucoid cells, Pearse) which they interpret as evidence of increased secretion of ACTH. When recovery from acute stress occurs the pituitary is restored first and the adrenal again begins to accumulate lipid in the zona reticularis and fasciculata but full restoration of the normal degree of storage takes some time; accordingly the appearances in the adrenal are very varied depending on the degree of stress inflicted and the duration of survival.

With regard to the part played by the cortical hormones in pathological processes in man it is as yet too early to evaluate the full significance of the individual cortical hormones, but the extraction of purified adrenocorticotrophic hormone, and the synthesis or extraction of various pure crystalline steroids from the cortex has enabled further analyses to be made on adrenalectomised as well as on intact animals.

Methods of estimating the pure hormones in the blood or their metabolites in the urine have also greatly added to our knowledge of the pathological physiology of the adrenals. Aldosterone can be assessed by its effect on the sodium/potassium ratio in the urine; the glucocorticoids by the urinary output of 17-ketogenic steroids and of 17-hydroxycorticosteroids, and the adrenal androgens by the output of 17-oxosteroids.

The effects of adrenalectomy

Removal of the whole of both adrenals is followed by death usually within a comparatively short time. The time of survival varies in different animals but is ordinarily a matter of several days; it may be prolonged by administration of sodium chloride. Rats may survive longer probably owing to the presence of accessory cortical tissue.

The symptoms and biochemical changes following ablation of both adrenals are due to the loss of cortical hormones, and in acute insufficiency two main types of change result:

(*a*) The most striking effect is that resulting from an increased rate of loss of sodium and chloride ions in the urine. This leads to progressive fall in the plasma sodium and to an increase in the permeability of cell membranes which results in the loss of potassium and magnesium from the intracellular fluids into the blood. There is also some delay in the absorption of sodium chloride from the gut and consequently there results a pronounced ionic imbalance in the blood with deficiency in sodium and excess of potassium. The glomerular filtration rate is reduced and there is marked deficiency in the renal tubular absorption of sodium. The greater loss of sodium leads to a relative excess of chloride ions and there is thus a considerable degree of acidosis. The excretion of urea is notably diminished and the blood urea rises. The effects are therefore those of acute salt depletion, with secondary extracellular dehydration (p. 179), which if uncorrected leads to death in oligaemic shock. These changes are the result of loss of the mineralocorticoids and can be corrected by administration of cortical extract or of aldosterone. Deoxycorticosterone acetate (DOCA), although not a naturally occurring adrenal steroid, is also effective and has been much used clinically on account of its ready availability.

(*b*) The metabolism of carbohydrates is interfered with, the blood sugar level is lowered and the sensitivity to insulin is much increased; this is largely due to inability to promote the synthesis of glycogen from glucose owing to failure of gluconeogenesis, i.e. provision of glucose from protein degradation, but also in part to excessive utilisation of glucose and diminished intestinal absorption. These changes are due to loss of glucocorticoids and can be corrected by administration of these or of whole cortical extracts.

Thus, none of the purified substances alone, e.g. aldosterone, corticosterone, cortisol, etc., compensates for total adrenalectomy in all respects but both aldosterone and cortisol prolong the life of adrenalectomised animals, and their effects are much enhanced by simultaneous administration of sodium chloride. The effects of such steroids are truly dramatic. An adrenalectomised animal in a state of collapse and with a temperature more than five degrees below normal may be brought to a practically normal state within twenty-four hours. Active cortical extracts have some effect when given by the mouth but are much more effective when given by parenteral injection.

All these symptoms and biochemical changes have their counterpart in human pathology in destructive lesions of the glands, the effects of which will be considered below.

The adrenal medulla is of neuro-ectodermal origin and contains two main types of cells. The mother cells are the sympathogonia and from these are derived, (*a*) the ganglionic cells, through the sympathoblasts, and (*b*) the phaeochromocytes or chromaffin cells, through the phaeochromoblasts. As will be described below, from both classes of cells tumours arise which exhibit endocrine activity.

Chromaffin cells, named from their property of reducing chrome salts, are the source of adrenaline and noradrenaline. It is now known that noradrenaline is the transmitter of the sympathetic nerve impulse. It is necessary to refer to only two aspects, namely, their relation to blood pressure and to sugar metabolism. It is clear that adrenaline and noradrenaline are not materially concerned in maintaining normal vascular tonus. In emergency conditions, however, such as emotion, fright, or exposure to cold, there is increased discharge of the two hormones into the blood, where they tend to raise the blood pressure by promoting vasoconstriction in the skin and increasing the cardiac output. Therapeutically, noradrenaline is superior to adrenaline in its power to restore pathologically low blood pressure, as in shock or postoperative collapse, for it constricts the vessels in the skeletal muscles and thereby exerts a pressor effect without increasing the heart rate. In addition to its effect on the cardiovascular system, adrenaline causes increased glycogeno-

lysis in the liver (but not in the muscles) and thus raises the level of the blood sugar: the combined effects of increased discharge of adrenaline and noradrenaline into the blood in times of stress bring about the immediate changes which fit the individual to respond to the emergency which has caused their discharge. Because the effects of administering adrenaline and noradrenaline are those induced by stimulation of the sympathetic nervous system, they belong to the class of "sympathomimetic" drugs.

In certain species, adrenaline has the additional property of stimulating release of ACTH by the pituitary, but in man this effect is uncertain.

So far as human disease is concerned the disturbances of adrenal endocrine function which are clearly defined are:

A. **Hypofunction**, (1) Chronic—Addison's disease; (2) Acute—Adrenal apoplexy.

B. **Hyperfunction**, (1) Cortical; (2) Medullary; the latter is known definitely to occur only in cases of neoplastic growth.

Certain aspects of adrenal participation in diseases of adaptation are considered on p. 916: their scientific basis is not clearly defined.

A. Adrenal hypofunction

(1) Chronic—Addison's disease

The description of Addison in 1855 of the symptom-complex which now bears his name, and of its relationship to the adrenal lesions, formed the first fundamental contribution to the pathology of the adrenals.

Clinical features. These comprise pigmentation of the skin and sometimes of the mucous membrane of the mouth, marked asthenia and low blood pressure, emaciation and anaemia in varying degree, and alimentary symptoms such as anorexia, vomiting and diarrhoea. Asthenia is often a well-marked feature, and the muscles become very readily exhausted by exertion. There is also diminution of sexual function. The nature of the pigmentation has already been described (p. 200); it is most marked in areas where pigment is normally abundant and in exposed parts, and it is increased by irritation, for example, at the site of application of irritants to the skin.

Increased excretion of sodium chloride by the

kidneys is invariably present because in the absence of cortical hormones the renal tubules fail to reabsorb enough sodium from the glomerular filtrate. Consequently the plasma sodium is unduly low and this finding is useful in diagnosis in doubtful cases.

In addition to these chronic symptoms and signs there also occur in Addison's disease acute exacerbations or crises, which are amongst the gravest emergencies in medical practice, demanding energetic investigation and therapy to prevent death. In these there occur severe vomiting, which aggravates chloride loss, fall in blood pressure and extreme asthenia with hypoglycaemia terminating in collapse. Such a crisis may be precipitated by even minor infections, indiscretions in diet, or by vomiting or diarrhoea, in fact by anything which depletes still further the blood sodium level. The resulting severe salt deprivation leads to excretion of extracellular water, and this preserves isotonicity, the plasma volume falls and haemoconcentration follows, with elevation of blood urea. Increased permeability of cell membranes permits release of potassium and magnesium ions into the plasma in increased amounts. Finally a state resembling oligaemic shock supervenes and leads to death. These facts show that the important functions of the cortex in relation to water and salt control have been destroyed in Addison's disease.

Pathological changes. The commonest cause of Addison's disease in Britain was formerly destruction of the adrenals by chronic tuberculosis, which usually involves both cortex and medulla and converts both glands into fibrocaseous masses. As the incidence of tuberculosis has fallen, cases of Addison's disease have in increasing proportion been of a non-tuberculous nature, due to selective chronic inflammation and atrophy of the adrenal cortex (Fig. 24.22). These changes are accompanied by lymphocytic and plasma-cell infiltration. The lesion is certainly not simply atrophy, as occurs in the adrenal cortex in hypopituitarism. The medulla is relatively unaffected and this shows that loss of the cortex is the main cause of the symptoms of Addison's disease. Antibodies to adrenocortical tissue were first detected in 1957 in this laboratory, in the serum of two patients with non-tuberculous Addison's disease, and their presence in approximately 50 per cent of cases has since been confirmed by various workers.

They have been shown to react with lipoprotein of the endoplasmic reticulum of the cortical cells, and are not formed in cases of tuberculous Addison's disease. This finding, and the well-established associations of "idiopathic" Addison's disease with chronic thyroiditis, thyrotoxicosis, atrophic gastritis and idiopathic hypoparathyroidism, indicate that it is one of the organ-specific auto-immune diseases (p. 111). Less commonly, fibrosis, amyloid, or hypoplasia

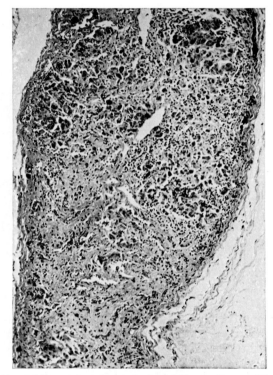

Fig. 24.22.—Adrenal atrophy in Addison's disease. The cortical tissue is represented by scattered groups of cells, with much fibrosis and lymphocytic infiltration. No medullary tissue is shown, but elsewhere it was well preserved. × 95.

of the adrenals are found in Addison's disease, while in very rare instances destruction of the glands by metastatic tumour is the cause. In all cases the syndrome of Addison's disease depends upon destruction or defective function of adrenal tissue.

It was also demonstrated in this laboratory that, while the adrenal antibodies of Addison's disease usually react specifically and solely with adrenocortical cells, in occasional cases antibody is present which reacts also with other steroid-producing cells, i.e. the theca-lutein and true lutein cells of the corpus luteum, the theca-interna cells of the Graafian follicle, placental trophoblast, Leydig cells and hilus cells of the ovary. In some female patients with Addison's disease accompanied by amenorrhoea and sterility, Irvine has demonstrated the presence of this steroid-cell antibody, and has shown destructive inflammatory changes in the ovaries.

In tuberculous Addison's disease the adrenals are enlarged, firm, and irregular. They are marked than in other wasting diseases, perhaps because of the low blood pressure. Atrophic change is present also in the gonads and breasts.

In Addison's disease there is a striking diminution of the basophil cells and a less severe loss of acidophil cells of the pituitary (Crooke and Russell), associated with pronounced degranulation in both types. The disturbance of carbo-

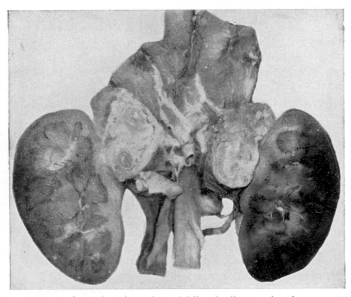

FIG. 24.23.—Adrenal glands in tuberculous Addison's disease, showing caseous destruction and enlargement.

changed into masses of putty-like caseous material, with dense fibrous tissue surrounding it (Fig. 24.23); calcification is frequent and may be visible in X-ray examination. Though the lesion is usually very chronic, tubercle bacilli may sometimes be found in large numbers. There are also cases where partial destruction by tubercle is associated with some of the symptoms of Addison's disease. Tuberculous lesions are usually present in other organs, e.g. the lungs or lymph nodes, though in a small proportion of cases the adrenals appear to be affected alone. Chronic tuberculosis usually affects both adrenals; in addition there is often much fibrous thickening of their capsules, and beyond, and this may involve the semilunar ganglia and the sympathetic plexus.

Apart from the adrenal lesions the main necropsy finding is marked wasting and this involves the muscles as well as the fat. Atrophy of the heart is also noteworthy; it is often more

hydrate metabolism results in a marked decrease in liver glycogen, the patients are highly sensitive to insulin and attacks of hypoglycaemia are fairly common.

Clinico-pathological correlation. In Addison's disease we have a picture of virtually complete destruction of a gland essential to life. Interpretation of the symptoms in relation to the structural changes is now, in part at least, possible.

The complete control of symptoms in adrenalectomised animals afforded by the known cortical hormones justifies the conclusion that the symptoms are due to loss of cortical tissue. The prompt elevation to normal of the blood pressure by such hormones is specially noteworthy. This view has been fully confirmed by the effects of cortical hormones in cases of the disease, cortisol being highly effective. The chronic symptoms have been diminished, and especially the acute symptoms of crisis have been relieved. The favourable results in the latter have been enhanced by the specific addition of sodium chloride to the diet, and in mild cases increased sodium intake alone will greatly ameliorate the symptoms. Synthetic deoxycorticosterone acetate has been much used to control the electrolyte balance and is highly effective when implanted into the subcutaneous tissues in the form of a pellet of the crystalline material. Aldosterone is also effective replacement therapy for the electrolyte imbalance. It does not, however, restore the dysfunction of carbohydrate metabolism, as this depends on the glucocorticoids, e.g. corticosterone and cortisol, etc. Of course, such therapeutic measures have no effect on the lesions in the adrenals.

In some cases there is hypoglycaemia and increased glucose tolerance which was attributed formerly to adrenaline deficiency; this is now known to be due to failure of gluconeogenesis from loss of glucocorticoid hormones. The failure of the usual effect of injection of adrenaline in causing glycosuria is probably due to lack of glycogen storage in the liver thus induced.

With regard to the pigmentation, it has been supposed that in Addison's disease, a substance, possibly tyrosine or an allied compound, accumulates in the skin and is changed into melanin by oxidation under the influence of the melanocyte-stimulating hormone of the pituitary acting excessively through lack of adrenal inhibition of the pituitary.

Apart from replacement therapy in states of chronic adrenal insufficiency cortisol may be administered over prolonged periods for its anti-inflammatory properties, e.g. in the so-called connective-tissue diseases or allergic asthma. The resulting reduction in the secretion of ACTH leads to simple atrophy of the adrenal cortices and a state of induced hypofunction which may constitute a serious risk to the patient subjected to some unforeseen emergency such as a major surgical operation. Accordingly ACTH has been given periodically with cortisol in order to maintain the adrenal cortices in an active condition.

(2) Acute hypofunction—adrenal apoplexy

Acute deficiency occurs sometimes as the result of haemorrhage into and necrosis of the substance of both adrenals—adrenal apoplexy (Fig. 24.24). In septicaemias, especially in fulminating meningococcal infections, haemorrhages into the adrenals occur in 2–4 per cent of cases in children. Sometimes the haemorrhage may be so extensive as to cause their complete disruption (Fig. 24.24). The haemorrhage is primarily in the medulla, and at the periphery of the glands the cortical tissue is stretched into a thin and irregular yellowish layer, and largely necrotic. Such an occurrence is usually accompanied by abdominal pain and marked collapse, and death occurs sometimes within a

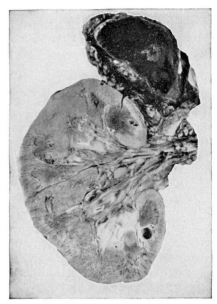

Fig. 24.24.—Adrenal haemorrhage from a case of septicaemia dying suddenly some days after operation. The other adrenal was similar. × ⅔.

few hours, or at most in a day or two; this is known as the **Waterhouse-Friderichsen syndrome**. Adrenal haemorrhage is also a feature of endotoxic shock (p. 190).

In view of the lesions found, it is clear that their effects correspond with those of bilateral adrenalectomy. It is, however, now thought that the fulminating infection bears greater responsibility for the rapid death than loss of adrenal function. If the haemorrhage occurs on one side only, a space or cyst containing altered blood may result. The toxaemia of diphtheria is associated with marked congestion of the adrenals and minute haemorrhages, but it is now regarded as unlikely that this is responsible for the fall of blood pressure in diphtheria and other infections, damage to the myocardium being probably responsible.

B. Adrenal cortical hyperfunction

As has been stated above adrenal cortical hormones are of three principal types, the mineralocorticoids, controlling electrolyte balance, the glucocorticoids regulating the intermediary metabolism of carbohydrate, fat and protein, and the ketosteroids which, by their predominantly androgenic and oestrogenic effects, participate in the regulation of sexual functions.

Three corresponding types of adrenal cortical hyperfunction are known to exist and a short account of these will now be given.

1. Primary hyperaldosteronism (Conn's syndrome)

The term primary hyperaldosteronism is often applied to a clinical syndrome first recognised in 1954–1955 and which, as later shown by Conn, may be due to an adrenocortical tumour. The tumour is usually unilateral and benign, but may be bilateral, and is rarely malignant. More recently it has become evident that the syndrome may occur in the absence of an adrenocortical tumour; in these cases the histological changes are those of bilateral hyperplasia of the zona glomerulosa with or without multiple nodules. The syndrome, which is due to the effects produced by an excess of aldosterone, and sometimes other corticosteroids, is characterised by the following features:

(a) Hypertension. The elevation of arterial blood pressure is usually moderate but cases of severe hypertension, even in the malignant phase, are recorded.

(b) Electrolyte disturbances. *Hypokalaemia.* In the first reported cases of this syndrome, the plasma potassium concentration was distinctly and consistently subnormal. It is now clear that the potassium values may fluctuate, with a varying proportion falling into the lower part of the normal range. The incidence of normokalaemic cases, first reported by Conn, remains unknown.

Extracellular alkalosis. As a result of the potassium depletion, plasma pCO_2 is normally raised.

Plasma sodium concentrations. The plasma sodium concentration in patients with this syndrome usually falls into the upper part of the normal range or even higher. A low plasma sodium concentration should be taken as evidence against the presence of an adrenocortical aldosterone secreting tumour and more in favour of hyperaldosteronism of other etiology (secondary hyperaldosteronism).

Plasma renin concentration. In this syndrome plasma renin concentration is low and often subnormal. This biochemical abnormality is probably due to the sodium retention, in turn produced by the effect of the excess aldosterone on the renal tubules.

The symptoms, apart from those caused by the hypertension, are due to the potassium depletion. They consist of neuromuscular symptoms, e.g. attacks of muscle weakness, paresis, muscle discomfort, paraesthesiae and tetany; and also nocturia and polyuria. All are reversible. Some cases remain symptom-free and may be diagnosed wrongly as essential hypertension.

The changes are reversed when the metabolic effects of the excess aldosterone are blocked by spironolactone or removed by excision of an adrenocortical tumour.

2. Cushing's syndrome

This condition was first described by Cushing who collected a number of cases where a group of changes was associated with a basophil adenoma, often remarkably small, of the anterior lobe of the pituitary. The significance of the basophil adenoma is uncertain, because many basophil tumours produce none of the associated symptoms. More rarely tumours of other endocrine glands have been present, e.g. thymus, pancreas, ovary. Carcinoma of the bronchus is also not uncommon: this is known as the *ectopic ACTH syndrome*; the degree of adrenal hyperplasia is especially marked and the symptoms of adrenal hyperfunction are often rapid in onset and severe in degree. In all cases, whether or not there is another endocrine tumour, adrenal cortical hyperfunction is present, resulting from either hyperplasia (Fig. 24.25) or neoplasia of the cortex. In about one-third of all cases the adrenals are not enlarged although they can be shown to be hyperactive. In most cases increased amounts of glucocorticoids can be demonstrated in the plasma, and this is confirmed by the increased output of 17-ketogenic and 17-hydroxysteroids in the urine. There is also a variable increase in the output of androgenic cortical steroids with the result that an element akin to virilism is present; the changes are, however, by no means identical with those of adrenal virilism but are of a mixed

be distinguished from that due to neoplasia by the marked elevation of 17-ketogenic and 17-hydroxysteroid output in the urine that follows administration of ACTH in cases of hyperplasia but not usually in neoplasia; in adrenal carcinoma the output of 17-oxosteroids is likely to be very high, whereas in hyperplasia and adenoma it is only moderately elevated.

Crooke's hyaline change in the basophil cells

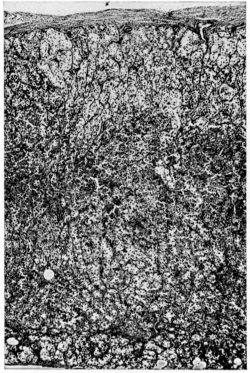
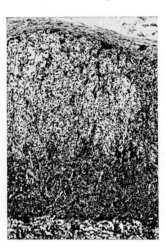

FIG. 24.25.—Hyperplasia of the adrenal cortex in Cushing's syndrome (left), compared with a normal adrenal cortex (right).

Note the increased width of the hyperplastic zona reticularis and the compact type of cell composing the fasciculata. × 45.

type. The significance of excessive glucocorticoid activity is not in doubt as a similar train of symptoms has been observed to follow prolonged therapeutic administration of cortisol or of ACTH.

Cushing's syndrome in children is nearly always due to an adrenal cortical tumour, usually carcinomatous, but in adults only about 15 per cent of cases are due to adenoma or carcinoma and 85 per cent to bilateral hyperfunction of which nearly one-half are within the normal weight range and appear histologically normal despite increased hormone output. Cushing's syndrome due to bilateral hyperplasia can usually

(p. 879) is usually present in such cases, and appears to result from the high level of circulating glucocorticoids. There is some evidence that cases of adrenal cortical hyperplasia may be attributable to increased secretion of ACTH but this has not been shown to be invariably present. It is, however, clear that the high level of circulating glucocorticoids fails to suppress ACTH secretion and there appears to be, therefore, a failure of the homoeostatic feed-back mechanism.

Clinical features. Cushing's syndrome is about five times more common in women than in men, but it also occurs occasionally in infants and children. The appearance is striking and the symptoms consist of painful adiposity of the body but not of the limbs, often accompanied by purplish striae on the skin of the abdomen (Fig. 24.26), excessive sweating and growth of hair (hypertrichosis) of the masculine type, impairment of sexual functions—amenorrhœa or impotence—high blood pressure, polycythaemia, osteoporosis and glycosuria. The prognosis in untreated cases is grave; of four cases of Cushing's syndrome observed personally within a brief period, one died from cerebral haemorrhage, two died from septic infections in the course of severe insulin-resistant diabetes, but one has been dramatically cured by X-ray treatment to the pituitary fossa, without treatment of any kind to the adrenals, an outcome which is not unique and, though difficult to reconcile with a primarily adrenal origin of the disorder, may fit into the hypothesis of disordered hypothalamic control of anterior pituitary function.

3. The adrenogenital syndrome: adrenal virilism

This condition is due to the over-production of adrenal androgens, either by hyperplastic adrenals or by adrenal adenoma or carcinoma. It may be present in the newborn causing pseudo-hermaphroditism in the female, or it may arise in childhood or in adult life, where it causes masculinisation of the female. The congenital variety appears to be an autosomal recessive genetic character resulting in an inborn deficiency of the enzyme necessary to hydroxylate the 21 position of adrenal steroids; accordingly 17-dihydroxyprogesterone is formed instead of hydrocortisone. This abnormal steroid does not inhibit the anterior pituitary; in consequence the absence of hydrocortisone leads to over-secretion of ACTH and this in turn induces adrenal cortical hyperplasia and increases the elaboration of androgenic oxosteroids. Administration of hydrocortisone promptly reduces the output of ACTH and the urinary excretion of 17-oxosteroids then falls, an observation that contributed greatly to our understanding of the essential nature of the abnormality. Hyperplasia affects chiefly the inner zone of the cortex, but occasionally it is associated with inadequate production of mineralocorticoids as well as of glucocorticoids, and symptoms resembling the crises of Addison's

disease may develop. Occasionally virilism is accompanied by hypertension. Much more rarely, adrenal cortical hyperplasia with excessive lipid storage has been observed also in infant male pseudo-hermaphrodites and it is presumed that the defect is again one of hormone synthesis.

Clinical features. In childhood, the adrenogenital syndrome in the male is characterised by

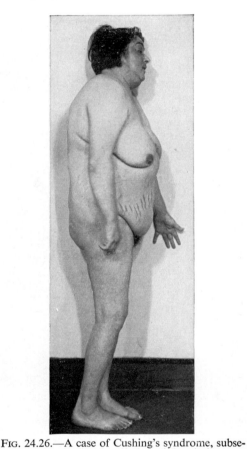

FIG. 24.26.—A case of Cushing's syndrome, subsequently cured by irradiation of the pituitary.

Note the characteristic adiposity, striae in the skin and dusky cyanosis with facial hirsuties.

precocious bodily growth associated with premature development of the secondary sexual characters—*macrogenitosomia praecox*. Growth of the genital organs and of facial and bodily hair occurs and the voice deepens. Such boys often show excessive muscular strength—the "infant Hercules" type. Adrenal cortical overactivity is more common in female children (about five to one, Glynn) but it does not induce a true iso-sexual precocious puberty.

There is at first precocious growth in height and in strength, but usually the secondary sexual characters do not appear even when the age of normal puberty is reached. The breasts remain undeveloped and menstruation fails to occur; instead, the body is of masculine habitus with excessive facial and bodily hair of male pattern and marked growth of the clitoris. This is known as *adrenal virilism*. In both sexes, premature closure of the epiphyses occurs so that the child, initially too large for its age, may ultimately be relatively dwarfed.

Pathological findings. In adult life adrenal hyperfunction is most frequently due to a single adrenal adenoma or carcinoma (Fig. 24.27),

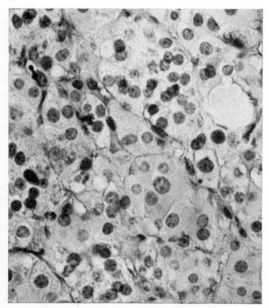

FIG. 24.27.—Section of adrenal cortical adenoma associated with virilism, showing trabecular structure with tendency to variation in the types of cells. × 375.

but in children and adolescents bilateral adrenal hyperplasia is the commoner lesion. Adrenal hyperfunction occurs especially in women, leading to masculinisation, i.e. atrophy of the breasts, enlargement of the clitoris, amenorrhoea, growth of bodily and facial hair of masculine distribution, and deepening of the voice. In post-menopausal women, hirsutism may be associated with diabetes mellitus (Achard–Thiers syndrome). Conversely, but much more rarely, males affected by adrenal hyperfunction may develop feminisation with atrophy of the gonads, enlargement of the breasts

GG

and even lactation. Removal of the neoplasm has in some cases been followed by a dramatic disappearance of the abnormal sexual characters; in cases of hyperplasia, cortisol therapy may be highly beneficial and unilateral or bilateral adrenalectomy is now less often necessary.

The diagnosis may be assisted during life by estimation of the amount of 17-oxosteroids excreted in the urine. These are derived largely from androgenic adrenal cortical hormones, and the amount excreted in the above neoplastic conditions exceeds that in any other condition, e.g. over 40 mg. per day; after successful operation the daily excretion rate is notably reduced but not always to normal levels. In hyperplasias the amount excreted is rarely so high, though often in excess of the normal 10–15 mg. per day; it can be suppressed by the administration of cortisol and failure to reduce the output by cortisol is strongly suggestive of a neoplasm as the source.

Adrenal cortical tumours and hyperplasias are associated both with true virilism and also with Cushing's syndrome and cases presenting mixed features are encountered.

C. Adrenal medullary hyperfunction

Repeated injections of adrenaline in rabbits lead to hyaline change and calcification of the media in the aorta and large vessels, and local aneurysmal dilatations may follow. Hypertrophy of the heart also may be produced, and may be accompanied by small areas of necrotic change and fibrosis in the myocardium. There is no evidence that essential hypertension is due to the production of adrenaline or noradrenaline in excess.

The only clear example of medullary hyperfunction is given by chromaffin adenomas (phaeochromocytomas) which release intermittently an increased supply of noradrenaline and adrenaline resulting in paroxysmal hypertension. These tumours are described below.

Inflammatory and degenerative changes of the adrenals

Acute inflammation of the adrenals is rare, but evidence of damage to the cortical cells, areas of necrosis, etc., is seen in acute infections, especially in diphtheria. In fevers and in septic conditions intense congestion and haemorrhages may be found, and the latter are sometimes large (p. 911). Embolic foci are occasionally found in pyaemic states and occasionally small abscesses are produced.

Tuberculous lesions of the more extensive kind are described in connection with Addison's disease (p. 909). In addition, however, one or two caseous nodules may sometimes be found in the adrenals in chronic tuberculosis. *Syphilitic lesions* both in the congenital and acquired types present the usual features; they are, however, rare. Giant cell granulomas, apparently neither tuberculous nor syphilitic, have also been described, both as independent lesions and associated with similar changes in the pituitary. In cases of general amyloid disease the adrenals are not infrequently involved; the amyloid change occurs especially in the capillaries of the cortex and causes atrophy of the cortical cells, affecting all zones, including the glomerulosa; it is a rare cause of Addison's disease.

The "adaptation syndrome". The importance of the adrenal cortical hormones in the reaction to unfavourable environmental conditions has been emphasised by Selye, who suggested that the response of the individual to stresses of all kinds follows a fairly uniform pattern, the "general adaptation syndrome". The first stage, the "alarm reaction", resembles oligaemic shock. The second stage resembles the counter-shock phase in which there is a rise in the blood volume and involution of the thymus and lymphoid tissues attributed by Selye to the increased discharge of adrenal cortical hormones under the influence of increased secretion of ACTH from the pituitary, provoked in part by outpouring of adrenaline. The adrenal cortex shows varying degrees of lipid depletion. Finally if the stress continues with sufficient severity the "stage of exhaustion", comparable with adrenal insufficiency, supervenes.

Selye has extended his theory to explain the pathogenesis of a group of disorders which he calls "diseases of adaptation"; these include hypertension, nephrosclerosis, peptic ulcer, rheumatoid arthritis and rheumatic disorders generally, polyarteritis and the "diffuse collagen diseases of allergic origin".

It remains to be seen to what extent Selye's interesting speculations reflect the true pathogenesis of these various disorders.

Adrenal tumours

Neoplasms of the adrenals are of much interest both from the functional and morphological points of view, and may originate in the cortex or in the medulla.

Of the *cortical* tumours the commonest are *adenomas*. They occur in the form of comparatively small, rounded nodules, well defined, and usually of yellow colour, owing to the large amount of fat and steroids in the cells; not infrequently they are multiple. In the smaller adenomas the cells are arranged in trabeculae and resemble closely those of the zona fasciculata; but in the larger examples, though the trabecular arrangement is retained for a time, there is a tendency towards alteration in the types of the cells. A cortical adenoma may be associated with abnormal sexual development as described above, causing either the adrenogenital syndrome or Cushing's syndrome, or it may, more rarely, secrete aldosterone in excess (p. 912). The majority, however, appear to be devoid of functional activity. The cells may become large, often contain more than one nucleus, and all transitions to distinctly aberrant forms occur. The tumour rarely becomes carcinomatous. Sometimes carcinoma is bilateral, although one may be a metastasis. Excessive hormone secretion may persist in spite of much cellular aberration.

The tumours originating from the *medulla* are of quite a different order, and three varieties have now been recognised. Two of these take origin from nerve cells, namely the *ganglioneuroma*, a simple growth containing ganglionic nerve cells and nerve fibres, and the *neuroblastoma* or *sympathicoblastoma* composed of embryonic nerve cells or neuroblasts. These tumours are described elsewhere (pp. 674–6). Neuroblastoma is much the commoner growth, in fact it is fairly frequent in children. It may reach a large size, is composed of soft cellular tissue, and is very haemorrhagic. Secondary growths are often widespread and occur both in other organs and in the bones, the skull often being affected. Similar tumours may arise also from other parts of the sympathetic system. Such tumours may secrete catecholamines other than adrenaline and noradrenaline, especially dopamine, which appears in the urine chiefly as vanillin mandelic acid (VMA) and homovanillic acid.

The third variety of tumour takes origin from

the chromaffin cells, and is the *phaeochromo-cytoma* or *paraganglioma*, the former term being used for growths of chromaffin tissue within the adrenals, and the latter for extra-adrenal growths. It is composed of polyhedral cells, many of which give the chromophile reaction, staining a brownish-yellow colour with chrome salts, and rich in glycogen (Fig. 24.28). When placed in formol-saline it imparts a brown colour to the fixative. The cells are arranged in solid masses which fill alveolar spaces; the stroma is somewhat scanty and vascular. The cells may show aberrant characters, but the growth is usually benign. It is sometimes associated with medullary thyroid carcinoma (p. 897).

Clinical features. A phaeochromocytoma, usually benign, may be associated with a definite group of symptoms which appear to have as their basis hyperfunction of the chromaffin tissue with over-production of noradrenaline and adrenaline, and the clinical symptomatology may vary, depending on which hormone pre-dominates. The symptoms are: hypertension which is often of a paroxysmal character at first, a tendency to profuse perspiration, glycosuria, and occasionally pulmonary oedema.

The hypertension is associated with arterio-sclerosis even in young subjects. Occasionally death has occurred from cerebral haemorrhage. The intermittent character of the hypertension is of interest in view of the supposed "emergency discharge" of adrenaline in normal conditions, but in some cases it becomes continuous. Neurofibromatosis has been present in some cases. Familial examples of bilateral phaeo-chromocytoma associated with medullary carci-noma of the thyroid and neurofibromas are en-countered. Early surgical removal of the tumour is followed by disappearance of the symptoms. The occurrence of such functioning tumours is of interest as affording a parallel to endocrine tumours elsewhere, e.g. in the islets of Langer-hans, pituitary, etc. One or two examples of paraganglioma with a similar syndrome have been noted in chromaffin tissues outside the adrenal, e.g. in the organ of Zuckerkandl, but the majority of such growths outside the adrenal are devoid of hormonal activity. The diagnosis may be assisted by estimation of the urinary catecholamines which are much increased in the presence of a secreting phaeochromocytoma and the response to adrenolytic drugs, e.g. phentol-amine, dibenamine, is also helpful.

Other tumours may originate from the stroma of the adrenals. Benign growths such as *lipoma*, *myelolipoma* and *haemangioma* have been observed, but all of them are rare. *Melanomas* also occur, as a rule bilaterally. Carcinomatous metastases are often present in the adrenals, particularly in bronchial carcinoma, in which both glands may be implicated, the ipselateral gland being first involved and usually the larger (Onuigbo).

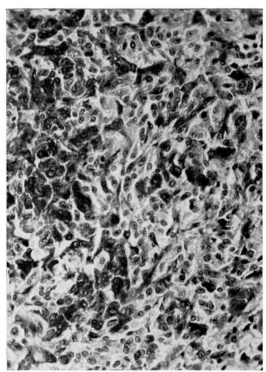

FIG. 24.28.—Phaeochromocytoma of the adrenal medulla. The darkly stained elements are cells giving the chro-maffin reaction. There was a high output of catechol amines prior to surgical removal. × 200.

Congenital abnormalities

Absence of both adrenals is a rare abnormality, incompatible with life; or one (the right only) may be absent. These abnormalities are intimately related to gross defects of the central nervous system, such as micrencephaly or anencephaly; in other cases of such cerebral lesions the adrenals may be hypo-plastic.

Accessory adrenals are comparatively common; they are small masses of cortical substance and can be readily recognised by their brownish-yellow colour. They occur in the surrounding tissues, on the surface or occasionally in the substance of the kidney or liver, and in the region of the ovary or testicle, and very frequently at the apex of congenital hernial sacs. Rarely tumour arises from them. The non-association of these structures with the so-called hypernephromas of the kidney has already been discussed (p. 738).

CHAPTER 25

HISTOPATHOLOGY OF THE SKIN

Skin pathology is often regarded as so specialised a subject that it is not suitable for inclusion in a general textbook. But the tissue responses in the diseased skin are basically the same as those that occur in other organs, and it is an ideal organ in which to study the correlation of naked-eye changes with microscopic, especially as the evolution of a lesion may be readily followed by repeated biopsy.

As in other tissues, local factors modify the basic responses, and the spectrum of possible changes is less than the number of causes of change. This is particularly true in the case of the inflammatory diseases: here however in making a diagnosis the distribution and naked-eye appearance of the lesion must be considered as well as the histology. The following account is intended only to cover a representative selection of dermatological conditions which have a characteristic pathology. Major omissions are the infective conditions (other than viral) and the granulomas, but some at least of these are dealt with in other chapters.

Some of the reactions peculiar to the epidermis are defined below.

Acanthosis. A generalised thickening of the *stratum malpighii*, which may or may not be associated with hypertrophy of the other layers. It may be closely imitated by oblique section, but this can be obviated by proper orientation of the tissue.

Acantholysis. In this the cells of the epidermis lose their cohesive properties, leading to the formation of clefts, vesicles and bullae within the epidermis. It is an important diagnostic feature of several diseases.

Dyskeratosis. Premature, abnormal or individual keratinisation of epidermal cells. These cells lose their prickles and become rounded off, their cytoplasm becomes strongly eosinophilic and the nucleus undergoes pyknosis. While this may be seen in a few rare benign diseases it is most common in malignant and premalignant lesions of the epidermis.

Hyperkeratosis is self-explanatory. It is usually associated with hypertrophy of the granular layer although the rete malpighii may be normal, acanthotic, or even atrophic.

Parakeratosis is an abnormal form of keratinisation. The cells of the stratum corneum retain their nuclei and are swollen. This results in a lack of cohesion which is apparent clinically as scaling. It is associated with an absence of the stratum granulosum and is caused by oedema or inflammatory infiltration of the underlying epidermis.

In mucous membranes composed of stratified squamous epithelium it is normal in some areas for the surface cells to retain their nuclei and to have no granular layer. This normal process is often loosely called parakeratosis but it must be differentiated from the pathological parakeratosis which occurs in the skin.

Biopsy. It is of the utmost importance that an early representative lesion be selected for biopsy and that this be taken carefully, with the minimum of trauma, together with a portion of adjacent normal skin. The most satisfactory biopsy is taken by ringing the lesion with local anaesthetic and excising a small ellipse with a scalpel. Forceps should not be used to grasp the tissue and their need is obviated by the use of a Gillies hook to elevate the portion to be removed. High speed punches have been advocated but these cause severe trauma and distortion of the tissues and they are not recommended.

To obtain maximum information it is necessary to orientate the specimen and this is aided by gently pressing the undersurface onto a small square of blotting paper before putting it into the fixative. Failure to do this results in warping of the tissue and may lead to errors in diagnosis.

HEREDITARY AND CONGENITAL CONDITIONS

There are many hereditary disorders in which the skin is involved as part of a general bio-chemical abnormality: excess or lack of pigment in haemochromatosis and albinism respectively and photosensitivity in some forms of porphyria are examples. In others the recognisable disorder appears to be confined to the skin itself. The exact origin of the defect is not known in any of the examples given below, but in the first three it appears self-evident that there is some inherent defect of the epidermal cells.

Ichthyosis or "fish-skin disease" is not as uncommon as is generally believed. Many individuals suffering from a dry skin are sub-clinical examples of the condition. In its most severe form the plaque-like scales impede respiratory movement and death ensues. Fortunately this degree of severity is rare.

Two main types of ichthyosis are encountered: (1) an autosomal dominant type and (2) a sex-linked recessive type confined to males. In the former, which is the commoner, the characteristic histological feature is hyperkeratosis with thinning, or often complete absence, of the granular layer. This finding is contrary to the usual hypertrophy of the granular layer when there is hyperkeratosis. The non-keratinised part of the epidermis is thin and the hyperkeratosis at the mouths of the hair follicles may eventually lead to atrophy and disappearance of the hair and its associated sebaceous glands. A mild perivascular infiltrate of chronic inflammatory cells may be present. In one rare variant of this condition, a defect of retinol (Vitamin A) metabolism has been demonstrated: it can be treated by oral or topical application of retinoic acid (Vitamin A acid).

In the sex-linked type there is marked hyperkeratosis, hypertrophy of the granular layer and acanthosis of the epidermis. Sebaceous glands are present in normal numbers and there is a moderate perivascular infiltrate of chronic inflammatory cells.

Darier's disease (Keratosis follicularis). A familial occurrence of this disease is now generally recognised. Though relatively rare, it is included because of its characteristic histological features and its confusion with other conditions. The epidermis shows considerable hyperkeratosis and acanthosis, and is thrown into folds.

This causes oblique cuts in the preparation of sections and gives rise to the appearance of a core of dermis surrounded by a single layer of epidermal cells, the so-called papillomatosis. Due to the process of acantholysis, clefts (lacunae) appear in the epidermis and in properly orientated sections these are found just above the basal layer. The two most striking features are, however, the presence of dyskeratotic cells in the epidermis called *corps ronds* and *grains* (Fig. 25.1). The *corps ronds*, which are enlarged squamous cells, are seen mainly in the upper epidermis in the region of the granular layer.

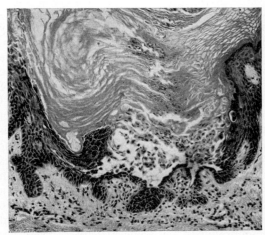

Fig. 25.1.—Darier's disease. The corps ronds are seen in the upper layers of the epidermis and the grains underlying the central hyperkeratosis. × 150.

They are easily recognised by their large size (two to three times that of the surrounding prickle cells) and in haemalum and eosin-stained sections by their hyaline-looking eosinophilic cytoplasm (premature keratinisation). The grains are found in the horny layer and differ only in size and shape from those found in the more usual type of parakeratosis. These changes are focal and may involve only very small areas of the epidermis.

This form of benign dyskeratosis must be differentiated from its malignant counterpart which is seen in some types of intra-epithelial neoplasm.

Benign familial pemphigus. This condition resembles Darier's disease in so far as acantholysis and papillomatosis occur (Fig. 25.2). The acantholysis is much more widespread and the epidermis has been aptly likened to a dilapidated brick wall. Dyskeratosis may be seen but is not so severe as in Darier's disease. Areas of grain-like parakeratosis are found overlying the acantholytic epidermis. In cases lacking dyskeratosis, differentiation from pemphigus vulgaris (*see below*) may be impossible on purely histological grounds.

Urticaria pigmentosa. This disorder is usually congenital, but may appear first in adult life. No familial background has been established. It usually presents clinically as widespread pigmented macules which urticate, although occasionally the entire cutaneous surface is involved.

Histological examination (Fig. 25.3) reveals a normal epidermis apart from an increase in melanin pigmentation of the basal layer. Depending on the severity of the condition part or all of the dermis contains closely packed mast cells. In routine haemalum and eosin preparations these are seen as polygonal or hexagonal cells with abundant eosinophilic cytoplasm and

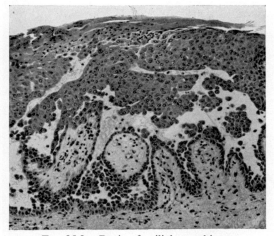

FIG. 25.2.—Benign familial pemphigus. Note the extensive acantholysis and "papillomatosis". × 150.

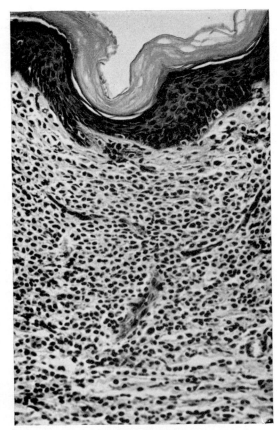

FIG. 25.3.—Urticaria pigmentosa. Closely packed mast cells occupy the upper dermis. × 200.

well defined, rather dense nuclei. Staining by toluidine blue or polychrome methylene blue brings out their typical granular appearance. A few eosinophil leukocytes are seen. In the urticated phase oedema is evident and may at times be so marked as to cause a subepidermal bulla.

The mast cell infiltration is not confined to the skin and may be seen in lymph nodes, spleen, liver and bone-marrow. Despite the enormous increase of mast cells no significant abnormality of clotting mechanism has been detected.

VIRUS DISEASES

Virus infections of the skin are common, and, as usual with virus infections, have clearly-defined features. They can be divided into the two sharply contrasted groups of those that cause cells to multiply (the tumour viruses) and those that cause necrosis of cells. Of the latter, only the most important infections, caused by the herpes–smallpox group, will be dealt with here.

Warts are by far the commonest virus disease of the skin. The histology of the vulgar wart usually seen on the hands and knees is essentially similar to the plantar wart found on the soles of the feet. The plane wart which is found on the face and dorsum of the hand is also similar histologically. This is not surprising as they are all caused by identical or closely related strains of the same DNA papovavirus.

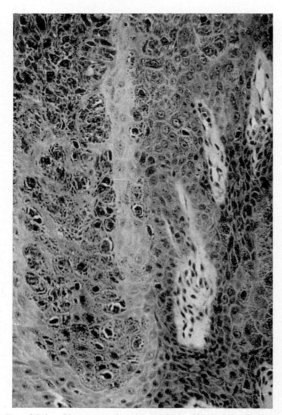

Fig. 25.4.—Verruca vulgaris. Margin of a lesion showing the eosinophilic cytoplasmic inclusions. × 200.

Verruca vulgaris and verruca plantaris. The epidermis is markedly acanthotic and thrown into folds. The rete ridges are elongated, those at the periphery of the lesion being the longest: they are curved inwards so that if projected they would converge on a central point. There is marked hyperkeratosis alternating with para-keratosis. Scattered throughout the upper layers of the rete malpighii and in the region of the granular layer are large cells with vacuolated nuclei (Fig. 25.4). The cytoplasm contains eosinophilic masses, and the vacuolated nucleus eosinophilic or basophilic inclusions, presumed to be virus aggregations. In older lesions these inclusions may not be prominent: they are usually best seen in plantar warts.

Verruca plana. In contrast to the verruca vulgaris, the acanthosis in this type is a gener-alised thickening without the formation of folds. There is hyperkeratosis of a peculiar type but no parakeratosis (Fig. 25.5). Numerous vacuolated cells with pyknotic nuclei are found in the upper layers of the stratum malpighii and in the stratum corneum. This gives the stratum corneum an open woven appearance which has been likened to basket weave: this appearance is normal in most parts of the body, where movement and stretching of the skin are of importance. On the palms, soles, and other pressure areas, however, the keratin is normally denser and of laminated structure. Intranuclear inclusions or cyto-plasmic masses are not usually seen although they have been reported by some observers.

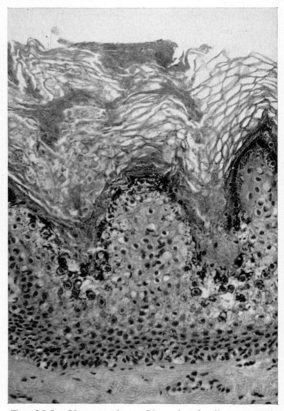

Fig. 25.5.—Verruca plana. Vacuolated cells are seen in the upper layers of the acanthotic epidermis.
Note the basket weave appearance of the stratum corneum. × 150.

Molluscum contagiosum. This relatively com-mon contagious condition, due to a DNA poxvirus, consists of an eruption of waxy skin-coloured papules or nodules with characteristic central umbilication. Pressure on the lesions causes expression of a small quantity of cheese-like material.

Section through a typical lesion shows a localised overgrowth of the epidermis into the dermis compressing the connective tissue to form a pseudo-capsule (Fig. 25.6). Small oval

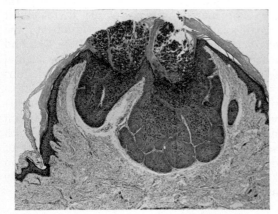

FIG. 25.6.—Molluscum contagiosum. The localised overgrowth of the epidermis is clearly seen. Numerous molluscum bodies are being extruded at the surface. × 30.

eosinophilic inclusion bodies are seen in the basal cells. These rapidly increase in size and push the nucleus to one side, the cells at this stage being considerably larger than normal squamous cells. As the degenerated cells approach the surface, the inclusions change their staining reactions and become basophilic. Electron-microscopic examination of these inclusions (molluscum bodies) reveals them to be made up of aggregations of virus particles.

The herpes–smallpox group. Herpes simplex, varicella (chickenpox), zoster, variola (smallpox) and vaccinia are very different diseases, and the DNA viruses which cause them belong to the structurally distinct poxvirus and herpesvirus groups. Despite these differences, the tissue reactions are closely similar in all these conditions, and they may conveniently be considered together.

In all of them excluding vaccination, the original natural infection is probably through the upper respiratory tract or mouth, with a viraemic phase before the definitive localisation to the skin. In all, some minor degree of proliferation of epidermal cells may occur at first. The characteristic skin lesion is, however, a blister, histologically an intra-epidermal vesicle or bulla. The individual epidermal cells attacked by the

virus become much enlarged and in the early stage are characterised by a rather homogeneous eosinophilic cytoplasm and one to several enlarged nuclei (Fig. 25.7). Profound degenerative changes with vacuolation then occur (balloon degeneration), the cells lose their adhesion to one another and lie loose in the bulla. Many cells enlarge and rupture so quickly that neighbouring cell walls remain adherent and these may be seen running across various parts of the bulla. This process is known as *reticular degeneration* and gives rise to a multilocular vesicle or bulla.

Inclusion bodies may be seen in the degenerate epidermal cells. In variola these are predominantly cytoplasmic while in herpes simplex, zoster and varicella these are mainly intranuclear. This feature, however, is not reliable

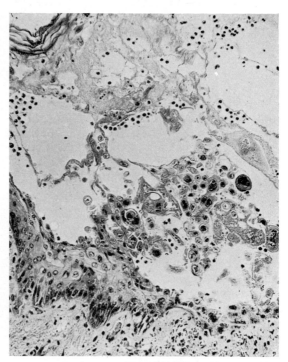

FIG. 25.7.—Zoster. Multilocular intra-epidermal bulla, showing large swollen cells (balloon degeneration) and strands of cell walls traversing the bulla (reticular degeneration). × 350.

enough to differentiate variola from the other three. In spite of their histological similarity, the diseases caused range from the major and frequently fatal variola to the mild and non-disabling herpes simplex. In *variola* the severity of the disease is due principally to the number and severity of the skin lesions: so much skin is damaged and so much virus produced that, though other tissues may be involved, this alone is enough to cause death. In *vaccinia* the lesions are individually similar, but nearly always remain localised to a small area of the skin, and therefore vaccination produces only a minor illness. Vaccinia virus is, however, sufficiently closely similar antigenically to variola virus to produce cross-immunity against smallpox.

Varicella is a disease remarkably similar to smallpox, but the lesions are smaller and fewer, and serious illness is rare. In spite of this the virus is widely disseminated in the body, producing mild pneumonitis fairly often and widespread visceral lesions in occasional subjects, particularly those with a congenital or acquired defect of delayed hypersensitivity responses (p. 115). The virus can survive in the body for long periods, for *zoster* is apparently produced by recrudescent activity of the same virus late in life, producing a recurrence of intra-epidermal vesicles within the area of distribution of one sensory nerve, combined with painful lesions of the corresponding posterior root ganglion (p. 641).

Herpes simplex is a ubiquitous infection. Most people acquire it asymptomatically via the oral mucosa when young: thereafter it remains latent, producing skin lesions of the characteristic type, usually around the lips, and often under the stimulus of some incidental febrile illness. Occasionally more severe lesions may occur, usually as part of the original infection, e.g. aphthous stomatitis, keratoconjunctivitis, or meningoencephalitis, the latter of which may be fatal (p. 643). Herpes simplex shares with vaccinia virus the ability to colonise areas of dermatitis in children, producing a condition known in both cases as *Kaposi's varicelliform eruption.*

INFLAMMATORY CONDITIONS

Because of the lack of knowledge of the etiology of skin disease many apparently different conditions are arbitrarily grouped under the heading of inflammatory diseases. This is not so irrational as it may seem because those varied diseases show different degrees and facets of the changes of inflammation.

Dermatitis

Much confusion has been caused by the use of the terms dermatitis and eczema in describing similar conditions but by common usage they are now regarded as synonymous. For the purpose of this discussion dermatitis will be used. The term covers the inflammatory response of the skin to a wide variety of etiological agents ranging from contact with external primary irritants to a hypersensitivity reaction to various antigens, both exogenous and endogenous.

The external primary irritants such as strong acids or alkalis produce an acute inflammatory response similar to that seen in other tissues and the dermatitis is self-limiting once the irritant has been removed.

The hypersensitivity group is however, more complex and as yet imperfectly understood. Most of the chemical substances causing this type of reaction are not in themselves complete antigens but are haptens and need to combine with an epidermal protein, most likely keratin, in order to become antigenic. Once induced the sensitivity, which is of the delayed type (p. 83), tends to be self-perpetuating and overlaps into the field of auto-immune skin disease by way of continued epidermal trauma from scratching or superadded infection.

Drugs which produce a dermatitis-type of skin eruption similarly act as haptens, in this instance combining with one of the plasma proteins to become antigens.

Whatever the causal factor the basic tissue response is similar and for this reason it is better to speak of a dermatitis reaction which, like any inflammatory process, may be classified as acute, subacute or chronic. As this basic reaction occurs in so many named skin diseases the pathologist can only report on the type of dermatitis reaction and is not in a position to give any indication as to the etiological factors.

Acute dermatitis. The initial lesion is an intercellular oedema which separates the prickle cells and is followed by lymphocytic infiltration. Then follows degeneration and liquefaction of the cells which leads to the formation of vesicles within the epidermis (Fig. 25.8). In the fully developed lesion the epidermis contains multiple vesicles many of which are separated by thin strands of epithelial cells. At a later stage these may rupture, giving rise to larger vesicles or

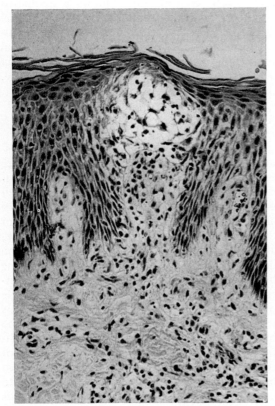

FIG. 25.8.—Acute dermatitis, showing an intra-epidermal vesicle containing leukocytes and degenerate epithelial cells. × 200.

bullae. The vesicles contain fibrin, degenerated epithelial cells, polymorphonuclear leukocytes and lymphocytes. Overlying these areas the nutrition of the stratum corneum is interfered with and parakeratosis results. Depending on the severity of the reaction the dermis shows varying degrees of oedema, vascular dilatation and congestion, and perivascular inflammatory cellular infiltration by lymphocytes, eosinophils and polymorphonuclear leukocytes.

As with other vesicular and bullous diseases of the skin an early typical lesion must be selected for biopsy.

While this histological picture may be seen in the acute phase of any dermatitis it is best observed in an acute contact dermatitis of hyper-

sensitivity type. The margin of the lesion of *pityriasis rosea* shows an acute vesicular reaction in the epidermis.

Subacute dermatitis. As the acute stage subsides the lesions become less vesicular and although oedema and vesiculation may persist, there are fewer and smaller vesicles. The epidermis is acanthotic and parakeratosis is marked. The surface is covered with a mixture of fibrin, degenerating leukocytes and bacteria. Where a vesicle has ruptured on to the surface a naked dermal papilla covered by fibrin and debris is seen (Fig. 25.9), the so-called *dermatitis pit*. There is less oedema and vascular congestion in the dermis, and while the amount of inflammatory infiltrate is greater, this is composed mainly of lymphocytes and histiocytes with only an oc-

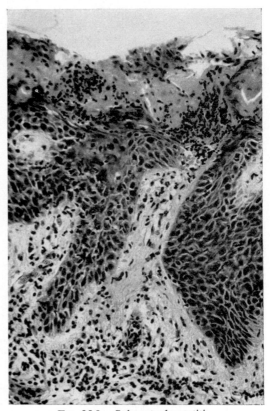

FIG. 25.9.—Subacute dermatitis.
Note the tip of the dermal papilla in contact with the serous exudate and debris on the surface. × 300.

casional neutrophil leukocyte. *Nummular dermatitis* is the classical example of this stage of dermatitis although it may be seen also as a phase of others, in particular atopic dermatitis. Stasis dermatitis, associated with inadequate venous return from the lower limbs, differs in that deposits of haemosiderin are found in the dermis.

Chronic dermatitis. The epidermis shows a marked acanthosis with elongation of the rete ridges. There is hyperkeratosis with areas of parakeratosis. Small foci of intercellular oedema may be seen but no vesicles (Fig. 25.10). There is a moderate inflammatory infiltrate in the upper dermis composed of lymphocytes, histiocytes, fibroblasts and eosinophil leukocytes. The walls of the dermal arterioles and vessels often

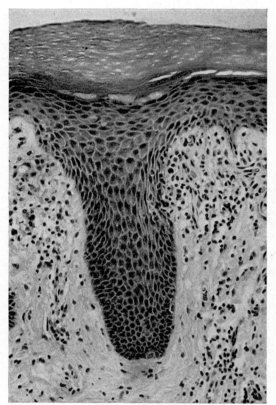

Fig. 25.10.—Chronic dermatitis. There is hyperkeratosis, elongation of the rete ridges and a perivascular inflammatory infiltrate in the upper dermis. × 300.

show a hyaline thickening with reduction in the size of their lumina. This histological picture is seen in the chronic phase of any dermatitic process when the skin is thickened and leathery in appearance (lichenified). The most characteristic clinical condition is, however, that of *neurodermatitis* or *lichen simplex chronicus*.

Some skin conditions, including parapsoriasis, erythema multiforme and annular erythema, are not clinically examples of dermatitis, and yet show the histological features of dermatitis: this may also be seen at times during the evolution of clinically atypical cases of diseases such as psoriasis or lichen planus, which normally have characteristic changes.

Generalised exfoliative dermatitis, a striking and serious clinical entity, shows a dermatitis reaction in either the subacute or chronic phase. As some 25 per cent of people with this condition develop a malignant reticulosis it is essential to examine repeated biopsies in order to detect any change in the quality of the dermal infiltrate.

Acne vulgaris

This extremely common inflammatory disorder affects adolescent males and females equally. Commencing at or about puberty, it runs a fluctuating course eventually burning itself out sometime in the mid-twenties. The disorder affects mainly the pilosebaceous follicles of the skin of the face, chest and upper back, although in severe cases it may extend over the deltoid region and downwards to involve the buttocks. The initial pathological process consists of a blockage of the pilosebaceous follicle opening by a mass of keratinous debris. This lesion is known as a comedo (blackhead) and the black coloration of its tip is due to the deposition of melanin pigment. The pathogenesis of comedo formation is imperfectly understood but recent work suggests that it may be related to androgen biosynthesis by the sebaceous glands themselves. Although the pilosebaceous follicle is blocked the secretion of sebum continues at least for some considerable time. In some cases the pilosebaceous follicle becomes increasingly distended until the pressure within it causes atrophy of the sebaceous gland. At this stage the lesion consists of a cystic dilatation of the follicle which contains a mixture of keratinous debris and sebum (cystic acne). More commonly, however, the contents of the pilosebaceous follicle become infiltrated by polymorphonuclear leukocytes and purulent material is eventually discharged on to the surface (pustular acne). The reason for the development of pustules is obscure. It is thought that the commensal anaerobic diphtheroid organism, *Corynebacterium acnes*, finds the occluded follicle suitable for growth. This organism produces a potent lipase which splits the neutral fat in sebum to

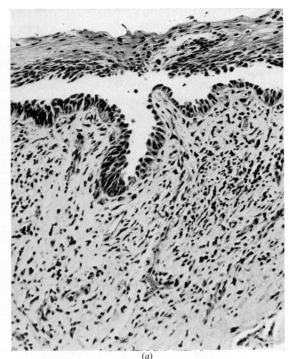

(a)

FIG. 25.11.—Pemphigus vulgaris.
(a) Acantholytic bulla in buccal mucous membrane.
× 150.
(b) Intra-epidermal bulla containing acantholytic cells,
best seen just above the basal layer of the epidermis.
× 150.

(b)

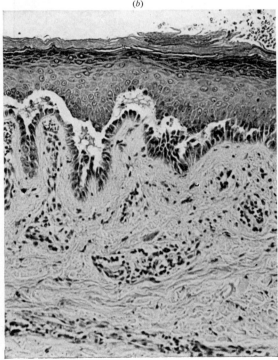

free fatty acids, which are extremely irritant to the tissue. Should fatty acids escape from the pilosebaceous follicle, either by spontaneous rupture or aided by pressure caused by the patient trying to express the lesions, an intense inflammatory reaction ensues with subsequent folliculitis and perifolliculitis. Disintegration of the follicular wall allows the altered sebum and keratinous debris into the tissue and this evokes further inflammatory changes, as evidenced by the formation of foreign body granulomas. The healing of the perifolliculitis and the perifollicular granulomas is by granulation tissue with subsequent scar formation. Such scarring is, of course, permanent and may be severe, progressing even to keloid formation.

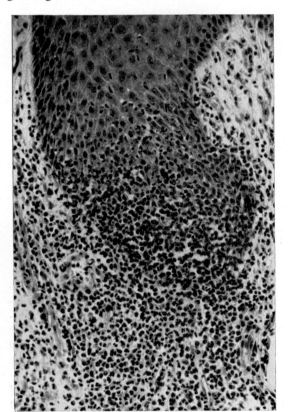

FIG. 25.12—Pemphigus vegetans. Intra-epidermal abscess composed of eosinophil leukocytes at tip of an elongated rete ridge. × 300.

The bullous group

This comprises pemphigus, pemphigoid, dermatitis herpetiformis and erythema multiforme. It is possible to separate these conditions by histological examination but only if an early representative biopsy is taken. Secondary infection and degenerative changes rapidly alter the histological features. Ideally a small lesion

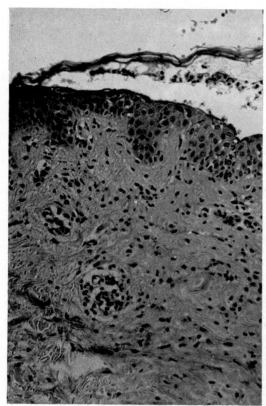

FIG. 25.13.—Pemphigus foliaceus. Subcorneal bulla containing occasional acantholytic cells and some leukocytes. × 200.

should be taken within 12 hours of its appearance. Three basic types of pemphigus are recognised, viz. pemphigus vulgaris, pemphigus vegetans and pemphigus foliaceous. In the latter two types bullae may not be in evidence clinically although histological examination will reveal the characteristic changes at the edge of the lesion.

The bulla of pemphigus is intra-epidermal and arises as a result of acantholysis of the epidermal cells which produces a horizontal plane of cleavage in the epidermis.

Pemphigus vulgaris. In pemphigus vulgaris (Fig. 25.11) the cleavage takes place above the basal layer, this layer remaining intact due to its attachment to the dermis by cytoplasmic processes. The bulla contains serum and somewhat condensed, rounded-off prickle cells. A few polymorphonuclear leukocytes and eosinophils

may also be present within the bulla. The underlying dermis shows slight oedema and a sparse infiltrate of polymorphs and eosinophils.

Pemphigus vegetans. In pemphigus vegetans the early lesion is identical with that of pemphigus vulgaris. As the disease progresses, however, the epithelium proliferates and the characteristic acantholysis is not seen. There is marked acanthosis of a verrucose type and intra-epidermal abscesses composed almost entirely of eosinophil leukocytes (Fig. 25.12). The inflammatory infiltrate in the upper dermis includes many eosinophil leukocytes and is much more pronounced than in pemphigus vulgaris.

Pemphigus foliaceus. In pemphigus foliaceus the acantholysis occurs high in the epidermis, usually just below the stratum corneum

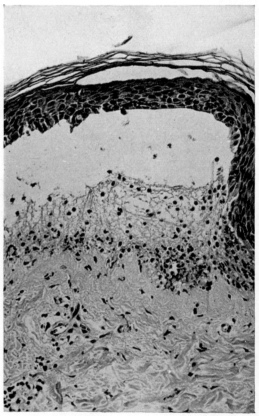

FIG. 25.14.—Dermatis herpetiformis. Subepidermal bulla containing fibrin and leukocytes. × 200.

(Fig. 25.13), and if the biopsy is not carefully taken or the tissue is roughly handled the superficial layer may be lost, making the diagnosis difficult. Careful examination of the surface, however, will reveal acantholytic cells.

Mucosal lesions of pemphigus. While all forms of pemphigus are usually regarded as skin diseases, many cases begin as "ulcers" of the mouth or genitalia. These may precede the skin lesions by as long as two years. The histological changes in mucous membranes are similar to those in the skin, viz. acantholytic bullae (Fig. 25.11*b*). Because of the moist condi-

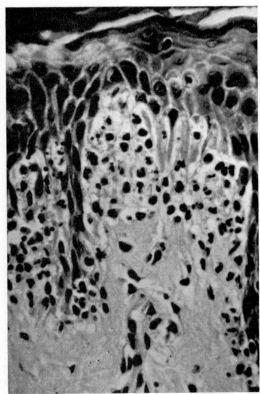

FIG. 25.15.—Dermatitis herpetiformis. "Eosinophil abscess" in an oedematous dermal papilla at the margin of a bulla. × 350.

tions within the mouth or on the vulva, maceration occurs rapidly and the roof of the bulla is quickly lost, making histological diagnosis extremely difficult. The recent finding that patients in the active stages of pemphigus have serum antibodies to an intercellular antigen of squamous epithelium, demonstrable by indirect immunofluorescence staining (p. 80), should greatly facilitate the precise diagnosis where histological methods fail.

Dermatitis herpetiformis. In this chronic condition the early lesion is a subepidermal vesicle (Fig. 25.14) which rapidly enlarges into a bulla. There is no acantholysis. Difficulty may

arise if an older lesion is biopsied as the epithelium regenerates rapidly and may give the impression that the bulla is intra-epidermal. The subepidermal bulla is filled with serous exudate and contains leukocytes, a high percentage of which are eosinophils. The underlying dermis is oedematous and there is a considerable leukocytic infiltration with a prominent eosinophil content. A useful diagnostic feature is the "eosinophil abscesses"—oedematous dermal papillae packed with eosinophil leukocytes at the margins of the bullae (Fig. 25.15). These abscesses are not present in all cases but are diagnostic.

A similar histological picture is seen in *bullous pemphigoid*; this has hitherto been regarded as

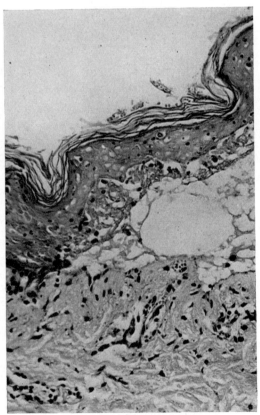

FIG. 25.16.—Erythema multiforme. Subepidermal bulla roofed by infarcted epidermis. Regenerating epidermis can be seen at the left of the picture. × 200.

a variant of dermatitis herpetiformis seen in the elderly, but the demonstration of an antibody reacting with epidermal basement membrane in this condition suggests that it is a distinct entity.

Erythema multiforme. This inflammatory disorder, as its name implies, presents a variety of clinical and histological appearances varying from a dermatitic reaction in the epidermis to

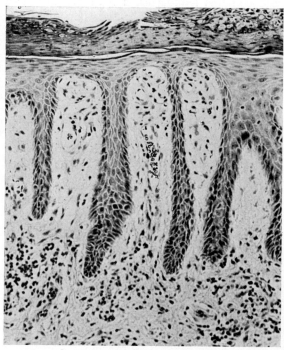

Fig. 25.17.—Psoriasis. The surface is covered by a parakeratotic scale containing numerous polymorphonuclear leukocytes. The rete ridges are elongated and the suprapapillary epidermis is narrowed. × 150.

subepidermal bullous formation and sometimes to an acute vasculitis. It represents a response in the skin of varying intensity to bacterial toxins and drug sensitivity. In the classical type, of moderate severity, the histological picture is diagnostic and consists of an area of coagulative necrosis of the epidermis, in fact an area of infarction (Fig. 25.16).

Regeneration of the epidermis from the edge is rapid and a single layer of epithelial cells is often seen growing under the necrotic epidermis. The dermis is oedematous and there may be an acute necrotising vasculitis with haemorrhage. More often there is a fairly dense perivascular cellular infiltrate composed of neutrophils, eosinophils, histiocytes and lymphocytes.

The frank bullous forms may be indistinguishable from dermatitis herpetiformis although the eosinophil abscesses, if present, will clarify the diagnosis.

Scaling disorders

Psoriasis. This common disorder has a characteristic histological picture (Fig. 25.17). There is parakeratosis, the extent and amount of which depends on the chronicity of the lesion. The granular layer is absent. The epidermis shows a peculiar type of acanthosis in which the rete ridges are greatly elongated. The portions of the epidermis overlying the papillary bodies are, however, narrowed to two or three cells. The papillae are oedematous and broadened at their tips and contain dilated and rather rigid looking capillaries. It is these features which are responsible for the bleeding points which are so easily produced when the psoriasis lesion is scraped. As a rule inflammatory infiltration of the dermis is slight and composed of lympho-

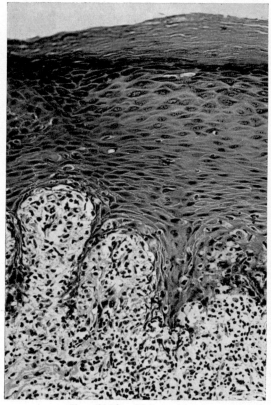

Fig. 25.18.—Lichen planus.
Note the hypertrophy of the granular layer and the saw-tooth appearance of the rete ridges. × 200.

cytes and histiocytes. In early lesions collections of neutrophil leukocytes are found in or just below the parakeratotic stratum corneum (*Munro micro-abscesses*).

Lichen planus. While relatively uncommon this condition is of importance as it may affect mucous membranes and may be misdiagnosed as leukoplakia.

The papule of lichen planus has characteristic diagnostic features (Fig. 25.18). There is marked hyperkeratosis with focal increase in the granular layer. The epidermis is acanthotic and the rete ridges assume a pointed outline, giving a sawtooth appearance. There is a dense inflammatory infiltrate composed of lymphocytes with a few histiocytes confined to the upper dermis. The upper border of this infiltrate is in contact with the epidermis and may actually invade the basal layers causing the dermo-epidermal junction to be indistinct. Lesions in the mucosa present a similar appearance although the hypertrophied granular layer is not so obvious. Normally there is no granular layer in some areas of mucous membranes.

VASCULAR DISORDERS

Erythema nodosum, nodular vasculitis and erythema induratum (Bazin's disease)

These three conditions are all characterised by nodular lesions on the lower extremities. While there are differences in etiology and clinical course they cannot, in our experience, be clearly separated histologically and the appearances vary with the age of the lesion. The reason for their histological similarity is that they produce areas of inflammation and fat necrosis with subsequent repair. In the early stages there is an infiltrate of polymorphonuclear leukocytes and lymphocytes in the subcutaneous fat. Inflammatory infiltration of the walls of small veins is seen and in the more severe cases endothelial

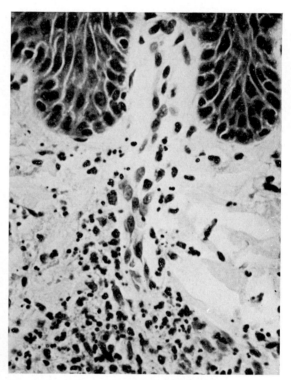

FIG. 25.20.—Henoch–Schönlein purpura. Small dermal vessel showing perivascular polymorphonuclear infiltration with invasion of the vessel wall. × 350.

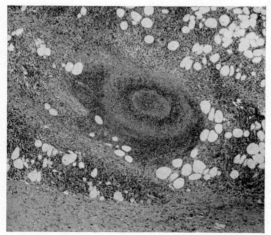

FIG. 25.19.—Erythema nodosum. Thrombophlebitis of subcutaneous vein with surrounding inflammatory reaction in adipose tissue. × 30.

proliferation and thrombosis may occur. It seems probable that this phlebitis is the basic lesion (Fig. 25.19). As the nutrition of the fat is impaired, foci of endothelioid cells and giant cells appear in response to liberated fat. In severe cases necrosis resembling caseation is seen. These changes gradually resolve and at a later stage the process of healing is observed.

It will be appreciated that the extent of the histological changes will be dependent on the severity or acuteness of the condition. In erythema induratum abscess formation may cause the lesion to ulcerate.

Anaphylactoid (Henoch–Schönlein) purpura

Most cases of cutaneous purpura show merely extravasation of red cells into the dermis with varying inflammatory cellular infiltrate as a result of this. In anaphylactoid purpura, however, there is a characteristic capillary lesion which may be of diagnostic importance.

The small dermal vessels show endothelial swelling and there is dense perivascular polymorphonuclear leukocytic infiltration which invades the vessel wall. Much nuclear dust is seen, being derived from disintegrating polymorphs (Fig. 25.20). Foci of haemorrhage are seen which in older lesions become converted to haemosiderin.

Necrotising or allergic vasculitis

Segmental necrosis of cutaneous vessels may be seen in the course of systematised polyarteritis nodosa (p. 280), and may even be confined to the skin for many years. There is also a group of necrotising vascular lesions which differ from polyarteritis nodosa, and to which the name acute necrotising or allergic vasculitis has been applied. The clinical presentation is usually that of a purpuric eruption, often widespread but usually worse on the lower legs. Haemorrhagic blisters may appear as lesions coalesce and necrosis with ulceration may follow. The lesions are confined to the vessels of the skin, and complete recovery is the rule. Etiological factors include drug sensitivity and haemolytic streptococcal infections but in many instances no etiological factor can be determined. Histologi-

cal examination reveals acute fibrinoid necrosis of the walls of the dermal arterioles and capillary loops with extensive fibrin seepage (Fig. 25.21). Dermal haemorrhage occurs and this may be followed by epidermal necrosis and ulceration. There is a considerable perivascular polymorphonuclear leukocytosis around the affected vessels.

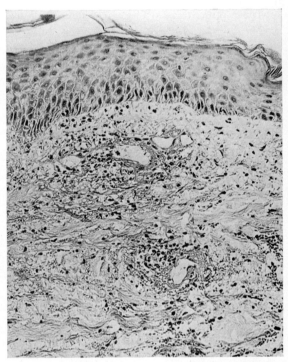

FIG. 25.21.—Acute necrotising vasculitis showing fibrinoid necrosis of dermal vessels. There is haemorrhage under the epidermis and a marked perivascular inflammatory infiltrate. × 200.

CONNECTIVE TISSUE DISEASES

Lupus erythematosus

Two basic types of this condition are recognised: (1) chronic discoid lupus erythematosus, which is confined to the skin, and (2) acute systemic lupus erythematosus, in which visceral lesions predominate (see p. 814) and which may run its entire course without cutaneous manifestations. Intermediate forms between these extremes are encountered and transition from one type to another, although rare, may occur.

Chronic discoid lupus erythematosus. The histological changes are usually sufficiently

characteristic to permit a firm histological diagnosis (Fig. 25.22). The epidermis is atrophic with loss of the rete ridges. There is moderate to severe hyperkeratosis which is most marked in relation to the follicular orifices, resulting in dilated orifices filled by keratin (*follicular plugs*). The basal layer of the epidermis shows degenerative changes causing vacuolation of the cells (*liquefaction degeneration*). This change is focal in nature and is always present (Fig. 25.23). A diagnosis of lupus erythematosus should not be made in its absence.

The dermis shows oedema and there is dense

patchy lymphocytic infiltrate in relation to the dermal appendages, in particular to the hair follicles.

Acute systemic lupus erythematosus. The histological appearances of the cutaneous lesions are not so striking as in the chronic variety. The

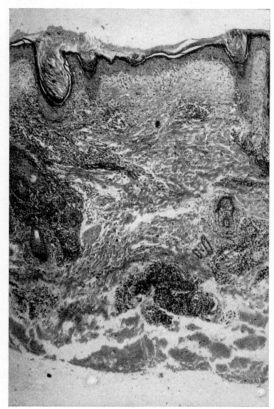

FIG. 25.22.—Chronic discoid lupus erythematosus. Flattening of rete ridges, follicular plugging and focal lymphocytic infiltration of the dermis are seen. × 40.

epidermis is atrophic and liquefaction degeneration of the basal layer is marked (Fig. 25.24). Small areas of fibrinoid degeneration of the collagen of the upper dermis may be seen and this may also affect the ground substance of the collagenous tissue of the cutaneous vessels, giving a vasculitis. Inflammatory infiltrate is minimal. In a proportion of cases, however, there are only mild inflammatory changes of a non-specific nature in the dermis.

Scleroderma

Much confusion has arisen over the nomenclature of this condition. As its name implies,

it is a hardening of the skin and its use should be limited to the cutaneous disease. The condition with which it is confused is *progressive systemic sclerosis*, a generalised disease in which there is sclerosis of the skin of the extremities and which is dealt with on p. 814. The histological features of the skin in these two conditions are quite different.

Clinically scleroderma occurs as localised patches (*morphoea*) or diffuse areas of thickening and hardening of the skin. In the early stages an inflammatory halo is seen at the margin of the lesion. After spreading for an indefinite period, involution occurs with resulting atrophy and depigmentation of the area involved.

In the fully developed lesion (Fig. 25.25) the epidermis is thin and there is loss of the rete

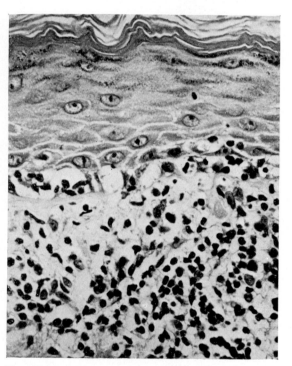

FIG. 25.23.—Chronic discoid lupus erythematosus. Liquefaction degeneration of the basal layer of the epidermis. × 300.

ridges due to stretching. The collagen bundles of the dermis are swollen and thickened and lie parallel to the epidermis. The distinction between the papillary and reticular layers of the dermis is lost. Sweat glands and hair follicles disappear but blood vessels remain intact. At the margin of an active lesion there is an

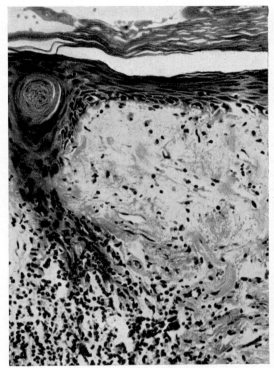

Fig. 25.24.—Acute systemic lupus erythematosus. Liquefaction degeneration of the basal layer with oedema and fibrinoid change in the collagen of the upper dermis. × 200.

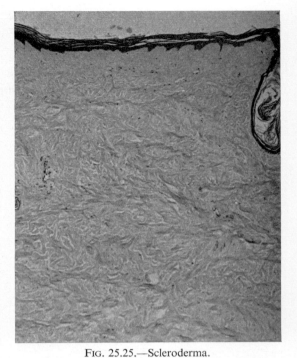

Fig. 25.25.—Scleroderma.
Note the flattening of the rete ridges and the increase in thickness of the dermal collagen. Dermal appendages are absent. × 40.

inflammatory infiltrate in the dermis composed of lymphocytes and histiocytes.

Sections from the sclerosed skin of an extremity in progressive systemic sclerosis show an entirely different picture (Fig. 25.26). Even in advanced cases the micro-anatomy of the skin is normal with retention of all the dermal appendages. The entire skin has, however, shrunk so that the subcutaneous fat is much nearer the surface. If ulceration or infection supervenes, then some fibrosis will result.

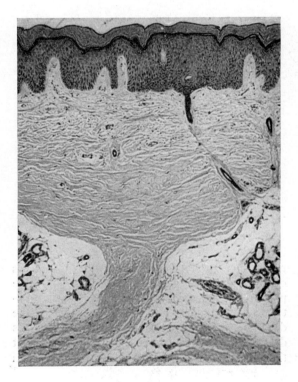

Fig. 25.26.—Systemic sclerosis. The general micro-anatomy of the skin is maintained but the sweat glands and subcutaneous fat are much nearer the surface. Although from different regions of the skin, this figure and Fig. 25.25 are taken at the same magnification, illustrating the difference between systemic sclerosis and scleroderma. × 40.

MALIGNANT RETICULOSES

In the course of the systematised malignant reticuloses such as lymphoid neoplasms and the leukaemias, skin lesions may occur. Specific lesions are most common in cutaneous lympho-sarcoma and reticulosarcoma and uncommon in the leukaemias. Involvement of the skin in Hodgkin's disease is rare. When present, the skin lesions show the histological structure of the parent condition. Pruritic eruptions occur in the leukaemias and Hodgkin's disease but the histological picture is that of a non-specific inflammatory reaction and is not diagnostic.

Mycosis fungoides is a malignant reticulosis peculiar to the skin which has certain clinical and histological characteristics. It has a prolonged course, being preceded for many years by various non-specific pruritic eruptions (premycotic phase) before the characteristic tumour stage is reached.

In the premycotic stage histological diagnosis may be difficult or impossible. The usual histological findings are those of a non-specific dermatitis but certain features should arouse suspicion and call for a repeat biopsy in three to six months' time. These include the presence, in the inflammatory infiltrate, of nuclear pyknosis (provided operative trauma can be excluded), a scattering of plasma cells, and occasionally an aberrant mitosis. Repeated biopsies may be necessary, however, before the diagnosis can be substantiated.

In the tumour stage the upper dermis is infiltrated by a pleomorphic infiltrate composed of histiocytes, lymphocytes, reticulum cells, plasma cells and eosinophil leukocytes (Fig. 25.27). The tendency to nuclear pyknosis is more marked and mitotic figures, although not numerous, are seen. Of diagnostic importance are the collections of mononuclear cells in the epidermis (Pautrier's "abscesses"). These are collections of tumour cells which have immigrated into the epidermis. Unfortunately these abscesses are not seen in every case but when present may be considered diagnostic.

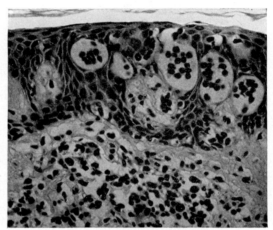

FIG. 25.27.—Mycosis fungoides. Several Pautrier "micro-abscesses" are seen in the epidermis. In the upper dermis there is a pleomorphic cellular infiltrate. × 265.

There is some confusion in the literature as to whether mycosis fungoides produces lesions in internal organs or not. Our experience is that it remains confined to the skin and that cases reported with visceral manifestations are other varieties of malignant reticulosis.

TUMOURS OF THE SKIN

The skin is a large and complex organ, and it is directly exposed to many carcinogenic agents in the environment: it is not therefore surprising that tumours are numerous and varied. They are soon detected and easily removed: the pathologist therefore sees many small and early tumours which would escape attention at less accessible sites. Early diagnosis and relatively early treatment account in part at least for the fact that a much smaller proportion of malignant tumours cause death of the patient than in any other organ.

Skin tumours can be classified readily according to the tissue of origin. Epithelial tumours may arise from the epidermis, the sweat gland or the hair follicle: dermal tumours may arise from the fibrous, vascular, nervous or reticulo-endothelial elements: and a third group arises from melanocytes. Some of the most important tumours, such as squamous carcinoma, have been dealt with already in Chapter 11 as local representatives of more general types, but many are peculiar to the skin.

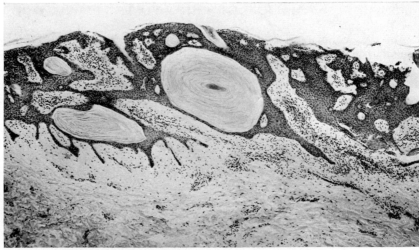

FIG. 25.28.—Basal cell papilloma. A flat papillary tumour composed of basal-like epidermal cells. Note the several "pearls" of keratin formation within the epithelium. × 40.

Epidermal tumours

Embryological studies have revealed that the keratinocytes of the skin undergo specific differentiation at an early stage in development; three distinct cell lines are produced relating to the surface epidermis, the pilo-sebaceous complexes and the sweat apparatus. This probably explains the differing biological behaviour of tumours arising from the epidermis.

Two sharply distinct types of tumour arise from the surface epidermis, the *squamous group* and the so-called *basal-cell group*, which includes rodent ulcer and basal cell papilloma (verruca senilis). Tumours of the sweat glands form a heterogeneous group and are discussed later.

Basal-cell papilloma (verruca senilis) is a fairly common warty growth seen most often on the trunk of older people. It produces a flattened papilloma consisting chiefly of basal-like cells, with relatively little differentiation into prickle cells unless irritated: keratin is however formed,

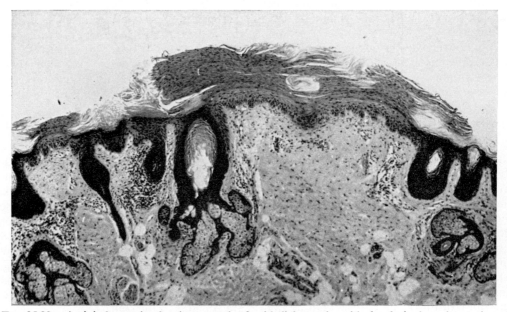

FIG. 25.29.—Actinic keratosis, showing a patch of epithelial atrophy with dysplasia, hyperkeratosis and parakeratosis. × 25.

often in fairly large amounts, characteristically in spherical masses (horn cysts) within the epithelium and sometimes reaching the surface (Fig. 25.28). Melanocytes are usually present among the basal-like cells and melanin is often abundant. This may give rise to diagnostic confusion with malignant melanoma. Mitoses are usually absent, growth is slow and malignancy so rare that cases can mostly be explained as coincidences or mistaken diagnoses. The

(plantar warts), and about the genitalia of those exposed to venereal infection (condyloma acuminata). If one excludes viral tumours, and the keratoses dealt with in the next section, the squamous papillomas (Fig. 11.1, p. 229) are probably very rare. Malignant change in a skin papilloma is extremely rare, though occasionally genital tumours show an exuberant growth hard to distinguish from malignancy.

Squamous keratosis. This is the best name for

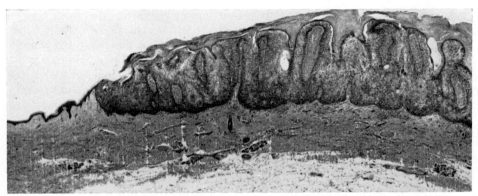

Fig. 25.30.—Bowen's disease, showing marked thickening and de-differentiation of epidermis and abrupt transition to normal skin. × 14.

name *seborrhoeic keratosis*, sometimes applied to these tumours, indicates their common occurrence on so-called seborrhoeic sites (forehead, chest and back).

"Squamous" group

These tumours consist of stratified squamous epithelium, and their mode of growth is clearly based on the ordinary process of growth of the epidermis. Normally multiplication occurs in the relatively undifferentiated basal cells, and differentiation occurs through prickle cells to keratin. In the benign tumours, the undifferentiated basal layer is only one cell thick, and the differentiated cells and the keratin more conspicuous than in normal skin, but with increasing malignancy the undifferentiated cells become more numerous and keratin and prickle cells diminish, though in skin tumours they hardly ever disappear altogether.

Squamous papilloma is the benign member of this group. It has already been mentioned in Chapter 11 and earlier in this chapter. Most are viral in origin, and seen usually on the hands of children (juvenile warts), on the soles of the feet of those who use communal changing-rooms

the premalignant lesions of this group. When the etiology is known, such terms as actinic or arsenical keratoses are commonly used, and in old people they may be called senile keratoses, but the lesions are identical. They are typically dry, rough-surfaced thickenings, arising usually in an area of skin which shows, by its thinness (Fig. 25.29), inelasticity and irregular pigmentation, the effects of prolonged exposure to sunlight or other carcinogen: the face and the back of the hands are the usual sites.

Histologically one sees all stages from the slightest thickening and irregularity of the epidermis to large lesions with gross irregular hyperplasia of the epithelium, a massive overlying layer of keratin, and greatly enlarged rete ridges apparently on the brink of invasion. The hallmark of these lesions is the presence of alternating columns of hyperkeratosis and parakeratosis. Nuclear pleomorphism, frequency of mitoses and cellular de-differentiation usually increase in parallel with the above changes. Sometimes, severe cytological changes occur in the presence of relatively minor general hyperplasia, and the term *carcinoma-in-situ* of the skin might reasonably include this condition.

Bowen's disease. This, though also an epidermal hyperplasia which may progress to squamous carcinoma, is a very different lesion. It may arise anywhere in the skin, but nearly always in non-exposed areas. While the keratosis blends into surrounding skin, which is itself abnormal, Bowen's disease is sharply circumscribed from normal skin (Fig. 25.30) forming

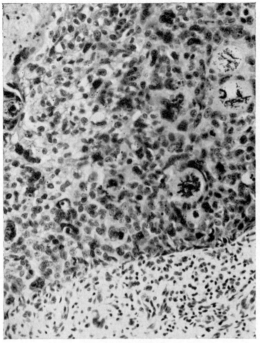

FIG. 25.31—Bowen's disease of the skin.
The epidermis is replaced by altered epithelial cells in which there are many aberrant cells and atypical mitoses.

rounded, reddish patches which spread slowly over a period of years. The epidermis in the affected area shows marked hyperplasia, with deep but fairly regular rete ridges and usually not much keratin: cellular de-differentiation is prominent, and large cells with multiple large clumped nuclei are a characteristic feature (Fig. 25.31). The importance of recognising Bowen's disease, which is another form of carcinoma-in-situ, is twofold. First, it may look like (and is often treated for years as) a patch of psoriasis or other chronic skin disease. Secondly, a degree of de-differentiation of the epidermis which in a squamous keratosis showing carcinoma-in-situ would mean imminent invasion, in Bowen's disease is compatible with many years of continued limitation to the surface—even though ultimate invasion is usual.

Squamous carcinoma. The description of squamous carcinoma in general in Chapter 11, and the many observations on its etiology in Chapter 10, make it unnecessary to say much of this important tumour of the skin here. The great majority are better differentiated than the average *mucosal* squamous carcinoma: this, combined with accessibility, makes for a relatively good prognosis. Dissemination, when it does occur, is by the same routes of local, lymph and blood spread as with other carcinomas. It may arise anywhere on the body surface, but in Great Britain the face (including the ears) and the backs of the hands are the commonest sites. The muco-cutaneous junctions are also important sites, but the bulk of these arise on the mucosal side of the junction: thus, most lip tumours arise from the red margin, most anal tumours within the canal, and most penile tumours from the glans; however, though some vulvar tumours arise from the modified skin of the labia minora, the majority appear in the true skin of the labia majora.

The tumours of the exposed surfaces presumably arise chiefly from the effect of ultraviolet light in sunlight. Industrial exposure usually produces tumours of the hands and forearms, but with carcinogens which penetrate the clothes, such as the lighter mineral oils and dusts like soot (Fig. 10.2, p. 214) and powdered arsenic, the scrotum becomes an important site, probably because its rugose surface traps dirt. Some carcinomas may result from prolonged contact with decomposing desquamated keratin: this is suggested by the occurrence of "dhoti cancer" under the waistbands of Indians living under poor sanitary conditions, and by the fact that early circumcision seems to prevent carcinoma of the glans penis. The relation of circumcision to cancer is a particularly interesting one. Among the Jews who circumcise at birth, cancer of the penis is all but unknown. Among Moslems, who circumcise at puberty, it is rare; but the occasional cases suggest that even before puberty some irreversible change may be induced —a fact that recalls the induction process in experiments on co-carcinogenesis. The majority of penile cancers are associated with an intact foreskin and a low standard of personal hygiene.

There is a small but clinically important group of squamous carcinomas which arise in the edges of long-standing ulcers (the so-called *Marjolin's ulcer*) and sinuses, presumably as a result of hyperplasia following prolonged attempts at healing.

Rodent ulcer (basal-cell carcinoma)

The typical rodent ulcer begins as a slow-growing, flattened nodule of the skin of the face. The centre breaks down, forming a shallow ulcer, but the periphery of the nodule persists to form a smooth, slightly raised margin to the

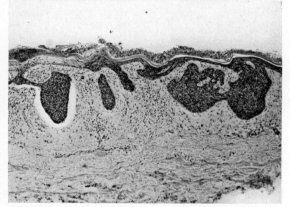

FIG. 25.32.—Rodent ulcer. Showing the apparently multicentric origin from the base of the epidermis. × 32.

ulcer which, as the latter spreads, becomes the characteristic rolled edge. If not successfully treated, the ulcer spreads slowly, and ultimately bites deeper and destroys the underlying structures of the face. Death results, if at all (for nowadays treatment is rarely so unsuccessful), from destruction of mouth and nose, or from invasion of the cranial cavity, most often via the orbit.

Neither lymph spread nor blood spread is seen except as the greatest of rarities. This is the only common malignant tumour other than those within the cranial cavity (where conditions are exceptional) which shows this extreme disinclination to metastasise, a finding that remains entirely unexplained.

Histologically, the tumour begins with groups of small, dark, basal-like cells, apparently sprouting from the undersurface of intact epidermis (Fig. 25.32). These cell groups enlarge and grow down into the dermis, forming clumps with an outer layer of columnar cells which resemble the basal layer of the epidermis. Instead, however, of the prickle cells which one would expect to see arising from this basal

layer, the centre of each clump is occupied by a solid mass of darkly-staining spheroidal cells (Fig. 25.33). The term basal-cell carcinoma indicates the similarity of the tumour cells to the basal cell layer of the surface epithelium.

Continued proliferation of the cell masses beneath the epidermis gives rise to a nodule: breakdown of the overlying epidermis gives rise to the ulcer (Fig. 25.34). The characteristic rolled border is due to lateral invasion of the tumour under the intact epidermis.

The detailed histology of these tumours varies considerably, but the well-defined single peripheral columnar layer ("palisading"—one of several different uses of this word in pathology), and the predominance of "basal" cells, are constant. The cell masses may be large and uniform, or narrow and ribbon-like. Small patches of squamous differentiation or even keratinisation may cause confusion with squamous carcinoma if one is not aware of their frequency in rodent ulcers. Small cystic spaces form at times, some genuine, some the result of stromal degeneration. Inclusion of a few melanocytes from the original epidermis is common, and rarely so much melanin may be formed that clinical confusion with melanoma may occur.

On the whole, the more complex the histology of the individual tumour, the less malignant; recurrence occurs most often with tumours consisting of relatively narrow burrowing columns of cells of uniform pattern. Little attention should be paid to the number of mitoses, which can be surprisingly numerous even in slow-growing examples. One variety meriting special mention is the *sclerotic* type, in which the tumour cells elicit a marked desmoplastic reaction: this results in the edges being ill-defined and may lead to incomplete excision or irradiation.

Sites. Though they can be found anywhere on the skin (except the palms and soles) the majority of rodent ulcers occur in a relatively restricted area of the face, in front of the ears, above the mouth and below the supra-orbital ridges. In this area, sunlight produces far more rodent ulcers than squamous carcinomas (in some parts of Australia it is the exception for a fair-skinned man to reach the age of 75 without having had at least one rodent ulcer on the face): elsewhere the reverse holds, and a radiation-induced rodent ulcer of the trunk, for instance,

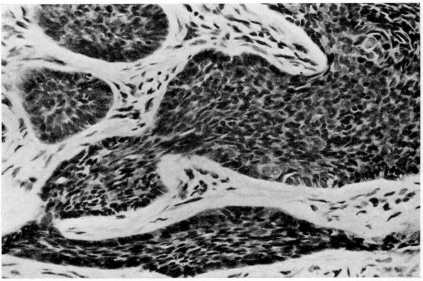

FIG. 25.33.—Rodent ulcer. The dermis is invaded by clumps of small, darkly-stained tumour cells resembling basal epidermal cells. The cells at the margin of some of the clumps present a palisaded appearance. × 250.

or one arising in the margin of a varicose ulcer of the skin is much less often seen than the corresponding squamous carcinoma. However, deep X-ray therapy, for example for ankylosing spondylitis, is sometimes followed many years later by a crop of rodent ulcers distant from the field of irradiation.

Tumours of sweat glands (hidradenomas)

These form a distinct group, of varied and often bizarre histological appearances, but characteristically they exhibit a two-layered epithelium and traces of mucin secretion. The superficial hidradenoma presents a papillary architecture within a duct (Fig. 25.35) and in the vulva, a frequent site, a cystadenomatous struc-

ture. Almost anywhere on the body one may see occasionally tumours resembling in structure the "parabuccal" mixed tumours of salivary glands: they are now thought to be hidradenomas arising from the glandular part of the sweat gland. Another variant of hidradenoma is the so-called turban tumour of the scalp. Like the salivary tumours hidradenomas show many histological variants. Malignant forms (hidradenocarcinomas) are rare.

Tumours of pilo-sebaceous follicles

True tumours are even less common than in the sweat glands. True sebaceous adenomas are very rare: the "tumours" of tuberose sclerosis (p. 666) are fibrous nodules, and "seborrhoeic

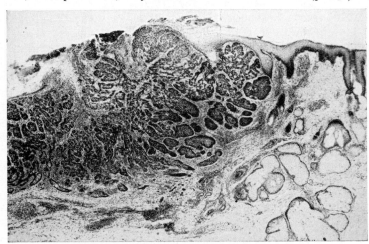

FIG. 25.34.—Rodent ulcer, showing the flat, shallow ulceration. Note the extension laterally which accounts for the "rolled" border. × 20.

keratosis" is a misnomer for the basal cell papilloma. An uncommon tumour which probably arises in the hair matrix is the so-called "benign calcifying epithelioma" of Malherbe. These form rounded masses lying under the skin, arising anywhere on the body surface and at any age, and growing slowly. In spite of the name, only about a quarter show calcification, though when present it may be extensive and spectacular, true bone being sometimes present. The epithelium of the tumours consists of small dark-staining regular cells, which form disproportionately large masses of keratin in which ghosts of the cells that have formed it can often be seen. Foreign body giant cell reaction to the keratin is frequent, and calcification when present seems to be a sequel of this reaction, though sometimes a curious direct calcification of ghost-cell areas of keratin seems to occur.

Molluscum sebaceum (kerato-acanthoma). This

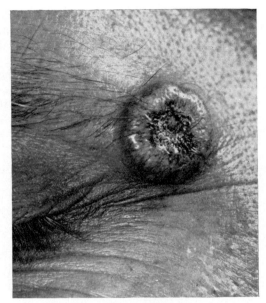

FIG. 25.36.—Molluscum sebaceum. Clinical photograph of an eight-week-old lesion near the eye. A firm rounded nodule with epidermis stretched over the edge, and a central crater where the keratin core is exposed. × 1·5.

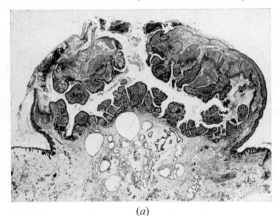

(*a*)

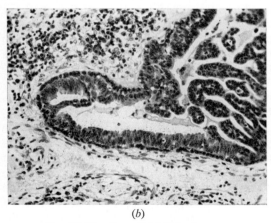

(*b*)

FIG. 25.35.—Superficial hidradenoma.
(*a*) Low power view to show general architecture. × 8.
(*b*) High power view to show the typical two-layered epithelium. × 150.

tumour-like but self-healing lesion is much commoner than any of the true hair follicle tumours. It occurs predominantly on the face of adults. A nodule in the skin appears and grows rapidly for about eight weeks, forming finally a rounded, slightly umbilicated mass, 10–20 mm. in diameter (Fig. 25.36). It stops growing, the central dimple enlarging and becoming dry and scaly, then the central plug is discharged and the lesion heals: the whole process usually takes about six months.

Histologically, the resemblance to squamous carcinoma is very close during the active phase, so much so that it was only after 1950 that it won general recognition as a distinct lesion that did not require to be treated as a carcinoma. The appearances which mimic invasion are however the result of rapid irregular overgrowth of a group of hair follicles (Fig. 25.37). During the stationary phase, the epithelium so formed is progressively keratinised, and the resulting mass of keratin is finally discharged. The whole appears to be a distortion of the normal cyclical process of growth and regression in the hair follicle: in rabbits, similar lesions can be produced by painting with a carcinogen at the right phase of the hair growth cycle. Recognition of this lesion is obviously of great importance in treatment. However, it is not always possible to differentiate it from squamous carcinoma, even after very careful correlation of the clinical and histological findings.

Self-healing squamous-cell carcinoma of the skin. This is a rare familial disorder, first described by Shaw Dunn and Ferguson Smith. It begins usually in early adult life, and is characterised by the appearance at intervals of tumours

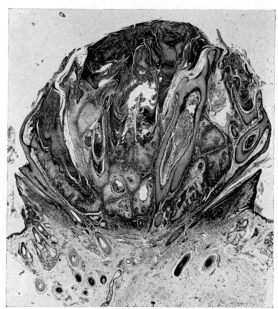

Fig. 25.37.—Molluscum sebaceum. A lesion about the same age as Fig. 25.36.
Note the resemblance to squamous carcinoma. × 12.

of the skin, mostly, but not exclusively, of the exposed parts, which are indistinguishable histologically from squamous-cell carcinomas. After some months of activity, each lesion in succession undergoes involution by keratinisation of the infiltrating columns of cells and discharge of the dead cells leaving shallow depressed pits. We have had the opportunity of studying several such cases and confirm the view of Currie and Ferguson Smith that they are indistinguishable from the ordinary solitary squamous carcinoma until regression sets in. The age and history are therefore very important. It is quite unrelated to molluscum sebaceum.

Melanocytic tumours

Histogenesis. The following account attempts to give a clear, if somewhat oversimplified, explanation of a complex series of phenomena, interpretation of which is still controversial.

Neural crest cells migrate into the epidermis in the fetus to form melanocytes. Occasionally some of them fail to reach the epidermis, developing in the dermis to form a "Mongolian spot" or a more compact mass termed a "blue naevus" (p. 946).

The epidermal melanocytes come to lie among the epidermal basal cells. As the fetus and in its turn the child grows, the melanocytes maintain a due proportion with the other elements of the skin. When a small patch of epidermis is lost, for example in a superficial abrasion or a small burn, epithelial cells and melanocytes may proliferate in proportion to restore the normal balanced epidermis. In deeper wounds, with destruction of dermis and skin appendages, the regenerated epithelium is devoid of melanocytes and the scar is unpigmented.

In nearly every child, at a few points on the skin surface the balance breaks down: the melanocytes multiply too rapidly and become too numerous to be accommodated in their normal position. At first, little collections of cells (junctional nests) form at the dermo-epidermal junction. When they become so numerous as to threaten to disrupt the epidermis, they pass down into the dermis. The process looks very like invasion of the dermis by tumour cells, but it has no sinister significance: the cells cease to proliferate or to produce melanin as soon as they lose contact with the epidermis. The lesion so formed is a *pigmented naevus*. During childhood the process of new formation of melanocytes in the epidermis continues, and the naevus grows: at puberty, growth of the naevus nearly always ceases, and it remains as a permanent inactive excrescence in most cases for the rest of life.

Melanocytes are subject, however, like any other cells of the body and particularly those on the surface, to a variety of carcinogenic stimuli, and may mutate to tumour cells. The unstable groups of melanocytes which produce naevi are naturally particularly susceptible to this, but other epidermal cells may also be affected. The change is exceedingly rare in childhood, and increases in frequency with age. The effect of the change is at first very similar to that of the naevus process: the abnormal melanocytes multiply to form junctional nests at the dermo-epidermal junction, and later are pushed down into the dermis. But these cells, unlike the cells of the naevus, are not dependent for the stimulus to multiply and to produce pigment on contact with the epidermis: having entered the dermis they continue to grow and to invade, and behave as a malignant tumour—*malignant melanoma*.

The principal lesions produced by this process are described below.

The pigmented naevus

This is an exceedingly common lesion, few people having none at all and some people very large numbers: the mean per person is said to be 18. Individually they vary greatly in appearance.

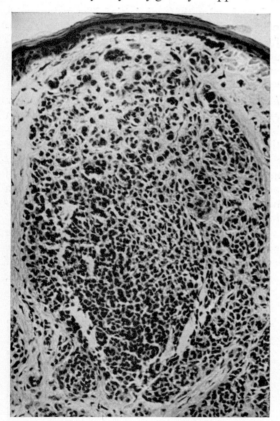

FIG. 25.38—Section through an intradermal naevus, showing collections of so-called "naevus cells" underneath the epithelium. × 220.

At one extreme is the extensive, deeply pigmented hairy lesion seen most often in the "bathing-trunk" area: this form of naevus is rare, and exceptional in that malignancy supervenes in a proportion of cases. At the other extreme are the smooth rounded lesions, usually not noticeably pigmented, which are prominent on the face of many elderly men: enlargement in adult life is unusual, and may mark the appearance of malignant change, but very much more often it is the result of inflammation of the hair follicles and sebaceous glands which are embedded in most naevi, or some similar extraneous event.

Histologically, the pigmented naevus consists of small rounded inactive-looking cells lying in loose masses in the dermis (Fig. 25.38). These cells are, of course, the misplaced melanocytes whose origin from the epidermal melanocytes has been described above. They are often called "naevus cells" although the fact that there are other kinds of naevi (e.g. angiomas) makes the usage somewhat illogical. Near the surface some of these cells contain melanin, and often phagocytic cells nearby also contain coarser granules of melanin, but most of the cells are not pigmented. There is a small layer of dermis between the naevus cell groups and the epidermis: the latter usually contains more melanocytes and is more deeply pigmented than surrounding normal skin, but the melanocytes in it are individually normal. The epidermis itself is usually distorted in some way, and not infrequently shows a grossly irregular pattern such as that seen in Fig. 25.39, produced apparently by the growth of junctional nests of melanocytes within the epidermis in the childhood phase. Hair follicles within naevi (especially in the face) are sometimes abnormally large and irregular in various ways (hairy naevi). There are also histological variants in which resemblances have been claimed to neurilemmal cells and to sensory nerve endings, both of which, like melanocytes, are of neural crest origin, but these are of little practical significance.

Juvenile melanoma. The histology of this lesion can be readily deduced from the account of "histogenesis" above. Because of the very active proliferation of melanocytes, they have often in the past been mistaken for malignant melanomas, and the mistake can still be made if the age of the patient is not known. A feature of value in histological diagnosis is the vascularity of many juvenile melanomas, which may give them a reddish appearance to the naked eye. Malignant melanoma before puberty, though not unknown, is exceedingly rare. Particular difficulty can be caused by the rare benign lesion in which a juvenile type of activity is retained into adult life.

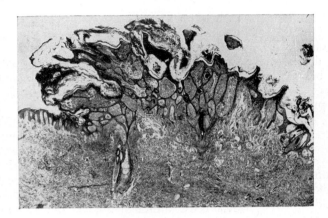

FIG. 25.39.—Pigmented naevus of warty type. The dermal papillae are filled with naevus cells which extend widely in the underlying dermis. × 12.

Junctional activity in pre-existing naevi. Resumption of growth of melanocytes at the dermo-epidermal junction in adult life sometimes occurs in naevi (Fig. 25.40). In most cases this is no more than a temporary phase, resulting probably from such stimuli as minor damage to the epidermis or UV light: careful search of most large naevi will reveal one or two junctional nests of this type, and little attention need be paid to them. Occasionally, however, junctional nests with obvious proliferation of melanocytes become prominent and numerous and this spontaneous overactivity of the melanocytes must be regarded as the result of a transformation in the direction of neoplasia, and considered premalignant. A lesion of this type, combining both old naevus cells and new junctional activity, is commonly called a *compound naevus* to distinguish it from the *simple* or *dermal pigmented naevus*, in which junctional activity is absent.

Junctional activity *ab initio*. The melanocytes of normal skin may undergo a similar transformation to neoplastic, but premalignant hyperactivity (Fig. 25.41). If the proliferation is moderate in degree, the appearance is merely that of a deeply pigmented spot on the skin, a *lentigo*. This is not the same as a freckle or *ephelis*, in which there is hyperpigmentation but no increase in melanocytes. If the proliferation is marked, and junctional nests become large and numerous, the lesion is called a *junctional naevus*—although, since it is a new lesion and not a birthmark, it is not strictly speaking a naevus at all. Such lesions are especially common on the legs.

Both lentigo and junctional naevus are potentially malignant, and require adequate excision, but so long as the proliferation of melanocytes is confined to the junctional nests, no question of dissemination arises.

FIG. 25.40.—Compound naevus. Some groups of proliferated melanocytes lie in the deeper part of the epidermis. Other groups have become separated from the epidermis and lie in the superficial dermis. × 100.

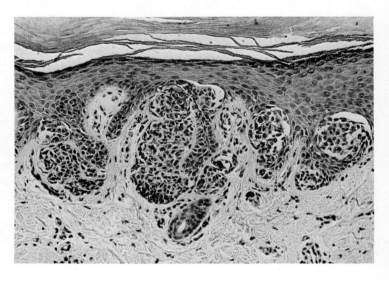

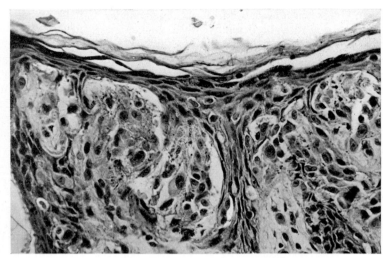

Fig. 25.41.—Junctional naevus. Note the groups of melanocytes lying in the deeper part of the epidermis. × 200.

Malignant melanoma

All malignant melanomas of the skin arise in either compound naevi (Fig. 25.40) or, more often, junctional naevi (Fig. 25.41), though the pre-existing lesion may be hard to demonstrate. The crucial event is the invasion of the dermis by pigmented tumour cells streaming down from the junctional nests (Fig. 25.42). Clinically there may be more rapid growth, increase or decrease in pigmentation and sometimes itching or pain, often followed soon by ulceration and bleeding. It should be emphasised, however, that clinical diagnosis of malignant melanoma at the early stage when they can best be treated is often very difficult. An adequate excision biopsy—that is to say excision of the whole lesion with a margin of 3 mm. on all sides—is essential in all cases in which there is any suspicion of this diagnosis: cutting into the tumour as in an ordinary biopsy may aid dissemination.

Microscopically, apart from the highly characteristic epidermal origin, malignant melanomas present a variable and not always characteristic pattern. The presence of melanin may make diagnosis easy, but it may be scanty and hard to see. It may even be totally absent from the area examined, or occasionally absent from all the tumour cells—"amelanotic melanoma". One must beware also of assuming that brown pigment in a tumour automatically

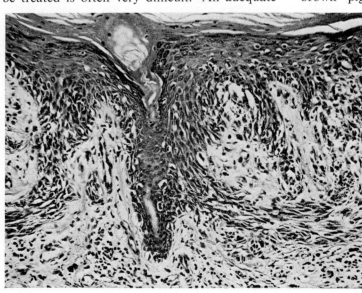

Fig. 25.42.—Malignant melanoma. There is junctional change, and the melanoma cells, which in this example are spindle shaped, have streamed into the dermis. Note also the numerous aberrant melanocytes with clear cytoplasm lying singly at various levels in the epidermis. × 100

means a melanoma: even if the pigment is melanin one may be dealing with a pigmented epithelial tumour or a blue naevus (see below) or, in the case of apparent metastasis to a lymph node, with melanin drained into the node in the course of a skin disease (*lipo-melanic reticulosis*). The haemosiderin in a very cellular sclerosing angioma has sometimes led to a hasty mis-diagnosis of melanoma.

The actual tumour cells vary considerably. They may be spindle-shaped, imitating a cellular fibrosarcoma, but most often they are spheroidal, fairly large, with abundant solid cytoplasm in which there may be a fine dusting of melanin. These cells form clumps such as are seen in carcinoma, but less compact and continuous, and never with any trace of gland formation or squamous differentiation. Cells containing coarse granules of melanin are usually phagocytes, and their presence should raise the suspicion of melanoma in the adjacent tissue.

Site and etiology. Melanomas may occur anywhere in the skin surface, but they have a higher incidence per unit area in the face, the genitalia and the feet than elsewhere. In general, they are less common in dark-skinned races, but in them are particularly often found in the feet. Any carcinogenic agent that increases the incidence of other skin tumours (sunlight in the fair-skinned, X-rays, tar) also increases the incidence of melanomas: of the tumours resulting from these agents, only a small proportion are melanomas, but they have, of course, a disproportionate effect on the mortality.

Metastasis. While *local spread* may include deep invasion, there is a special tendency to superficial spread in the skin itself, producing satellite nodules. This may be the result of spread in dermal lymphatics, but there is sometimes seen a curious intra-epidermal migration of tumour cells similar to that in Paget's disease of the nipple (p. 870). The first distant metastases usually appear in the local *lymph nodes*. Blood spread may be long delayed, but when it occurs is often rapid and extensive, with the spectacular black (or mixed black and white) metastases appearing in large numbers in a short time in many organs.

Malignant melanoma is the most malignant of the skin tumours, and has a curiously sinister reputation. But in fact if properly treated before the appearance of metastases, more than half of all cases are cured. The very long delay that often occurs between excision of the primary melanoma and the appearance of metastases makes exact figures difficult to arrive at. Prognosis is better in females, especially if young, than in males: there is also evidence that some cases develop specific antibodies against the surface membrane of tumour cells, and that this substantially improves the prognosis (p. 226).

Blue naevus or "melanophoroma"

In these lesions there are accumulations of deeply pigmented cells in the dermis. These are melanocytes in the sense that they produce melanin: they correspond to no normal human cell but have some homology with the frog melanophores—hence the alternative name. The lesions are blue in colour as a result of an optical effect due to their depth beneath the surface. Occasionally elements of blue naevi and ordinary pigmented naevi occur together in one

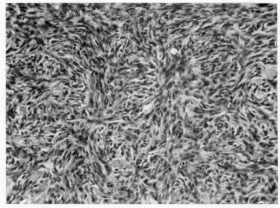

Fig. 25.43.—Sclerosing angioma, showing the characteristic whorled pattern, with inconspicuous capillaries. × 154.

tumour, producing a very confusing histological picture. Malignancy in blue naevi is very rare.

Dermal tumours

With a few exceptions, these are less common and less important than the epithelial tumours. They are, however, too numerous in variety for any systematic treatment here and what follows consists only of notes on some of the more interesting kinds. Reference should be made to

Chapter 12 for fibromas (p. 244), lipomas (p. 247) and angiomas (p. 250) and their variants, which include several important skin tumours. Neurofibromas will be found in Chapter 20 (p. 679). Lymphoid tumours and their precursors have been mentioned earlier in this Chapter (p. 935).

The sclerosing-angioma/dermatofibroma group

This group contains at least three seemingly distinct tumours (or apparent tumours) which often show transitions and are believed to

endothelial cells and the haemosiderin disappear and one is left with a collagenous nodule in the dermis containing numerous lipid-laden histiocytes: this stage is called a *histiocytoma*.

Finally, the histiocytes also disappear, and the result is a fibrous nodule, a *dermatofibroma*. Like its predecessors, this is a benign lesion, and commonest on the limbs. They can usually be readily distinguished from true fibromas: in the earlier stages by the persistence of some histiocytes, in the later stages by very low cellularity and a general pattern suggesting rather a thickening or distortion of the dermis than new fibroblastic proliferation.

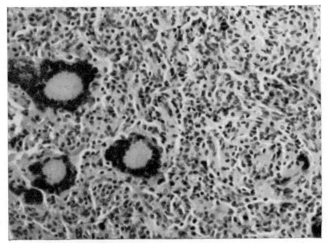

Fig. 25.44.—Juvenile xanthogranuloma. The dermal mass consists of histiocytes and giant cells with multiple peripheral nuclei. × 240.

represent stages of one process, though this is not certain. The name *subepidermal nodular fibrosis* may be used for the whole group.

The process begins with a hypothetical *angioma*, perhaps too small to be clinically evident. This may undergo, as a result of trauma, a brief phase of haemorrhage and endothelial cell proliferation. The result is a brownish protruding mass, the so-called *sclerosing angioma*, which may reach 25 mm. in diameter, though 10–15 mm. is more usual, and which may readily be mistaken clinically for a malignant melanoma. Histologically, they show dense masses of proliferating endothelial cells with numerous but inconspicuous angiomatoid vessels (Fig. 25.43) and numerous histiocytes and giant cells containing haemosiderin and lipid, both derived presumably from breaking-down erythrocytes.

Left alone, these lesions regress, most of the

HH

True fibroma of the dermis is probably rare, but confusion is possible not only with dermatofibroma but with neurofibroma.

Dermatofibrosarcoma protuberans

Fibrosarcoma of the skin is represented by this lesion, which arises usually *de novo* from the skin of the trunk. It has the histology of any low-grade fibrosarcoma, and when small a characteristic hour-glass shape, with a base in the dermis and two nodules, one superficial pressing the epidermis outwards (hence "protuberans") and one larger invading the deeper tissues. It is slow growing and rarely metastasises but recurs persistently after any but the most ruthless excision.

Xanthogranuloma (naevoxantho-endothelioma)

The various types of lipid infiltration of the skin (xanthomatosis) have been dealt with in other chapters as part of the systematised lipidosis.

There remains one very rare form which occurs in infancy and is dissociated from generalised abnormal lipid metabolism. It may present as multiple yellowish-brown nodules on the ex-tensor aspect of the limbs, or as a solitary tumour-like nodule in the dermis.

They contain large giant cells with a peripheral or nearly peripheral ring of nuclei and having a finely foamy cytoplasm aptly likened to ground glass (Touton giant cells), surrounded by masses of histiocytes with vacuolated cytoplasm (Fig. 24.44). The lesions usually heal spontaneously: the cause is unknown.

SUGGESTIONS FOR FURTHER READING AND CONSULTATION

The following list consists mainly of textbooks and review articles: their suitability as reading material or for consultation is indicated by the title and length. References to most of the original reports mentioned in the text of this book will be found in the appropriate items listed below, and separate references to original papers are provided only for a few recent reports of outstanding interest.

HISTORICAL

Cohnheim's Lectures in General Pathology. Vol. 1. Introduction. pp. 1–15. English translation. New Sydenham Society, London, 1889.

Classic Descriptions of Disease. R. H. Major. 3rd ed., 3rd printing, pp. 679. Blackwell Scientific, Oxford, 1948.

A History of Pathology. E. R. Long. pp. 291. Williams and Wilkins, Baltimore, 1928. (Also published by Dover Publications, Inc., New York, pp. 199, 1965.)

GENERAL

General Pathology. Ed. Lord Florey. 4th ed., pp. 1259. Lloyd-Luke, London, 1970. (A more detailed account of many topics in general pathology, with a good historical introduction and bibliography.)

An Introduction to Pathology. G. Payling Wright. 3rd ed., pp. 660. Longmans, Green & Co., London, 1958. (Despite its age, this is still of great interest as further reading in general pathology.)

Biochemical Disorders in Human Disease. Ed. R. H. S. Thompson and I. D. P. Wootton. 3rd ed., pp. 875. Churchill, London, 1970.

The Physiological Basis of Medical Practice. Ed. C. H. Best and N. B. Taylor. 8th ed., pp. 1793. Williams and Wilkins, New York, 1966.

Human Genetics. V. A. McKusick. 2nd ed., pp. 221. Prentice Hall, Englewood Cliffs, 1969.

The Metabolic Basis of Inherited Disease. J. B. Stanbury, J. B. Wyngaarden and D. S. Fredrickson. 2nd ed., pp. 1434. McGraw Hill, New York and London, 1966.

Medical Terms: their Origin and Construction. Ffrangcon Roberts. 4th ed., pp. 96. Heinemann, London, 1966.

The Principles of Medical Statistics. Sir A. Bradford Hill. 8th ed., pp. 381. Lancet, London, 1966.

INDIVIDUAL CHAPTERS

Chapter 1

The Megaloblastic Anaemias. I. Chanarin, pp. 9–39. Blackwell, Oxford, 1969.

Dible *et al.*, 1941. See *Pathology.* J. H. Dible and T. B. Davie. 2nd ed., pp. 68–77. Churchill, London, 1945.

Lysosomes in Biology and Pathology. J. T. Dingle and Dame Honor Fell. 2 vols. pp. 543 and 689. North Holland Publishing Co., Amsterdam, 1969.

Fredrickson, D. S., Levy, R. I. and Lees, R. S. (1967). Fat transport in lipoproteins—an integrated approach to mechanisms and disorders. *New Eng. J. Med.*, **276**, 34–44, 94–103, 148–156, 215–225.

Cellular Injury. Ciba Symposium. Ed. A. V. S. de Reuck and Julie Knight. pp. 403. Churchill, London, 1964.

Chapter 2

The Inflammatory Process. Ed. B. W. Zweifach, L. Grant and R. T. McCluskey. pp. 931. Academic Press, New York and London, 1965.

The Pharmacology of Inflammation. W. G. Spector and D. A. Willoughby. pp. 123. English Universities Press, London, 1968.

Chapter 3

Tissue Repair. R. M. H. McMinn. pp. 423. Academic Press, London, 1969.

Sevitt, S. (1970). Bone repair and fracture healing. *Brit. J. hosp. Med.*, **3**, 693–710.

Wound Healing. Ed. W. Montagna and R. E. Billingham. pp. 251. Pergamon Press, London, 1964.

Chapters 4 and 5

Immunology for Students of Medicine. J. H. Humphrey and R. G. White. 3rd ed., pp. 757. Blackwell Scientific, Oxford, 1970.

Clinical Aspects of Immunology. Ed. P. G. H. Gell and R. R. A. Coombs. 2nd ed., pp. 1356. Blackwell Scientific, Oxford, 1968.

Autoimmunity, Clinical and Experimental. J. R. Anderson, W. W. Buchanan and R. B. Goudie. pp. 485. Thomas, Springfield, 1967.

Chapters 6 and 7

Bacteriology and Immunology for Students of Medicine. F. S. Stewart. 9th ed., pp. 603. Ballière, Tyndall and Cassell, London, 1968.

A Short Textbook of Medical Microbiology. D. C. Turk and I. A. Porter. pp. 335. English Universities Press, London, 1969.

Principles of Microbiology and Immunology. R. B. Davis *et al.*, pp. 853. Harper and Row, New York, 1968.

The Biology of Animal Viruses. F. Fenner. Vol. 2. The Pathogenesis and Ecology of Viral Infections. pp. 845. Academic Press, New York and London, 1968.

Chapter 8

Blood Transfusion in Clinical Medicine. P. L. Mollison. 4th ed., pp. 863. Blackwell Scientific, Oxford, 1967.

Blood Groups in Man. R. R. Race and Ruth Sanger. 5th ed., pp. 599. Blackwell Scientific, Oxford, 1968.

The Pathology of Trauma. Ed. S. Sevitt and H. B. Stoner. pp. 214. *J. clin. Path. Suppl.* (Coll. Path.) 4, 1970.

Burns: Pathology and Therapeutic Applications. S. Sevitt. pp. 364. Butterworths, London, 1957.

Chapter 9

Pigments in Pathology. Ed. M. Wolman. pp. 551. Academic Press, New York and London, 1969.

Amyloidosis. D. A. Price Evans and J. Price. pp. 183–93 in *Selected Topics in Medical Genetics.* Ed. C. A. Clarke. Oxford University Press, London, 1969.

J. A. Boyle. (1969). Hyperuricaemia. *Brit. J. hosp. Med.*, 2, 1984–8

Chapter 10

Pathology of Tumours. R. A. Willis. 4th ed., chapters 1–12, pp. 1–207. Butterworths, London, 1967.

The Spread of Tumours in the Human Body. R. A. Willis. 2nd ed., pp. 447. Butterworths, London, 1952.

Racial and Geographical Factors in Tumour Incidence. A. A. Shivas. University Press, Edinburgh, 1967.

Systemic Effects of Neoplasia. J. G. Azzopardi. pp. 98–184 in *Recent Advances in Pathology.* Ed. C. V. Harrison. 8th ed., Churchill, London, 1966.

The Virology and Immunology of Cancer. L. A. Zilber and G. I. Abelev. pp. 474. Pergamon Press, Oxford, 1968.

Oncogenic Viruses. L. Gross. 2nd ed., pp. 991. Pergamon Press, London, 1970.

Jarrett, W. F. H. (1971). Feline leukaemia. *Internat. Rev. exp. Path.* (in press).

Jarrett, W. F. H. (1971). Viruses and leukaemia. *Brit. J. Cancer* (in press). (A review of the role of viruses in animal leukaemia and the possible relevance to human leukaemia.)

Chapters 11 and 12

Histological Appearances of Tumours. R. Winston Evans. 2nd ed., pp. 1256. Livingstone, Edinburgh, 1966.

Pathology of Tumours. R. A. Willis. 4th ed., pp. 209–1019. Butterworths, London, 1967.

Atlas of Tumour Pathology. (Numerous "Fascicles" on tumours of particular organs, tissues and regions. A valuable source of detailed information on the histology and behaviour of individual tumours.) U.S. Armed Forces Institute of Pathology, Washington, D. C.

Chapters 13 and 14

Cardiovascular Pathology. R. E. B. Hudson. Vols. 1 (pp. 1190) and 2 (pp. 933), 1965; Vol. 3 (Supplement, pp. 1166), 1970. Edward Arnold, London.

Paul Wood's Diseases of the Heart and Circulation. By various authors. 3rd ed., pp. 1164. Eyre and Spottiswoode, London, 1968.

Arterial Disease. J. R. A. Mitchell and C. J. Schwartz. pp. 411. Blackwell Scientific, Oxford, 1965.

Smith, J. P. (1956). Hyaline arteriolosclerosis in spleen, pancreas and other viscera. *J. Path. Bact.*, 72, 643–56.

Chapter 15

Pathology of the Lung. H. Spencer. 2nd ed., pp. 1106. Pergamon Press, London, 1968.

The Lung. Ed. A. A. Liebow and D. E. Smith. pp. 400. Williams and Wilkins, Baltimore, 1968.

J. Stark (1969). Respiratory viruses. *Brit. J. hosp. Med.*, 2, 1791–1804.

D. A. J. Tyrrell (1968). Respiratory viruses. *J. clin. Path.*, 21, Suppl. 2., pp. 6–9.

Chapter 16

Atlas of Haematology. G. A. McDonald, T. C. Dodds and Bruce Cruickshank. 3rd ed., pp. 226. Livingstone, Edinburgh, 1970.

Clinical Haematology. M. M. Wintrobe. 6th ed., pp. 1287. Kimpton, London, 1967.

Disorders of the Blood. Whitby and Britton. By C. J. C. Britton. 10th ed., pp. 860. Churchill, London, 1969.

The Megaloblastic Anaemias. I. Chanarin. pp. 1000. Blackwell Scientific, Oxford, 1969.

Practical Haematology. J. V. Dacie and S. M. Lewis. 4th ed., pp. 568. Churchill, London, 1968.

Chapter 17

Diseases of Lymphoid Tissue. C. V. Harrison. In *Recent Advances in Pathology.* Ed. C. V. Harrison. 7th ed., 1960, pp. 35–53; 8th ed., 1966, pp. 207–36. Churchill, London.

Leading Article (1969). Lymphoma and Glandular Fever. *Brit. med. J.*, 4, 445–6.

Lukes, R. J., Butler, J. J. and Hicks, Ethel B. (1966). Natural history of Hodgkin's disease as related to its pathologic picture. *Cancer* (*Philadelphia*), 19, 317–44.

Young, M. and Turnbull, H. M. (1931). An analysis of the data collected by the status lymphaticus investigation committee. *J. Path. Bact.*, 34, 213–58.

Niederman, J. C., McCollum, R. W., Henle, Gertrude and Henle, W. (1968). Infectious mononucleosis. Clinical manifestations in relation to EB virus antibodies. *J. Amer. med. Assoc.*, 203, 205–9.

Chapter 18

Clinical Gastroenterology. F. Avery Jones, J. W. P. Gummer and J. Leonard-Jones. 2nd ed., pp. 888. Blackwell Scientific, Oxford, 1968.

Diseases of the Digestive System. S. C. Truelove and P. C. Reynell. pp. 696. Blackwell Scientific, Oxford, 1963.

Modern Trends in Gastroenterology. Series 4. Ed W. I. Card and B. Creamer. pp. 362. Butterworths, London, 1970.

Peptic Ulcer. C. F. W. Illingworth. pp. 287. Livingstone, Edinburgh, 1953.

Chapter 19

Diseases of the Liver and Biliary System. Sheila Sherlock. 4th ed., pp. 809. Blackwell Scientific, Oxford, 1968.

Progress in Liver Disease. Ed. H. Popper and F. Schaffner. Vol. 1, pp. 363, 1961; Vol. 2, pp. 554, 1966; Vol. 3, pp. 562, 1970. Grune and Stratton, New York.

Liver Biopsy Interpretation. P. J. Scheuer. pp. 138. Ballière, Tyndall and Cassell, London, 1968.

Virus Diseases of the Liver. A. J. Zuckerman. pp. 174. Butterworths, London, 1970.

The Liver and its Diseases. H. P. Himsworth. 2nd ed., pp. 238. Blackwell Scientific, Oxford, 1953.

The Effects of Hepatotoxic Agents. K. Weinbren. pp. 197–206 in *Recent Advances in Pathology*. Ed. C. V. Harrison. 8th ed. Churchill, London, 1966.

Himsworth, H. P. and Glynn, L. E. (1944). See *The Liver and its Diseases*, Himsworth, 1953.

Lancet (London). (Leading articles on the hepatitis virus.) Australia antigen and hepatitis (1969) **2**, 143. Hepatitis virus (1969) **2**, 557. More on hepatitis virus (1970) **1**, 706.

Chapter 20

Atlas of Neuropathology. W. Blackwood, T. C. Dodds and J. C. Sommerville. 2nd ed., pp. 234. Livingstone, Edinburgh, 1964.

Cole, F. M. and Yates, P. O. (1967). The occurrence and significance of intracerebral micro-aneurysms. *J. Path. Bact.*, **93**, 393–411.

Greenfield's Neuropathology. Ed. W. Blackwood *et al*. 2nd ed., pp. 679. Edward Arnold, London, 1963.

The Pathology of Mental Retardation. L. Crome and J. Stern. pp. 403. Churchill, London, 1967.

The Pathology of Tumours of the Nervous System. D. S. Russell and L. J. Rubinstein. 3rd ed., pp. 429. Edward Arnold, London, 1971.

The Pathology of Trauma. Ed. S. Sevitt and H. B. Stoner. pp. 214. *J. clin. Path Suppl.* (Coll. Path.) 4, 1970. (For head injuries.)

Virus Diseases and the Nervous System. Ed. C. W. Whitty, J. T. Hughes and F. O. MacCallum. pp. 259. Blackwell Scientific, Oxford, 1969.

Chapter 21

Pathology of the Kidney. R. H. Heptinstall. pp. 836. Churchill, London, 1966.

Experimental Glomerulonephritis: Immunological Events and Pathogenetic Mechanisms. E. R. Unanue and F. J. Dixon. pp. 1–90 in *Advances in Immunology*. Ed. F. J. Dixon and J. H. Humphrey, Vol. 6. Academic Press, New York and London, 1966.

Renal Disease. Ed. D. A. K. Black. 2nd ed., pp. 798. Blackwell Scientific, Oxford, 1967.

Autoimmunity, Clinical and Experimental. J. R. Anderson, W. W. Buchanan and R. B. Goudie. pp. 485. Thomas, Springfield, 1967.

Long term results of intensive steroid therapy of childhood nephritis. G. C. Arneil and C. N. Lam. pp. 95–107 in Vol. 3 of *Proceedings of the 3rd International Congress of Nephrology*. Karger, Basel and New York, 1966.

Hawkins, D. and Cochrane, C. G. (1969). Glomerular basement membrane damage in immunological glomerulonephritis. *Immunology*, **14**, 665–81.

Horster, M. and Thurau, K. (1968). Micropuncture studies on the filtration rate of single superficial and juxtamedullary glomeruli in the rat kidney. *Pflügers Archiv.*, **301**, 162–81.

The validation of fibrin, and its significance in the story of hyalin. A. C. Lendrum. pp. 159–83 in *Trends in Clinical Pathology*. British Medical Association, London, 1969.

Lerner, R. A., Glassock, R. J. and Dixon, F. J. (1967). The role of anti-glomerular basement membrane antibody in the pathogenesis of human glomerulonephritis. *J. exp. Med.*, **126**, 989–1004.

Lever, 1969. See Brown, J. J. *et al.* (1970). Renin and acute renal failure: studies in man. *Brit. med. J.*, **1**, 253–8.

Chapter 22

Calcium Metabolism and the Bone. P. Fourman *et al.*, 2nd ed., pp. 656. Blackwell Scientific, Oxford, 1968.

Diseases of Bone and Joints. L. Lichtenstein. pp. 211. Mosby, St. Louis, 1970.

Pathology of Bone. D. H. Collins. pp. 248. Butterworths, London, 1966.

Bone Tumors. D. C. Dahlin. 2nd ed., pp. 280. Thomas, Springfield, 1967.

Diseases of Muscle. R. D. Adams, D. Denny-Brown, and C. M. Pearson. 2nd ed., pp. 717. Cassell, London, 1962.

Pathology of the Connective Tissue Diseases. D. L. Gardner. pp. 441. Edward Arnold, London, 1965.

Chapter 23

Novak's Gynaecological and Obstetrical Pathology. E. R. Novak and J. D. Woodruff. 6th ed., pp. 696. Saunders, Philadelphia and London, 1967.

Chapter 24

Endocrine Pathology. Ed. J. M. B. Bloodworth. pp. 750. Williams and Wilkins, Baltimore, 1968.

Textbook of Endocrinology. Ed. R. H. Williams. 4th ed., pp. 1258. Saunders, Philadelphia, 1968.

Functional Pathology of the Human Adrenal Gland. T. Symington. pp. 551. Livingstone, Edinburgh and London, 1969.

Chapter 25

An Introduction to the Diagnostic Histopathology of the Skin. J. A. Milne. Edward Arnold, London. (in preparation).

A Guide to Dermatohistopathology. H. Pinkus and A. H. Mehregan. pp. 546. Butterworths, London, 1969.

INDEX

Page numbers in heavy print indicate the main accounts of topics which also receive attention on the other pages indexed.